Exotic Animal Medicine for the Veterinary Technician

Exotic Animal Medicine for the Veterinary Technician

Fourth Edition

Edited by

Bonnie Ballard DVM
and
Ryan Cheek LVTg, VTS (ECC)

WILEY Blackwell

Library of Congress Cataloging-in-Publication Data

Names: Ballard, Bonnie, editor. | Cheek, Ryan, editor.
Title: Exotic animal medicine for the veterinary technician / edited by
  Bonnie Ballard and Ryan Cheek.
Description: Fourth edition. | Hoboken, New Jersey : Wiley-Blackwell,
  [2024] | Includes bibliographical references and index.
Identifiers: LCCN 2023049049 (print) | LCCN 2023049050 (ebook) | ISBN
  9781119863144 (paperback) | ISBN 9781119863168 (adobe pdf) | ISBN
  9781119863151 (epub)
Subjects: MESH: Animals, Exotic | Animal Diseases | Veterinary
  Medicine–methods | Animal Technicians
Classification: LCC SF997.5.E95 (print) | LCC SF997.5.E95 (ebook) | NLM
  SF 997.5.E95 | DDC 636.089–dc23/eng/20240105
LC record available at https://lccn.loc.gov/2023049049
LC ebook record available at https://lccn.loc.gov/2023049050

Cover Design: Wiley
Cover Images: © Kate Lafferty; Nia Chau & Austin James; Jody Nugent-Deal; Ashley McGaha

Set in 9.5/12.5pt STIXTwoText by Straive, Chennai, India

SKY10068242_022724

Contents

Contributors

Bonnie Ballard, DVM has worked in veterinary medicine since 1974, starting as a veterinary assistant, becoming a technician in 1979, and earning a DVM in 1994 from the University of Georgia College of Veterinary Medicine. After graduation, she worked at a small animal hospital where she introduced exotic and fish medicine to the practice. Later she did relief work in the Atlanta metro area. In 1997, while doing relief work, she started the Veterinary Technology Program at Gwinnett Technical College. The program has been AVMA accredited since 2000. Dr. Ballard served as the program's director and one of two full-time faculty members. She retired in 2018 and moved to Pensacola, Florida. She has had a lifelong interest in exotic animals and has owned many different types over the years. She currently works with the Escambia County Sea Turtle Beach Patrol.

Ryan Cheek, LVTg, VTS (ECC), BS, graduated from Gwinnett Technical College with an Associate of Applied Veterinary Technology where he focused his studies on exotic animal medicine. From there, he worked at Zoo Atlanta and then at a small animal/exotic animal practice for four years and has worked in emergency and critical care since 1998. He completed his Veterinary Technician Specialist in emergency and critical care in 2005 and his Bachelor of Applied Science in Veterinary Technology from St. Petersburg College in 2007. He also earned a MS and PhD in Instructional Technology from Georgia State University. He has spoken at state and national conferences on the topics of exotic animal medicine. Ryan is currently the Dean of Health Sciences at Gwinnett Technical College where he teaches many subjects including exotic, wildlife, zoo, and laboratory animal medicine. Ryan's life as a reptile hobbyist began in 1986 when he purchased his first pet lizard and has since owned more than 40 different species of reptiles.

Pia Bartolini, CVT, VTS (CP-Exotics) graduated from Front Range Community College in 2008 with an Associate of Applied Science in Veterinary Technology. She started her career in shelter medicine and wildlife rehabilitation, then went into small animal emergency and critical care until she accepted the veterinary technician intern role at White Oak Conservation Center in Yulee, Florida. After completion of her internship, she was employed at the University of Florida Zoological Medicine Service. During her time at University of Florida Zoological Medicine Service, she completed her VTS application for the Academy of Veterinary Technicians in Clinical Practice. In 2015, she spent a year in Arizona where she sat and passed the VTS Exam in Clinical Practice for Exotic Companion Animals while at the Arizona Exotic Animal Hospital. Currently, her primary role is a CVT at Disney Animal Health, Science and Environment. She is co-owner of Fishhead Diagnostics, as well as co-founder of a 501c3 reptile conservation center; the Reptile Preservation Institute.

Denise I. Bounous, DVM, PhD, Diplomate ACVP, graduated with her DVM and PhD in Veterinary Science/Immunology from Oklahoma State University College of Veterinary Medicine. She became a Diplomate of ACVP in 1992. She then became a professor of clinical pathology at LSU and later at the University of Georgia College of Veterinary Medicine before moving to the pharmaceutical industry. She retired from Bristol–Meyers Squibb Company in 2020.

Nia Chau, RVT, VTS (Exotic Companion Animal) received a BS in psychology and biology from the University of Georgia and an AAS in veterinary technology from Gwinnett Technical College in 2014. She started as a veterinary assistant in small animal and emergency medicine. As her career progressed, she worked in exotic animal medicine in practices in the Atlanta, Georgia area. Her career changed to solely exotic animal medicine when she went to work at the University of Georgia Veterinary Teaching Hospital in 2015 and has been there ever since.

Sarah Camlic, DVM graduated from Louisiana State University School of Veterinary Medicine in 2019. Since graduation, she has completed a small animal rotating internship at BluePearl Tampa, an avian and exotics specialty internship at Red Bank Veterinary Hospital in New Jersey, and an emergency and critical care specialty internship at the University of Georgia College of Veterinary Medicine. She spent a year practicing small animal emergency medicine in a specialty and emergency hospital in the Atlanta metro area prior to returning to the University of Georgia for her current position as an anesthesia resident.

Cheryl B. Greenacre, DVM, DAVBP (Avian and ECM) earned her DVM from the University of Georgia College of Veterinary Medicine and is boarded in both Avian Medicine and Exotic Companion Mammal Medicine through the American Board of Veterinary Practitioners. She has taught avian and exotic animal medicine at both the University of Georgia and the University of Tennessee for over 30 years. She has held past leadership positions as an AVMA Delegate, Chair of the AVMA Avian Working Group on the Panel of Euthanasia, Chair of the UT IACUC, and president of the Association of Avian Veterinarians. Currently, she holds a position as a Laboratory Animal Veterinarian with the University of Georgia. She is editor of the book, "Backyard Poultry Medicine and Surgery – A Guide for Veterinary Practitioners."

Tarah Hadley, DVM, graduated from Tufts University School of Veterinary Medicine. After graduation, she completed a rotating Medicine and Surgery Internship at Rowley Memorial Animal Hospital in Springfield, MA, followed by a residency in Avian Medicine at the University of Tennessee. Dr. Hadley spent several years as an exotic animal private practitioner in Georgia. She also worked part-time at Zoo Atlanta, worked as an avian and exotics consultant for IDEXX, and served as Executive Director of AWARE Wildlife Center outside of Atlanta. Dr. Hadley currently resides in Texas where she serves as Assistant Director of Veterinary Care at the San Antonio Zoo.

Melanie Haire, VMT, received an AS degree in veterinary technology from Wilson College, Chambersburg, PA, and worked as a veterinary technician in an Atlanta small animal clinic following graduation. She has spent the last three decades on the staff of Zoo Atlanta where she is the senior veterinary technician and serves as the hospital manager. She is federally licensed to rehabilitate migratory bird species, including raptors, and has a GA state DNR permit to rehabilitate all native GA wildlife with specialties in songbird and river otter care.

Jan Hooimeijer, DVM, MSc has been a birdwatcher and a veterinarian since 1982 focusing on health, behavior, and welfare problems in birds. He has presented more than 75 presentations at international conferences and contributed to different textbooks. Since 2013, he has joined Dr. Irene Pepperberg in presenting lectures for veterinary students at universities in the United States, South America, Europe, Australia, and Asia about behavior, intelligence, cognition, and preventing and solving behavioral problems in birds.

Micah Kohles, DVM, MPA, earned his DVM from Kansas State University in 2001 and a Master's Degree in Public Administration from the University of Nebraska–Omaha in 2010. Dr. Kohles joined Oxbow Animal Health in 2006 and currently serves as the Veterinary Medical Officer for Compana Pet Brands. Additionally, he owns and actively practices at Woodland Animal Hospital and serves as an adjunct professor appointment at the University of Nebraska School of Veterinary Medicine and Biomedical Sciences. Dr. Kohles is a frequent lecturer at veterinary schools and conferences domestically and internationally and has been chosen as both VMX and Western States Veterinary Conference Exotic speaker of the year.

Katrina Lafferty, BFA, CVT, VTS is a 2001 graduate of DePaul University with a Bachelor of Fine Arts in Theatre. Katrina received her degree in Veterinary Technology in 2005, her Veterinary Technician Specialty (VTS) in anesthesia/analgesia in 2009, and her registered laboratory animal technician certification (RLAT) in 2019. Katrina has worked at the University of Wisconsin–Madison since 2005, with time spent at both the School of Veterinary Medicine and the National Primate Research Center. She is also involved in the education of veterinary and veterinary technician students. Katrina is involved in the education of all members of the veterinary community and she has written numerous articles and textbook chapters. She has presented at dozens of continuing education seminars on an international level. Her passion is anesthesia and pain management, most particularly in exotic species.

Vanessa K. Lee, DVM, DACLAM obtained her veterinary degree from University of Georgia in 2005. After practicing in a small animal and exotics clinic for two years, she went to Emory University for a laboratory animal medicine residency. She stayed at Emory after finishing her residency in 2009 and is currently serving as an Assistant Director and Associate Professor in the Division of Animal Resources.

David Martinez-Jimenez, DVM was born in Spain where he completed his veterinary degree in 2002. After graduation, he performed several externships in exotic pet, zoo, and wildlife medicine. In 2004, Dr. Martinez completed a Master's degree in Wild Animal Health at the Royal Veterinary College and Institute of Zoology in London, UK. He then completed an internship in exotic, zoo, and wildlife medicine and surgery at the College of Veterinary Medicine, University of Georgia. He is currently a side-liner beekeeper and works in private practice in the out skirts of Atlanta, GA.

Ashley McGaha, BAS, RVTg, VTS (Exotic Companion Animal), received a BS in veterinary technology from Fort Valley State University. She has been working at the University of Georgia as a Zoological Medicine Technician since August 2010. She is very active in her specialty and sits on the board as an exotic member at large. She has trained many veterinary students, technicians, and technician students in exotic animal handling and nursing care. She also has Avian Fear Free certification.

Deborah Mook, DVM, Diplomate ACLAM, received her DVM from the University of Wisconsin–Madison in 1998 and became board certified in laboratory medicine in 2004. She worked with pet rabbits in the clinical setting and rabbits as research models in the medical school setting. Her primary expertise lies in the field of laboratory animal medicine with a focus on murine infectious disease and laboratory animal program management.

Jody Nugent-Deal, RVT, VTS, is a Registered Veterinary Technician and Veterinary Technician Specialist (VTS) in Anesthesia/Analgesia and Clinical Practice – Exotic Companion Animal. She has worked for the UC Davis Veterinary Medical Teaching Hospital since 1999, working in the Companion Exotics Department for 10 years and currently in the Anesthesia Department where she is the supervisor. Jody is passionate about teaching and life-long learning. She recently started her own company where she provides CE via online webinars and in-clinic hands-on training as well as teaches for VSPN and VetMedTeam on topics including anesthesia, analgesia, and exotic animal medicine. Jody has had the opportunity to lecture throughout North America since 2000 on anesthesia and various exotic animal topics as well as publishing numerous articles and book chapters for both canine/feline and exotic animal medicine and anesthesia topics.

Rachel Parchem, AAS, always knew growing up that she wanted to be involved in veterinary medicine and species conservation. While working as an assistant in general practice in 2014, she attended Joliet Junior College's veterinary technician program, graduating with an AAS in Veterinary Medical Technology in 2016. While in school, she interned at a specialty hospital with exotics and the Shedd Aquarium. She remained a volunteer at the Shedd Aquarium from 2016–2017 and eventually became a full-time employee in 2017. She is currently working at the Lincoln Park Zoo. She enjoys working with the unique species, the staff, and being able to make an impact by being involved in conservation and research as well as educating the public and future veterinary technicians.

Janet L. Pezzi-Jones, LVMT, is a Licensed Veterinary Medical Technician at University of Tennessee-Knoxville, Veterinary Medical Center and has been working there since 2010 in the Avian/Exotics/Wildlife/Zoo department. She has had speaking engagements at Exotics Con and local conferences and instructs clinical veterinary students in reptile, avian, and small mammal husbandry and nursing techniques. She is pursuing her master's degree in educational psychology concentrating on Adult Education.

Samuel Rivera, DVM, MS, DABVP (avian practice), DACZM, DECZM (ZHM) graduated from Kansas State University College of Veterinary Medicine in 1996. After graduation, he practiced in a small animal/exotics practice in the Atlanta metro area for nine years prior to accepting a full-time position at Zoo Atlanta. He currently serves as the Vice President of Animal Health at Zoo Atlanta. Sam also serves as an adjunct faculty at the University of Georgia College of Veterinary Medicine.

April Romagnano, PhD, DVM, ABVP graduated from McGill University with a BSc in Agriculture in 1982, obtained a PhD from Université de Montréal in 1987, and a DVM from University of Florida in 1992. She completed an internship in Wildlife/Small Animal Medicine at UF in 1993, a residency in non-domestic avian medicine at NCSU in 1995, and became ABVP boarded in avian practice in 1996. In 1995, she was staff veterinarian at ABRC, the largest avicultural collection in the United States until it closed in 2001. Since 2001, she has been an avian specialist, exotic veterinarian, practice owner, and manager. In 2001, she opened the Small Animal, Bird, and Exotic Clinic then sold it in 2017. A second clinic, Avian and Amphibian Exotic Clinic opened in 2011 and third in 2018 for Small Animal and Large Exotic Cats. From 2007 to 2011, she also worked at Scripps Florida, first as the Clinical Veterinarian and then the Director of Animal Resources. Since 1996, she has been a courtesy clinical assistant professor in the Wildlife and Zoological Medicine Service, Dept of SACS, College of Veterinary Medicine, University of Florida.

Colleen Roman, DVM, RVT, BS, was a registered veterinary technician of small animals and exotics medicine for 10 years and obtained her DVM from the University of Georgia in 2021. She has been an associate veterinarian at a busy small animal and exotics practice in Atlanta, Georgia since graduation. She has studied under some of the most prominent leaders in exotic animal medicine at UGA, Zoo Atlanta, North Carolina's Avian and Exotic Animal Care Hospital, and Florida's Broward Avian and Exotic Animal Hospital with aspirations to achieve American Board of Veterinary Practitioners (AVBP) in Exotic Companion Mammal Practice, Avian Practice, and Reptile and Amphibian Practice. Her long-term goal is to establish a high-quality private practice for small animal and exotic medicine in the state of Georgia.

Serina Scott, RVT, received her AAS in veterinary technology from Ogeechee Technical College in Statesboro, Georgia in 2019. After completing an internship at the Avian and Exotic Animal Hospital of Georgia, she was hired on as a technician. She continues to work exclusively with exotics and wildlife.

Jodi Seidel, RVT, CCRP, has been working in the veterinary industry for 20 years. She worked as a kennel and veterinary assistant through tech school and graduated from Kirkwood Community Technical College in

2005 with an associate degree in applied technology in veterinary technology. After graduation and licensing, she pursued a full-time position at the University of Missouri Veterinary Teaching Hospital in the small animal orthopedics service. In 2008, Jodi was certified in physical rehabilitation through the University of Tennessee and helped develop the small animal rehabilitation service at the University of Missouri. In 2010, Jodi continued her passion for patient care working in both rehab and surgery in a private referral practice before eventually returning to academia. Jodi has been responsible for the growth and development of the small animal physical rehabilitation service at the University of Georgia since its inception in 2015. Jodi is passionate about teaching DVM and technician students about all things related to full body medicine (especially posture!) and educating owners on how to help their pets (no matter the species) live their best pain-free and independent lives.

Sandy Skeba, LVMT, received her AS degree from Harcum College in 1987. She has always had an interest in exotic animals. After working with both large and small domestic species at the University of Pennsylvania she was hired at the Philadelphia Zoo, where she worked for ten years. Since then, she has worked in various roles, including an exotics-only private practice in Miami, raptor rehabilitation in Arizona, an avian field biologist in New Mexico, lab tech at the Alaska SeaLife center, and most recently at the Nashville Zoo, where she was hospital manager. She is currently working on finishing her bachelor's degree in Fisheries and Wildlife Conservation at Oregon State University.

Douglas K. Taylor, DVM, received his DVM degree from Michigan State University in 1995. Following five years in general veterinary practice, he studied wildlife toxicology at Clemson University and then entered the laboratory animal medicine training program at the University of Michigan in 2002. While at the University of Michigan, Dr Taylor earned his MS degree and became a Diplomate in the American College of Laboratory Animal Medicine in 2006. He is currently the Director of the Division of Laboratory Animal Services, Attending Veterinarian, and Clinical Professor of Physiology at Augusta University in Augusta Georgia.

Liz Vetrano BS, CVT, VTS, received her BS in biology from Towson University in 2009. During that time, she took an internship with the Philadelphia Zoo and was able to land a job after graduation as a Children's Zookeeper and bird show trainer. She continues her bird training with Animal Behavior and Conservation Connections today. During the following years, she worked for an ABVP avian-boarded veterinarian and received her CVT in 2015 and her VTS (Exotic Companion Animals) in 2022. After 12 years working with exotic companion animals, she is now the exotics department supervisor at Mount Laurel Animal Hospital.

Stacey Leonatti Wilkinson, DVM, AVBP, graduated with her DVM from the University of Tennessee in 2006. From 2006–2015, she worked as an associate veterinarian at Avian and Exotic Animal Care in Raleigh, NC. In 2013, she became a diplomate of the American Board of Veterinary Practitioners in Reptile and Amphibian Medicine. In 2015, she opened Avian and Exotic Animal Hospital of Georgia, a practice exclusively dedicated to the care of exotic pets. Dr. Wilkinson is also an adjunct assistant professor at North Carolina State University College of Veterinary Medicine. She has been published in scientific and non-scientific journals, written multiple textbook chapters, and lectures nationally on exotic animal medicine and care. She is Treasurer of the Association of Reptile and Amphibian Veterinarians and is active in the Association of Exotic Mammal Veterinarians and Association of Avian Veterinarians as well.

Brad Wilson, DVM, is a veterinarian and partner in two private practice veterinary clinics in north Atlanta. He received his BS in zoology and his DVM from the University of Georgia. He is a consulting veterinarian for the largest wholesale importer and distributor of fish, reptiles, amphibians, pocket pets, ferrets, and birds in north Georgia as well as for the Atlanta Botanical Garden, which has an extensive collection of dendrobatid and Central and South American hylid frogs. He has personally maintained and captively bred many species of snakes and frogs.

Preface

The fourth edition was written to provide the veterinary technician with important updated information about a variety of species commonly seen in exotic practice reflecting changes in this branch of medicine that have occurred since the third edition. This text will be beneficial to technicians who are just now entering the exotic animal field, have been in the field for a while, or for those brave individuals who are preparing for the VTS (Exotic Companion Animal) examination. While it was not written for veterinarians, they may find it beneficial as well.

With the help of this book, the technician will know what questions to ask to obtain an adequate history, be able to educate the client about husbandry and nutrition, be able to safely handle and restrain common species, and be able to perform necessary procedures when needed. Because the field of exotic animal medicine is a dynamic one, new knowledge is constantly emerging about many of the species kept as pets and new information can in some cases contradict what was thought to be true before. For many species, exotic animal medicine could be said to be in its infancy. We realize that for some of the species featured in this book, the information presented may need to be modified in the future. Because what is known about exotic animal medicine is forever changing and much has not been scientifically proven, it is common to find contradicting information from one reputable source to the next. This can create frustration but also provides the challenge of working in a cutting-edge area of medicine. This is the major reason why obtaining continuing education in this area of medicine is paramount. Veterinary technicians working in exotic medicine need to engage in lifelong learning to be up to date on the latest information.

New contributors have been added to this edition as well as new chapters. While some of the contributors provided drug dosages and formularies, we do not take responsibility for what is provided. We also realize that while technicians do not make decisions about what drugs to use in any animal, they are required to be familiar with different pharmaceuticals, know where to find a dosage, know how to calculate it, and what to expect when the drug is given.

This book was written with the assumption that the technician already is educated in topics such as anatomy, physiology, medical terminology, pathology, and pharmacology. Only what is unique to the species featured is presented.

We hope this book proves to be beneficial to all technicians interested in exotic animal medicine.

Bonnie Ballard
Ryan Cheek

Acknowledgments

We would like to extend our gratitude to the following individuals who were contributors to the first edition of the book. Without their help, this book would not have become a reality.

Anne E. Hudson, LVT, LAT
Trevor Lyon, RVT
Julie Mays, LVT
James R. McClearen, DVM
Shannon Richards, CAT

We would like to thank following individuals who contributed to the 2nd and/or 3rd editions of the book.

Susan Coy, CVT
Maria Crane, DVM
Lilian Gerhardt, LVT
Tarah Hadley, DVM
Michael Huerkamp, DVM
Michael Duffy Jones, DVM
Jill Murray, RVT

Disclaimer

As exotic animal dosages are based largely on empirical data and not researched facts, the editors and contributors make no guarantee regarding the results obtained from dosages used in this textbook.

About the Companion Website

This book is accompanied by a companion website:

www.wiley.com/go/ballard/4e

The website includes:
- Supplementary mock tests and history forms

Section I

Introduction

1

Exotic Animals in Clinical Practice
Bonnie Ballard

Welcome to the world of exotic animal medicine! For those who practice it, it is the variety that provides the spice to veterinary life. In a practice that sees exotics, it would not be uncommon to see a dog for vaccines, a diabetic cat, an iguana with pathologic fractures, a ferret for a physical examination, and a feather-picking cockatoo all in one day. The challenge for those who work in this field lies in the vast differences in the species seen and the rapid increases in knowledge related to this field (Figure 1.1).

While not as common as small animal practices, more exclusively exotic animal practices are cropping up across the country. It is not surprising that just as a small animal practice may have a clinic cat, practices that see exotics exclusively may have a bird or an exotic companion mammal as their clinic pet (Figure 1.2).

In veterinary medicine, an exotic animal is any animal that is not a dog, cat, horse, or cow. Exotic animals include wildlife species, animals commonly used in research that are kept as pets, and animals native to various regions of the world, such as South America, Australia, and Africa. The interest in exotic animal medicine continues to grow, and this is related to the fact that the number of people who own exotic pets increases year after year. Based on data from the AVMA 2022 Sourcebook, it is estimated that 9.4% of households in the United States own "exotic pets," meaning pets other than dogs and cats. With respect to exotic companion mammals, rabbits are the most popular at 1.2% of households. It was estimated that 1.4% of households own pet reptiles. Households owning birds in the United States are estimated to be 2.5% (AVMA 2022). These statistics are evidence that there is a need for veterinarians and veterinary technicians to provide care for these animals. It should come as no surprise that the client who brings their dog or cat into a small animal hospital also has one of the aforementioned pets and would welcome the chance to bring that pet to the hospital if exotic animal care was offered.

Many households that own dogs and cats also have an aquarium. In 2022, it was estimated that 2.7% of US households owned aquarium fish (AVMA 2022). Fish owners may have many aquariums, and some may even breed certain types of fish. Historically, fish owners have relied on other fish enthusiasts and Internet sites to learn about fish care because other than a local pet shop there may not have been any reliable resources for information and treatment of their fish. Having a veterinarian willing to treat fish would be a welcome idea once a client learns that services are available.

Continuing education is an important part of a veterinary technician's professional enhancement, and its importance in exotic medicine cannot be overemphasized. What is known about the care and treatment of exotic animals is forever changing as more and more is learned. What one may have heard is the proper diet for a particular lizard one year may be something different the next year. More and more drugs are being tried in exotics. The use of analgesics continues to be an important topic in exotic animal medicine as more and more drugs have been tried and shown to be effective. This is largely because veterinary professionals are acknowledging that these species feel pain and because many owners no longer consider them to be expendable pets. This type of cutting-edge information is presented at conferences and in professional publications. This presents an added challenge to practices that see exotic animals, as information is forever changing.

With an increase in exotic pet ownership comes an increase in the amount and variety of continuing education available for veterinary professionals at veterinary conferences both in person and virtually. In recent years, there has been an increase in the number of continuing education hours related to exotic analgesia, behavior, and enrichment. Each summer, Exoticscon, a conference that features continuing education exclusively toward exotic

Exotic Animal Medicine for the Veterinary Technician, Fourth Edition. Edited by Bonnie Ballard and Ryan Cheek.
© 2024 John Wiley & Sons, Inc. Published 2024 by John Wiley & Sons, Inc.
Companion Website: www.wiley.com/go/ballard/4e

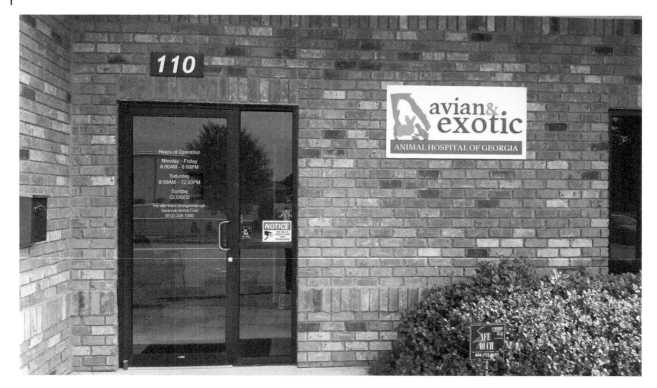

Figure 1.1 An exclusively exotic animal medicine practice near Savannah, Georgia. This practice sees all types of exotic animals including reptiles, birds, exotic companion mammals, amphibians, and fish. (Courtesy of Dr. Stacey Wilkinson.)

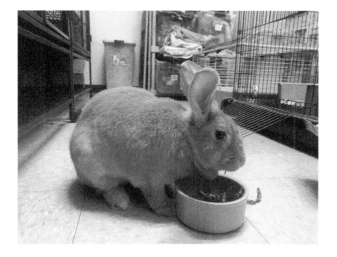

Figure 1.2 Red, the New Zealand Red rabbit is the clinic pet at an exclusively exotics practice. (Courtesy of Dr. Stacey Wilkinson.)

Table 1.1 Summary of requirements and application process to become a VTS (Zoo).

1.	Be a credentialed veterinary technician in your state of practice
2.	Obtain 10,000 hours of clinical experience within the field of zoological medicine within 7 years prior to application
3.	Obtain a minimum of 40 hours of CE related to zoological medicine or appropriate related topics within 5 years of application
4.	Case log comprising a minimum of 40 cases within 3 years of application
5.	Completion of mastery of skills list
6.	Write five case reports
7.	Two letters of recommendation
8.	Submit application by deadline
9.	Sit for examination

For the most current application packet, details, and information, visit www.avzmt.org/AVZMT-Candidate.

animal medicine, is held. This conference is open to veterinarians and veterinary technicians. VMX, held annually in January in Orlando, Florida, includes an extensive exotics program open to veterinary professionals.

There are now two veterinary technician specialties available for those interested in exotics. The Academy of Veterinary Zoological Medicine Technicians provides an avenue for becoming credentialed in zoo animal medicine

(Table 1.1). Currently, there are 16 active and 2 emeritus zoo VTS'. The newest exotic specialty can be obtained through the Academy of Veterinary Technicians in Clinical Practice (Table 1.2). This academy has a concentration in exotic companion medicine. Currently, there are 15 veterinary technicians with this specialty.

Table 1.2 Summary of requirements and application process to become a VTS (Exotic Companion Animal).

1. Be a credentialed veterinary technician in your state of practice
2. Obtain 10,000 hours of clinical experience within the field of exotic animals within 5 years prior to application with a minimum of 7,500 hours in exotic companion animals
3. Obtain 50 hours of CE with 37.5 hours related to exotic animals related to advanced clinical practice within 5 years of application
4. Case log comprising a minimum of 50 cases related to advanced clinical practice in the calendar year of the application
5. Completion of mastery of skills list
6. Write four case reports
7. Two letters of recommendation
8. Submit application by deadline
9. Sit for examination

For the most current application packet, details, and information, visit avtcp.org/exotic-companion-animal.html.

There are three associations and specialties available to veterinarians related to exotic animal medicine. The Association of Exotic Companion Mammals, established in 2000, and the related ABVP Exotic Companion Mammal Specialty were created to meet the needs of those who seek more education in these animals. This specialty had its first diplomats in 2010. The AEMV currently has over 900 members. Similarly, the Association of Reptile and Amphibian Veterinarians was established in 1992, and the related ABVP Reptile and Amphibian specialty was established in 2009. Additional evidence of increasing interest in exotic animal medicine is found in the number of veterinarians who have pursued a specialty in exotic medicine. As of 2019, there are 16 veterinarians with the ABVP specialty in reptiles and 32 in exotic companion mammals. Additionally, there are over 100 veterinarians with the ABVP specialty in avian medicine. These numbers do not reflect the many veterinarians who are members of the associations, desiring to gain valuable information in exotic animal medicine.

The Association of Avian Veterinarians, established in 1980, has roughly 1,700 members, but very few see avian patients exclusively. Approximately 135 veterinarians are boarded in avian medicine by the ABVP. For technicians who enjoy working with birds, it still remains difficult to find a practice that sees them for anything more than a beak, nail, or wing trim.

Because of the increase in interest in exotics evidenced by the number of members in these associations, more opportunities for technicians to work with exotics continue to increase. Opportunities to expand a technician's knowledge base also exist as these three exotic associations allow technicians to become members.

While there has not been an explosion in exotic-only practices, many small animal practices have expanded their scope of practice to include more species. For example, a small animal clinic that may have only seen rabbits in the past may expand the number of species they are willing to see to include many or all of the exotic companion mammals. Conversely, there are small animal practices that will see reptiles.

There are several scenarios in which a technician interested in exotics may find this book helpful. A technician may take a job in a practice where exotics are seen but knows little about them. This book will help that person get up to speed with what one needs to know about popular exotic species. A technician may work for a veterinarian who wants to add exotics to the practice but does not have hands-on experience with them. Alternatively, a technician may find employment working with a wildlife rehabilitator and need to brush up on current information about exotics. Knowledge of exotic animals, their treatment, and their care is desirable when pursuing employment in the zoo and public aquarium environment.

For a technician who works for a veterinarian who would like to add exotics to the practice, the technician can play a key role in helping to establish them as patients. It is essential that the technician help the veterinarian understand how the practice will need to change to accommodate these species. A veterinarian must accept the fact that a 15- or 20-minute appointment will not suffice. In many cases, appointments of 30 minutes or longer will be required. Because husbandry and nutrition are typically the two most common causes of illness in exotic animals, a thorough history in these areas is essential. Also, because of the delicate nature of some of the species seen, more time may be required to perform a physical examination. In many cases, the owner will require client education to keep his or her pet healthy, so adequate time to do so will be required.

One of the challenges in treating exotic animals is that many will keep the appearance of health as long as they can, as this is what is beneficial in the wild to prevent becoming attractive to a predator. A bird is a great example of this. A bird can be incredibly ill and even be in actuality dangerously thin, but the owner will think it is fine because its feather appearance is still being maintained. A patient like this is very fragile, so handling it in a stressful clinical environment may be just what could tip them over the edge, resulting in death. Because one may have a very limited time to perform a physical examination or perform a procedure, it is the technician's job to make sure that all supplies and instruments needed for the examination

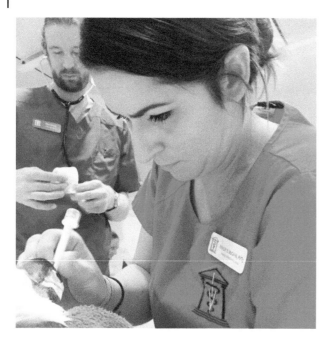

Figure 1.3 A veterinary technician intubating a cockatoo. (Courtesy of Ashley MaGaha.)

and/or treatment are ready prior to handling the animal. With many patients, time is of the essence.

Anesthesia for exotic patients poses a huge change from small animal medicine in that a veterinary technician who is experienced with exotics will be required to monitor anesthesia on ALL patients for ALL procedures. These patients require second-to-second monitoring. This is especially true for avian patients (Figure 1.3).

A veterinary technician who has an interest in exotic animal medicine will be expected to be a trusted expert in restraint techniques, which can vary from species to species. Different types of lizards require different restraint techniques, for example. Proper restraint ensures the safety of the veterinary staff and the patient whether dealing with a cockatoo or a chinchilla.

The front office staff must be knowledgeable and interested in exotic pets as they will be the first people the pet owner comes in contact with. The worst thing that can happen is for a snake owner, for example, to come to the front desk and the receptionist recoils in fear at the sight of it. This is not only unprofessional behavior but one that puts the knowledge of the doctors into question. Likewise, if a receptionist does not know the difference between a macaw and a cockatoo, the bird owner may question the knowledge of the doctors, as it may appear that the clinic does not see many birds. When an appointment is made, it is crucial that the exact species of animal is obtained. For example, a "lizard appointment" is not enough information. What type of lizard is important, especially since it is possible that

the patient coming in is not one the veterinarian or technician is familiar with. In this case, research about the specific lizard coming in can be done before it arrives.

Another consideration when deciding to see exotic pets is where they are going to be housed in the hospital. Because many of the exotic companion mammals seen are prey animals, where they are housed in relation to dogs and cats must be taken into account. For example, a rabbit should not be caged where a cat patient can watch it. This alone can create undue added stress for a rabbit patient, who is already stressed being in the hospital environment. An exotic pet should not have to add the fear of being eaten to its worries during a hospital stay.

One of the most important roles of the veterinary technician is that of a meticulous history-taker. As each chapter illustrates, a simple history will not do. It is not uncommon for a practice that sees exotics to have a separate history form from those used for dogs and cats. For example, the practice may have a history sheet for reptiles, another for exotic companion mammals as well as one for avian patients. Having history forms such as these not only ensures that all necessary questions are asked, but it also saves time. Wild-caught species can have different health problems than captive-raised ones, so the origin of the pet needs to be ascertained. How the pet is housed is vitally important, and this means not only asking what it is housed in but also the cage size, construction, substrate used, and where it is kept at the home. If the animal is not brought in the cage it is housed in, the technician, after gathering the history, should be able to create a mental picture of what the cage at home looks like. In a world in which most people carry a cell phone, it would be possible to have the receptionist who schedules the appointment ask the owner to take a picture of the cage prior to their visit to the practice.

For practices that see fish, a specific history sheet for them is important as well. Questions similar to those asked in other exotic patients should be asked. Knowing the aquarium size, whether the fish are in fresh or salt water, what diets are fed, how many fish are in the tank or pond, and where it is in a household or yard is important information. Having the owner provide pictures of their tanks/ponds is beneficial for these patients as well.

The same is true for gathering adequate information about the pet's diet. It is not good enough to ask what is fed as what is fed may not be what is consumed. For example, an owner may report that their Amazon parrot's daily diet is made up of fruits, vegetables, and seeds. When asked how much of each is consumed each day, the answer may be mostly seeds, which is an inadequate diet. For the practice that sees reptiles that are insectivores, a veterinary technician must be knowledgeable about what insects are safe and nutritious to feed and what ones are not.

In many cases, owners of exotics may have gained misinformation about their pet's care from the pet shop where it was purchased. While some may be knowledgeable, many pet shop employees simply do not know the correct information about the species they sell. The veterinary technician should be able to give owners the correct information about husbandry and nutrition without chastising them for their mistakes. Many honestly may not know that what they were doing was wrong. Owners may have obtained books that are not written by reputable sources or found information on the Internet that is inaccurate. In a clinic that sees fish, the veterinary technician can offer advice on how to set up a tank and avoid common pitfalls that happen to new fish owners, such as buying too many fish for a brand-new tank, or not quarantining new additions. Owners value information on how to keep their pets healthy and their veterinary clinic should be the source of that information.

The veterinary technician can also be of value when helping a client make a decision about what type of exotic pet to buy. For example, an iguana is considered to be a difficult reptile to keep as its housing and nutrition requirements are demanding. A bearded dragon may be a better choice. A budgie may be a better choice for a first-time bird owner than a macaw, which can be noisy and messy as well as requiring a lot of behavioral enrichment. Because a macaw would require a larger cage than a budgie, the size of the client's home may factor into the decision. The size of a client's home can be a consideration with certain reptiles as well.

The topic of conservation of species is also important. New exotic pet owners should be encouraged to acquire captive-raised species rather than wild-caught if possible. With many exotic species, numbers in the wild are diminishing. Captive-raised species can also be a benefit as they may have fewer disease and behavioral problems. For example, wild-caught snakes typically have more parasites than captive-raised ones. Most exotic species desired as pets can be obtained from captive-raised sources.

The veterinary technician can also provide the veterinarian who wants to add exotics to the practice ideas on how to market this change. It is easy for a clinic to advertise this addition by putting a sign up at the reception desk and mentioning it on the clinic's website and on social media sites. If a clinic produces a periodic newsletter, the technician can add an item related to exotics. A simple, low-cost service to offer to fish-owning clients is water testing. By using a professional water testing kit rather than one found in a pet shop, clients can see the value in what they are paying for. If a veterinarian wants to add fish to the practice, offering house calls to evaluate fish in their environment can be offered. The veterinary technician can do water testing and obtain a history while the veterinarian evaluates the fish. With the help of good marketing, the practice soon can become the go-to resource for their clients and the community to obtain information about the ins and outs of keeping and caring for exotic animals as pets.

Offering services for exotic patients does not require a large amount of money, as the average animal hospital will have most of the necessary supplies and equipment needed to treat exotics. There are some items that will need to be purchased, however. For example, a gram scale will be required to weigh many of the very small patients. Microtainer blood collection tubes are also essential. For the veterinarian who desires to see fish, the good news is that it does not require a huge expenditure to add them. Many items needed to treat fish are those that a clinic already has. Appendix 12 provides a list of equipment useful in exotic practices.

One should never underestimate the strength of the human–animal bond that exists between owners and their exotic pets. An owner can be as bonded to a mouse or a snake as another owner would be to a dog or horse. Just as one should never assume what an owner is willing to spend for medical care on dogs, cats, and horses, one should never assume what exotic pet owners would be willing to spend for their pets. The low cost of some exotic companion mammals does not mean that owners will not seek quality veterinary care. It is not uncommon to see a devoted owner spend hundreds of dollars on a surgical procedure for a pet rat. For those who keep fish, they can range in cost from around $3 for a fancy guppy to $100 or more for some marine species (Noga 2010). There are fish kept in ponds, such as koi, which can cost several thousands of dollars. Fish owners can and do become very attached to their fish and may even have names for them. These owners will be willing to spend money to treat them and learn how to properly care for them.

Practices seeing exotic pets must be aware of and provide current standards of care as these have advanced in exotic animal medicine. For example, during anesthesia, monitoring devices used in dogs and cats can and should be used, such as pulse oximetry and ECGs. Providing analgesia is an important consideration as well. Multimodal techniques as well as regional nerve blocks are used in exotic animals including reptiles. In recent years, there has been an emphasis on creating stress/anxiety-free clinical environments and techniques for dogs, cats, and horses. These practices can and should be used with exotic patients when possible.

There are veterinary practices that see exotic pets that will also see primates and venomous species. Because of the dangers to humans from these animals, veterinarians will typically set the "rules of engagement" regarding the care and treatment of these animals. For example, the veterinarian may only see a primate or a venomous snake after hours, when all other employees and clients have left the premises. Likewise, a veterinarian may require that the owner of a venomous snake provide in-date antivenom along with the snake.

Some veterinarians will not see large exotic cats in practice due to safety concerns. And yes, there are people who have permits to keep them. Others will see these animals on the owner's premises as long as handling equipment, such as a squeeze cage, is provided. It will be important that **all** employees know the clinic's protocol for seeing primates, venomous species, and large cats.

Every state has its own laws regarding which species are legal to keep as pets and which are not and changes in these laws happen frequently. It is up to the practice to be apprised of the current laws involving ownership of exotic animals in the municipality and state in which the clinic is located. It is up to the veterinarian to decide whether they will see pets that may in fact be illegal pets and to communicate this information to the technicians and other staff (Figure 1.4).

Because many veterinary technicians who work with exotics have an interest in working in a zoo or aquarium,

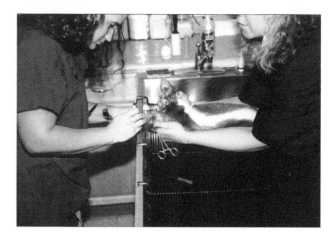

Figure 1.4 A technician drawing blood from a skunk. (Courtesy of Ryan Cheek.)

included are two chapters devoted to explaining the technician's role in these environments.

In response to the increasing interest in exotics, this book provides a compilation of the most recent practices in the area of exotic animal care. Exotic animal medicine provides a veterinary technician with the opportunity to utilize all of their skills and knowledge in a way that has a direct benefit to the practice and the patients.

References

AVMA. 2022. U.S. Pet Ownership & Demographics Sourcebook. American Veterinary Medical Association.

Noga, E. 2010. Fish Disease-Diagnosis and Treatment. Ames: Wiley.

Section II

Analgesia and Anesthesia

2

Exotic Anesthesia and Analgesia

Jody Nugent-Deal

Anesthetic and analgesic techniques in exotic animals have had many advances over the past several years. While exotic animal patients are not little dogs and cats, many of the same anesthetic drugs, anesthetic monitors, and multimodal anesthetic techniques are used in both groups of patients. When working with dogs and cats, it is generally easy to place an intravenous catheter, provide fluid therapy, intubate, hook up an ECG, place a blood pressure cuff, and keep track of the core body temperature. This can be much more difficult in many exotic animals. How does one compensate for the potential lack of monitoring? In some cases, we may not be able to, but as highly trained anesthetists we can do our best to monitor the anesthetic patient by looking at trends, using visual assessments, and being able to anticipate the needs of the patient.

Pre-anesthetic Assessment

The pre-anesthetic assessment in exotic animals is very similar to that in dogs and cats. Patients should have a full physical examination and baseline blood work performed prior to general anesthesia. A complete blood count (CBC) and biochemistry panel are ideal to help assess organ function and overall health. In some cases, a full panel may not be possible, either due to the species or the size of the patient. Ideally, a minimum baseline should be established, and this generally includes a packed cell volume (PCV), total solids (TS), blood glucose (BG), and BUN via a reagent Azostix® (the latter in mammals only).

A physical examination should be performed prior to choosing an anesthetic protocol. Drug protocols are not black and white. They should be chosen based on several factors including, but not limited to, the following: the species being anesthetized, the procedure performed, anticipated pain of the procedure, ASA status of the patient (see Table 2.1), age, drugs available, and experience of the anesthetist. Although the final decision on the drug

protocol is up to the veterinarian, it is important that the veterinary technician has a full understanding of the drugs being used and why they were chosen.

A basic physical examination will vary slightly by species. All equipment needed for the examination should be out and within arm's reach prior to capturing the patient. Common items needed for a physical examination include a pediatric or infant stethoscope, light source, oral specula, otoscope, ophthalmoscope, species-specific restraint gear such as gloves and towels, and supplies needed for venipuncture. Having supplies prepared ahead of time will decrease the time in hand and reduce the overall stress placed upon the patient.

A visual assessment should occur prior to removing the patient from the cage. The respiratory rate can be obtained as well as the overall attitude and mentation of the animal. Capture and restraint will be dependent upon the species and type of enclosure in which it is housed.

Physical Examination

The hands-on physical examination should start at the head and end at the tail. This will help ensure that nothing is overlooked. Regardless of species, all instruments, tools, and diagnostic supplies (Figure 2.1) should be out and within hand's reach prior to ever capturing the patient. This reduces the time in hand and the overall stress placed upon the animal.

Obtaining the patient's weight and core body temperature (if possible) should be the first part of the physical examination. Since many exotic animals are small, it is best to use a scale that weighs to the nearest gram. It is also important to note that most ear thermometers do not work well in exotic pets, often due to aural anatomy. It is best to use a digital rectal thermometer.

The primary deviation from the "head to tail" method of a physical examination in exotic small mammals is the oral

Exotic Animal Medicine for the Veterinary Technician, Fourth Edition. Edited by Bonnie Ballard and Ryan Cheek.
© 2024 John Wiley & Sons, Inc. Published 2024 by John Wiley & Sons, Inc.
Companion Website: www.wiley.com/go/ballard/4e

Table 2.1 ASA physical status classification system.

ASA Physical Status 1—A normal healthy patient

ASA Physical Status 2—A patient with mild systemic disease

ASA Physical Status 3—A patient with moderate to severe systemic disease, but the patient is able to compensate

ASA Physical Status 4—A patient with severe systemic disease that is a constant threat to life

ASA Physical Status 5—A moribund patient who is not expected to survive without the operation

Based on the Physical Status Classification System of the American Society of Anesthesiologists, 520N Northwest Highway, Park Ridge IL 60068-2573; www.asahq.org. ASA, American Society of Anesthesiologists.

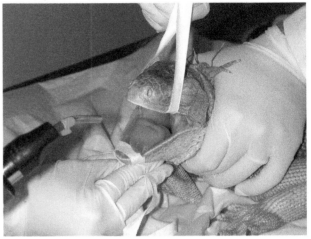

Figure 2.2 Oral examination of a lizard.

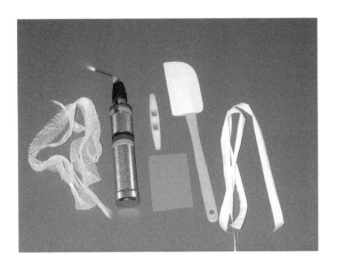

Figure 2.1 Instruments and supplies necessary for a physical examination of an exotic animal.

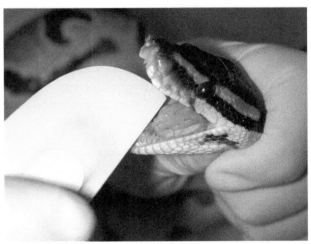

Figure 2.3 Oral examination of a snake using a kitchen spatula.

examination. In other exotic species, the mouth is usually examined when the head is examined. Damage can easily occur in many species of reptiles and birds during the oral examination. It is suggested that an atraumatic tool is used to open the oral cavity. The author suggests tape (Figure 2.2), gauze stirrups, or a plastic spatula (Figure 2.3) over the commercially available metal specula.

The oral examination can be stressful for exotic small mammals (ferrets are the exception) and therefore is generally performed last. The oral examination can be difficult in an awake patient, therefore sedation or general anesthesia may be required in patients that are not cooperative. Common drugs used for sedation include a benzodiazepine such as midazolam and an opioid such as butorphanol, buprenorphine, or full mu opioids such as morphine, hydromorphone, or methadone. Acepromazine or dexmedetomidine can also be used in most species of exotic small mammals. Isoflurane or sevoflurane are the two inhalant anesthetics used to provide general anesthesia

when necessary. Ferrets are an exception. The oral examination of the ferret can be performed when the head is being examined (very similar to oral examination in a dog or cat). One great thing about ferrets is that when you scruff them, they usually open their mouth! This is an easy way to get a quick oral examination.

A mouth speculum with a light source is one of the most helpful instruments that can be used when performing an oral examination (for rodents and rabbits only). There are a few different mouth specula that can be used (Figure 2.4). A long otoscope cone attached to the otoscope handle can be used to examine the mouth. A small vaginal speculum and a penlight can also be used. A rigid endoscope along with a mouth speculum can be used to examine the mouth. One of the most effective ways to perform an oral examination on an exotic small mammal is with a bivalve nasal speculum. This instrument (manufactured by

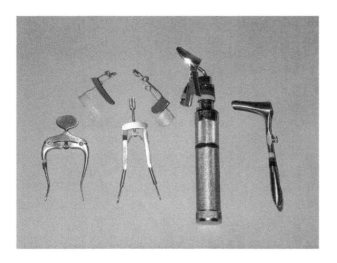

Figure 2.4 Instruments used to perform an oral examination.

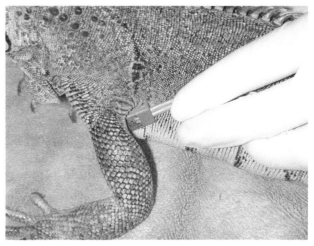

Figure 2.5 Use of a Doppler as a way to get a heart rate on a lizard.

Welch Allyn®) has a light source and attaches to a Welch Allyn® battery handpiece. The bivalve speculum is ideal because it has the light source attached to the speculum. This combination frees up one hand.

It is important to examine the gingiva, tongue, and all dental arcades including the incisors. Look for any dental abnormalities such as malocclusion, tongue entrapment (generally seen in guinea pigs with severe dental disease), incisor overgrowth, fractured teeth, or points on the lingual or buccal surfaces of the premolars and molars (common in guinea pigs, rabbits, and chinchillas). If dental disease is present, a further workup may be necessary, including blood work, radiographs, etc.

Although exotic animal patients are quite different from dogs and cats, the physical examination is fairly similar. The examination is generally started by looking at the eyes, ears, and nares. They should be clean, clear, and free of any discharge. Any signs of discharge or debris can be a sign of an underlying disease process and should be investigated further.

It is important to palpate the limbs (if present) as well as the abdomen or celom. Palpation should include checking for any masses, wounds, lesions, and any other potential abnormalities on the body. The palmar and plantar surfaces of the feet should also be closely examined. Lastly, examine the skin and look for any signs of dermatophytes or ectoparasites.

The heart and lungs should be auscultated using an infant or pediatric stethoscope. It is important to note the presence of any potential heart murmurs, arrhythmias, harsh lung sounds, or anything that may sound abnormal. Heart murmurs are graded using the standard scale of 1 to 6 (I to VI). Auscultation with a stethoscope is difficult in most reptilian species due to the thickness of the scales or, in chelonians, the presence of the shell. The heart rate is generally

obtained using a Doppler ultrasonic unit (Figure 2.5) or simply watching the heartbeat when possible.

A body condition score should be assigned to each patient during the examination. The same system used in dogs and cats is also used with exotic small mammals. Scales vary based on species and many examples are currently available for use.

The hydration status of the patient should be evaluated during the physical examination. In most species, the mucous membranes should be moist and pink. The capillary refill time should be between 1 and 2 seconds and is most accurately used in mammalian patients. In birds, venous refill time can be used to assess overall hydration. This is done by gently pulling the wing away from the body and quickly depressing the cutaneous ulnar vein (basilic vein). Refill of the vessel should be instantaneous. Extended refill time suggests dehydration.

A common sign of dehydration is dry or tacky mucous membranes, sunken eyes, extended venous or capillary refill time, and lack of skin turgor. In mammals and reptiles, the skin should be tented or pulled upward to assess dehydration. In birds, the skin over the keel can be pulled gently to the side. The longer the skin stays in place, or stays tented, the more dehydrated the animal. Percentages of dehydration can be assigned to the patient. This is done in the same manner as for dogs and cats. For example, a slightly dehydrated patient with a capillary refill time of about 2.5 seconds and skin that is only slightly slow (instead of immediate) to return to normal can be assigned a 5% dehydration status. If the patient has very tacky, dry mucous membranes, sunken eyes, a capillary refill time of 3 to 4 seconds, and skin that stays in a tented position, a 10% to 12% dehydration status can be assigned. A dehydration status of 10% to 12% is an emergency and should be treated immediately.

Once a complete physical examination has been performed and the animal is stable, diagnostics can be performed as needed.

Venipuncture

Blood volume is generally not taken into account when obtaining pre-surgical blood work in the canine and feline patient. Many companion exotic patients are quite small, therefore total circulating blood volume, the amount of blood needed for sample submission, and the amount of blood loss anticipated during surgery must be considered. Table 2.2 demonstrates approximate circulating blood volume and how much blood loss can occur safely.

Blood collected from small exotic species should be placed in BD Microtainer® collection tubes. These tubes are made specifically for small sample sizes (preventing dilution of sample). CBC samples are placed in the purple top tube (EDTA) and the biochemistry sample is placed in the green top tube (heparin). Blood can be placed in a non-additive red-top tube, but heparin yields a larger volume of plasma compared to the serum in the red-top tube after centrifugation. If blood work is not being processed in-house, check with the commercial lab to see what requirements they have. Every lab is a little different. Many people suggest placing reptilian (and some avian) blood samples in a heparinized syringe or heparin tube, but this can cause blue-tinged staining to the cells and clumping of the thrombocytes and leukocytes, making interpretation of the CBC results more difficult (Bounous 2010). To avoid this, the author suggests taking a blood sample via a clean syringe and first making a blood smear before placing the remaining blood into the EDTA and/or heparin or non-additive tubes.

EDTA can cause hemolysis in some reptilian and avian species. If this occurs, heparin will need to be used for both the CBC and biochemistry panels.

Table 2.2 Indicative blood volumes and safe blood loss.

	Circulating blood volume (% total body weight)	Total blood volume safe to lose (% total body weight)
Reptiles	~5–8%	~1%
Exotic small mammals	~5–8%	~1%
Birds	~10%	~1% (healthy) ~0.5% (sick)

Preparing for Anesthesia

Whether the animal requires general anesthesia for a routine procedure such as a castration or it has presented on emergency for a fractured limb, the same protocols and procedures are usually followed. A general rule of thumb (although there are exceptions) is that all animals under anesthesia obtain some sort of fluid therapy whether it is intravenous (IV), intraosseous (IO), or subcutaneous (SC). IV catheters are preferred over other fluid therapy routes. Emergency drugs should be pre-calculated and drawn up prior to an animal being anesthetized for any length of time. This may seem wasteful because most of the time the drugs are not used and need to be discarded once the animal has fully recovered. Drugs are always pre-drawn prior to induction because, under many circumstances, there is not a lot of time to figure out doses and draw up drugs once the patient starts doing poorly under anesthesia. A cheat chart can be hung on the wall for quick reference or a spreadsheet program can be created. Spreadsheets are helpful as one can be created for each major group of animals commonly seen in practice (i.e., chinchillas, rabbits, and rats) The spreadsheet should remain simple and contain the common drugs used during emergency situations. Spreadsheet programs are ideal because they can be used over and over again. Just input the patient's weight, and the program will calculate the proper drug dosages.

It is important to have everything set up and within hand's reach before starting the anesthetic procedure. This includes all equipment that may be needed such as an ECG (Tables 2.3 and 2.4), blood pressure cuff and sphygmomanometer, $ETCO_2$, pulse oximetry, endotracheal tubes, catheter supplies, fluids, drugs, syringe pump, etc. Being prepared will help the procedure move along in an organized fashion. It is important to have pediatric items such as 26-gauge and 24-gauge IV catheters, 4.0 mm

Table 2.3 Common ECG electrode placement in chelonians, snakes, and lizards.

Snakes	Chelonians	Lizards
Cranial electrodes—place one probe 2 heart lengths cranial to the heart and 2 heart lengths caudal to the heart	Cranial electrodes—cervical region or forelimbs	Cranial electrodes—cervical region or forelimbs
Caudal electrode—caudal portion of the left side of the body	Caudal electrode—left side of the celom, inguinal area, or hindlimb	Caudal electrode—left side of the celom, inguinal area, or hindlimb

Table 2.4 Common problems often noted on the reptile ECG.

Improper probe placement

Scales too thick

Low electrical impulses causing small amplitudes making it
difficult to read the ECG waveform

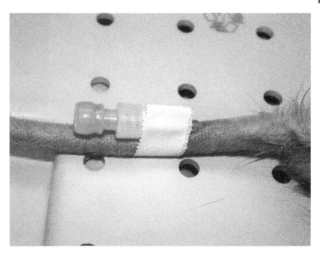

Figure 2.7 IV catheter in the tail of a rat.

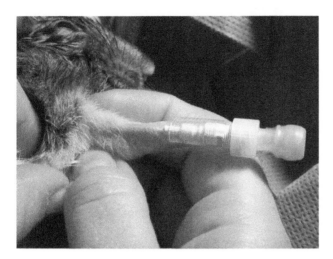

Figure 2.6 IV catheter in the cephalic vein of a rat.

uncuffed and cuffed endotracheal tubes, and smaller (18 to
14-gauge catheters can be adapted into tiny endotracheal
tubes), mini volume IV lines, pediatric T-ports, etc.

Fluid therapy routes in exotic animals under anesthesia include subcutaneous, intravenous, and intraosseous
administration. Vessels used for IV catheterization include
the cephalic (Figure 2.6) and lateral saphenous in most
small mammals. In rabbits, the auricular (lateral ear) veins
can be used, but the cephalic and lateral saphenous should
be attempted first. The lateral auricular veins are small,
can blow easily, and in rare cases, the ear can slough when
certain drugs are given perivascularly. In rats, the lateral
tail veins (Figure 2.7) can be used to place an IV catheter.
Multi-lumen catheters can be placed when necessary in
rabbits and ferrets. This is done using the same technique
used in canine and feline patients.

Common sites used for IV access in avian patients
include the medial metatarsal, cutaneous ulnar, (Figure 2.8)
and jugular veins. The medial metatarsal vessel is often
the easiest site to secure a catheter and maintain patency
during the peri- and postoperative periods. The cutaneous
ulnar vein (also known as the basilic vein) is generally easy
to catheterize but needs to be sutured in place. The wing
must be bandaged using a figure of eight if the catheter
needs to stay in place after recovery. Lastly, the jugular
vein can be used for IV catheter placement. The catheter
must be sutured in place and bandaged upon recovery to
maintain patency.

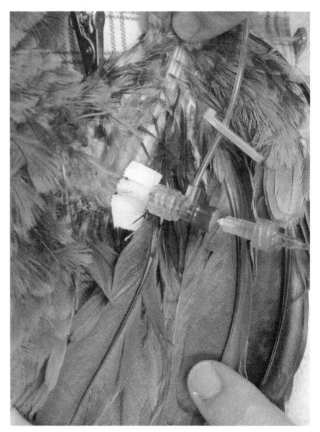

Figure 2.8 IV catheter in the cutaneous ulnar vein of parrot.

Catheter sites in reptiles will vary by species and size of
the patient. Snakes are generally difficult. The first choice
for catheter placement is the tail vein (Figure 2.9). Due
to the transverse processes of the vertebrae, the ventral
approach is much easier than the lateral approach, but both
can be done. The second IV catheter site used in snakes

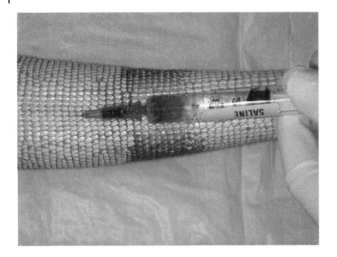

Figure 2.9 IV catheter placement in the caudal tail vein of an iguana.

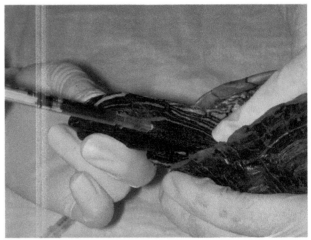

Figure 2.10 Jugular catheter in a chelonian.

is the jugular vein. A surgical cut-down is necessary for jugular catheterization in snakes.

Catheters can be placed into the jugular and cephalic vessels of lizards. These vessels require a surgical cutdown for placement, and in many species, these veins are often quite small, therefore they are not utilized very often. The most common vessel used for IV catheter placement is the caudal tail vein. As with snakes, either the lateral or ventral approach to the vessel can be used, but the ventral approach is generally much easier.

Some people advocate IV catheter placement into the abdominal vein of lizards. This can certainly be done, but a surgical cutdown is necessary. It is hard to maintain, especially postoperatively and is often in the way. This site is not used very often as it really is just not practical.

Intravenous catheters can be placed in the tail vein of chelonians. The tail vein is often difficult to catheterize and maintain patency, therefore the jugular vein is generally the first choice (Figure 2.10).

In some cases, an IV catheter may be impossible to place. This may be due to several reasons including, but not limited to, poor perfusion, phlebitis, blown vessels, anatomy, or vessels that are just too small. Under these circumstances, an intraosseous catheter should be considered.

It is best to use a spinal needle for IO catheterization. There is a lesser chance of the lumen becoming clogged with a bone core during placement. A regular hypodermic needle can be used when needed. IO catheters are placed using aseptic technique. The area should be aseptically prepared prior to catheter placement and sterile gloves should be worn during the procedure.

Placing an IO catheter is painful and should ideally be done under anesthesia or, at the minimum, heavy sedation with preemptive analgesic administration. If the patient is

crashing and systemic access is needed immediately, the catheter can be quickly placed without the aid of any drugs. In these cases, aseptic technique is often not possible. This is not ideal, but a quickly placed IO catheter can save the patient's life.

The size of the spinal needle will depend on the bone it is being placed in and the size of the patient being worked on. Most commonly a 25- to 20-gauge spinal needle is used.

In mammals, the IO catheter is usually placed in the proximal femur (Figure 2.11) or the tibial crest (Figure 2.12) if the patient is large enough. This is performed in the same manner as in dogs and cats.

It is not possible to place an IO catheter in snakes. In lizards, an IO catheter is often placed in the femur (Figure 2.13), humerus, or tibial crest. The technique used in lizards is opposite to what is done in mammalian species. The catheter is placed in the distal femur as the femoral

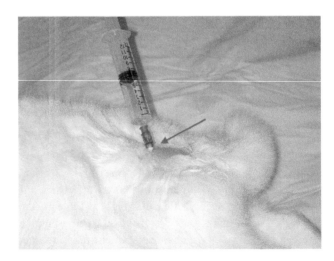

Figure 2.11 IO catheter in the femur of a rabbit.

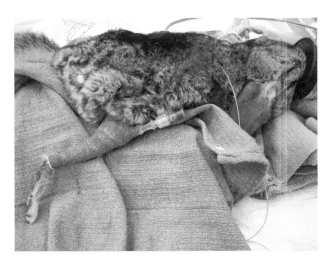

Figure 2.12 IO catheter in the tibial crest of a chinchilla.

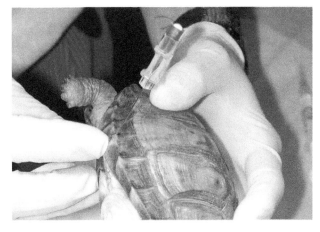

Figure 2.14 IO site for a chelonian patient. The needle is placed at the plastrocarpacial junction also known as the plastrocarpace bridge.

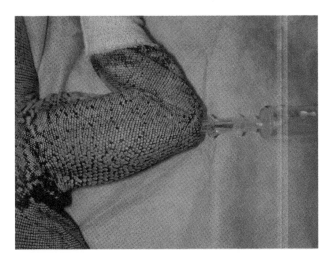

Figure 2.13 IO catheter in a lizard.

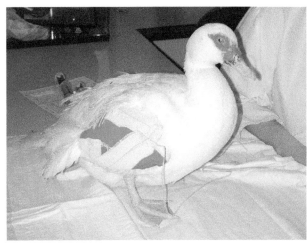

Figure 2.15 An avian patient with a figure-of-eight bandage to secure a catheter.

head and greater trochanter are not easily palpated. It is easier to secure the catheter in place and maintain it over longer periods of time when the femur is used.

There are several sites that can potentially be utilized for IO catheterization in chelonian species. Sites include the distal humerus, femur, cranial portion of the gular scute, and the cranial plastrocarapacial junction (Figure 2.14).

The most common IO catheterization sites in the avian patient include the distal ulna and proximal tibiotarsus (tibial crest). A figure-of-eight bandage (Figure 2.15) can be used to secure both an IV and IO catheter (see Chapter 30 for the steps in placing this bandage). The humerus and femur are **never** used in the avian patient because these bones are pneumatized (filled with air) and have a direct connection to the respiratory system. Administering fluids and medications into these sites can drown the patient. Another common site for IO catheter placement in birds is the tibiotarsus (tibial crest).

All catheters should be cared for on a daily basis. The bandage wrap should be removed and the area cleaned at least once daily. If the catheter site is reddened, irritated, or shows signs of phlebitis or infection, the catheter should be pulled and moved to another site.

Fluids

Fluids are generally administered to patients under general anesthesia to help replace both sensible and insensible losses. Insensible fluid losses include fluids lost through the skin, normal feces, and respiratory tract. Sensible losses include fluids lost via urination, diarrhea, and vomiting. Since most exotic patients are small, it is suggested that a syringe pump or a fluid pump is used to administer IV or

IO fluids. This is much more accurate and a lot safer for these small patients.

Anesthetic fluids include common crystalloids and synthetic colloids. With the exception of colloids (dose will vary by species and drug), anesthetic maintenance in small exotic mammals and birds for most fluids is 5 to 10 mL/kg/hour. Reptile fluid maintenance is generally lower at 2 to 5 mL/kg/hour. It is important to monitor the patient receiving IV or IO fluids as some patients can experience fluid overload. If the anesthetic procedure is long, the fluids can be given at the higher end of the dose range for the first hour and then decreased to the lower end of the range to help prevent fluid overload. Fluid rates should be adjusted based on the needs of the individual patient. If subcutaneous fluid therapy is chosen then fluids are generally given at a rate of 50 to 60 mL/kg/day for exotic small mammals and birds and 10 to 30 mL/kg/day for reptiles. Subcutaneous fluids are only given either when a procedure is very short and an IV catheter is not necessarily needed (i.e., ultrasound or radiographs under anesthesia) or an IV/IO catheter is unable to be placed (i.e., the animal is very small or the vessels have been blown).

If an IV or IO catheter cannot be placed or the procedure was very quick and only a small volume of fluids was delivered, the remaining daily maintenance of fluids is generally administered subcutaneously or intracelomically (reptiles only). This is done to help keep patients hydrated during recovery. Even the shortest period of anesthesia can affect how the patient eats and drinks for the rest of the day or days to come.

Anesthetic Induction

Most animals are administered premedications prior to anesthetic induction, although this will depend on the preference of the clinician and will vary with each patient. A current exotic animal formulary should be consulted prior to drug adminstration. Drugs dosages are generally much higher compared to canine and feline patients. Drugs are often injected directly into the muscle because uptake is generally quicker, although most drugs can be given subcutaneously or intravenously too. After premedications have been given, the animal should be placed in a clean, empty cage while the drugs become effective. This generally takes 10 to 20 minutes but depends on the species (reptiles generally take up to 1 hour or more), the drug combination used, and the disposition and mentation of the patient. After the premedications have taken effect, general anesthesia can be induced.

There are a few different techniques that can be used to induce anesthesia. When at all possible, it is suggested to pre-place a catheter, pre-oxygenate the patient, and induce anesthesia with an appropriate injectable drug combination. This is the same technique as used in canine and feline patients.

Reptiles

Drugs protocols will vary by species, procedure, ASA status, age, comorbidities, etc. Common premedicants include the use of dexmedetomidine, alfaxalone, ketamine, Telazol, midazolam, and various opioids such as morphine, hydromorphone, and butorphanol. These drugs are often used in various combinations with each other in order to reach a synergistic effect of sedation and analgesia. In some cases, sedation will be heavy enough for direct intubation. The use of anticholinergics as premedicant is somewhat controversial in many species. Either glycopyrrolate or atropine can be used as deemed necessary and when appropriate.

Although the reason is controversial, most drugs are still given cranial to the kidneys. It is believed that some drugs given caudal to the kidneys can potentially be shunted by the renal portal system to the kidneys before being systemically absorbed. If this occurs, drugs may not be metabolized correctly.

Common IV induction agents used in reptiles are alfaxalone and propofol. In snakes, propofol can also be given into the heart. Intravenous catheters are often difficult to place prior to anesthetic induction in most reptiles, therefore a single injection is titrated slowly to effect. The term "slowly to effect" in reptiles is much different than mammals. In mammals, a single calculated dose of propofol is titrated to effect over about 2 to 4 minutes (when given properly) and alfaxalone is titrated over about 1–2 minutes. In reptiles, a single calculated dose given to effect can take up to 10 minutes. Ideally, propofol should be administered ¼ increment doses to effect. Each ¼ increment dose in a reptile should be given over about 2 to 3 minutes. If the volume is just too small to administer in this manner, it can be diluted with regular saline. Drug metabolism in reptiles tends to be much slower compared to birds and mammals, therefore anesthetic induction (regardless of the drug used) will take longer.

Reptiles can also be induced using inhalant anesthetics such as isoflurane or sevoflurane in oxygen although it can be lengthy to achieve a surgical plane of anesthesia and is often not recommended over other injectable options.

An induction chamber, plastic garbage bag, or any other non-permeable container can be used for an inhalant induction. Masks can also be used, but are often more difficult due to the size and shape of many species. Masks used for dogs and cats can be adapted for use in reptiles. In some cases, one will need to be inventive when dealing with patients with tiny heads, those with shells, or aggressive animals. Ideally, the seal on the mask should be tight so the staff is not breathing in anesthetic gases. The author believes that mask induction is generally safer compared to chamber induction because the patient can be monitored more closely. The anesthetist should ideally monitor the patient's heart rate using a Doppler ultrasound unit from the time of induction until the patient is extubated. Isoflurane and sevoflurane are potent vasodilators and can have a dose-dependent effect on hypotension. These inhalants act rapidly and are only minimally metabolized by the liver. Changes in anesthetic depth can occur rapidly. Minimal alveolar concentration (MAC) is the concentration of anesthetic that produces anesthesia in 50% of patients who are given a noxious stimulus. MAC is influenced by anesthetic drug protocol, temperature, disease processes, species, stress, and age. In simple terms, MAC is the lowest percentage of inhalant anesthetic that can be administered to the patient without it moving in response to being stimulated (Muir 2007). Only a few MAC studies have been performed in reptilian species: MAC in monitor lizards is around 1.6% (Bertelsen et al. 2005) and in green iguanas around 2.1% for isoflurane (Barter et al. 2006; Brosnan et al. 2006). More research and pharmacokinetic studies need to be undertaken.

Anesthetic induction can occur about 30 to 45 minutes after the patient has been premedicated. In an ideal world, all patients would be intubated during any anesthetic procedure. There are several reasons why a patient may not be intubated during anesthesia, including patient size, anesthetist skill level, species, and the reason for anesthesia. Even if a patient is not intubated, it is ideal to be ready to intubate in the event of respiratory or cardiac arrest. Apnea is extremely common during general anesthesia in reptiles. It is highly recommended that intubation is performed after anesthetic induction and intermittent positive pressure ventilation (IPPV) is started via either mechanical or manual methods. A variety of tubes should be available including IV catheters and small rubber feeding tubes adapted into an endotracheal tube as well as small non-cuffed and cuffed endotracheal tubes (2.0 to 4.0 mm or larger as needed).

Non-cuffed endotracheal tubes are generally used in most reptiles due to the overall size of the trachea. Snakes and lizards have incomplete tracheal rings similar to those found in mammals. A cuffed endotracheal tube can be used in these species. Chelonians have complete tracheal rings similar to those found in birds. To avoid tracheal damage, a non-cuffed endotracheal tube should be used.

Most reptiles are extremely easy to intubate. Reptiles lack an epiglottis and the opening to the trachea sits at the base of the tongue (Figure 2.16). A laryngoscope is helpful in not

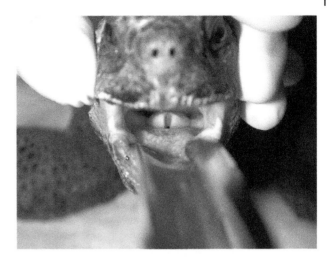

Figure 2.16 The glottis of a chelonian.

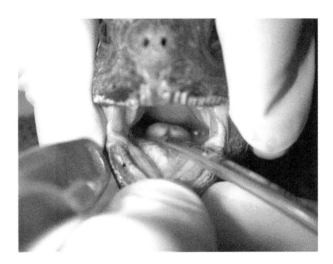

Figure 2.17 Intubation of a chelonian.

only holding the mouth open, but also pushing the tongue out of the way. Placing a drop of lidocaine onto the glottis will also help facilitate intubation. Lidocaine takes about 60 seconds to become fully effective.

There are times when reptiles breath-hold after anesthetic induction. Unfortunately, most reptiles can hold their breath for several minutes. This can make it difficult to pass an endotracheal tube into the glottis. In cases such as this, a tomcat catheter or polypropylene urinary catheter can be used as a stylet. Once the stylet is seated in the glottis, the endotracheal tube can be fed over the top of it and into the trachea (Figure 2.17).

Once the endotracheal tube is placed into the glottis, it will need to be properly secured. This can be tricky since it is almost impossible to tie around the nose or base of the skull as for dogs and cats. Many reptiles have strong jaws and sharp teeth. If they become light during anesthesia, some species can bite or puncture the endotracheal tube. To help prevent this, a plastic speculum or tongue depressor is placed under the tube. This also provides something to tape the endotracheal tube too. Creative taping is often the key to success!

In some cases, the patient will not need to be induced using an inhalant or IV injectable anesthetic. Certain drug combinations can cause enough sedation to intubate without the use of additional drugs. This is often referred to as "direct intubation." Direct intubation should only be performed when the patient allows an anesthetist to open the mouth or beak without resistance. Forcing a tube into the trachea in an awake patient can cause undue stress and trauma.

Birds

Analgesic options for birds vary by species. Until recently, full mu opioids have not been widely used in a clinical setting in the avian patient. Recent studies have suggested some promising results for hydromorphone and fentanyl in some avian species, primarily certain species of falcons and hawks (Guzman et al. 2013; Guzman et al. 2014; Pavez et al. 2011).

Buprenorphine is a partial agonist opioid. This opioid is a partial mu agonist and a partial kappa antagonist. Only a few studies have been performed to date and have shown that buprenorphine may be effective in species where full mu opioids are efficacious and not effective in species where butorphanol provides more superior analgesia.

Butorphanol is a mixed agonist/antagonist opioid that is best used for sedation or mildly painful procedures unless the species being worked on is known to have primarily kappa receptors throughout the body (likely several avian species). Butorphanol is a kappa agonist opioid which is why it works better in patients with mostly kappa pain receptors. It is very short-acting (likely only 30 to 60 minutes in many species), therefore it will be important to re-dose the patient as needed. A constant rate infusion of butorphanol can be administered as needed during and after a painful procedure.

Premedications are commonly used in the avian patient and most often include the use of midazolam and an appropriate opioid. These drugs are generally given IM in the pectoral muscles. The use of anticholinergics as premedication is somewhat controversial in many species. Either glycopyrrolate or atropine can be used as deemed necessary.

Birds have a renal portal system. It is believed that some drugs given caudal to the kidneys may potentially be carried directly there before systemic absorption can take place. If this occurs, drugs may not be metabolized correctly.

Injectable induction agents such as ketamine, benzodiazepines, alfaxalone, and propofol are not commonly used in the avian patient. Most commonly, general anesthesia is obtained via mask induction or chamber (box) induction. More research is needed on injectable anesthetics in the avian patient.

Most general anesthesia is induced and maintained via an inhalant such as isoflurane or sevoflurane in oxygen. Mask induction is most commonly performed, but chamber or box induction can be used as well. Masks used for dogs and cats can be adapted for use in birds. In some cases, it requires one to be inventive when dealing with patients with long or large beaks. Ideally, the seal on the mask should be tight so the staff is not breathing in anesthetic gases. Mask induction is often considered safer compared to box induction because the patient can be monitored more closely. The anesthetist should ideally listen to the patient using either a stethoscope or Doppler probe from the time of induction until the patient is extubated. Isoflurane and sevoflurane are potent vasodilators and can have a dose-dependent effect on hypotension. These inhalants act rapidly and are only minimally metabolized by the liver. The depth of anesthesia can change rapidly. Birds do not have an alveolar lung, therefore it is inappropriate to use the term "minimal alveolar concentration" in these species. Instead, MAC in birds is referred to as "minimum anesthetic concentration." MAC in the avian patient is defined as the minimum anesthetic concentration required to keep the patient from purposeful movement to a noxious stimulus (Ludders & Matthews 2007). In simple terms, MAC is the lowest percentage of inhalant anesthetic that can be administered to the patient without it moving in response to being stimulated. Isoflurane and sevoflurane do not provide analgesia, therefore an analgesic drug must be used if performing a painful procedure.

Anesthetic induction can occur about 20 to 30 minutes after the bird has been premedicated. Again, injectable drugs are not generally used due to the lack of studies in avian species and the difficulty of pre-placing an IV catheter (but they can be used). Once the bird has entered the appropriate plane of anesthesia, it should be intubated with an uncuffed endotracheal tube and either hand ventilated or placed on a ventilator and provided IPPV (Figure 2.18). Birds are very easy to intubate. They do not have an epiglottis and the glottis is located at the base of the tongue. Once the mouth is opened, the glottis can be visualized. The use of a laryngoscope and a small blade (even in small birds) aids in quick intubation of the patient. Birds have a thickened, muscular tongue. The laryngoscope not only provides a light source, but also helps push down the tongue, making it easier to correctly pass the endotracheal tube. The endotracheal tube should be secured by taping

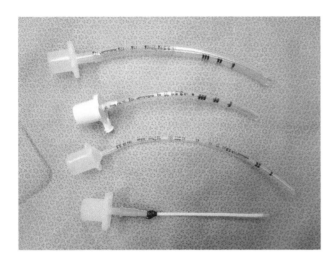

Figure 2.18 Examples of endotracheal tubes used in avian patients.

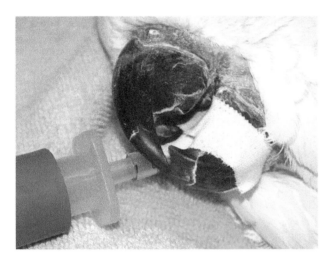

Figure 2.19 An intubated avian patient with the endotracheal tube taped in.

it to the lower beak (Figure 2.19) or taping it around the head (similar to what is done in dogs and cats).

Most birds do not ventilate adequately under anesthesia therefore providing ventilation is often a must. A non-cuffed endotracheal tube is used because birds have complete tracheal rings and lack elasticity in the trachea, unlike dogs and cats. Using a cuffed, endotracheal tube can cause trauma and pressure necrosis to the tracheal tissue. This could eventually lead to the need for a tracheal resection or potentially death.

The avian trachea seems also to be sensitive to dry air forced through the endotracheal tube. Dry, forced air can cause irritation to the trachea leading to transtracheal membrane formation. Transtracheal membranes are not common and there is not a lot of information about them. Clinically, if they form, development occurs about

5 to 10 days after intubation. Most cases occur in small birds maintained on a pressure-driven ventilator, but they can certainly be seen in large birds as well. These membranes are usually fatal. Treatment often requires a tracheal resection and anastomosis. To help prevent transtracheal membranes, the use of ventilators with ultra-low-pressure settings or handbagging of smaller birds is suggested. Adding a Humidvent® to the endotracheal tube can also help as this disposable device provides humidity to the respiratory tract while the patient is intubated.

Air Sac Cannulas

Birds have a unique respiratory system that includes nine air sacs (four pairs and one singular air sac). These air sacs are beneficial because they provide the anesthetist with an additional way to induce and maintain anesthesia. An air sac tube or cannula can be placed into the caudal thoracic or abdominal air sac. This allows for direct exchange of air through the air sac cannula, into the air sac and lung (Figure 2.20). Air sac cannulas are generally placed in an emergency situation when a bird presents to the clinic for severe dyspnea. Proper placement of the air sac cannula can provide immediate relief for patients with

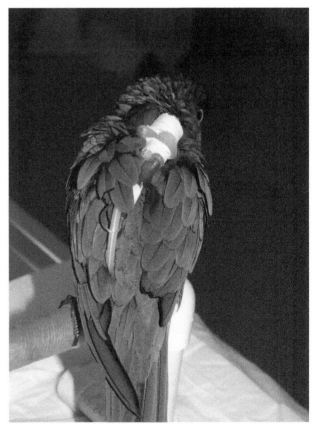

Figure 2.20 An avian patient with an air sac cannula.

upper airway obstruction caused by masses, foreign bodies, fungal plaques, etc.

Air sac cannulas are advantageous for surgical procedures of the head, neck, and trachea. A shortened endotracheal tube, rubber feeding tube, or intravenous catheter (very small birds only) can be used for air sac cannulation. The diameter and length of the tube will vary based upon the species. The bird should be placed in lateral recumbency, the feathers plucked, and the area aseptically prepared. An incision is made in the skin and mosquito forceps are used to bluntly dissect through the muscle wall and penetrate the air sac. Once the air sac is penetrated, the cannula is inserted into the air sac through the opened jaws of the forceps. If the cannula has been properly placed, air movement will be easily observed in the tube with each breath. A down feather can also be placed at the opening of the cannula. If it moves in and out with each breath, the cannula has been correctly placed. To properly secure the tube, a "butterfly" piece of tape is placed around the diameter of the cannula and sutured to the skin using a finger trap suture technique. If a cuffed endotracheal tube has been placed, the cuff can be slightly inflated to help hold the cannula in place. Ideally, this procedure should be done under general anesthesia, but if a patient is literally dying, the cannula will need to be placed straight away. Because this is a minor surgical procedure, it must be performed by a veterinarian.

The bird will begin breathing immediately if the cannula has been placed properly. If the bird is anesthetized, the end of the cannula will need to be covered or the anesthetic breathing circuit moved to the cannula to prevent the patient from entering a light plane of anesthesia (due to the gas inhalant escaping from the cannula). The cannula will act as an endotracheal tube. This will allow the anesthetist to induce and maintain inhalant anesthesia as well as provide IPPV as needed. When the cannula is not being used for anesthetic purposes, a piece of HEPA filter should be placed over the opening to prevent large particles or debris from entering the air sacs.

Exotic Companion Mammals

As with other species, drug protocols will vary by species, age, ASA status, procedure performed, drugs available, and experience of those involved. Common premedications used in exotic small mammals include dexmedetomidine, midazolam, ketamine, alfaxalone, acepromazine, and various opioids such as full mu opioids, partial agonist opioids, and mixed agonist opioids. These drugs are generally used in combination for a synergistic effect of sedation and analgesia. The use of anticholinergics as a premedicant is somewhat controversial in many species. Either glycopyrrolate or atropine can be used as deemed necessary. It is important to note that a high percentage of rabbits have circulating levels of atropinesterase which makes the use of atropine less effective. In an emergency, atropine should be administered first to treat severe bradycardia. If the heart rate does not increase quickly, a dose of glycopyrrolate should be administered.

Many drug combinations can be used for induction of exotic small mammals. Common drugs include propofol with or without a benzodiazepine; ketamine and a benzodiazepine; alfaxalone with or without a benzodiazepine; and lastly, etomidate and a benzodiazepine. Propofol can be used as an induction agent in ferrets but is not suggested in other small mammals as they are often difficult to intubate and apnea is a potential side effect of injecting propofol too quickly. If a catheter cannot be pre-placed (which is sometimes the case in small exotic mammals such as guinea pigs, chinchillas, and other small rodents), the patient can either be masked down or placed in an induction chamber using a gaseous inhalant anesthetic such as isoflurane or sevoflurane. A small mask can be placed over the face, as with a dog or cat, or the animal can simply be placed in an induction chamber. The heart and respiratory rates should be monitored from the time the animal is induced until the time it awakes from anesthesia. This will help prevent any anesthetic-related problems including death. In some cases, placing a facemask on the patient's head can be stressful, therefore an induction chamber should be used. Induction chambers potentially provide a less stressful induction for the patient; however, the heart rate cannot be monitored during the time induction is taking place.

Regardless of species, there are advantages and disadvantages to the induction method and drug protocol chosen. The author prefers using an injectable anesthetic induction protocol whenever feasible. Both the drug protocol and how the patient is induced should be based on the needs of the patient. Assessing the plane of anesthesia is accomplished in the same manner as for a dog or cat. The most common assessments include eye position, jaw tone, palpebral reflex, and toe pinch.

It is important to remember that many exotic animals are prey species. Holding them down for a mask induction can be extremely stressful and can increase the potential of death. Good sedation prior to induction is imperative.

Establishing a patent airway is ideal although there are several reasons why a patient may not be intubated during anesthesia, including patient size, anesthetist skill level, species, reason for anesthesia, etc. Even if a patient is not intubated, it is important to be ready to intubate in the event of respiratory or cardiac arrest. A variety of tubes should be available in the clinic including an IV catheter adapted into an endotracheal tube and small noncuffed and cuffed endotracheal tubes (2.0 to 4.0+ mm).

It is important to remember that most of the exotic small mammals (except ferrets) have moderate amounts of foodstuff in their mouths at any given time. These species do not normally undergo long periods of fasting, therefore they commonly have a mouth full of food. After sedation, it is a good idea to gently swab out the mouth until it is clean as this can help prevent aspiration. If the patient will not let you, you can wait until after anesthetic induction, but it is ideal to remove food debris prior to induction.

Small Rodents

Under most circumstances, small rodents are maintained on an inhalant anesthetic via a facemask. It is possible to intubate them (especially rats), but their small size makes it difficult and potentially time-consuming to achieve. Intubation in rats is very similar to that in a cat. The use of a laryngoscope will aid in visualization of the tracheal opening. Once the glottis is within view, the endotracheal tube can be inserted into the trachea. Even the smallest endotracheal tube (2.0 mm) is usually too large, therefore an 18-and a 14-gauge IV catheter should be available for intubation. Since these patients are difficult to intubate, a time limit should be set for trying (this is true for any species of exotic small mammal). If a patient cannot be intubated during that time limit, the patient will be maintained on a tight-fitting mask for the duration of the procedure. A piece of suture can be attached to the upper or lower incisors and strung out of the circuit attachment portion of the mask (Figure 2.21B). This technique is helpful for keeping masks in place, not only in small rodents, but also in guinea pigs, chinchillas, and rabbits.

Most exotic small mammals are very small and often one will need to be creative with in making anesthesia masks (Figure 2.21A).

It is important to be gentle with any exotic small mammal during the intubation process. Trauma can occur easily and lead to laryngeal edema, trauma, and a potential airway obstruction. Maintaining endotracheal tube placement can be tricky. The tube can be tied or taped into place. In some cases, tape can be placed around the endotracheal tube and stapled or sutured to the mandible. As a cautionary note, these endotracheal tubes are small and can kink or clog easily. The use of capnography can help identify airway obstruction or kinking of the tubes before it becomes a problem.

Guinea Pigs

Guinea pigs are difficult to intubate due to an anatomical structure called the palatal ostium. The palatal ostium is a centralized opening located between the caudal portion of the tongue and the soft palate. The palatal ostium is small, making it difficult to pass an endotracheal tube through it and into the trachea. There are a few ways endotracheal intubation can be attempted. Blind intubation, the use of a laryngoscope, and the use of rigid endoscopy are all options. These techniques are accomplished in the same manner as in a rabbit and are described in detail within this chapter under the heading "Rabbits."

The use of an otoscope cone, light source, and stylet is one technique employed for the guinea pig intubation technique (Figure 2.22A,B). The patient should be in sternal recumbency with the head and neck hyperextended. Hyperextension helps align the oral cavity and glottis. The otoscope cone is placed into the oral cavity. The light source

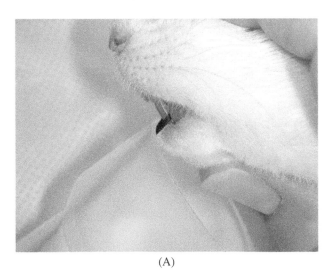

(A)

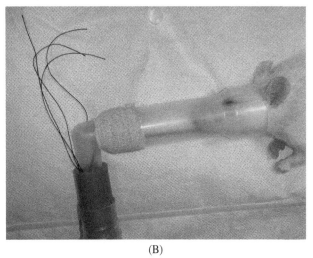

(B)

Figure 2.21 (A) A rat with an anesthetic mask made out of a syringe case. (B) A piece of suture can be attached to the upper or lower incisors and strung out of the circuit attachment portion of the mask. This provides a tight fit.

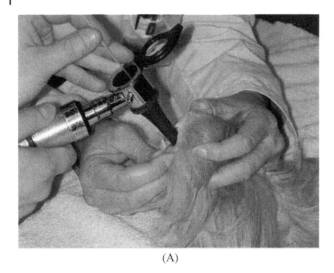

(A)

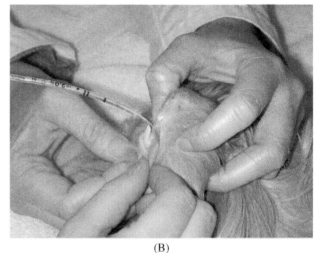

(B)

Figure 2.22 (A) Guinea pig intubation. (B) Guinea pig intubation using a stylet.

attached to the otoscope cone will help with visualization of the palatal ostium and the tracheal opening as well. Once the glottis is in sight, a small-diameter flexible stylet can be placed into the trachea. The otoscope cone is now removed and the endotracheal tube is fed over the stylet. Once the endotracheal tube is properly placed, the stylet is removed and the patient is hooked to the anesthetic circuit. A capnograph can be used to confirm proper placement of the endotracheal tube.

Chinchillas

It is possible to intubate chinchillas but it is also difficult due to size as well as the palatal ostium. The procedure is similar to that in guinea pigs.

It is important to remember that the hindgut fermenters such as rabbits, guinea pigs, and chinchillas are obligate nasal breathers. This means that they will not breathe out of their mouths unless they have no choice. As an anesthetist, this is helpful because a patient can be maintained on a mask for an oral examination or even dental or oral surgery. Again it is ideal for the patient to be intubated in order to help prevent aspiration of fluid or food, to decrease staff's exposure to gas, and to maintain a patent airway in the event of an emergency.

Ferrets

Ferrets are among the easiest of the exotic small mammals to intubate. Their anatomy is very similar to that of a small cat. Once the patient is in an appropriate plane of anesthesia the mouth is opened by the restrainer and the tongue is extended outward. Extending the tongue will help the anesthetist visualize the glottis. A gauze sponge will help the restrainer a traumatically extend the tongue. Pulling or extending the tongue with forceps or hemostats

is not recommended. A laryngoscope should be used to visualize the tracheal opening. Once the glottis is visualized, lidocaine should be placed around the opening (same procedure as in a cat). Lidocaine takes about 60 seconds to become effective, therefore a facemask with oxygen should be placed over the face until intubation is attempted. Ferrets can weigh between 500 and 1500 grams depending on age, sex, disease status, etc. Endotracheal tube size will vary greatly based on overall size of the patient. It is ideal to place a cuffed endotracheal tube, but this is not always possible due to patient size. Cuffed tubes will help prevent aspiration, keep staff from unnecessary exposure to anesthetic gases and provide a more even plane of anesthesia. A 500 g ferret may require a 2.5 mm non-cuffed endotracheal tube whereas a 1500 g ferret may use a 3.0 or 3.5 mm cuffed endotracheal tube. Having multiple sizes available during induction is ideal.

Once the ferret has been intubated, the tube is tied into place around the back of the skull behind the ears. Since the ferret's skull is somewhat tube-shaped, tying the tube to the mandible and wrapping it back around the neck is often necessary. Tie gauze lacks grip and can easily slip away from the endotracheal tube, leading to extubation. An old piece of IV tubing that will cling to the endotracheal tube can be used in place of the tie gauze (Figure 2.23).

Rabbits

Rabbits can be tricky to intubate but with experience and good technique, it can be done in about 1 to 2 minutes. There are several techniques that can be used to intubate a rabbit including the use of laryngoscope, rigid endoscopy, blind intubation (multiple techniques), nasotracheal intubation, and the rabbit v-gel® device.

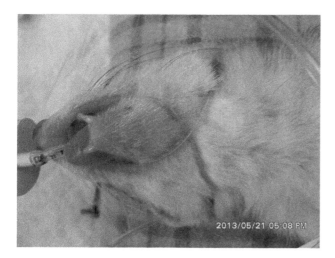

Figure 2.23 Ferret intubation using IV tubing to secure the endotracheal tube in place.

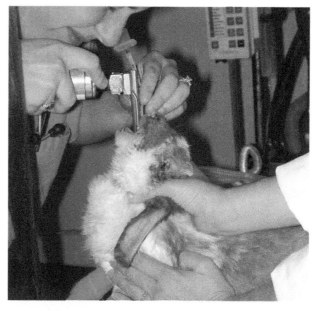

Figure 2.24 Rabbit intubation using a laryngoscope.

Having an established airway can save the patient's life in an emergency situation and provides a more stable and reliable plane of anesthesia. Rabbit intubation can be intimidating and frustrating, but once one is comfortable with a specific technique, it can be achieved with very high success rate. The author suggests choosing one technique and becoming an expert at that technique. Technicians and veterinarians who do this can have upward of a 99% success rate.

The size of the endotracheal tube will depend on the size of the patient. A small rabbit such as a Netherland Dwarf (800 g to 1.3 kg) will generally require a 2.0 or 2.5 mm non-cuffed tube while a large Flemish Giant (4 to 6 kg) can usually be intubated with a 3.5 to 4.5 mm cuffed endotracheal tube. A cuffed tube is preferred, but the cuff may not pass through the tracheal opening in smaller patients.

Laryngoscopes are commonly used in canine and feline patients to aid in successful intubation. The same technique used with dogs and cats can also be used in rabbits (Figure 2.24). The patient is placed in sternal recumbency with the head and neck hyperextended. Hyperextension helps align the endotracheal tube with the glottis. The glottis is very caudal in the oral cavity with a lot of fleshy tissue in the surrounding area. The laryngoscope should be used to visualize the glottis while the blade pushes down the tongue. Lidocaine should then be placed onto the glottis. Use of a tomcat catheter to more accurately apply the lidocaine is suggested. Once the lidocaine is placed, the oxygen mask should be placed back onto the rabbit's face for about 60 seconds while the lidocaine takes effect. Lidocaine is really a must for rabbit intubation due to the high occurrence of laryngospasms. After the lidocaine has taken effect, the patient can be repositioned and then intubated. The laryngoscope can be used to visualize the glottis and

pass the tube or it can be used to visualize the glottis and pass a stylet prior to passing the endotracheal tube. After successful intubation, the endotracheal tube is tied in place using either a tie gauze or IV tubing. As mentioned previously, IV tubing is often preferred because it seems to hold the small endotracheal tube in place better than gauze.

Rigid endoscopy can also be used for intubation. This technique requires expensive equipment and highly trained staff to maintain it. There are advantages and disadvantages to any technique. A positive attribute for rigid endoscopy is that the oral cavity and tracheal opening can be visualized very well. In some cases, the scope can be used as a stylet to help pass the endotracheal tube into the trachea. The disadvantages are that expensive equipment can break easily if mishandled and, in an emergency situation, there may not be time to pull out a bunch of equipment, turn everything on, and proceed with intubation. If this technique is going to be used, the patient should always have a mouth speculum in place to help prevent biting down on the scope (should the patient become light).

Another technique often used for establishing a patent airway in rabbits is nasotracheal intubation. This technique generally works well in larger breeds. The patient is placed in sternal recumbency again with the head and neck hyperextended. The endotracheal tube is passed through the nasal passage and hopefully into the trachea. There is a chance that the tube can be placed into the esophagus, therefore proper placement is confirmed with the passage of air through the tube and/or a normal capnograph reading. This technique is useful if the tube is obstructing

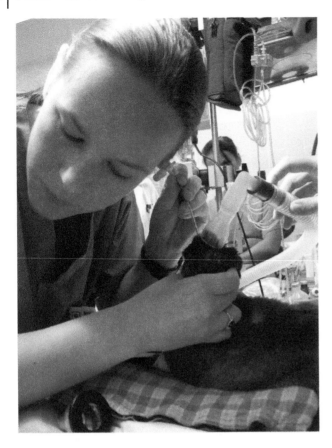

Figure 2.25 Blind intubation of a rabbit.

the oral cavity during a dental procedure or during oral surgery. Rabbit nares are small so unfortunately the tube used to pass through the nasal passage is generally smaller than what can be used orally. Rabbits are also obligate nasal breathers, therefore irritation or trauma caused to the nasal passage can cause the patient undue stress.

Blind intubation (Figure 2.25) is one of the most common techniques used for rabbit intubation. There are several different ways to perform intubation blindly. The first technique is the use of a modified esophageal stethoscope attached to the endotracheal tube. The rabbit is placed in sternal recumbency with the head and neck hyperextended. The endotracheal tube is attached to the modified esophageal stethoscope and placed into the mouth. The tongue is generally left in the mouth, but it can be gently pulled out of the mouth if needed. The tube is used to first flip open the soft palate. Once this is accomplished, air will enter into the endotracheal tube. At this point, the tube should be just slightly above the glottis. The esophageal stethoscope is removed from the tube (keep tube in place) and lidocaine is then injected down the tube using a 1.0 mL syringe and tomcat catheter. The tomcat catheter is long and helps place the lidocaine directly onto the glottis. The tube is then removed for about 60 seconds and an oxygen

mask is placed over the face while the lidocaine is taking effect. Once the lidocaine has taken effect, the endotracheal tube is placed back onto the esophageal stethoscope. With the ear pieces in place, breath can be heard every time the patient inhales and exhales. The endotracheal tube should be inserted into the trachea as the patient inhales. The anesthetist should not poke around the tracheal opening as excessive trauma can cause laryngeal edema and respiratory distress.

The other blind intubation technique that can be used is very similar to the esophageal stethoscope technique (basically just minus the stethoscope; Figure 2.26). The rabbit is placed in sternal recumbency with the head and neck hyperextended. The tube is placed into the oral cavity and is used to flip the soft palate. Once the soft palate is flipped, air will enter and exit the tube with each breath. Again, a tomcat catheter is placed into the endotracheal tube and deposited directly onto the glottis. The endotracheal tube is removed, and the oxygen mask is placed over the patient's face. Once the lidocaine takes effect, the tube is reinserted into the oral cavity. The author prefers to place an ear near the endotracheal tube opening so the breath can be felt as the patient inhales and exhales. On inhalation, the tube is gently inserted into the trachea. Another method is to just watch the breath move in and out of the tube rather than listen to it. Once the tube is in the trachea, it is tied in placed with either tie gauze or IV tubing.

The use of a rabbit v-gel® device (Figure 2.27) is also another option for securing a patent airway. The v-gel® uses a non-inflatable, atraumatic, and anatomically shaped cuff that creates a seal around the pharyngeal, laryngeal, perilaryngeal, and upper esophageal structures. These devices are easy to use and are great for those who are not comfortable using traditional endotracheal intubation

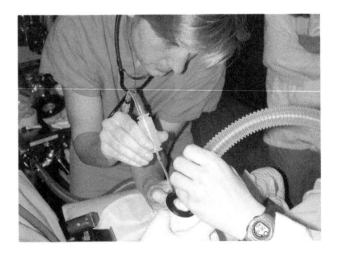

Figure 2.26 Intubation of a rabbit without the use of an esophageal stethoscope.

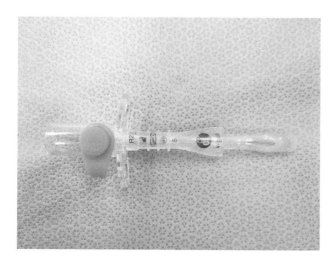

Figure 2.27 Rabbit v-gel device.

techniques. The v-gel®, like any product, has advantages and disadvantages. In the author's experience, it cannot be used for oral surgery or dental procedures because it is often too large. It does not allow for providing IPPV via a mechanical ventilator, but can provide very light IPPV via manual ventilation if necessary. This generally precludes the use of advanced analgesic techniques such as constant rate infusion (CRI) of fentanyl. If the head or neck is manipulated a lot, the v-gel® can become dislodged. The author primarily uses the rabbit v-gel® in very specific cases. These cases include, but are not limited to: a crashing rabbit where intubation would be difficult due to apnea; an endotracheal tube pulled out during surgery and cannot be easily replaced; and as a stylet guide. The v-gel® can be placed over the glottis and a stylet can be placed through the v-gel®. Once the stylet is in place, the v-gel® is removed and an endotracheal tube is placed over the stylet.

Multimodal Anesthetic Techniques

Advanced pain management techniques such as local and regional blocks, analgesic CRIs, and epidural anesthesia/analgesia can be incorporated into almost any clinical setting. One does not need to work in a specialty referral hospital or academic institution to utilize and effectively perform advanced pain management techniques. Controlling pain in exotic animals is extremely important. Not many pharmacokinetic studies exist to date for multimodal techniques in these species. Many common techniques are currently extrapolated from canine and feline techniques.

The use of epidural analgesia and anesthesia and CRIs of analgesic drugs in dogs and cats are commonly used in practice today. Many people do not use these techniques

on exotic small mammals but they should be taken into consideration. The species, type of procedure, and status of the patient must be taken into consideration prior to administration. Epidural anesthesia and analgesia should be considered for painful abdominal surgeries, urogenital procedures, and orthopedic procedures (especially of the pelvic limbs).

Epidurals

Epidural supplies are illustrated in Figure 2.28. Epidural placement is performed in the same manner as in canine and feline patients. The patient is placed in sternal recumbency (although it is possible to administer an epidural in lateral recumbency when necessary). The spine should be straight and symmetric. The hind legs should be pulled forward and positioned against the sides of the abdomen. Pulling the legs forward will open the epidural space. The wings of the ilium should first be palpated. The lumbosacral space can be palpated between vertebral bodies L7 and S1 (Figure 2.29). Prior to placing the epidural needle, the area should be shaved and aseptically prepared. Sterile gloves must be worn when administering the epidural. A 25- or 22-gauge spinal needle should be used for drug administration (Figure 2.30). Spinal needles contain a stylet which keep the lumen of the needle free of tissue upon placement. The spinal needle should be placed on the midline, perpendicular to the skin, and slowly inserted into the epidural space. A "pop" will often be felt as the needle passes through the ligamentum flavum and enters the epidural space. If the needle touches bone, it has been advanced too far and needs to be backed out a little bit. A sterile glass syringe containing a small amount of air can be placed on the spinal needle and injected into the space. This is called the "loss of resistance" technique

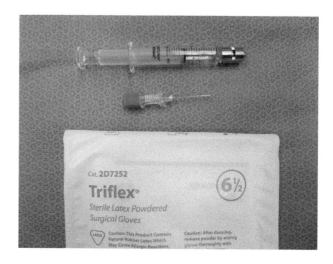

Figure 2.28 Epidural supplies.

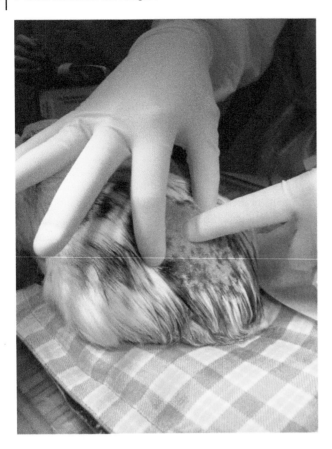

Figure 2.29 A guinea pig being palpated for proper placement of an epidural needle in the space between vertebral bodies L7 and S1.

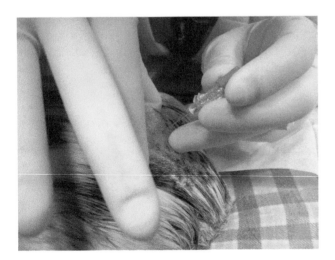

Figure 2.30 Placement of a spinal needle.

(Figure 2.31). If the air injects easily then the needle has been properly seated within the epidural space. If there is a vacuum on the syringe, the needle is likely not in the correct space and needs to be repositioned.

The hanging drop technique can also be used in place of a glass syringe. Once the spinal needle has been inserted

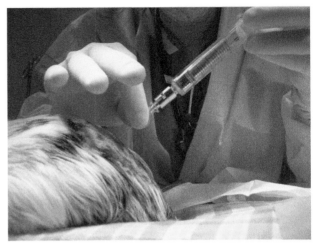

Figure 2.31 The use of a glass syringe containing a small amount of air using the "loss of resistance" technique.

just under the skin, the stylet can be removed. A drop of saline is placed into the hub of the spinal needle. The spinal needle is then very slowly advanced. If the drop of saline is sucked into the hub of the spinal needle, the needle is in the epidural space. If the drop of saline is not sucked into the spinal needle, or if the needle touches bone, the needle is not in the correct spot and will need to be repositioned. Once the needle has been correctly placed, the syringe with the drugs in it is attached to the spinal needle (Figure 2.32). This technique is not as effective in small patients. Regardless of the techniques used, the syringe should always be aspirated prior to injection to ensure there is not any blood or spinal fluid present. If blood is aspirated, the needle should be pulled out and the process started over. If spinal fluid is aspirated, approximately only 1/4 of the initial calculated dose should be administered.

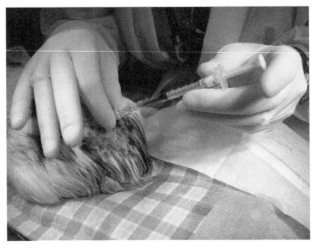

Figure 2.32 Administering epidural drugs.

Common drugs used for epidural administration include preservative free morphine, lidocaine, bupivacaine, and preservative free buprenorphine.

Epidural anesthesia/analgesia should not be administered if the patient is septic, has a clotting disorder, or has signs of pyoderma or a skin infection around the epidural site.

Epidural dosages for exotic patients can be found in Figure 2.33. An example of an epidural calculation can be found in Figure 2.34.

Common Epidural Drug Dosages for Exotic Small Mammals

Preservative Free Morphine – 0.1 mg/kg diluted to 0.33 mL/kg with sterile saline, administered epidurally (with a maximum volume of 6.0 mL regardless of patient size)

Buprenorphine – 12.5 mcg/kg diluted to 0.33 mL/kg with sterile saline administered epidurally (with a maximum volume of 6.0 mL regardless of patient size)

Lidocaine – 0.5 mg/kg to 1.0 mg/kg diluted to 0.33 mL/kg with sterile saline administered epidurally (with a maximum volume of 6.0 mL regardless of patient size)

Bupivacaine – 0.5 mg to 1.0 mg/kg diluted to 0.33 mL/kg with sterile saline administered epidurally (with a maximum volume of 6.0 mL regardless of patient size)

Preservative Free Morphine & Bupivacaine – 0.1 mg/kg of preservative free morphine mixed with 0.5 to 1.0 mg/kg bupivacaine (with a maximum volume 6 mL regardless of patient size)

Buprenorphine & Bupivacaine – 12.5 mcg/kg buprenorphine mixed with 0.5 to 1.0 mg/kg bupivacaine (with a maximum volume 6.0 mL regardless of patient size)

**It is important to note that the maximum dose of lidocaine and bupivacaine should not exceed 2 mg/kg and 1 mg/kg respectively. You must take into account any lidocaine and/or bupivacaine administered not only in the epidural, but also given in other local blocks such as ring blocks, line blocks, or even small amounts administered onto the tracheal opening to prevent laryngospasms (this is especially true for small exotic mammals and very small kittens, puppies, toy breeds, etc.).

Figure 2.33 Epidural dosages.

Epidural Calculation Example:

You have been asked to administer a morphine and bupivacaine epidural to a 3.5 kg rabbit.

Step 1 – Calculate total volume to administer:

(wt.) x (0.33 mL/kg) = total volume therefore (3.5 kg) X (0.33 mL/kg) = 1.2 mL total epidural volume

Step 2 – Calculate the drugs dosages for the patient:

Preservative Free Morphine ((wt.) × (dose)) / (concentration of drug) = morphine dose in mL

Therefore ((3.5 kg) × (0.1 mg/kg)) / (1 mg/mL) = 0.35mL

Preservative Free Bupivacaine ((wt.) × (dose)) / (concentration of drug) = bupivacaine dose in mL

Bupivacaine ((3.5 kg) × (1 mg/kg)) / (5 mg/mL) = 0.7 mL

Step 3 – Add preservative free saline to equal total volume needed for delivery:

Total calculated volume subtracted from volume of calculated drugs = Amount of saline needed
1.2 mL – (0.35 mL + 0.7 mL) = 0.15 mL

Step 4 – Add all the components from steps 2 and 3 together in one syringe

Figure 2.34 Example of an epidural drug calculation.

Constant Rate Infusions

Delivering CRIs during general anesthesia is an excellent way to provide additional analgesia to the patient. Common drugs used for analgesic CRIs in exotic small mammals include ketamine and fentanyl. Using one or a combination of the two drugs not only helps provide additional analgesia but, depending on the species, may also help reduce the percentage of gas anesthesia (MAC) needed to keep the patient in a surgical plane of anesthesia. Reducing the amount of gas anesthesia has many benefits including helping reduce the hypotension commonly experienced with inhalants such as isoflurane and sevoflurane. If fentanyl is used as a CRI, the patient should be intubated and placed on IPPV (either manual or mechanical) as this drug can cause severe respiratory depression, especially at higer doses.

In many instances, analgesic CRIs require a loading dose given at the onset of CRI delivery. A loading dose will quickly increase the drug plasma concentration levels, enabling the low-dose CRI to become effective quickly.

If the patient is being induced with ketamine, for example, the induction dose can be used as the loading dose as long as the CRI is within a few minutes after induction.

An example CRI calculation can be found in Figure 2.35.

Local Anesthetic Techniques

Local and regional anesthetic techniques are the only way to provide a complete blockade of peripheral nociceptive input, therefore they are the most effective way to prevent sensitization of the central nervous system and development of pathologic pain. The onset and duration of local anesthesia will vary based on the drug chosen.

However, the preoperative use of local anesthetics will reduce inhalant anesthetic requirements and can often help patients have a smoother and less painful recovery. It is important to note that lidocaine has a quick onset but a short duration of action while bupivacaine has a longer onset and longer duration of action. Lidocaine will become effective in as little as 5 minutes and will last about 1 to 2+ hours. Bupivacaine will become effective in about 15 to 20 minutes and lasts about 4 to 6+ hours.

Nocita is an injectable liposome bupivacaine suspension that can provide up to 72 hours of postoperative pain relief at a surgical site. The use of Nocita in exotic animals is considered off-label at this time and research is needed to help develop appropriate dosing regiments.

Side effects of local anesthetics can be fatal. Common side effects include local tissue irritation, nerve damage, sedation, ataxia, disorientation, convulsions, muscle tremors, respiratory depression, depression of myocardial contractility, peripheral vasodilation, profound hypotension, ventricular arrhythmias, and cardiovascular collapse. When dealing with small patients, it is imperative that local anesthetics are properly calculated prior to administration.

Topical Anesthetics

Topical anesthetics such as 2.5% lidocaine and 2.5% prilocaine (EMLA cream) can be applied to skin for minor procedures such as intravenous and arterial catheter placement. It is advisable to shave the area of interest, spread on a thin layer of cream, and place an occlusive dressing over the area of application for at least 10 minutes. This technique works well for placing arterial catheters in the auricular arteries of rabbits' ears.

CALCULATING A CONSTANT RATE INFUSION

Calculating a CRI is very easy once you understand what formula to use. For example, let's say you are about to anesthetize a patient that requires a fracture repair of the right femur. How would you calculate a CRI of fentanyl?

The formula for calculating a CRI is as follows:

[(Patient's weight) × (Dosage of the drug) × (*Time factor)] / Concentration of the drug

*The time factor for this equation is 60 minutes/hour

Let's say the patient weighs 2.0 kg and the dose of fentanyl that we are going to administer is 0.7 mcg/kg/min. Since my dose is given as mcg/kg/min, I will want to convert this to mL/h. The concentration of fentanyl is 50 mcg/mL.

I now have all the information I need to calculate the CRI. How will I calculate this?

[(2.0 kg) × (0.7 mcg/kg/min) × (60 min/h)] / 50 mcg/mL = 1.68 mL/h
This standard equation can be used for other CRIs such as ketamine, hydromorphone, and dopamine or dobutamine, etc.

Figure 2.35 CRI calculation.

Local anesthetics can be administered into existing wounds or open surgical sites. This is generally accomplished by "splashing" the local anesthetic into the surgical site.

Infiltration of Local Anesthetics

Local anesthetics are commonly used to provide additional anesthesia and analgesia for procedures such as minor laceration repair, skin biopsies, and removing small tumors lying just under the skin. Local anesthetics such as lidocaine and bupivacaine can be injected into the tissue, preferably around the nerve where blocking the pain sensation is desired.

Infiltration of local anesthetics is generally quite easy and relatively quick. The area should be shaved and aseptically prepared prior to administering any drugs. Aseptic technique will help prevent accidental contamination of the tissues with skin bacteria when the local anesthetic is injected. Generally, a small 25- to 27-gauge needle attached to a 1 or 6 mL syringe is used to prevent tissue damage and allow for more precise administration of the drug. The volume of drug to be administered will vary based on the area of interest and size of patient. If the patient is very small and the volume to be delivered is tiny, it may be necessary to dilute the local anesthetic prior to administration. Sodium chloride 0.9% is the most common fluid used for dilution. The syringe should always be aspirated prior to giving the injection. If blood is aspirated, the needle should be repositioned and placed again (this is true for any injection of a local anesthetic).

Ring Blocks

Ring blocks in exotic animals (Figure 2.36) are performed using the same techniques as in canine and feline patients. The area is shaved and aseptically prepared prior to the administration of the drugs. Generally, a 25- to 27-gauge needle is used. The same technique as outlined above is employed.

Testicular Blocks

Testicular blocks can be performed prior to neutering exotic small mammals. The testicle is first aseptically prepared and then isolated. The local anesthetic is often administered in a 1 mL syringe with a 25-gauge needle. The needle is placed into the testicle. Once the needle is in place, the syringe plunger is aspirated. If blood is aspirated, the needle should be pulled out and the procedure started over. If the syringe is free of blood, the local anesthetic can be administered. This is repeated into the other testicle.

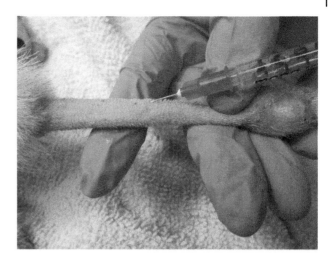

Figure 2.36 Ring block on a ferret.

Since the total maximum volume is going to be small, it is ideal to dilute out the local anesthetic with saline. This block is extremely helpful for perioperative and postoperative pain management. Providing a local blockade should be MAC reducing as well.

Recovery and Postoperative Management

The patient should continue to be monitored until it is awake and extubated (if intubated). If a painful procedure was performed on the animal, appropriate postoperative pain medications should be administered. Common postoperative pain medications include opioids such as butorphanol, buprenorphine, full mu opioids, and/or NSAIDs such as meloxicam. If the patient was on a fentanyl CRI during anesthesia the CRI can be maintained at a lower dose postoperatively. This is true for a ketamine CRI, too. Exotic animals recover poorly and often will become anorexic when in pain. The IV or IO catheter should not be removed until the animal is fully awake, and it is no longer needed.

Birds and exotic small mammal patients generally recover quickly from general anesthesia. Reptiles often have a much slower recovery and can take hours to extubate. Reptile respiratory physiology is extremely complicated. The drive to take a breath can be influenced by several factors including, but not limited to, oxygen and carbon dioxide levels, diving reflex in aquatic species, and increased temperature. It is often normal for a reptile to inhale, hold their breath (sometimes for several minutes), exhale, and then quickly inhale again. Hypoxemia is well tolerated in reptiles. During periods of apnea, reptiles are able to convert to anaerobic metabolism, the heart rate reduces, and cardiac shunting of blood often switches from left-to-right to right-to-left. Right-to-left shunting bypasses pulmonary circulation. Reptiles can also tolerate acid-base disturbances produced during hypoxemia.

For the most part, reptile respiratory physiology is quite different compared to that in a mammal. In mammals, a build-up of carbon dioxide in the body stimulates the brain telling it to take a breath. This is why when mammals are hyperventilated, they remain apneic until the CO_2 builds up again. Reptiles are different in that low levels of oxygen are often the stimulating factor for respiration. High levels of oxygen generally lead to a decreased respiratory rate and tidal volume or apnea. This means that not only will reptiles need to be ventilated under general anesthesia, but they will likely have a prolonged recovery if they are kept on increased percentages of oxygen. It is suggested that reptiles are recovered from anesthesia on room air using an Ambu bag (Longley 2008). Commonly, 2 to 4 breaths per minute are delivered to the patient during the recovery period.

Patients should be recovered in a warm and quiet environment. Incubators often provide the ideal environment for postanesthetic patients (Figure 2.37) because they are small, easy to pad, provide environmental temperature control, and in many cases oxygen.

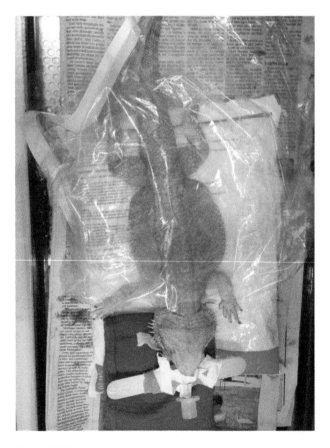

Figure 2.37 A bearded dragon recovering from anesthesia.

Postoperative recovery is obviously an extremely important part of the peri-anesthetic period. Each species often has special considerations that should be taken into account for optimal care and management during this time. Reptiles metabolize drugs more quickly when they are kept within their preferred optimum temperature zone (POTZ). Each species has a slightly different POTZ, therefore it is important to know the specific POTZ for the species being worked with.

Most exotics are fairly small and have a high surface area to volume ratio. This means that they can become hypothermic quickly; luckily, it also means that they will warm up fast as well. Patients can be kept warm using multiple types of traditional heating source such as forced warm air blankets, heating pads, heat lamps, warm water gloves, plastic/bubble wrap, and/or the HotDog® heating unit. Increasing the ambient temperature of the room is also helpful.

Certain species-specific considerations should be taken into account during the recovery process. Aquatic species should not be returned to the water until they are completely recovered from anesthesia. This can take 24 hours or even longer in some cases. Returning patients to the water too quickly can cause aspiration pneumonia or drowning. Aquatic species should also be restricted postoperatively if submersion may cause a problem with healing, and to help prevent infection. Patients can be kept hydrated by lining the cage with moist towels, administering fluids, and/or increasing the overall humidity of the environment.

All patients, regardless of species, should have large water bowls removed from the cage during the recovery period to reduce the chance of drowning.

Other considerations for postoperative care including removing branches from arboreal reptile species and perches from birds so that they do not fall and injure themselves. Lastly, direct basking spots should be turned off until the patient is fully recovered. Thermal burns can occur if the patient cannot move away from the basking spot.

Postoperative nutrition in any exotic animal is extremely important. Proper nutrition helps the body heal more quickly. There are several ways to approach postsurgical nutrition. If the animal can eat on its own, it is best to offer a normal, species-specific diet as soon as possible. For patients that are anorexic, hand or tube feeding may be necessary. Various commercial diets are available. Common examples include Oxbow Carnivore and Critical Care and Lafeber hand-feeding formulas. Appropriate baby food mixtures can also be used on a more short-term basis.

Exotic animal anesthesia can be difficult and stressful for the anesthetist. It is important to remember to be prepared for the procedure prior to anesthetic induction. A full physical examination should be completed, an patient specific anesthetic protocol planned out, and all items needed for induction, maintenance, and recovery organized and ready for use. Anesthetic protocols and monitoring equipment will vary depending on species and procedure being performed. Although pharmacokinetic and even basic anesthetic studies are lacking in many species of exotic animal, it is still important to take what is known about anesthesia in other species and apply what we can to exotic animals. Looking at trends over time can yield valuable information. Lastly, the author encourages the use of advanced anesthetic techniques in exotic animals. Local blocks, analgesic CRIs, and epidurals can be successfully used in many species of exotic animal.

References

Barter LS, Hawkins MG, Brosnan RJ, Antognini JF, Pypendop GH. 2006. Median effective dose of isoflurane, sevoflurane, and desflurane in green iguanas. *AJVR* 67(3): 392–397.

Bertelsen MF, Mosley CA, Crawshaw GJ, Dyson D, Smith DA. 2005. Minimum alveolar concentration of isoflurane in mechanically ventilated Dumeril monitors. *JAVMA* 226(7): 1098–1101.

Bounous DL. 2010. Avian and reptile hematology. In: *Exotic Animal Medicine for the Veterinary Technician* (eds B Ballard, R Cheek), 2nd edn, pp. 387–393. Ames, IA: Wiley-Blackwell.

Brosnan RJ Pypendop GH, Barter LS, Hawkins MG. 2006. Pharmacokinetics of inhaled anesthetics in green iguanas (*Iguana iguana*). *AJVR* 67(10): 1670–1674.

Guzman DS, Drazenovich TL, Olsen GH, Willits NH, Paul-Murphy JR. 2013. Evaluation of thermal antinociceptive effects after intramuscular administration of hydromorphone hydrochloride to American kestrels (*Falco sparverius*). *AJVR* 74(6): 817–822.

Guzman DS, KuKanich B, Drazenovich TL, Olsen GH, Paul-Murphy JR. 2014. Pharmacokinetics of hydromorphone hydrochloride after intravenous and intramuscular administration of a single dose to American kestrels (*Falco sparverius*). *AJVR* 75(6): 527–531.

Longley LA. 2008. Reptile anesthesia. In: *Anaesthesia of Exotic Pets*, pp. 185–241. London: Saunders Elsevier.

Ludders JW, Matthews NS. 2007. Birds. In: *Lumb and Jones' Veterinary Anesthesia and Analgesia* (eds WJ Tranquilli, JC Thurmon, KA. Grimm), 4th edn, pp. 841–868. Ames, IA: Wiley-Blackwell.

Muir WW. 2007. Considerations for general anesthesia. In: *Lumb and Jones' Veterinary Anesthesia and Analgesia* (eds WJ Tranquilli, JC Thurmon, KA Grimm), 4th edn, pp. 17–30. Ames, IA: Wiley-Blackwell.

Pavez JC, Hawkins MG, Pascoe PJ, Knych HK, Kass PH. 2011. Effect of fentanyl target-controlled infusions on isoflurane minimum anaesthetic concentration and cardiovascular function in red-tailed hawks (*Buteo jamaicensis*). *VAA* 38(4): 344–351.

3

Anesthetic Equipment and Monitoring for Exotic Patients

Katrina Lafferty

Introduction

Exotic animal pets, or "pocket pets" are increasingly common members of pet-owning households in the United States. With the increasing awareness of veterinary medical needs of all pets, these exotic animal pets are coming to veterinary clinics with increasing regularity for both wellness and emergency care. Ovariohysterectomies, castrations, laparotomies, fracture repairs, and dental procedures are becoming more commonplace. The expectation for those "pocket pet" owners is that these pets receive the same level of care as their canine and feline counterparts. Veterinary medicine is always moving forward and veterinary professionals have more tools and knowledge than ever before about the care and maintenance of exotic pets. That being said, even those veterinary professionals having a high comfortable level working with exotic species may not feel confident regarding exotic animal anesthesia. The number of exotic pet owners is increasing dramatically, with more exotic patients presenting for general anesthesia than ever before. This chapter provides information on anesthetic circuits, systems, intubation equipment and techniques, and monitoring tools specifically related to exotic animal patients.

Breathing Systems

Anesthetic breathing systems exist to fulfill three primary needs:

1. Deliver all inhaled gases (including anesthetics, oxygen, nitrous oxide, and medical-grade room air) to the patient.
2. Allow for assisted or controlled ventilation of intubated patients.
3. Provide a method by which to remove carbon dioxide from the system.

Breathing systems are categorized by circuit function as either a *rebreathing circuit* or *non-rebreathing circuit*. The non-rebreathing circuit is further divided into several types of non-rebreathing systems. Table 3.1 lists the advantages and disadvantages of rebreathing and non-rebreathing circuits.

Rebreathing Circuits

The rebreathing system utilizes oxygen flow rates of 5 to 30 mL/kg/min. The inspiratory and expiratory one-way valves and canister containing carbon dioxide absorbent allow for removal of carbon dioxide from the system and safe recycling of anesthetic gases to the patient (Figure 3.1). Reuse of anesthetic gases allows for decreased inhalant costs, delivery of warm, humidified air to the patient, and reduced exposure of personnel to waste gases. However, these components add weight, bulk, and resistance to breathing within the anesthetic system. Rebreathing circuits are generally too cumbersome for use on patients less than 3 kg.

Non-rebreathing Circuits

Non-rebreathing circuits rely on fresh gas flow to force carbon dioxide through the system and into a waste absorption container or active scavenging system. The flow rates are much higher than those required by rebreathing circuits. The systems discussed in this section all require minimum oxygen flow rates of 100 to 150 mL/kg/min. Non-rebreathing systems are used for patients under 3 kg, which will comprise most exotic animal patients seen in a clinical setting. The non-rebreathing circuit has less mechanical dead space and little resistance to breathing. The components are relatively inexpensive and lightweight. Despite this, overall costs for non-rebreathing circuits may be elevated as they require higher fresh gas

Exotic Animal Medicine for the Veterinary Technician, Fourth Edition. Edited by Bonnie Ballard and Ryan Cheek.
© 2024 John Wiley & Sons, Inc. Published 2024 by John Wiley & Sons, Inc.
Companion Website: www.wiley.com/go/ballard/4e

Table 3.1 Advantages and disadvantages of rebreathing and non-rebreathing circuits.

	Advantages	Disadvantages
Rebreathing system	Low oxygen flow requirements (decreased cost)	Components more expensive initially
	Reuse of inhalant anesthetics	Slow change to inhalant levels
	Less desiccation of patient airway	Increased mechanical dead space
	Less gas exposure to personnel	Increased resistance to breathing
		Heavier/bulker components
Non-rebreathing system	Components less expensive initially	Higher oxygen flow requirements (increased cost)
	Quick change to inhalant levels	More heat loss/airway desiccation
	No carbon dioxide absorbent needed	More personnel exposure to waste gases
	Little resistance to breathing	
	Little mechanical dead space	
	Lightweight components	

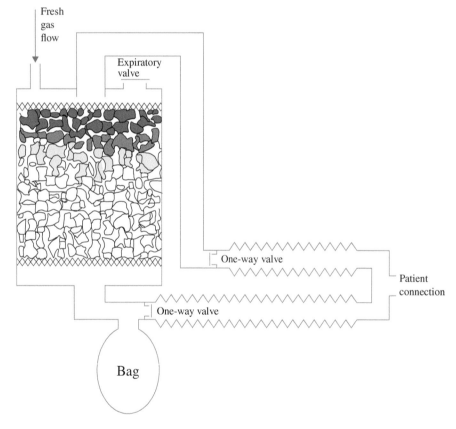

Figure 3.1 Rebreathing or "circle". (Image by Craig Johnson. Reprinted with permission.)

flows and more inhalant gases than does a rebreathing circuit. Non-rebreathing circuits deliver cold, dry air to the patient, which will desiccate the airway and lead to hypothermia and increased fluid losses.

Non-rebreathing valveless systems are broken down into several categories, each type serving a different purpose. The classifications often have several names and can be confusing. The most common systems will be discussed here.

Non-rebreathing systems are categorized as "Mapleson" systems, each with a letter attached for further classification. Mapleson systems are described as A to F; in veterinary medicine, the most commonly used systems are Mapleson A, D, and F.

Figure 3.2 Magill non-rebreathing system. (Image by Craig Johnson. Reprinted with permission.)

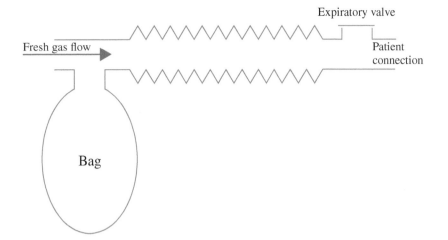

Mapleson A (Magill, Lack, and Modified Mapleson A)

The Modified Mapleson A has two systems within that designation. In the Magill system, (Figure 3.2) fresh gases enter the system at a junction between the rebreathing bag (also called the reservoir bag) and the anesthetic hose. Waste gases leave the system through the pressure relief valve on the patient end of the anesthetic hose. The Lack system delivers gas through coaxial tubing. Fresh gases are introduced to the system in the large outer tube; the inner tube transports waste gas to the pressure relief valve. Both of these systems allow for efficient spontaneous breathing but poor controlled ventilation.

Mapleson D (Bain, Modified Mapleson D)

Most commonly referred to as the Bain circuit (Figure 3.3), the modified Mapleson D utilizes coaxial tubing. The interior tube delivers the fresh gas and the outer tube transports waste gas to the pressure relief valve. In theory, the coaxial system warms and humidifies the inhalants being delivered, but the required high fresh gas flows do not allow time for warming or humidification of the gases passing through the tubing.

One significant advantage to using the Bain or modified Mapleson D is that it allows for usage of a "bain block" or "Armstrong arm." The bain block allows for two immutable safety features: (i). An integrated manometer and (ii) A pop-off occlusion safety valve. The bain block consists of standard attachments and allows for use of any size rebreathing bag as well as universal scavenge system attachments. The integrated manometer is calibrated in standard cmH_2O and gives the anesthetist an accurate gauge of pressure delivered in a manually administered breath. The bain block can be used to facilitate mechanical ventilation in patients when used in conjunction with an anesthetic ventilator and pediatric settings. Figures 3.4 and 3.5 show the bain block from the front and aerial views, respectively. The bain block has a built-in clamp on the back of the device. It can be mounted to an anesthetic machine or medical IV pole. Figure 3.6 shows the bain block attached to an anesthetic machine (Robertson et al. 2018).

Figure 3.3 Bain non-rebreathing system. (Image by Craig Johnson. Reprinted with permission.)

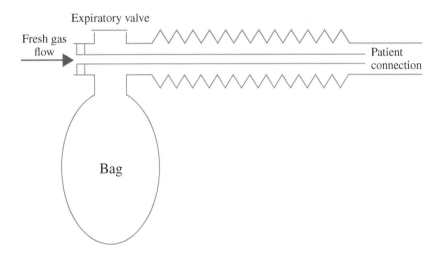

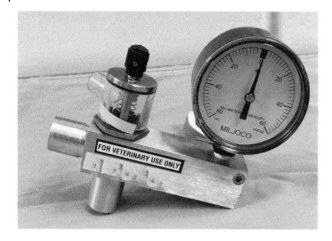

Figure 3.4 Bain block front view. Rebreathing bag, hose, and scavenge attachments visible. (Courtesy of Katrina Lafferty.)

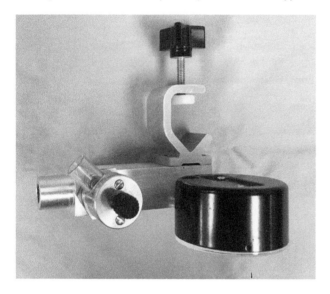

Figure 3.5 Bain block aerial view. Attachment clamp is visible. (Courtesy of Katrina Lafferty.)

Mapleson F (Jackson–Rees Modified Ayre t-piece)

In this system, fresh gas is introduced to the system near the patient and exits from the reservoir bag. This is a very lightweight, low-resistance system, often preferred for very small patients. This system has the highest level of personnel gas exposure due to inefficiencies in the scavenging system (Johnson 2009; Muir et al. 2007).

Intubation

Intubation of patients allows for:

1. Obtaining and maintaining a patent airway.
2. Introduction and maintenance of oxygen and/or anesthetic gases.

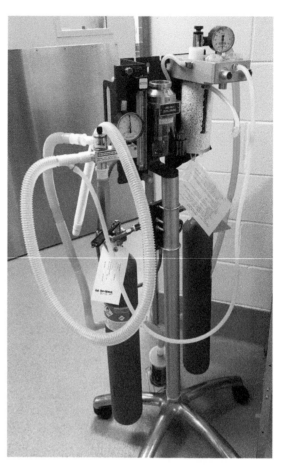

Figure 3.6 Bain block mounted to the anesthetic machine. Complete view with hose, scavenge, and fresh gas attached. (Courtesy of Katrina Lafferty.)

3. Protection of the airway and respiratory system from aspiration of fluid and/or debris.
4. Assistance or control of ventilation.
5. Reduction in exposure to waste gases.
6. Delivery route for some emergency drugs.
7. Additional monitoring (via capnometry).

With very few exceptions, anesthetized patients should be intubated regardless of species or duration of procedure. The technicalities of intubation are discussed in the species-specific chapters and will not be included here. This section will cover various types of endotracheal tubes (Figure 3.4) and laryngoscopes. This section will also cover laryngeal mask airway (LMA) equipment.

Murphy-style Endotracheal Tubes

There are two styles of endotracheal tubes serving as the mainstay in veterinary medicine. Murphy-type endotracheal tubes are outfitted with a standard 15 mm connector on the machine end, pilot balloon for cuffed tubes, a radiopaque marker (in the event placement confirmation is required), balloon, beveled end, and "Murphy eye." The Murphy eye is an adaption specific to Murphy-style endotracheal tubes. The eye, or side hole, is located directly across from the bevel and allows for continued gas flow and ventilation should the bevel side opening become occluded. Cuffed Murphy tubes range in size from 3 mm inner diameter (ID) to 35 mm ID. Murphy tubes less than 3 mm ID are not cuffed. There are manufacturers that produce non-cuffed Murphy-style endotracheal tubes up to size 10 mm ID.

Cole-style Endotracheal Tubes

Cole-style endotracheal tubes are a cuffless style of endotracheal tube. Cole tubes are shorter and identified by "shoulders" at the distal end of the tube. The narrow portion is inserted in the trachea, with the shoulders placed against the arytenoids. It is easy to cause trauma to the laryngeal cartilage if the tube is pressed against the larynx.

Uncuffed tubes are required for avian intubation as birds have complete tracheal rings and cuffed endotracheal tubes can cause tracheal necrosis. The cuff on an endotracheal tube adds increased bulk and may "catch" on intubation. Nasal intubation or intubation in more difficult species such as rabbits may benefit from use of uncuffed endotracheal tubes. Keep in mind that, without a cuffed tube, there is no ability to create a complete seal within the trachea. There will be increased waste gas, leading to greater exposure to gases for staff. Inhalant and oxygen levels may have to be kept higher to compensate for leakage within the system. The airway is not sealed against foreign material or liquid.

Reinforced (armored) Endotracheal Tubes

Endotracheal tubes reinforced with wire or plastic are useful for cases where the head and neck are positioned such that the airway could be compromised. The reinforcing material prevents the endotracheal tube from bending, which could lead to airway obstruction. Situations where reinforced tubes are warranted include ophthalmic procedures, neurologic diagnostics and/or surgeries, oral surgeries, and more extensive dental procedures.

Reinforced tubes are quite flexible and may require a stylet or other guide for placement. The stylet should not be allowed to extend beyond the end of the endotracheal tube as it could lead to tracheal damage. The additional material within an armored tube decreases the internal diameter, leading to increased resistance to breathing. If metal wire is used as the reinforcing material, such tubes

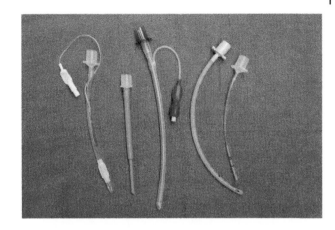

Figure 3.7 From left to right: Murphy-style endotracheal tube, Cole-style endotracheal tube; reinforced/armored endotracheal tube; special order uncuffed Murphy-style endotracheal tube; standard uncuffed Murphy-style endotracheal tube. (Courtesy of Katrina Lafferty.)

would not be appropriate for radiographic diagnostics such as magnetic resonance imaging, computed tomography, or radiographs. Figure 3.7 contains examples of several different endotracheal tubes.

Laryngeal Mask Airway Tubes

Laryngeal masks are supraglottic airway devices (meaning they sit over the glottis) and are heavily utilized in human medicine, particularly in pediatric cases. In some exotic species, namely rabbits, guinea pigs, and chinchillas, using an LMA may increase the likelihood of successful intubation and decrease the incidence of oropharyngeal trauma.

LMA devices may allow for more successful intubation in exotic patients, specifically rabbits, but ease of placement will depend on several factors. Level of sedation, patient size, and technical skill will influence the success rate of blind or oroscopic intubation techniques. LMA device intubation requires less technical skill for placement, but this does not negate the need for hypervigilant monitoring and placement confirmation.

LMA devices may cause less trauma to mucosa and lingual tissues. This is especially useful for situations where a patient may require multiple days of intubation or have existing damage to lingual or mucosal tissues. One significant drawback to the LMA devices is the relative size of the device. This can be prohibitive in cases where the primary site is in the oral cavity. Figures 3.8 and 3.9 show the V-gel, the most common of the commercially available LMA devices marketed towards rabbits. Figure 3.10 shows a rabbit intubated for surgery (Photo courtesy of Rebecca Johnson).

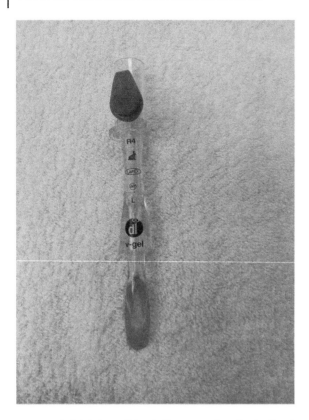

Figure 3.8 Arial view of V-gel. (Courtesy of Katrina Lafferty.)

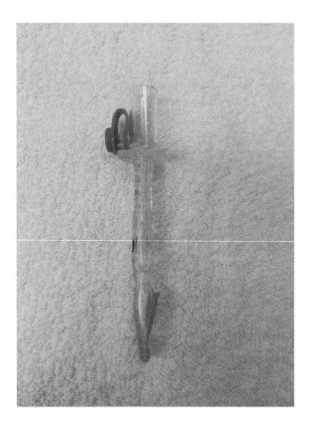

Figure 3.9 Side view of V-gel. (Courtesy of Katrina Lafferty.)

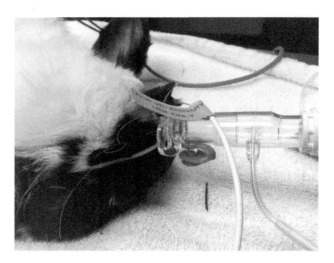

Figure 3.10 Surgical patient intubation with V-gel. (Courtesy of Rebecca Johnson.)

It is possible to monitor end-tidal carbon dioxide (ETCO$_2$) through the use of a side stream adapter. It is also possible to ventilate the patient, both manually and mechanically. Caution must be taken with using mechanical ventilation as there may not be a perfect seal with the LMA and it is possible to force gas into the esophagus and stomach.

Currently, LMAs are marketed towards canine, feline, and rabbit patients. There are research and development projects looking toward LMA devices in other exotic species (Engbers et al. 2017).

Miscellaneous Endotracheal Tubes

In some cases, it may be necessary to use non-traditional materials to intubate exotic patients. Very small exotic patients—some species of bird, reptile, non-human primates, etc.—will need tubes smaller than the standard sizes available. Red rubber catheters can serve as endotracheal tubes when cut to correct length; 20-, 18-, and 16-gauge intravenous catheters, with the stylet removed and attached to a 3.5 mm ID tracheal tube adaptor, also serve as reasonable endotracheal tubes. Small tubes are more prone to kinks and blockage, so the anesthetist must be vigilant. Figure 3.11 shows intravenous catheters converted into endotracheal tubes for an 80g cockatiel.

Laryngoscopes

Use of a laryngoscope allows for:

1. A good light source that facilitates correct endotracheal tube placement.
2. A good light source that in some species will allow for thorough oral examination at the time of intubation.

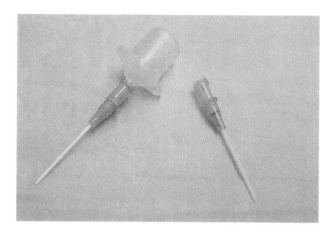

Figure 3.11 18g and 20g Intravenous catheters converted into endotracheal tubes. (Courtesy of Katrina Lafferty.)

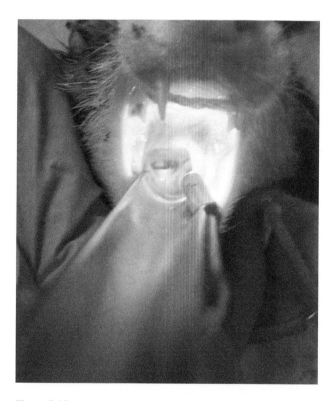

Figure 3.12 Proper use of a laryngoscope for visualization and intubation of a ferret. (Courtesy of Katrina Lafferty.)

3. A blade of correct length that can be used to *gently* maneuver oral structures such as the tongue, soft palate, and epiglottis. Figure 3.12 shows use of a laryngoscope for visualization and intubation of a ferret.

There are many types of laryngoscope blades available. Blades are available in several lengths. Short blades, used in human medicine for neonatal intubation, work well for many exotic species including rabbits, mustelids, non-human primates, and reptiles (Tranquilli et al. 2007).

Monitoring

Adequate monitoring is an integral and essential part of safe anesthesia for any patient, regardless of species. In traditional small-animal anesthesia, there would be no question as to how best to monitor an anesthetized patient. When asking "what monitoring equipment should be used" the answer would be "everything available." In exotic animal anesthesia, the monitoring techniques become more complicated. Standard canine/feline monitors are confounded by the extremely high (or in the case of reptiles, extremely low) heart rates, small size, as well as the unique and widely varying anatomy and physiology of exotic animals. For exotic patients, nothing is equal to a pediatric stethoscope, digital pulse palpation, and a watchful anesthetist. Commercial equipment can be used to supplement hands-on monitoring, providing information on circulation, oxygenation, ventilation, and temperature. Much can be gathered when conscientiously monitoring with pulse oximetry, capnography, ultrasonic Doppler flow detectors, ECG, and temperature probe. In larger patients, it is possible to add non-invasive blood pressure monitoring (Bailey & Pablo 1998).

Pulse Oximetry

Pulse oximetry serves as a rapid and non-invasive method of obtaining heart rate and arterial oxygenation saturation levels. It is inexpensive, easy to use, and works in real-time. A pulse oximeter calculates oxygen saturation of circulating hemoglobin using infrared light transmitted and reflected in areas of pulsatile blood flow. In most species, saturation readings at or above 95% are acceptable.

Pulse oximetry probes come in a variety of shapes and sizes. There are numerous locations suitable for placement of a pulse oximetry probe. Table 3.2 lists locations for probe placement. Figure 3.13 shows several styles of pulse oximetry probes. Clamp or clip-style probes can have a tourniquet-like effect which may be damaging on small toes, tails, legs, and tongues. Probes left in one place for too long can cause tissue necrosis. Figure 3.14 shows a ferret following tongue debridement. The tip became necrotic after a pulse oximetry clamp-style probe was left on for an extended time period. Figures 3.15 and 3.16 show examples of pulse oximetry placement.

Accuracy of some standard pulse oximetry monitors can be challenged by heart rates below 50 or above 300 bpm. A study in chickens found pulse oximetry monitors over estimated saturation levels when compared to arterial blood samples (Schmitt et al. 1998). Pulse oximeters serve as a quick, easy-to-use monitoring tool, but should not be the

Table 3.2 Placement locations for pulse-oximetry probe.

Probe type	Avian	Reptile	Mammal
Clamp	Toes	Toes	Tongue
	Legs	Legs	Toes
	Wing	Tail	Legs
	Tongue	Tongue	Tail
			Scrotum
			Vulva
			Ears
Flat reflectance	Esophagus	Esophagus	Esophagus
	Mouth	Mouth	Mouth
	Cloaca	Cloaca	Rectum
			Ear canal

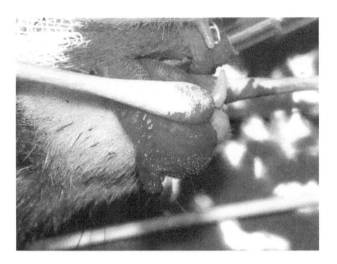

Figure 3.14 A ferret requiring tongue debridement after using a large pulse-oximetry probe. (Courtesy of Katrina Lafferty.)

only benchmark for quantifying stability of anesthetized patients (Nevarez 2005; West et al. 2007).

Capnography

Capnography provides early warning for a number of life-threatening situations such as cardiovascular collapse, endotracheal tube blockage or misplacement, hyper- or hypoventilation, and hyper- or hypocarbia. Capnometry is the measurement of carbon dioxide—displayed as a single number. Capnography is an all-inclusive measurement that gives numbers and a real-time display of the CO_2 waveform, providing additional information.

Normal $ETCO_2$ values should be within 20 to 40 mmHg in the anesthetized exotic patient (Lierz & Korbel 2012). $ETCO_2$ is usually closely reflective of arterial CO_2, though $ETCO_2$ tends to underestimate by 5 mmHg in a normal patient with appropriate ventilation and perfusion (Nevarez 2005). A capnograph will give information on the four main phases of a complete exhalation: phase one—exhalation of anatomic dead space; phase two—end of expiration; phase three—expiratory pause/exhalation of alveolar gases; phase four—beginning of inspiration.

Carbon dioxide monitoring is directly related to ventilation. It provides a respiratory number for any patient that

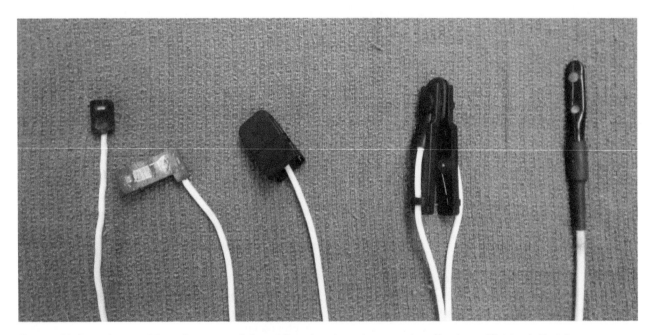

Figure 3.13 Several types of flat reflectance and clamp/clip style pulse oximetry probes. (Courtesy of Katrina Lafferty.)

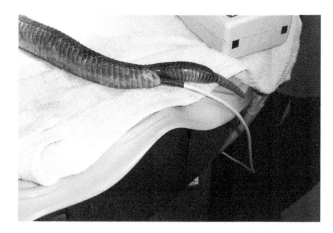

Figure 3.15 Cloacal pulse-ox placement in a snake. (Courtesy of Katrina Lafferty.)

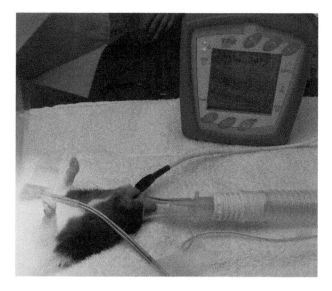

Figure 3.16 Pulse-ox probe in the mouth of a rat; Doppler crystal placed over thorax for auditory heart rate monitoring. (Courtesy of Katrina Lafferty.)

is intubated or utilizing a tight-fitting anesthetic mask. Carbon dioxide that is exhaled (or inhaled in the case of CO_2 rebreathing) is given a number and provides information about how well the patient is breathing. It provides a respiratory rate which is helpful in cases where there is little movement of the bag, or the patient is covered by drapes and actual respiration is difficult to observe. Carbon dioxide production and cardiovascular function are inextricably linked. For CO_2 to be removed from tissues, delivered to the lungs, and exhaled from the body, adequate blood flow is required. If a patient becomes hypotensive with decreased perfusion, less CO_2 is carried to the lungs. A CO_2 monitor can be one of the earliest alerts to a failing cardiovascular system.

Capnography can also be an early alert to failure within the anesthetic system. If the inspiratory or expiratory one-way valve is obstructed or incorrectly placed, it will alter the waveform on the capnograph. If the CO_2 absorbent has been exhausted, it will be reflected in rising inspired CO_2. One reason for a cessation in the capnograph waveform can be disconnection of the anesthetic hosing (Tranquilli et al. 2007).

There are two types of capnographs on the market: mainstream sampling monitors and sidestream sampling monitors.

Sidestream, or diverting, monitors involve a small adapter connected between the endotracheal tube and the anesthetic hoses. A sampling line then draws a sample of the gas and carries it to a unit where it will be analyzed. The main advantages to the sidestream monitors are the light weight of the sampling adapter and the lower cost of the monitor versus the mainstream monitors. Sidestream adapter pieces are easily cleaned and can therefore be used for any wet or messy procedures such as dental procedures, rhinoscopies, or endoscopies. Sidestream monitors can also be connected to nasal cannulas to obtain readings. There are unfortunately many disadvantages to using sidestream sampling monitors compared with mainstream monitors. Sidestream monitors pull approximately 200 mL/min from the system. In very small patients, this can be a large volume to remove. The sample has to be carried through a line to the analyzing unit and thus the sample can be a few breaths behind real time. This large volume draw may give inaccurate readings in small patients. There are commercially available small-volume sidestream analyzers that sample less than 50 mL/min and may be more accurate for small animals (Hawkins & Pascoe 2012; Tranquilli et al. 2007).

Mainstream monitors are also called inline or non-diverting monitors. The sampling box is placed directly between the endotracheal tube and the anesthetic hoses. There are several advantages to mainstream monitors. They provide a very fast response time and can be used on any size patient as there is no sample being removed through an external line. There are fewer pieces with a mainstream monitor—no sampling line and no water traps. The disadvantages to mainstream monitors are primarily cost: they are much more expensive than sidestream monitors. The sampling box can also be heavy and may be too much weight for small patients—leading to inadvertent extubation. As all the sampling pieces are immediately in line with the endotracheal tube, they are more susceptible to damage by water and blood and should not be used for wet or bloody procedures.

A capnograph should be used on every patient. However, if a choice must be made, patients benefitting most from

Table 3.3 Advantages and disadvantages of sidestream and mainstream capnographs.

	Advantages	Disadvantages
Sidestream (diverting) capnograph	Light weight	Large sampling volume
	Inexpensive	Most accurate on larger patients
	Easily cleaned	Several second delay in readings
	Can be used with wet/bloody cases	More pieces to replace (line, filter, adapter)
Mainstream (in-line or non-diverting) capnograph	Immediate, real-time readings	More expensive
	No sampling draw (accurate for any size patient)	Heavy sampling box
	Fewer pieces	Sampling equipment sensitive to damage by liquids

capnographic monitoring include those with respiratory disease, neurologic disease, and cases with metabolic dysfunction. Procedures benefitting from use of a capnograph are those involving the respiratory system—thoracotomy, lung lobectomy, diaphragmatic hernia, or cases where positioning could cause obstruction of the endotracheal tube—cervical neck procedures, ophthalmic cases, etc. (Bryant 2010; Greene 2002; Tranquilli et al. 2007). Table 3.3 lists the advantages and advantages of sidestream versus mainstream capnographs.

Non-invasive Blood Pressure Monitoring

The ability to monitor blood pressure in exotic patients varies widely by species. Avian patients have anatomy and physiology designed for different activities when compared to mammalian or reptilian patients. Birds have larger, thicker hearts, and arteries with denser walls. The heart comprises a larger percentage of total body weight in exotics when compared to equally sized mammals. This "high perfusion" system is set up for a species that routinely endures the atmospheric pressure changes occurring during flying and diving. The parameters for avian blood pressure are much higher than mammalian counterparts, with mean arterial pressures ranging from 100 to −250 mmHg to handle the increased demands on the cardiovascular system created by their unique anatomic abilities (Lierz & Korbel 2012; Strunk & Wilson 2003).

In birds, it is possible to use a Doppler flow detector to obtain fairly accurate blood pressure readings. Oscillometric readings are also possible in larger avian species. Oscillometric blood pressure monitors are non-invasive, easy to use, allow for "set it and forget it" monitoring, and are relatively affordable. They provide at least three parameters: systolic, diastolic, and mean arterial pressures. Some non-invasive blood pressure monitors also provide

a number for heart rate. Oscillometric pressure monitors are only as good as the anesthetist placing them. They can be easily confounded or confused by the physiologic differences in avian patients. A 2009 study in red-tailed hawks looked at the validity of oscillometric blood pressure readings and Doppler blood pressure readings when compared to directly obtained arterial pressures. The study found the non-invasive oscillometric pressure readings to be incorrect more than 50% of the time. In comparison, the non-invasive Doppler pressure readings were generally consistent with the directly obtained pressure readings (Zehnder et al. 2009).

For most species, the goal is to maintain mean or systolic arterial pressures between 70 and 100 mmHg. There is a dearth of studies into the minimum pressure requirements for various exotic species to provide adequate organ and tissue perfusion while under anesthesia. In birds, citing a study done involving pigeons, mean arterial pressure should be kept between 70 and 100 mmHg under anesthesia (Strunk & Wilson 2003). In mammalian species, such as ferrets, rabbits, rats, etc., it is recommended to maintain systolic arterial pressures above 90 mmHg (Bailey & Pablo 1998).

It is difficult to obtain and measure blood pressure parameters in reptiles. Readings vary significantly based on individual species. Reptile anatomy and physiology are quite different from the avian or mammalian groups and different parameters and environmental factors influence heart rate and blood pressure. Some reptilian groups are classified as "three-chambered" hearts, others as "four-chambered" hearts. Within those groups, there is debate as to which species actually qualify as three- or four-chambered. Heart location varies between species, as does the effect of ventilation (both voluntary and involuntary apnea) on heart rate (Kik & Mitchell 2005). Even though it may not be possible to use non-invasive blood pressure monitors to obtain pressure parameters, a Doppler

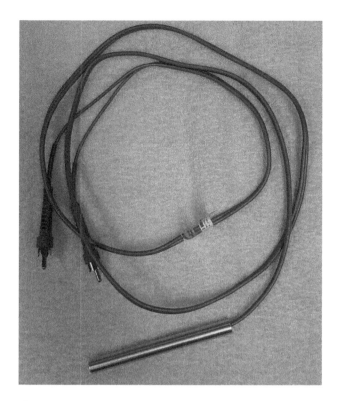

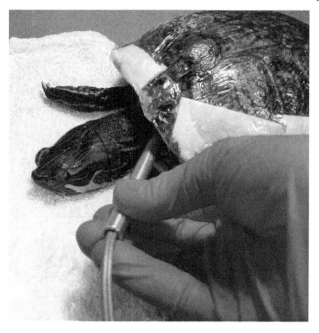

Figure 3.18 Use of pencil-style Doppler probe to confirm heart rate in a red-eared slider. (Courtesy of Katrina Lafferty.)

Figure 3.17 Pencil-style doppler probe. (Courtesy of Katrina Lafferty.)

is an essential tool when attempting to obtain a heart rate or confirm life in many reptile patients. There are a variety of types of Doppler probes that extend beyond the traditional ones used in canine and feline patients. The pencil probe is a style particularly suited to reptilian patients. Figure 3.17 shows a pencil-style Doppler probe. Figure 3.18 shows use of the pencil probe to confirm heart rate in a red-eared slider.

For most avian species, a Doppler pressure reading can be obtained using the brachial or medial metatarsal arteries. Note: it is not required to pluck feathers when placing the Doppler crystal. In rabbits, the carpal artery is preferred; in ferrets, large rodents, larger marsupials, and limbed reptiles, the carpal, tarsal, or tail arteries can be used. The crystal is placed distal to the blood pressure cuff. Proper cuff measurement is 30% to 40% of the circumference of the appendage being used. In patients too small to obtain blood pressure readings, the Doppler can still be a useful monitor. The crystal can be placed over any artery, including the palatine artery, and can be used as a real-time auditory monitor for heart rate and rhythm. In very small patients, or critical or shocked cases, the crystal can be placed directly over the heart. Caution should be used when securing the crystal on the thorax; it is possible to restrict ventilation with over-zealous taping. The Doppler can be used to verify accuracy of the pulse oximetry

provided heart rate. In some instances, respiratory sounds can be heard on the Doppler. It is extremely subjective, but it can be possible to detect, but not verify, pressure changes when listening to the Doppler sound. Changes in the volume of the "whoosh" can indicate a change in blood pressure (Bailey & Pablo 1998). Figure 3.19 shows a Doppler crystal placed against the palatine artery in a bald eagle. Figure 3.20 shows placement of a Doppler crystal on the thorax of rat. Also shown is a flat pulse oximetry probe placed against the tongue and giving accurate readings.

Electrocardiography

Electrocardiography does have some uses in exotic animal anesthesia. In most exotic species, an ECG complex is made up of the same components (P, QRS, T) as a canine or feline complex. Unfortunately, there is limited information on normal and abnormal references. ECG placement can still allow for further confirmation of heart rate and in some cases respiratory waves. Placement of the leads mimics that of any other species.

Exotic species are generally small in size and often have delicate skin. To minimize trauma, alligator clips with flattened teeth can be used. The preferred method is to use 25g needles pierced through the skin with an alligator clip attached to the needle end. This technique is less damaging than using alligator clips on the skin. There are also many types and brands of conductive adhesive ECG patches.

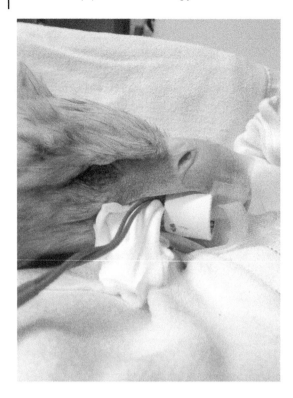

Figure 3.19 Doppler crystal placed against the palatine artery in a bald eagle. (Courtesy of Katrina Lafferty.)

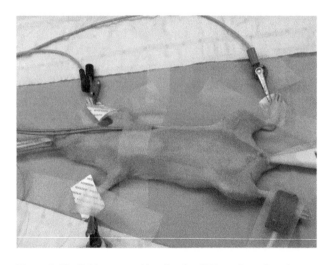

Figure 3.20 Hairless rat with adhesive ECG patches placed on the feet, Doppler crystal over the thorax, pulse-ox probe on the foot, and rectal digital thermometer. (Courtesy of Katrina Lafferty.)

Patches can be trimmed to an appropriate size and placed on the feet (Hawkins & Pascoe 2012). Figure 3.12 shows a hairless rat with adhesive ECG patches placed on the feet. This particular patient also has a Doppler crystal secured over the thorax, pulse oximetry probe on the foot, and digital thermometer placed rectally.

Temperature and Thermal Support

Normal core body temperatures vary greatly depending on species. Some avian species have normal temperatures as high as 109°F (43°C). Some reptile species have preferred environmental temperatures as low as 68°F (20°C).

There are four primary categories of heat loss that occur before and during the anesthetic period:

1. Evaporative (clipping, plucking, prepping, and dry/cold anesthetic gases).
2. Conductive (contact with cold surfaces).
3. Convective (open abdominal surgeries, cold flush).
4. Radiant (open abdominal surgeries, cold flush, and uncovered patients).

Exotic patients are at a greater risk of hypothermia due to small size and increased ratio of surface area to mass. Many negative situations can result from prolonged hypothermia including extended elimination of anesthetic drugs, depressed cardiovascular parameters, depressed respiration and ventilation, and an increased risk of mortality. At a certain point, patients become so chilled they are unable to shiver to warm themselves. Recovery can be prolonged and the central nervous system may be affected. In extreme cases, hypothermia can lead to bradycardia, arrhythmias, hypoxemia, thrombosis, and death.

It is a requirement to monitor temperature and provide necessary thermal support. Esophageal temperature monitors are the most reliable way to track core temperature changes, but rectal or cloacal temperature readings can be used. If using a rectal probe, a soft, flexible variety should be chosen. There are many forms of thermal support that can be used during anesthesia:

- Increasing ambient temperature of preparation room and surgical suite.
- Using clear plastic drapes to provide an extra layer of insulation.
- Minimizing surgical time or time involving open abdominal cavity.
- Minimizing time for surgical preparation—especially when involving alcohol or water.
- Using warmed fluids when lavaging open body cavities.
- Using warm water bottles, wrapping in towels to minimize burns.
- Using circulating hot water blankets.
- Using radiant heat lamps (with EXTREME caution).
- Using convective forced-air warming units.

In the same way that small patients cool quickly, they can just as easily become hyperthermic. Patients can warm by several degrees within minutes of initiation of thermal support. One must be vigilant with temperature monitoring for any patient under anesthesia (West et al. 2007).

Recovery

A survey covering "anesthesia-related" deaths in small animals (Brodbelt et al. 2008) discovered that more than half of such deaths occurred during the recovery period. Postoperative monitoring of all patients is a necessity, with special attention being paid to patients during the first 3 to 4 hours post-anesthesia. It can be a challenge to appropriately monitor many exotic species while maintaining enough of a distance to avoid distressing the patient.

Post-anesthesia, all patients should be restrained with gloves or towel until righting reflexes have fully returned and the patient is able to stand or perch unsupported. Animals released before they are fully recovered are at increased risk of fractures, dislocations, or other injuries. The exception to this statement would be any exotic animal patient that could pose a danger to personnel if restrained until full recovery. Patients should be placed in a warm, quiet, dim area where they can be monitored without being disturbed (Wenger 2012).

Incubators

Incubators or "brooders" are one piece of equipment essential in an exotic animal recovery ward. Incubators come in many sizes, shapes, and prices. It is worth purchasing the best incubator the clinic can afford. Incubators have the ability to warm, humidify, oxygenate, ventilate, and even nebulize patients. Incubators can serve many functions:

- "Acclimation" chamber for stressed exotic patients on intake
- Pre-warming for surgical cases
- Providing a warm, safe, easily monitored environment for recovery
- Warming chamber for surgical or intravenous fluids
- Providing an oxygen chamber for challenged patients
- Serve as an isolation chamber for compromised patients

Incubator construction can be as simple as an insulated box with a heating unit or as complicated as digital incubators with timers and humidity level controls.

Recovery Room

The recovery space should be an area that is species-specific—in particular, the patient should be kept away from other animals that could be viewed as predatory. The area should be quiet, with lights dimmed, and patients caged separately from other recovering animals. If possible, cages or incubators should be only large enough for the patient to turn around. Oversized cages allow for too much movement, particularly with ataxic patients. Once a patient is moved to a recovery cage, all monitoring equipment will likely need to be removed, with the possible exception of a pulse oximeter with an unobtrusive probe. Patients should be closely monitored for at least 3 hours. Assessment of

Table 3.4 Recovery room emergency kit.

Equipment supply list	Drug and supplements supply list
Pediatric stethoscope	Epinephrine
Towels/gloves for restraint	Atropine
Cuffed and uncuffed endotracheal tubes size 2–10	Glycopyrrolate
Miscellaneous small endotracheal tubes (18/16g IV catheters, red rubber catheters, etc.)	Lidocaine
	Dobutamine
	Vasopressin
Ties/tape/suture for endotracheal tubes	Dextrose
	Flumazenil
Laryngoscope with long and short blades	Naloxone
	Yohimbine
Tracheostomy kit	Atipamezole
Suction equipment	IV fluids, several types
Various syringes and needles	
Facemasks, several sizes/shapes	Synthetic colloids
Reservoir bags, several sizes	
Rebreathing hoses	
Non-rebreathing hoses	
Anesthetic machine and/or oxygen source	
IV catheters size 18g–26g	
IV lines, extension sets, caps	
Tape, several types	
Gauze squares	
Cotton tip applicators	
Chart with emergency drug doses	
Examination gloves	
Rapid digital thermometer	
Pulse oximeter	
Doppler/crystal/gel	

parameters should occur every 15 to 30 minutes, or as often as can be safely tolerated by the patient (Welsh 2009).

Assessments should include:

- respiratory rate
- respiratory character
- heart rate
- pulse quality
- mucous membrane color
- capillary refill time
- locomotion

- mentation
- food and water consumption (if able to offer).

Recovery Room Emergency Kit

In order to successfully handle emergency situations that may arise, there must be a fully stocked and well-organized recovery room emergency kit. Table 3.4 includes a comprehensive list of supplies—both equipment and drugs—that should be stocked in the recovery area. Many of the pieces of equipment and emergency drugs are the same as for canine or feline emergency cases.

References

Bailey JE, Pablo LS. 1998. Anesthetic monitoring and monitoring equipment: application in small exotic pet practice. *Semin Avian Exotic Pet Med* 7(1): 53–60.

Brodbelt DC, Blissitt KJ, Hammond RA, et al. 2008. The risk of death: the confidential enquiry into perioperative small animal fatalities. *Vet Anaesth Analg* 35: 365–373.

Bryant S. 2010. *Anesthesia for Veterinary Technicians*, 1st edn. Ames, IA: Wiley.

Engbers S, Larkin A, Rousset N, et al. 2017. Comparison of a supraglottic airway device (v-gel) with blind orotracheal intubation in rabbits. *Front Vet Sci* 4(49): 1–8.

Greene SA. 2002. *Veterinary Anesthesia and Pain Management Secrets*, 1st edn. Philadelphia, PA: Hanley & Belfus.

Hawkins MG, Pascoe PJ. 2012. Anesthesia, analgesia, and sedation of small mammals. In: *Ferrets, Rabbits, and Rodents: Clinical Medicine and Surgery* (eds KE Quesenberry, JW Carpenter), 3rd edn, pp. 429–451. St. Louis, MO: Elsevier Saunders.

Johnson C. 2009. Breathing systems and airway management. In: *Anaesthesia for Veterinary Nurses* (ed E Welsh), 2nd edn, pp. 90–120. Ames, IA: Wiley.

Kik MJL, Mitchell MA. 2005. Reptile cardiology: A review of anatomy and physiology, diagnostic approaches, and clinical disease. *Semin Avian Exotic Pet Med* 14(1): 52–60.

Lierz M, Korbel R. 2012. Anesthesia and analgesia in birds. *J Exotic Pet Med* 21(1): 44–58.

Muir WM, Hubbell JAE, Bednarski RM, et al. 2007. *Handbook of Veterinary Anesthesia*, 4th edn. St. Louis, MO: Mosby Elsevier.

Nevarez JG. 2005. Monitoring during avian and exotic pet anesthesia. *Semin Avian Exotic Pet Med* 14(4): 277–283.

Robertson SA, Gogolski SM, Pascoe P, et al. 2018. AAFP feline anesthesia guidelines. *J Feline Med Surg* 20(7): 602–634.

Schmitt PM, Gobel T, Trautvetter E. 1998. Evaluation of pulse oximetry as a monitoring method in avian anesthesia. *J Avian Med Surg* 12(2): 91–99.

Strunk A, Wilson GH. 2003. Avian cardiology. *Vet Clin North Am: Exotic Anim Pract* 6(1): 1–28.

Tranquilli WJ, Thurmon JC, Grimm KA. 2007. *Lumb and Jones' Veterinary Anesthesia and Analgesia*, 4th edn. Ames, IA: Wiley.

Welsh L. 2009. *Anaesthesia for Veterinary Nurses*, 2nd edn. Ames, IA: Wiley.

Wenger S. 2012 Anesthesia and analgesia in rabbits and rodents. *J Exotic Pet Med* 21: 7–16.

West G, Heard D, Caulkett N. 2007. *Zoo Animal and Wildlife Immobilization and Anesthesia*, 1st edn. Ames, IA: Wiley-Blackwell.

Zehnder AM, Hawkins MG, Pascoe PJ, et al. 2009 Evaluation of indirect blood pressure monitoring in awake and anesthetized redtailed hawks (*Buteo jamaicensis*): effects of cuff size, cuff placement, and monitoring equipment. *Vet Anaesth Analg* 36: 464–479.

4

Physical Rehabilitation

Jodi Seidel

Introduction

Veterinary technicians are educated on how to care for a variety of species. Regardless of the species, physical rehabilitation should always be considered standard of care for every patient. The American Physical Therapy Association (APTA) describes that physical therapists (PTs) and physical therapy assistants (PTAs) are movement experts who help maximize movement in order to manage pain, avoid surgery and prescription drugs, manage chronic conditions (such as osteoarthritis), and recover from and prevent injury. This is synonymous to what physical rehabilitation does for our veterinary patients, exotic species included.

According to the American Association of Rehabilitation Veterinarians, physical rehabilitation is defined as "the diagnosis and management of patients with painful or functionally limiting conditions, particularly those with injury or illness related to the neurologic and musculoskeletal systems. The goal of rehabilitation is to achieve the highest level of function, independence, and quality of life possible for the patient."

This chapter introduces how to integrate physical rehabilitation into the care of exotic animal patients by performing some basic techniques and how to educate clients on the best long-term physical care for their pets.

Why Rehab?

- Improvement of post-op recovery—return to normal activity or return to the wild more quickly with fewer complications (Tomlinson 2018).
- Simple to add to daily routine—some of the most effective rehab techniques are simple to add to an already busy daily routine. One of the most challenging aspects of veterinary rehabilitation is owner compliance.

Keeping things simple will make it more likely that there will be proper owner follow-through.

- Noninvasive—this is what can be done when surgery is not an option either from a financial standpoint or other restrictions from the client (schedule, post-op recovery, etc.). Since surgery is not always on the table, discussing rehabilitation ensures the client has heard all the options.
- Aids in the maintenance of function and health of joints—studies have shown that regular exercise is successful at decreasing lameness in patients with chronic pain/orthopedic disease (Geneen et al. 2017; Greene et al. 2013).
- Decreases dosage or need for pain medications—not all patients with acute or chronic joint disease will need to be on pain medications long-term if they are getting the appropriate amount of exercise. Rehabilitation techniques may be able to help improve a patient's function while on medications and then as the patient is improving the veterinary technician should work with the client and the overseeing veterinarian to find the lowest effective dose without disrupting the patient's activity schedule/exercise routine.
- Improves endurance and function—from mental health benefits to cardiac endurance, regular exercise can help improve overall patient function and improve long-term quality of life. Most evidence is limited to human, canine, or rat studies but there is an easy argument that all species can benefit from regular exercise/controlled activity (Callaghan 2004).
- Improves the human–animal bond and help improve overall quality of life—encouraging owners to take a more active role in their pet's life can significantly improve the human–animal bond and reflect positively on the patient's overall quality of life (Goldberg and Tomlinson 2018).

Where to Start—Asking the Right Questions

Evidence has shown that regular daily exercise is not only beneficial to a human's physical health, but also to their mental health (Sharma et al. 2006). The same statement can be applied when talking about veterinary medicine and the overall health of veterinary patients, especially small, exotic patients, who may spend a large amount of their day in a small habitat. Discussing activity is an important puzzle piece for the thorough history taker but it is a topic that tends to be under discussed in veterinary medicine, even for our more common canine species (Marcellin-Little et al. 2005). The answer to this question aids in making a realistic plan for the pet owner when the technician and veterinarian are aware of how much (or how little) the clients exercise their pet currently. Clients may appear confused when asked what their iguana or caged bird does all day, but those clients who are active in their pet's health will be quick to explain how much they exercise their pet and all the care that goes into their daily routine.

Author tip: Develop new and returning client forms for every species the practice sees. A cockatoo and a guinea pig will have very different requirements with housing and activity and forms with pre-thought questions and checkboxes to ensure that neither the client nor the technician forgets to discuss an important part of the pet's history. This will improve the efficiency of every appointment and standardize the care given to every patient who walks through the veterinary clinic door.

Examples of questions that would be part of a rehabilitation client form

1. What size of enclosure does your pet stay in?
2. What type of exercise does our pet get throughout the day? (i.e., Supervised play in larger enclosure or home? Exercise wheel? Interactive toys?)
3. If litter box trained, is your pet still able to get in/out of the litter box?
4. What physical challenges do you notice your pet having lately? (i.e., Off balance? Difficulty walking, turning, stepping, etc.?
5. Is there anything your pet used to be able to do that they are no longer able or willing to do (i.e., climb/crawl/hop on furnishings in enclosure, play with toys, etc.?)

Other important information to gather when getting a thorough history about exotic patients:

- Housing/habitat size, perches, rocks, etc.
- Nutrition
- Chief complaint/reason for appointment
- Any recent history of lameness, injury, changes in activity, posture, food/water consumption, etc.
- What has the client tried so far? Did it help? Medications vs. rest, vs. other?

The Rehab Examination

Using objective measurements is important when looking for a pattern in improvement or regression of the patient's overall function. However, using a goniometer (joint measuring device) on every joint in a bird or ferret may not be very practical during a stress-free-based exam and may not be necessary for the success of the treatment plan/recommendations. Documenting function and joint health using descriptive terminology combined with photography and videography can significantly decrease the placebo effect when not using objective measuring tools.

Regardless of what tools are used, even if it is just the technician or veterinarian's hands, describing and properly documenting in the medical record exactly what is felt during palpation and joint movement is key to helping the next veterinary team member who may be examining that patient, especially if a new medication has been prescribed or a new treatment was recommended (Millis and Levine 2014a).

The key to a good physical examination is consistency. Performing physical examinations, the same way each time (this could be different for each species) is important to ensure no detail is missed. This is another time when forms (electronic or paper) are very helpful to the veterinary technician, so that any important observations or measurements are not forgotten.

The rehab examination does not have to complicate or add too much time to the already delicate exotic animal physical examination. For example, when getting a TPR and palpating pulses, symmetry in muscle mass on each side of the body can be quickly checked. If the patient does not like to be handled, they can be observed as they move around the room (or cage). One should be mindful of how they step on/off perches, blocks/rocks (looking at the range of motion of each joint), and how they get up/down from a lay or stand (are they using their body appropriately). The normal relaxed position for the species and how they are holding that posture should also be observed. Are they shifting weight more forward, supporting more weight on one limb vs. the other, keeping their head low or tilted to the side, do they have any facial grimace changes?

Pain assessments should be part of every veterinary visit no matter what species is treated or what the reason for seeing the patient is (Goldberg 2019). Discussing pain and the behavioral signs associated with pain for our exotic patients is extremely important, especially for a new owner. These clients may not have much, if any, experience caring for an exotic pet and it is the veterinary technician's job to make sure the client understands what to look for in order to help their pet maintain a healthy lifestyle with a good quality of life.

> Tip: One should not get tunnel vision, think of the entire patient, beak/nose to tail. Compensatory injuries are common in any species recovering from illness or injury. Older patients who may be compensating for chronic arthritic changes in their pelvic limbs may be shifting excessively forward causing strain on shoulder and neck muscles. Or if a patient has an injury in thoracic and pelvic limbs the spine could be taking some extra strain causing spasms in accessory muscles

Everything needs to be documented! Notes should be taken about the standing examination vs. the lateral examination vs. postural and transition observations. Taking photos and videos to make for easier follow-up and to collect as much subjective data as possible when discussing the history with the client is an important part of the documentation process (Guskiewicz and Perrin 1996).

All exotic species are at risk for orthopedic and neurologic diseases and may benefit from rehabilitation, but one of the most common diseases that can affect all species is osteoarthritis. Risk factors for getting osteoarthritis include but are not limited to age, breed, obesity, congenital deformities, and previous injury. Osteoarthritis causes "degradation of the articular cartilage, thickening of subchondral bone, osteophyte formation, variable degrees of synovial inflammation, degeneration of ligaments, hypertrophy of the joint capsule, and changes in the periarticular muscles and nerves" (Loeser et al. 2012). Untreated osteoarthritis can cause debilitating changes in function. The patient may compensate for joint pain by not using the affected limb normally. This will cause muscle atrophy of the affected limb(s) and create increased strain on the rest of the body. The affected joints will also undergo even more joint remodeling creating more arthritic changes in the joint when not being used, making it even more challenging to encourage the patient to start using that limb, even with proper pain management. The saying "if you don't use it, you lose it" really applies in the scenario of describing

osteoarthritis. It is important to encourage patients with osteoarthritis to maintain a consistent level of daily activity to help modulate the inflammatory processes within the joint. This will help keep the joint healthy by improving joint fluid production and natural lubrication of the joint making it more comfortable for the patient to support weight on the affected limb. This ultimately improves function and overall quality of life. Allowing an arthritic patient to stay sedentary due to fear of causing more pain is counterintuitive. The amount of activity does not need to be extreme, but for the health of the joints they must keep moving (Ritzman and Knapp 2002).

Other common diseases and injuries that exotic pets suffer from that can benefit from rehabilitation include vertebral fractures and luxations (especially in rabbits), spondylosis, patella or elbow luxations, post-op repair of long bone fractures, congenital or acquired spinal defects, and intervertebral disc disease (Huynh and Piazza 2021).

Special considerations when thinking about physical rehab for the exotic patient include locomotion of species, patient's response to stress, bone and muscle strength, type and location of injury, and owner capabilities. It is important that the entire healthcare team and client have a realistic goal for the patient and that the quality of life of both the patient and the client is considered.

There is common terminology the veterinary technician should be comfortable with when performing or assisting with a physical rehab examination. Below are examples of brief documentation of observations or findings on a physical written in italics.

- Flexion: During flexion, the limbs on either side of a joint are moved toward each other creating a smaller angle.
  - *Decreased flexion of the stifle was observed during examination of the geriatric parrot. This could explain why the patient has difficulty stepping up on the higher perch.*
- Extension: Extension is the movement that brings the bones/joints toward a straight position.
  - *Client reports rabbit has a harder time hopping. On examination, the stifle joint appears stiff preventing normal extension which could be causing the change in movement the client is seeing at home.*
- Abduction: "Movement of a body part away from median plane"
- Adduction: "Movement of a body part toward the median plan"
  - *Normal side shuffling observed when watching an avian patient move on a perch.*
- Circumduction: Movement of a limb or joint in which the segment outlines a circle
  - *The ferret is circumducting his right thoracic limb due to limited shoulder joint movement caused by osteoarthritis.*

- Pronation: Internal rotation of the limb such that the ventral surface of the wing or paw is facing laterally
- Supination: External rotation of the limb such that the ventral surface of the wing or paw is facing medially.
  - *Palpable pectoralis muscle atrophy may explain the change in the patient's flight performance as this muscle helps control the twisting/rotating of the wing during flight.*
- Valgus: twisting outward, deformity of limb with angulation away from the midline of the body. *Tip: The L in valgus can help you think of the word lateral (away from midline)*
- Varus: Twisting inward, deformity of limb with angulation toward midline of the body
  - *The patient has a history of a fracture that healed abnormally resulting in a varus deformity of the femur.*

Putting It All Together

After obtaining a thorough history and having an understanding of the overall function and joint health of the patient, the next step for the veterinary technician is to present the patient to the veterinarian overseeing the case and work together with the client to come up with a treatment plan. This does not need to be looked at strictly as a rehab plan but more of a full-picture, multimodal approach to the best overall long-term care of the patient. These plans and recommendations typically include activity modification (increasing or sometimes decreasing the amount of a certain activity), nutritional recommendations, medications and/or supplements, and adding controlled exercise/activity.

Caspersen et al. (1985) reports that "exercise is a subset of physical activity that is planned, structured, and repetitive and has as a final or an intermediate objective for the improvement or maintenance of physical fitness." This is important to differentiate between physical activity and day-to-day activity as many clients do consider what their pet does day to day as exercise. That said, there is a lot of success to be had by taking the patient's "normal daily physical activity" and turning it into an exercise.

This could be as simple as asking a parakeet to sidestep on a perch for a few minutes back and forth for their favorite treat or placing a small obstacle in the way of a patient's food dish, or favorite resting spot to encourage slightly more active range of motion (AROM) to the joints of an arthritic (and maybe lazy) patient. The side-stepping exercise would help improve the patient's hip adduction and abduction strength and overall balance while also sneaking in a little cardiovascular exercise depending on the speed at which the patient was moving. Having patients step over obstacles

also encourages more AROM and challenges their balance as compared to a patient who walks on a flatter surface throughout the day. Creativity is the only limiting factor when helping to design a home exercise plan.

When looking at joint health, controlled activity is the best way to help protect the joint cartilage as it is more receptive to slow loading. Understanding the composition of a joint and what happens as pets age is important when recommending certain activities. Preventative medicine is an important aspect of all species. Preventing health problems and/or treating them early leads to greater strength/function, better full body health, and significantly improves overall long-term quality of life. Annual or biannual checkups with the veterinarian should be standard of care for all exotic species, and it is important to share all exam findings with the client so that they may help monitor their pet's health and function from home. It would not be recommended to wait a year between visits to the veterinary clinic if a patient is found to have any acute or chronic joint disease or signs of neuropathies. Veterinary clients are not always astute at the small details or changes in their pet's function or daily routine that the experienced veterinary technician may observe. Waiting too long between visits could be detrimental to the patient's physical function as chronic postural changes (how a patient stands, walks, sits, etc.) are difficult to reverse, especially once the joint capsules tighten and muscles shorten. It can also be challenging to break bad habits in posture which can occur rapidly when a patient is compensating for pain. This reinforces the importance of proper pain management and consistent follow-up.

From a physical rehabilitation standpoint, geriatric medicine is not that different than the acutely injured young patient and should be focused on maintaining or restoring normal movement. However, as mentioned previously, severely chronic changes in posture and function will limit the success of rehab regardless of how aggressive the treatment is. Once a patient reaches the geriatric age they likely have, at minimum, some mild signs of degenerative joint disease, sarcopenia, or polyneuropathies (Volpi et al. 2004). Keeping the patient active will help maintain some level of endurance and strength despite the obstacles to their overall health. A common misconception of aging patients is that their age defines what they can or cannot do. All patients should always be able to perform the basic postures for living a normal life. This means being able to stand, sit, step up, walk, etc.; all movements that are important in allowing a patient to get to and from their food/water bowls and to eliminate normally. Geriatric patients who lose too much muscle mass and strength may have a difficult time urinating or defecating. This could cause them to strain and ultimately shift their weight even more abnormally than they already are doing throughout the day. Ensuring patients maintain at least the minimal amount of joint movement to get into normal postures is beneficial to the long-term quality of life of the patient.

Physical Rehab Techniques: The Why and The How

Passive range of motion (PROM) is used to help maintain joint health, prevent joint contracture, and soft tissue adaptive shortening, decrease pain, improve blood and lymphatic flow, and increase synovial fluid production and diffusion. Special considerations before considering PROM include type of injury, number of days post-op, species, temperament of patient, and how much do they like to be handled. It would be contraindicated to perform PROM on an unstable fracture or luxated joint (Figures 4.1–4.4).

How to Perform PROM

Mammals: Gentle flexion and extension of affected joint or all joints depending on patient needs. Limbs should be supported in a neutral position and motion should be slow and continuous. Repetitions and frequency will depend on patient and ailment but are typically started with 10–20 repetitions 2–4x/day (Millis and Levine 2014b), (Figures 4.5 and 4.6).

Avian Species

Contraindications for performing range of motion exercises include but are not limited to joint luxation, unstable fractures, and osteopenia. Performing AROM may be more successful when trying to improve joint movement in a bird (Figures 4.7–4.12). However, considerations need to be evaluated when a patient is recovering from surgery. Wing PROM is typically performed under inhalant gas anesthesia +/– analgesic. Pollock (2002) recommends:

- A minimum of 10 gentle flexion and extension 2x/week for ~3 weeks.
- Gentle pronation and supination to prevent radioulnar synostosis.
- Leg PROM and AROM are more challenging. If the patient likes to be handled and can be properly restrained without causing too much stress, gentle flexion, and extension of the stifle joint could be performed similarly to how it is described in mammals.
  - Example of AROM—forced wing flapping would be the next step in the rehab/recovery process after successfully improving range of motion with passive movement.
    - Can use rocking perch or hand

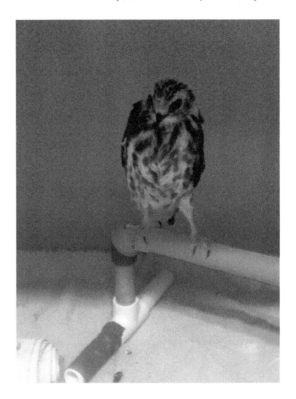

Figure 4.1 Abnormal perching stance post femur fracture repair on a small raptor.

Massage

Massage is well documented in providing benefits for all aspects of the body. Increased blood flow for the post-op recovery patient and stimulating the parasympathetic system to calm an anxious patient are examples of how massage has great uses in veterinary medicine. Contraindications include but are not limited to shock (due to massage helping lower blood pressure), fever, acute inflammation, skin problems (ringworm), infectious diseases, and acute stages of viral disease (herpes). Other special considerations before starting massage on an exotic patient are the location that will be massaged, the number of days post-op/injury, and the species—can they handle being touched or will this cause unnecessary stress?

Massage is typically used in conjunction with PROM to help prevent contractures (especially post-op). Massage can be used as a warmup or a cool down. It is important to maintain a steady rhythm and start light. Pending what the patient can tolerate, friction massage can help break down adhesions (Gasibat and Suwehli 2017). For birds, tarsitis and pododermatitis typically respond well to massage. The reader can be directed to other sources for additional reading on the benefits of massage. While most publications talk about the benefit of massage for canine patients, it can be

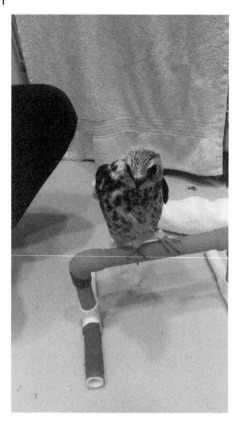

Figure 4.2 Small raptor post femur fracture repair wearing hobbles during passive weight shifting exercises to encourage more normal placement and use of left pelvic limb.

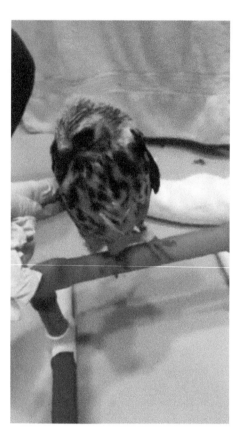

Figure 4.3 Passive weight shifting exercise on a small raptor—note two fingers on the right side of the patient pushing gently to shift weight to the left pelvic limb.

easily extrapolated to all species (Hourdebaigt 2004; Rychel et al. 2011) (Figure 4.13).

> Tips: Go slow. Have patience. Do not stress your patient! Get creative: consider using a small ice cube for an ice massage over an inflamed joint, or an electric toothbrush on the tight hamstrings of a rabbit, or a cotton-tipped applicator to give an avian patient a relaxing head massage!

Cryotherapy causes vasoconstriction and is an easy way to help decrease pain and inflammation in post-op and chronic pain patients (Millard et al. 2013). Care should be taken when considering cryotherapy for small exotic patients. While the author is not aware of any studies documenting a decrease in core body temperature with peripheral cold applications, it is important to monitor the patient during the treatment to ensure there are no negative side effects. Cold therapy should be applied during the acute inflammatory stage, the first 72 hours post-injury/surgery for 5–20 minutes depending on patient needs/size. Cold therapy can also be used for chronic joint

pain after exercise. Considerations: patient's tolerance to cold, is there a barrier between skin and cold compress/ice, does the patient have hypertension (cold could increase blood pressure)?

Superficial heat therapy has the opposite effect of cryotherapy in that it causes vasodilation. Both cold and heat can help with decreasing pain, but heat should not be applied during the acute inflammatory stage. Superficial heat can be used to help increase blood flow and improve the extensibility of the soft tissues allowing for better/easier joint movement. For therapeutic treatment, heat should be applied for at least 15 minutes. Considerations for application should be location, patient skin and use of barriers, and heat should not be used in areas of decreased sensation, acute inflammation, or poor circulation.

Therapeutic exercises can be used to improve balance, posture, and to retrain normal body movements after injury. As previously mentioned in this chapter, taking normal daily activity for the exotic patient and increasing the intensity (time, repetitions, etc.) may be the most successful form of controlled exercise. Activities can include walking, climbing, hopping/jumping, and flapping. This is where creativity plays a large role in the success of the

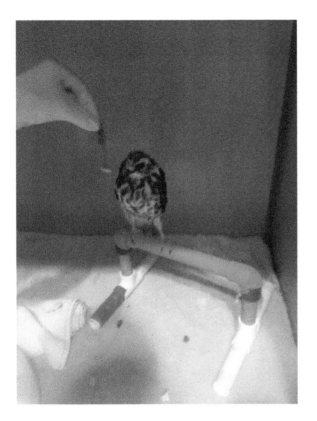

Figure 4.4 Small raptor post femur fracture repair, hobbles removed, using food for motivation.

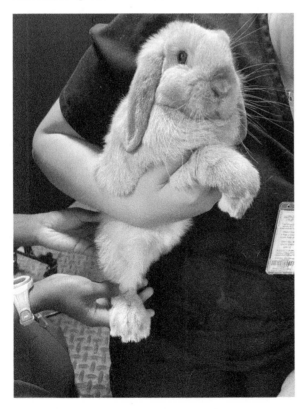

Figure 4.5 Pelvic limb range of motion assessment of a rabbit.

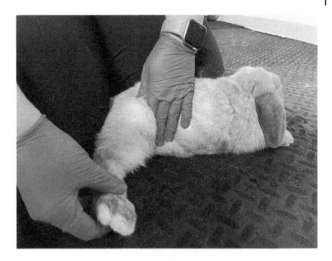

Figure 4.6 Pelvic limb range of motion assessment of a rabbit.

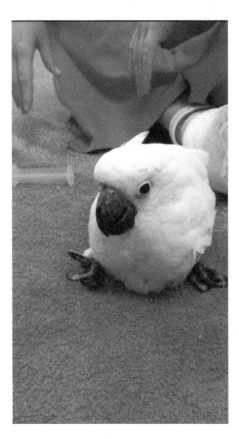

Figure 4.7 Talon deformity in a young Umbrella cockatoo.

rehab program and recommendations. Exercise equipment may also be beneficial, such as utilizing balance discs, wobble boards (perch on wobble board for avian patients), stepping over obstacles, or exercise wheels to improve a patient's coordination, balance, proprioception, and increasing (and hopefully evening out) their muscle mass.

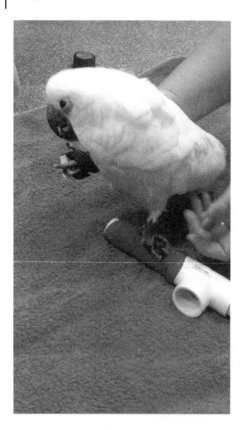

Figure 4.8 Perch/grip retraining in young Umbrella cockatoo with talon deformity. Patient is gripping the perch.

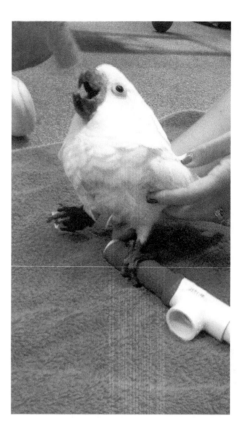

Figure 4.10 Positive reinforcement with food from syringe to get patient to reach while gripping perch.

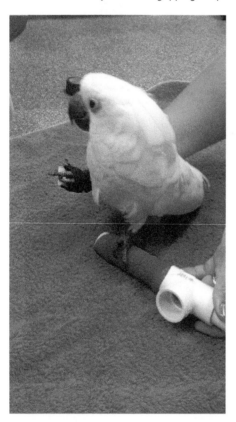

Figure 4.9 Perch/grip retraining in young Umbrella cockatoo with talon deformity. Patient is also wearing a custom talon orthotic.

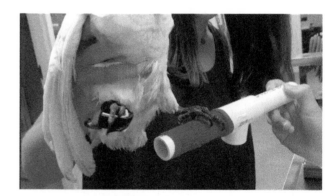

Figure 4.11 A closeup of grip training.

Common Rehab Modalities Used in Exotic Medicine

Photobiomodulation Therapy (PBMT): PMBT is typically applied using a class III or IV therapeutic laser. Application of PMBT for musculoskeletal disorders is highly referenced in both human and veterinary medicine to aid in the pain management of chronic joint disease and to improve healing of post-op patients (Mayer and Ness 2017). It is recommended that any personnel using the therapeutic laser undergo proper safety and equipment

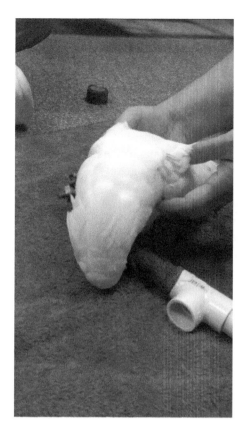

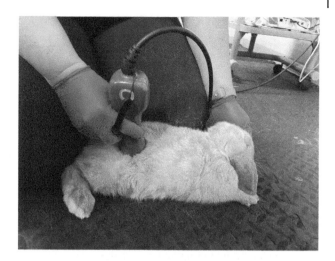

Figure 4.14 Photobiomodulation of proximal hip flexors and medial hip joint of the right pelvic limb (on a tripod rabbit).

Figure 4.12 The patient is tired and unable to keep thorax lifted, resting with beak on towel.

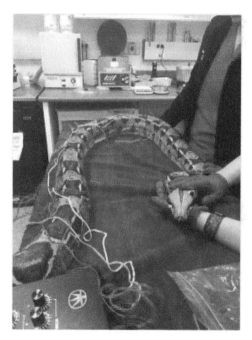

Figure 4.15 Acupuncture on a red-tailed boa. (Courtesy of Jennifer Good.)

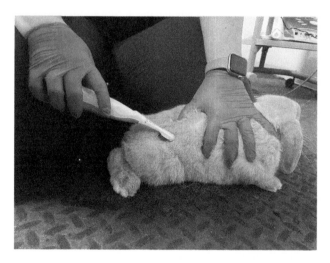

Figure 4.13 Electric toothbrush massage to pelvic limb musculature on a rabbit.

training prior to treating any patient. Safety precautions must be observed for all personnel and patients in the treatment area, including protective eyewear that is specific to protecting the retina from damaging effects of the infra-red laser (Figure 4.14).

Acupuncture: Acupuncture can help the body restore normal homeostasis by stimulating specific acupoints with acupuncture needles, laser acupuncture, or acupressure (Marziani 2018). Stimulating these points is based on a Traditional Chinese Veterinary Medicine (TCVM) pattern diagnosis to have a local and systemic effect on the body. Acupuncture must be performed by a veterinarian whereas acupressure and laser acupuncture can be performed by a veterinary technician under the guidance of the prescribing veterinarian (Figure 4.15). Veterinary technicians interested in TCVM are encouraged to research their state regulations regarding participation in this specific part of veterinary medicine.

Adaptive Devices Used in Exotic Patient Medicine

Adaptive devices can be wonderful tools in helping a handicapped patient live their best life. However, it is important for the veterinary technician to understand that adaptive devices are not quick fixes and are not recommended to be used as the only form of treatment. If a patient requires an adaptive device, the patient should also be receiving other rehabilitation treatments at home or at a dedicated facility. As with most of the rehabilitation recommendations in this chapter, there are special considerations that should be discussed before considering an adaptive device for the exotic patient. These considerations are similar to many that were listed previously, including how much the patient likes to be handled, type of and location of injury, etc., but cost of treatment should be discussed. Unlike most of the rehab recommendations that were discussed previously, which included minimal, if any, extra equipment or cost, adaptive devices may come with a hefty price tag. Sometimes the smaller the patient is, the more custom the device needs to be. This requires more time and attention to detail which typically comes with a steeper price tag. Adaptive devices that have been used successfully in exotic medicine include orthotics, prosthetics, and wheelchairs.

Wheelchairs can help patients with pelvic or thoracic limb weakness get around more easily by using wheels on a frame that are ergonomically attached to the patient to allow for normal body mechanics. Quad-carts are wheelchairs with wheels placed near all 4 limbs to allow for easier movement in patients with full-body weakness. Quad-carts are less utilized in exotic medicine as compared to canine medicine.

Orthoses and prostheses are less commonly used in exotic animal medicine, but the veterinary technician should still be aware of their usage and how these devices may help the patient. Due to the small size of exotic patients and their anatomy/conformation, custom orthoses would be required.

Orthotics are used to protect and support injured joints, while prosthetics are used to replace a limb. Typically comprised of a hard thermomoldable plastic lined with supportive foam, these devices can be useful in helping limit pain with ambulation, protecting weak joints, and preventing future injury. There are many considerations the veterinary technician should discuss with the client and the overseeing veterinarian before recommending an orthosis or prosthesis (see Figure 4.9). These considerations include: how much the patient likes to be handled? Client capabilities—can the client safely apply the device at home? Can they come for appropriate follow-up? And the reason for needing the adaptive device. Does the patient always need some sort of support to ambulate without causing sores? If so, then the veterinary technician needs to have the foresight to recommend a soft brace for when the patient is not in the hard support device. Special care also needs to be considered if the patient has protruding bony prominences as these areas are easily subjected to developing wounds or sores.

Soft custom braces may also be used to aid a patient in their recovery from injury. These would also require a custom design but may be more manageable for the client and the patient, even if they do not provide the full rigid support that the patient may need.

Below are a few examples of companies to investigate when considering an adaptive device.

https://www.handicappedpets.com/
https://eddieswheels.com/
https://orthopets.com/
https://www.aocpet.com/
https://www.therapaw.com/

Conclusion

This chapter demonstrates that ingenuity and creativity are the only limiting factors when considering adding rehabilitation to exotic animal medicine. The veterinary technician should have a base knowledge of how rehabilitation can help their patient improve or maintain their quality of life and how to communicate this with the client.

However, it is still important to consider expanding the veterinary team by utilizing your local rehab practitioner. Rehabilitation veterinarians and technicians can help improve a patient's overall health while also sharing some of the workload when it comes to managing an exotic patient's chronic orthopedic or neurologic disease.

Resources to locate rehab professionals are listed below.

https://www.ncsuvetce.com/canine-rehab-ccrp/ccrp-
    practitioners/
https://www.caninerehabinstitute.com/Find_A_Therapist
    .html
https://vsmr.site-ym.com/search/custom.asp?id=5595
https://www.aprvt.com/find-a-member.html

References

Callaghan P. 2004. Exercise: a neglected intervention in mental health care? *J Psychiatr Ment Health Nurs* 11: 476–483.

Caspersen, C., Powell, K., Christenson, G. 1985. Physical activity, exercise and physical fitness: definitions and distinctions for health-related research. *Public Health Reports*, 100 130-134.

Gasibat Q, Suwehli W. 2017. Determining the benefits of massage mechanisms: a review of literature. *J Rehabil Sci* 2: 58–67.

Geneen LJ, Moore RA, Clarke C, Martin D, Colvin LA, Smith BH. 2017. Physical activity and exercise for chronic pain in adults: an overview of cochrane reviews. *Cochrane Database Syst Rev* 1(1): CD011279.

Goldberg ME, Tomlinson J. 2018. Chapter 7/Supporting the client and patient. In: *Physical Rehabilitation for Veterinary Technicians and Nurses* (eds ME Goldberg, JE Tomlinson). Wiley.

Goldberg ME. 2019. A walk on the wild side: a review of physiotherapy for exotics and zoo animals. *Vet Nurs J* 34(2): 33–47. 10.1080/17415349.2018.1529547.

Greene LM, Marcellin-Little DJ, Lascelles BD. 2013. Associations among exercise duration, lameness severity, and hip joint range of motion in Labrador Retrievers with hip dysplasia. *J Am Vet Med Assoc* 242(11): 1528–1533.

Guskiewicz KM, Perrin DH. 1996. Research and clinical applications of assessing balance. *J Sport Rehabil* 5: 45–63.

Hourdebaigt J-P. 2004. *Canine Massage: A Complete Reference Manual*. Dogwise Publishing.

Huynh M, Piazza S. 2021. Musculoskeletal and neurologic diseases. *Ferrets, Rabbits, and Rodents*, pp. 117–130. doi: 10.1016/B978-0-323-48435-0.00010-1. Epub 2020 May 29. PMCID: PMC7258713.

Marziani JA. 2018. Nontraditional therapies (traditional Chinese medicine and Chiropractic) in exotic animals. *Vet Clin North Am Exot Anim Pract* 21, pp. 511–528.

Loeser RF, Goldring SR, Scanzello CR, Goldring MB. 2012. Osteoarthritis: a disease of the joint as an organ. *Arthritis Rheum.* 64(6): 1697–707. doi: 10.1002/art.34453. Epub 2012 Mar 5. PMID: 22392533; PMCID: PMC3366018.

Marcellin-Little DJ, Levine D, Taylor R. 2005. Rehabilitation and conditioning of Sporting Dogs. *Vet Clin N Am Small Anim Pract* 35(6), 1427–1439. doi: 10.1016/j.cvsm. 2005.08.002.

Mayer J, Ness RD. 2017. Laser therapy for exotic small mammals. In: *Laser Therapy in Veterinary Medicine* (eds RJ Riegel and JC Godbold). doi: 10.1002/9781119220190.ch26.

Millard RP, Towle-Millard HA, Rankin DC, Roush JK. 2013. Effect of cold compress application on tissue temperature in healthy dogs. *Am J Vet Res* 74(3): 443–447. doi: 10.2460/ajvr.74.3.443. PMID: 23438121.

Millis DL, Levine D. 2014a. Chapter 13/Assessing and measuring outcomes. In: *Canine Rehabilitation and Physical Therapy*, p. 220. Elsevier.

Millis DL, Levine D. 2014b. Range of motion and stretching exercises. In: *Canine Rehabilitation and Physical Therapy*, 2nd edn, pp. 431–438. Elsevier.

Pollock C. 2002. Postoperative management of the exotic animal patient. *Vet Clin N Am Exot Anim Pract* 5: 183–212.

Ritzman TK, Knapp D. 2002. Ferret orthopedics. *Vet Clin North Am Exot Anim Pract* 5(1): 129–155 vii. doi: 10.1016/s1094-9194(03)00050-1.

Rychel JK, Johnston MS, Robinson NG. 2011. Zoologic companion animal rehabilitation and physical medicine. *Vet Clin North Am Exot Anim Pract*, 14(1), 131–140. doi: 10.1016/j.cvex.2010.09.008.

Sharma A, Madaan V, Petty FD. 2006. Exercise for mental health. *Prim Care Companion J Clin Psychiatry* 8(2): 106. doi: 10.4088/pcc.v08n0208a. PMID: 16862239; PMCID: PMC1470658.

Tomlinson, J. 2018. The veterinary technician and rehabilitation pain management. In: *Physical Rehabilitation for Veterinary Technicians and Nurses*, Wiley.

Volpi E, Nazemi R, Fujita S. 2004. Muscle tissue changes with aging. *Curr Opin Clin Nutr Metab Care* 7(4): 405–410. doi: 10.1097/01.mco.0000134362.76653.b2. PMID: 15192443; PMCID: PMC2804956.

Additional Resources

http://www.rehabvets.org/
https://www.handicappedpets.com/
https://eddieswheels.com/
https://orthopets.com/
https://www.aocpet.com/
https://www.therapaw.com/

Section III

Avian

5

Psittacine and Passerine Birds

Cheryl B. Greenacre and Janet L. Pezzi-Jones

Introduction

The Class Aves consists of over 8,500 different species of birds and 29 orders of birds. Two orders commonly kept as pets in the United States are the Psittaciformes (parrots; Figures 5.1 to 5.3; Table 5.1) and the Passeriformes (canaries and finches; Figures 5.4 to 5.7; Table 5.1).

Anatomically and physiologically, there is no generic bird, meaning that each species is different in its anatomy, hematology (lymphocytes may predominate in some species), and drug metabolism. Avian medicine has many similarities to canine and feline medicine, but also some definite differences. The similarities include the use of similar, albeit smaller, equipment, similar drugs, and similar techniques. Most differences encountered in caring for birds relate to the drastically different anatomy and physiology, especially respiratory physiology, and this in turn dictates a different approach to supportive care and restraint, such as allowing the sternum to move up and down so the bird can breathe. Once these differences are recognized, then avian medicine is quite straightforward and rewarding.

Anatomy and Physiology

The anatomy and physiology of birds are drastically different from mammalian anatomy and physiology and are usually due to an adaptation that helps enable flight or development within an egg.

Integumentary System

Feathers are made of keratin and are used for flight, insulation, and attracting a mate. There are various types of feathers including primaries, also known as wing remiges and tail rectrices (very large feathers that originate from

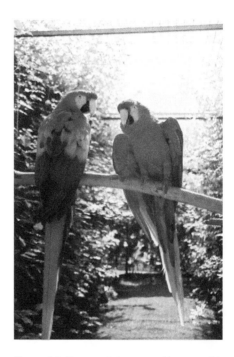

Figure 5.1 Two scarlet macaws (*Ara macao*) in an outdoor aviary. This is an example of a psittacine bird or parrot.

the carpus and metacarpus, and pygostyle, respectively), secondaries (large feathers that originate from the radius and ulna), contour (over the body), and down feathers (produce powder down). Feathers lie in feathered tracts called pterylae, and the non-feathered tracts are called apterylae. The main shaft of the feather is called the rachis, with barbs attached to the rachis, and then barbules attached to the barbs at a 45° angle that hook with nearby barbules at a 90° angle (Figure 5.8).

A developing blood feather, called a blood or pin feather, has a blood supply, and in the case of large wing feathers, it is attached to the bone (periosteum). Pigmented blood feathers have a black shaft, and non-pigmented blood feathers have a pink shaft (Figure 5.9).

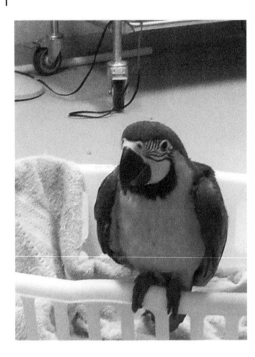

Figure 5.2 A 6-month-old blue and gold macaw (*Ara ararauna*). Note the dark-colored iris. The iris will gradually lighten to a corn-yellow color as the bird matures.

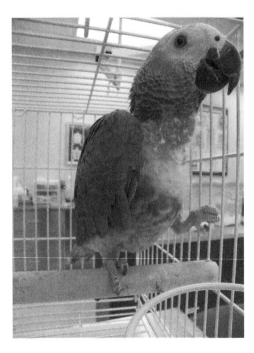

Figure 5.3 Adult African Grey parrot (*Psittacus erithacus*) with evidence of feather picking around the neck.

Table 5.1 Examples of common species of birds encountered in practice.

Common name	Scientific name	Figure number
Cockatoo		
Moluccan	*Cacutua moluccensis*	
Umbrella[a]	*Cacatua alba*	Figure 5.1
Sulfur-crested	*Cacatua sulphurea*	
Macaw		
Blue and gold[a]	*Ara ararauna*	
Scarlet	*Ara macao*	Figure 5.1
Hyacinth	*Anodorhynchus hyacinthinus*	Figure 5.7
Military	*Ara militaris*	Figure 5.8
Green-winged	*Ara chloroptera*	
Amazon parrot		
Yellow-naped[a]	*Amazona ochrocephala*	Figure 5.10
Red-lored	*Amazona autumnalis*	
Orange-winged	*Amazona amazonica*	
Double yellow-headed	*Amazona ochrocephala*	
Blue-fronted	*Amazona aestiva*	Figure 5.11
Mexican red-headed	*Amazona viridigenalis*	
Lory, Rainbow	*Trichoglossus haematodus*	
Conures		
Blue-crowned	*Aratinga acuticaudata*	
Sun	*Aratinga solstitialis*	
Half-moon	*Aratinga canicularis*	
Maroon (Red)-bellied	*Pyrrhura frontalis*	
Nanday	*Nandayus nenday*	
Green-cheeked	*Pyrrhura molinae*	
Mitred	*Aratinga mitrata*	
Lovebird, Peach-faced	*Agapornis rosicollis*	
Cockatiel[a]	*Nymphicus hollandicus*	Figure 5.3
Parakeet		
Standard budgerigar[a]	*Melopsittacus undulates*	
Gray-cheeked	*Brotogeris pyrrhopterus*	
Monk (Quaker parrot)	*Myiopsitta monachus*	
Finch		
Zebra	*Poephila castanotis*	Figure 5.4
Lady Gouldian	*Poephila gouldiae*	
Parrot		
African Grey[a]	*Psittacus erithacus*	Figure 5.4
Eclectus	*Eclectus roratus*	Figure 5.2

a) Most commonly encountered species.

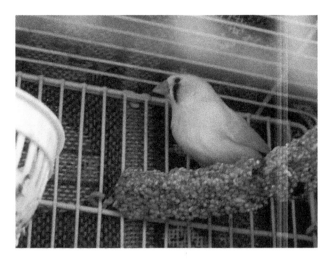

Figure 5.4 Female fawn-colored zebra finch (*Poephila castanotis*). This is an example of a passerine, or soft-billed, bird.

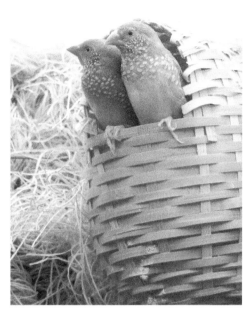

Figure 5.6 A male (left) and female star finch (*Neochmia ruficadua*) protecting their nest.

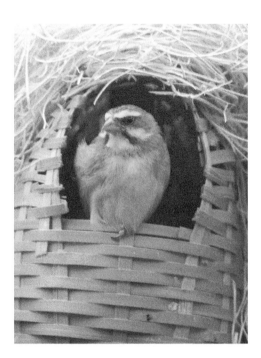

Figure 5.5 A male yellow-fronted canary finch, also known as green singing finch (*Serinus mozambicus*).

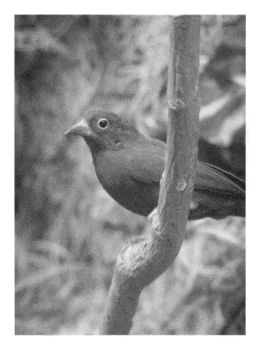

Figure 5.7 A male red-billed fire finch (*Lagonostica senegala*).

If a blood feather is broken, the bird can slowly bleed to death because the blood supply at the proximal end of the feather does not vasoconstrict to stop bleeding. This is why a damaged, bleeding blood feather needs to be gently pulled out.

The very thin skin (two to four cell layers thick in feathered areas) is difficult to suture, usually requiring 4/0 or 5/0 suture. There is very little, if any, subcutaneous tissue. The feet are an exception in that they usually have thick, prominent scales in the non-feathered regions to protect them from trauma. The wing web of a bird is called a patagium. There are only two proper glands in birds: the bilobed uropygial (preen) gland that helps waterproof the feathers, which is absent in some birds (such as Amazon parrots), and the ear gland, which is absent in most birds.

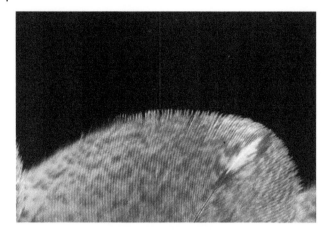

Figure 5.8 The central main shaft of the feather is called the rachis. Barbs extend from each side of the rachis at a 45° angle. Microscopically, barbules extend from each side of the barb at a 45° angle. Barbules on the leading edge of a barb hook onto the barbules of the trailing edge. When birds preen their feathers, they are realigning these barbules.

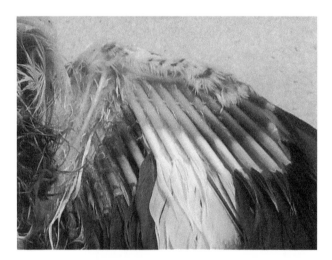

Figure 5.9 Growing feathers have an active blood supply and are called blood or pin feathers. Pigmented blood feathers have a black shaft and non-pigmented blood feathers have a pink shaft.

Birds have no external ear pinna and no sweat glands. Birds bruise green since they lack biliverdin reductase, an enzyme that converts biliverdin to bilirubin. About three days after trauma, a bright green bruise can form that should not be confused for gangrene.

Musculoskeletal System

Unlike mammals, birds can have a variable number of cervical vertebrae; 8 to 25 instead of 7 (King & McLelland 1984). Birds use their long, flexible necks to access food and to reach the uropygial (preen) gland to preen their feathers. The remainder of the spine is fused in many areas to provide a stable body part for flight (see Figure 5.10). The notarium is a fusion of the first thoracic vertebrae. The synsacrum is a fusion of the caudal thoracic, lumbar, sacral, and caudal vertebrae. The pygostyle is a distal fusion of the caudal vertebrae for tail muscle attachment. The sternum has a prominent keel for large pectoral (flight) muscle attachment. The pectoral girdle consists of the unique coracoid bone that acts as a strut enabling flight, the clavicle, and the scapula. Bones of the wing from proximal to distal include humerus, radius, ulna, ulnar and radial carpal bones, and major and minor metacarpals, alula (remnants of a thumb), and the major and minor digits. Bones of the hindlimb from proximal to distal include femur, tibiotarsus, tarsometatarsus, and phalanges. Most important clinically is that the femur, humerus, and some vertebrae are pneumatic bones—bones filled with air—which connect directly to the respiratory tract to lighten the bones for flight. Intraosseous catheters should not be placed in pneumatic bones because any fluid administered could go directly to the lungs and drown the bird.

Cardiovascular System

Birds, like mammals, possess a four-chambered heart, but unlike mammals, birds lack a diaphragm; therefore, the apex of the heart is directly surrounded by liver (Figure 5.11).

The avian heart is comparatively 1.5 to 2 times larger than a mammalian heart (Table 5.2). Unlike in mammals, the mean electrical axis of birds is negative 90° (in dogs it is positive 90°). Birds do not possess lymph nodes, but they do have lymph vessels. Phlebotomy sites in birds include the right jugular vein (the right one is 2/3 larger than the left), the basilic (or cutaneous ulnar) vein, and medial metatarsal vein. The cutaneous ulnar vein, as it crosses the proximal ulna, is an excellent vein for determining vein refill time; if the vein can be seen to refill, this is considered slow and suggestive of dehydration or shock. Through a renal portal system (see "Renal system"), birds can choose to shunt blood from the caudal half of the body through the kidneys first before going through the heart; therefore, it is better to give parenteral medications in the front half of the body (i.e., give intramuscular injections in the pectoral muscles rather than in the leg).

Renal System

Birds possess a renal portal system, where blood from the caudal half of the body may pass through the kidneys first before reaching the heart, meaning any drug administered in the caudal half of the body may go undiluted

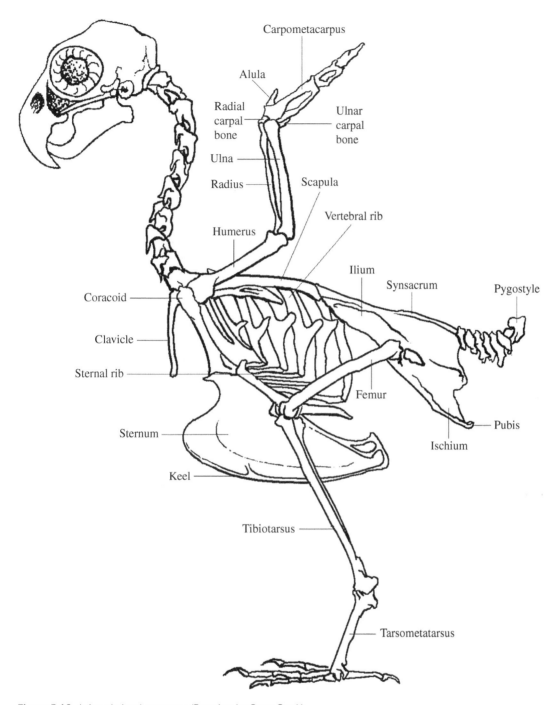

Figure 5.10 Avian skeletal anatomy. (Drawing by Scott Stark).

directly to the kidneys before going to the heart. Parrots have three divisions to their kidneys (cranial, middle, and caudal), and the kidneys are located dorsally in a concavity of the sacrum. Avian kidneys produce both urine (from their mammalian-type nephrons) and urates (from their reptilian-type nephrons that lack the loop of Henle). Urates consist of uric acid. Therefore, to determine renal function in birds, uric acid concentrations are evaluated, not BUN.

Neurology and Ophthalmology

Birds possess a large optic nerve compared to mammals. In fact, the two optic nerves together are larger than the bird's spinal cord. Olfactory lobes are small in most birds since the sense of smell is not an important sense in most birds. The eyes of a bird constitute approximately 15% of the body weight (whereas in humans they constitute 1%). The avian iris consists of voluntary, striated muscle, not smooth

Table 5.2 Representative heart and respiratory rates for various species of birds.

Species	Weight (grams)	HR (rest)	HR (restraint)	RR (rest)	RR (restraint)
Cockatiel	100	200	500–600	40–52	60–80
Amazon	400	150	200–350	25–30	40–60
Macaw	1000	125	150–350	15–20	25–40

Ritchie et al. (1994).
HR, heart rate; RR, respiratory rate.

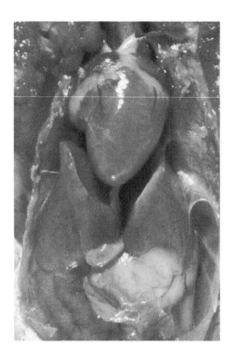

Figure 5.11 Birds, like mammals, possess a four-chambered heart, but since birds lack a diaphragm, the apex of the heart is directly surrounded by liver.

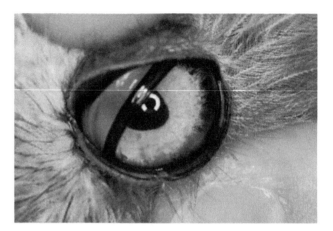

Figure 5.12 Birds have a well-developed third eyelid that closes over the eye in a craniodorsal to caudal ventral direction.

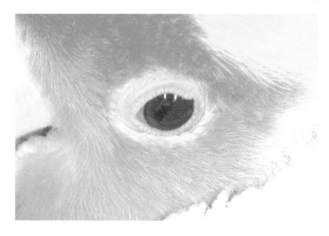

Figure 5.13 The pecten can be seen in the posterior chamber of this peach-faced lovebird as a black worm-shaped structure. This normal structure supplies nutrients to the vitreous.

muscle as in mammals; therefore, atropine is ineffective at dilating the pupils. Birds have a well-developed third eyelid that closes over the eye in a craniodorsal to caudal ventral direction (Figure 5.12).

A unique pigmented structure called the pecten attached to the retina supplies nutrients to the vitreous. Birds have no tapetum and have an avascular retina (Figure 5.13).

Respiratory System

The cere is an area at the base of the upper beak that surrounds the nostrils (nares) (see Figure 5.29). Just inside the nares in parrots is a keratinized flap of tissue called the operculum. Birds possess an extensive infraorbital sinus; in fact, most of their head is sinus. Compared to mammals, birds have a very large trachea, allowing them to inhale more air than mammals. The opening to the trachea is called a glottis (Figure 5.14).

Birds have complete tracheal rings; therefore, uncuffed ET tubes must be used to avoid pressure necrosis inside the trachea. Birds lack a diaphragm; therefore, they must be allowed to move their sternum up and down or they will suffocate. Old stories of birds dying right after being restrained were probably due to accidental sternal compression and secondary suffocation. The syrinx is responsible for sound generation in birds, not the larynx

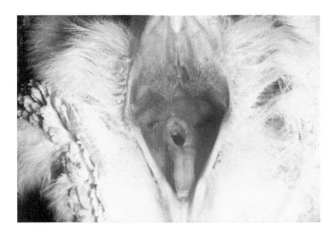

Figure 5.14 Open mouth of a barn owl showing the opening to the trachea that in birds is called a glottis. The glottis is usually located directly caudal to the base of the tongue in most birds. Also note the V-shaped opening on the roof of the mouth called the choana.

as in mammals. Since the syrinx is just past the tracheal bifurcation, birds can still vocalize even though intubated. The path of air through a bird is very different than that of mammals, and air can take 1–2 breath cycles to travel through a bird. After air passes through the cere, the trachea, and the primary bronchi, approximately half the air goes directly to the lungs during inspiration, and the other half goes to the "caudal" air sacs (caudal thoracic and abdominal air sacs) to be temporarily stored before it goes to the lungs during expiration. Expired air is temporarily stored in the "cranial" air sacs (cervicocephalic, clavicular, and cranial thoracic air sacs) before it goes back out of the trachea. The air sacs also warm the air (Figure 5.15). Bird lungs have air capillaries that are 3 microns in diameter, whereas the smallest mammals have alveoli that are approximately 10 microns in diameter. Therefore, birds have a comparatively greater lung surface area than mammals. The term "Minimum Alveolar Concentration" or MAC in birds means "Minimum Anesthetic Concentration" instead.

Because air can go from the caudal air sacs to the lungs, as well as from the trachea to the lungs, oxygen exchange occurs on both inspiration and expiration, increasing oxygen use in birds compared to mammals. See "air sac cannula placement" section regarding making it possible for a bird to breathe room air through an air sac cannula if the trachea is compromised.

Digestive System

Since birds lack a diaphragm, they possess a coelomic cavity, not an abdominal cavity. Birds do not have teeth, instead, they have a beak that is variable between species.

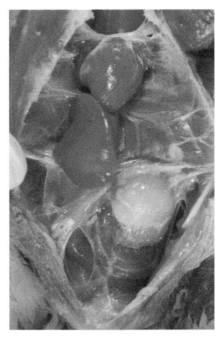

Figure 5.15 Necropsy of a parrot demonstrating clear, normal air sacs. Air sacs warm and store air. Since air from the caudal air sacs shown here goes directly to the lungs, air, oxygen, or anesthesia can be delivered through a tube (air sac tube) placed into one of these air sacs.

Parrots are sometimes called hookbills because of their strong, hooked beak. The tongue is quite variable among bird species; parrots have a muscular tongue. The esophagus in birds is divided into two sections (cervical esophagus and thoracic esophagus) by an outpouching of the esophagus called the crop (ingluvies). The ingluvies stores food and undergoes waves of peristalsis that occur at least one per minute. Birds possess a proventriculus (true glandular stomach) and a ventriculus (or gizzard) (Figure 5.16).

Some birds (e.g., chickens) possess a cecum, while others (e.g., parrots) lack one. Some birds possess a gallbladder, while others lack one (parrots). The feces of parrots contain mainly (90% or more) Gram-positive organisms (staining purple); waterfowl, raptors, and poultry can have mostly Gram-negative organisms (staining pink). Typically, passerine birds have very little bacteria in their feces, and it is Gram-positive.

Clostridium spp. should not be seen in parrot feces and is characterized by a septic tank smell to the feces and the characteristic safety-pin or racket shape seen on Gram stain (Figure 5.17). The cloaca is the end point for three systems: the gastrointestinal, reproductive, and urinary systems. The cloaca is divided into three parts: the copradeum receives feces from the rectum; the urodeum receives urine and urates from the ureter, and sperm or eggs from the vas deferens and uterus/vagina, respectively;

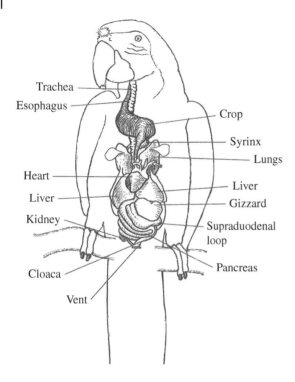

Figure 5.16 Avian viscera. (Drawing by Scott Stark).

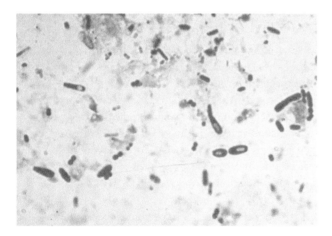

Figure 5.17 Clostridial overgrowth is apparent in this fecal Gram stain from a parrot. *Clostridium* spp. shown here is a large Gram-positive rod with no spore, a clear central spore (safety-pin shape), or clear end spore (racket shape).

and the proctodeum is the area just before the opening (vent).

Reproductive System

The male bird possesses two intra-abdominal testes and a phallus (a rudimentary fold of tissue that is either intromittant or non-intromittant). The female bird usually possesses only one left ovary (the right ovary usually fails to develop). The female reproductive tract consists of an

Table 5.3 Approximate average lifespan and approximate longevity in captivity of commonly kept psittacine birds.

Species	Average lifespan (years)	Approximate longevity record (years)
Budgie	5–7	18
Cockatiel	5–10	32
Lovebird	10	13–34
Conure	10	25
Amazon	15–50	22–66
African Grey	15–40	55
Cockatoo	15–30	82–103
Macaw	15–30	63–92
Lory	7	17–30

infundibulum, magnum, isthmus, uterus (or shell gland), and a very short vagina. Parrots are not usually or obviously sexually dimorphic (the exception being Eclectus parrots where the male is green and the female is red); therefore, in order to determine the gender of a bird, surgical sexing, or blood sexing must be performed. Surgical sexing involves visualizing the gonads and reproductive tract via a rigid endoscope placed in the abdominal air sac. Blood sexing involves evaluating 0.2 mL of blood via an ELISA test for a heterogamete (female is ZW) or homogamete (male is ZZ).

Lifespan and Longevity

Lifespan refers to the period of time that an individual is alive. Therefore, the average lifespan is the life expectancy for a particular group or breed (Table 5.3).

Longevity is the maximum lifespan that can be expected under ideal conditions (Young et al. 2012). Unfortunately, ideal conditions are not present in all captive situations and an individual's lifespan may not reach the maximum, or even get close. The lifespan of an individual bird depends on many factors including species, amount of genetic inbreeding, size, concurrent disease, diet, and environment. Chronic malnutrition, specifically hypovitaminosis A, can lead to a decreased lifespan.

Comparative Clinical Pathology

The blood glucose of birds is twice that of mammals. Birds possess heterophils instead of neutrophils; they are called heterophils due to the different, eosinophilic staining of the rod-shaped cytoplasmic granules. Birds, like reptiles, have nucleated RBCs and thrombocytes (Figure 5.18). Some parrots are lymphocytic species like cows (Amazon parrots,

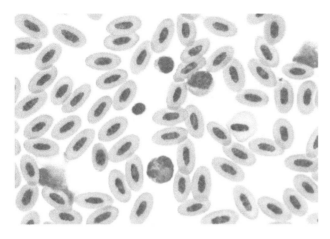

Figure 5.18 A Diff-Quick stained blood smear from a parrot. Note that birds have nucleated red blood cells. The cell at the 12 o'clock position is a lymphocyte, at the 2 o'clock position is a monocyte, at the 6 o'clock position a heterophil (like a neutrophil), and at the 9 o'clock position a normally occurring nucleated thrombocyte.

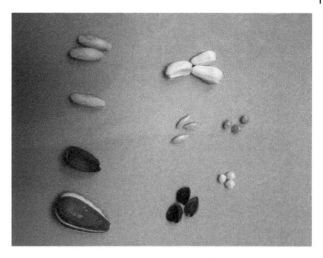

Figure 5.19 Examples of seeds found in seed diets. The left column from top to bottom is wheat, oat groat, small black sunflower seed, and large white-striped sunflower seed. The right column from top to bottom is safflower seeds, canary seeds, red millet, buckwheat, and white millet.

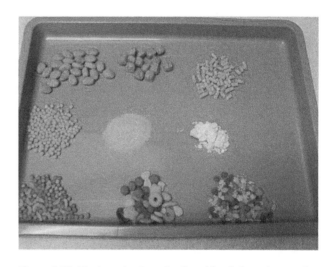

Figure 5.20 The introduction of pelleted foods for avian species has made it possible to dramatically improve the overall health of companion and caged birds. Shown are various brands of natural and artificially colored pelleted food marketed for birds. Finely ground formulas are available to mix with water for hand or tube feeding.

cockatiels, budgies, eclectus, etc.) Birds can normally have up to 8% polychromasia since their RBC lifespan is so short (38 days compared to 120 days for most mammals).

Nutrition

Species of birds kept as pets come from all over the world. Their diets are as varied as they are and the environments they come from. The specific dietary requirements for all these species are not well known.

Historically, psittacines (hooked-billed birds or parrots) and passerines (canaries and finches) kept in captivity readily accepted seed diets, which then became the basis of diets available for pet birds (Figure 5.19). Seed-based diets provide poor nutrition, being low in calcium, vitamins, and protein, and high in fat.

Consequently, birds on all-seed diets commonly present with hypovitaminosis A, especially older (>15 years) Amazon parrots. Most nutritional research is still based on the dietary requirements of chickens (Brue 1994).

The introduction of pelleted foods for avian species has made it possible to dramatically improve the overall health of companion and caged birds (Figure 5.20).

Balanced nutrition can be provided with the same ease of feeding as a seed diet. Two methods are used to manufacture pelleted diets. "Bound" pellets are not usually cooked and are finely ground. The pellet is mixed under pressure with a substance that when pressed forms the pellets. Much of the color and smell of the food used is retained in bound pellets. "Extruded" pellets are made of food ingredients that have been cooked and mixed together. The mixture moves

through a processing machine that presses the food into various shapes. Color and vitamins are added afterwards to the shapes and many have a sweet smell.

The current recommendation is to feed parrots a quality pelleted food that makes up 80% of their total intake. Fresh dark-green and dark-yellow vegetables (carrots, sweet potatoes, and leafy greens) should make up the other 20%. Fruits and seeds are to be offered as treats. Some quality nuts (preferably in their shells) such as almonds, Brazil nuts, or pine nuts can also be offered. Avoid peanuts since they all contain some degree of aflatoxins, which over time cause liver disease, specifically bile duct hyperplasia. Budgerigars and cockatiels seem to be the exception and the current recommendations are that they be provided some seed as part of their daily diet (up to 50%). Pellets alone may provide protein levels that are too high for these species.

Passerine birds (songbirds, i.e., canary and finches) eat seed as part of their basic diet (up to 50%). Canary/finch diets will contain millet, rape, hemp, sesame, and linseed, among other types of seeds. These seed mixes, along with pellets and fresh vegetables, will form a complete diet. Many of the rarer species of finch not commonly kept as pets will also require insects or fruit as part of their regular diet.

Special-need diets have been created for some species. Lories and lorikeets from Australia and the South Pacific Islands eat mainly nectar, fruits, and pollen. Fresh fruits and powdered diets are commercially available for lories and should be the basic diet for these species. Toucans, mynah birds, and some lories are predisposed to iron storage disease of the liver (hemochromatosis). Diets with low iron composition have been specially formulated for these species. Care must be taken with the choice of vegetables and fruit added for these species. For example, grapes are high in iron and should not be fed to mynah birds or toucan and others susceptible to iron storage disease (Tully 2009). Also, food high in vitamin C should be avoided since vitamin C enhances absorption of iron.

Some foods can be toxic to birds. Do not feed chocolate (toxic theobromine) or avocados. Foods high in salt, sugar, or caffeine should also be avoided. Peanuts should also be avoided for the aflatoxins that are invariably present.

Birds in the wild spend long hours foraging for food. They eat a wide variety of foods that change with each season and have many colors, textures, and tastes, creating a diverse diet that stimulates a bird psychologically and provides a lifetime of health. In the hospital setting, a variety of diets should be kept on hand, such as the commonly used pelleted foods, as well as seeds of various sizes for various species. During hospitalization, it is not advisable to change diets. During illness and the stress associated with a hospital stay, it is often difficult to keep a bird eating enough to maintain its weight. Having familiar diets available can encourage the avian patient to eat. This will include fresh vegetables and fruits.

Should a bird's appetite decrease or cease during hospitalization? It will become necessary to supplement nutrition via gavage feeding. Gavage tubes come in a number of sizes. There are various critical care diets available to readily pass through a gavage tube (see the "Techniques" section). Hand-feeding formulas designed for neonates also work well. Weighing the bird becomes a critical part of care

to assess that enough nutrition and calories are provided to maintain body weight. Ideally, the patient should be weighed every morning before food or treatments are given.

Fresh clean water should be provided daily. Birds are able to tolerate municipal tap water. Well water may be clean coming out of the ground but may be easily contaminated by bacteria colonizing the pipes leading to the faucet. Some owners may choose bottled water. Spring or drinking water can be used, but do not use distilled water, since this lacks electrolytes and minerals.

History, Restraint, and Physical Examination

Often a bird's illness has been developing much longer than the owner realized, and by the time signs are noticed, the problem may be advanced. As with all species of animals, acquiring a thorough history is the first step. Obtaining an adequate avian history may involve more time than that of a dog or a cat patient. Ideally, develop a questionnaire for clients to fill out. Birds should always be enclosed in a carrier or travel cage when arriving for their appointments (Figure 5.21).

There are many opportunities for harm to come to the bird in an unfamiliar environment. The owner should be made aware of this when they are making the appointment.

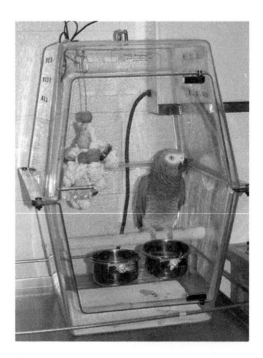

Figure 5.21 Birds should always be enclosed in a carrier or travel cage when arriving for their appointments. A towel can be used to cover a cage, especially a clear one such as this to provide visual security for the bird as well.

History

The following are questions to be asked about the bird:

- How old is the bird?
- How long has it been owned and where was it acquired (breeder/pet store/bird fair)?
- Have there been any previous problems?
- Has the bird been tested for chlamydiosis or psittacine beak and feather disease?
- Has it been vaccinated against polyomavirus?
- Have there been any changes in the bird such as voice change, attitude or weight change, or a change in the droppings (increase or decrease, color changes, more or less urine or urates) (Figures 5.22–5.26)?
- When was the last molt and has the bird been given any medications or herbal supplements?
- What is the problem today?
- How long has the illness been occurring?
- When, if ever, has the bird been to a veterinarian?

Next questions should be asked about the animal's environment:

- What is the bird fed and what does he/she actually eat out of what is offered?
- What is the cage like: size, perching?
- What materials are used to make the cage (lead/zinc)?
- What type of substrate is used, how often is it cleaned, and with what?
- Does the bird spend time outdoors?
- What is the temperature where the cage is kept and are there any drafts?
- Is the bird let out of the cage and is it supervised during that time?
- What type of enrichment is used (toys)?
- How much sleep does the bird get?

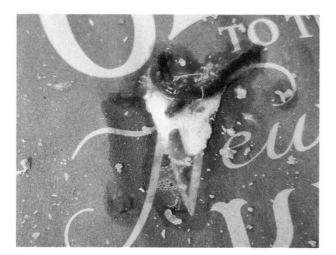

Figure 5.22 Normal feces.

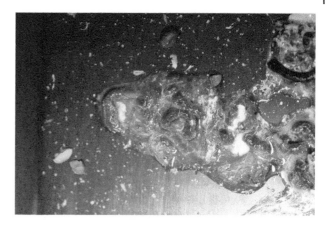

Figure 5.23 Normal feces.

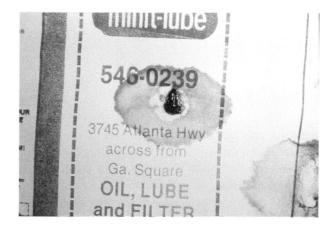

Figure 5.24 Hematuria and melena.

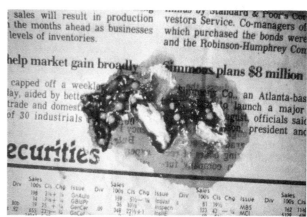

Figure 5.25 Undigested seeds.

Sleep is very important to a bird and approximately twelve hours of sleep each night is required for good health. This should not be in a covered cage in a room where the television is on or family members are still talking but somewhere where there is quiet. With these

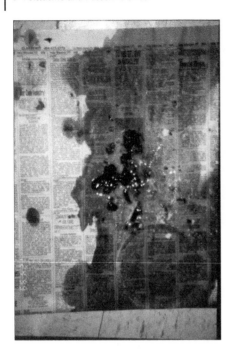

Figure 5.26 Polyuria.

questions, one can also develop an idea of the general knowledge that the owner has regarding bird care.

When a complete history has been attained, the physical examination should be performed. It should begin by observing the bird from afar. Birds are prey animals and will work at looking normal, especially in an unfamiliar environment. A bird in the hospital should never be sitting fluffed or closing its eyes. This would indicate a very sick animal. Observe the bird's behavior, attitude, posture, breathing, skin and feather quality, and neurologic status.

Look for symmetry. Look at the droppings in the cage bottom, or for regurgitated food. Dyspnea in a bird usually manifests as a "tail bob" movement of the tail up and down with each breath. After observing the bird from a distance, a physical examination can be performed with the bird restrained in a towel.

Restraint

After the bird has been observed and deemed able to withstand a hands-on examination, it can be restrained in a towel. To perform a thorough examination on a bird, restraint is needed. Capture and restraint are perhaps the most traumatic events for the avian patient, and one should strive to have this procedure be as stress-free as possible (see stress free options in Chapter 6). There are many methods advocated to capture and restrain a bird. The use of a towel and, talking in a calm voice and moving calmly, show the bird the towel and then wrap it around its wings to get a hold around its neck while the hands are protected under the towel. Some prefer to have the bird step up on a perch to remove it from the cage or carrier, then set the bird on the floor in a corner, and then catch it up using a towel. The authors prefer not to do this since it lets the bird out of the carrier, out of your control, and invites potential injury, as well as exposes the bird to possible contaminants that could be on the floor. The towel is used to help protect the hands and to have the bird associate being restrained with the towel, not the hands. Never attempt to capture a bird when it is being held by the owner, who could get bitten, and this could possibly affect the bond between owner and bird (Figure 5.27).

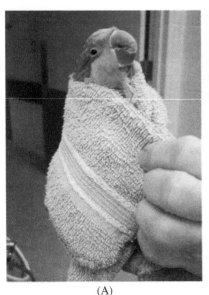

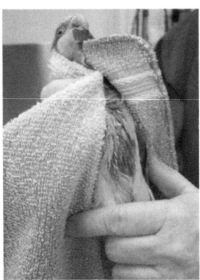

(A) (B)

Figure 5.27 (A) A bird properly restrained within a towel. The neck and wings are under control. (B) The towel can be manipulated to gain access to various areas while still restraining the bird.

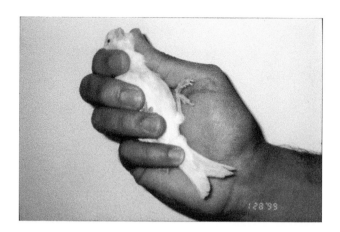

Figure 5.28 Restraint of a small bird.

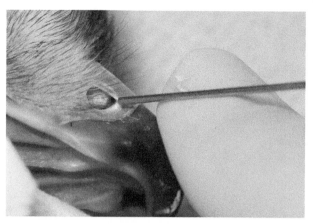

Figure 5.29 Just inside each naris (nostril) is a fleshy part called the operculum that warms and regulates air. Most birds, including this red-tailed hawk, have an operculum and it should not be mistaken for something that needs to be removed since disturbing this structure causes bleeding.

The parrot should be approached with a towel-covered hand and attempt to quickly wrap the fingers around the bird's neck. An ideal opportunity to grasp the neck is when the bird is attempting to move away from the towel, using its beak to hold onto the cage or carrier.

Coming from behind, the fingers can be wrapped around the neck, forming a collar. When the head is secured, the towel can be brought around the body with the other hand, meeting the two ends of the towel across the front of the bird. This will control flapping of the wings. Remember that birds move the sternum up and down to breathe and to move air through the respiratory system (they lack a diaphragm) and therefore care must be taken not to put pressure on the sternum as suffocation can occur. The towel can be moved to expose sections of the bird as the examination progresses. When dealing with small cage birds (canaries, budgerigars; Figure 5.28), it is helpful to have one person at the light switch while another puts their hand into the cage. Make note of where the bird is just before the lights are turned off and then grab the bird quickly before it has time to adjust to the darkness.

Restraint time needs to be kept to a minimum (preferably less than 2 to 4 minutes). Before the bird is caught up, all material needed for diagnostic sample collection, examination, and grooming should be anticipated and in place. During the restraint, it is commonly the responsibility of the holder to monitor the well-being of the bird. When signs of excessive stress appear, including panting, eye closing, weakness, and generally any change from when the bird was initially restrained, the bird should be released and given an opportunity to recover. Speaking to the bird in a soothing voice can help reduce the stress during handling.

Physical Examination

Once the bird has been restrained, the physical examination of the avian patient is not any different than that of any other animal. The examination begins at the head and ends at the vent. Look straight on at the head and beak. Examine for symmetry and normal alignment of the beak, check for swelling or bruising, pitting on surface of beak, or fractures (Harrison & Ritchie 1994). Look at the nares (nostrils) to note symmetry and any discharge, debris, or blood. Since most birds have feathers near the nares, matting of the feathers above the nares will occur with a discharge. Note: It is normal for a structure to be present just inside the nares: it is called the operculum (Figure 5.29). Disturbing this structure can cause bleeding.

The eyes are also checked for discharge (again the matting of feathers will be present), lens opacity, blood, or disruption of normal anatomy. Hydration can be assessed using ocular parameters, such as tenting of eyelid skin, moisture of the cornea (dull appearance when dehydrated), and the position of the globe (will be recessed when dehydrated). Hydration can also be assessed by evaluating cutaneous ulnar vein refill time (it should refill instantaneously).

Seldom is there disease in the ears of birds, but they should be examined. There is no external pinna and the ears are located caudal and ventral to the lateral canthus of the eye. By moving the feathers, the ears may be observed (Figure 5.30).

The oral cavity and choanal slit can be viewed with the help of an avian speculum. The choanal slit is the V-shaped opening on the roof of the mouth. Care must be taken when using a speculum, to prevent iatrogenic trauma to the beak (Figure 5.31 A,B).

A normal choanal slit is lined with papillae (pointed projections). Lack of vitamin A can cause the papillae to become blunted or to disappear completely in severe cases.

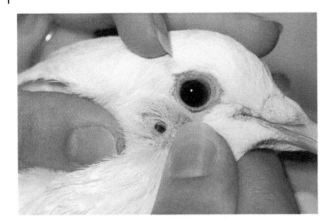

Figure 5.30 Birds do not have an external ear pinna. The ears are located caudal and ventral to the lateral canthus of the eye. By moving the feathers cranially the ears may be observed, as is shown on this white Carneaux pigeon.

The tongue is a prominent feature in the oral cavity. The glottis, which is the opening to the trachea in birds, is at the base of the tongue. The tissue in the oral cavity should be dry and smooth. Abnormal findings can include abscesses, fungal plaques, and excessive moisture. Next, palpate the thoracic inlet. Check the crop for foreign objects, crop burns (in young birds being hand-fed), distention, or crop stasis. Crop stasis can be noted by parting feathers and watching for movement (regular contractions occur in the crop). There should be at least one wave of movement across the crop per minute.

Palpating the pectoral muscles can determine the body condition of the avian patient (Figure 5.32). A score of 1 to 5, or 1 to 9, is used, where 1 signifies a very emaciated animal, 3 is normal, and 5 is considered to be overweight, or 9 is considered obese and 5 is normal if using the 1–9 scale.

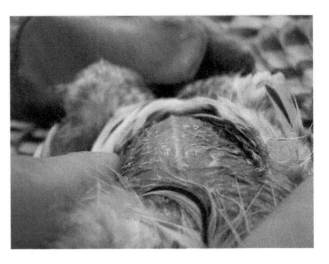

Figure 5.32 A cooper's hawk restrained with gloves in dorsal recumbency showing normal pectoral muscle mass on either side of the bony keel forming a slight V-shape. This view is from the head of the bird looking caudally. Less pectoral muscle mass and a more prominent keel would have suggested a thin bird.

Normally, the edge of the keel can be palpated between the rounded pectoral muscles that slope slightly on either side. The feathers should be examined over the body. Feathers should have a bright iridescent appearance. Wings and legs should be gently flexed and extended to evaluate joint function. Check the plantar surface of the feet. Erosion of the bottom of the feet may be associated with a diet deficient in vitamin A and/or improper perches. Erosions can lead to ulcerative dermatitis, commonly known as bumblefoot (Figure 5.33).

Also look for necrotic areas, swelling, abscesses, or gout (which is an accumulation of white uric acid under the skin). Examine the cloaca (vent), looking for masses,

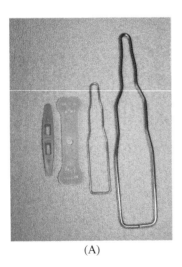

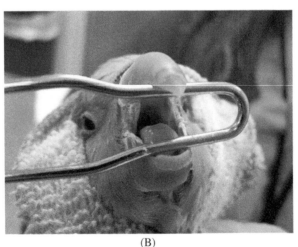

(A)   (B)

Figure 5.31 (A) A variety of specula are available. (B) Care must be taken when using any speculum in a bird since beak damage can occur.

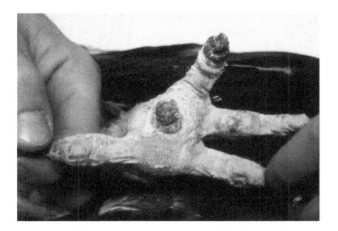

Figure 5.33 Plantar surface of a raptor foot demonstrating ulcerative pododermatitis, also known as bumblefoot. This lesion can start as a smooth, pink, erosive, or flattened area on the plantar surface of the foot. In psittacine birds, this can be due to poor-quality perches or vitamin A deficiency.

irritation (hyperemia), prolapse of the tissue, and the presence of matted fecal material (the feathers around the vent should be clean).

The caudal coelomic cavity can be palpated. Due to the sternum extending over most of the coelomic cavity, organs cannot be easily palpated; however, a large liver or the presence of an egg can be palpated and should be considered abnormal findings. Normally, the liver does not extend past the level of the sternum. At the extreme caudal dorsal surface, the uropygial gland (preen gland) can be found and should be examined for symmetry and overall appearance. Remember, not all birds kept as pets have a uropygial gland.

The bird should be auscultated to assess heart health and respiratory condition. Using a pediatric stethoscope placed over the cranioventral body wall will allow auscultation of the heart. Auscultating over the craniodorsal body wall is best to assess the respirations. Hydration can be assessed with a "vein refill time" using the basilic (cutaneous ulnar) vein (Figure 5.34). In a normally hydrated bird, this vein should instantaneously refill and, by the time a finger is lifted off the vein to see it, it should have refilled. If the basilic vein can be seen refilling then it is estimated that the bird is about 5% dehydrated. If the vein requires one second to refill, the bird is severely dehydrated (10%) or is in shock (low blood pressure). Dehydration can also be associated with tacky oral mucous membranes or decreased eyelid turgor.

At the end of the examination, before the bird is placed back into the carrier, it should be weighed. A digital gram scale should be used that has a maximum weight of 4 to 5 kilograms and should weigh in 1-g increments (Figure 5.35).

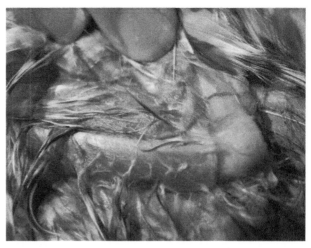

Figure 5.34 Elbow area of a bird showing the cutaneous ulnar (basilic) vein crossing superficial to the proximal ulna. This vein is used to determine hydration status in a bird, and used for phlebotomy and for IV injections.

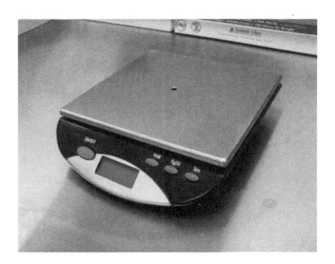

Figure 5.35 A digital gram scale should be used to accurately determine the weight of birds. The scale should be able to weigh in 1-g increments.

Common Diseases

Infectious Diseases

Avian Chlamydiosis

Avian chlamydiosis is one name given the disease in birds caused by the organism *Chlamydia psittaci* (formerly known as *Chlamydophila psittaci*); other names include ornithosis, chlamydiosis, and chlamydophilosis. The term "psittacosis" refers to the disease in humans originating from a parrot (a psittacine bird), whereas the term ornithosis refers to the disease in humans originating from any species of bird. Note that *Chlamydia psittaci* should not be confused with a related organism in people, *Chlamydia trachomatis*, a sexually transmitted disease of humans or another related organism, *Chlamydia pneumoniae*, a common respiratory pathogen of people.

The organism has been found in over 130 species of birds worldwide and a variety of mammals, including humans, and is therefore a zoonotic disease. There are numerous potential avian species that may act as a source of infection for humans. The most common source of infection (70% of all cases in the 1980s) is exposure to a recently acquired psittacine bird. Other birds can be a potential source of infection, such as domestic or wild pigeons, passerines (soft-billed birds), or poultry. People at occupational risk include pet store employees, veterinarians, veterinary technicians, laboratory workers, workers in avian quarantine stations, farmers, wildlife rehabilitators, zoo workers, and employees of poultry slaughtering and processing plants (usually turkey). Occasionally, exposure to wild pigeon roosts is a source of infection to the general public.

The *Chlamydia psittaci* organism is transmitted by either inhalation or ingestion of the spore-like elementary body phase of the organism. Shedding in birds can be activated by stress, such as shipping, crowding, chilling, and breeding. Person-to-person transmission has been suggested by one study (Zhang et al. 2022). Individuals who are immunosuppressed are more susceptible to the disease and its effects. The organism *Chlamydia psittaci* is relatively resistant, surviving in the soil for 3 months or within a bird dropping for up to 1 month.

Clinical signs can differ based on the species of bird. Some birds present quite ill, whereas others exhibit very subtle signs of disease. Generally, the parrot with psittacosis presents with depression, lethargy, anorexia, dyspnea, nasal or ocular discharge, conjunctivitis, and biliverdinuria (green urates). Rarely, birds present comatose, which has been observed in sensitive species such as macaws. Commonly, both the spleen and liver are enlarged. Pigeons and passerines seem to exhibit little if any clinical signs of disease while infected with the *Chlamydia psittaci* organism and therefore are sometimes referred to as asymptomatic carriers of the disease.

A *suggestive* diagnosis can be made by radiographic evidence of splenomegaly, hepatomegaly, and air sacculitis, and a complete blood count (CBC) showing heterophilic, monocytic, leukocytosis, and mild non-regenerative anemia. A plasma electrophoresis may indicate either acute or chronic disease.

A *definitive* diagnosis requires various diagnostic tests, sometimes in combination. There are tests to detect antibodies in the serum (elementary body assay [EBA] and immunofluorescent antibody [IFA]) and tests to detect antigen in the feces or blood (enzyme-linked immunofluorescent antibody assay [ELISA] and polymerase chain reaction [PCR]). It is best to perform a panel of three tests including PCR of blood, PCR of feces, and IFA of serum. Also, a fluorescent antibody (FA) test can be performed on tissue such as liver tissue from a biopsy or necropsy. For legal purposes, cell culture from the feces is the best test, but the organism does not consistently grow, shedding of the organism in the feces is intermittent, and there is also a risk to laboratory personnel when the organism is grown in the lab. Currently, there is one lab commercially offering culture and that is the Texas Medical Diagnostic Laboratory. Addresses and phone numbers of laboratories that test for *Chlamydia*, and the following definitions that have been accepted by the American Veterinary Medical Association (AVMA) and the Association of Avian Veterinarians can be found in the *Compendium of Measures to Control* Chlamydophila psittaci *(formerly* Chlamydia psittaci*) Infection Among Humans (Psittacosis) and Pet Birds (Avian Chlamydiosis)* (2010) by the National Association of State Public Health Veterinarians (NASPHV) at http://www .nasphv.org/documentsCompendiaPsittacosis.html. There is a 2017 updated version that was published in the Journal of Avian Medicine and Surgery (Balsamo et al. 2017).

Treatment of birds should be supervised by a licensed veterinarian and consists of doxycycline for 45 days. A lower dose is used in macaws to prevent regurgitation. Avian chlamydiosis is usually a reportable disease, but it depends on the state. If a veterinarian diagnoses psittacosis in a bird, then most states require that the case be reported to the state veterinarian or public health department.

Other Bacterial Infections

Bacterial infections in birds can be localized or systemic and can involve any system, but commonly involve the liver, gastrointestinal, or respiratory systems. Usually, Gram-negative organisms are involved, such as *E. coli*, *Klebsiella*, *Enterobacter*, or *Pseudomonas*, but infections involving Gram-positive organisms or anaerobes can occur as well. Treatment is based on culture, sensitivity, and cytologic findings (such as an in-house Gram stain) but usually involves the use of broad-spectrum, bacteriocidal antibiotics, such as enrofloxacin, trimethoprim-sulfa, and cephalosporins. Macaws commonly regurgitate after trimethoprim-sulfa or doxycycline administration.

Canary Pox

Poxviruses are the largest of viruses, and the genus *Avipoxvirus* is found worldwide in over 20 families of birds. There are many species of *Avipoxvirus*, such as psittacine pox, canary pox, pigeon pox, falcon pox, and fowl pox. Each species of pox has varied host specificity, but typically the most severe clinical signs are seen in its natural host.

The virus is transmitted via mosquito or via mechanical means through broken skin. Ten to fourteen days post-infection, birds can show blepharitis, ocular discharge, rhinitis, and conjunctivitis associated with raised papules. Clinical signs can be divided into "dry" pox, which consists of cutaneous papular lesions, and "wet" pox, which consists of mucosal papular lesions of the oropharynx. Occasionally birds may display neurologic signs.

Diagnosis is based on typical clinical signs and histologic findings of dermal, which are intracytoplasmic inclusion bodies (Bollinger bodies). Treatment consists of providing supportive care. Prevention consists of using a canary pox vaccine (Poximune® C, Biommune, Ceva Animal Health, Lenexa, KS).

Polyomavirus

Polyomaviruses are rather host-specific and cause sub-clinical disease in mammals but can cause severe clinical disease in a wide variety of psittacine and other species of bird. Immature psittacine birds commonly present with acute disease with an approximate mortality rate of 27 to 41%, and includes 12 to 48 hours of depression, anorexia, delayed crop emptying, regurgitation, diarrhea, dehydration, subcutaneous hemorrhage, dyspnea, and polyuria. The subcutaneous hemorrhages are most easily seen over the crop, carpi, or cranium. Transmission of polyomavirus is through exposure to excretions and secretions, especially urine. Since it is a non-enveloped virus, it is very stable in the environment and difficult to destroy. A DNA probe (PCR) test is available to detect viral DNA in tissue or feces. Antibody tests are available and a positive denotes that exposure has occurred and that the bird probably sheds virus intermittently. Many birds in aviaries are subclinically affected, are a constant source of infection for all birds in the aviary, and are a particular danger for young birds. Therefore, all birds should be vaccinated. There is a commercially available, licensed vaccine for use in psittacine birds (Psittiumune APV, Huvepharma, Lincoln, and NE). It is an inactivated vaccine; therefore, optimum protection occurs 2 weeks after the second dose of vaccine. There is no treatment for the disease. The prognosis in a young bird is grave if clinical signs are present.

Proventricular Dilation Disease

An organism has been found associated with this disease, a Bornavirus. The route of transmission is via fecal–oral and appears to affect birds of many orders, including psittacine birds (Figure 5.36 A,B). Clinical signs include severe, chronic weight loss, regurgitation, delayed crop emptying, ravenous appetite, undigested food in stool, and neurologic signs (i.e., falling off perch) in an adult bird. The

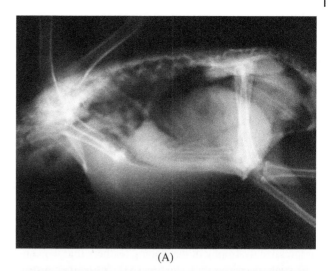

(A)

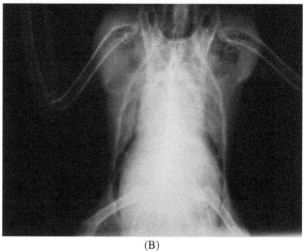

(B)

Figure 5.36 (A, B) A parrot with proventricular dilation disease (PDD), caused by a virus that can paralyze the nerves of the proventriculus. Suggestive diagnostic testing includes radiographs (lateral and ventrodorsal) demonstrating proventricular dilation.

virus paralyzes the nerves in the proventriculus and other areas, and the bird essentially starves to death despite a good appetite, due to the inability to process its food. Suggestive diagnostic testing includes radiographs demonstrating proventricular dilation and whole undigested food particles or seeds in the feces. Note that many diseases can cause proventricular dilation including disease from parasites, yeast, avian gastric yeast, *Mycobacterium*, foreign bodies, neoplasia, and lead and zinc toxicosis. Definitive diagnostic testing includes a crop biopsy demonstrating lymphoplasmocytic ganglioneuritis. Birds usually die within 2 years of developing clinical signs, but treatment can be attempted with the NSAID celecoxib (Celebrex®, a COX-2 inhibitor). The mechanism against the virus using the NSAID is unknown but is thought to decrease an autoimmune inflammation. Prevention currently consists of avoiding exposure to known infected birds.

Psittacine Beak and Feather Disease

This now rare disease of captive parrots in the United States is caused by a circovirus. The disease is now a problem in wild parrots of Australia. The Psittacine Beak and Feather Disease (PBFD) virus is shed in feces, feather dander, and various excretions and secretions. Asymptomatic birds can shed the virus for years before exhibiting any clinical signs. Because the virus is non-enveloped, it is very stable and can survive years in the environment and is resistant to destruction by common disinfectants. Most birds present with chronic PBFD characterized by symmetrical, slowly progressive dystrophy of developing feathers that worsens with each successive molt (Figure 5.37). The feather dystrophy includes retained feather sheaths, hemorrhage within the pulp, curled feathers, and circumferential constrictions of the feather shaft. Birds can go on to develop complete alopecia and sometimes beak abnormalities consisting of progressive elongation of the beak and necrosis of the palate rostrally, near the upper beak. These birds are often immunocompromised and die of secondary bacterial or fungal infections.

Diagnosis is based on PCR tests performed on whole blood. Alternatively, a feather follicle biopsy and DNA in situ hybridization can be performed in addition to the PCR blood test. Treatment consists of supportive care and antimicrobials for secondary infections. Once clinical signs develop, the disease is always fatal.

Papillomatosis Caused by Psittacine Herpesvirus 3

Papillomatosis, or wart-like gastrointestinal/cloacal lesions caused by a herpesvirus, should not be confused with facial warts caused by papillomavirus. Species most commonly

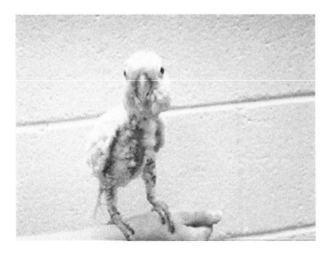

Figure 5.37 Bird with psittacine beak and feather disease (PBFD).

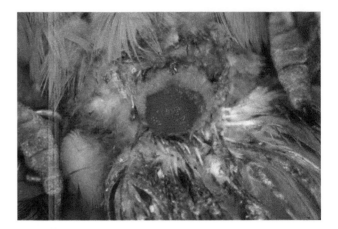

Figure 5.38 Clinical signs of papillomatosis (caused by a herpes virus) include wart-like masses observed anywhere along the gastrointestinal tract, but most commonly in the cloaca, as seen in this Amazon parrot, and oropharynx.

affected include the Amazon parrots and macaws. Amazon parrots are prone to developing concomitant bile duct adenocarcinoma that has recently been associated with Psittacid herpesvirus (PHV-1), genotype 3.

Clinical signs of papillomatosis include wart-like masses observed anywhere along the gastrointestinal tract, but most commonly in the cloaca (Figure 5.38) and oropharynx.

Birds may exhibit weight loss, signs of straining to defecate, soiled vent, or blood in stool. Some cases have a gastrointestinal obstruction with associated clinical signs. Because the virus is latent, birds that have been previously treated may have recurrence of lesions and signs with stress. Amazon parrots need to be checked for concomitant bile duct carcinoma due to this virus. They may exhibit biliverdinuria and lethargy, and bile acid levels may be high. Diagnosis is suggestive based on gross appearance and location. Definitive diagnosis is based on histology. Treatment involves removing the wart-like growth. In the author's experience, it is best to apply silver nitrate to the lesion, or half the lesion if it is circumferentially involving the cloaca, and deactivate the chemical burning one minute after application. This treatment is repeated every week under anesthesia until gone. Butorphanol is also administered at 1 to 2 mg/kg IM once before the procedure.

West Nile Virus

West Nile virus disease is caused by a flavivirus. West Nile virus is endemic in many countries, and in the late 1990s, it was found within the eastern United States and has since spread across the United States. Crows, jays, raptors, and horses are susceptible species, whereas poultry are considered resistant. The virus is spread by mosquitoes. If people or dogs are affected, they are usually older or immunosuppressed. Clinical signs range from none in resistant species such as poultry to neurologic signs (ataxia, circling, head tilt, and seizures) and death in susceptible species. A CBC is usually normal or a lymphocytosis is present. A serum antibody test is available. Treatment consists of supportive care. In humans, the use of alpha interferon has seemed to result in better success. A licensed vaccine is available for use in horses that is currently being used extra-label in birds at the same or a reduced dose rate.

Avian Influenza

Avian influenza is caused by a type A influenza virus and affects many species of birds (Fulton 2021). Since influenza viruses so easily mutate there is concern that someday this virus could acquire the ability to spread from human to human rather than just from bird to human. There are low pathogenic forms (LPAI) and highly pathogenic forms (HPAI). Clinical signs of LPAI include anorexia, decreased egg production, and mild respiratory disease. Clinical signs of HPAI may include respiratory distress, facial swelling, subcutaneous bruising, diarrhea, and neurological signs, but often times, it is associated with sudden high mortality with few clinical signs. HPAI is a highly contagious, reportable disease in the United States.

Until recently, HPAI was only sporadically seen in the United States, but since 2022, there has been a Eurasian HPAI that is spreading via migration routes in wild waterfowl and other birds and HPAI is now being seen more frequently in wild birds, commercial poultry flocks, and backyard flocks. If a high mortality rate is seen in any type of bird, contact your state veterinarian immediately. They will want to know sooner rather than later and they can help determine if the cause is HPAI or not. State diagnostic laboratories are accredited to conduct screening testing for HPAI. Backyard poultry owners can work with the National Poultry Improvement Plan (NPIP) in their state to become certified as an AI-negative flock. Currently, there is no vaccine available in the United States, but one is being developed and may be available in the future. Depopulation is the only control currently in the United States for this highly contagious disease, and the sooner and quicker this is done, the less likely the disease is to spread and cause further deaths.

Fungal Diseases

Aspergillosis

The two most common etiologic agents associated with aspergillosis in birds are *Aspergillus flavus* and *A. fumigatus*. Predisposing factors associated with the disease are immunosuppression, including hypovitaminosis A, and being exposed to and inhaling massive quantities of fungal spores, which can easily occur when corn cob, wheat, or pine straw is used as bedding or substrate. Aspergillosis is more common in African grey parrots, macaws, and raptors. The location of the infection is most commonly at the bifurcation of the trachea near the syrinx or in the caudal thoracic air sac, and occasionally the sinuses. A suggestive diagnosis is based on a very elevated CBC (above 40,000 usually), with a heterophilic leukocytosis and monocytosis. Tests for serum antigen, antibody, galactomannan, and gliotoxin are available but are just suggestive of the disease. A definitive diagnosis is usually obtained by direct visualization and sampling via endoscopy of either the trachea or the air sac, and cytology or culture of those samples. Treatment consists of antifungals such as conazoles, including ketaconazole, itraconazole, and fluconazole. Itraconazole is the best but should not be used in African grey parrots (or only used at very low doses). Also, amphotericin-B can be used, but can only be given intravenously, topically, or through nebulization; it is quickly renal-toxic. Months of treatment are necessary, so early and proper diagnosis is imperative. Any underlying cause of immunosuppression or overexposure to fungal spores should also be corrected.

Candidiasis

Candidiasis is caused by the yeast organism *Candida albicans*, or the recently identified, difficult to treat, *Candida glabrata*. Clinical signs include regurgitation, delayed crop emptying, and white plaques in the oral cavity. The crop is the most common organ affected and the crop contents will have a yeasty, sweet smell. Young birds or neonates are the most severely affected. If adults have clinical signs of candidiasis, then look for some cause of immunosuppression. Diagnosis is easily done by identifying the organism on a Gram stain of crop or fecal material. Treatment of mild cases consists of antifungal therapy with oral nystatin, which acts topically in the gastrointestinal tract. If the candidiasis is severe and invading the mucosa then, in addition to nystatin, a systemic antifungal such as one of the conazoles is necessary to attack the infection from the vascular system as well as topically.

Non-infectious Diseases

Heavy Metal Toxicosis

Heavy metal toxicosis is usually caused by ingestion of lead or zinc. Sources of lead include fishing weights, curtain weights, bullets, paint, and costume jewelry. Sources of zinc include pennies minted after 1982, Monopoly® game pieces, powder coating, paint, and costume jewelry. The ventriculus (gizzard) of birds retains heavy particles for grinding food, but in the case of heavy metal particles,

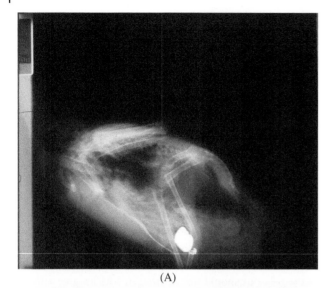

(A)

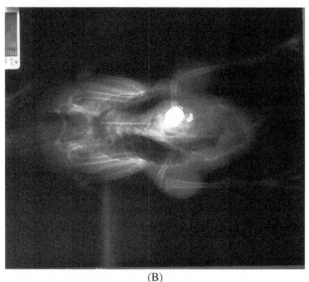

(B)

Figure 5.39 (A) Lateral standing radiograph in a duck showing heavy metal in the ventriculus. Later 97 cents worth of various coins were removed endoscopically. (B) Ventrodorsal view of the same duck. This particular radiograph was taken awake and standing since perfect positioning was not required to just confirm the presence of heavy metal.

they are retained and slowly digested allowing constant absorption of the toxins. Clinical signs include depression, weakness, regurgitation, and sometimes neurologic signs. Diagnosis is usually made by visualizing the metal-dense particles on radiographs (Figure 5.39 A, B), but a definitive diagnosis can be made on only 0.2 mL of blood for lead, or 0.2 mL of serum for zinc at the Louisiana Veterinary Medical Diagnostic Laboratory or with an in-house lead analyzer.

Toxic levels of lead in the blood are greater than 0.2 ppm, and for serum zinc, greater than 2.0 ppm. Treatment consists of a chelating agent such as injectable CaEDTA,

dimercaptosuccinic acid (DMSA), or d-penicillamine to bind with the heavy metal rendering it harmless, which then can be urinated out of the body. Note that CaEDTA does not cross the blood–brain barrier and is not as useful once neurological signs are evident. Stressful procedures such as surgery or endoscopy to remove a large particle should be done after some chelation therapy since stress can cause lead to move suddenly from the bone where it is stored to the blood and worsen the clinical signs. Other products such as lactulose to assist the liver with toxicosis, or lubricants such as corn oil or peanut butter, or bulking agents such as psyllium, can also be given.

Hypovitaminosis A

A diet deficient in vitamin A, such as an all-seed diet, can lead to hypovitaminosis A. Clinical signs include choanal papillae in the oral cavity that are blunted, plantar erosions on the feet, and poor-quality skin and feathers (darkened areas on the feathers of the wings). A diagnosis is made based on history and clinical signs. Secondary bacterial or fungal infections involving the respiratory tract are common. Sometimes a Gram stain of a choanal swab will show increased epithelial cells and basophilic staining. Treatment includes an increase in dietary vitamin A by providing the bird with dark yellow vegetables (sweet potato, carrot, and commercial bird pellets). One injection of vitamin A could be given, but one should avoid giving too much vitamin A as it is a fat-soluble vitamin that can result in hypervitaminosis A.

Hypocalcemia of African Grey Parrots

Adult African grey parrots, especially those on a low-calcium seed diet, rather than a healthy pelleted diet, can present with seizures due to hypocalcemia. An ionized calcium will diagnose the disease. Treatment consists of intramuscular calcium gluconate. Later, oral calcium can be administered in the form of calcium glubionate. Of course, treatment also includes improving the diet by supplementing with calcium, usually with calcium carbonate, and slowly changing to a pelleted diet.

Non-stick Cookware Toxicosis

Non-stick cookware, such as Teflon®, is made with poly-tetrafluoroethylene (PTFE). If burned and heated to over 540°F, the PTFE fumes are released which causes immediate pulmonary hemorrhage and death in birds anywhere in the household. Rarely, immediately supplied fresh air and steroids will prevent death.

Egg Binding

Some birds, such as cockatiels, can chronically lay eggs. Birds on an all-seed diet that is low in calcium can present with egg binding. The egg is basically stuck in the uterus because the uterine muscles lack enough calcium to contract and push the egg out. In this position, the egg puts pressure on the kidneys, causing the bird to go into shock, and the bird can die within hours to days without removal or implosion of the egg. Other birds may have dystocia due to an abnormally large egg, blockage, or partial blockage along the path of the egg. If the egg is of normal size and there are no obstructions such as scarring of the uterus, then hormones, such as oxytocin or prostaglandin F2 alpha, can be given to stimulate contractions, but only after calcium has been administered IM and has had time to be absorbed so the uterine muscles have enough calcium to contract. If the egg cannot be laid with medical management, then it can be imploded by creating negative pressure within the egg by suctioning out the contents with a needle and syringe placed either through the egg exposed at the cloaca or through the coelomic wall and uterus on the ventral coelom. This is an emergency procedure, called ovocentesis, and is performed under anesthesia; it is not without risk of hemorrhage or infection. If these procedures are unsuccessful, then surgery to perform a salpingohysterectomy (removal of uterus) can be performed. Supportive care, fluids, antibiotics, pain relievers, anti-inflammatories, etc., are also necessary.

Crop Burns

Juvenile birds being hand-fed by humans may sometimes be offered gruel that is too hot (>105°F), usually heated in a microwave, which causes a burn of the thin crop and overlying skin. It is not until 10 days later usually that the effects of the burn are noticed with the sudden appearance of gruel pouring out of a hole in the crop and running down the breast of the bird. It is only at this ten-day point, after a scab has formed, and the body has been determined dead from healthy tissue, that surgery should be performed to close the hole. Supportive care, including antibiotics or the mild antifungal, nystatin, and fluids, etc., is usually needed.

Radiology

Radiographs can be taken awake or under anesthesia depending on goals. Usually, the bird is under anesthesia so that the bird is absolutely still and in the proper position for accurate evaluation, and producing the least amount of stress. A bird can be placed in a cardboard box awake to determine if an egg is present, or if metal is present. In the case of a barium series, this can also be done awake or under anesthesia to see the location and speed of barium travel. Most radiographs are taken at 500 mAs and 50 kVp for 1/120 of a second, but each machine is different. Two views are taken, the ventrodorsal with the keel of the sternum perfectly aligned with the spine (Figure 5.40), and the lateral, with the coxofemoral joints and shoulder

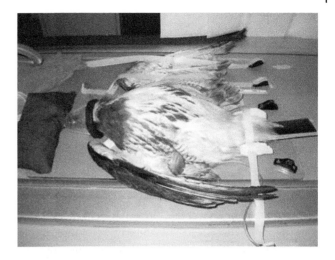

Figure 5.40 A red-tailed hawk properly positioned for a ventrodorsal radiograph.

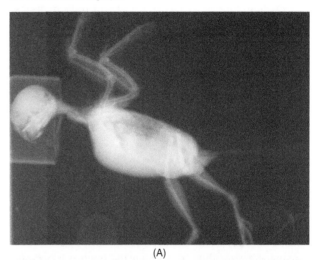

(A)

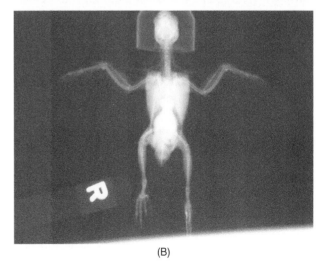

(B)

Figure 5.41 (A) An example of a parrot well positioned for a lateral radiograph. Note how the shoulder joint is aligned, but how the femoral heads could be better aligned. (B) An example of a parrot well positioned for a ventrodorsal radiograph. Note how the keel and spine are aligned (superimposed).

joints superimposed (McMillan 1994; Figure 5.41A,B). This positioning allows evaluation of the radiographs.

Anesthesia and Analgesia

Isoflurane and sevoflurane are the safest gas anesthetics available for birds (Curro et al. 1994). Sevoflurane has been shown to be just as effective and recovery is slightly faster than with isoflurane (Quandt & Greenacre 1999). Birds are usually restrained in a towel in a standing position so they are most comfortable. Healthy birds are mask induced starting at about 2%, at 2 L/mins oxygen flow rate. For short procedures such as immobilization for radiographs that require less than 15 minutes, most birds are not intubated. For longer procedures, birds can be intubated with an uncuffed endotracheal tube. Once intubated, the oxygen flow rate must be reduced to 1 L/min or less so as not to damage the delicate air sacs. The best method to secure an endotracheal tube in a bird is to tape it to the bottom beak so the mouth can be opened to wipe out excess wetness if necessary. The head and glottis should always be kept above the level of the crop, since liquid from the crop can enter the trachea, resulting in aspiration pneumonia or drowning of the bird. Since birds have complete tracheal rings, an inflated cuffed tube can exert too much pressure on the lumen of the trachea that cannot expand; this can cause pressure necrosis and a subsequent diphtheritic membrane. Also, it is important to realize that birds, especially cockatoos, have a trachea that narrows a few centimeters past the glottis, causing an endotracheal tube to initially seem the appropriate size but then after passing it a very short way down the trachea it becomes lodged, causing pressure necrosis (often not clinical until weeks later). Therefore, pick an appropriate-sized tube and reintubate if it feels to be lodged. Also, do not force the tube or place it further than needed. It is very easy to intubate a parrot because the glottis is very rostral at the base of the tongue.

Birds generally do not do well after one hour of anesthesia due to hypothermia, hypoventilation, and respiratory acidosis. The use of forced heated air blankets has greatly improved the attempted maintenance of normal body temperature (~105°F) in birds under anesthesia (Rembert et al. 2001). It is imperative that adequate lubrication is applied to the eyes to prevent dry eye with forced heated air blankets. Also, the laterally placed eye of birds should not be allowed to rest on any surface or the anterior chamber can collapse, which is usually temporary, but may be a permanent condition.

Common monitoring equipment includes constantly watching the respirations, using a stethoscope, pulse

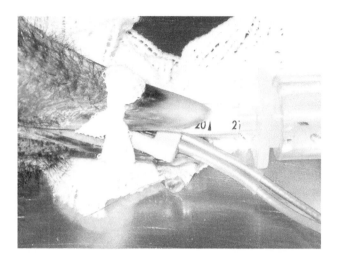

Figure 5.42 A wild turkey intubated and under anesthesia, showing the placement of a Doppler probe on the roof of the mouth over the palatine artery to monitor heart rate. This can be performed on any species of bird.

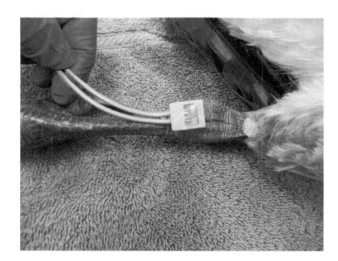

Figure 5.43 A wild Canada goose intubated and under anesthesia showing the placement of a Doppler probe on the medial metatarsal artery on the anterior surface of the hock. This can be taped in place and can be performed in any species of bird.

oximeter on the toe or leg (Figure 5.43, Doppler probe (Figure 5.46) over the radial artery (Figure 5.45) or palatine artery (Figures 5.42 and 5.44), end-tidal CO_2 with respiratory monitor, and ECG.

Simply listening with a stethoscope and CONSTANTLY watching the respiratory rate and depth are the absolute minimum in monitoring birds under anesthesia.

When assessing an avian patient for signs of pain, or deciding on which pain reliever to use, or what dose and how often to administer, it must be taken into account that there is NO GENERIC PARROT, and one must be familiar with the very limited scientific research that has

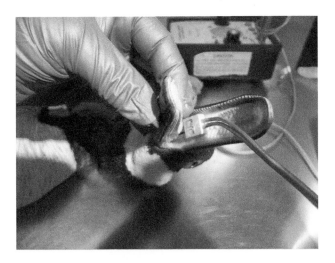

Figure 5.44 A wild Canada goose under anesthesia showing the placement of a Doppler probe on the roof of the mouth over the palatine artery in order to monitor heart rate. This is then secured with tape around the upper beak. This can be performed in many of the larger species of birds.

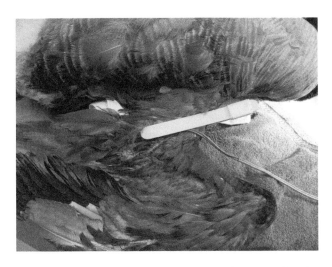

Figure 5.45 A wild Canada goose under anesthesia showing the placement of a Doppler probe on the radial artery in order to monitor heart rate. It is secured with two tongue depressors taped together to form a clothespin-type apparatus. This can be performed in any species of bird.

Table 5.4 Analgesic doses for psittacine birds

Drug	Dosage
Lidocaine	1 mg/kg at site, dilute 1:10; 4 mg/kg or higher is toxic
Butorphanol	0.5–2.0 mg/kg IM (1–2 mg/kg IM every 2–4 h as needed)
Carprofen	1–10 mg/kg IM/PO (most use 2 mg/kg)
Celecoxib	10 mg/kg PO (used for proventricular dilatation disease)
Meloxicam	0.1–1.0 mg/kg IM/PO (0.5 mg/kg)

Guzman et al. 2022; Crespo & Petritz 2022.

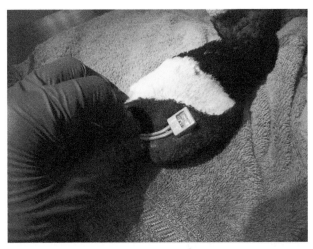

Figure 5.46 A wild Canada goose under anesthesia showing the placement of a Doppler probe on the cornea (with plenty of eye lube) in order to monitor heart rate. This can be performed in any species of bird.

been conducted regarding pain management in psittacine birds (Table 5.4). Also, each patient must be evaluated and reevaluated individually and constantly. Unlike mammals, birds have more kappa than mu opiate receptors; therefore, a partial agonist/antagonist such as butorphanol has been shown to provide pain relief, but at much higher than mammalian doses at 1 to 2 mg/kg IM (Paul-Murphy et al. 1999). Buprenorphine has not been shown to work as well (Paul-Murphy et al. 2004).

It is very difficult to assess pain in birds and there are no standard methods or assessments available to assess the level of pain in birds. Therefore, one is left with past experience, observation, and anthropomorphism (if I had a fractured bone I would want an opiate). Birds are very stoic and do not cry out in pain despite the fact that they can be very loud when they want to be. Birds have a flock mentality, meaning that they are a prey species, and if they make their illness conspicuous to the rest of the flock, they risk being ostracized by the rest of the flock (so as not to attract the attentions of a predator). It is best to observe the patient before they are aware of someone observing them. When they realize someone is there, it is likely you will observe them straightening up, opening their eyelids more and they may even turn to partially face the observer in an attempt to look alert.

Birds do not seem to become profoundly depressed on opioid analgesics; therefore, the author tends to give analgesics at any hint of pain in a bird. In most cases, an opiate will be given prior to surgery, then both an opiate (butorphanol) and an anti-inflammatory (meloxicam) after surgery and during the first 6 to 48 hours, and then use only the anti-inflammatory for about 3 to 5 days post-surgery. It is necessary to constantly reassess the level of pain in birds. A pain scale has yet to be developed for birds, so observe for normal behaviors or lack thereof.

Surgery

There is a wonderful chapter on general principles of surgery, instruments, and equipment in the new surgery book edited by Drs. Bennett and Pye that is a great overview of this subject. Remember it is best to use analgesics before pain occurs, to prevent "wind up." Butorphanol is the most commonly used opioid in birds (see above) (Bennett 2022).

Preparation of the skin is similar as in mammals with three applications in succession of chlorhexidine scrub or iodine scrub and either alcohol or sterile saline, but there are some differences, including the use of sterile saline or very sparing amounts of alcohol, patting the skin rather than rubbing so as not to cause subcutaneous petechial hemorrhaging, and plucking of feathers under anesthesia before preparing the skin. Birds can become excessively cold when using alcohol. Plucking feathers is very painful and usually requires a surgical plane of anesthesia and should be done one feather at a time, pulling in the direction in which they grow. Clear, see-through drapes are a necessity for the anesthetist to be able to assess breathing in the patient. Sterile adhesive surgical drapes or sterile clear plastic wrap can be used. A radiosurgical unit is preferable to an electrosurgical unit in birds, especially since the plate does not need to be in direct contact with the bird. Radiosurgical units can be used in monopolar or bipolar modes. There is a special "Harrison tip" which is a bipolar tip used in birds (Figure 5.47).

Ideally, birds should be under anesthesia for less than one hour, so it is essential in avian surgery to have everything possible prepared and ready for use to shorten surgery time. If the coelomic cavity is going to be breached, remember that birds do not have a diaphragm and that anesthetic gases will escape the surgery site, causing the bird's anesthetic depth to lighten. Also, be aware that it will be easier to "bag" a bird or administer intermittent positive pressure ventilation once the air sac is incised. If at any time the bird's breathing cannot be assessed, it is the anesthetist's responsibility to stop the surgeon in order to assess the breathing. Fluids, such as Lactated Ringer's Solution, Plasmalyte, or Normosol-R, are usually administered intravenously at 10 mL/kg/hour for the first hour and then at 5 mL/kg/h thereafter. A bolus of fluids or hydroxyethyl starch may need to be given if blood loss

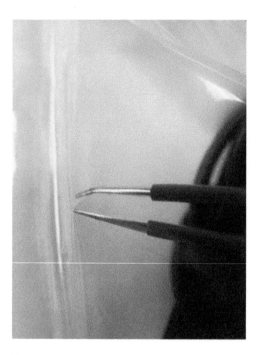

Figure 5.47 Radiosurgical or electrocautery tips used in birds. A bipolar "Harrison tip" is specifically designed for birds, with one bent tip for better access. Do not straighten.

is greater than 10% of the blood volume. Suture used is typically 4/0 to 5/0 PDS.

Common surgeries include accessing the crop for a biopsy to definitively diagnose proventricular dilation disease (PDD), repairing a crop burn in a neonate, or removing a foreign body, or accessing the proventriculus with an endoscope through the crop. Common surgeries requiring coelomic cavity access include salpingohysterectomy (removing the uterus in a bird, not the ovary), liver biopsy (either directly or endoscopically), proventriculotomy to remove a foreign body, or an exploratory laparotomy.

Strictly follow the manufacturer's directions on cleaning, maintaining, and handling endoscopes to ensure long life of this expensive equipment.

Parasitology

Ascaridosis is uncommon now, but the clinical signs are none or diarrhea; rarely, a gastrointestinal impaction can occur. A diagnosis is easily made on fecal flotation. The most used antihelminthics include ivermectin, selamectin, fenbendazole, and piperazine. Giardiasis is caused by the protozoal organism, *Giardia* spp. Clinical signs can be none, or diarrhea, and weight loss. A diagnosis can be made on a fecal Gram stain in severe cases, but the motile protozoa are easier to visualize on a direct saline smear, especially with the addition of iodine. An ELISA for *Giardia* antigen is the best current test. Treatment is with metronidazole.

Trichomoniasis is caused by *Trichomonas* spp. of protozoa and is called "canker" in pigeons and "frounce" in raptors eating pigeons and is associated with white plaques in the oral cavity. Diagnosis is based on demonstration of the protozoal organisms on direct saline smear of the oral cavity. Treatment is metronidazole. *Syngamus* is also known as "gape worm" since the birds gape their mouths open, trying to breathe around the physical presence of the large worm in their trachea. The worms are thick-bodied, dark red, and the male and female join to form a permanent "Y" shape. Gape worm is common in waterfowl and robins and is treatable with parasiticides; some have even used endoscopy to retrieve the worms. *Knemidokoptes pilae*, known as the scaly leg and face mite, causes pitting and scaling of the keratin of the skin and beak of parakeets

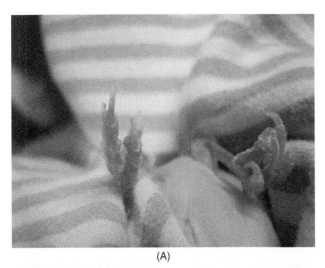

(A)

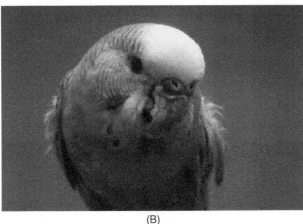

(B)

Figure 5.48 (A) *Knemidokoptes* mite infestation in a canary manifesting as flaking of skin on feet. (B) Deformed beak from *Knemidokoptes* mites.

and other birds, and causes scaling on the legs and feet of canaries and finches (Figure 5.48 A,B).

Although the diagnosis can be made by the typical appearance of the skin and beak, a scraping of the affected area onto a slide with mineral oil will reveal the round-shaped mites. The treatment is *topical* ivermectin, or similar products, given twice, 10 to 14 days apart. Do NOT give ivermectin IM in birds, especially small birds, because they can die from an anaphylactic reaction presumably from the propylene glycol in the product.

Gender Determination

Most parrots do not exhibit obvious signs of sexual dimorphism. The gonads in both male and female are internal. If a client wishes to know the gender of their pet bird, a blood test should be recommended. This involves taking a small amount (0.2 mL) of blood or pulling a feather, which is DNA checked for chromosomes. There are several companies that offer this test. Surgical sexing by visualizing the gonads directly endoscopically is typically only offered to owners who plan on breeding their birds or if a reproductive problem is being investigated. With the use of a sterile rigid endoscope, the gonads are visualized. Any abnormalities of the gonads or other structures can then be identified. This of course carries the low risk of anesthetic complications, hemorrhage, and infection.

Grooming (Beak, Nail, and Wing Trims)

Nails

Often when a bird presents for a nail trim, the nail is not overgrown but the points have begun to traumatize the skin of the owner's arm. Using a stone tip on a roto-tool or an emery board will quickly round and dull the points. If nails are overgrown, a human nail clipper or guillotine-type nail trimmer can be used to take the length back. This should then be followed with the roto-tool or emery board to round off any sharp edges created during clipping the nails (Figure 5.49). If the nail extends in an arc that is more than half a circle, it is probably too long.

The quick will differ in length between individuals. Always have silver nitrate sticks or ferric subsulfate powder available to stop hemorrhage if it occurs.

Beak

Knowing the normal beak shape and length for various species is a must before any trimming takes place (Figure 5.50). Some species of parrots possess a longer beak

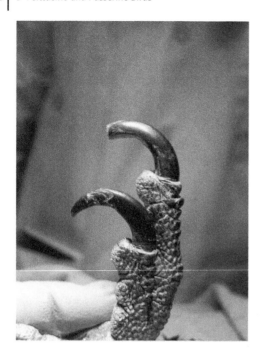

Figure 5.49 A clipped and unclipped nail.

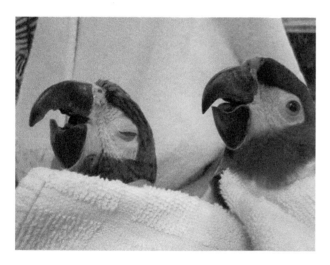

Figure 5.50 Most birds do not need their beak trimmed. The Severe macaw on the right has a normal beak, while its clutch mate on the left has an abnormal, thickened beak.

than others (compare a macaw to an Amazon parrot). Beak trims can be performed when the bird is awake. A roto-tool (larger parrot) or nail file (birds smaller than a cockatiel) can be used. The tip can be blunted. If the bill tip organ becomes visible (as a row of white dots on the occlusal surface of the beak), do not trim further or hemorrhage and pain will occur. The flaking on the external surface of the beak can be removed with the roto-tool/nail file. When using the power tool, be sure to never stop moving, using long, gentle strokes to avoid going too deep and cutting into

bone. The beak is a bony structure covered with keratin. Some individual parrots maintain their beak length and never need a trim. A bird with a maloccluded beak will need corrective trimming on a regular schedule. Also, a bird with a fast-growing beak that is constantly in need of trimming may have underlying liver disease that needs to be addressed.

Wing

Wing trims are performed in order to help prevent the bird from flying freely (Figure 5.51). Indoors, free-flying birds have encounters with ceiling fans, windows, getting squeezed into doors, and flying out through an open door or window. An ideal wing trim will be performed symmetrically and allow the bird to gently glide to the floor. Too severe a wing trim can cause trauma, most commonly resulting in damage to the keel or incite feather-picking behavior. A correct wing trim depends on the weight of the bird (i.e., obese compared to a normal-weight bird), body type of bird (i.e., heavy-bodied bird compared to an elongated, long-tailed bird), and the number of pin (blood) feathers that are growing in at the time of the trim. Only primary feathers should be trimmed (consisting of the first ten wing feathers counting from the tip). So, depending on the body shape of the bird a wing trim consists of cutting four to ten primary feathers on each side.

If, for example, one were trimming an Amazon parrot, which is a heavy-bodied, short-tailed bird, then approximately 4 or 5 feathers would be trimmed on both wings. A cockatiel, built very differently than an Amazon, most likely will need all ten primary feathers trimmed. To clip the feathers, the wing must be gently extended, incorporating the carpus and propatagial ligament in the hold. This will support the wing if the bird should struggle and help to avoid injury to the wing. Before cutting, check for pin feathers. These are feathers that have not finished growing and still have a blood source. If pin feathers are present, leave a mature feather on either side of the pin feather to protect the growing feather. If several blood feathers are present, it would be best to reschedule the trim when they have finished maturing. The feathers are trimmed just longer than

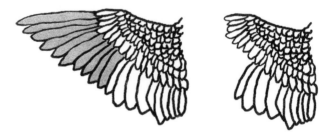

Figure 5.51 Wing trim. (Drawing by Scott Stark).

the tips of the lateral coverts. Care should be taken not to clip the covert feathers as this will leave an unsightly cut line. Sharp scissors should always be used and care should be taken to not cut toes straying into the field of the scissors. Birds with properly trimmed wings will live a safer life indoors. Owners must be made aware that even a bird with properly trimmed wings can fly away. Some owners elect not to have their bird's wings trimmed to allow the bird to exercise. Exercise is good but warn owners of potential dangers such as ceiling fans, doors closing on the bird, open windows and doors, and hot foods cooking on the stove.

Emergency and Critical Care

The causes for a bird to have an emergency visit to the veterinarian are similar to those for mammals but may vary slightly. Examples of cases seen as an emergency include trauma (hit by ceiling fan, toe closed in door, big bird/little bird incidents, dog/cat attack, burns), toxins (lead, zinc, PTFE fumes from Teflon), metabolic disorders (chronic hypovitaminosis A, hypocalcemia in African Grey parrots), or infection (due to bacteria, virus, fungus, or *Chlamydia* usually involving the liver, gastrointestinal or respiratory tract). There is an excellent book available, Exotic Animal Emergency and Critical Care Medicine, that has 18 chapters just on birds and is very thorough with many useful pictures and diagrams (Graham et al. 2021).

Unlike mammals, birds usually present with a terminal manifestation of chronic disease that has just recently shown overt acute signs. Subtle clues of disease have often gone unrecognized by the owner. This is because birds hide signs of disease to avoid being ostracized by the flock, i.e., the flock does not want to be around a bird that is attracting a predator. Common avian emergencies include egg binding (dystocia) due to low total body calcium from a long-term calcium-deficient diet (such as a seed diet) and trauma. The first approach to an emergency should include, if possible, obtaining a history over the phone so as to be as prepared as possible when the bird arrives. Be familiar with common species problems (i.e., for a seizuring African Grey parrot, hypocalcemia would be at the top of the rule-out list). Evaluate the history, cage, husbandry, and droppings and observe the bird for clues as to the etiology before pursuing stressful restraint.

A rapid but thorough physical examination is of most importance. Collection of diagnostic samples (± CBC, profile, radiographs, fecal Gram stain) may need to wait until supportive care makes it so the bird does not die during sampling. Sometimes the bird may be so stressed that the examination may need to be performed in less than one minute or performed in stages. Obtain an accurate

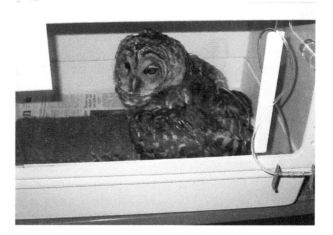

Figure 5.52 A hospitalized barred owl in a heated oxygen cage. The bird is receiving fluids through an intraosseous catheter.

weight with a gram scale so as to administer accurate drug dosing. Provide therapy to stabilize the patient including providing warmth (85–90°F) (Figure 5.52) and place in a stress-free environment (no barking dogs), ± oxygen. Offer familiar/favorite foods and water that are elevated to sit right in front of the bird, provide 10 hours of daylight and 14 hours of dark, and provide a low perch or none at all (birds insist on perching on the highest available perch, even when severely debilitated).

During the examination for an emergent bird, first check to see that the patient has a patent airway. Is the airway patent or is there a mass or foreign body in the trachea? Examples of a mass include an *Aspergillus* granuloma, neoplasia, and diptheritic membrane. Examples of a foreign body include a millet seed in a cockatiel's trachea (this can be directly visualized in the trachea with a semi-rigid 1.1 mm endoscope). Second, check to see if the animal is breathing, and if not then intubate with an uncuffed endotracheal tube, provide intermittent partial pressure ventilation in birds at 1 breath per 5 seconds. Due to the unique respiratory system in birds, an air sac tube (canula) can be placed in caudal thoracic or abdominal air sac and oxygenated air will flow through the lung. An air sac tube can be connected to oxygen or anesthesia and left in place for 5 days. Third, check to see if there is a heartbeat. If a bird experiences cardiac arrest, then the prognosis for reversing this situation is poor to grave due to a bird's high metabolic rate and oxygen demands. The following treatments can be attempted to reinitiate heartbeat: rapid heart massage and ventilation (100 beats per minute and 1 breath/5 seconds), intravenous or intratracheal (IT) epinephrine, atropine (usually used to prevent bradycardia though), doxapram IV or IT (stimulates respirations), bolus IV fluids with ±2.5 to 5% dextrose, and/or hydroxyethyl starch.

Blood Loss

The average blood volume of a bird is approximately 10% of its body weight. For example, a 1.0 kg blue and gold macaw has an average blood volume of about 100 mL. A healthy bird can lose up to 10% of their blood volume (or 1% of body weight) without any adverse side effects. Therefore, a healthy 1.0 kg blue and gold macaw could lose up to 10 mL without any adverse side effects. Unlike mammals, a healthy bird can usually lose up to 30% of its blood volume without dying, due to compensatory mechanisms. In one study, half of healthy mallard ducks lived despite acutely losing 60% of their blood volume (Lichtenberger et al. 2009). Because of these compensatory mechanisms, it is important to realize that the PCV in a bird is not accurate (i.e., not equilibrated) for 24 hours after a hemorrhagic incident because birds can compensate their PCV during blood loss by shunting blood from large skeletal muscle capillary beds and away from the kidneys via the renal portal system to increase blood flow to central areas. Therefore, an equilibrated PCV <15% and an immediate PCV <20% are similar and serious enough to contemplate a blood transfusion. Fluids, hetastarch, oxyglobin (not currently available), or a blood transfusion (5% of body weight) will help a bird with severe blood loss. The anemic patient may require vitamin B complex, iron dextran, and vitamin K_1.

Dehydration

Most sick birds are 5–10% dehydrated. Severe dehydration is usually >10%. Clinical signs of dehydration include depression, reduced skin elasticity over digits or eyelids, sunken eyes, cool digits, and decreased refill time of the basilic (cutaneous ulnar) vein. A general rule of thumb is that a normally hydrated bird will have a basilic vein refill time that is instantaneous, such that when a finger occluding the vein is lifted quickly the vein cannot be seen refilling. If the vein refill can be seen, then the bird is at least 5% dehydrated. If the vein takes 1 second or more to refill, then the bird is over 5% dehydrated.

Maintenance fluids are the same for birds as they are for mammals at 50 mL/kg/day. For example, maintenance fluid calculations for a 500 g Amazon parrot would be 0.5 kg × 50 mL/kg/day = 25 mL/day. Fluid replacement for a 500 g Amazon parrot that is 6% dehydrated would be calculated as follows: dehydration replacement in liters is body weight (in kg) × % dehydration (expressed as a decimal amount), 0.5 kg × 0.06 = 0.030 L = 30 mL. The calculated dose for dehydration replacement (30 mL) should be administered over a 48-hour period. For example, the schedule for administration of maintenance and dehydration fluids given to the above bird in 48 hours would be as follows: day 1: 25 mL for maintenance + 15 mL for half

the dehydration replacement = 40 mL; day 2: 25 mL for maintenance + 15 mL for the second half of dehydration replacement = 40 mL. Fluid therapy is a critical component of emergency therapy. The most commonly used fluids are Lactated Ringer's Solution or Normosol-R since they most closely resemble the fluid lost. WARM FLUIDS (about 100°F) are imperative, realizing that the body temperature of most birds is 104–109°F. Sometimes 2.5% dextrose is added to the subcutaneous or intravenous fluids. Mild dehydration may only require conservative management such as oral or subcutaneous fluids. Subcutaneous fluids are generally administered into the inguinal area in birds. Severe dehydration or shock requires rapid circulatory expansion with intravenous or intraosseous fluids since oral or subcutaneous fluids are inadequate in these cases due to lack of absorption at the administration site. Peripheral indwelling catheters have been avoided in birds since they have small, fragile veins that easily form hematomas, their dermis is highly mobile causing difficulties in stabilizing the catheter, and they have refractory temperaments and a powerful beak. Repeated intravenous bolusing can be attempted, but it is stressful to the birds to be repeatedly restrained and it is damaging to the veins. Switching to oral fluids should be done as soon as possible.

Clinical Techniques

Blood Feather Removal

If a blood or pin feather is bleeding, then it should be removed to prevent further blood loss. Ideally, the bird should be anesthetized, but this procedure can be performed awake with opioid pain relievers such as butorphanol. The follicle is supported with the thumb and forefinger of one hand while a hemostat is used to firmly grasp the feather as close to the follicle as possible. The blood feather is then pulled gently but firmly in the direction it grows. Check to ensure that the entire feather has been removed—it should be narrow at the tip. Hold the follicle for a few seconds to prevent any bleeding.

Catheter Placement

Intraosseous Catheters

Intraosseous (IO) catheters allow continuous access to peripheral circulation, and they provide the ability to administer drugs, fluids, or total parenteral nutrition (TPN). The use of IO catheters is safe, rapid, and practical. IO catheters are most commonly placed in the distal ulna (Figure 5.53 A,B) or proximal tibiotarsus. IO catheters should not be placed in a pneumatic bone as this may drown the bird when fluids are administered,

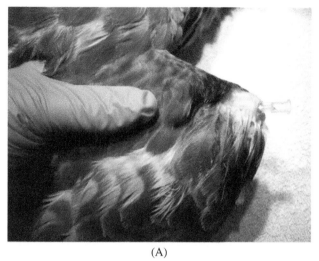
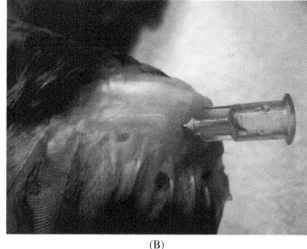

(A)   (B)

Figure 5.53 (A, B) Intraosseous catheter placement into the distal ulna of a Cooper's hawk. A 22-gauge needle or spinal needle can be used. A catheter cap will fit on the end. Sterile technique should be used to place a catheter.

since pneumatic bones communicate directly with the respiratory system. Likewise, intracoelomic fluids should not be administered as this may also drown the bird if fluids get into an air sac. To place an IO catheter, feathers should be plucked and an area of the carpus aseptically prepared. The needle should be positioned in the center of the distal ulna. With the ulna supported, the catheter can be rotated. Once past the cortex, the catheter passes easily. Aspiration should produce a small amount of blood. The catheter is anchored to the soft tissue of the carpus and a figure-of-eight bandage is applied.

Air Sac Tube

To place an air sac tube (canula), make a skin incision over the sternal notch area (borders are the last rib, the femur, and the lateral processes of the vertebrae) and use a pair of hemostats to penetrate the body wall, and then insert an endotracheal tube (usually about the same size that would be used to intubate the bird). This can be sutured in place and the bird can breathe room air through the end of the tube or can be placed in an oxygen cage to breathe oxygenated air through the tube. If the tube is attached to an anesthesia machine for direct oxygen or anesthetic delivery, the flow rate should be about 1 liter/minute as if the bird was intubated.

Blood Collection

The blood volume of birds is approximately 10% of their body weight. The amount of blood that can be collected safely from a healthy bird is approximately 10% of their blood volume or 1% of their body weight (1 mL per 100 g of body weight in a healthy bird). This amount should

be reduced in a sick patient. For example, a maximum of 1.0 mL of blood can be removed from a healthy 100-gram (0.10 kg) cockatiel without adverse effects. For a 1000-gram (1.0 kg) healthy macaw, a maximum of 10 mL can be removed.

$$\text{cockatiel } 0.100 \text{ kg} \times 0.01 = 0.001 \text{ L} = 1 \text{ mL}$$

$$\text{macaw } 1.0 \text{ kg} \times 0.01 = 0.010 \text{ L} = 10 \text{ mL}$$

There are a variety of sites from which blood can be collected in the avian patient. These include the right jugular vein (preferred since it is 2/3 larger than the left jugular vein), left jugular vein, basilic vein (cutaneous ulnar vein), and the medial metatarsal vein. The size and species of the bird may influence the site chosen. For example, pigeons do not have distinct jugular veins, but a network of small vessels in the neck; therefore, the medial metatarsal vein is the best choice for phlebotomy in pigeons.

Jugular Vein

The right jugular vein (Figure 5.54) is the vein of choice for parrots kept as pets. The right jugular vein is chosen over the left since it is two-thirds larger. To collect from the jugular vein, the bird must be restrained in right lateral recumbency with the head and neck gently extended. When collecting blood, the vein should be visible. The jugular vein is found in a featherless tract or aptera (featherless area) on the ventrolateral aspect of the cervical area. By lightly wetting the skin with alcohol and parting the feathers in the lateral cervical aptera, the vein can be seen. Bird veins are mobile under the skin and have very elastic vessel walls, which can make needle punctures a challenge. Light digital pressure at the level of the thoracic inlet should be used when holding off the vein. A 1- or 3-mL syringe with a 22- to 25-gauge needle is commonly used.

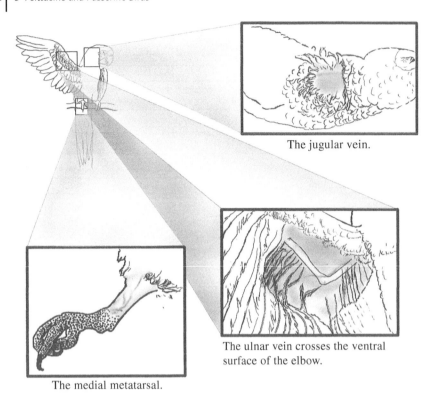

Figure 5.54 Venipuncture sites. (Drawing by Scott Stark).

The jugular vein.

The ulnar vein crosses the ventral surface of the elbow.

The medial metatarsal.

Basilic Vein

The basilic vein (cutaneous ulnar vein) is also a choice for blood collection on medium to large birds (Figure 5.54) and courses over the medial surface of the proximal ulna. This vein is superficial, lacks support tissue, and is often small, making it prone to collapse and hematoma formation. The bird should be restrained on its back. The wing should carefully be extended, making sure that it is supported by grasping the carpus and patagium.

Medial Metatarsal Vein

The medial metatarsal vein is another venipuncture choice. The larger the bird, the more developed the vein. This vein lies in a groove on the medial side of the tibiotarsus, near the tiobtarsaltarsaometatarsal joint (hock joint). This vein is a good choice for small amounts of blood, for an IV injection or IV catheter placement. The bird can be restrained in a towel, held upright, and the leg gently extended. Poultry and waterfowl have a large metatarsal vein, making it an excellent choice for blood collection. Small blood tubes (Figure 5.55), including serum separator tubes, are available for use in small patients.

Administration of Medications

Most infections in parrots are due to Gram-negative organisms. Most drugs are used empirically, since very few

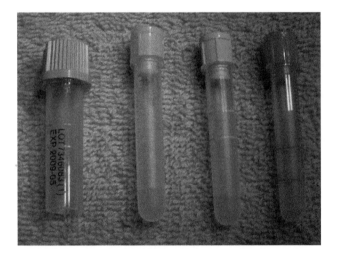

Figure 5.55 Small blood collection tubes are available for small patients.

pharmacodynamic and pharmacokinetic studies have been performed in any species of bird, and those in only a few species of bird (there is no generic bird, and different parrot species react differently to different drugs, so research on every species would take impossibly long). The most popular book/formulary for doses of medications in birds is Carpenter's Exotic Animal Formulary with a chapter on birds and a separate chapter that covers backyard poultry, gamebirds, and waterfowl (Guzman et al. 2022, Crespo & Petritz 2022).

The goal is to achieve antimicrobial tissue levels at the site of infection that are greater than the MIC (minimum inhibitory concentration) while realizing that drug excretion is rapid in birds compared to mammals. Antibiotics can cause immunosuppression and change normal flora, producing a secondary fungal infection; therefore, antibiotics should only be used when indicated so as not to upset the delicate balance of normal flora in the bird. Choose bactericidal instead of bacteriostatic antibiotics.

Additives to Water

The advantages of adding medication to the drinking water are ease of administration, the bird medicates itself, restraint is not required, and it may reduce specific waterborne diseases. The disadvantages, which far outweigh the advantages, of adding medication to the water include inexact dosing, poor palatability that reduces water and drug intake, instability of some medications in water, the likely possibility of underdosing, increasing organism resistance, and medication being poorly or slowly absorbed. Since sick birds are often anorexic, this route is usually not a good choice.

Additives to Food

The advantages of adding medication to the food include ease of administration, food consumption may be fairly consistent, and it is easier to treat hand-fed nestlings in this way. The disadvantages of adding medication to food again outweigh the advantages and include the same reasons discussed above for adding medication to water. Since sick birds are often anorexic, this route is usually not a good choice.

Direct Oral Medication

The advantages of giving medications orally (Figure 5.56) include the fact that a precise dose is given (unless the patient spits the drug out or does not swallow), many pediatric suspensions are available, and these medications can be given when a bird is gavaged or tube-fed at same time. The disadvantages of medicating directly orally include the stress of capture and restraint, the risk of aspiration of the drug, the drug may be poorly or slowly absorbed through the gastrointestinal tract of very ill birds, or malabsorption (if, for example, the bird is in shock or has a gastrointestinal disorder).

Intramuscular Injection of Medication

The advantages of giving medication via an intramuscular injection into the pectoral muscle of a bird (Figure 5.57)

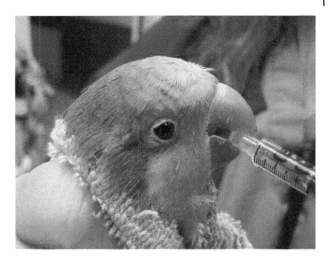

Figure 5.56 Oral medications being given to a Quaker parrot. One drop at a time should be given under the tongue to avoid aspiration.

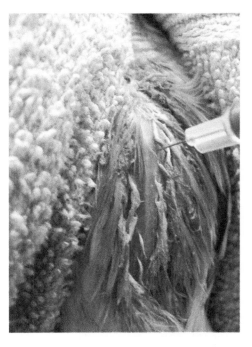

Figure 5.57 Intramuscular injection given into the left pectoral muscle of a bird. The pectoral muscles are found on either side of the bony keel. Use a 25- to 26-gauge needle.

include the knowledge that the bird will get an exact dose, it is quick and easy to administer, meaning less stress of handling, and it is quickly absorbed. The disadvantages of using intramuscular medication include that not all drugs are available for intramuscular use, and pain and necrosis may occur at the injection site. In critically, ill birds that cannot initially absorb oral medications, the bird can be started on intramuscular medications and then switched to oral forms later.

Intravenous Medications

The advantage of intravenous medications via the jugular or medial metatarsal or basilic vein is that an exact dose is given, it is rapidly absorbed, and rapidly reaches therapeutic levels. The disadvantages of intravenous medications are the stress of prolonged restraint while giving a bolus, or if on an IV drip the risk of the bird chewing the IV line, and the fragile veins of birds.

Intraosseous Medication

The advantages of giving medications via an intraosseous catheter in the distal ulna or proximal tibiotarsus include a precise dose is given, and like IV administration, it is rapidly absorbed, and the catheter can be left in place up to 5 days.

The disadvantages of intraosseous administration include discomfort or, if not bolus treating, the bird chewing the IO line.

Subcutaneous Medication

The advantages of giving medications via the subcutaneous route (Figure 5.58) in the inguinal region include that a precise dose can be given and it is quick and easy to administer. The disadvantages of giving medications via the subcutaneous route include the fact that some drugs are irritating

when given SQ, and some severely debilitated birds may not absorb SQ fluids or drugs. If fluids pool in the subcutaneous space and are not absorbed within 1 to 2 hours, then IV or IO fluids are necessary.

Topical

In birds, greasy topical compounds should be avoided because this reduces the insulation of the feathers. If ointments must be used in birds, then they should be used sparingly. It is better to use water-soluble creams.

Nebulization

Nebulization is used to deliver medications for respiratory infections. Nebulization is a process in which atomization of a liquid into small (<3 microns) droplets occurs so that it can be inhaled. Usually, nebulization is performed for 10 to 30 minutes by forcing oxygen through a solution containing antibiotics or antifungals, etc.

Sinus/Nasal Flushing

Sinus flushing (Figure 5.59) can be diagnostic (cytology, culture) and/or therapeutic. WARM saline should be used. Also, it is imperative to hold the bird completely vertically upside-down so as to avoid aspiration of fluid into the trachea. Flushing can be performed in an awake bird or an anesthetized, intubated bird.

Tube feeding

Tube feeding is controversial in critically ill patients (will they process it?). The bird must be hydrated first. Feeding

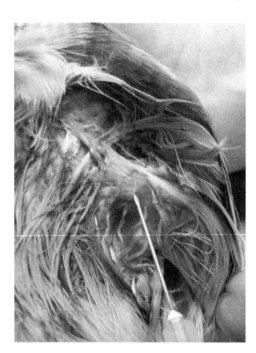

Figure 5.58 Subcutaneous fluids being given to a bird with a 22-gauge needle into the left inguinal area. The left leg is gently pulled caudally. Care should be taken to not abduct (pull laterally on) the leg since bird legs do not naturally abduct.

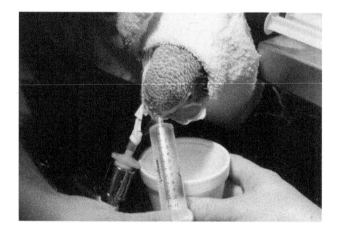

Figure 5.59 Example of a nasal flush being performed in an African grey parrot.

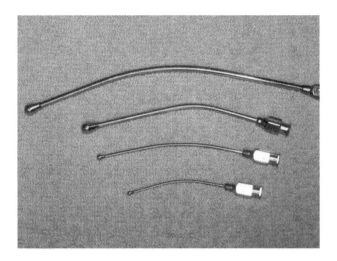

Figure 5.60 Variety of sizes of stainless steel ball-tipped feeding needles used to gavage food directly into a bird's crop.

should begin with a thin carbohydrate supplement and later use a juvenile parrot hand-feeding formula or specially made avian critical care diet (high calorie, easy to digest).

Birds have a high basal metabolic rate with very little in reserve; therefore, if a bird is losing weight, it needs to be tube-fed. While hospitalized, a bird is weighed daily in the morning on a gram scale. Tube feeding is necessary if a bird is not maintaining or gaining weight in the hospital. Generally, birds are tube-fed 1 to 4 times/day. The technique consists of restraining the bird in a normal upright position so as to avoid regurgitation and aspiration. Some prefer a stainless steel feeding needle with ball tip (Figure 5.60), while others use a red rubber catheter and a speculum to prevent the bird from biting the tube in two. If using a speculum, care must be taken to not traumatized the beak.

The tube is aimed from the left commissure to the right crop area (Figure 5.61). Care must be taken to avoid the large trachea and avoid excessive force so as not to puncture the esophagus and deposit food into the neck of the bird. Confirm placement of the tube by palpating or visualizing tube in the crop before administering the formula. If the bird regurgitates at any time, then set it down and let go immediately to allow the bird to concentrate on not aspirating.

Approximate Feeding Quantities (start with small amounts, then increase to amount below)

Budgerigar: 1 mL
Cockatiel: 3–5 mL
Amazon parrot: 15–30 mL
Cockatoo: 20–40 mL
Macaw: 30–60 mL

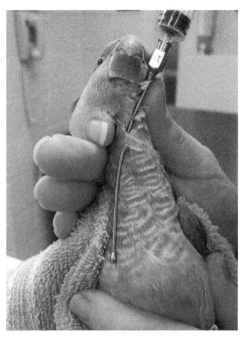

Figure 5.61 A metal ball-tipped feeding or gavage tube is held external to the bird to show the proper placement of the tube internally. The tube should gently enter from the bird's left commissure and aim for the right shoulder area. The crop of a bird is on the right side of the neck and is very thin and subject to puncture.

Diagnostic Sampling

Blood is drawn from the right jugular vein since it is two-thirds larger than the left. No more than 10% of the blood volume, or 1% of the body weight, can be removed from a healthy bird without adverse effects. If a bird is sick or debilitated in any way, then less should be taken. Generally, whole blood is placed in a lithium heparin tube for a CBC, or a CaEDTA tube can be used for most avian species. However, some bird's blood, such as crow's blood, will hemolyze in CaEDTA. Plasma from a lithium heparin separator tube is ideal, but other tubes producing plasma or serum can be used. Microtainer tubes that hold less than 1 mL are ideal for small bird patients. The newer benchtop analyzers can provide a complete chemistry profile including bile acids using only 0.1 mL of blood in a lithium heparin tube. Research has shown that these benchtop analyzers give comparable results to laboratory methods (Greenacre et al. 2008).

Many references are available regarding normal or expected reference ranges for CBC, chemistry panel results, and other diagnostic testing in a variety of avian species. Two such resources include the easy-to-use Exotic Animal Formulary and the very thorough Exotic Animal

Laboratory Diagnosis which includes specific chapters on raptors, Psittaciformes, Galliformes, pigeons and doves, passerine birds, seabirds, and waterfowl (Heatley & Russell 2020).

Wound Care and Bandaging

Wound care is very similar to mammals, except that birds are very sensitive to steroids, so topical or parenteral steroids should be avoided. Also, if the bird is a food animal species such as a chicken or turkey, then care must be taken to not use prohibited drugs. The FDA's list of prohibited drugs in chickens and turkeys can be found at: www.farad.org. The FDA rules apply whether the bird or its eggs are eaten or not. Bandaging is also similar except for those below which pertain to the special anatomy of birds. Typical bandage materials just need to be cut smaller. Ball or snowshoe bandages are used to protect the plantar surface of the foot and evenly distribute the bird's weight in cases of ulcerative pododermatitis, or bumblefoot. The interdigitating bandage is wrapped around the entire foot between the toes.

The ball bandage (Figure 5.62) is more ball-shaped, the snowshoe bandage being flatter. Figure-of-eight bandages (Figure 5.63) are used to immobilize the wing distal to and including the radius and ulna. It is not used for humeral fractures unless a wrap about the body is included. This bandage is usually for temporary use since after 5 to 7 days the propatagial ligament that extends from the shoulder to the carpus becomes severely contracted. A good rule of

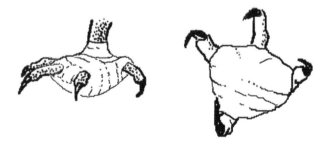

Figure 5.62 Ball foot bandage. (Drawing by Scott Stark).

thumb to follow is that for every week in a bandage there is a month of rehabilitation.

Elizabethan or tube collars (Figure 5.64) about the neck are not recommended in birds because they are invariably heavy, make eating and preening difficult, and stress the bird. Exceptions are made for collar use when a bird self-traumatizes, i.e., bites its own flesh and bleeds.

Euthanasia

Ideally, all animals should be rendered unconscious prior to euthanasia, regardless of the species. Birds are easily anesthetized and rendered unconscious either by being masked under anesthesia with isoflurane or sevoflurane, or by injectable anesthetics (Greenacre 2016). Then, once unconscious, the euthanasia solution can be given via the intravenous or intracardiac route, or in the cisterna magna. AVMA Euthanasia Guidelines 2020 includes information on all possible forms of euthanasia in a variety of bird

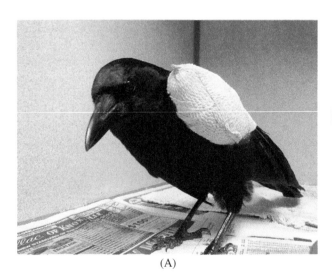

(A)

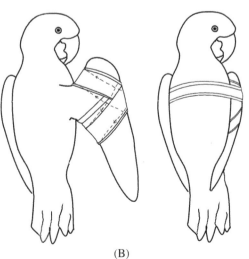

(B)

Figure 5.63 (A) Figure-of-eight bandage on a crow. (B) Figure-of-eight bandage wrapped around the body for stabilization of a humeral fracture. (Drawing by Scott Stark).

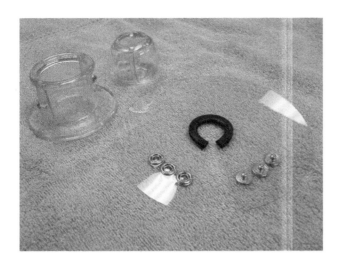

Figure 5.64 Examples of Elizabethan and tube collars used in birds. Generally, they are not recommended for use in birds because they are invariably heavy, make eating and preening difficult, and stress the bird. Exceptions are made for collar use when a bird self-traumatizes, i.e., bites its own flesh and bleeds.

species and can be found at https://www.avma.org/sites/default/files/2020-02/Guidelines-on-Euthanasia-2020.pdf (AVMA 2020).

There are also documents available online through the AVMA to address methods of humane slaughter in the AVMA Guidelines for the Humane Slaughter of Animals: 2016 Edition and to address methods of depopulation in times of emergency, such as during highly pathogenic avian influenza (HPAI) outbreak, in the AVMA Guidelines for the Depopulation of Animals: 2019 Edition. (AVMA 2016, AVMA 2019).

Acknowledgment

The authors thank Lillian Gerhardt, LVT, for her contributions on the previous editions of this chapter.

References

AVMA. 2019. *AVMA Guidelines for the Depopulation of Animals: 2019 Edition*. Schaumburg, IL: American Veterinary Medical Association. Website accessed 12-8-2022. https://www.avma.org/sites/default/files/resources/AVMA-Guidelines-for-the-Depopulation-of-Animals.pdf.

AVMA. 2020. *AVMA Guidelines for the Euthanasia of Animals: 2020 edition*. Schaumburg, IL: American Veterinary Medical Association. Website accessed 12-8-2022. https://www.avma.org/sites/default/files/2020-02/Guidelines-on-Euthanasia-2020.pdf.

AVMA. 2016. *AVMA Guidelines for the Humane Slaughter of Animals: 2016 edition*. Schaumburg, IL: American Veterinary Medical Association. Website accessed 12-8-2022. https://www.avma.org/sites/default/files/resources/Humane-Slaughter-Guidelines.pdf.

Balsamo G, Maxted AM, Midla JW, et al. 2017. Compendium of measures to control *Chlamydia psittaci* infection among humans (psittacosis) and pet birds (avian chlamydiosis). *J Avian Med Surg* 31(3): 262–282.

Bennett RA. 2022. General principles, instruments, and equipment. In: *Surgery of Exotic Animals* (eds RA Bennett, GW Pye), pp. 1–10. Hoboken, NJ: Wiley.

Brue RN. 1994. Nutrition. In: *Avian Medicine: Principles and Application* (eds BW Ritchie, GJ Harrison, LR Harrison). Lake Worth, FL: Winger's Publications.

Crespo R, Petritz OA. 2022. Backyarsd poultry, gamebirds, and waterfowl. In: *Carpenter's Exotic Animal Formulary* (eds J Carpenter, CA Harms) 6th edn, pp. 444–495. St. Louis, MO: Elsevier.

Curro TG, Brunson DB, Paul-Murphy J. 1994. Determination of the ED_{50} of isoflurane and evaluation of the isoflurane-sparing effect of butorphanol in cockatoos (*Cacatua* spp.). *Vet Surg* 23: 429–433.

Fulton RM. 2021. Avian influenza and viscerotropic velogenic (exotic) newcastle disease. In: *Backyard Poultry Medicine and Surgery: A Guide for the Veterinary Practitioner* (eds CB Greenacre, TY Morishita) 2nd edn, pp. 229–233. Hoboken, NJ: Wiley.

Graham JE, Doss GA, Beaufrere H (eds). 2021. *Exotic Animal Emergency and Critical Care Medicine*. Hoboken, NJ: Wiley. [Part 2 – Avian chapters with multiple authors, pp. 431–694].

Greenacre CB, Flatland B, Souza MJ, Fry MM. 2008. Comparison of avian biochemical test results with Abaxis VetScan and Hitachi 911 analyzers. *J Avian Med Surg* 22(4): 291–299.

Greenacre CB. 2016. Euthanasia. In: *Current Therapy in Avian Medicine and Surgery* (ed B Speer), pp. 714–718. St, Louis, MO: Elsevier.

Guzman DSM, Beaufrere H, Welle KR, Heatley J, Visser M, Harms CA. 2022. Birds. In: *Carpenter's Exotic Animal Formulary* (eds JW Carpenter, CA Harms), 6th edn, pp. 222–443. St. Louis, MO: Elsevier.

Harrison GJ, Ritchie BW. 1994. Making distinctions on the physical examination. In: *Avian Medicine: Principles and Application* (eds BW Ritchie, GJ Harrison, LR Harrison).

Lake Worth, FL: Winger's Publications. Or access free downloadable book in PDF format at: https://avianmedicine.net/publication_cat/avian-medicine/.

Heatley JJ, Russell KE (eds). 2020. *Exotic Animal Laboratory Diagnosis*. Hoboken, NJ: Wiley.

King AS, McLelland J. 1984. *Birds, Their Structure and Function*, 2nd edn. Eastbourne, UK: Baillière Tindall.

Lichtenberger M, Orcutt C, Cray C, Thamm DH, et al. 2009. Comparison of fluid types for resuscitation after acute blood loss in mallard ducks (*Anas platyrhynchos*). *J Vet Emerg Crit Care* 19(5): 467–472.

McMillan MC. 1994. Imaging techniques. In: *Avian Medicine: Principles and Application* (eds BW Ritchie, GJ Harrison, LR Harrison). Lake Worth, FL: Winger's Publications.

Paul-Murphy JR, Brunson DB, Miletic V. 1999. Analgesic effects of butorphanol and buprenorphine in conscious African grey parrots (*Psittacus erithacus erithacus* and *P. erithacus timneh*). *Am J Vet Res* 60(10): 1218–1221.

Paul-Murphy J, Hess JC, Fialkowski JP. 2004. Pharmacokinetic properties of a single intramuscular dose of buprenorphine in African grey parrots (*Psittacus erithacus erithacus*). *J Avian Med Surg* 18(4): 224–228.

Quandt JE, Greenacre CB. 1999. Sevoflurane anesthesia in psittacines. *J Zoo Wildlife Med* 30(2): 308–309.

Rembert MS, Smith JA, Hosgood G, Marks SL, Tully TN. 2001. Comparison of traditional thermal support with the forced air warmer system in Hispaniolan Amazon parrots (*Amazona ventralis*). *Assoc Avian Vets Annual Conf*, 215–217.

Ritchie BW, Harrison GJ, Harrison LR (eds). 1994. *Avian Medicine: Principles and Application*. Lake Worth, FL: Winger's Publications.

Tully TN. 2009. Birds. In: *Manual of Exotic Pet Practice* (eds Mitchell MA, Tully TN), pp. 250–298. St Louis, MO: Elsevier.

Young AM, Hobson EA, Bingaman-Lackey L, Wright TF. 2012. Survival on the ark: life-history trends in captive parrots. *Anim Conserv* 15(1): 28–43.

Zhang Z, Zhou H, Cao H, Ji J, et al. 2022. Human-to-human transmission of *Chlamydia psittaci* in China, 2020: an epidemiological and aetiological investigation. *Lancet Microbe*.

6

Psittacine Behavior, Husbandry, and Enrichment

April Romagnano, Tarah Hadley, Ashley McGaha, and Jan Hooimeijer

Introduction

Psittacine bird species account for approximately 350 of the 18,000 + known avian species. Psittacine birds (commonly referred to as parrots), which are primarily found in tropical regions of the world, are classified into three families: the Loriidae (includes lories and lorikeets), the Cacatuidae (cockatoos), and the Psittacidae (includes parakeets and parrots) (Forshaw 1977). Birds in each of these families demonstrate distinct physical and behavioral characteristics. One should keep in mind that what constitutes normal and abnormal behavior may be heavily influenced by the species, the individual bird, and the environment. In many situations, behavior of captive birds does not always equate with the behavior of those birds in the wild. At the same time, it is not unusual that birds may show behaviors that are normal under natural circumstances in nature (Luescher 2006).

Behavior in the wild is based on innate behavior and founded on **observational** learning, experience, intelligence, and cognitive abilities. This key concept of observational learning is important to understand. Birds learn like human children. They are visual learners. Bird behavior is driven by the urge to survive as an individual and as a species. When working with parrots in captivity, one needs to understand that the behavior of parrots is determined by different factors including hereditary factors, as well as being determined by living in captivity under extremely unnatural circumstances (Pepperberg and Hooimeijer 2018).

Interestingly, after 45 years of scientific research, Dr. Irene Pepperberg has shown that parrots have a level of intelligence that can be compared with a 6–7-year human child. Acknowledging this intelligence and the highly developed cognitive capacities is showing respect for parrots (Pepperberg and Hooimeijer 2019).

Respected avian behavior expert, Dr. Jan Hooimeijer, who established his Consultancy Practice for Birds in 2013, has developed the "Five Steps to Positive Parrot Behavior" which is useful during veterinary examinations, diagnostics, treatment, and beyond.

The most important aspect of dealing with parrots is the attitude of the person or persons caring for the parrot. A basic protocol for technicians, veterinarians, and caregivers of parrots, creating mutual respect and mutual trust, can be summarized in five steps. This protocol can also be used with any parrot exhibiting a behavior problem. It will reduce the stress and will make the bird feel comfortable.

Using this 5-step protocol, coupled with understanding the following descriptions listed below this section of different parrot species' behavior, diets and particularities, the veterinary technician, veterinarian, and parrot caretaker should be better equipped to mitigate interactions with the different parrot species encountered.

Step 1: When approaching a parrot, the person should convince the parrot that they have no negative intentions, by showing nonintimidating posture and body language. This acknowledges the fact that parrots are prey animals. Acting comfortably in the presence of the parrot and initially not looking at the bird, lets the parrot observe the person. The person should be vocal, playful, and silly. Parrots feel comfortable with people who are comfortable with parrots and with themselves. The person's behavior is demonstrating respect for the parrot, resulting in mutual respect. Being positive, creating **desired** behaviors is the goal.

Step 2 **Desired** behaviors achieved in step 1 should be rewarded. The key is that one should make an intellectual connection, letting the parrot know its intelligence is appreciated.

Step 3 The person needs to establish oneself as the best teacher the parrot can wish for. Showing respect for his/her intelligence can be achieved by saying out loud, in detail, what there is to see around him/her pointing out toys, colors, shapes, foods, objects, etc. and praising the bird. Parrots love observing and learning. Acknowledging the

Exotic Animal Medicine for the Veterinary Technician, Fourth Edition. Edited by Bonnie Ballard and Ryan Cheek.
© 2024 John Wiley & Sons, Inc. Published 2024 by John Wiley & Sons, Inc.
Companion Website: www.wiley.com/go/ballard/4e

intelligence is rewarding the bird for their intelligence, again in a nonintimidating way.

Step 4 After acknowledging/rewarding the intelligence, the bird should be allowed to touch something the person is holding such as a pen, toy, paper, or towel and praise the bird enthusiastically. The parrot should only be allowed to touch items when they have been told that they may touch. They are in general very gentle when touching objects with their tongue. The bird can be encouraged to participate in the learning process by offering new, small, nonthreatening objects. Telling the bird they may touch and feel the objects allows the bird to investigate that object. Each positive move should be praised. At step 4, a person can also present their hand and tell the bird that they may step up and praise the bird for doing so. This is the opposite of giving a command or making the bird step up motivated by a treat.

> **The goal is to create a relationship based on mutual trust and respect.**
> It is vital because it will enhance the welfare and prevent behavior problems and is a tool to solve behavior problems.
> It is vital to reward **desired** behaviors.
> It is vital not to reward normal behaviors.
> It is vital not to reward **undesired** behaviors.

Step 5 This shows the parrot that accepting new situations is okay because it can trust the person and the circumstances that have been created. If the parrot shows fear, one should not reassure the bird. Reassurance can easily create more fear and insecurity. Typically, after Steps 1 through 4 mutual respect and mutual trust have been established. When the parrot fears a place or object like the towel, one needs to be understanding and start over again with step 1 of the protocol and follow through. With time and patience, a parrot can be convinced that there is no reason for fear. Telling the parrot how intelligent he/she is will help to reinforce the self-esteem that all parrots need to be able to develop normal behaviors. The outcome is to create a situation in which a parrot can accept novel situations without fear. These situations can be a physical examination, taking a blood sample, holding a bird for anesthesia, taking radiographs, grooming, nail trimming, wing clipping, beak trimming with a Dremel tool or other medical procedures, toweling, or other medical procedures (Hooimeijer 2022).

The veterinary profession has come a long way over the years in the way patients are handled in the hospital setting. Large strides have been made in the way an animal's behavior is approached in this setting in an effort to create a less stressful experience for the pet and their owner.

Historically, an animal in fear has been a very large part of a visit to a veterinary clinic. New smells, new people, loud predatory animals, and being carried around in a box are just some of the environmental factors that can cause fear, and that is all before the handling even begins.

Birds, especially those that are not used to being handled, can become very fearful, which can lead to stress, which may cause open-mouth breathing, tachycardia, hyperventilation, and in some extreme cases, death. If a veterinary professional is not accustomed to handling a bird, or understanding their behavior, handling a bird can be a very daunting task.

Anxiety/stress-free techniques have been developed to make veterinary visits less daunting for animals large and small as well as for the staff. In 2016, the Fear Free® approach was introduced for small animal practice. The Fear Free® courses offered to veterinary and pet professionals alike, were created by Dr. Marty Becker. The Fear Free® program was created to alleviate fear, anxiety, and stress in patients.

Being trained in the Fear Free® approach allows the veterinarian or veterinary technician to think like the animal, get to know different species' body language, and how to work with the animal, rather than against it. This approach now includes avian patients in an effort to enhance the veterinary experience for the avian patient (Demaline 2018).

As previously explained, avian handling can be challenging for a multitude of reasons. Since most captive pet parrots are also considered prey species, they may perceive any new place, thing, or person as a threat. This can cause a fight or flight reaction, which is the consequence of a fear response. When handling any species of bird, large or small, prey or predator, ensuring the safety of the veterinary team, as well as the animal, should be the top priority.

The use of Fear Free® practices in clinics that see exotic animals may be a newer concept, but it has great potential to create a trusted environment from both the animal's and client's perspective. Having clients involved in the training of their animals can also have a significant impact on how the exam goes (Demaline 2018).

When handling a bird for the first time, one should take a brief moment to recognize any fear-provoking environmental factors that may be eliminated. This may include other animals nearby, loud noises in the exam room and/or too many strange people. In the past, handling included strictly overpowering the bird for manual restraint. This method while not ideal in all situations, has not been completely eliminated as each patient and circumstance is different. However, for birds that are willing and with veterinary personnel trained in stress-reducing techniques, taking the time to get to know the animal and have them interact with personnel without creating a fearful event,

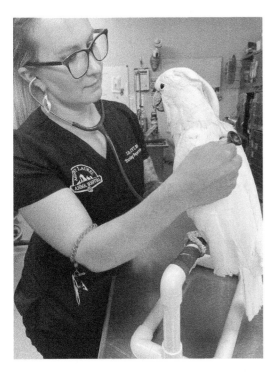

Figure 6.1 A Moluccan cockatoo being auscultated while sitting on a perch. (Courtesy of Liz Vetrano).

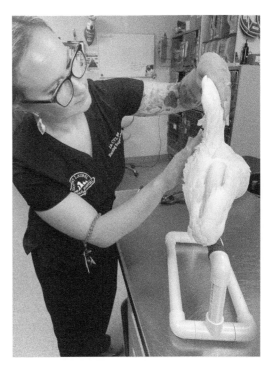

Figure 6.2 The Moluccan cockatoo undergoing a physical examination while sitting on a perch. (Courtesy of Liz Vetrano).

can create a healthy relationship between the veterinary professional and the patient (Figures 6.1 and 6.2).

Examples of Techniques for Fear Free® and How They Can Be Implemented:

1. Minimal restraint/ or no restraint physical exams. If the bird is comfortable, this can be performed in the exam room with the client while the bird is on a perch. If they allow, you can collect a respiratory rate, heart rate, a CRT to assess hydration status, auscultate lungs and air sacs, perform an ophthalmic exam, and collect a BCS.
2. Keeping healthy treats in the clinic for food-motivated animals may be very helpful during the exam. Ask the client if they have a special treat that their bird enjoys and offer that treat while you are letting the animal acclimate to their new surroundings. However, this may not work with animals that are nervous and not willing to take the treat that is offered.
3. Using towels for handling can be a scary new experience for a bird that is not acclimated to them. Desensitizing the bird to towels prior to their veterinary visit is something a client can work on, which can be a great tool to help create a stress-free environment during a veterinary examination.

A veterinary technician can become Fear Free® certified by enrolling in the online certification program.

Behavior of Common Pet Psittacine Species

Lories and Lorikeets

These birds are extremely energetic and intelligent. They are not good talkers but when excited or stressed they may emit an ear piercing, high-pitched screech. In the home environment, these birds tend to be very curious and may get into trouble going into places they should not. Many of these birds do well in at least a group of two. As individual pets, they can attach themselves to one favorite owner and be very nippy toward anyone else.

In general, due to their wet diet of fruit, nectar, and pollen, these birds are also very messy eaters and it is not unusual to see food splashed around the cage or on floors and walls. Note that lory diets must be low in iron and thus grapes are contraindicated, as are citrus fruits. Acidic fruits are contraindicated as they increase iron absorption. Lory commercial diets of nectar, mash, or pellets are available, and their iron content should be under 40–60 PPM.

Lories seen in the pet trade include the Black Lory, Red Lory, Rainbow Lory, and the Chattering Lory. The brilliance and beauty of their plumage have made these birds attractive as pets and aviary display birds in zoos, butterfly gardens, and private collections. However, they may also be extremely territorial, which may contribute to unwanted biting behaviors, especially when kept as pets.

Cockatoos

Like all birds, cockatoos are very intelligent (see Figure 6.3). Most cockatoos, especially the larger varieties, also tend to be very sweet-natured. This behavioral tendency may encourage some owners to treat them like babies or small children instead of birds. Likewise, many of these same birds become very attached to their owners, contributing to the development of abnormal behaviors such as feather picking, screaming, and biting.

Smaller cockatoos tend to bite even their owners, but some may also be sweet-natured. Cockatoos are decent talkers. They are also prone to screaming loudly at certain times of the day such as dusk or dawn, when they are tired and ready for sleep, or when they get excited. If left unattended or sometimes in plain view, their curiosity may get the best of them and lead to their chewing on wood, such as baseboards, other wooden items or unsafe items, like electrical cords.

Cockatoos cannot distinguish between safe and unsafe items, so it is essential to bird-proof the home environment from the unsafe items like electrical cords, metallic items, stained glass, or jewelry.

The cockatoo species most commonly kept as pets include the umbrella cockatoo, salmon-crested cockatoo (also known as the Moluccan cockatoo), galah (the rose-breasted cockatoo), sulfur crested cockatoos (Lesser, Medium, and Greater varieties), Citron cockatoo, Goffin's

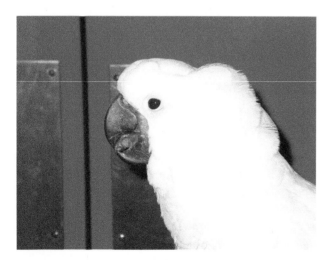

Figure 6.3 Umbrella cockatoo. (Photo courtesy Dr. Tarah Hadley).

cockatoo, the Ducorp's cockatoo and the exquisite very quiet tool using Black Palm cockatoo.

In general, the temperament of these pet birds may quickly change from very quiet and observant to very noisy and active, with the exception of the Black Palm cockatoo. These birds also produce a large amount of dander which coats their beaks with a visible layer of fine powder down. In addition, a large amount of feces is normally produced daily by these birds.

Budgerigar

These small birds are very active and social, especially when grouped together with other birds. It is not unusual to see preening or food-sharing behavior between birds. As with other birds, they may be trained to step up and follow other commands. If they are not trained, they tend to be very flighty when approached and can sometimes be a challenge to capture. These birds may also become nippy during restraint. In most other areas, the behavior of budgerigars is similar to other birds. For this reason, it is important to avoid promotion of these birds as "starter birds" for new enthusiasts since their intelligence requires enrichment equal to that of other birds. Considering a life expectancy of 15–20 years, it does not make sense to talk about a "starter bird." They need very knowledgeable caretakers to prevent the common behavior problems.

Eclectus

These birds are one of the few sexually dimorphic psittacine species (males are green and females are red) (Figure 6.4). Eclectus differs very much from all other psittacines. During the breeding season, one female can have up to 3 males as her partners for mating and for feeding her, while she produces her eggs, lays her eggs, and feeds her chicks. Having a female and a male together in a cage is basically a very unnatural situation and the reason for many behavior problems seen in captivity in this species. The male *Eclectus* tends to have a sweeter and calmer disposition compared to the female *Eclectus* whose behavior seems more cautious and suspicious, especially toward people they do not know. The females also are more aggressive in some situations and are more likely to bite than males. They are also the only female parrot that initiates mate trauma in captive one-female and one-male breeding situations, where they may attack and bite their male mates. Female *Eclectus* are also the most fecundate and nurturing of the psittacine species.

In general, *Eclectus* birds are quieter and less active than other birds. Like most birds, however, they are very intelligent and curious about their surroundings. As pets,

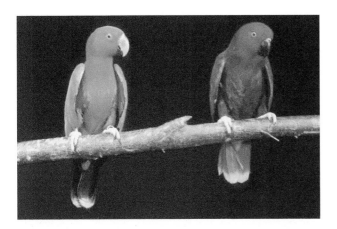

Figure 6.4 Pair of Eclectus parrots, one of several sexually dimorphic psittacine species. (Photo courtesy Dr. April Romagnano).

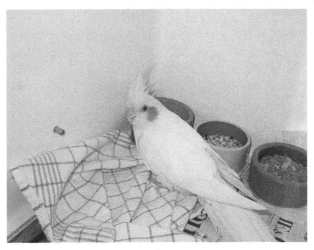

Figure 6.5 Bright orange cheek patches are often more prevalent in male cockatiels, such as the one pictured here. (Photo courtesy Dr. Tarah Hadley).

these birds thrive with owners who have a patient hand. With time and practice, they may become adequate talkers. Like the cockatoos, these birds may also develop feather-destructive behaviors, especially the males. Hence the males need extra enrichment, such as foraging toys and attention from their owners, to avoid this aberrant behavior. Males also tend to have long, overgrown maxilla tips. Liver problems are considered an important reason for overgrowth caused by malnutrition. Birds having an overgrown beak are basically not healthy. Overgrown beaks are uncommon in nature. Hence their beak growth needs to be closely monitored. Affected birds have significant maxilla tip growth, which could progress to a self-trauma or difficulty in eating and mastication.

Cockatiel

Cockatiels are sweet feisty birds with a very active social life (Figure 6.5). They may also be very vocal at times and can be good talkers and singers. They are very trainable to the hand and make good avian pets for first-time bird owners. They enjoy interacting with other cockatiels or with people. Female birds kept in a group or alone may be prone to chronic egg-laying, which can be detrimental to their overall health. Cockatiels can live as long as 30–35 years.

African Grey

These birds are extremely intelligent and also very good talkers (see Figure 6.6). They tend to be friendly birds but also may be somewhat cautious depending on the environment. African Grey parrots are also one of a few species that are commonly present for feather-destructive behaviors. Respiratory diseases like sinusitis and aspergillosis also seem to be prevalent in this species (Figure 6.7). Hence

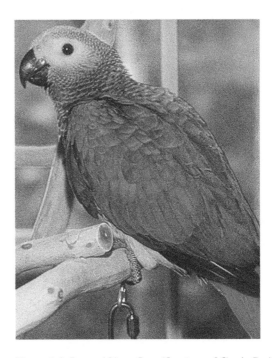

Figure 6.6 Congo African Grey. (Courtesy of Cherie Fox).

many of these birds may be more sensitive to aerosolized toxins and other agents. Like other birds, interaction with the owner and environmental enrichment, such as foraging toys, etc. are just some of the ways these birds may be kept stimulated. These birds normally produce a small amount of feather dander that lightly coats their beaks with a fine white powder. Malnutrition and lack of sunlight are the main reasons for respiratory problems in African greys. As with all parrots, they should be outside as much as possible.

Senegal

These smaller parrots make good pets and seem to thrive in an environment supported by interaction with the owner. They are fairly good speakers and may also be trained to perform small tricks.

Lovebirds

Owners may form close and friendly relationships with these birds on an individual basis. They may learn to vocalize some and tend to be fairly active singers. When paired up with one or more other lovebirds, these birds may sometimes become less friendly with their owners to the point of biting and become overly protective of their cage mates.

Macaws

These birds make up some of the largest members of the Psittacidae family. They are very active and vocal and may be adequate to fairly good talkers with encouragement. Sometimes their vocalizations can be ear-piercing. Behavior of these birds may range from friendly to cautious or unfriendly, depending on the background of the bird (see Figures 6.8–6.10).

On occasion, macaws in stressful environments may exhibit feather-destructive behaviors. Due to their large size and particularly long feathers, large cages that permit activity are required to house these birds. Owners should also be aware that they produce large amounts of feces on a daily basis.

Their large beaks, another common characteristic of these birds, are used to crack open nuts with the largest

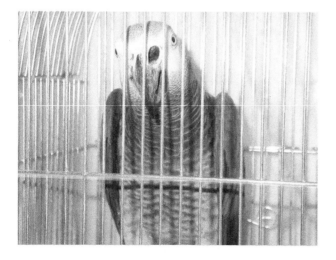

Figure 6.7 Congo African Grey parrot with an enlarged left nare most likely caused by chronic upper respiratory infections and sinusitis. (Photo courtesy Dr. Tarah Hadley).

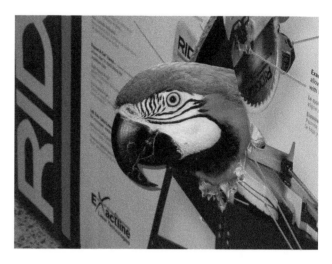

Figure 6.8 Blue and gold macaw that has chewed its way partly out one side of a cardboard box. (Photo courtesy Dr. Tarah Hadley).

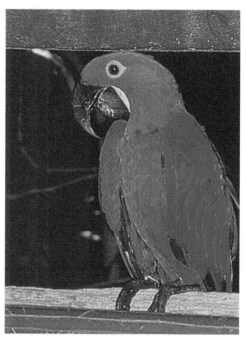

Figure 6.9 Hyacinth macaw (Courtesy of Cherie Fox).

and hardest of shells. Many species exist in the pet population, including the hyacinth macaw, blue and gold macaw, scarlet macaw, green-winged macaw, and military macaw.

Conures

These species of bird comprise some of the small to medium-sized parrots. They are extremely active birds and very active singers or talkers. They may sing or screech for

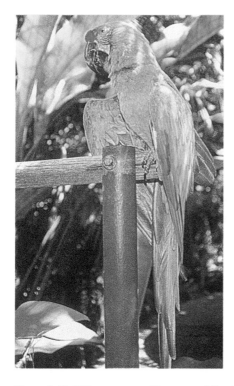

Figure 6.10 Military macaw. (Courtesy of Cherie Fox).

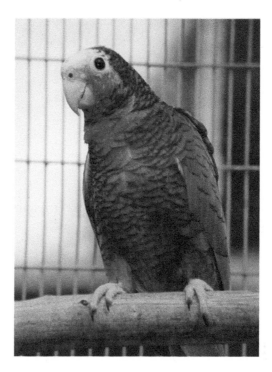

Figure 6.11 Cuban Amazon in outside aviary on a natural wood perch. (Courtesy Dr. April Romagnano).

several minutes or more at a time. Hence, the best households are those that can tolerate the loud vocalizations. They may form close relationships with owners and they can also be nippy or bite in certain situations. Common species seen in the pet industry include the mitred conure, sun conure, maroon-bellied conure, and green-cheeked conure.

Parrotlet

Parrotlets include some of the smallest species in the Psittacidae family. They are also extremely intelligent birds with a feisty temperament that belies their body size. They have been known to challenge or defend their territory from birds that are many times larger, which can sometimes get them into trouble. They are not considered very good talkers but will vocalize with encouragement. Parrotlets lead a very active life and tend to be very good fliers. Owners should always be aware of the location of non-caged birds as they can sometimes get underfoot.

Amazon

Amazon bird species are big-bodied birds that are medium in size (see Figures 6.11, 6.12, and 6.13) but very strong physically. They may be trained to become very good talkers, wonderful singers, and may be friendly pets, depending

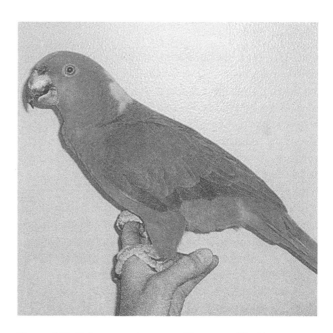

Figure 6.12 Yellow-naped amazon. (Courtesy of Dr. Sam Rivera).

on the individual bird and the environment. They enjoy the interaction with owners as well as playing on their own with toys in their environment. Amazons have a tendency to become obese and need to have a healthy diet including lots of fresh fruits and vegetables.

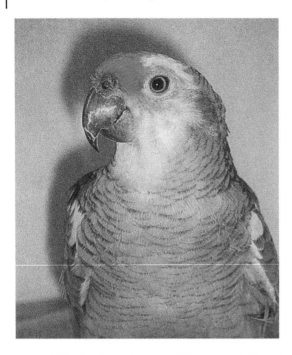

Figure 6.13 Blue fronted amazon. (Courtesy of Dr. Sam Rivera).

Husbandry

The Cage Environment

After and sometimes before the acquisition of a pet bird, many owners consider the habitat that the bird will live in when it is not outside of the cage. One of the most important considerations will be the size of the cage. The size of the cage obtained should be appropriately matched to the size of the bird. If the cage is for a large parrot species, such as a macaw, the cage should be at least a bit wider than the birds' wingspan.

An even wider cage will also provide plenty of room for play and other antics. At the same time, the height of the cage must also be evaluated such that the long tail feathers of perched birds have adequate room to prevent damage when the bird moves around. Likewise, smaller birds will require cages that are proportional to their wingspans, tail feathers, and sizes.

Other considerations include the thickness of the bars and the width between bars. While larger birds may be safely enclosed in cages with wide spaces between bars, owners of small birds need to be careful that the bar width is not so large that the bird may be able to easily slip through or get caught between the bars. Precautions should also be taken to ensure that the cages are properly manufactured and do not contain materials, such as zinc or lead, that are toxic to birds. For instance, the powder coating of painted cages made abroad may contain zinc. Stainless steel cages are the safest and the easiest to properly clean and disinfect.

Cages should have the ability to separate the bird from the fecal droppings so that birds who like to go to the bottom of their cages may do so without risk of stepping in their feces. Ideally, the grate above the bottom of the cage would be removable for ease of cleaning.

Placement of food bowls within cages should also be considered. Some cages have built-in brackets that hold food and water bowls. Other cages are flexible and allow the owners to decide where they should be located. Keep in mind that many smaller birds do a good job by leaving the food bowls alone and do not try to remove them from their holders. However, many larger birds will continually attempt to dislodge bowls from their holders. For these birds, a system where the bowl sits in a permanent bracket and cannot be removed when the bowl is inside the cage is a good solution. This will also prevent birds from creating more cage mess by wasting food or water on the floor.

There is a tremendous variety of cage styles and designs to choose from. The actual style chosen may depend on multiple factors. Owners should consider the space available for the cage. The shape of the cage is also a major consideration as some birds prefer dome-shaped cages over flat-topped cages. The shape of the cage will also affect the inside space available to the bird. The owner should wisely choose the preferred height of the cage so that birds on top of cages are not unreachable by the owner. Owners may choose from a variety of cage designs that could include external play and perching areas.

Perches

The appropriate choice of perches is often poorly understood by many owners. There are also many opinions on what is the best type of perch and size of perch for birds. Many owners forget that birds stand on their feet all day while they are awake and all night while they sleep. Hence, what the bird stands on may have a serious impact on their overall well-being in addition to their health. That being said, there are a variety of perch sizes and types available for sale for owners to choose from. Here are a few considerations for choosing the best perch.

As a general rule, the best perch allows the bird's toes to wrap around about three-quarters of the diameter of the perch. The best perches are also typically made out of natural wood. Owners will often ask whether wooden dowels or concrete perches are acceptable kinds of perches. The answer is that neither type is acceptable nor safe. Wooden dowels are uniform, exactly the same diameter from one end to the other, repeatedly putting pressure on the bird's toes and feet in the same spots. This can lead to pododermatitis secondary to repeated pressure lesions. Cement perches of all sizes definitely lead to pododermatitis; the roughness and firmness of these perches cause both topical lesions and pressure lesions.

Additionally, dowels that are flat are sometimes slippery and lack good texture for gripping. Although they are a reliable form of transport for birds traveling between water and food bowls at mealtimes, they are not comfortable for long-term perching. Pet stores also sell plastic dowels which will fit nicely inside prefabricated cages; however, they tend to be more slippery than wooden dowels. Smaller and lighter-weight birds will do better on plastic dowels but will also likely encounter the same problems with toe and foot discomfort and pododermatitis after a period of time.

Concrete perches, like sandpaper perch covers sold for smaller bird perches, are often touted as a good alternative to nail trimming in birds of any size. Based upon experience, these perches do not dull the nails of birds. For many birds, particularly those with foot or ankle problems, and heavier birds, the concrete wears away the normal skin layer on some parts of the foot. In its place, the skin may become callused, worn, and unnaturally smooth. This may also lead to extreme discomfort and, as stated above, pododermatitis.

Natural wood perches, such as manzanita, may provide the best source of comfort for a bird's feet. These perches come in varying diameters. As long as part of the perch length is an appropriate diameter for the foot size of the bird, changes in the diameter within the same perch provide the best opportunity for a bird to exercise its feet. Foot problems may lead to poor health and increased risk for systemic disease. Healthy feet will lead to healthy skin, allow for increased activity and movement, and permit the bird to get a better-quality rest in the evenings. The number of perches provided will be affected by the size of the cage. Avoid having too many perches as that will crowd the cage and decrease available living space.

The Cage Bottom

Bird owners far and wide have all received a similar warning: when your bird goes to the bottom of the cage, it is extremely sick. While that is true in some cases, it is not true in all cases. In fact, the cage bottom is just another place where birds may play. Many birds will routinely go to the bottom of the cage to play with toys or shred inkless paper or newspaper and this is completely normal. Not all birds will do this. Some birds are completely terrified of the bottom of the cage. Do not force them to go to the cage bottom.

It is important to provide birds that do play on the cage bottom with appropriate toys or enrichment. If a bird likes to shred paper, place a layer of paper on top of the grate for the bird to have access to. Do not scold birds that like to play with paper for making a mess. That is just part of being an active bird. Some birds may also enjoy paper balls or cardboard boxes. Birds that were previously scolded for shredding paper may enjoy accidental access to paper. In this scenario, owners may make it a little easier for birds to grab paper through the grate while the birds still see it as a challenging and forbidden activity. Offering paper of any kind or boxes for shredding is not ideal for broody adult female pet birds, as shredding encourages other broody behaviors and may lead to unwanted egg laying.

Upkeep of the cage bottom is especially important to the overall cleanliness of the cage. Options for substrate include white paper towels, inkless newspaper, bleached or natural butcher paper, recycled cardboard, and ash wood shavings. Never should corncob bedding be used as it fosters bacterial and especially fungal growth, nor pine shavings as the oils can cause skin contact and respiratory compromise. Ideally, the substrate on the cage bottom should be changed once daily. This is easier to do when newspaper or butcher paper are used as substrates. The advantage of daily cleaning is that it limits the growth of bacteria, fungus, and parasites.

Daily cleaning is not so easy or cost-efficient when wood shavings or corn cob bedding are used. Many owners that use these substrates prefer to scoop away fecal piles on a daily basis rather than replace the substrate. The likelihood that bacteria or fungus will grow in these scenarios is higher. Owners should also be aware that wood shavings with added treatments, such as cedar wood shavings, can also be harmful to birds. Young birds that do not know any better, or older birds that have a tendency to eat things they should not, have also been known to ingest the substrate so it is essential that it be relatively safe.

Toys and Non-toy Enrichment Items

Birds are extremely intelligent animals that need an active fulfilling environment to match their intensity. Toys tend to be the most common way that owners provide fulfillment to the inner and outer environment of their bird's cage. Toys come in a variety of shapes, sizes, colors, and noise options. Many birds love bells, so it is always best to offer stainless steel bells with stainless steel clackers. Stainless steel cowbells are available in many sizes suitable for parrotlets to Macaws. Avoid painted bells and less expensive silver bells made of toxic metals like zinc (the bell) and lead (the clacker).

The best toy for a bird depends on the size of the bird, the space available for the toy, and the personality of the bird. Many birds are afraid of new additions to their cages and may need time to get used to new toys. Owners should also avoid the temptation to crowd the cage with several toys. Crowded cages do not allow enough room for birds to stretch or play with toys and may pose an environmental hazard. Toys should be individually assessed for practicality and safety. Toys made of cloth and/or string or hanging huts or tents made of cloth are extremely dangerous. Birds can get their feet, toes, or other body parts entangled in the cloth or string. Birds entangled in hanging string toys will flap about violently, resulting in critical to fatal rhabdomyolysis if not rescued and treated immediately in hospital. Birds that get their feet and toes entrapped in the material of the hanging huts or tents try to free their feet by biting on them. This often results in the birds eating their skin, muscles, tendons and even bone in attempt to free themselves. Typically, when rescued and presented to their avian veterinarian these birds have lost toes or their entire foot or even both feet.

Toys created from safe household items are always good choices, such as ink-free cardboard boxes or paper, natural rope, and paper towel rolls. These items are usually cheap to create and are easily replaced. They may also be tailor-made to suit the activity level of the bird. Toys that encourage curiosity on the part of the bird, particularly those that encourage foraging or searching for food, may also provide great stimulation to the bird's environment. Like covering the birds' food bowl with white paper, that it has to break through or wrapping healthy nuts or pellet treats in small pieces of white paper that the bird has to open. Other items of enrichment that birds may enjoy include music, television, or videos.

Cage Location

The location of the cage is also important. Owners should choose a location for their birds that will allow daily interaction with owners and provide quiet in the evening for rest. It is not enough to simply cover a bird's cage in the evening and expect that complete rest will occur. As long as activity, noise, and bright light occur in the environment, birds may also continue to stay awake and not sleep. For this reason, many owners will have a separate cage in a quiet place to put their bird at night. Typically, multiple places, five are recommended for pet birds to be within the home is best. For instance, main day cage, night cage, perch, play gym, and a flat bottom carry cage for transport and/or trauma or illness situations.

As a general rule, birds usually need between 9 and 12 hours of sleep each night to be well-rested for the following day. Birds that do not get enough sleep may become anxious, nippy, or resort to feather-destructive behaviors. Safety should also be a consideration. For instance, a kitchen location for a cage may expose birds to undesirable fumes.

Normal Behavior of Psittacine Bird Species

What constitutes normal behavior tends to be similar across many psittacine bird species, with some minor differences. Many of these behaviors are particular to birds in captivity although some may be exhibited by birds in the wild that have not had the influence of a captive experience. Bird owners also come to learn that differences in behavior, activity level, and temperament occur among their individual pet birds. Environment and husbandry will likely play strong influences in the development of certain behaviors.

Bathing

Some birds enjoy bathing themselves in their water bowl. Bathing may be triggered by loud noises, such as music or a vacuum cleaner, by the appearance of natural sunlight on certain portions of the cage, or may just occur at some time known only to the bird. When a bird is self-bathing, it is not uncommon for it to dunk its head, beak, feet, legs, or parts of its tail in the water bowl. After dunking parts of its body, the bird usually shakes off the water and then the behavior is repeated. A bird that is allowed more free flight in the home may fly to the sound of running water and immerse itself underneath the running spout or sprayer.

Playing on the Cage Bottom

The old adage that a bird that goes to the bottom of the cage is a sick bird is not necessarily true. Some birds actually enjoy spending time on the cage bottom as much as they do on perches near the top of the cage. The cage bottom is where "illegal" access to inkless newspaper or other substrates may occur, which seems to be thrilling for many birds.

Owners are encouraged to place toys, inkless newspaper, or other items on the bottom grate so birds will have activities. The healthy bird that plays on the cage bottom may still vocalize and will continue to be very active—all normal behaviors for birds.

Preening and Molting

Preening is a normal grooming activity that birds perform on a daily basis. As part of the normal preening behavior, it is not unusual to see a few old or loose feathers drop from the body. Birds will use their beaks to smooth down rough erratic-looking feathers all over their body. Often, owners may see birds reaching to the hidden preen gland (uropygial gland) at the lower back near the base of the tail. The oily substance taken from this area is used by the birds to get their feathers back in shape, provide some waterproofing and when the birds are exposed to natural sunlight it also provides a major source of Vitamin D3. Not all species have an uropygial gland, for instance, all Amazon species do not.

Molting is another behavior that occurs in birds. As new feathers come in, old feathers are pushed out. Newer feathers may come in singly, as in the case of large wing and tail feathers, or may come in groups, such as is the case with head feathers. Newer feathers may be surrounded by an opaque sheath that the bird removes during the preening process. When a large tail or wing feather molts on one side of the body, the same feather on the opposite side of the body usually molts at the same time. In general, it is normal for large feathers to molt twice yearly and small feathers such as those covering the chest and head to molt several times yearly. Malnutrition and stress are major reasons for molting disorders. Every new feather can be used to determine the health condition at that time. When birds are sexually active the molting can be delayed.

Sleeping

Many birds will sleep through the evening for about 9–12 hours, depending on the environment and the lighting conditions. Birds will also take naps periodically during the day. Most birds that are sleeping for an extended period of time will usually sleep on their most comfortable perch with one foot clinched and held up near their abdominal area. Their heads will often be turned backward a full 180° and their beaks tucked into the feathers of their back near their wings. Any loud noises or other disturbances may disrupt a bird from this position. Some birds, such as cockatoos, may get upset about disruptions to their sleep time and may start to vocalize loudly until things in their environment quiet down. Many birds respond well to having a cover placed around their cages at sleep time. In nature, birds sleep at a very different location from where they eat or drink. Creating a separate sleeping spot where they can sleep in total darkness is a way to mimic their natural day-night rhythm.

Regurgitation

Parents who raise chicks in the nest provide nutrition to them in the form of regurgitated food. However, juvenile and adult birds have been known to regurgitate to their owners. Often no food material is expelled but the birds are going through the motion of regurgitating food into their mouths and re-swallowing it. This may simply be a sign of a bird's close attachment with an owner and does not necessarily mean that the bird is sick. Feeding another adult bird in nature is typically a behavior that is associated with pair bonding and ends up in mating and raising chicks together. It is important to prevent a bird human relationship that is based on this kind of pair bonding. Birds that do this with an owner will become insecure, territorial and develop a one-person relationship.

Eye Movements

Owners often marvel at how quickly and easily birds are able to change the way their eyes look. In most other animals, the size of the colored iris is affected by the amount of light coming into the eye. Hence, these animals have involuntary control of their iris muscles. Birds are uniquely able to directly control the movement of their irises due to the presence of voluntary muscles. Often, birds that are excited or angry will make the openings of their irises smaller. This is often referred to as "flashing" their eyes. When they look at a person with one eye, **the** excitement can be considered as positive. When they look at person with two eyes and the beak pointing toward the person, the excitement will turn into aggressive behavior.

Body Shivering

Many birds will give the appearance of being cold when their bodies start to quiver or shake. Although this is a possibility for birds exposed to cold weather, in most situations birds will quiver or shake when nervous or exposed to new environments or people. Some birds appear to do this for no reason in environments where they have been completely comfortable.

Vocalizations

The time of day or situation during which a bird will vocalize depends upon many factors. The species of bird and the personality of the individual bird usually plays a role. Stimuli that cause vocalizations by birds may be natural or artificial in origin. Common stimuli for vocalization by birds include bathing time, loud noises such as music or the vacuum cleaner, feeding time, or during dawn and dusk.

Abnormal Behavior

There are some very obvious signs that veterinary staff may pick up on to determine whether a bird is not feeling well. More subtle clues are usually detected by the owner. That is why it is so important to get a thorough and complete history, which should include asking the same background questions of every avian owner.

Feather Destructive Behaviors

Feather destructive behaviors include medical and non-medical causes of injury to the feathers and surrounding tissue. Malnutrition, lack of sunlight, lack of exercise, and insecurity because the bird is not treated with respect are major reasons for self-mutilation. Birds may destroy parts or all of a feather. They also may directly cause trauma to the underlying skin and muscle. Some birds will just pull-out feathers. Behaviors that involve feather and tissue destruction are not normal and potential causes should start to be investigated as early as possible to try to minimize trauma. Any trauma that causes excessive bleeding and/or tissue damage will need immediate attention (see Figure 6.14).

Sitting on the Cage Bottom

Birds that are extremely ill will often be too tired or weak to perch and will go to the bottom of the cage. These birds may be distinguished from their healthy counterparts by their dull attitude and overall depression. Sometimes they will lean against the side of the cage and keep their eyes closed for extended periods of time even when you attempt to stimulate them. This appearance of a bird is considered a medical emergency and requires immediate attention by a veterinarian. It should never be forgotten that egg binding should always be part of the differential diagnosis. It can occur in females at any time and after many years. Typically **a** single pet bird may produce her very first egg in her late teens or in her 20s or 30s or beyond.

Fluffed Feathers and Shivering

Often one of the first signs of illness that owners will notice is when their bird's feathers become fluffed and they look puffy (see Figure 6.15). Many birds will often shiver. These

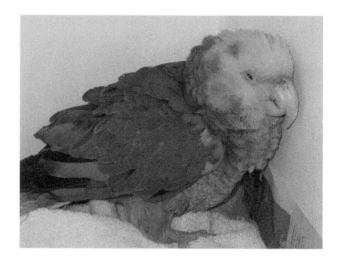

Figure 6.15 Yellow-headed Amazon that presented lethargic with eyes closed and fluffed feathers. (Photo courtesy Dr. Tarah Hadley).

are signs that the bird is unable to properly regulate its body temperature and the bird is doing everything it can to trap heat for warmth. Birds in this condition should be evaluated as soon as possible by a veterinarian.

Regurgitation and Vomiting

Regurgitation can be a sign of illness in a bird. Birds will often make bobbing motions with their heads as food is moved from the lower gastrointestinal tract to the beak. If the food material is unable to be re-swallowed, the bird will vomit the contents. A sick bird will make these motions repetitively. Causes of regurgitation and vomiting include an obstruction in the gastrointestinal tract, inflammation, infection, heavy metal toxicosis, and cancer.

Mean Bird Turned Friendly

This is a classic sign observed by owners who notice that their bird is not acting like it usually does. Owners who inquire further will interact with a usually mean bird and are surprised to see that the bird will come out of its cage and onto the owner's hand easily. These birds are likely sick and tend to be quieter and act more docile than usual. In addition, some previously unapproachable birds may permit you to touch them.

Decreased or No Fecal Production

Fecal production is one of the best indicators of how well or how poorly a bird is eating. That is why it is a good idea for owners to change the substrate at the bottom of cage frequently so that the amount of fecal production may be

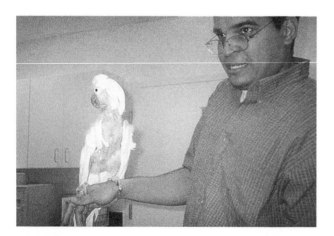

Figure 6.14 A feather picker. (Courtesy of Dr. Sam Rivera).

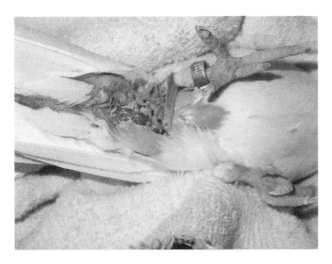

Figure 6.16 Cockatiel with fecal staining of vent area secondary to egg binding. (Photo courtesy Dr. Tarah Hadley).

regularly evaluated. A bird that is anorexic or has decreased appetite will have scant or no feces in its droppings. In an anorexic bird fecal color will progress from green to dark green and finally to charcoal black when the bird's body starts to digest the inner lining of its gastrointestinal tract which causes it to bleed. Some birds may also have multiple droppings (which contain urine, urates, and feces) stuck to the underside of their tails, usually caused by general weakness and an inability to properly posture to defecate and raise their tail releasing their droppings away from the body (see Figure 6.16). The opposite of this is a bird that is producing a large volume of feces in the morning instead of producing feces all night. This morning feces may be malodorous. In nature, this occurs when birds (typically female) are sitting in their nests on their eggs or on their babies. In order to incubate the eggs properly and/or protect the babies, birds cannot leave the nest and therefore store their feces in their cloaca. So when pet birds are hormonally active and act as if they are having eggs or chicks, they will store their feces until the morning, even when they are simply sleeping on a perch.

Open Mouth Breathing and Tail Bobbing

A bird that is breathing abnormally will breathe with its mouth open and often its tongue will move in and out of the mouth as it inhales and exhales. Many birds having difficulty breathing will also bob their tails up and down as they struggle to bring air into their bodies. These signs should also be treated as a medical emergency, and oxygen supplementation is required as part of the initial treatment.

Falling Off Perch

It is not unusual for most birds to fall off their perches at some point while they are sleeping. However, birds that do this consistently while asleep or awake are not normal. This may actually be a sign of neurologic disease, a nutritional abnormality such as hypocalcemia, or some other illness. Causes of falling off the perch may need further investigation. Until then, it may be safer to lower the perches in these birds' cages or use a smaller cage where the perches are closer to the bottom and also put a thick towel under the bird for added safety.

Inappropriate Molting

Most birds should molt their large wing and tail feathers at least twice yearly, while their small covert or covering feathers usually molt more frequently. Birds that fail to molt these feathers on a regular basis may have issues with their nutrition or some other illness affecting their metabolism. Long-standing feathers may become tattered, broken, or dull. Regular baths should be part of the hygiene for all birds to assist them in the maintenance of their plumage. Evaluating the molt and the molted feathers is one of the most important tools to evaluate the health of a bird. It tells whether the bird is healthy and can help differentiate an acute problem from a chronic one. In falconry, for over 5000 years, feather and molt evaluation have been the most important tool to determine the health of birds of prey.

References

Demaline B. 2018. Fear in the veterinary clinic: history and development of the Fear Free[SM] initiative. *Conspec Borealis* 4(1): 2.

Forshaw JM. 1977. *Parrots of the World*. Neptune: Doubleday & Company.

Hooimeijer J. 2022. How to create mutual respect and mutual trust in the examination room. In: Proc Exoticscon Conference, Denver, USA, p. 550–559.

Luescher AU (ed). 2006. *Manual of Parrot Behavior*. Ames, IA: Wiley-Blackwell.

Pepperberg IM, Hooimeijer J. 2018. Understanding and appreciating Avian cognition to address behavioral issues. In: Proc Exoticscon conference, Atlanta, USA, p. 239–247.

Pepperberg IM, Hooimeijer J. 2019. Cognitive Abilities of Grey Parrots (Psittacus erithacus) and Dealing with Parrot Intelligence.

Further Reading

Bradley Bays T, Lightfoot T, Mayer J. 2006. *Exotic Pet Behavior*. Philadelphia: Saunders.

Exoticscon 2019. Cognitive abilities in daily practice. In: Proc Exoticscon conference, St. Louis, USA, p. 291–292.

Stanford TL 1981. Behavior of dogs entering a veterinary clinic. *Appl Anim Ethol* 7(3), 271–279. 10.1016/0304-3762(81)90083-3.

7

Aviary Design and Management

April Romagnano

Introduction

The avicultural veterinary team, consisting of the avian technician and avian veterinarian, must know the avian collection, including its size and culture, and be aware of the importance of avicultural management and pediatric care. Good hygiene and impeccable sanitation are important for successful pediatrics and breeding of adult birds, but sound avicultural management must precede it.

This primarily includes good sanitation, effective nutritional protocols for birds of all ages, and preventive avicultural and pediatric medicine. In larger aviaries, this is more of a challenge. Second, proper quarantine for new acquisitions is imperative, as are necropsy and histopathology of those lost to the collection. The latter procedures, necropsy, and histopathology are important because a complete preventive medicine program incorporates a thorough pre- as well as postmortem evaluation.

Aviculture

In order to ensure a successful avicultural collection, the avicultural veterinary team must first be aware of the importance of cleanliness, husbandry, avicultural and pediatric medicine, and common sense in aviary management. The best way to achieve the above is to follow a strict set of rules to protect the entire avicultural collection as a whole.

In an aviary:

- The number of birds to be acquired must be considered in advance.
- The species of birds to be acquired must be considered in advance.
- Birds must be acquired from a reputable source. Strict quarantine must be followed at all times.

- Extensive testing is required at pre- and post-purchase examination, as well as yearly for the health of the collection.
- Proper management and nutrition must be implemented (Figures 7.1 and 7.2).
- Good hygiene and impeccable sanitation must be practiced routinely (Figure 7.3).

Infectious disease prevention is best achieved by following the principles mentioned above. Hence the avicultural veterinary team must first make sure that good medicine, management, husbandry, and hygiene practices are in place. The team must then implement proper quarantine, vaccination, disinfection, necropsy, and histopathology procedures. The latter two procedures are important because a complete preventive medicine program incorporates thorough postmortem evaluation.

Quarantine

Newly introduced birds should undergo strict quarantine in a separate designated quarantine building where extensive testing and a minimum quarantine period of 45 days are required. Although testing can be cost-prohibitive to some, an outbreak would be devastating to all. Management must decide if new acquisitions are worth the risk.

Quarantine is indeed one of the best methods of infectious disease control. When a separate building is unavailable, an alternative plan must be instituted. Hence, regardless of the collection size, location, or value, a separate quarantine facility, even if it is a friend's bird-free home, is imperative.

Collections vary and may include large or small psittacines, soft bills, and passerines. All collections warrant constant consistent flock management. A complete health history of all breeding birds in a collection, including baseline blood work and endoscopy, is imperative for

Exotic Animal Medicine for the Veterinary Technician, Fourth Edition. Edited by Bonnie Ballard and Ryan Cheek.
© 2024 John Wiley & Sons, Inc. Published 2024 by John Wiley & Sons, Inc.
Companion Website: www.wiley.com/go/ballard/4e

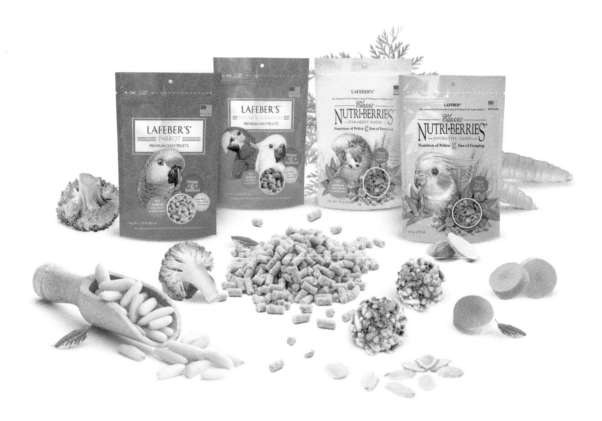

Figure 7.1 High-quality bird pellets are an important part of a nutritious diet for the majority of breeding, weaning, and juvenile parrot species when coupled with species-specific fresh vegetables, fruits, nuts, grains, and flax seeds. (Courtesy of Nadine Lafeber/Lafeber Company).

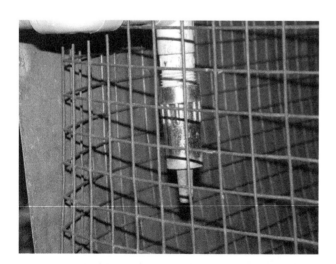

Figure 7.2 Aviary watering system that constantly provides fresh water from a central system into individual cages. Aviary birds learn to operate and drink water from the nozzle, which minimizes bacteria buildup.

ensuring proper reproductive management and optimal reproductive performance. Consideration for maintaining an open or closed aviary is important for the health of the collection. Open aviaries are defined as those in which new birds (thus new potential diseases) can be introduced directly into the collection.

The "closed aviary concept" where strict quarantine procedures are practiced is a must in an effective preventive medicine program. A closed aviary means no new direct introductions without strict quarantine, although birds may leave the collection. Traffic within the aviary should be managed and controlled, and new introductions must immediately be put into a separate quarantine building. Only dedicated staff who have no contact with other birds in the collection or general staff who are at the end of their day and about to leave the property should enter this building.

Further, before entering employees must gown, put on booties, masks, and gloves. The building should be self-sufficient with its own caging, nets, towels, protective clothing, water sources, bowls, and washing facilities. Nothing should ever leave the quarantine building to be reintroduced into the main collection as it may act as a fomite. The only exception should be garbage going directly off the property.

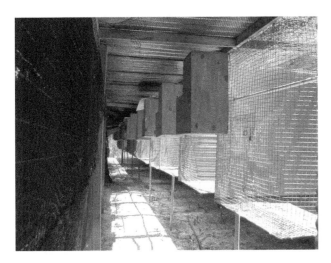

Figure 7.3 Longitudinal aviary cage design permits quick visualization of multiple cages. The cage design provides barriers between individual cages to minimize contact. Mesh cage bottoms permit release of unwanted food, water, and feces away from the cage and onto the ground where appropriate removal may take place. Wooden nest boxes, located for easy access by the veterinary team, may be easily replaced as needed.

Examinations and Diagnostic Testing

Neonates, Juveniles, Breeders, and New Acquisitions

Neonates and juveniles are examined daily and tested on a case-by-case basis (Figure 7.4). A crop and cloacal culture and fecal Gram stain are considered routine tests in young

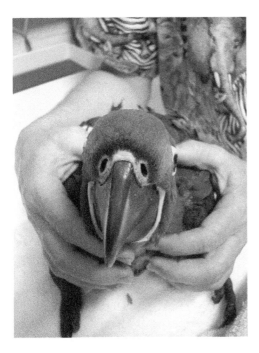

Figure 7.4 Young hyacinth macaw during examination by the veterinary team.

and very young birds. Yearly examination and testing of breeders and immediate testing of new acquisitions should include a complete blood count, serum chemistries, fecal float, fecal direct examination, fecal Gram stain and cytology, cloacal culture, polyomavirus swab DNA probe test, PBFD whole blood DNA probe test, chlamydophila PCR, and indirect, plus or minus direct, screening for proventrical dilatation disease (PDD). Additional or alternative testing may be performed and is determined on a case-by-case basis. Again, although testing can be cost-prohibitive to some, an outbreak would be devastating to all.

Vaccination protocols are limited in avian medicine, because very few vaccines are available, safe, and effective in psittacine birds. Presently only the polyoma vaccine (Avian Polyoma Virus vaccine, Biomune) is recommended for routine use and is USDA-registered.

Disinfection and Disease Prevention

Disinfection and infectious disease prevention are very important in an effective preventive medicine protocol because organic matter inactivates most disinfectants. A disinfectant is defined as an agent that will destroy many disease-causing microorganisms present on the surface of inanimate objects. Hence, first clean the area, removing all organic debris prior to disinfectant application. The easier an object is to clean, the more likely it can be adequately disinfected.

Wood is the perfect example of a difficult-to-clean material, hence, all wooden perches, nest boxes, and toys should be destroyed and replaced yearly, or immediately if an infectious disease is suspected (see Figure 7.3). Enveloped viruses are the most easily inactivated and are susceptible to quaternary ammonia products. Note that chlorhexidine has limited activity against some bacteria, especially *Pseudomonas* spp. and certain Gram-negative bacteria, and although it can kill some enveloped viruses, it cannot be considered a reliable viricide. Non-enveloped viruses require phenolic compounds and sodium hypochlorite (bleach) or stabilized chlorine dioxide for inactivation.

Glutaraldehydes will inactivate most bacteria, including mycobacteria, many viruses, and chlamydophila even in the presence of organic debris. Hence this product is particularly useful for endoscopy disinfection and sterilization. Overall, the most widely recommended and economical disinfectant in avian establishments is bleach (at the dilution of 1 part bleach to 20 parts of water). Bleach, in any strength, should never be sprayed around birds, as it can be fatal. Bleach, however, is often used to disinfect floors

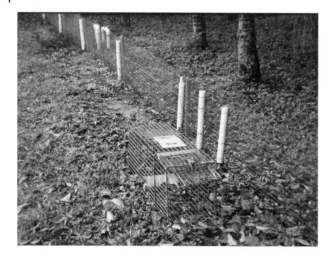

Figure 7.5 Metal traps and hot-wire fencing are just some of the methods used to minimize the introduction of disease into an aviary via indigenous vectors like opossums and raccoons.

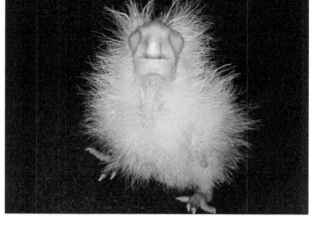

Figure 7.6 Psittacine neonate.

and bowls in aviculture, once they have been pre-washed with hot water and soap.

The geographic location and whether the birds are housed in or out of doors reflect disease potential and susceptibility. For example, sarcocystosis, Eastern equine encephalitis, and poxvirus are diseases introduced by indigenous vectors, such as opossums, cockroaches, mosquitoes, rats, raccoons, and snakes in southern states like Florida. An effective pest prevention program is required in any aviary (Figure 7.5).

Pediatrics for the Aviculturist

Pediatric History Evaluation

Note that a chick's health depends on many historical factors, such as its parents' health and breeding history, the condition of its siblings, and any problems the chick may have had during its incubation and hatching. The pediatric diet, its preparation, and the amount and frequency of feedings delivered are also part of the history. Whether the chick's crop is empty for each feeding, especially the first feeding of the day is also part of the history. It is important to know whether its environment, housing, and substrate were and are clean, safe, and warm choices. A chick's behavior, especially its feeding response, and the colors, consistency, and volume of its feces, urine, and urates are all important historical factors.

Frequent Examination of Young Birds

Physical examination of the chick entails evaluation of available weight charts for daily gain, assessing overall appearance, proportions, and behavior. In neonates, this examination should be performed in a warm room with pre-warmed hands. Knowledge of growth rates, development, and behavioral characteristics of different species is helpful.

Psittacine neonates are altricial (hatched with eyes closed, down minimal to absent, and limited mobility), hence nourishment, warmth (93–98°F), and a safe place must be provided (Figure 7.6). Neonates normally have a visible liver, duodenal loop, yolk sac, ventriculus, and occasionally lung through their body skin. The lungs and heart should be ausculted. Assess body mass by palpation of elbows, toes, and hips, as keel muscle mass is an unreliable indicator of weight in the very young.

Crops should be examined visually for size and color, and carefully palpated for thickness, tone, burns, punctures, or the presence of foreign bodies. Skin should be evaluated for color, texture, hydration, and the presence of subcutaneous fat. Normally, psittacine chicks should have beige-pink, warm, and supple skin. Dehydration causes a chick's skin to become dry, hyperemic, and tacky. In juveniles, feathers should be examined for stress marks, color bars, hemorrhage, or deformities of shafts and emerging feathers.

The musculoskeletal system should be palpated and assessed for skeletal defects or trauma in chicks of all ages. Until weaning, cockatoo chicks sit back on their hocks and are balanced forward on their large abdomens; macaws prefer to lie down. Chicks normally have prominent abdomens, due to a food-filled proventriculus, ventriculus, and small intestine. Beaks should be examined for malformations at rest. Examine the beak's pump pads for wounds.

Eyes should be examined for swelling, discharge, crusting, or blepharospasm. Normally a clear discharge is noted in the eyes when they are first opening, which typically occurs unilaterally. Nares and ears should be examined for discharge and aperture size. The oral cavity should be examined for plaques, inflammation, or injuries. Generally, a healthy chick or baby bird should elicit a vigorous feeding response when stimulated at the beak's lateral commissures or pump pads.

Pediatric Diagnostics

Clinical Pathology

- PCV, TP = lower
- WBC = may be higher
- Albumin, uric acids = lower
- ALP, CPK = higher

Microbiology

Gram-Positive Bacteria Normal
- Cloacal cultures
- Crop cultures
- Gram stain

Radiology

Gastrointestinal tract enlarged

Endoscopy

- Foreign body retrieval
- Syrinx examination
- Surgical sexing

Pediatric Problems

Common Pediatric Problems

- Unretracted yolk sac
- Stunting
- Leg and toe deformities
- Constricted toe syndrome
- Beak malformations
- Regurgitation
- Esophageal or pharyngeal punctures
- Crop stasis
- Crop burns
- Foreign body ingestion or impaction

Less Common Pediatric Problems

- Intestinal intussusception
- Hepatic hematomas
- Gout
- Wine-colored urine
- Hepatic lipidosis

Diseases in the Nursery

Viral Diseases

- Polyomavirus
- Psittacine beak and feather disease
- Proventricular dilatation disease
- Pacheco's disease
- Poxvirus

Microbial Diseases

Microbial Alimentary and Respiratory Infections
Gram-negative or yeast infections are abnormal.

Chlamydia

Zoonotic disease

Conclusion

Aviculture: Breeder and Pediatric Care

The aviculture care of breeders and pediatric patients are tightly associated disciplines. A neonate that gets off to a good start has the best chance of becoming a thriving juvenile, and eventually a reproductively successful adult (Figure 7.7). The majority of pediatric problems are associated with avicultural husbandry and hand feeding. Nursery management and veterinary preventive medicine are both equally important in the production of healthy baby birds.

Crop stasis is the most common pediatric problem seen, and if managed correctly, it need not be a fatal condition. Immediate intervention should include a thorough history, physical examination, crop culture, medical and mechanical therapy, and blood work to help reverse this condition. Daily fluids are critical in this reversal process, and probiotics including *Lactobacillus* are also helpful.

Antibiotic and antifungal medications, although important, need to be used cautiously in baby birds. When used correctly, antimicrobials can halt infection and decrease the chance of sepsis. Along with dehydration, sepsis is the most common killer of pediatric patients.

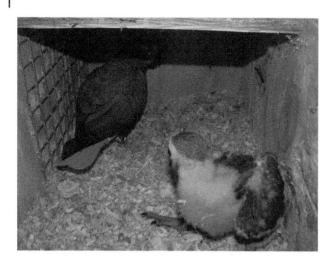

Figure 7.7 Healthy Congo African grey chick (right) and parent in nest box.

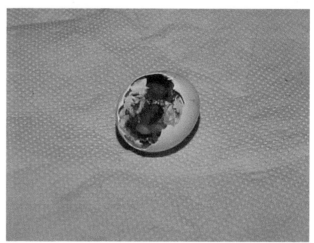

Figure 7.8 A psittacine embryo deceased in egg. Necropsy will often include assessment of the embryo's position in the egg, evaluation of anatomy, and culture when infection is suspected.

Preventive avicultural medicine and pediatrics are an ongoing interactive process that incorporates thorough routine avicultural team visits as a method of data collection. The aviculturist and the avian veterinarian and technician must know the pet bird and/or the collection (large or small) intricately and be aware of the importance of psittacine husbandry and management. The team must evaluate, diagnose, and treat the individual pet bird, as well as the entire collection. The necessity of diagnostic testing and therapeutic protocols are established based on the patient's history, the veterinarian's overall observations of the collection, and the physical examination of the individual patient.

Thus, premortem tests are chosen on a case-by-case basis, but postmortem examination is imperative and should be performed in all cases. Hence, necropsy and histopathology are also necessary for infectious disease prevention, as are quarantine, vaccination, and disinfection (Figure 7.8).

Additional Reading

Romagnano A. 2006. Mate trauma. In: *Manual of Parrot Behavior* (ed AU Luescher), pp. 247–253. Ames, IA: Wiley-Blackwell.

Romagnano A, Wolf S, Garner MM. 2000. Management of diseases and syndromes in a closed psittacine nursery. In: Proc 21st Annual Conf Assoc Avian Vet, Portland, OR.

Schubot RM, Clubb KJ, Clubb SL. 1992. *Psittacine Aviculture*. Loxahatchee, FL: Avicultural Breeding and Research Center.

8

Sex Differentiation and Reproduction

April Romagnano and Tarah Hadley

Introduction

Veterinary clinics that see birds as patients are likely to have owners who want to know if their pet is male or female, if it is not visually obvious. Veterinary technicians must be educated in the methods of sexing a bird and able to discuss these options with owners. Veterinary technicians also must be knowledgeable about normal reproductive anatomy and problems that can arise. These topics are addressed in this chapter.

Sex Differentiation

Most psittacines are sexually monomorphic—the male and female are visually indistinguishable from each other. Although a few general characteristics may help the aviculturist guess a bird's sex, they are only indicators that are incapable of accurate sexual determination. Such indicators include the size of the head and beak, overall size of the bird, feather color, and aggressive behavior.

Sexual differentiation is paramount for successful psittacine aviculture because the first requirement for successful captive breeding is a heterosexual or true pair. Sexual differentiation is also important for the client who is struggling with his pet bird's identity—should "it" be named Jack or Jill? Whatever the reason, accurate sexual differentiation is important because the clinician is making a diagnosis when providing the veterinary service of sexing. Various options for sexing are now available, so the avian veterinarian can choose the method most suitable to the patient, the client, and the practice.

Visual Sexing

A handful of psittacine species are sexually dimorphic and can be definitively sexed by visual examination. These species include:

Eclectus parrot: Male is green and female is vibrant red and purple.

White-fronted Amazon parrot: Male has red versus green feathers on the upper wing coverts, the edge of the carpus, and the alula.

Pileated parrot: Males have red feathers on head; females have green.

Red-tailed black cockatoos: Females have spots on head, body, and wing feathers, and tail is barred with yellow-orange feathers. Males lack spots and the tail has red bars.

White-tailed black cockatoos: Females have white ear coverts and light horn-colored beak. Males have gray ear coverts and dark gray beaks.

Yellow-tailed black cockatoos: Females have white ear coverts and light, horn-colored beak. Males have gray ear coverts and dark gray beaks.

Gang–gang cockatoos: Males have red head and crest feathers; females are totally gray and barred with grayish white (Figure 8.1).

White cockatoos: In some of the white cockatoo species, iris color is reddish/light brown/tan or gold at maturity in females and dark brown to black in males.

Pesquet's parrot: Males have red feathers behind the eye, which are absent in females.

Australian king parrot: Males have scarlet red feathers on the head, neck, and underparts. Female has green feathers on the head and chest and red feathers on the lower abdomen. The beak is red-orange and black-tipped in the male and black in the female.

Vent Sexing

Vent sexing is an accurate sexing method for some avian species, such as the vasa parrot, poultry, waterfowl, ratites, and canaries during the breeding season.

Exotic Animal Medicine for the Veterinary Technician, Fourth Edition. Edited by Bonnie Ballard and Ryan Cheek.
© 2024 John Wiley & Sons, Inc. Published 2024 by John Wiley & Sons, Inc.
Companion Website: www.wiley.com/go/ballard/4e

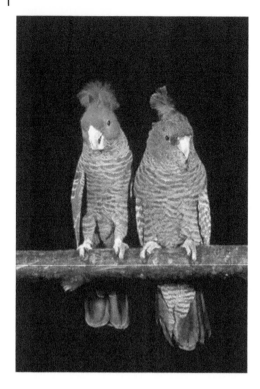

Figure 8.1 Pair of gang–gang cockatoos. Note the distinction between the male (left) and the female.

Surgical Sexing

Surgical sexing was first performed in the 1970s. The fasted bird is masked down with isoflurane. The endoscope is inserted through an incision in the left flank between the ribs and the femur. Typically, the caudal thoracic air sac is entered first; the lungs are straight ahead, the abdominal air sac is to the right, and the cranial thoracic air sac is to the left. The abdominal air sac is entered next, and the gonads are visualized and evaluated, sexing the bird immediately. A traditional protocol is to tattoo the ventral wing web of the sexed bird; males are tattooed on the right, and females on the left. Tattoos must be performed with the minimal amount of sterile ink, as wing webs are composed of thin sensitive tissues that can stricture, impeding flight permanently.

During surgical sexing, the abdominal air sac, kidneys, adrenals, spleen, and gastrointestinal tract are also examined. Organs visible through the caudal thoracic and cranial thoracic air sacs, including the proventriculus, liver, heart, and great vessels, should also be assessed. The main disadvantage of surgical sexing is the inherent, though minimal, surgical risk.

Feather Sexing

Feather sexing was first performed in the 1980s as a non-surgical alternative for sexing birds. Blood feathers are plucked and placed in media for overnight mailing to a cytogenetic laboratory. Chromosomal analysis is performed on cells cultured from the growing blood feathers.

Advantages of cytogenetics include complete karyotype evaluation and identification of chromosomal defects. Cytogenetic defects identified in psittacines include chromosomal inversions, chromosome translocations, triploidy, and ZZ ZW chimerism. These defects significantly reduce fertility. Disadvantages of feather sexing include a two-week turn-around time and the remote possibility of culture failure.

DNA or Blood Sexing

DNA or blood sexing tests, the newest means of non-surgical sex determination in avian medicine, became commercially available in the 1990s. This technique involves acquiring and submitting a very small amount of whole blood preserved in saline and EDTA or more recently simply blotted onto paper, to a DNA sexing laboratory. The DNA is run on an electrophoretic gel (Southern blot) and the resulting bands are probed and compared with male and female controls. The main disadvantages of blood or DNA sexing are the one-week turn-around time and the requirement of species-specific probes in some cases.

Reproduction

Female

In most avian species, the female reproductive tract consists of a left ovary and oviduct because the right side regresses before hatching. Exceptions include some raptors and the brown kiwi. In raptors, the right ovary and oviduct may be present and even active post-hatch. In the brown kiwi, both ovaries are active, but only the left oviduct receives the ovum by spanning the width of the celomic cavity with its fimbria.

The avian ovary is located at the cranial pole of the kidney and is flat and small in young birds and bumpy and large in mature birds. Normally it contains numerous follicles when active and it may be melanistic depending on the species. During lay, the left oviduct enlarges and occupies most of the left abdomen; in the nonbreeding season, it shrinks considerably in size.

The oviduct consists of five microscopically distinguishable regions: infundibulum, magnum, isthmus, uterus (shell gland), and vagina. Peristaltic activity moves the ovum down and the sperm up. The infundibulum has a funnel shape near the top. Fertilization occurs in the lower tubular part of the infundibulum as does the production of the chalaziferous layer of the albumen and the paired chalazae, which suspends the yolk at both ends of the egg.

In the magnum, the largest part of the oviduct, the egg takes on albumin, sodium, magnesium, and calcium. In the isthmus, it acquires the inner and outer shell membranes. The uterus, or shell gland, produces the egg's shell and its pigment. It also gives the egg salts and water. The vagina is the thickest portion of the oviduct and terminates in the cloaca.

Male

The male reproductive tract consists of paired "tic tac" shaped internal testes located ventral to and near the cranial border of the kidney and the abdominal air sac. Both testes are functional, although one may be larger than the other. Like the ovaries, the testes may be melanistic depending on the species. During the breeding season yellow testes may turn white and black-gray testes turn gray–white. Some species of birds have a phallus or phallus-like protrusion. These include the vasa parrots, various waterfowl, and ratites.

Reproductive Medicine and Surgery

Normal Oviposition

Oviposition includes the processes that occur when the egg is expelled from the body. The muscular uterus pushes the formed egg into the vagina. The bearing down reflex is started when the vagina "senses" the presence of the egg, forcing the egg into the cloaca and then out of the body.

The length of time for oviposition and the time of day, when oviposition occurs, is different between bird species. However, in most birds, the egg-laying interval ranges from 24 hours to 5 days. The brown kiwi lies at the opposite end of the spectrum with a laying interval up to 44 days.

Post-incubation and Hatching

At the end of incubation, the beak of the embryo breaks through the inner shell membrane into the air cell. The lungs start to work at this time. After several hours, the beak "pips" or cracks the outer shell membrane and shell to begin the active part of hatching.

Abnormal Oviposition or Dystocia

Some birds experience difficulty in laying eggs. Many of these birds are first-time layers. Others may be chronic egg layers. Avian species overrepresented as problem layers include budgerigars, cockatiels, cockatoos, and eclectus.

Amazon species may lay their first egg well into their prime and experience multiple problems as a result. Of key importance is that the presence of a male bird is often not required to stimulate egg-laying behavior in a female bird.

Improper diets, which tend to be low in calcium and other needed nutrients, are in part to blame for dystocia. Female birds that have been on all-seed diets, which are low in calcium and other needed vitamins and minerals, have the greatest risk of egg-laying difficulties. Inappropriate husbandry may also play a role, including the lack of a proper nesting area and proper temperature and humidity. The requirements vary between avian species. Some, such as cockatoos, may experience heightened reproductive behavior due to an inappropriate relationship with the human caretaker.

Signs of dystocia in a bird may include decreased or absent fecal production, watery or bloody droppings, anorexia, regurgitation, difficulty breathing, tail bobbing, fluffed feathers, swollen celomic (abdominal) area, abdominal straining, leg lameness, and sitting on the cage bottom. These signs occur for many reasons. The egg may put pressure on the gastrointestinal tract, preventing the passage of ingesta. This blockage may lead to regurgitation. Other times only liquid products may pass through, resulting in watery droppings.

A large egg may also put pressure on the air sacs, making it difficult for the bird to breathe. Likewise, pressure from the egg on the sciatic nerve unilaterally or bilaterally can cause lameness. Similar pressure on the kidneys may lead to life-threatening renal compromise. Abdominal straining may lead to prolapsed tissues, such as a prolapsed cloaca or prolapsed oviduct (Figure 8.2). Other signs seen in these patients may be due to general illness. A basic blood panel can provide the first step in determining the underlying health status of the patient.

Palpation of the abdominal area often reveals skin that is stretched and edematous. A firm egg-shaped swelling can usually be felt beneath. Care must be taken not to stress the patient and to avoid cracking what may be a fragile egg. Radiographs of the bird usually show the outline of an egg in the area of the pelvic canal (Figure 8.3). The egg may also be just cranial to the pelvis and unable to pass through the canal because it is very large. Sometimes the egg is soft-shelled and difficult to detect radiographically.

A bird in dystocia is considered a medical emergency as the patient may die while attempting to pass the egg. The mass effect of the egg impairs breathing and the pressure of the egg on the nerves and the vessels can cause serious neurologic and cardiovascular impairment. These patients usually require humidity and a warm incubator heated to 87–90 °F. The patient in respiratory distress also requires supplemental oxygen. Other medical treatments include

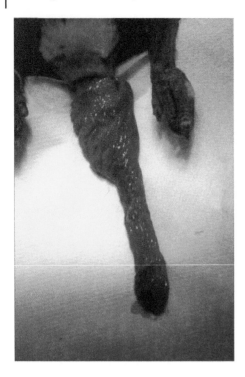

Figure 8.2 Parrot with prolapse of the oviduct.

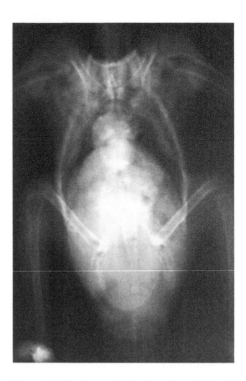

Figure 8.3 Radiograph showing dystocia in a bird. (Courtesy of Ryan Cheek, RVT).

nutritional supplementation, calcium supplementation, antibiotic medication, anti-inflammatory medication, and fluid therapy. Diagnostics are also necessary to properly treat these patients.

A patient who is early in the dystocia process may successfully pass the egg with this minimal supportive care. An egg that is close to passing, and already exteriorized, may also be lubricated with a water-based lubricant. Sometimes gentle massage of the area may assist with passage of the egg, but anesthesia is always highly recommended. More critical patients require faster intervention and possibly more invasive therapy under anesthesia. Large eggs that will not pass on their own may be pushed out under anesthesia after various treatments, including NSAIDs. Larger eggs may need to be collapsed after their contents are aspirated under anesthesia with a needle attached to a syringe. The needle is preferably inserted directly into the egg. This can occur once the egg is visualized within the vent, during celomic cavity exploratory surgery, or through the body wall as a last resort. The collapsed egg may be gently removed under anesthesia whole or carefully in pieces. Allowing a collapsed egg to pass on its own is never recommended and can lead to uterine rupture.

Other patients, particularly those suspected of having severely infected reproductive tracts, may require surgery to remove an egg that has formed adhesions with the

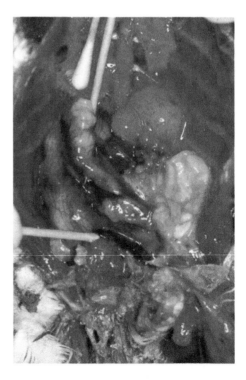

Figure 8.4 Egg yolk peritonitis in a parrot. Note the yellow-tinged coelomic cavity contents caused by a ruptured egg.

oviduct/uterus/vagina. One of the most challenging circumstances is a patient with soft-shelled eggs. Sometimes the back-up of soft-shelled eggs behind a calcified egg causes parts of the reproductive system to become necrotic. The breakdown of egg components and/or associated soft tissues often leads to egg yolk peritonitis, a severe inflammation of the celomic cavity (Figure 8.4). The risk of sepsis, or a systemic infection, is increased in these patients.

Care of the patient after treatment for dystocia is just as important. These birds may need additional supportive care to help them feel better prior to discharge from the hospital. In particular, a plan of action must be formulated for chronic egg layers to break the reproductive cycle. Some birds have experienced successful treatment with Cabergoline orally, Lupron injections or Suprelorin F (deslorelin acetate) implants. An avian veterinarian can help determine the best course of action for these birds. Surgery is also an option, where the oviduct is removed and the ovary remains. Modifications in diet, light cycle, and relationship with the human caretaker may also go a long way toward improving the bird's reproductive function.

Additional Reading

King AS, McLelland J. 1984. Female reproductive system. In: *Birds: Their Structure and Function*. Philadelphia: Baillière Tindall.

Romagnano A. 2012. Psittacine incubation and pediatrics. Special issue on Pediatrics of common and uncommon species (ed K Kuchinski Broome). *Vet Clin North Am Exot Anim Pract* 15(2): 163–182.

Romagnano A. 2005. Reproduction and pediatrics. In: *BSAVA Manual of Psittacine Birds* (ed N Harcourt-Brown), 2nd edn. BSAVA.

Section IV

Reptiles

9

Lizards

Stacey Leonatti Wilkinson and Brad Wilson

Introduction

From the seemingly impenetrable spines of *Moloch horridus*, the gliding pseudo-wings of *Draco* spp., the color-changing chromatophores of *Chamaeleo* spp., the cryptic cutaneous fimbriations of *Uroplatus* spp., the venomous bite of *Heloderma* spp., to the bipedal water-walking *Basiliscus* spp., the adhesive glass-climbing Gekkonidae, and the legless snake-like Anguinidae, lizards, of the order Squamata in the class Reptilia, exhibit tremendous anatomic, physiologic, nutritional, and behavioral variations that make them the hallmark of diversity among all modern reptiles. When distributed among 6,000 known species (www.reptile-database.org), it becomes obvious that the diagnostic challenge presented to the veterinary clinician and technician can be overwhelming (Figures 9.1–9.5).

Though the details may be overwhelming, differentiating lizards into some basic categories based on natural history leads to a basic understanding of their husbandry requirements. Technicians familiar with reptile medicine soon learn that many health disorders arise from improper husbandry; therefore, recognizing and correcting improper husbandry techniques may hasten the recovery from disease and prevent unnecessary medicating of debilitated patients.

Representatives of many families of lizards are commonly seen in the pet trade (Table 9.1). The bearded dragon (*Pogona vitticeps*) is the most popular of all reptile pets, replacing the green iguana (*Iguana iguana*) which historically had been the first reptile pet of many people new to the hobby of herpetoculture—the care and maintenance of captive reptiles and amphibians. In the past 30 years, the reptile pet industry has exponentially increased in popularity, and in recent years, the popularity of lizards has approached, if not exceeded, that of snakes as reptile pets. This leads to the question: why keep reptiles as pets? To the dedicated pet owner, the answer is

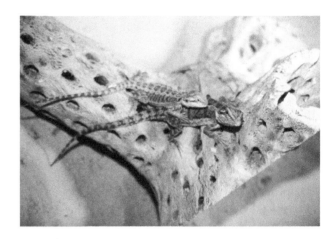

Figure 9.1 Bearded dragons. (Courtesy of Ryan Cheek).

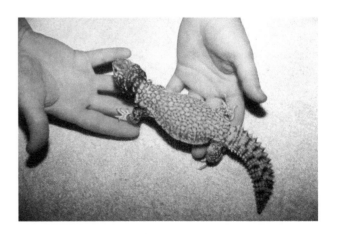

Figure 9.2 Mali uromastyx. (Courtesy of Ryan Cheek).

the same as if the question were about keeping a spider, fish, bird, cat, dog, goat, or horse as a pet. For avid reptile pet owners, however, a quote from de Vosjoli (1997) is most appropriate: "the current philosophy in herpetoculture strives towards establishing viable self-sustaining

Exotic Animal Medicine for the Veterinary Technician, Fourth Edition. Edited by Bonnie Ballard and Ryan Cheek.
© 2024 John Wiley & Sons, Inc. Published 2024 by John Wiley & Sons, Inc.
Companion Website: www.wiley.com/go/ballard/4e

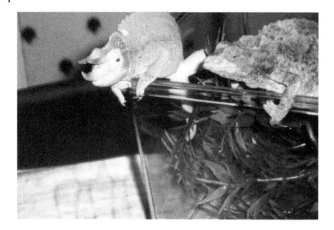

Figure 9.3 Jackson chameleons. The one on the left is a male, and the one on the right is a female. (Courtesy of Dr. Sam Rivera).

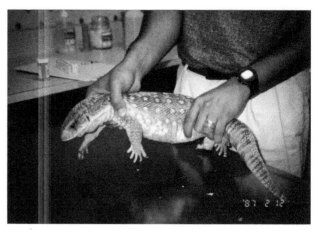

Figure 9.5 Savannah monitor. (Courtesy of Dr. Sam Rivera).

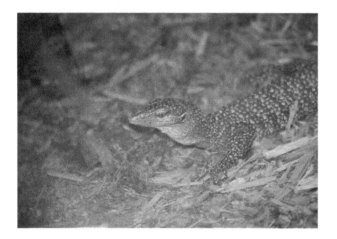

Figure 9.4 Mangrove monitor. (Courtesy of Ryan Cheek).

captive-breeding populations through managed field culture and/or through more controlled systems of indoor and outdoor vivaria."

Anatomy and Physiology

Integument

Lizard scales commonly overlap and are created by a many-layered epidermis that is shed at regular intervals during the life of the lizard. The shedding of skin, ecdysis, occurs in multiple pieces in lizards, as opposed to snakes, in which the skin is usually shed in one piece. Many lizard species eat the shed skin. Factors that influence ecdysis are age, growth rate, temperature, humidity, and nutrition (Barten and Simpson 2019). Dysecdysis is commonly associated with low humidity and poor nutrition among other health abnormalities.

Reptilian epidermis does not have a respiratory function and contains very few glands (Barten and Simpson 2019). The skin and scales are relatively impermeable in normal health. The mucous membranes (oral cavity, cloaca, and conjunctiva) are quite permeable, however. This consideration is important when considering potential absorption of topical medications applied to these regions (Barten and Simpson 2019, Perry and Mitchell 2019). Some reptile vitamin supplements are marketed as sprays to be applied to the skin. These products, though not likely harmful, have little to no systemic physiologic value to reptiles.

Chamaeleo spp. and *Anolis* spp. have chromatophores in the skin that allow change in the reflectivity of visible light, resulting in color change. These changes are influenced by light, heat, and social factors, but not by surrounding environmental color (Barten and Simpson 2019). Many herpetoculturists who raise chameleons can predict color changes of particular species or individuals based on a variety of environmental or behavioral influences.

Some gecko species can autotomize, tear, or release the entire skin in response to capture by a predator. These species include the fish-scale geckos (*Geckolepis* spp.) and the day geckos (*Phelsuma* spp.) (Glaw & Vences 1994, McKeown 1993). Skin regeneration occurs in these species but may result in unsightly scars and secondary bacterial or fungal infections.

Foot and toe adaptations are diverse. Integument specialization is quite notable in the fan-like adhesive disks of Gekkonidae. These species are capable of climbing glass and inverted smooth surfaces. Large arboreal and terrestrial lizards usually possess sharp sturdy claws. Lizard claws are similar to those of birds; they have a pulp containing a blood vessel and nerve that is sensitive to short trimming.

Table 9.1 Lizards commonly seen in captivity.

Common name, species name	Origin	Habitat	Size (cm)[a]	Temp. (d/n)[b]	Reproduction[c]	Feed[d]	Rest[e]	Handling concerns[f]
Agamidae								
Agamas, *Agama* spp.[j]	Africa	Arid, desert, terrestrial	30–40	30°C/20°C	Oviparous	O/a	Yes, no	Occasionally aggressive, sturdy
Bearded dragon, *Pogona* spp.[j,p]	Australia	Arid, terrestrial	to 50	30°C/20°C	Oviparous	O/a	Yes	Docile, sturdy
Frilled lizard, *Chlamydosaurus kingii*[j,p]	Australia	Dry, forest, terrestrial	to 100	30° C/20° C	Oviparous	C/a,v	Yes	Occasionally aggressive, sturdy
Water dragon, *Physignathus cocincinus*[j]	SE Asia	Humid, rainforest, arboreal	100	26°C/20°C	Oviparous	O/a,v,n	No	Occasionally aggressive, sturdy
Uromastyx, *Uromastyx* Spp.[l]	NW Africa, SW Asia	Arid, desert, terrestrial	30–50	37°C/22°C	Oviparous	H,O/a	Yes	Docile, sturdy
Anguidae								
Glass lizards, *Ophisaurus* spp.[j]	Worldwide	Dry, rocky forest, terrestrial	to 140	26°C/20°C	Oviparous	C/a,g	Yes	Docile, fragile, tail autotomy+
Chamaeleontidae								
Veiled chameleon, *Chamaeleo calyptratus*[m]	E Africa	Montane forest, arboreal	50	30°C/20°C	Oviparous	I	No	Docile, fragile to sturdy
Flapneck chameleon, *Chamaeleo dilepis*[j,n]	Africa	Tropical savannah, arboreal	30	30°C/20°C	Oviparous	I	No	Docile, fragile to sturdy
Three-horned Chamaeleon, *Ch. jacksonii*[m]	E Africa	Montane forest, arboreal	30	25°C/20°C	Viviparous	I	No	Docile, fragile to sturdy
Panther chameleon, *Chamaeleo pardalis*[m]	Madagascar	Coastal forest, arboreal	60	30°C/20°C	Oviparous	I	No	Occasionally aggressive, sturdy
Gekkonidae								
Day geckos, *Phelsuma* spp.[h]	Indian Ocean islands	Tropical rainforest, arboreal	to 25	30°C/25°C	Oviparous	O/a,n	No	Docile, tail autotomy, skin slough
Crested gecko, *Correlophus ciliatus*	New Caledonia	Temperate rainforest, arboreal	to 15	26°C/22°C	Oviparous	O/n,a	No	Docile, tail autotomy
Leaf-tailed geckos, *Uroplatus* spp.[f,j,n]	Madagascar	Tropical rainforest, arboreal	to 25	28°C/22°°C	Oviparous	I	No	Docile, fragile, tail autotomy+

(*continued*)

Table 9.1 (Continued)

Common name, species name	Origin	Habitat	Size (cm)[a]	Temp. (d/n)[b]	Reproduction[c]	Feed[d]	Rest[e]	Handling concerns[f]
Leopard gecko, *Eublepharis macularius*[i]	Asia	Desert, terrestrial	to 20	30°C/25°C	Oviparous	I	Yes	Occasionally aggressive, tail autotomy[+]
Tokay gecko, *Gekko gecko*[j]	SE Asia	Tropical rainforest, arboreal	to 30	27°C/20°C	Oviparous	C/a,v	No	Aggressive, sturdy
Iguanidae								
Green anole, *Anolis carolinensis*[j]	N America	Temperate forest, arboreal	20	26°C/20°C	Oviparous	I	Yes	Docile, tail autotomy
Green iguana, *Iguana iguana*[g]	Central, S America	Tropical rainforest, arboreal	200	31°C/22°C	Oviparous	H	Yes	Very aggressive, tail autotomy
Horned lizards, *Phrynosoma* spp.[j]	Central, N America	Arid, desert, savannah, terrestrial	to 20	35°C/20°C	Viviparous, oviparous	I/t	Yes	Docile, sturdy
Spiny lizards, *Sceloporus* spp.[j,n]	N, S, Central America	Dry, rocky, forest, arboreal/terrestrial	to 30	26°C/20°C	Viviparous, oviparous	I	Yes	Docile, sturdy
Lacertidae								
Jeweled lizards, *Lacerta* spp.[j]	Europe, Africa	Dry, forest, arboreal/terrestrial	to 40	25°C/15°C	Viviparous, oviparous	O/a,n	Yes	Occasionally aggressive, sturdy
Scincidae Skinks, *Eumeces* spp.[j]	Worldwide	Forest, terrestrial, occasionally arboreal	to 30	26°C/20°C	Viviparous, oviparous	I	Yes	Docile, tail autotomy
Blue-tongued skinks, *Tiliqua* spp.[j,n]	Australia	Forest, desert, terrestrial	to 50	30°C/20°C	Viviparous	O/a,g	Yes	Docile, sturdy
Prehensile-tailed skink, *Corucia zebrata*[o]	Solomon Islands	Tropical forest, arboreal	to 60	30°C/24°C	Viviparous	H	Yes	Occasionally aggressive, sturdy
Teiidae								
Ameivas, *Ameiva* spp.[j]	Central, S America	Forest, fields, terrestrial	to 50	26°C/20°C	Oviparous	O/a,n	Yes	Docile, sturdy
Tegus, *Tupinambis* spp.[j,k]	S America	Forests, terrestrial	to 140	30°C/20°C	Oviparous	C/a,v,e	Yes	Occasionally aggressive sturdy
Varanidae								
Nile monitor, *Varanus niloticus*[k]	Africa	Stream, riverbank, terrestrial	to 200	30°C/20°C	Oviparous	C/e,g,v	Yes	Very aggressive, sturdy

Table 9.1 (Continued)

Common name, species name	Origin	Habitat	Size (cm)[a]	Temp. (d/n)[b]	Reproduction[c]	Feed[d]	Rest[e]	Handling concerns[f]
Savannah monitor, *V. exanthematicus*[k]	Africa	Desert, dry grassland, terrestrial	to 100	30° C/20°C	Oviparous	C/a,g,e,v	Yes	Occasionally aggressive, sturdy

a) Average maximum adult size.
b) Average day and night temperatures for adults of species or typical of genus.
c) Oviparous = egg laying; viviparous = live birth.
d) Diet of the adult lizard *in nature*: O = omnivore, I = exclusive insectivore, C = primary carnivore, H = exclusive herbivore, H,O = some spp. exclusively herbivorous, some spp. omnivorous. Specializations or primary food consumed listed in order of importance for each species: a = arthropods, e = eggs, g = gastropods, n = nectar or ripe fruit, t = termites and ants, v = vertebrates.
e) Does lizard seasonally hibernate or brumate? Yes = successful captive breeding may require cooling/rest period. No = successful breeding does not require cooling/rest period.
f) Typical response of patient to handling:
   Docile: lizards will allow handling with minimal resistance.
   Occasionally aggressive: lizards may attempt to bite or claw when handled and can inflict injury upon handler.
   Aggressive: lizards will routinely bite, claw, or struggle during or before handling. The Tokay gecko is not particularly dangerous to handle, but is aggressive.
   Very aggressive: lizards may bite, scratch, or whip tail *prior* to handling. Large monitors and iguanas should be considered dangerous at all times and handled only by experienced staff.
   Sturdy: little to no stress or trauma results from routine handling when healthy.
   Fragile: may stress easily when handled for routine examination. Bodily injury to lizard may result from routine restraint or handling.
   Tail autotomy: lizards may lose tail when handled (not all spp. capable of autotomy are marked). [+]Tail autotomy in some species may occur even if lizard is not handled, but merely stressed.
   Skin slough: lizards with skin that tears easily when minimally restrained or touched.
g) de Vosjoli (1992).
h) McKeown (1993).
i) de Vosjoli et al. (1997).
j) Obst et al. (1989).
k) Balsai (1997).
l) de Vosjoli (1995).
m) de Vosjoli & Ferguson (1995).
n) de Vosjoli (1997).
o) de Vosjoli (1993).
p) de Vosjoli et al. (2001).

Skeletal System

The general lizard skeletal system is quadruped consisting of an ossified skull, vertebral column, ribs, and pelvic and pectoral girdles (Figure 9.6). The ribs of lizards connect ventrally to a cartilaginous sternum, which is absent in snakes and turtles (Barten and Simpson 2019). Lizard teeth are either acrodont or pleurodont. Acrodont teeth attach to the masticating surface of the mandible or maxilla and have no socket. These teeth are not replaced when lost and are characteristic of true chameleons and agamids. Pleurodont teeth are attached to the inner or lingual surface of the mandible or maxilla and have no socket. These teeth are replaced throughout the life of the lizard and are characteristic of iguanas and monitors.

Locomotion for lizards is apodal, bipedal, or quadrupedal. Most lizards have four legs and five toes on each leg, though there are species that are snake-like with no functional legs (*Anguis* spp., *Anniella* spp., *Lialis* spp., *Ophisaurus* spp.) and others with greatly reduced limbs (*Chalcides chalcides, Neoseps reynoldsi, Chamaesaura* spp.). Bipedal locomotion is observed in basilisks (*Basiliscus* spp.) and frilled dragons (*Chlamydosaurus kingii*) when excited or during escape behavior. This behavior is rarely observed in small enclosures. Old-world chameleons (*Chamaeleo* spp.) are zygodactylous, having two toes and three toes fused into a claw-like foot, creating a strong gripping foot for climbing on limbs and branches (Barten and Simpson 2019).

Tail autotomy, the loss or release of the tail, occurs in many species (Iguanidae, Gekkonidae, and some Scincidae). This adaptation (coupled with certain behaviors) creates distraction and allows the tailless lizard to escape as a potential predator investigates the released yet still-moving tail. Transverse cleavage plates are present in each caudal vertebra of these species, allowing release of

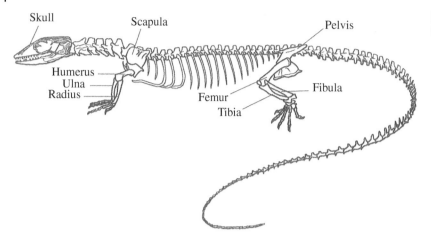

Skull   Scapula   Pelvis

Humerus
Ulna
Radius   Femur   Fibula
Tibia

Figure 9.6 Lizard skeletal anatomy. (Drawing by Scott Stark).

the tail at multiple locations (Barten and Simpson 2019). Hemorrhage is minimal with tail loss because vertebral vessels are quick to constrict. If the tail stump is undamaged, species capable of autotomy can usually regenerate tails that are usually smaller with irregular scalation and darker color than the original tail. However, crested geckos (*Correlophus ciliatus*) and other *Rhacodactylus* spp. cannot regenerate a tail if lost. If species that are not capable of autotomy (Chamaeleontidae, Varanidae) suffer traumatic tail loss, the tail cannot regenerate. Some lizards (some Chamaeleontidae and *Corucia zebrata*) use a prehensile tail for stabilization or movement between branches.

It is important to note that touching or manipulating the tail is not necessary to cause its release in some species. The leaf-tailed geckos, *Uroplatus* spp., can only autotomize the entire tail from the first one or two caudal vertebrae so the entire tail is always lost (Glaw & Vences 1994). A common escape behavior in these species is to wave the tail to distract the potential predator and then release it from the body without the lizard being touched or manipulated. Similar behavior can occur in the terrestrial leopard and African fat-tailed geckos (*Eublepharis macularius, Hemitheconyx caudicinctus*), along with the crested gecko and other *Rhacodactylus* spp. (Barten and Simpson 2019, de Vosjoli 1997).

Cardiovascular System

The heart has three chambers consisting of two atria and one ventricle. Despite the absence of an interventricular septum, the majority of deoxygenated blood is directed to the lungs via the pulmonary aorta, and oxygenated blood is directed to the right and left aortic arches to perfuse the body tissues (Barten and Simpson, 2019).

Lizards, like amphibians, possess a large ventral abdominal vein that is intracoelomic along the ventral midline

several millimeters dorsal to the body wall. This vein is secured by a thin mesovasorum and travels adjacent to the ventral midline from one-fourth the distance from the cranial aspect of the pubis cranially to the umbilicus and then courses dorsally to join the hepatic vein. Venous collateral circulation parallels the ventral abdominal vein via the caudal vena cava. The ventral abdominal vein is routinely avoided during coelomic surgery, though accidental or intentional transection and ligation of this vessel are compensated by collateral circulation (Mader 2002).

The caudal tail vein is the optimal site for blood collection from lizards. It is located along the ventral midline of the tail and is accessed approximately one-third (or less) the distance from the cloaca to the tail tip.

Respiratory System

The respiratory system of lizards consists of external nares, internal nares, glottis, trachea, and lungs. The internal nares are located rostrally in the dorsal oral cavity and are contiguous with the external nares. Some species, such as Iguanidae, have salt glands inside the nares which excrete excessive salt, sneezing it out the nose. The glottis, located at the base of the tongue, fits into the common opening of the internal nares when the mouth is closed to enable nasal respiration.

The trachea of most lizards bifurcates into the lungs, which in some lizards may more resemble air sacs of birds than the familiar mammalian lung. Lizards do not have a diaphragm and therefore have a common coelomic cavity rather than separate thoracic and abdominal cavities. Ventilation in lizards is accomplished with rib expansion by contraction of intercostal muscles.

The lungs of lizards are not as highly derived as those of mammals. The cranial portions of the lungs are more vascular and serve for most respiratory functions whereas the caudal lungs are more sac-like and may extend to the pelvis (Barten and Simpson 2019, Knotek and Divers 2019). Unlike birds, lizards do not have pneumatic bones.

Digestive System

The digestive system of most lizards is quite basic and, with the exception of the teeth, follows the design of higher vertebrates. The oral cavity contains several glands that aid in the lubrication of food items for swallowing. The Gila monster and Mexican beaded lizard (*Heloderma suspectum*, *H. horridum*) have modified bilateral sublingual glands that produce venom that is chewed into the prey item rather than hypodermically injected as with venomous snakes (Barten and Simpson 2019).

The tongue of some lizards serves in both scent collection and swallowing. The tongue of anguimorph (legless) lizards serves almost exclusively a sensory function, and the tongue of some Chamaeleontidae serves an exclusive food prehension and swallowing function (Barten and Simpson 2019). Most carnivorous lizards (Varanidae) have snake-like tongues to track prey items, and the majority of herbivorous lizards have thick fleshy tongues to aid in swallowing. The sensory tongue retracts into a lingual sheath that lies ventral to the glottis.

The alimentary tract consists of an esophagus, stomach, small and large intestine, and cloaca. The alimentary, respiratory, reproductive, cardiovascular, and reproductive tracts are not separated by a diaphragm and are contained within a pleuroperitoneum or coelomic cavity (coelom). The proximal portion of the esophagus is the only opening to the back of the oral cavity. Thus, by visualizing and avoiding the opening to the glottis on the floor of the mouth, feeding or sampling tubes may be safely passed into the digestive tract with no risk of accidental respiratory intubation. The stomach in most lizards is quite large and does not serve as a gizzard or grinding organ (Barten and Simpson 2019). The small intestine has histologically discrete duodenum, jejunum, and ileum (Barten and Simpson 2019). A cecum-like sacculation of the colon is present in herbivorous lizards (*Corucia zebrata*, *Iguana* spp., *Uromastyx* spp., and others). The cloaca is the common collecting chamber of the digestive and genitourinary tracts. These openings are the coprodeum and urodeum, respectively. The proctodeum is the common chamber opening to the vent. (Figures 9.7 and 9.8).

The liver and gall bladder are present in lizards and located cranial to the stomach in the cranio-ventral abdomen. The liver has a right and left lobe. The gall bladder in anguimorph lizards is observed in a more caudal position and is usually found in close proximity to the

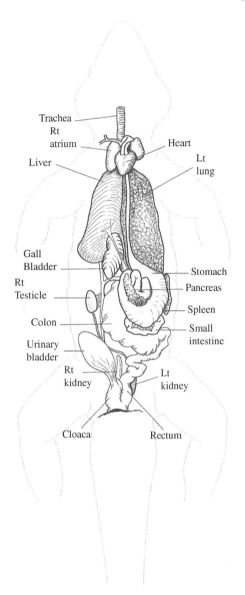

Figure 9.7 Lizard visceral anatomy. (Drawing by Scott Stark).

pancreas, as seen in snakes. The pancreas in lizards has both endocrine and exocrine glandular functions.

Large, paired fat bodies in the left and right caudal coelomic cavity are not digestive structures but may be commonly confused with pathologic lesions. These are particularly palpable in bearded dragons and are commonly observed in dorsoventral radiographs.

Excretory System

Paired kidneys are located in the caudal coelom and in most lizard species the kidneys are completely within the pelvic canal. Lizards are uricotelic; the majority of nitrogenous waste from purine digestion is excreted from most lizards as insoluble uric acid (Barten and Simpson 2019).

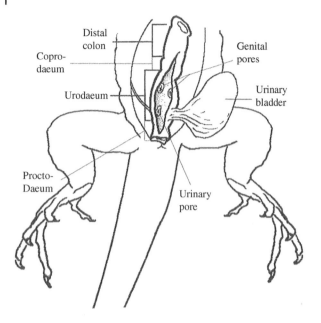

Figure 9.8 Lizard cloaca. (Drawing by Scott Stark).

A mesonephric duct collects and transports nitrogenous wastes from each kidney to a urinary bladder, in species where a urinary bladder is present. The urinary bladder empties into the cranio–ventral urodeum. In larger lizards, the urinary bladder may be catheterized from the cloaca via this opening. Species lacking a urinary bladder include the bearded dragon (*Pogona vitticeps*), some agamids, some varanids, some *Crotophytus* and *Scleroporus* spp., teids, and some geckos (Barten and Simpson 2019).

The renal portal system in reptiles is well documented (Barten and Simpson 2019; Divers and Innis 2019, Holz et al. 1997). The system allows blood to flow from the caudal portion of the body directly to the kidneys prior to returning to the heart. Historically, this physiology led to the conclusion that the reptile kidney may reduce the concentration of chemotherapeutics injected into the caudal body prior to their entry into the general circulation, thus leading to a decreased concentration in the blood and tissues. Also, suspicion was raised that injections of potentially nephrotoxic drugs should be avoided in the region. Several pharmacologic studies in turtles have revealed that the presence of this system does not necessarily indicate that all blood flow follows this theorized pathway and there may be no impact on drug metabolism when injected into the caudal body of tortoises (Divers and Innis 2019, Holz et al. 1997, Perry & Mitchell 2019). Pharmacokinetic studies have shown that some medications have variable levels of absorption whether they are given in the cranial or caudal half of the body. In most cases, these effects are not clinically significant, though there are some anesthetics that produce greater sedative effects when given in the cranial half of the body; this seems to be due more in part to the hepatic portal system than the renal portal system (Fink et al. 2018). Even though with most drugs, there is no significant difference, it remains common practice to avoid injections in the caudal half of the body for medications with possible renal side effects (e.g., aminoglycosides) (Divers 2019, Perry & Mitchell 2019, Holz et al. 1997).

Reproductive System

Lizards have intracoelomic paired testes or ovaries, and oviducts. Female lizards have no true uterus, but in live-bearing (ovoviviparous or viviparous) lizards, the oviduct may serve a similar function to the non-placental uterus of mammals by providing nutrients for the developing non-shelled embryo (Stahl and DeNardo 2019). The term "ovoviviparous" has become obsolete (Stahl and DeNardo 2019). The eggshell is secreted in the oviduct of oviparous lizards in an area called the "shell gland." The eggshell of many lizards (except Gekkonidae) is somewhat pliable, as seen in snakes, rather than rigid, as seen in tortoises and birds.

Male lizards have paired hemipenes that are invaginated into the proximal ventral tail slightly lateral and caudal to the vent. During mating, one hemipenis is everted by relaxation of the retractor muscle and the filling of vascular spaces of the hemipenes with blood. Following mating, fertilization is internal and occurs within the oviduct. No urinary structures are present within the hemipenes of lizards.

Sexual dimorphism occurs in some species of lizards, while in others determining sex may be difficult. For most juvenile lizards of all species, there is no reliable method to determine sex. For adult lizards, the technique of sex determination is determined by species.

External sex characteristics may be applied to many lizards. These characteristics include the presence of obvious sexual dimorphism such as the horns of *Chamaeleo jacksonii*, precloacal pores of many Gekkonidae, femoral pores of many Iguanidae and Agamidae, and post-cloacal tail bulging of the hemipenes in many species. Many species of male lizards have larger heads and jowls than females. Researching the anatomy of the species in question is the best method to determine if external sex characteristics are applicable.

Cloacal probing, the primary technique used in sex determination of snakes, may be applied to some lizards but is not 100% accurate in all species. A blunt or ball-tipped smooth metal sexing probe designed exclusively for this purpose is used. The only other acceptable instrument may be a sovereign red rubber urinary catheter or feeding tube. This procedure carries the risk of causing trauma to the patient; therefore, proper restraint and proficiency are required. The probe is inserted into the vent and directed caudally just lateral to the ventral midline in a position parallel to the surface of the tail. In males, the probe enters the inverted sheath of the hemipenis and travels a distance into the tail. This distance is subjective and variable by species. In some female lizards, the distance the probe travels is shorter when compared to the male.

Radiographic sex determination is possible in some monitors. This technique is based on the presence of calcifications in the hemipenes of some species (Barten and Simpson 2019). These mineralizations are absent in males of both Nile and savannah monitors. Contrast radiography has been employed in skinks to determine sex by infusing contrast material into the hemipenal canals (McKenzie et al. 2022). Ultrasound can also be used to identify ovaries or testes with greater success during the species' natural breeding season.

Surgical or endoscopic sex determination is obviously definitive. Surgical scar tissue formation, difficult visualization, and availability of equipment are potential complications. Anesthesia is required for either procedure.

Manual and hydrostatic eversion of the hemipenes are possible techniques but are not recommended. Both techniques can have serious complications if performed improperly, and since other techniques are available these are no longer recommended. Manual eversion is more common in neonate snakes.

Nervous System

The central nervous system consists of a cerebrum, cerebellum, brainstem, and spinal cord. The spinal cord extends to the tip of the tail as opposed to mammals, in which the cord terminates proximal to the sacral vertebrae. The peripheral nervous system consists of 12 cranial nerves and numerous peripheral nerves to the viscera, trunk, and limbs.

Pain receptors and pain responses in reptiles are still poorly understood (Sladky and Mans 2019). It is apparent that lizards have a withdrawal response or reflex from traumatic wounds such as punctures, lacerations, or surgical incisions; however, expected withdrawal reflexes and responses from potentially traumatic heat are not observed (Sladky and Mans 2019). Captive management of lizards must take into account these apparent behavioral and/or neurologic reflex differences from mammals with regard to cage heating (see section on "Husbandry").

Sense Organs

The majority of lizards have movable eyelids and a nictitating membrane. Those without movable lids (some Gekkonidae, and *Ablepharus* spp.) have a clear spectacle as seen in snakes. The spectacle is a scale-like structure formed by the fusion of the upper and lower eyelids. As with snakes, the spectacle is impermeable to topical medications. True chameleons possess turret-like eyelids and eyes that are capable of independent movement. Glands are present in the eyelids of lizards and may become swollen in cases of hypovitaminosis A.

The muscles of the iris are striated and under conscious control; thus, pupillary light reflexes are not predictable and the use of standard mammalian mydriatics is not possible (Barten and Simpson 2019). The pupil may be circular or elliptical.

The parietal eye, or "third eye," is apparent in some species (Iguanidae, Agamidae, tuatara [*Sphenodon punctatus*]). This structure is located on the dorsal head and is connected via the parietal nerve to the pineal body in the brain. The parietal eye is a photoreceptor that is integral in hormonal production and thermoregulatory behavior (Barten and Simpson 2019).

The lizard ear consists of an external acoustic meatus, tympanic membrane, middle ear cavity, and inner ear cavity. Within the middle ear cavity is the columella bone, which receives vibrations from the tympanic membrane via the extracolumellar cartilage (Barten and Simpson 2019). The tympanic membrane of some lizard species is clear and in others it is covered with scales and not visible.

The vomeronasal organ, or Jacobson's organ, is present in many lizards and located in the dorsal oral cavity ventral to the nasal cavity but not continuous with the nasal cavity (Barten and Simpson 2019). Scent particles collected on the tongue are transferred to sensory cells when the tongue is retracted into the mouth. This organ is primarily used by lizards to track prey items and possibly to detect mates or enemies by detecting pheromones.

Husbandry

Understanding the natural history (anatomy, physiology, habitat requirements, reproductive habits, behavior, longevity, etc.) of the patient in question is the greatest diagnostic tool in differentiating between normal health and disease. Combining this knowledge with the presenting complaint, medical history, physical examination, and laboratory data is necessary for the treatment and rehabilitation of the diseased patient. For instance, understanding the differences in dietary and habitat requirements of two common similarly sized lizard pets, the green iguana (*Iguana iguana*) and savannah monitor (*Varanus exanthematicus*), is essential even to obtain an appropriate history. It is not possible for even the most educated zookeeper to know every aspect of natural history of every lizard, nor is it expected that the veterinary technician can become educated in the feeding habits of every species of lizard kept in captivity. There are, however, several fundamental aspects of knowledge regarding lizards with which to simplify the approach to understanding natural history. There is an excellent discussion of current recommended husbandry practices for common species in Rossi (2019).

The following are general categories and associated specific questions with which the technician and practitioner should be familiar regarding every lizard patient:

Native habitat and microhabitat: Does the patient inhabit tropical rainforest, desert, mountain slope, estuary, beach, and so forth? Is the patient arboreal, terrestrial, aquatic, or subterranean?

Anatomy and physiology: What is normal coloration and can the patient change coloration in response to environmental, seasonal, health, reproductive, or behavioral influences? Are there size or other physical differences based on sex? What is the normal mucous membrane color? Does the patient normally have four limbs and a certain number of digits? Does the patient normally have secretions from the eyes or nostrils? What are the characteristics of normal feces and urates? How long does the patient normally live?

Diet: Is the patient insectivorous, carnivorous, herbivorous, or omnivorous, and does the diet change with respect to life stage or seasonality? If insectivorous, does the patient have a preferred food item or size of food item (ants, centipedes, spiders, etc.)? How does the patient prehend food and at what time of day does it normally feed? How does the patient normally obtain water?

Behavior: Is the patient diurnal, nocturnal, or crepuscular? Is the patient solitary or communal? Does the patient experience climatic seasonality? Does the patient hibernate or estivate? Does the patient use different microhabitats during different seasons or life stages? How does the patient reproduce and how often?

These natural history parameters for all species of lizards would require volumes to list and these are questions to which the technician or veterinarian may not always know the answer. There are many similarities among genera, but even within the same genus there are marked differences between species in husbandry requirements.

Looking again at the green iguana and the savannah monitor: the green iguana is a tropical, arboreal, diurnal, somewhat communal (though not in captivity), generally non-seasonal, and non-hibernating lizard (de Vosjoli 1992; Obst et al. 1989), whereas the savannah monitor is a temperate, semi-arid, terrestrial (and burrowing), crepuscular (to diurnal), solitary, somewhat seasonal, and occasionally

hibernating lizard (Balsai 1997; Obst et al. 1989). The diet of green iguanas is herbivorous, though as with other species, in their native habitat they may be opportunistically insectivorous. For the savannah monitor, the diet is carnivorous or insectivorous (depending on the life stage and food availability). Remember, however, that one can only speak of living systems in generalities; adaptation is the key to survival, and many captive lizards "adapt" to the captive environment. Thus, behavior observed in nature may not occur in captivity.

Reptile hobbyists who pride themselves on maintaining and breeding common and rare lizards in captivity have learned that recreating the native environment in almost every aspect is the key to success. These achievements are accomplished by observing the animals in their native habitat, corresponding with other hobbyists or zoologic professionals, and logging countless hours of trial and error. Occasionally substantial investment is made in the construction of suitable habitats that far exceeds the monetary value of the lizard in question.

Enclosures and Environment

Cages

There is no way to generalize a basic lizard cage. There are, however, categories of habitats from which the foundation for housing most species can be derived. In general terms, lizards are categorized as arboreal or terrestrial. Remember that some arboreal lizards are occasionally both terrestrial and arboreal. Therefore, suitable cage design may not be exclusive for either habitat. Native habitat use is listed in Table 9.1 for common species. Key requirements for all enclosures include security from escape, protection from injury, access for cleaning, and environmental control of light, heat, humidity, ventilation, and water and food availability.

True chameleons (*Chamaeleo* spp.) and day geckos (*Phelsuma* spp.) are good examples of primarily arboreal lizards. Though these species vary greatly in size and in microhabitat distribution, most species benefit from a vertically spacious cage that offers visual security on three sides and from above. Typically, enclosures for arboreal lizards contain numerous limbs, branches, or plants in both a vertical and horizontal orientation. The cage is typically rectangular and may range from $0.3 \times 0.3 \times 0.5\,m$ to $1 \times 1 \times 2\,m$. The primary, if not exclusive, construction material should be plastic screen with metal or plastic frame for chameleons and a glass or plastic aquarium for geckos. Screen allows for good ventilation and is relatively non-abrasive to the lizard. Wire mesh can lead to skin abrasions and may be more difficult to clean. Glass or plastic (e.g., Plexiglass) offers no ventilation and may lead to overheating but allows for maintenance of higher humidity. The cage floor may be solid (wood, glass, or plastic) or mesh. Though a mesh floor with removable tray beneath may be most accessible for cleaning, it potentially allows escape of insect food items or may cause injury to the lizard. A solid floor with removable indoor/outdoor carpet is relatively easy to clean and provides security for chameleons. A well-sealed cage and lid are required for geckos because they are masters of escape. The cage ceiling is typically screen for both chameleons and geckos to allow adequate ventilation and humidity control (Figure 9.9).

Substrate for chameleons should be simple: newspaper or indoor/outdoor carpet is best. Soils, mulches, and shavings are messy and not essential for housing chameleons. Glass enclosures for arboreal lizards requiring higher humidity, such as day geckos, may contain soil in which plants are grown. The great majority of arboreal captive lizards do not use the substrate except to oviposit, and this substrate may be provided in the form of a nesting box or potted plant when required. Though aesthetically pleasing, particulate substrates such as soil, sand, gravel, and wood chips pose a great risk to small (<20 cm) lizards because accidental ingestion may result in gastric or intestinal obstruction or impaction.

The leopard gecko (*Eublepharis macularius*) and the savannah monitor (*Varanus exanthematicus*) are good examples of primarily terrestrial lizards. As opposed to the arboreal cage design, terrestrial enclosures are horizontally spacious to accommodate a large cage floor and may contain one or several diagonal or horizontal perches of relatively large diameter. Smaller cages range from $0.2 \times 0.3 \times 0.5$ m to many meters in length, width, and height. Because many terrestrial lizards are relatively strong, more durable construction materials may be required for cage design. Though the glass aquarium is the standard enclosure for most small terrestrial lizards, it is more difficult to maintain heat and humidity in glass enclosures with a screen top. Enclosures that are solid on all sides and open in the front with slots for ventilation are often easier for keepers to maintain properly. Larger lizards, such as monitors, commonly require custom-built enclosures made from wood, glass or plastic, or wire mesh. Commonly these larger lizards are housed in outdoor enclosures where climates are favorable (Figures 9.10 and 9.11).

Lighting
Lighting requirements vary greatly among species. Some lizards require ultraviolet light (specifically UVB) for vitamin D_3 (cholecalciferol) synthesis and subsequent calcium absorption from the gastrointestinal tract (Baines and Cusack 2019, Boyer and Scott 2019, Raiti 2019) UVB

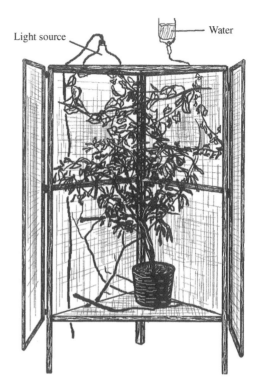

Figure 9.9 Arboreal habitat. (Drawing by Scott Stark).

should be provided for all lizards, but the type of bulb, output, distance to the bulb, hours of exposure daily, etc. may vary between species. Many lizard owners provide artificial lighting in the form of various incandescent and fluorescent fixtures.

Additionally, for some species of lizards, UVA radiation is considered part of the visual spectrum and may impact environmental and social interactions and behaviors. The addition of full-spectrum lighting to enclosures may be required for some species to thrive in captivity. UVA will be provided by most lamps used for heat as well.

A common historical notion is that primarily nocturnal species do not require UVB radiation. This is likely incorrect, in spite of continued promotion of this information throughout the pet industry. Field observations and UVB measurements in highly shaded areas of forest reveal that low levels of UVB radiation (1 to $2\,\mu W/cm^2$) penetrate all areas where visible light is observed (Baines and Cusack 2019, B. Wilson, personal observation). Additionally, some species of lizard are capable of synthesizing vitamin D_3 with very low levels of UVB exposure (Carman et al. 2000). Even nocturnal lizards can benefit from UVB exposure (Gould et al. 2018). Interesting research investigating the variation of UVB passage through shed skin indicates that lizards exposed to higher amounts of natural light in nature have more resistance to UVB passage through the epidermis (http://www.uvguide.co.uk/skintests.htm).

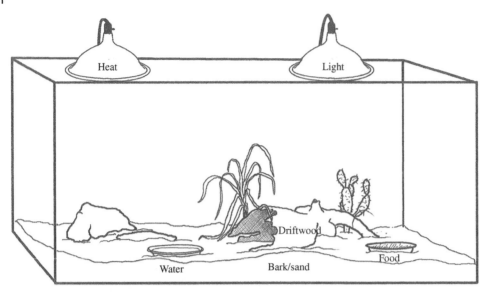

Figure 9.10 Terrestrial habitat. (Drawing by Scott Stark).

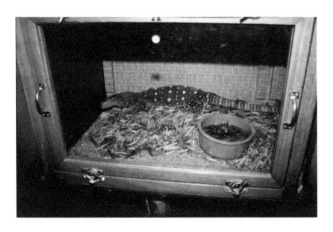

Figure 9.11 An inappropriate size cage for a lizard.

Therefore, investigation of the natural history of the lizard species should dictate the amount and type of lighting provided in captivity with the understanding that some species may require very low levels of UVB exposure on a routine basis.

An additional consideration regarding UVB exposure and vitamin D$_3$ synthesis is the ability for some species to absorb and utilize dietary vitamin D$_3$. It is theorized that many carnivorous lizards that eat primarily a vertebrate diet ingest and utilize vitamin D$_3$ that has already been synthesized by their prey. This phenomenon may account for the fact that many monitors and other large carnivorous lizards are rarely clinically observed with nutritional secondary hyperparathyroidism (NSHP). However, one can certainly see cases of monitors with NSHP, so keepers should err on the side of always providing UVB for these species as well, especially when they are young and

growing. Research on several closely related species of *Anolis* support the potential variation among species with regard to utilization of dietary vitamin D$_3$ (Ferguson et al. 2005). Excessive oral supplementation of vitamin D$_3$ can also be harmful, as it can lead to soft tissue mineralization.

As with other environmental parameters such as temperature and humidity, light should be provided in the captive environment as a gradient. The captive lizard may then behaviorally regulate exposure to UVB radiation.

It is important to understand that ultraviolet light does not penetrate glass or plastic; therefore, sunlight through windows and fluorescent lighting filtered by glass is inadequate to meet ultraviolet light requirements. Direct sunlight is the best source of ultraviolet light for lizards and may be provided periodically to lizards that otherwise are maintained indoors. Most if not all lizards become stimulated when exposed to direct sunlight and may become aggressive and very quick, making escape possible. Lizards should never be housed in enclosed or open-top glass or plastic containers when in direct sunlight to avoid life-threatening hyperthermia. Some nocturnal lizards, such as leaf tail and flat-tail geckos (*Phyllurus* spp., *Uroplatus* spp.), avoid bright light and are not active by day when in good health.

Heating elements for lizards should be mounted outside the enclosure so that the lizard cannot directly contact the light (or heating element). Ultraviolet light sources should be mounted at the proper distance from the animal based on the type of bulb being used. UVB decreases the further from the bulb; some bulbs are designed to be closer than 12 inches to the animal, while some are designed to be much further away. Measurement of UVB output is best achieved with a handheld UVB meter. There is tremendous manufacturer variation among bulbs with UVB output, and there is no oversight or central regulation of these devices or the claims made by their manufacturers. One can also increase the output of a UVB bulb by mounting it in a fixture with a reflector, while various screen tops will block a portion of UVB reaching the animal (Baines and Cusack 2019).

Recent research (Baines and Cusack 2019; Mitchell 2009) indicates that the newer coiled "screw-in" type fluorescent bulbs manufactured specifically for reptile enclosures provide adequate UVB radiation for lizards in enclosures, but only in a narrow area directly under the bulb. As such, these are not the best choice for most lizards. Some of these higher-powered compact fluorescent UVB-producing bulbs that are not full spectrum may be responsible for keratitis and skin damage, and any UVB bulb must be placed appropriately in order to prevent this problem. Historically, the long "tube-type" fluorescent bulbs were considered the standard of artificial lighting for reptiles. The newer T5 fluorescent lighting systems are proving to provide higher output UVB and can penetrate deeper into an enclosure. Mercury vapor bulbs provide full spectrum UVB, UVA, and heat radiation and can be useful as well, but also put out UVB in a smaller area than a fluorescent tube. Currently in development are LED lighting systems that may be capable of UVB emission in the physiologic spectrum for reptiles.

Heating

Most common pet lizards require additional heating during some portion of their captive existence. Because lizards are ectothermic, they seek microhabitats that meet their preferred optimal temperature zone (POTZ). The POTZ is the temperature range in which normal physiology is most efficient (Rossi 2019). It is important for the client to understand that a lizard uses a range of temperatures, not a uniform cage temperature, to create the POTZ; in the cage setting, this range is commonly referred to as the thermal gradient. It is also important to understand that various physiologic conditions such as pregnancy or disease may change the POTZ for a given animal. Observing the natural history and behavior and the study of lizard physiology is important for deriving the POTZ of each species. These values are available in many books, manuals, and journals for the species in question (see Table 9.1). Lizards achieve their POTZ by thermoregulation. By altering their exposure to light, orientation to light, and reflectivity of light (coloration), and by radiating heat (gaping, respiration), lizards are able to regulate body temperature within a few degrees.

Heating a lizard cage is generally not as difficult as providing an adequate thermal gradient. The ideal heat sources should be located outside the cage so that the lizard cannot directly contact the heating element. In-cage heating elements such as hot rocks are poor choices for heating reptiles and should never be recommended by veterinary staff. Similarly, ceramic radiant heating elements and light bulbs, which mount into incandescent fixtures, should not be placed inside the enclosure unless the animal cannot get up near them. Lizards have a poor sense of conductive heat and do not necessarily avoid contact with hot surfaces (Sladky and Mans 2019). Ideally, cage heating should be provided through radiant heat from an overhead light or ceramic heating element. Commonly heating tape or heating blankets are placed outside and beneath the cage, but these should not be used as a single heat source. Care must be exercised to avoid regions of the substrate or cage floor where heat is excessive. Additionally, below-cage heating may lead to increased evaporation of water sources and increased cage humidity.

Some desert species such as *Uromastyx* spp. may require daytime basking temperatures that range from 37 to 49°C (100 to 120°F) to nighttime temperatures of 25°C (77°F) (de Vosjoli 1995). Montane forest lizards such as Jackson's chameleon (*Chamaeleo jacksonii*) require daytime temperatures of 25°C (77°F) and night temperatures near 17°C (62°F) (de Vosjoli & Ferguson 1995). Arboreal lizards generally do not benefit from under-cage or substrate heating. Certain temperate and some subtropical lizards may require cooler temperatures during winter months to induce brumation or hibernation, which is essential for successful breeding. Temperature is best measured with thermometers or temperature probes placed inside the enclosure at various locations. Non-contact infrared temperature guns also work well, and it is important for the keeper to measure the temperature where the lizard actually sits in the cage.

Humidity and Ventilation

Humidity can be a difficult parameter to regulate in the lizard enclosure, especially in smaller enclosures. As with temperature, many lizards' benefit from a humidity gradient—another example of microhabitat use by lizards. In larger cages, this gradient is created by the interface between substrate and cage ornaments such as rocks or logs. Small covered plastic containers containing moistened substrate such as vermiculite or moss may be provided. These are called humidified shelters or moist hide boxes (de Vosjoli 1997) and are particularly useful to assist shedding in some species such as leopard geckos and blue-tongued skinks.

In well-ventilated cages, such as those for true chameleons, hand misting or electronic misters, vaporizers, or humidifiers are useful for increasing humidity. These are easily regulated by automatic timers. Regulating ventilation with screen lids or the addition of small fans is helpful to control humidity for glass aquariums or terrariums. Humidity is an important factor in both the respiratory and epidermal health of some lizards. Hygrometers are used to measure humidity in the lizard cage.

Ventilation is primarily controlled to indirectly regulate heat and humidity. Ventilation can be modified by cage design or may be controlled by external and internal cage accessories. Small fans, such as computer cooling fans, are quiet, and capable of moving large quantities of air. To a lesser extent, moving water such as small waterfalls, misters, and passive evaporation create some air circulation for more humid enclosures. It is important with any electrical devices that all wires be fully insulated from contacting water or metal in or on the cage and that they cannot be altered by cage inhabitants. Also, fans must be housed outside the enclosure so that the lizard cannot contact the turning blades.

Water and Food Availability

Water availability and water quality must be closely controlled. Some desert species such as *Uromastyx* spp. do not require standing water to be available in the cage (de Vosjoli 1995). Instead, these animals may be removed from the cage and soaked in water once weekly, or they may be misted in an enclosure separate from their cage once weekly. Some tropical lizards such as true chameleons may drink only water dripping off leaves or other cage ornaments. In time, these lizards may learn to drink from containers or from hand misting. The client should be educated that not all lizards readily accept water from containers or are physically capable of ingesting standing water. If water is not provided in the form in which these lizards typically drink, they will dehydrate rapidly. Water containers for all lizards should be cleaned at least weekly. Soaking with a 10% bleach solution for 15 minutes is sufficient for disinfection. Because some lizards may defecate or otherwise contaminate larger water containers, more frequent cleaning of water containers may be required.

Feeding stations for lizards are preferred over the random introduction of food items into the enclosure. Carnivorous lizards should be fed pre-killed food items such as small mammals from a container within the cage, or the lizard may be moved to a separate cage for feeding. Most insectivores only eat moving insects and therefore must be fed live food items. These food items may be introduced into small bowls within the enclosure. Many lizards readily adapt to eating from containers. Invariably some food items will escape into the cage and are usually consumed by the lizard. Presenting food in containers can reduce the risk of accidental substrate ingestion. It also may provide a central location at which the lizard may be observed while feeding to evaluate appetite and health. However, allowing the lizard to chase live insect prey also has benefits as it encourages normal behaviors (enrichment) and promotes exercise. Feeding live foods such as small mammals and crickets increases the risk of bodily damage to the lizard by the food item. Crickets, just as mice and rats, may feed on the flesh of lizards if deprived of food or water for more than a day in the enclosure.

Herbivores are generally fed prepared meals in containers. Most healthy herbivorous lizards consume their daily share of food at one feeding, though in nature these animals generally browse throughout the day. Uneaten food should be removed from the cage on the day of feeding to prevent spoiling. Prepared foods such as powdered, frozen, or otherwise processed herbivore foods should be provided with strict attention to the manufacturer's recommendations for rehydration, thawing, and feeding frequency. For herbivorous lizards, freshly prepared vegetable diets are preferable over processed diets.

Quarantine

The most important consideration often overlooked by the owner of new pet lizards is quarantine. Many clients who own one lizard eventually increase their collections, establish breeding colonies, or expand their interests to other reptiles. In their excitement to introduce new pets to the home, they ignore the potential for contagious infectious diseases that may affect their entire collection of animals.

Acariasis is a significant contagious disease seen in reptile collections (see section on "Parasitology"). Mite infestations can lead to reduced fertility, multisystemic disease, and death in captive reptile collections, and may be extremely difficult to eradicate once established in large collections (Wellehan and Walden 2019). Intestinal parasitism is a prime concern in lizards housed together. Other diseases that are generally not contagious but may opportunistically spread are bacterial and fungal dermatitis, pneumonia, and infectious stomatitis (primarily from fighting).

Though recommendations on quarantine vary, a minimum of 90 days of isolation in addition to physical exams and clinical laboratory tests, especially fecal exams, are recommended (Rossi 2019). In the absence of fecal parasites, prophylactic deworming may be indicated in wild-caught animals, and many herpetoculturists routinely medicate new animals without the diagnosis of parasitism. Clients who prophylactically deworm their pets should be thoroughly informed of the potential side effects of medications and the potential side effects of killing parasites in the patient's body, along with the effects of massive parasite die-off in a stressed, wild-caught animal. Prophylactic treatment with antibiotics is not recommended unless clinical signs of bacterial or protozoal infections are observed or clinical disease is diagnosed.

Housing during quarantine should consist of an enclosure that provides comfort and visual security for the lizard, but also provides visualization of every aspect of daily (or nightly) activity. Substrate, when possible, should be paper to visualize and collect feces, urates, and urine. Feedings should be provided at a consistent feeding station and supervised to observe all aspects of feeding behavior and quantify food intake. Impeccable sanitation and cage hygiene are essential.

Ornaments, hide boxes, and water bowls should be simple and either disposable or easily cleaned. Minimizing accessories and having duplicates for each cage aids in cleaning. Safe and effective disinfectants for home use are chlorine bleach at a 1:10 dilution of the commercially available concentration, and ammonia at 5% solution. However, these two products should never be mixed to prevent the release of poisonous chlorine gas. Soaking surfaces for 15 minutes is adequate for disinfection with chlorine bleach at a 1:10 dilution (Wellehan and Walden 2019). When cryptosporidiosis is a concern, soaking accessories with 5% ammonia and allowing them to dry for a minimum of 3 days is advised (Boyer et al. 2013; Wellehan and Walden, 2019).

Record keeping by the client is essential for both long-term captive lizards and new arrivals. Recording dates of feeding and ecdysis, environmental parameters, and especially weekly or monthly weight (in grams) are all helpful in monitoring for disease. With the exception of hibernation or parturition, lizards rarely lose weight as part of normal physiology. Juvenile lizards that fail to grow or adults that progressively lose weight are usually diseased. Casual observations such as the frequency and consistency of defecation and urination and daily activity patterns should also be recorded.

Nutrition

One adaptation that has allowed lizards to colonize nearly all terrestrial (and some aquatic) habitats on earth is their variation in dietary preference. Consequently, their prime vulnerability in captive management becomes nutritionally related disease when the proper diet is not provided. Lizards are commonly classified as herbivorous, insectivorous, carnivorous, or omnivorous. Though the differentiation between insectivorous and carnivorous may seem subtle, some species are so highly specialized to eat specific arthropods and gastropods that they refuse to eat and fail to thrive in captivity if offered any substitutes.

Just as there is no way to describe the basic lizard cage, it is impossible to generalize lizard diets. Each species has specific dietary requirements and variations in food availability in their native habitats that dictate dietary preferences on a seasonal or even monthly basis. Carnivorous lizards (monitors, tegus) ingest other vertebrates (fish, reptiles, birds, and mammals) as their primary diet, but remain opportunistic and usually attempt to eat anything that moves and anything that will fit into their mouth. Some carnivorous and omnivorous species may also eat carrion or may be cannibalistic (Balsai 1997; Boyer and Scott 2019). Carnivorous lizards that are not fed whole prey are more likely to develop nutritional disease (Boyer and Scott 2019). Some herbivorous lizards are opportunistically carnivorous or insectivorous, which, with some species in captivity, may cause serious nutritional disease when animal protein is fed in abundance (see section on "Common Disorders").

The ultimate paradox with some "nutritional diseases" in lizards, however, is that the causes of disease may have nothing to do with food. Temperature, humidity, landscape, water, infectious organisms (intestinal parasites, bacteria), and especially light (specifically ultraviolet light) commonly factor into nutritional health despite the provision of proper diet. Thus, proper husbandry becomes the key to providing proper nutrition.

Nutritional requirements pertain to all lizards. Feeding behavior, digestion, absorption and assimilation of nutrients, and cellular physiologic activity are all somewhat dependent on temperature for all reptiles (Barten and Simpson 2019; Boyer and Scott 2019). The POTZ and thermal gradient must be provided for each species to optimize the nutritional value of foods. Improper humidity also impacts overall patient health and may lead to a decreased feeding response. Boyer and Scott (2019) provide an excellent discussion of the nutrient requirements and daily energy needs of various reptiles, and the nutrient values of various animal, plant, and commercial food items.

The quality and variety of food offered are important for all lizards. Food items should be fresh or provided promptly after thawing if frozen. Foods offered once to lizards should be disposed of and not refrozen or preserved and offered again. Protein content and quality are generally met with whole animal diets and insects. For herbivores, the entire protein requirement should be plant origin.

Calcium is an essential element for all captive lizards and its deficiency is the cause of NSHP which encompasses a vast syndrome of physiologic disorders. Calcium absorption and excretion are regulated by several factors. Calcium absorption in the small intestine is regulated by an activated metabolite of vitamin D_3, cholecalciferol, which occurs in some animal tissues (Raiti 2019). Vitamin D_2, ergocalciferol, occurs in plants and does not apparently facilitate the uptake of calcium in the gut of lizards and does not appear to be beneficial as a dietary supplement for reptiles regarding calcium metabolism (Boyer and Scott 2019). Therefore, supplements claiming to contain vitamin D should be scrutinized as to which form of vitamin D is provided. Vitamin D_3 may be exogenously consumed in the form of dietary animal tissues and some dietary supplements or it may be endogenously produced when the lizard is exposed to appropriate ultraviolet (UV) radiation. Cholecalciferol is synthesized in the skin of lizards, and then is hydroxylated first in the liver and then the kidney to become 1,25-dihydroxycholecalciferol, the active metabolite of vitamin D_3 (Raiti 2019). The consequence of this pathway is that in spite of adequate dietary calcium, lizards may be prone to NSHP in the absence of adequate vitamin D_3. Clinically this is most commonly the result of insufficient exposure to UVB radiation.

Ultimate control of blood calcium homeostasis rests with the parathyroid glands and their production of parathyroid hormone (PTH). The occurrence of hypocalcemia or hyperphosphatemia results in increased production of PTH. Calcium is removed from bone (calcium resorption) to increase calcium ions in the blood. Additionally, PTH stimulates the production of the active metabolite of cholecalciferol (vitamin D_3) to increase intestinal calcium absorption (Raiti 2019). When calcium levels in the blood are adequate, the thyroid hormone calcitonin inhibits the effects of PTH and bone resorption slows or reverses.

Excess phosphorus in the diet is also a nutritional concern. High-phosphorus diets can induce NSHP, which ultimately depletes calcium stores in bone (Raiti 2019, Boyer and Scott 2019). In addition to the overall content of calcium in the diet, attention must be given to the calcium to phosphorus ratio (Ca:P). This ratio should be 1:1 to 2:1 for the entire diet (Boyer and Scott 2019). Whole animal diets (rodents and chicks) provide this ratio. Organ meats such as heart, liver, and muscle without bone are excessively high in phosphorus. Most commonly fed insects have a Ca:P of 1:9 and thus require periodic to routine vitamin and mineral supplementation (Boyer and Scott 2019). Salads containing leafy greens such as beet greens, outer green cabbage leaves, collards, dandelion leaves, and mustard greens are calcium-rich (Boyer and Scott 2019).

Nutritional supplements abound for reptiles and are required for optimal nutritional health of insectivorous and herbivorous lizards Supplements containing calcium carbonate are most commonly used and recommended and should never contain phosphorus. Calcium with vitamin D3 can be used for nocturnal species or those who are not exposed to UVB lighting, but oral D3 is not a replacement for UVB lighting. Some species cannot utilize oral D3 effectively, and it is always preferable to allow the animal to synthesize what it needs through UVB exposure rather than risk overdose of oral D3 and soft tissue mineralization. Multivitamin supplements should be provided as well but are typically given less often (once every 1–2 weeks) depending on the species. Insectivores require a multivitamin that contains preformed vitamin A as they are not able to convert beta-carotene or other carotenoids into vitamin A as herbivores and omnivores can (Boyer and Scott 2019). Without this, signs of hypovitaminosis A develop in these species. Supplements are applied to insects by "dusting," in which the prey items are placed in a container and the powder added. With gentle swirling of the container, the supplement is attached to the insect and then fed to the lizard. They must be consumed fairly quickly as the supplements will fall off or be groomed off by the insect if dusted on ahead of time. For herbivores, the supplements are sprinkled over or mixed with the salad. Supplementation schedules vary by species, but in general, young growing lizards need more frequent calcium supplementation than adults. Problems associated with mineral supplements include decreased palatability or refusal of supplemented food items; disproportionate distribution, improper ratio, or decomposition of nutrients within supplements; toxicities from overdosing or ingestion of high levels of certain nutrients; and false claims made by manufacturers. Supplements do not compensate for the feeding of imbalanced or poor-quality diets.

Herbivorous Lizards

The primarily or exclusively herbivorous lizards seen in practice include green iguanas (*Iguana iguana*) and other iguana species, chuckwallas (*Sauromalus* spp.), prehensile-tailed skinks (*Corucia zebrata*), and spiny-tailed agamids (*Uromastyx* spp.).

Omnivores can eat the same plant material as herbivores for that portion of their diet. All protein in the diet of herbivorous lizards should be derived from plant sources. The staples of the diet should be dark leafy greens (about 70–80%) with a variety of other shredded vegetables. Typically, fruit should be fed only as a treat, and edible flowers are often a favorite treat as well. Herbivores should typically be fed daily. Boyer and Scott (2019) is an excellent resource for the nutritional content of various food items.

Most herbivores conserve water well and obtain the majority of their water needs from plants. The salads can be heavily misted with water before feeding to help encourage water intake.

Insectivorous Lizards

Insectivorous lizards are among the most popular pet lizards today and have nutritional and feeding needs similar to herbivorous lizards. The insectivores comprise the majority of all modern lizards, and because of their dietary diversity their nutritional needs are the least known of captive lizards. The likely key to understanding insectivorous lizard nutrition is probably not in the food items themselves, but in the food *of* the food items themselves (de Vosjoli 1997; Boyer and Scott 2019). Lizards in nature eat insects that browse on numerous plants, detritus, feces, soil, and other animals. The assimilation of these nutrients may be crucial for the health and survivability of some species. Providing the insects with a healthy diet before feeding them to the lizard is also important and makes the prey item more nutritious. Various commercial diets for insects exist, both as maintenance and "gut loading" diets. The insects can also be fed the same produce being fed to the lizard (Boyer and Scott 2019).

The diet for captive insectivorous lizards should be varied and supplemented with vitamin and mineral powders (Boyer and Scott 2019). A variety of insects should be offered to most species including crickets, various feeder roaches, black soldier fly larvae, hornworms, mealworms, superworms, waxworms, flies, etc. Because most domestically raised insects are low in calcium and have an improper Ca:P ratio, calcium supplementation is crucial. Little is known about the dietary needs for amino acids, vitamins, other minerals, and trace elements. Generally, these are supplemented in addition to calcium. Boyer and Scott (2019) provide an extensive overview of the nutritional value of various captive-raised insects as some are better staple choices and some should be fed more sparingly.

The patterns by which animals choose their prey are described by optimal foraging theory (OFT) (Helfman 1990). It is theorized that animals choose between energetic costs and energetic gains when selecting food items. Insectivorous lizards have been observed to choose certain species of insects even when multiple species of a similar size are present, or the lizard chooses a certain size of insect when different sizes of the same species are available. For example, the energetic costs involved in prehending, swallowing, and digesting 10 crickets that are 10-mg each may exceed the energetic costs of capturing and eating a single 100-mg cricket for a particular lizard. Therefore, the lizard ignores the smaller food items and searches or waits for a larger item. This behavior is seen in captivity as the refusal of certain-sized foods. Lizards that are incapable of dismembering or shredding large food items usually avoid catching and eating them. Similarly, large lizards typically ignore small food items that the lizard may have eaten as a juvenile. Both the size and type of food items must be considered when feeding captive lizards.

Some lizards eat only one or two specific prey items and may or may not accept crickets or other domestic insects at the expense of anorexia—*Moloch horridus*, some *Phrynosoma* spp. (ants), *Dracaena* spp. (snails) (Obst et al. 1989). Most other insectivores accept domestic insects such as crickets, mealworms, waxworms, superworms, and roaches. Field sweepings for wild insects can also be offered to smaller insectivores, though the owner must be cautious of pesticides and potentially venomous or dangerous insects. Insects are offered in an amount that the lizard can consume in one feeding, which is typically several hours in a day or overnight in the case of nocturnal lizards.

Insects loose in a cage can be as much a hazard to insectivorous lizards as live rodents are to carnivorous lizards. Adult crickets are capable of chewing through skin, digits, and eyes of lizards that cannot escape from the enclosure. Mealworms are also similarly implicated in trauma or death to otherwise healthy lizards (de Vosjoli 1997). Feeding stations that restrict the movement of these insects can reduce the health risk to caged lizards. Most insectivorous lizards should be fed daily, though as with adult herbivores, every other day feedings are appropriate (de Vosjoli 1992, 1997). Dusting with vitamin and mineral supplements is done as with various life stages of herbivorous lizards.

Carnivorous Lizards

Clinically carnivorous lizards typically present less often with nutritional diseases than herbivorous or insectivorous lizards. Carnivores are generally fed whole animal vertebrates such as small mammals or birds, which, when fresh, are generally well balanced with nutrients (Boyer and Scott 2019). These lizards also are more likely to accept a wide variety of food items, which allows for more variety in nutrients. There are several reasons for the nutritional stability of carnivorous lizards in captivity, based on their natural history; these include a generally wider POTZ than herbivores and insectivores, less specific humidity requirements; and with proper diet less specific light requirements, all of which make habitat management less time consuming and less expensive for the owner. There are also some intangible reasons for the nutritional stability of carnivorous lizards; these include: they are less shy about eating in captivity, and the availability of food as whole animals requires less work by the owner to prepare the meal and provide balanced nutrition. Though some of these reasons suggest owner non-compliance, they are unfortunately substantial causes for the prevalence of nutritional disease in many herbivorous reptiles in the pet trade.

Consideration must be given to the quality of the carnivorous diet. To prevent rodent bites, live foods should never be fed to carnivorous lizards. Similarly, live wild-caught vertebrates and most purchased "feeder" reptiles and amphibians should not be fed so as to prevent the transmission of certain parasitic, bacterial, and viral diseases. Fresh-killed prey items have equal nutritional value to live prey (Boyer and Scott 2019). Frozen vertebrate food items are commonly offered after complete thawing. These items should have been frozen immediately after death, thawed only once, and disposed of if not consumed within hours after feeding. Frozen tissues decompose rapidly after thawing, and the author has observed regurgitation by lizards within days after the ingestion of apparently rancid food items. Adult monitors and tegus are fed rodents or other whole prey once weekly. Obesity is common in these species, and overfeeding is the primary cause. This feeding schedule may be adjusted for obesity or leanness.

Prepared foods such as poultry meat, beef, and dog and cat foods are not substitutes for whole animal meals and should not be offered. Exceptions may be made for short periods if rodents are unavailable or if assisted feeding is required for health-compromised individuals. A variety of prepared diets specifically for lizards are available through pet suppliers. Veterinarians and herpetoculturists should thoroughly research dietary claims and scrutinize research for these products before recommending them as a sole source of nutrition. Lizards fed diets primarily of fish may be susceptible to thiamine and vitamin E deficiencies (Boyer and Scott 2019).

Hatchling and juvenile carnivorous lizards can present a few nutritional challenges to their owners. Because of their smaller size, these lizards may not accept whole vertebrate food items early in life. Therefore, insects are commonly offered to smaller lizards, and newborn or "pinkie" mice are offered to larger juvenile lizards. Because insects have a relatively poor Ca:P (1:9) ratio, dusting of these insects with calcium powders is recommended (Boyer and Scott 2019). Pinkie mice (1:1) have a lower calcium content than do weanling (1.1:1) or adult mice (1.4:1), though the Ca:P ratio is suitable, and due to the relatively short term over which these food items are offered, calcium supplementation is not likely required (Boyer and Scott 2019). Hatchling and juvenile carnivorous lizards should be fed at least every 2 to 3 days.

Finally, *never feed large adult carnivorous or herbivorous lizards by hand.* The potential consequence to fingers and hands is obvious, but more serious is the conditioned response that is created by this behavior. Lizards are wild animals whose behavior is driven by instinct and conditioning, not by reasoning. A lizard cannot discern between the end of the food item and the beginning of the human hand until after the bite occurs. The client should also be instructed to exercise caution when removing uneaten food items from cages.

Common Disorders

Diseases of lizards include many diseases common to reptiles in general and a few that are unique to particular species or families of lizards. Many disorders are husbandry-related. Some diseases are more common in imported lizards than in domestically captive-raised lizards; therefore, it is important to inquire or discern the origin of the patient.

Not all disorders require medications, and many diseases are treated by correction of improper husbandry and supportive care. The author advocates increasing quality caloric intake for all traumatic injuries and many infectious diseases to strengthen the immune response and speed tissue repair in reptiles. Observation of POTZ and humidity is essential for the healing of all reptilian diseases.

Integument

Rostral abrasions are a common skin disorder of many lizards including *Iguana* spp., *Physignathus* spp., *Chlamydosaurus kingii*, and some *Varanus* spp. Abrasions are less common in gekkonids or in deliberate or slow-moving species such as *Uromastyx* spp. and *Chamaeleo* spp. The most common cause of rostral abrasions is facial impact with glass walls of aquariums, or pacing and rubbing the nose on cage walls. Many larger imported iguanas and water dragons develop these abrasions from handling during the importation and distribution process to pet stores. Animals not adjusted to captivity commonly attempt escape by incessantly rubbing on cage walls or lids or crash into walls when startled by movement in the room around them (Figure 9.12).

Recovery from rostral abrasions may be prolonged and the patient may be subject to recurrent injury. Treatment must include altering the enclosure to prevent further injury. Creating visual security such as a paper covering or the painting of glass walls or adding other visual barriers, even if temporary, is mandatory. Various antibiotic ointments may be used if indicated for infection. Note: Inform the client that treatment through habitat or behavioral modification is more important than medicating the lesion.

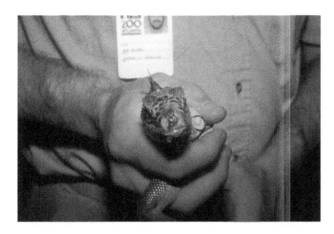

Figure 9.12 Rostrum abrasion. (Courtesy of Zoo Atlanta).

Trauma

As with any animal, trauma may be an emergency. Many cases of trauma present ambiguously because the patient is found in a compromised state and the owner did not observe the inciting cause. Trauma should be suspected whenever the onset of clinical signs is acute; that is, within hours of the patient being observed in a normal state and with no history of gradual onset of lethargy, anorexia, weight loss, or other abnormal physiology. The presence of a thin or dehydrated animal or any history of anorexia should indicate the presence of another or an additional underlying disease process. Infectious or metabolic diseases rarely show acute clinical signs in lizards.

Diagnosis of trauma may be speculative because no external clinical abnormalities may be apparent. Radiography is the desired diagnostic test to evaluate for abnormal anatomy. Hematocrit and blood profile parameters may be normal, though creatine kinase (CK) values are commonly elevated with skeletal muscle injury. Radiographically suspected intracoelomic fluid may be aspirated for analysis.

With a high degree of suspicion of traumatic injury, providing a proper thermal gradient is extremely important. Warmed intravenous, intraosseus, or subcutaneous fluids are indicated for hypotension. Analgesia is often indicated, and any wounds can initially be covered and antibiotics administered until the patient is stable enough for further wound care. Stabilization of fractures or luxations is performed following cardiovascular and thermal stabilization.

Traumatic injury may occur from bite wounds, thermal burns, and skin autotomy. Both burns and bite wounds (cage mate or prey item) commonly require surgical debridement of damaged or necrotic tissue and primary or delayed secondary closure. Secondary bacterial and/or fungal infections are common, and systemic antibiotics are indicated in most cases. Bacterial culture and sensitivity are indicated for all slow- or non-healing wounds that do not respond to empiric therapy. Topical cleansers such as chlorhexidine (Perry and Mitchell 2019) or chloroxylenol (B. Wilson, personal observation) (Vet Solutions, Fort Worth, TX) are excellent topical antimicrobial agents. Silver sulfadiazine cream or medical grade honey also works well for reptile wounds and stimulating healing. These injuries invariably result in scar tissue formation and occasionally disfiguration. Reptile skin is slow to heal, and open wounds require sequential shedding to fully close Note: Inform the client to expect prolonged (months) healing and to expect permanent scarring to the affected skin.

Bacterial and fungal dermatitides may occur as primary or secondary infections and are typically the result of improper husbandry. It is essential to know if the patient is captive-raised or wild-caught and if any cage mates are similarly affected. Clinically these diseases are more common in terrestrial species. Improper hygiene and increased humidity are suspected as the primary causes of infection (Pare et al. 2021). Other potential causes include acariasis, trauma from cage ornaments or accessories, immunosuppression from a variety of factors (temperature, nutrition, metabolic disease, overcrowding, capture, and importation), prolonged exposure to water or sitting in water bowls, and dysecdysis. Histologic microscopy, fungal culture, and bacterial culture are all indicated for diffuse or focally extensive disease. Treatment is based on diagnostic testing and may include enteral or parenteral antibiotics or antifungals, topical antibiotics or antifungal agents, and most importantly identification and correction of improper husbandry. Note: Inform the client of prognosis based on diagnostic testing and response to treatment. Correcting any existing defective husbandry is essential for both healing and prevention of recurrence.

Of particular concern in captive collections, especially among bearded dragons is the fungal disease caused by *Nannizziopsis* spp. (previously known as the *Chrysosporium* anamorph of *Nannizziopsis vriesii* (CANV). *N. guarroi* is most common in bearded dragons but various species have been diagnosed in a multitude of lizard species and is a contagious disease with high morbidity (Pare et al. 2021). Physical exam findings are relatively consistent as focal to focally extensive coalescing crusts on the skin, particularly, but not restricted to, the head and limbs. Fungal infection can also spread internally and cause severe systemic illness. This disease is commonly referred to as "yellow fungus disease," though the yellow or amber coloration is not a consistent finding. Diagnosis is made based on histopathology, or more commonly PCR testing as the organism does not grow well on culture. Clinical history and physical exam is often highly suggestive. This debilitating mycosis may be cured when diagnosed early and treated aggressively with a combination of oral and topical antifungal agents and occasionally surgical debridement for deeper skin lesions. However, in the majority of cases, treatment is long term and the condition is only managed, never cured; recurrence is common. Cleaning and disinfection of the habitat and removal of all organic materials that may serve as refugia for infectious spores are essential. Affected individuals must be isolated until clinical resolution occurs. Euthanasia is commonly required for patients that fail to respond rapidly to initial therapy, and may also be recommended in homes with multiple reptiles as the disease is quite contagious. Disinfection with bleach is required.

Dysecdysis is more a clinical sign of disease rather than a disease itself. Shedding problems are most commonly the result of underlying diseases or improper husbandry, particularly low humidity and malnutrition (often hypovitaminosis A). Low humidity may not be an entire enclosure phenomenon as much as a lack of humidity gradient. Even some desert-dwelling lizards benefit from microenvironmental humidified shelters to aid in shedding. Occasional misting for some species is beneficial. Other diseases that may contribute to dysecdysis are external parasitism and possibly thyroid disorders (Barten and Simpson 2019, Raiti 2019).

Complications that arise from dysecdysis are extremity necrosis, particularly toes and tails. This process arises from portions of the extremities that incompletely shed (occasionally more than once in several layers) and form a tourniquet to the distal extremity. Devitalization is quick and necrosis follows slowly over days or weeks. Lizards with thick skin or heavy scales may show no apparent signs of necrosis for weeks. Amputation of the affected extremity to the next proximal viable joint is required. Similar treatment is required for tails (see consideration of ascending tail necrosis, later in the text).

Broken tails resulting from tail autotomy and not from traumatic amputation usually do not require medical treatment. In rare cases, hemorrhage may be profound or last for more than one minute. In these cases, pressure bandaging may be used. An appropriately sized syringe casing packed with gauze is taped to the tail for one day if needed. The lesion should be cleaned if indicated and the patient maintained on a clean surface with no substrate for several days following the injury. Topical or systemic antibiotics are indicated only if wound contamination has occurred and only then for several days. Surgical repair is contraindicated in autotomous species because this inhibits or prevents tail regeneration. Note: Inform the client to maintain a clean environment and report any signs of inflammation; the less manipulation of the wound, the better; regeneration will occur over months resulting in a smaller and often darker regenerated tail.

Tail amputation in non-autotomous species or ascending tail necrosis in all species may require surgery and antimicrobial therapy. Traumatic tail amputation, though uncommon, may occur in chameleons, prehensile-tailed skinks, and rarely monitors. Also common is ascending tail necrosis, which results from trauma to the tail such as bite wounds, handling injuries, enclosure injuries, or dysecdysis. Gradually ascending darkening and devitalization of the tail distal to the injury characterizes this disease. Skin may slough at times, revealing devitalized vertebrae. Surgical tail amputation at a level proximal to the devitalized tissue is required. The gangrenous nature of this disease may lead to sepsis, and systemic antibiotics are indicated. For non-autotomous lizards, the tail stump can partially regenerate and is generally not sutured, though hemorrhage control with pressure is essential. Note: Inform the client to observe diligently for any signs of continued ascending devitalization and to be aware of signs of lethargy or anorexia that may result from sepsis.

Skeletal System

NSHP is a syndrome with variable manifestations. The pathophysiology of NSHP (previously referred to as metabolic bone disease[MBD]) is described in the section on "Nutrition." Clinically one of the most common signs of NSHP is generalized or hindleg weakness or paralysis, therefore, should also be considered a neurologic disorder. NSHP is the primary rule-out for lizards presented with this clinical sign. Other common signs include failure to grow, generalized weakness, anorexia, soft or pliable mandible or long bones on palpation, palpably swollen or thickened long bone(s), bowing or fractures of long bones, spinal curvature, and occasionally tremors or fine muscle fasciculations or seizures. In profoundly weak lizards, the pupils may appear to dilate and constrict erratically, possibly an ocular manifestation of muscle fasciculations (B. Wilson, personal observation). Presentation of a lizard with flaccid paralysis is an emergency. These clinical signs are most common in species of the Iguanidae, Agamidae (especially bearded dragons), Chamaeleontidae, and Varanidae.

A detailed history of diet, dietary supplementation, and lighting is essential. As discussed previously, even if calcium supplementation is adequate, without proper UVB lighting the patient cannot produce Vitamin D3, and NSHP results. Diagnostic testing includes blood chemistry and radiographs to evaluate bone density and fractures. Ionized calcium is particularly important as some patients will have a normal total calcium on a biochemistry panel. If hypocalcemia is detected, the patient should be considered critical, and intramuscular calcium gluconate 10% should be administered at a dose of 100 mg/kg every 6–12 hours until weakness and/or muscle tremors resolve After the patient is stable, it can be transitioned to oral liquid calcium (typically calcium glubionate). This treatment may continue for several weeks to months until normal appetite returns. Nutritional support is required in hypocalcemic patients and fluid therapy may be necessary as well (see section on "Techniques"). In addition to correcting the diet, supplementation, and providing proper UVB lighting, exposure to unfiltered sunlight as often as possible is extremely beneficial as well. Oral or parenteral vitamin D_3 is no longer recommended due to the risk of soft tissue mineralization when given with high doses of supplemental calcium. Fracture management is conservative for patients with NSHP. Traction and immobilization of forelimb and hindlimb fractures with external coaptation are performed (see section on "Techniques").

NSHP is physiologically a gradual onset disease, but from the client's perspective, the clinical signs of NSHP are rapid. Prognosis can be grave to good depending on the extent of disease at the time of presentation. Note: Educate the client about the basics of NSHP pathophysiology with emphasis on the interrelationships among diet, dietary supplements, and UV light exposure. Explain that a deficiency in one of these factors can lead to NSHP. Most importantly stress the fact that recovery from NSHP may require months and may result in some permanent debilitation or disfiguration in the patient who presents with a advanced disease.

Cardiovascular System

Cardiovascular disease in reptiles is still poorly described in the literature and is mainly limited to case reports. Much of what is known or treatments attempted are extrapolated from small animal patients. Clinical signs of cardiovascular disease in lizards can include cardiomegaly (more visible in snakes), gular or pharyngeal edema, cyanosis, peripheral edema, pulmonary edema, ascites, or exercise intolerance. They can also experience weakness, syncope, or neurologic signs from lack of oxygen and perfusion to certain tissues, often secondary to atherosclerosis (Schilliger and Girling 2019). Auscultation is difficult; typically only specialized electronic stethoscopes are useful in ausculting the heart in lizards, especially because in most species it lies within the bony pectoral girdle. A Doppler probe can be used to listen to rate and rhythm but only evaluates blood flow.

Multiple diagnostics can be used to evaluate the heart. Indirect blood pressure and pulse oximetry measurements are unreliable but can be used to monitor trends (Chinnadurai et al. 2010, Schilliger and Girling 2019). Electrocardiography is useful though lead placement can be challenging and electric amplitudes are low in reptiles, resulting in readings that can be difficult to interpret. Schilliger and Girling (2019) provide an excellent description of ECG placement and interpretation with some established reference ranges. Radiography is most useful to evaluate the heart and lungs in clinical practice, though echocardiography with Doppler flow will provide the most information, similar to small animal patients. Again Schilliger and Girling (2019) provide an excellent description of how to perform this exam along with established references for the bearded dragon (Silverman et al. 2016). Because bacterial endocarditis and myocarditis are common, a blood culture can be useful to help determine the cause.

A variety of causes of cardiovascular diseases have been reported in reptiles, with the most numerous involving snakes. These include cardiomyopathy, septic endocarditis, myocarditis, valvular insufficiency, pericardial effusion, infarcts, thrombus, atherosclerosis or arterial calcification, aneurysms, visceral gout, parasitic infections, congenital heart defects, and neoplasia. Every effort should be made to identify and treat the underlying cause if possible. Other cardiac medications like positive inotropes (pimobendan), ACE inhibitors, and diuretics have been used in reptiles as well and seem to help, though no pharmacokinetic studies exist (Schilliger and Girling 2019). Even though reptiles lack a Loop of Henle, the loop diuretic furosemide is commonly used and does help, so it is possible it works through other mechanisms (Parkinson & Mans 2018).

Respiratory System

The most common true respiratory disease in lizards is pneumonia. In lizards, etiologic agents of pneumonia are bacteria, fungi, and parasites (see section on "Parasitology"). Viruses have been reported as well but are less common in lizards (Knotek and Divers 2019). Clinically pneumonia develops with improper husbandry and rarely as contagious disease, and generally presents in the advanced stages of the disease. Pneumonia associated with pulmonary parasitism commonly occurs as a secondary bacterial infection (Knotek and Divers 2019).

The most prominent clinical sign of pneumonia is dyspnea. The posture may be altered with the neck held in extension and the mouth held open. Owners will often report hearing wheezing, crackling, or popping noises. Occasionally oral and nasal mucoid secretions are observed, though neither of these signs is pathognomonic for respiratory disease. Secretions originating from the mouth or esophagus can appear foamy in lizards with normal respiratory health. Thoracic auscultation may reveal crackles or popping sounds with pneumonia. The absence of any air sounds may indicate lung consolidation and advanced disease.

Radiographs are the diagnostic test of choice for pneumonia. Tracheal wash (see section on "Techniques") with cytology and bacterial culture with sensitivity of the wash are diagnostic for the etiology of pneumonia. For seriously compromised patients, a swab of the glottis or aspiration of tracheal exudate without flushing can be performed, but significant oral contamination may be present and must be taken into consideration when interpreting results. A fecal exam is indicated to diagnose lungworm infection.

Treatment is initiated upon diagnosis of pneumonia and modified based on cytology and culture and sensitivity results if indicated. Pneumonia in lizards frequently presents as an emergency and treatment must not be delayed. Antibiotics commonly used are broad-spectrum and bactericidal. These include aminoglycosides, beta-lactam antibiotics (cephalosporins), fluoroquinolones, and advanced-generation semisynthetic penicillins, all of which should be administered parenterally either IM or SC (Knotek and Divers 2019).

Recovery from pneumonia is prolonged physiologically by the accumulation of pulmonary exudates in recesses of the lungs (particularly caudally), and an inability to achieve the minimum inhibitory concentration (MIC) of antimicrobial agents in these relatively poorly vascularized regions. Nebulization with bacterial antimicrobial agents may be beneficial. Aerosolized particles must <5μm to reach the lungs (Knotek and Divers 2019, Perry and Mitchell 2019). Treatment periods are 10 to 30 minutes at a frequency of every 6 to 12 hours. Duration of treatment may be several days to one week pending clinical improvement.

Note: Meticulous investigation of all aspects of husbandry and correction of improper husbandry are required to develop a complete treatment plan. Inform the client of the seriousness of the disease and be realistic regarding prognosis. Treatment of pneumonia often requires protracted hospitalization, repeated diagnostic testing, moderate to marked financial investment, and tremendous patience.

Digestive System

Anorexia is the one of most common presenting complaints for digestive disorders, the cause of which can be a challenge to diagnose. Though anorexia is not a disease, it is both a clinical sign of nearly all reptilian diseases and a contributor to several other diseases. Comprehensive history is required because improper husbandry often contributes to the cause of anorexia. If history and physical exam fail to uncover improper husbandry issues or clinical disease, a series of diagnostic tests is indicated, including fecal exam, blood chemistry, complete blood count, radiography (including positive contrast), and ultrasound. Treat the diagnosed underlying disease and provide nutritional support.

Infectious stomatitis occurs as a secondary disease in lizards (De Voe 2019). This disorder may be unobserved by clients because the patient is presented for anorexia, lethargy, weight loss, or occasionally oral or nasal exudate. Oral exam may reveal focal or diffuse gingival erythema, petechiae, swelling, erosion, ulceration, and mucoid or purulent exudate (Figure 9.13).

The glottis mucosa may be involved in diffuse disease. In severe cases, aspiration of infectious exudates may lead to pneumonia (Knotek and Divers 2019). Because the oral cavity communicates with the nasal cavity dorsally through the choana, exudates may be observed bubbling from the nose in the absence of true respiratory disease.

Immunosuppression resulting from a myriad of underlying causes contributes to the development of infectious stomatitis. Improper temperatures, poor nutrition, and trauma from fighting with cage mates or oral cavity manipulation may be implicated. The infectious agent is determined through bacterial culture and sensitivity and is commonly identified as normal oral cavity bacterial flora including *Aeromonas* spp. or *Pseudomonas* spp., bacteria which are opportunistic pathogens.

Treatment is based on the degree of involved tissues, husbandry parameters, and sensitivity values. Small (2–3 mm) focal regions of stomatitis may require only warming of the environment and no antibiotic treatment or a single topical antiseptic or antibiotic application. Generalized or deep infections may require sedation, debridement, and a combination of topical and systemic therapy. Note: Inform the client that recovery may be protracted in severe cases

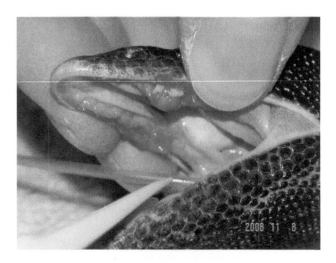

Figure 9.13 Stomatitis in a black tree monitor.

of stomatitis. Routine rechecks are necessary to monitor progress of healing of infection. Correcting improper husbandry is of primary importance.

Obstruction and impaction are common and may present days or weeks after the onset of the actual disease. The usual presenting complaint is anorexia, but bloating, lethargy, weight loss, diarrhea, constipation, and rarely regurgitation may be observed. Diagnosis may be suspected based on history alone. Investigating the patient's enclosure substrate, feeding habits, and normal defecation habits is important. Confirmation of obstruction can occasionally be made on physical exam, but commonly radiographs, contrast radiography, and/or ultrasound are required for definitive diagnosis. Complete foreign body obstruction commonly results in gas bloating, which is evident radiographically; the causative item, however, may not be radiographically visible. Complete obstruction with gas bloating is an emergency.

Impaction is often the result of particulate substrate, rodent hair, arthropod exoskeleton, or other food item accumulation in the intestines and may develop independently, in association with, or secondary to foreign body obstructions. Impactions are commonly palpable and visible on radiographs. If the lizard is alert and marked gas accumulation is not observed on radiographs, enemas and/or oral laxatives are indicated (see section on "Techniques"). Soaking in tepid water for 10 to 15 minutes may also stimulate defecation. Assess for dehydration and treat as indicated. Impaction may occur secondary to a number of husbandry issues, dehydration, improper diet, and hypocalcemia. Weak lizards with diagnosed or suspected obstruction should have blood chemistry analyzed. Surgical correction is required when laxatives, enemas, or other conservative therapy fails.

Intestinal parasitism is very common if not ubiquitous in imported lizards (Wellehan and Walden 2019), but even captive-bred lizards can suffer from parasitism as well. Signs of intestinal parasitism include anorexia, diarrhea, feces with mucous or blood in it, weight loss, failure to gain weight, and weakness. Treatment is based on diagnosis (see section on "Parasitology"). Quarantine, fecal screening, and cage hygiene are essential in limiting reinfection. Some parasites are zoonotic (see section on "Zoonoses") (Johnson-Delaney & Gal 2019, Wellehan and Walden 2019).

Cloacal prolapse may occur as a digestive, reproductive, or excretory disorder. The prolapse may occur secondary to straining from enteritis (for various reasons), egg laying, and uroliths, among other causes, and may comprise the cloaca, colon, oviduct, or urinary bladder, or a combination. Treatment is based on which organ is prolapsed, the

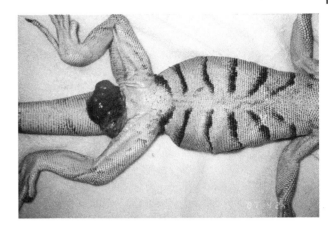

Figure 9.14 Cloacal prolapse in an iguana.

duration of the prolapse, and resultant trauma to involved tissues (Figure 9.14).

The colon is a tubular, smooth structure with a lumen. Fecal material may or may not been seen within the lumen. The oviduct is a thin-walled, longitudinally banded structure with a lumen and no fecal material will be present. The urinary bladder is a globular, thin-walled, smooth structure with no lumen and may be fluid-filled. Prolapse of these organs originates from the coelomic cavity cranial to the vent. Paraphimosis, or prolapse of the hemipenes, originates from the proximal aspect of the tail caudal to the vent. The prolapsed hemipenis is a solid, fleshy structure with no lumen. All organs may be darkened in color from devitalization or necrosis. Cloacal prolapse of coelomic structures is an emergency.

In cases in which prolapse is recent, tissues may be cleaned and lubricated with a water-based lubricant and gently reduced through the cloaca (McArthur & Machin 2019). A horizontal mattress suture can be placed at the lateral aspects of the cloaca on each side to maintain the reduction yet still allow the passage of urates and feces. If swelling of the tissue is present in the absence of necrosis, swelling may be reduced with hypertonic sugar solutions followed by manual reduction. Necrosis of prolapsed tissue requires surgical resection in the case of coelomic structures or amputation of the hemipenis (see section on "Anesthesia and Surgery"). Depending on the degree of prolapse, reduction of tissue may also be combined with coeliotomy to replace, pexy, or remove prolapsed tissue. The underlying cause of the prolapse must be addressed and treated as well, otherwise, the prolapse will just recur once the sutures are removed.

Excretory System

Renal failure is especially common in lizards and can occur at any age, though it is more common in older animals. Potential causes include chronic dehydration, NSHP, hypovitaminosis A, excessive dietary protein, excessive Vitamin D3 supplementation, various infections, toxin ingestion, or neoplasia. Common symptoms include lethargy, weakness, anorexia, dehydration, weight loss, polyuria and polydipsia, and constipation if renomegaly is present. Sometimes enlarged kidneys can be palpated cranial to the pelvis in lizards or can be seen on radiographs, and swollen joints can be seen with articular gout. Renal secondary hyperparathyroidism can also develop. A CBC and chemistry panel will often show elevated uric acid, phosphorous, potassium, or sodium levels with anemia and sometimes normo- or hypocalcemia. Articular and/or visceral gout can also develop with hyperuricemia. Aspirates of swollen joints will often demonstrate uric acid crystals. Other advanced diagnostics can be used as well. Treatment involves fluid therapy, medications such as allopurinol and phosphate binders, and supportive care and analgesia. Long-term prognosis is often poor by the time the condition is diagnosed.

Reproductive System

Lizards are presented with several reproductive abnormalities. Dystocia in females and paraphimosis in males are most common. Other disorders include cloacal prolapse of oviducts, ectopic eggs, and neoplasia. It is possible for lizards to ovulate and deposit infertile shelled eggs in the absence of a male. When gravid, most lizards do not eat but remain alert and active for a period of several days prior to egg laying, and many retain eggs until a suitable substrate or nest box is provided. Any dystocia accompanied by weakness or non-responsiveness despite the presence of a suitable nesting area is a critical emergency.

Dystocia in lizards can be pre-ovulatory (as follicles on the ovary) or post-ovulatory (as follicles or shelled eggs in the oviduct) (Stahl and DeNardo 2019). Differentiation of the two is made by radiography as the pre-ovulatory eggs are non-shelled and located dorsally in the abdomen whereas post-ovulatory eggs may be shelled and are more caudo-ventral in the abdomen, or with ultrasound where it is easy to differentiate follicles from shelled eggs, and follicles can be staged. Conservative management is advised when the lizard is alert and active with pre-ovulatory or post-ovulatory dystocia. Environmental modification, such as providing a suitable nesting area or more visual security, may be curative. However, if a patient has well-developed follicles and is exhibiting signs of gravidity (digging, pacing, decreased appetite, etc.), then they should lay eggs within 2–4 weeks. If no eggs are seen and their condition is not progressing, intervention is needed.

Traditional mammalian treatments for post-ovulatory dystocia refractory to conservative management include oxytocin and calcium injections to stimulate smooth muscle contractions. Calcium gluconate at a dose of 100 mg/kg IM followed in 1 hour by oxytocin at a dose of 5–30 IU/kg IM are given (Stahl and DeNardo 2019). Oxytocin may be repeated within 30 minutes of the first injection or can be given at regular intervals every 6–12 hours over the next 1–2 days. Efficacy is unpredictable and may only be effective in the first few days after starting to lay (Stahl and DeNardo 2019). If there is no progression with oxytocin, then surgery to remove the eggs will be needed. Manual reduction of retained eggs may be attempted for one or two eggs in close proximity to the cloaca and distal to the pelvic canal. Tremendous care must be exercised to avoid prolapse, oviductal rupture, or trauma to the kidneys. If the eggshell is not clearly visible emerging from the cloaca, manual reduction is contraindicated. Lizards with distal oviductal or cloacal dystocias following normal oviposition may be hypocalcemic.

Many cases of dystocia require surgical management. These are weakened and visibly distressed animals or those in which a radiographic diagnosis of obstruction is diagnosed. Obstruction may result from eggs too large to pass through the pelvic canal or from coelomic masses or enlarged kidneys that prohibit the passage of eggs. Surgery is also indicated for animals that do not lay with oxytocin, or with those who develop follicular stasis. If the ovaries are not removed, eventually the yolk material within the follicles will start to leak leading to egg yolk coelomitis which is a life-threatening condition.

Paraphimosis is managed similarly to cloacal prolapse (Stahl and DeNardo 2019). The prolapsed hemipenis is assessed for viability and replaced or amputated as indicated. Transverse cloacal suturing is indicated by reduction of paraphimosis.

Nervous System

Various conditions affecting the nervous system are possible in lizards. Neurologic symptoms such as ataxia, paresis, paralysis, tremors, and seizures are common emergency presentations. The primary differential, especially in lizards, is hypocalcemia, usually due to NSHP. Other differential diagnoses include hypocalcemia due to renal secondary hyperparathyroidism or reproductive activity, other nutritional deficiencies (thiamine, etc.), toxin exposure (especially from OTC mite treatments), infection (bacterial, viral, fungal, and parasitic), metabolic disorders (hepatic disease, xanthomatosis), genetic, trauma, vascular, and neoplasia (Platt 2019).

A complete history should be obtained, including anything the owner may have given the animal along with

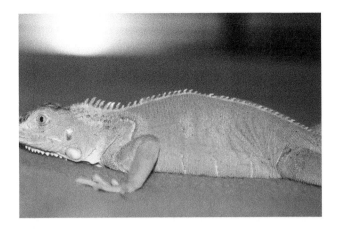

Figure 9.15 Spinal cord injury with vertebral column fracture due to trauma. Note the dorsal displacement caudal to the forelimbs.

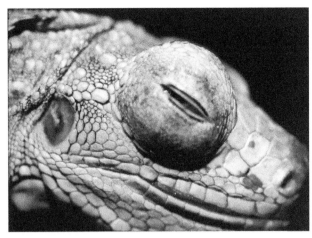

Figure 9.16 Retrobulbar abscess in an iguana.

detailed husbandry information, and a complete physical examination performed. Initial diagnostic tests include a complete blood count and chemistry panel, including an ionized calcium level. A fecal exam, radiographs, and additional blood testing (Atadenovirus testing, blood culture, etc.) may be recommended based on history and exam (Platt 2019). More advanced diagnostics such as CT and MRI may be needed if initial tests do not reveal the cause of the problem (Platt 2019). Treatment is directed at the primary cause and may include parenteral and oral calcium, antibiotics, antiparasitics, fluid therapy, correcting metabolic derangements, and addressing organ dysfunction (Figure 9.15).

Ophthalmology

Periocular inflammatory diseases are clinically the most common ophthalmic disorders in lizards. Infectious agents do not cause all periocular diseases, but many inflammatory diseases do result from or give rise to secondary bacterial infections.

One nutritional disorder that affects the eye is hypovitaminosis A. This disease is not specific to the eye, but also affects glandular mucous membrane epithelium including the respiratory and digestive tract. Clinically hypovitaminosis A is most commonly seen in turtles and insectivorous lizards such as leopard geckos and chameleons. Insectivores cannot convert carotenoids and other compounds into Vitamin A, and as such need to have preformed Vitamin A provided in the diet (Boyer 2019). Clinical signs include blepharitis, chemosis, and epiphora. Secondary bacterial infection is often observed in these cases, and topical ophthalmic antibiotics are commonly indicated in addition to supplemental Vitamin A (Boyer 2019). Often semi-solid keratinaceous debris will need

to be removed from under the eyelids. Recovery may be prolonged to several months. A thorough review of diet is recommended.

Several species of gecko have spectacles (see section on "Anatomy"). Subspectacular abscesses and retained spectacles occur as in snakes. The abscesses may be unilateral or bilateral and often are the result of ascending bacterial infection from the mouth. Treatment consists of surgical drainage and irrigation of the abscess along the ventral margin of the spectacle as well as treatment of associated stomatitis. The surgical incision remains open to drain, but commonly seals in a matter of days. Subsequent shedding of the spectacle results in complete closure of the surgical incision and resolution of the abscess. The spectacle revealed following shedding may appear wrinkled and typically requires several shed cycles to return to normal appearance.

Foreign bodies and trauma commonly result in blepharospasm. Evaluation of the globe and periocular tissues may require sedation. Treatment of lesions depends upon thorough examination of the globe, eyelids, and conjunctiva (Figure 9.16).

Neoplasia of periocular tissues is frequently reported, especially in the bearded dragon. Squamous cell carcinoma of the eyelids has been described in this area on multiple occasions (Hannon et al. 2011).

Behavior

The primary reported behavior disorder of lizards is aggression and is categorized as dominance or fear aggression, as seen in dogs and cats. Dominance aggression may be conspecific (same species) or intraspecific (different species) among lizards housed together, and it may be difficult to separate from fear aggression in cases of lizard–human interactions. Aggression is most often observed against humans in cases of large lizards such as iguanas, monitors, and tegus, especially during the breeding season, and is likely hormonally induced. This behavior is variable and may be directed at only one person in the household (B. Wilson, personal observation). The possibility of pheromonally induced aggression in iguanas against women who are in their estrous cycle has been suspected. Aggression in large lizards directed against humans is a serious and dangerous problem (see section on "Zoonoses"). Seasonal aggression can potentially be managed with ovariectomy or orchidectomy, but is not always successful.

Toxicity

Toxicities occur from a variety of substances including pharmaceuticals, insecticides, dietary supplements, chemicals, and cigarette smoke. Pharmaceutical toxicities are most commonly seen from injectable aminoglycosides and ivermectin, oral metronidazole, and topical pyrethrin or organophosphate compounds. A thorough history is required for diagnosis of toxic exposure, because there are rarely pathognomonic clinical signs for exposure to any of these compounds. Treatment is supportive depending on the underlying exposure. Fluid therapy is indicated for virtually any toxin exposures, and activated charcoal can be given PO depending on the toxin. Diazepam or midazolam can be used to control seizures. IV intralipid emulsions have been used in sporadic reports of reptiles for toxicities, so this therapy may be useful for reptiles suffering from toxin exposure or ingestion in the future (Cocilova et al. 2019, Perrault et al. 2021).

Nutritional Disorders

Nutritional disorders leading to neurologic signs of disease include vitamin B_1, vitamin E, and selenium deficiencies. Thiamine (B_1) deficiency is seen in carnivorous lizards fed raw egg diets in which the compound avidin inhibits vitamin B (Boyer and Scott 2019). It is also seen in patients fed a large amount of or exclusively frozen fish, as many fish contain thiaminase. Vitamin E deficiency is seen in lizards fed high-fat fish diets (Boyer and Scott 2019). Treatment consists of dietary correction and injectable vitamins as indicated.

Hypovitaminosis A is a common and likely much-underdiagnosed disease of many species of captive exotic animals. Herbivorous and insectivorous vertebrates appear to be most susceptible. Lizard species that clinically may

have a high incidence of this disorder are leopard geckos (*Eublepharis macularius*) and *Chamaeleo* spp. Other than the previously discussed ocular signs, recurrent hemipene infections or impactions, skin and shedding disorders, and decreased reproductive success may be clinical manifestations. Commonly blood testing is inadequate to make a definitive diagnosis in the living animal. Presumptive diagnosis is made based on physical exam, review of diet, and response to vitamin A dietary supplementation. Because the clinical manifestations of hypovitaminosis A develop slowly as a result of total body depletion of vitamin A, resolution following treatment may require months.

Gout is a disease of lizards and other animals with several potential etiologies. In lizards, gout can originate both from improper nutrition or secondary to various causes of renal disease (Wilkinson and Divers 2020). In vertebrates, the pyrimidine amino acids are metabolized into CO_2 and NH_3 and eliminated from the body. Purine amino acids are metabolized into various degradation products of which uric acid is the final product in reptiles (Divers and Innis 2019). Uric acid in high concentrations in the blood becomes insoluble. Simplistically, gout is the result of excessive uric acid in the blood that crystallizes and precipitates in tissues prior to elimination from the body via the kidneys. Common sites of this deposition are serosal surfaces of internal organs and synovial membranes. A common presenting complaint of gout is swollen joints or white to yellow nodules of the oral mucous membranes.

Gout is seen in lizards on diets high in purines, most commonly in herbivorous lizards fed a primarily animal rather than plant protein diet. Gout may also be renally induced secondary to dehydration or renal disease, which can occur for various reasons. Nutritionally, chronic NSHP or excessive Vitamin D3 in the diet can also lead to renal disease. Gout is a managed disease and not curable in most cases. Medications to lower blood uric acid concentrations and analgesia and supportive care are recommended (Innis and Divers 2019, Wilkinson and Divers 2020). In cases of advanced gout palliative therapy may be insufficient. This disease is best prevented before it occurs, with proper client education regarding diet and the judicious use of potentially nephrotoxic medications.

Zoonoses

Client education regarding zoonotic diseases must be a priority for all veterinary health professionals. Unfortunately, popular literature, television/radio, and the Internet are saturated with misinformation regarding reptile zoonotic diseases. The threats posed to humans, however, should not be underestimated. This information gap is prevalent within human medicine as well, and human physicians fall victim to the lack of education reflected by the popular press regarding disease in many domestic pets.

All veterinary staff should take the following steps to understanding zoonotic disease:

1. Gain a complete understanding of the pathophysiology and method of transmission (direct or indirect and vector) of the disease in question, both in the potential source animal and in humans.
2. Have a complete understanding of risk factors for humans to contract the disease in question, including immunosuppression and human behaviors when handling the pet.
3. Know which pet species are more likely to harbor particular zoonotic pathogens.
4. Gain a thorough knowledge of laws governing the possession and treatment of exotic species in a given jurisdiction.

Human behavior is likely to be a primary cause or facilitator of contracting zoonotic diseases from reptiles. Because many lizards are particularly sociable and exhibit behaviors that are commonly anthropomorphized, their owners form a human–animal bond that is similar to that seen with other domestic animals. Therefore, reasoning regarding the potential for zoonotic diseases is commonly ignored because of emotional considerations.

Behaviors that greatly increase the risk of contracting infectious diseases from lizards include:

- Housing or handling of lizards in or near food preparation or storage areas.
- Allowing lizards to soak in bathtubs, basins, or containers used for human hygiene.
- Allowing any part of the lizard to contact a human mouth or face.
- Allowing lizards to roam free in any facility of human habitation.
- Allowing young children to handle or have access to pet lizards when not under direct adult supervision.
- Handling of lizards by any person under treatment of immunosuppressive medication(s) or having contracted any immunosuppressive disease.
- Not washing hands and exposed skin following handling of pet lizards.

Other risk factors include possessing aggressive or potentially dangerous lizard species, disregarding the proper handling techniques for any lizard, feeding pet lizards by hand, and failing to maintain proper cage sanitation.

Bacterial diseases are most commonly implicated among reptilian zoonoses. Of these diseases, salmonellosis (*Salmonella* spp.) is most notorious for causing disease in humans. See Johnson-Delaney and Gal (2019) for a comprehensive discussion of salmonellosis. Salmonellosis is directly transmitted by a fecal–oral route. Transmission of infective serotypes does not require the direct contact of fecal material by a human. Because lizards are commonly maintained in enclosures where they defecate, invariably bacterial organisms from feces may contact the skin of the pet. Handling the pet can transfer infective organisms to human skin. It is likely that disease transmission will not occur given the combination of a relatively low number of infective organisms and an immunocompetent host; with zoonotic diseases, however, there is no acceptable level of risk.

Other bacterial infections may occur in humans from fecal–oral contamination or from penetrating wounds such as bites or scratches. *Aeromonas* spp., *Pseudomonas* spp., and other Gram-negative bacteria may be normal flora in the mouths of lizards. *Mycobacterium* spp. infections may occur in reptiles and are potentially infectious to humans through direct contact with skin defects and inhalation. This infection in reptiles may appear in any organ. *Chlamydophila psittaci* has been identified in infections of various species of lizards (Jacobson 2002). Direct transmission of *Chlamydia* from reptiles to humans is unknown. Several fungal infections (mycoses) that have the potential to infect humans have been reported in reptiles.

Reptiles are the definitive host for tongue worms (pentastomids) of various genera that are known to infect humans incidentally (Johnson-Delaney & Gal 2019, Wellehan and Walden 2019). Transmission is direct and fecal–oral by ingesting eggs or larvae. Because humans are incidental "dead-end" hosts, they do not pass infective stages of pentastomids. Larval forms of these worms may migrate and then die in humans, resulting in a localized immune response and calcification or granulation of lesions.

There are a variety of indirectly transmitted diseases for which lizards may be reservoirs of disease or carry the vectors of zoonotic disease. A variety of ticks, mites, and biting insects are implicated in transmitting viral, rickettsial, and bacterial diseases. Lizards have not been implicated in acting as a reservoir host for these diseases, but they may harbor ticks and mites that can bite and infect humans (Johnson-Delaney & Gal 2019, Wellehan and Walden 2019).

An often overlooked yet significant risk to humans from captive reptiles is trauma from bites and scratches. Besides the risk of infectious diseases, there is no excuse for humans to incur bite wounds from pet lizards. Some species are simply poor choices for the average hobbyist. These include *Heloderma* spp., adult green iguanas, large monitors, and some adult tegus. There is a risk of bite wounds or other injuries from these species when simply performing routine maintenance and a minimal amount or even no handling. Generally, however, injuries occur from careless interaction with the animals.

The importance of this issue becomes evident when legal authorities attempt to strip the rights of pet owners to possess these animals because of accidental bites or the irresponsible behavior of a few people. Many local ordinances restrict or prohibit the sale or possession of certain exotic animals, particularly venomous reptiles and large snakes or lizards, because of the perceived danger to humans. Accidental bites that occur at zoological parks and large snake escapes that are reported by the media contribute substantially to the hysteria that enables much kneejerk improper legislation. Veterinary staff have a critical role in educating clients about the proper handling of exotic animals and in advising clients about exotic animals that are unsuitable as pets.

Additionally, however, veterinary staff must be aware of these laws when admitting or treating pets that are illegal to possess. Injuries sustained to staff or clients by these pets (and others) are the responsibility of the practice owners when on the premises. Similarly, advising clients regarding the home treatment of potentially dangerous animals should be approached with great discretion. For a somewhat complete but already outdated overview of laws regarding reptiles in the United States see Lewbart and Lewbart (2019).

History, Restraint, and Physical Examination

History

In the practice of exotic animal medicine, as much can be learned about a patient from the history as from any other diagnostic procedure. With lizards, a veterinary technician, assistant, or customer service representative educated with a basic understanding of the patient's husbandry needs can often develop a working diagnosis well before the veterinarian examines the patient. It is the very diversity of husbandry requirements among species of lizards that demands a fundamental knowledge of all natural history aspects of the patient.

It is essential not to dismiss any observation by the client as trivial or inconsequential. The client may be the most educated person in the exam room with regard to the natural history of the patient, and with long-term captive lizards, the client is usually aware of a pattern of "normal" behavior. Discovering the deviations from normal behavior is essential to obtaining a complete history.

The following are fundamental questions for clients to answer regarding their lizard pets:

1. What is the presenting complaint(s), what is the duration of the problem, how rapidly has the problem developed, and does the client believe that the problem is related to any external influence(s) on the lizard?
2. What is the species, age, and sex? How long has the lizard been in the client's possession, and are there any known previous disease or health problems? Has the client or anyone else medicated the lizard or been instructed to medicate the lizard, and if so, by whom and for what reason?
3. Is the lizard captive-born or wild-caught? Where did they get it? This is not essential to the diagnosis but can be very helpful in developing a diagnostic plan for infectious disease.
4. In the area of general husbandry, in addition to obtaining a general overview of housing, lighting, temperature and heating, humidity, substrate, water availability, cage cleaning, and cage accessories, it is essential to ask the following: Does the lizard ever roam free in the house or in any area other than the cage or enclosure or has the lizard ever escaped from its enclosure? Does the lizard have any direct or indirect exposure to any other animals presently or in the past, and are those animals similarly affected? Is the lizard ever handled or observed by anyone except the client? Where is the cage located in the house? Is it ever moved? What are potential exposures to noxious materials such as cleaning agents, cigarette smoke, fuel exhaust, and so forth, and are there temperature, light, humidity, or ventilation fluctuations?
5. Regarding nutrition, determine *exactly* what the lizard is fed and the origin of the food (i.e., does the client collect food in the environment to feed or purchase the food at a pet store or grocery store?). How often is food offered, at what time of day is food offered, and in what quantities is food consumed? In cases in which a variety of food items are offered, which portions are usually consumed? Does the client use any commercially available foods or vitamin and mineral supplements and if so, how often and in what quantity? Does the client actually observe the lizard eating the food items or just notice that food is missing after a period of time?

Restraint

Portions of the physical exam, most diagnostic procedures, and many treatments require restraint. The veterinary staff must be aware that every species of lizard can bite. Most, however, will not bite or scratch unless restrained, and the more firmly they are restrained, the more they will struggle and attempt to bite or scratch the handler. Lizards with delicate skin should not be handled for physical examination unless absolutely necessary. These species include the Malagasy geckos *Geckolepis* spp. (fish-scale geckos) and *Phelsuma* spp. (day geckos) that may autotomize both tails and skin with minimal physical restraint. This behavior rarely results in death of the lizard, but it may cause permanent disfigurement. These patients can be observed through clear enclosures such as plastic pet carriers or they can be placed inside a 5 to 6-cm diameter clear plastic tube for examination (Figures 9.17–9.19).

There are some lizards that *at all times should be considered dangerous to handle*. These include all lizards greater than 1 m length, especially all large species of iguanas and monitors. Large lizards may be calmed by covering the head and eyes with a towel in addition to wrapping the body in a large towel or blanket to prevent clawing. The head, however, must be fully and firmly immobilized at all times. Occasionally these lizards cannot be safely restrained and examined without sedation (see section on "Surgery and Anesthesia"). Other species, though smaller and typically docile, are capable of inflicting digit amputation, disfiguration, or extremely painful bites on humans. These include prehensile-tail skinks (*Corucia zebrata*) and some adult tegus (*Tupinampis* spp.). Some smaller lizards such as the Tokay gecko (*Gecko gecko*) tend to be aggressive and will attempt to bite without being handled. Even small lizards such as fat-tailed geckos (*Hemitheconyx caudicinctus*) are capable of producing painful bites when handled and may be reluctant to release when biting a hand or finger (see Figure 9.19).

Veterinary staff should refrain from inappropriate contact with pet lizards. This includes kissing the patient, placing the patient near a human face, placing fingers or hands within the mouth of the patient, or allowing the patient to cling to clothing or hair in an unrestrained fashion. This behavior is both irresponsible and unprofessional and may result in serious injury to either the patient or veterinary staff. Clients should also be informed of the potential health risks that may result from these behaviors. The veterinary staff should never allow the client to assist in the restraint of a potentially dangerous patient during examination or when performing a treatment or diagnostic procedure. Though lizards may become somewhat tame, there are no domesticated lizards and their behavior may not be predictable.

Physical Examination

The traditional physical exam for most companion animals is a hands-on affair. More can be learned, however, by simple observation of the lizard patient at rest in a cage while in the exam room or waiting area. These observations can commonly be made during the traditional question-and-answer session and may quickly uncover

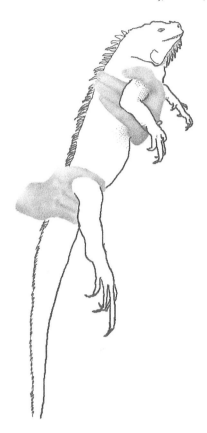

Figure 9.17 Proper restraint of a lizard. (Drawing by Scott Stark).

potential emergencies that have not been realized by the client. First observe the posture (again, the technician must first be familiar with normal posture of a particular species). Quadruped lizards generally hold the head somewhat erect and may have a portion (if not all) of the body held suspended above the ground. For diurnal lizards, assess alertness. Does the lizard follow the observer in the room with eyes or head? Healthy chameleons, for example, are constantly surveying their environment with turret-like eyelids and generally do not sit still except when restrained or confined. For lizards with movable eyelids (all but some geckos), are both eyes open and are they clear?

Observe general body condition, paying particular attention to the muscle mass of the dorsal tail, dorsal pelvis, and dorsolateral scapular region. Emaciation results in diminished subdermal fat and muscle mass and the skin may have a concave contour to one or all of these body regions. Additionally, the eyes may have a sunken or recessed appearance from diminished retrobulbar fat or from dehydration. Species that routinely present with signs of emaciation include the green iguana, spiny-tailed lizards (*Uromastyx* spp.), prehensile-tailed skinks (*Corucia zebrata*), bearded dragons (*Pogona* spp.), and monitors (*Varanus* spp.). It is important to understand that the

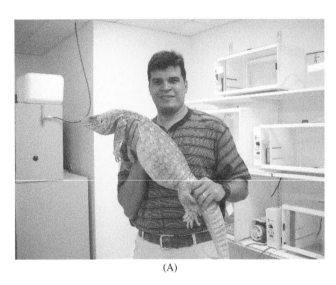

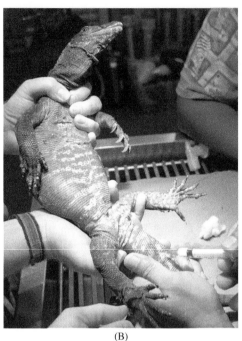

(A)   (B)

Figure 9.18 (A) Manual restraint of a large savannah monitor. (B) Manual restraint of a rough-necked monitor for an intravenous injection of propofol. (Photos courtesy of Dr. Sam Rivera).

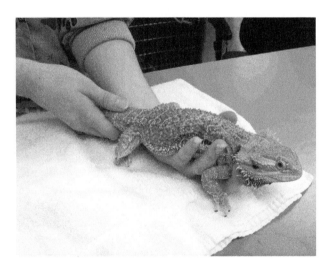

Figure 9.19 Restraint of a smaller lizard, a bearded dragon. (Courtesy of Dr. Bonnie Ballard).

physical changes associated with emaciation are chronic and do not occur over several days. Some lizards, which are laterally or dorsally compressed, may appear thin or underweight but they are in fact normal. Some of these species include leaf-tailed geckos (*Uroplatus* spp.), some true chameleons (*Chamaeleo* spp.), and spider geckos (*Agamura* spp.). Observe for symmetry, particularly of skeletal structures. Except for some skin appendages, the external and skeletal anatomy of lizards is bilaterally symmetric.

As with general body condition, the skin can be observed without handling the lizard. There is great structural variation among lizards in skin and scale texture. Lizards such as bearded dragons and horned lizards (*Phrynosoma* spp.) have roughly textured and armored skin. Others, such as some geckos (*Phelsuma* spp.), have relatively small granular scales and thin, delicate skin. Observe for missing scales, abnormal skin coloration, crusts, dysecdysis (incompletely shed skin), subdermal swellings, and external parasites including mites and ticks. Pay particular attention to skin folds, flaps, nostrils, eyelids, axillae, and ears for mites and ticks. Observe for signs of trauma such as rostral abrasions, necrotic or missing toes, damage to the tail, bite wounds, and signs of thermal or chemical burns, which may appear as erythema or tissue necrosis. Inspect for missing, damaged, or discolored toes or toenails. Remember that not all lizards have four legs and five toes per leg. *Ophisaurus* spp. and *Lialis* spp. are two examples of legless lizards. *Chamaeleo* spp. have five toes, which are fused into two gripping bundles per foot.

While observing the lizard, systematically pay attention to respiration and the respiratory effort. As with caged birds, respiration for most lizards at rest is relatively effortless and nearly imperceptible from a distance. Gaping (holding the mouth open) associated with dyspnea may be the result of upper or lower respiratory disease. Overheating, defensive posturing, and stress or anxiety may also lead to this behavior. Similarly, mucoid oral and nasal secretions are not normal, though crystalline or salt secretions may be normal in some species such as *Uromastyx* spp. and *Iguana* spp. Thoracic auscultation should be performed over the entire dorsal and lateral thoracic regions. When performing auscultation, a moistened paper towel or thin cloth may be wrapped over the diaphragm of the stethoscope to reduce noise from rough skin or scales.

An essential part of the physical exam for most lizards is the oral exam. This examination may require physical or chemical restraint and must be performed with consideration to safety of the veterinary staff and health risk to the patient. Some lizards (*Iguana* spp., *Varanus* spp., *Chamaeleo* spp., *Pogona* spp., and some *Gecko* spp.) may voluntarily open their mouth when approached in the cage or when restrained, making oral examination less physically challenging. In these species, (excluding *Gecko* spp.) the mouth may be opened with gentle retraction of the dewlap while the maxilla is secured with the other hand. This approach is contraindicated in patients that have normally fragile skin (most species of Gekkonidae) or those with diseased skin as with hypovitaminosis C. The author has observed the dewlap skin tear easily in malnourished *Chamaeleo* spp. suspected of having hypovitaminosis C among other malnourishment-related diseases. The gentle introduction of a rubber spatula into the mouth is useful as a speculum. Metal and wooden speculums should be avoided because they may result in damage to gums and teeth as well as damage to or accidental ingestion of the speculum (or portions thereof) with stronger lizards. For very small lizards, plastic spoons or plastic credit cards may be used as a speculum. For large lizards or those with dark-pigmented oral epithelium an otoscopic or laryngoscopic illuminator is useful to visualize the oral anatomy.

Chemical restraint may be required to examine the oral cavity with some species because of their strong jaws and a reluctance to open the mouth. Similarly, lizards with NSHP or those with thin mandibles may suffer traumatic iatrogenic fractures from manipulation of the mouth. Tremendous caution and attention must be used when manipulating the mouth of adult iguanas and monitors. Any distraction or a mistake in handling may result in serious injury or amputation of a digit to the handler. The bodies of larger lizards must be fully immobilized prior to opening the mouth to prevent the patient from exerting any leverage by thrashing or spinning the body, should an accidental bite occur.

Examination of the oral cavity includes observation of the choanae, dentition, glottis, and mucous membranes. While manipulating the head, palpate for the firmness and symmetry of the mandible and maxilla. Bones that compress or bend in a lateral fashion may signify NSHP. The mandibular symphysis is fused in lizards. Abscesses and granulomas may occur in the mandible with no apparent mucous membrane abnormalities. The oral cavity should be bilaterally symmetric. The mucous membranes of the oral cavity are generally uniform in color. Many lizards have a pink to pinkish–white color to the oral epithelium with a somewhat glistening surface. Some lizards may have pigmented oral epithelium. The oral mucous membranes of some old-world chameleons (*Chamaeleo* spp.) and bearded dragons (*Pogona* spp.) are yellow and should not be interpreted as icteric or jaundiced. In a healthy lizard, there is little to no mucus, blood, pus, or other exudates in the mouth. The glottis should be observed through several respiratory cycles of inspiration both to observe normal movement of glottis cartilages and to observe for any exudates from within the glottis. The choanae should be clear of any exudate. The dentition and gingiva should be free of erythema or exudate. Similar to snakes, some *Gecko* spp. have a spectacle which covers the eye. Subspectacular abscesses are commonly observed in conjunction with and may arise from infectious stomatitis (DeVoe 2019); an oral exam is always warranted with the presence of subspectacular abscesses. Periodontal disease is common in agamid lizards. The dental arcades should be examined for the presence of staining or calculus along with secondary infection.

Examination of the external cloaca or vent also requires physical restraint. The vent should have an appearance consistent with that of the remaining dermis with the exception of specialized scales, which vary among species. Some lizards possess femoral pores that extend laterally from the vent onto the ventral aspect of the hindlegs or pre-femoral pores cranial to the vent. The vent and surrounding integument should be bilaterally symmetric. As with the integument, observe for signs of trauma, swelling, exudates, and crusts, and observe for prolapse of cloacal tissue or hemipenes.

Coelomic palpation is a non-invasive method to evaluate gastrointestinal, reproductive, and urinary systems. Palpation is performed gently with the fingertips to create minimal stress and reduce the risk of internal damage to delicate or diseased patients. If gastrointestinal obstruction or bloating is suspected, caution must be exercised to prevent iatrogenic rupture to dilated gastrointestinal structures. Kidneys are located within the pelvis and thus are only palpable on coelmic palpation if they are enlarged and extending out of the pelvic canal. Uroliths, follicles, eggs, or masses of various types may be palpable. It is also difficult to impossible to differentiate gastrointestinal structures on palpation other than by extrapolating their location. Paired fat bodies are present in the caudal celom. These are bilateral and may be confused with kidneys or masses in the coelom. The fat bodies are particularly evident in dorsally compressed lizards such as bearded dragons and *Uromastyx* spp.

Small lizards, particularly many gekkonids, have semi-transparent ventral body walls and skin. This allows for visualization of some coelomic structures while the lizard is contained in a clear plastic or glass container. This technique is particularly useful for visualizing eggs in these species. An oviparous lizard carrying eggs is termed gravid, whereas a viviparous lizard carrying embryos is termed pregnant. But both terms are used interchangeably for both conditions. Eggs are generally visible against the body wall or are palpable in many gravid oviparous lizards. Pregnancy in viviparous lizards is suspected with generalized coelomic swelling, though developing embryos may not be palpable.

Radiology

Radiographic imaging is particularly useful in evaluating skeletal disorders in lizards. Evaluation of respiratory disorders and gastrointestinal disorders is also possible, though gastrointestinal imaging must commonly employ contrast media. Other coelomic structures that are evident on radiographs are kidneys (only if enlarged), liver, coelomic masses, fat bodies, the heart, and occasionally uroliths. During ovulation, ovaries and shelled or non-shelled eggs as well as developing embryos may be observed; otherwise, gonads are not visible on radiographs in lizards.

Radiographic equipment should have several capabilities. A milliampere (mA) setting of 300 mA and exposure times approaching 1/60 second (5 mAs) with relatively low kVp (45 to 60 kVp) produce excellent exposures using high-detail, rare-earth intensifying screens (Silverman & Janssen 1996). A collimator is essential to prevent scatter radiation when taking exposures on small patients. The radiographic machine should have horizontal beam capabilities, though without this, and through creative positioning of the patient, acceptable imaging is possible. A minimum of two exposures of the coelomic cavity are desired: dorsoventral and laterolateral (lateral). Similarly, extremities should be imaged in at least two planes.

For many lizards, a table-top technique is employed without a grid. Exposure techniques vary widely with different radiology units. With the advent and widespread use of digital radiography, this make it far easier to adjust settings for proper exposures of small patients. Most machines will have recommended setting for certain centimeter thickness of the patient, but the veterinary staff can develop their own technique chart based on what settings give the best images for patients of a certain size or species. The standard dorsoventral and lateral positioning techniques may not reveal the true nature of coelomic structures or abnormalities. Therefore, partial rotation of the patient to a 30-degree or 45-degree lateral exposure can be useful as a third exposure when evaluating the coelom as can the administration of contrast agents.

The difficulty with radiology in lizards is restraint and positioning. Large, healthy, or aggressive lizards may need to be sedated. The vasovagal maneuver can be used for restraint for large iguanas by placing a cotton ball over each eye and wrapping the head with vetwrap to hold them in place. This minimizes bite risk and radiation exposure risk to the handler(s). Small lizards that are slow-moving or calm may be allowed to rest unrestrained on the cassette for the dorsoventral vertical beam exposure. Lateral horizontal beam exposures are possible without restraint for some still or chemically restrained lizards. Small, fast-moving, or delicate lizards may be placed inside a clear plastic container or tube or cloth bag and positioned appropriately for exposure. Though some details of the image may be lost, this may be the only option to obtain radiographs of these patients. When sedated, gauze ribbons or masking tape may be used to extend limbs as needed.

Contrast media are commonly employed when non-skeletal imaging is required. Gastrointestinal contrast studies not only are beneficial for evaluating complete or partial obstructions, but also are particularly useful for evaluating extraintestinal coelomic masses. Barium sulfate is the standard contrast material for gastrointestinal contrast imaging. Barium for gastric and small intestinal imaging is administered via an oral ball-tip dosing needle or flexible, non-rigid rubber catheter (see section on "Techniques"). Unless the imaging of the esophagus specifically is required, administration of barium via a gastric tube is best. Oral cavity dosing may result in partial aspiration and loss of barium through the mouth or nostrils. In diseased lizards, gastric to colonic transit times may be delayed substantially.

Retrograde or percloacal barium administration is indicated when distal intestinal obstruction or caudal abdominal coelomic masses are suspected. Barium is administered via a flexible, non-rigid rubber catheter. In small lizards, (<200 g) rigid or metal catheters should be avoided to prevent iatrogenic cloacal or colonic perforation (see section on "Techniques"). The clinician should approximate the amount of barium required for the desired image (Banzato et al. 2013). Diseased colon or intestine may rupture with even the slightest pressure; therefore, resistance on the syringe is not good practice for approximating dosing for administration of oral or percloacal barium.

Anesthesia and Surgery

Once uncommonly performed, coelomic cavity surgery or coeliotomy is now routine for many pet lizards. These procedures include ovariectomy, orchiectomy, salpingotomy/salpingectomy, gastrotomy, enterotomy, cystotomy, biopsy, and tumor excision. Other surgeries that do not require coeliotomy include amputation (digits, limbs, tails, and hemipenis), enucleation, fracture repair, laceration repair, mass removal, prolapse (intestinal, oviductal) repair, and reconstructive surgeries.

Anesthesia

Injectable and inhalant anesthetics are commonly employed for surgery and sedation for diagnostic or treatment procedures and analgesia. Significant advances have been made through the years in the field of reptile anesthesia and analgesia. Each veterinarian and technician will develop their favorite anesthetic protocols they are most comfortable with but choices often vary between species, the procedure being performed, health status of the animal, etc.

In recent years, the preferred injectable anesthetic for reptiles (especially lizards) has become the neuroactive steroid alfaxalone (Alfaxan; Jurox, Kansas City, MO). Alfaxan has benefits over propofol in that it may be injected intramuscularly, may be redosed to effect, and offers brief immobilization and anesthesia (Bertelsen & Sauer 2011). Though analgesia is not sufficient for most incisional surgical procedures, it is particularly useful as an induction agent with inhalant anesthesia or as a sole sedative agent for brief procedures in conjunction with analgesics if pain control is needed. Alfaxalone is given most often in lizards at 5–15 mg/kg IV, IM, or SQ (Mans et al. 2019). Apnea is the most common side effect.

An additional injectable anesthetic, propofol (PropoFlo), is also used in reptiles for anesthetic induction and restraint. Propofol must be administered IV or via intraosseus catheter (IO) at a dose of 3 to 10 mg/kg (Mans et al. 2019). The drug is administered slowly over 30 to 60 seconds or until the desired sedation is achieved. Propofol is eliminated rapidly from the blood and therefore is suitable for short diagnostic procedures or to achieve intubation for inhalant anesthesia. Its anesthetic effects may be extended by slow constant rate or intermittent infusion. Unless an indwelling catheter exists in the patient to be sedated, other injectable or inhalant anesthetics are preferred.

Other injectable agents such as ketamine and telazol are commonly used as well, though their main disadvantage is a significantly prolonged recovery time over alfaxalone or propofol. These combinations are more commonly used in larger species (especially large chelonians, snakes, and crocodilians) where the volume of alfaxalone or propofol needed would be cost-prohibitive or impossible to administer. The alpha-2 agonist dexmedetomidine and benzodiazepine midazolam are commonly used in various protocols with other agents as well and produce reliable sedation (Mans et al. 2019). These have the benefit of being reversible with atipamezole, and flumazenil, respectively.

Opioids provide a smoother induction when administered as a premedication for injectable or inhalant induction and are the preferred agents for analgesia in reptiles. Pure mu-agonist opioids such as hydromorphone and morphine seem to be most effective for reptiles based on pharmacokinetic and pharmacodynamic studies (Greenacre et al. 2006, Kanui et al. 1990, Kanui & Hole 1992, Mans et al. 2012, Sladky et al. 2007, Sladky et al. 2008, Wambugu et al. 2010). Fentanyl patches show promise as studies show the drug is absorbed readily, but efficacy has not been proven (Gamble 2008, Kharbush et al. 2017). While historically butorphanol was used most commonly, more recent research has not demonstrated any analgesic effects (Greenacre et al. 2006, Olesen et al. 2008, Sladky et al. 2007, Sladky et al. 2008). Respiratory depression is the most common side effect of opioids. Tramadol appears to have greater analgesic effect in reptiles than in mammals with less respiratory depression and has become a preferred post-operative pain medication (Baker et al. 2011, Giorgi et al. 2015, Norton et al. 2015).

While non-steroidal anti-inflammatory drugs (NSAIDs) are popular in most other species, their benefit in reptiles is still unproven. Clinicians routinely use NSAIDs for pain management and post-operative pain as part of a multi-modal analgesic protocol in reptiles, particularly meloxicam as its safety and effectiveness have been proven in other exotic species (exotic companion mammals and birds). However, in reptiles, while multiple pharmacokinetic studies have been performed that demonstrate NSAIDs like meloxicam and ketoprofen reach therapeutic levels known in other species, minimal reports exist of their efficacy (Di Salvo et al. 2015, Divers et al. 2010, Greenacre et al. 2006, Lai et al. 2015, Olesen et al. 2008, Sladky and Mans 2019, Tuttle et al. 2006, Uney et al. 2016). The author routinely uses a single injection of meloxicam at 0.2–0.3 mg/kg post-operatively in most lizard surgeries (if there are no contraindications) in the hopes that it may help and is unlikely to hurt, but opioids are most reliable for analgesia in reptiles.

A common protocol for most lizard surgeries is hydromorphone 0.5 mg/kg + midazolam 0.5–1 mg/kg IM as a premedication, followed by induction with alfaxalone at

10–15 mg/kg IV or IM, but every veterinarian and technician will develop their own comfort level with various protocols. Most often tramadol at 5–10 mg/kg PO every 48–72 hours is prescribed post-operatively. Refer to Mans et al. (2019) and Sladky and Mans (2019) for extremely comprehensive discussions of anesthesia and analgesia in reptiles.

The benefits of the anticholinergics atropine or glycopyrrolate as pre-anesthetic medications in lizards are questionable and in general are not used. Atropine is typically only given in cases of emergency (severe bradycardia or cardiopulmonary resuscitataion). Atropine is administered IM at a dose of 0.01 to 0.04 mg/kg.

Local anesthetics can be used alone or in combination with other drugs as part of a multimodal anesthesia/analgesia protocol. Lidocaine, bupivacaine, or mepivacaine are most commonly used. These can be administered as in mammals locally at the site of surgery given subcutaneously or as ring blocks or direct nerve blocks. Typically one should not exceed 2–4 mg/kg dosing, and for small patients, the anesthetic can be diluted with saline in order to administer a safe dose or to create enough volume to block the entire site needed. For minor procedures like a digit amputation, skin biopsy, or pharyngostomy tube placement, sedation with alfaxalone combined with a local anesthetic block works extremely well. Intrathecal administration can be extremely useful for procedures of the tail, hind limb, cloaca, and hemipenes/phallus. Preservative-free lidocaine, bupivacaine, and/or morphine can be administered between coccygeal vertebrae into the intrathecal space. So far, intrathecal analgesia has mainly been used in chelonians, but can be extrapolated to lizards (da Silva et al. 2016, Rivera et al. 2011).

Inhalant anesthetics are preferred for maintenance of general anesthesia in lizards. The inhalant anesthetics of choice for lizards are isoflurane or sevoflurane. Isoflurane and sevoflurane provides relatively rapid induction if used alone for short sedation procedures. Because ventilatory suppression is common during anesthesia, recovery, though smooth, is prolonged compared to the typical recovery of mammals of similar size induced and maintained on isoflurane (Figure 9.20).

Lizards should be intubated for inhalant anesthesia whenever possible. Intubation is relatively easy for the sedated lizard. The glottis is visible in the floor of the mouth at the base of the tongue. Cuffed tubes should not be used (or the cuff not inflated) in species with complete tracheal rings. Cole-style endotracheal tubes (if the patient is large enough) are recommended as the tapered end fits into the glottis with the larger portion sitting against the glottis, creating a seal. Commercial tubes are made down

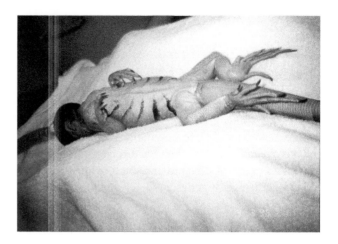

Figure 9.20 Mask anesthetic induction of a lizard.

to 1 mm in diameter, and ET tubes can also be modified from intravenous catheters or red rubber catheters with an adapter at the end. Most lizards will not breathe on their own under anesthesia, so maintenance on a mask is not a recommended option.

Reptilian respiratory physiology differs from that of mammals. In reptiles, the spontaneous ventilation rate is directly related to temperature and the partial pressure of oxygen (pO_2), whereas in mammals respiration, it is driven by carbon dioxide (pCO_2) (Mans et al. 2019). Thus, in high-oxygen environments spontaneous ventilation is suppressed because the demand for oxygen by tissues is met by the oxygen saturation of inhalant anesthesia. As with mammals, control of the airway during anesthesia is helpful for the control of depth of anesthesia and is essential for assisted ventilation. Breathholding is a common problem during the induction phase of inhalant anesthesia in some lizards. For this reason, mask induction is not typically recommended or feasible. Because lizards experience profound respiratory depression during general anesthesia, assisted or intermittent positive pressure ventilation (IPPV) ventilation is commonly required.

IPPV is performed at two to four breaths per minute at a pressure of less than 10 cmH$_2$O in medium to large lizards, and much less in smaller lizards (Mans et al. 2019). Ideally, the anesthetist should visualize rib expansion for several cycles of IPPV to discern the ideal pressure or ventilatory volume before the patient is draped. To avoid excessive pulmonary pressure and possible pulmonary rupture, the pop-off valve should never be fully closed when ventilating reptile patients. The great majority of lizards are maintained on a non-rebreathing anesthetic circuit; lizards over 10 pounds are maintained on a rebreathing circuit, similar to mammals. An oxygen flow rate of 300 to 500 mL/kg/min is indicated.

Anesthetic monitoring is essential during reptilian sedation. Unlike snakes, cardiac movement may not be detectable through the chest wall because of the presence of a cartilaginous sternum. A Doppler monitor is most useful for monitoring heart rate audibly as often pulse oximetry and ECG are more challenging to set up or get a consistent reading. The Doppler should be placed with lubricant and taped over the heart for continuous monitoring. Pulse oximetry can be used but more often for heart rate rather than for accurate oxygenation levels. Often this is used to monitor trends more than for specific readings. For small lizards, the finger probe may be placed across the dorsal head with the infrared transducer above the head and the receiver in the mouth. For larger lizards, the orientation is reversed on the mandible or may be placed across the tongue. The advantage of pulse oximetry is the detection of blood flow that is reflective of mechanical cardiac activity as opposed to simply the detection of electrical cardiac activity, which may continue after mechanical activity is compromised. Electrocardiography (ECG) is also valuable and is used with a three-lead system, but to obtain a reading, typically needles will need to be placed in the skin and the clips attached to these needles rather than directly to the skin. Blood pressure can be monitored by placing the cuff around the tail (in large enough species) but levels are not accurate when compared with direct blood pressure readings; they can, however, be used to monitor trends (Mans et al. 2019).

Reptile patients are warmed during surgical anesthesia with water-recirculating heating pads or commercial patient warmers such as a Hot Dog warmer (Hot Dog veterinary warming system, Eden Prairie, MN) or Bair Hugger (3M, St. Paul, MN). Electrical heating pads put the patient at risk for thermal burns. Surgical temperature should match the POTZ for a given species, but a range of 78 to 85°F (25 to 29°C) is sufficient for most patients. Supplemental heating is also indicated during the entire phase of anesthetic recovery.

Lizards sedated with injectable anesthetics may require hours to recover. In debilitated animals, this time is prolonged. For ketamine and telazol, recovery times from 1 to 96 hours are reported in reptiles. Because of this, alfaxalone and propofol have become the preferred agents for reptiles where recovery is typically less than 1 hour or even faster. During recovery, IPPV should be continued. The patient should be ventilated using an Ambu bag and room air and oxygen discontinued. Because a reptile's stimulus to breathe is low oxygen, if the patient is maintained on 100% oxygen this can prolong recovery. All injectables that can be reversed should be. Epinephrine given intramuscularly at a dose of 0.1 mg/kg upon recovery and an acupuncture needle placed at the point GV26 (ventral to the nose) has been shown to significantly shorten recovery time in crocodilians and snapping turtles (Gatson et al. 2017, Goe et al. 2016); this technique has been used in lizards as well.

Surgery

Celiotomy is commonly performed in lizards for the surgical procedures already listed. Surgical preparation for lizards is similar to that of small mammals. The lizard is placed in dorsal recumbency with legs and tail restrained by tape to the surgical table. The surgical site should be scrubbed with mild detergent if necessary to remove dirt or debris. Standard surgical preparation is performed. Surgical draping is required. A fenestrated paper drape or a combination of clear plastic and fenestrated paper drape is used. The benefit of clear plastic drape is visualization of the patient for anesthetic monitoring during the surgical procedure.

Surgical incisions are made with consideration for skin and abdominal musculature lines of force, trauma to tissues, visualization of the desired surgical field, and wound healing. The long-accepted standard approach to celiotomy is the ventral paramedian incision in an effort to avoid transection or manipulation of the large ventral abdominal vein (see section on "Anatomy"). This incision requires the transection of ventral abdominal muscle, which increases surgical bleeding, may decrease surgical field visibility (both from bleeding and from left versus right coelom access), and may increase postsurgical pain when compared to a ventral midline incision through the linea alba. In larger lizards, the ventral abdominal vein may be gently retracted during the ventral midline incision.

The most common procedures performed during celiotomy are ovariosalpingectomy or salpingotomy for dystocia, ovariectomy, orchiectomy, and enterotomy. In most cases, hemostatic clips are used for ligation of ovarian and oviductal vessels as indicated by surgical procedure. Great care must be exercised when handling all reproductive and mesenteric tissues in lizards, because they are delicate and quite friable. Sterile cotton swabs and fine instruments are commonly used for this. Hemostasis is extremely important in small patients, so in addition to hemostatic clips; radiosurgery, laser, or additional cautery methods are often employed to control bleeding. Closure of the celiotomy incision is in two layers consisting of abdominal musculature or linea with absorbable suture, followed by the skin. The skin is closed in an everting pattern with absorbable or non-absorbable tissue or skin staples. Reptilian skin heals significantly slower than mammalian skin. Suture removal is delayed until a minimum of 4 to 6 weeks post-surgery and until after the patient has shed at least once (Divers 2019). The patient should not be allowed to soak for at least 2 weeks after surgery.

A common non-celiotomy surgical procedure is digit or limb amputation. This procedure is indicated when trauma sustained from bites of cage mates or of rodents, or fractures result in non-healing wounds or ascending limb infection. Surgical preparation is standard as in celiotomy. Amputation is performed at the most distal non-infected joint for limbs, and preferably at the metacarpal or metatarsal-phalangeal joint for digit amputation. General anesthesia is required for limb amputations. Peripheral nerve blocks with sedation may be performed for some digit amputations.

Amputation of the hemipenes is indicated in cases of paraphimosis complicated by trauma, infection, or necrosis. This procedure may be performed with appropriate sedation using only injectable anesthetics. Aseptic preparation is standard. Amputation of one hemipenis does not sterilize the lizard because the hemipenes are paired. No compromise of urinary function will result from amputation, because there is no incorporation of urinary structures in the hemipenes or penis of reptiles (Barten and Simpson 2019).

Percloacal prolapse of colon, oviducts, or urinary bladder may require amputation or resection of the affected tissues. Exposure of affected tissues or severe trauma may result in necrosis if the prolapse is not reduced promptly after occurrence. Necrosis of large portions of these tissues may require celiotomy to evaluate viability and repair the affected organ.

Open reduction and internal fixation of long bone fractures in reptiles are performed following the surgical approach and principles applied to mammals. Intramedullary pins, orthopedic wire, external skeletal fixation, and bone plating are employed as indicated.

Orthopedic devices are removed following the principles used in mammals, though healing of fractures in reptiles is slow and hardware may require removal prior to radiographic evidence of complete bone healing (Knafo and Karlin 2019).

Parasitology

Many reptile owners are unaware of the prevalence of parasitism in their animals. It is safe to assume that all wild-caught reptiles are parasitized (Wellehan and Walden 2019). Commonly many captive-born reptiles are subclinically parasitized. In wild animals, internal parasites maintain a homeostasis with the host animal, because the host is essential for the survival of the parasite and a means of transporting future generations of the parasite to suitable areas for transmission to another host. Factors that maintain homeostasis include the host's immune system and the dilution of infective stages of the parasite in the environment that the host occupies. Thus, in many cases, the captive environment offers a prime opportunity for imbalances in favor of the parasite through the stress and subsequent immunosuppression of the host, and through the increased risk of reinfection of the host due to concentration of infective stages of the parasite.

Based on an awareness of parasites in some reptiles, however, some herpetoculturists advocate the prophylactic treatment of all reptiles with antiparasiticides for the more common intestinal parasites (de Vosjoli & Ferguson 1995). It is interesting, however, that the majority of hobbyists do not prophylactically treat for external parasites. This is perhaps because of an understanding of the potential side effects of pesticides applied to the animals. The side effects of oral deworming are similar. Though some therapeutics may be relatively safe at high doses, the potential effects of killing massive loads of intestinal parasites in an already immunocompromised animal can be severe. The safer alternative to prophylactic treatment of parasites is quarantine, serial parasite screening, and treatment of specific clinically identified diseases.

Techniques for identifying reptilian endoparasites are the same as those for small mammals. Flotation of fresh fecal material in concentrated salt or sugar solutions and wet mount direct smears in saline are essential to screen for reptilian endoparasites. Smaller infective stages of some parasites may only be observed by direct smear. Stains such as Lugol's iodine solution (5 g iodine crystals and 10 g potassium iodide in 100 mL distilled water) both kills motile protozoans and stains cysts to make identification easier. It is recommended to examine both stained and unstained direct smears in addition to the fecal flotation.

External Parasites

External reptilian parasites consist of ticks, mites, chiggers, leeches, and biting flying insects. Acariasis (mite, tick, or chigger infestation) is a serious disease of reptiles. Clinically tick infestations are most common in imported lizards. Wellehan and Walden (2019) report that there are seven genera of ticks and more than 250 species of mites that parasitize reptiles. Chiggers, also called red bugs, are the larval stage of trombiculid mites and are more common in lizards. Snake mites (*Ophionyssus natricis*) are mobile and highly transmissible and are capable of infesting multiple animals in a room or household without direct contact between hosts. While these most commonly affect snakes, they can spread to lizards as well. These mites may be transmitted between hosts on the skin or clothing of people, though human infestation is supposedly rare.

Reptile skin provides many sites for attachment and protection for both mites and ticks. Ticks are commonly found beneath scales or in crevices such as the junction of the limbs and body or around the eyelids. Mites may be seen crawling freely over the lizard, but commonly concentrate in protected skin folds. It is not uncommon to diagnose mites after handling a lizard and then observing them on the handler's skin, or seeing dead mites in water bowls of lizards that soak themselves routinely. Lizards that increase soaking behavior are commonly infested with mites.

Eradicating mites from individual animals is easier than eradicating them from the premises. Infestation of one animal indicates the possibility and likelihood of widespread infestation. Thus, prevention through quarantine of new animals is imperative (see section on "Husbandry") and treating the cage and cage accessories and maintaining cleanliness of the surrounding environment are imperative.

Treatment consists of physical removal of ticks and inspection for the presence of ticks over several weeks. The author's preferred treatment for mites is fipronil spray. This treatment appears to be safe and is extremely effective. The spray is applied to a towel, and the towel is used to wipe the animal down head to tail. At the same time, the enclosure must be broken down and cleaned, any particulate bedding discarded, and anything made of wood either discarded or soaked and bleached. The animal should be kept on paper towels or newspaper along with a water bowl and hide box and anything in the enclosure made of smooth, non-porous surfaces. Every 7–10 days, the fipronil treatment is repeated along with cleaning the cage and everything in it. If the owner is diligent about environmental cleanup, typically three treatments are effective at eliminating the infestation. Unfortunately, fipronil spray may be difficult at times to obtain due to a lack of availability of products on the market. Some newer antiparasitics for dogs and cats are being explored for reptiles. Fluralaner (Bravecto, Merck & Co., Inc., Rahway, NJ) has been used for snake mites in ball pythons (Gobble 2022). The introduction of parasitic mites and/or ladybugs that will feed on the reptile mites but not harm the reptile can also be used for environmental control (Schilliger et al. 2013).

Ivermectin (Ivomec, Merck; and generics) is reported as both a topical and systemic treatment for mites in reptiles (Wellehan and Walden 2019). The topical formulation is 0.5 mL ivermectin 1% (5 mg) added in 1,000 mL water and applied as a spray. The systemic administration is 0.2 mg/kg ivermectin 1% SC or PO. Clinical experience reflects unpredictable results and variable degrees of toxicity or side effects on a species-to-species basis with the injectable protocol, though no lethality has been observed in lizards by the author. Topical administration is absolutely not reliable. The miscibility and stability of ivermectin in water as a spray is questionable.

Many over-the-counter pet industry products are available for mites. These are generally "soap and water" mixtures designed to reduce the surface tension of water and allow water to penetrate the spiracles or airways of mites, which essentially drowns the mite. The active ingredients are generally fatty acids (listed by scientific name) in an aqueous base. Most of these compounds are not effective. One over-the-counter product that is effective and commonly used is Provent-A-Mite (Pro Products, Mahopac, NY) which is a permethrin spray. This can be used in the environment but should not be applied to the animal (Wellehan and Walden 2019, Perry and Mitchell 2019).

Other home remedies include the use of pest strips. These products are also quite effective in killing reptiles. Unfortunately, if used in a safe manner (or by sheer luck), these products have been effective in environmental control of mites in large collections. The narrow safety margin, however, prohibits recommendation of these products.

Note: Prepare the client for a long duration of treatment and for the strong possibility of both the contagious nature and high relapse rate of reptilian mite infestations. Also inform of the potential side effects of treatments both to lizards and humans from pyrethrins, pyrethroids, and organophosphates.

Internal Parasites

Internal parasites comprise many families and induce the majority of parasitic diseases in lizards. It is possible for many parasites to remain latent in the body and manifest disease during host immunosuppression from stress or other concurrent disease. Intestinal parasites consist of protozoa, coccidia, cestodes, trematodes, acanthocephalans, nematodes, pentostomes, and hemoparasites.

Protozoans

Many protozoans inhabit the gastrointestinal tract of lizards as non-pathogenic or commensal organisms. The technician and veterinarian must learn to identify various species and determine which are pathogens and which are not. Some may be non-pathogenic in low numbers, but if the patient is immunosuppressed or otherwise compromised, can replicate and become a problem.

Amoebiasis is directly transmitted by a fecal–oral route in reptiles and is pathogenic and highly virulent to some snakes and lizards. Amoebiasis is non-pathogenic in turtles and crocodilians but may be transmitted by both (Wellehan and Walden 2019). The life cycle of the amoeba *Entamoeba invadens* is as follows: passing of infective cysts from a host;

ingestion of cysts by a suitable host; multiplication into trophozoites in the intestinal tract; invasion of trophozoites into host tissues; formation of infective cysts; and shedding of infective cysts.

The pathogenesis of clinical disease is multifactorial and is caused by the tissue invasion of trophozoites and cellular destruction, and from secondary bacterial infection. Clinical signs include diarrhea or loose mucoid stools, anorexia, dehydration, and weight loss. Infective trophozoites may spread to other organs hematogenously, causing inflammation and potentially organ failure (Wellehan and Walden 2019).

Diagnosis is made by fecal examination. Cysts are identified by fecal flotation or direct saline smear, and trophozoites are identified only by direct smear. For direct saline smears, a drop of Lugol's iodide is helpful to immobilize and stain the organisms.

Treatment of amoebiasis consists of antibiotics and antiprotozoal medications. Antibiotics are administered to treat potential secondary bacterial infections or potential septicemia. Metronidazole is administered at varying doses depending on species while checking fecal samples for cysts or trophozoites (Wellehan and Walden 2019). Strict hygiene and sanitation are required to prevent horizontal transmission.

Numerous flagellates and ciliates can be present in lizards, especially hindgut fermenters. *Nyctotherus* and *Balantidium* are ciliates that do not cause disease. *Trichomonas* is present in almost all lizards in small amounts, and does not typically cause disease, yet it can overgrow in young or immunosuppressed animals and cause illness. *Hexamita* and *Giardia* are always considered pathogens. *Giardia* is relatively uncommon in reptiles, while *Hexamita* can ascend the urinary tract and cause renal infection and damage (Juan-Sallés et al. 2014). The most common symptoms of protozoal enteritis are diarrhea, foul odor of the feces, blood or mucous in the feces, and sometimes anorexia or regurgitation or stunted growth/failure to thrive in young animals. Treatment is with metronidazole.

Cryptosporidium is a highly virulent pathogen of snakes and lizards. *C. serpentis* affects snakes while *C. varanii* affects lizards. Cryptosporidium can affect any species of lizard, but leopard geckos are significantly overrepresented. Some animals remain asymptomatic carriers. In lizards, *C. varanii* causes a proliferative enteritis which interferes with digestion and absorption of nutrients (Deming et al. 2009, Wellehan and Walden, 2019). Affected lizards typically lose weight despite a good appetite and become very thin; signs can progress to regurgitation, diarrhea, anorexia, and eventually emaciation and death. Diagnosis is with acid-fast stain or PCR of feces, regurgitated material, cloacal swab (lizards), or gastric swab (snakes). The organisms are shed intermittently, so repeated tests are often needed and a negative test does not rule it out. Histopathology is the gold standard for diagnosis. Treatment is unrewarding as nothing has been shown to eliminate the parasite, though some treatments have been shown to reduce shedding (Boyer et al. 2013; Wellehan and Walden, 2019). Euthanasia is recommended because of the poor prognosis and to reduce the risk of transmission to other animals. Most common disinfectants are ineffective. All caging and furnishings should be discarded or cleaned with 5–10% ammonia and allowed to air dry; it can also be inactivated by heat (Boyer et al. 2013; Wellehan and Walden, 2019).

Coccidia

Coccidiosis is directly transmitted via the fecal–oral route and is caused by organisms of the genera *Eimeria*, *Isospora*, and *Caryospora*. The life cycle of coccidia in lizards is similar to that seen in mammals: oocysts passed in the stool sporulate outside the body and are ingested by a suitable host; sporozoites are released to invade host epithelial cells and mature; and the epithelial cell ruptures and releases merozoites, which infect other cells and then can either multiply to infect yet other cells or form intracellular gametocytes; the latter eventually become infective oocysts, which are passed in the stool. Clinical disease results from cellular destruction and from secondary bacterial infection. Detection of oocysts is made by fecal flotation or direct smear.

Understanding the pathophysiology is important because infective oocysts are shed intermittently; thus, clinical disease can occur in the absence of a detectable infectious agent. Clinically lizards may be asymptomatic or have diarrhea, blood in the feces, anorexia, weight loss, or failure to gain weight. Bearded dragons are significantly overrepresented and are affected by the organism *Isospora amphiboluri*. Many adult lizards with coccidiosis appear to be asymptomatic carriers, but neonates and juveniles with coccidiosis are usually clinically diseased. Coccidiosis can cause death in small or young lizards if undetected and untreated.

The preferred treatment for coccidia currently is ponazuril 30 mg/kg PO q48 h for 3 doses (Bogoslavsky 2007). Sulfa drugs seem to be less effective clinically at clearing infection. Strict hygiene and sanitation are required to prevent horizontal transmission. Repeat fecal examinations are imperative.

Cestodes

Tapeworms are infrequently encountered in captive lizards. Transmission is indirect, typically through an arthropod intermediate host as seen in dogs and cats. Diagnosis is made by observations of proglottids in the stool or identification of oocysts on fecal flotation. Treatment consists of praziquantel (Droncit) 5 to 8 mg/kg PO or IM, and treatment is repeated after 2 weeks (Wellehan and Walden 2019).

Nematodes

Various nematodes infect lizards. Those infecting the gastrointestinal and respiratory tracts include various species of the familiar roundworms and hookworms; pinworms (*Oxyuris* spp.); hepatic worms (*Capillaria* spp.); strongyles (*Strongyloides* spp.); and lungworms of the genus *Entomelas*. Treatment for all intestinal and respiratory nematodes follows descriptions.

Roundworms in lizards are similar to those in mammals. Transmission is indirect and diagnosis is made by fecal flotation and identification of the typical thick-walled round to ovoid oocysts. Diagnosis may also be made by identification of the adult worm in feces or vomitus. Because they require an indirect life cycle, these parasites are most commonly observed in carnivorous lizards and occasionally in omnivores.

Hookworms (*Oswalsocruzia* spp.) undergo direct transmission via the fecal–oral route or through skin penetration. Diagnosis is made by fecal flotation and identification of the typically thin-walled oval eggs. Hookworms are responsible for more clinical disease in lizards than roundworms because of the mucosal attachment of adult worms in the intestines. Clinical signs may include diarrhea, anorexia, and weight loss.

Pinworms (*Oxyuris* spp.) undergo direct transmission by the fecal–oral route and are found as adults in the large intestine of lizards. Diagnosis is made by fecal flotation and identification of the typically embryonated cigar-shaped larvae. Mammalian pinworm ova or larvae may be passed in the stool of carnivorous lizards but do not infect the lizards themselves. Typically pinworms are an incidental finding on fecal examination, as they are commensal organisms. However, in cases of very heavy burdens, often treatment is needed. In large numbers, they can cause anorexia, unthriftiness, impaction, and cloacitis.

Hepatic worms (*Capillaria* spp.) have both direct and indirect transmission by the fecal–oral route or through infected prey ingestion, and the oocysts somewhat resemble those of whipworms (*Trichuris* spp.) of dogs. *Capillaria* spp. typically inhabit the intestinal tract but may also migrate to other organs. Pathology due to these species is unclear. Diagnosis is made by fecal flotation and treatment is indicated on identification.

Strongyloides spp. have a somewhat complex life cycle with direct transmission by a fecal–oral route or through skin penetration. *Strongyloides* spp. inhabit the gastrointestinal tract and greatly resemble the lungworms of *Rhabdias* spp. on fecal flotation. Diagnosis for either species is made by fecal flotation and identification of larvae or embryonated eggs. Diarrhea, anorexia, or weight loss may be seen with *Strongyloides* infection. Increased respiratory secretions, pneumonia, anorexia, and weight loss may be seen with *Rhabdias* infections.

Filarid worms have been reported in various agamid and chameleon species, the most common of which is *Foleyella furcata*. As with filarid worms of mammals, the larvae live in the blood vessels of the animal and are transmitted by mosquitoes, while the adults are typically found within the body cavity or subcutaneous tissues. They are often diagnosed when the patient is presented for a subcutaneous swelling from which the worm can be removed. Historically treatment had been attempted with Ivermectin, but the die-off of the worms can result in anaphylaxis which can be fatal for the patient.

Treatment of all intestinal and respiratory nematodes consists of fenbendazole (Panacur) at a dose of 50 mg/kg PO once daily for 3 days, then repeated in 2 weeks followed by repeat fecal flotation, but various protocols exist (Wellehan and Walden 2019). The author typically uses fenbendazole 50 mg/kg PO once, then repeat in 2 and 4 weeks. Because the majority of nematode parasites have direct transmission, proper hygiene and sanitation are imperative.

Treatment of intestinal parasites in lizards is not without potential side effects. Anecdotal reports of sudden deaths in *Chamaeleo* spp. treated with standard single doses of fenbendazole and ivermectin (Stahl 1999) are known. Over several years, similar observations have been made of a dramatic decline in health following the deworming of some individuals of wild-caught *Uromastyx* spp., *Varanus* spp., and *Chlamydosaurus* spp. at a reptile wholesale distribution facility (Brad Wilson, personal communication). Some of the affected animals had no apparent compromised health prior to treatment but were housed with conspecifics in relatively small cages, experienced repeated movement of humans around the enclosures, and may not have been on the optimal plane of nutrition (Figures 9.21–9.32). Wild-caught animals are often adapted to low parasite burdens, but the stress of captivity and conditions described above alone can lead to high parasite loads, then the inflammation caused by the die-off of these parasites when treated can prove fatal.

Clinical Techniques

Intravenous and Intraosseous Catheter Placement

Intravenous (IV) catheter placement is generally limited to the medium to large lizards due to the difficulty in accessing

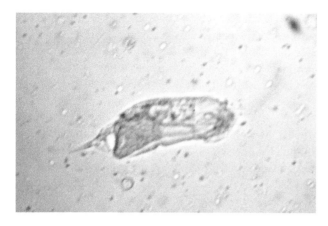

Figure 9.21 Ciliate protozoan, original magnification 40×. (Courtesy of Zoo Atlanta).

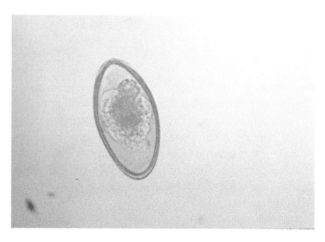

Figure 9.24 Oxyurid, original magnification 40×. (Courtesy of Zoo Atlanta).

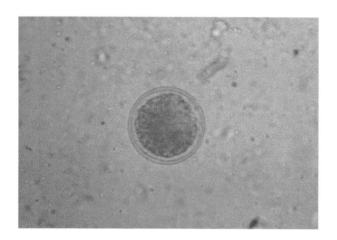

Figure 9.22 Roundworm, original magnification 40×. (Courtesy of Zoo Atlanta).

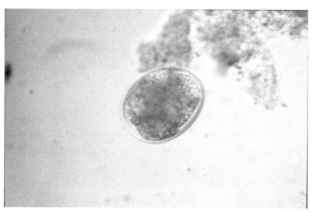

Figure 9.25 Ascarid, original magnification 40×. (Courtesy of Zoo Atlanta).

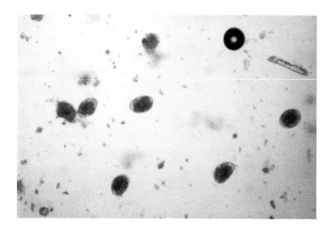

Figure 9.23 Ascarid, original magnification 40×. (Courtesy of Zoo Atlanta).

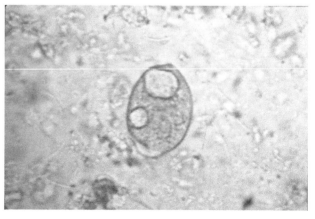

Figure 9.26 . Nyctotherus species cyst, original magnification 40×. (Courtesy of Zoo Atlanta).

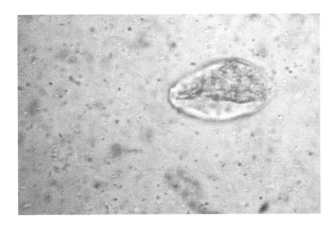

Figure 9.27 Nyctotherus, original magnification 40×. (Courtesy of Zoo Atlanta).

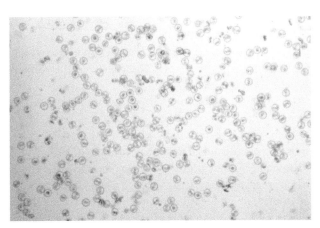

Figure 9.30 Eimeria, original magnification 40×. (Courtesy of Zoo Atlanta).

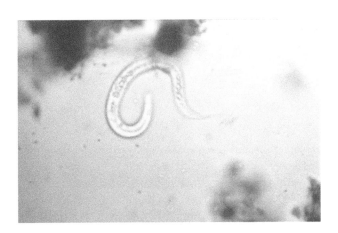

Figure 9.28 Strongyle larva, original magnification 40×. (Courtesy of Zoo Atlanta).

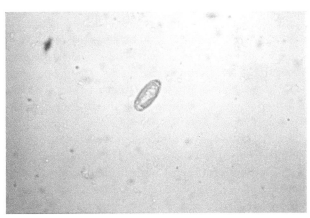

Figure 9.31 Capillaria, original magnification 40×. (Courtesy of Zoo Atlanta).

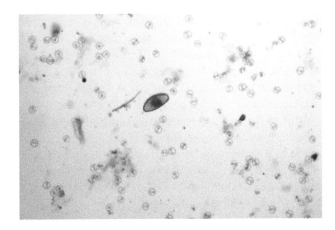

Figure 9.29 Pinworm and Eimeria, original magnification 40×. (Courtesy of Zoo Atlanta).

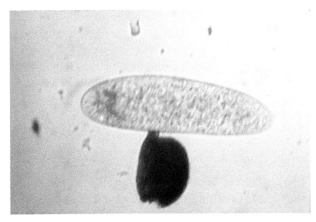

Figure 9.32 Rodent mite ova, original magnification 40×. (Courtesy of Zoo Atlanta).

a peripheral vein. The cephalic vein can be used in larger lizards, and the ventral coccygeal vein is a commonly used site as well. The ventral abdominal vein can be used but is difficult to maintain in an awake animal, so is more useful during anesthetic procedures. The jugular vein is difficult to access in most lizards.

Standard sterile preparation of the catheterization site is performed and a cutdown procedure is required for cephalic vein catheterization. A transverse skin incision is made across the dorsal distal aspect of the antebrachium, just dorsal to the carpus. In smaller lizards, the incision can be made with the sharp angle of a hypodermic needle, or in the case of larger lizards, with a scalpel blade. Once the vein is identified, standard catheterization technique is used with an appropriately sized intravenous catheter. The catheter is secured with tape or suture. Tail vein catheterization can be achieved without a cutdown and placement starts about 1/4 to 1/3 of the way down the tail distal to the cloaca.

Intraosseous (IO) catheters are indicated in smaller lizards or those with anatomy or disease that prohibits intravenous catheter placement. The bones of choice for intraosseous catheterization are the distal femur, proximal tibia, or distal humerus. Consideration must be given to the location with respect to the ability of the patient to interfere with or manipulate the catheter while hospitalized.

For IO catheterization, standard sterile preparation is performed over the catheter site and typically a local block with lidocaine is performed. A spinal needle or hypodermic needle of appropriate size is passed through a cutdown in the skin. The needle is advanced through the cortical bone of the distal diaphysis and then directed proximally into the medullary cavity of the bone. The tip of the needle should rest in the medullary cavity approximately one-third the distance from the proximal femur (Pardo and Divers 2019). The catheter is then secured with taping, which will also somewhat immobilize the stifle. Two-view radiographs can be taken to confirm correct catheter placement.

Intravenous and intraosseous fluid therapy is performed with standard balanced electrolyte solutions as for mammals at a rate of 1–3 mL/kg/hour (Wilkinson and Divers 2020) (Figure 9.33).

Venipuncture

Blood collection in lizards is performed from the ventral coccygeal vein or rarely from the ventral abdominal vein or jugular vein. Small patients are placed in dorsal recumbency and may be wrapped in a towel to ease restraint. Large lizards may remain in ventral recumbency with the tail supported off the edge of a table. Fractious, dangerous,

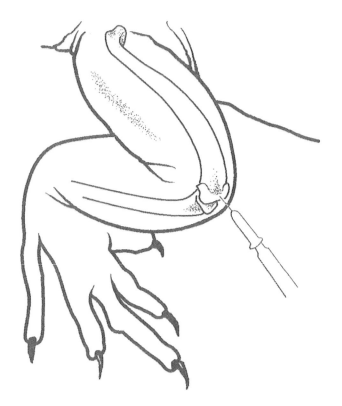

Figure 9.33 IO catheter placement. (Drawing by Scott Stark).

or very small and delicate lizards may require brief sedation for blood collection.

A portion of the proximal third of the tail from the vent is selected and aseptically prepared as if for surgery. A needle of appropriate length and gauge is selected for the patient. For lizards greater than 60 cm total length, a 22-gauge 1- to 1.5-inch needle on a 3-cc syringe is appropriate. For lizards less than 60 cm total length, a 22- to 25-gauge 0.5- to 0.75-inch needle on a 1-cc syringe is appropriate. For lizards less than 25 cm total length, a 27-gauge 0.5-inch needle on a 1-cc or smaller syringe is appropriate. Insulin syringes are commonly used for these smallest patients.

Blood collection is performed in a manner similar to that of venipuncture of the tail vein of a cow. The needle is advanced through the skin along the ventral midline in a perpendicular to slightly cranially directed angle until the tip of the needle contacts the vertebral body. Slight vacuum is applied to the syringe as the needle is slowly withdrawn until blood is seen entering the needle hub. Blood collection is slow and may require 15 to 30 seconds for large lizards and up to 45 seconds for smaller lizards.

Care is taken to slowly expel blood into the collection tube(s) to prevent hemolysis from narrow-gauge needles. Lithium heparin (green top) tubes are often the collection tube of choice for reptile biochemistry and complete blood count (CBC) as EDTA may lyse reptilian erythrocytes when used for CBC (Heatley and Russell 2019). However, for certain species, EDTA is preferred to heparin. A list of published recommendations is available in Heatley and Russell (2019). Whenever possible, the needles of 25-gauge or smaller should be removed from the syringe prior to transferring blood. Most labs that perform reptilian blood chemistries are capable of using samples as small as 25 µL (0.025 mL). The CBC may be submitted as a blood smear instead of whole blood when only a small sample is available for serum chemistry.

The ventral abdominal vein may be accessed in very small lizards or in those in which tail autotomy is likely. These patients should be sedated or anesthetized. The blood collection site is prepared with the patient in dorsal recumbency and accessed along the ventral midline at a point between the sternum and one-third the distance proximal to the pelvis. The bevel of the needle is directed dorsally and the needle advanced just beneath the skin while applying slight suction (Pardo and Divers 2019).

Blood collection may be faster when compared to collection from the ventral tail vein. Cardiocentesis is not recommended for blood collection in lizards because of the risk of trauma and the relative lack of access to the heart in lizards (Figure 9.34). The jugular vein can be used in some lizards, though is difficult to access in most. A technique is described in chameleons (Eshar et al. 2018). The cranial vena cava can also be accessed for venipuncture in small lizards such as crested and leopard geckos (Mayer et al. 2011). The patient is held in dorsal recumbency with a finger underneath the neck extending it dorsally and the head slightly ventrally. The needle is inserted at the sternal notch similar to a cranial vena cava blood draw in a mammal (such as ferrets).

Tracheal Wash

Microbiology and cytology specimens may be collected from the lungs in a manner consistent with that used for

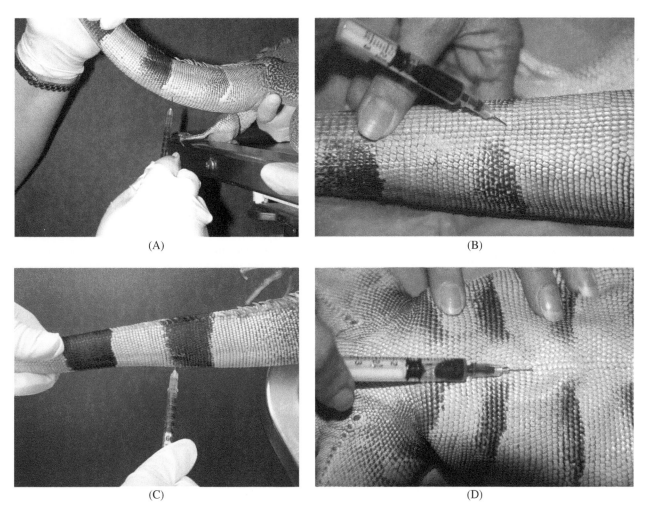

(A)

(B)

(C)

(D)

Figure 9.34 A, B, & C demonstrate the sternal, dorsal, and lateral approach to venipuncture of the tail vein. D demonstrates venipuncture of the ventral abdominal vein. (Photos courtesy of Jody Nugent-Deal and Ryan Cheek).

mammals. The glottis is easily visualized in patients that cooperate in opening the mouth. Sedation will be required for patients that are reluctant to open the mouth. Following a diagnosis of pneumonia, a sterile catheter of appropriate diameter and length is advanced through the glottis and directed into the right or left lung as indicated by radiographs. A sterile wire may be inserted into the catheter and molded (using sterile technique) to aid the direction of the tip into the left or right mainstem bronchus (Knotek and Divers 2019). At no time should the tube be forced if resistance is encountered. A speculum is employed to keep fingers out of the mouth and aid in visualization during the procedure.

Following placement of the catheter, warmed (to ambient temperature of the patient) sterile saline solution is infused at a dose of 5–10 mL/kg body weight and then retrieved into the syringe (Knotek and Divers 2019). Repeated flushing of the saline, gentle coupage, or gentle rolling of the patient following infusion, increases the return of diagnostic material. Following collection the patient is carefully monitored for normal respiration and heart rate. Samples should be submitted for appropriate culture and sensitivity and cytology. Portions of the sample may be preserved in EDTA or fixed on a microscopic slide for cytologic analysis.

When a tracheal wash is contraindicated, bacterial culture and sensitivity may be obtained from pulmonary exudates swabbed from the glottis by culturette. By observing the patient's respiratory cycle, a microtip culturette is carefully inserted into the glottis and then retrieved in a matter not to retrieve oral secretions. This method may not reflect the bacterial population present in the lower respiratory tract and may be contaminated by oral bacteria, so is less ideal.

Cloacal and Colonic Wash and Enema

Techniques for cloacal and colonic wash are applicable for microbiologic and cytologic sample collection, enema, and barium administration for contrast radiography. Colonic wash is performed in the absence of a fresh fecal sample for parasite analysis. Retrograde percloacal colonic catheterization of lizards is not as routine and as simple as performed in mammals, and improper technique can result in severe health consequences to the patient. Sedation is not commonly required except in fractious patients.

A clean catheter similar to that used for tracheal wash, a saline-filled syringe, and water-based lubricant are used. Dosage for colonic wash is approximately 10 mL/kg (Schumacher 2002b). Copious lubrication of the tube is recommended for all procedures. Careful and slow advancement of the catheter in a retrograde fashion through the cloaca will reach the colon. On occasion,

the urinary bladder may be accessed accidentally. The urodeum lies ventrally and the coprodeum lies dorsally in the cranial cloaca. Resistance should never be achieved upon the syringe plunger with the administration of any colonic solutions.

It is imperative not to force the catheter if any resistance is encountered upon advancement. The coelomic tissues may be ruptured easily, and the technician or clinician may not perceive a rupture based on the resistance encountered. Occasionally, the slow infusion of fluid upon advancement of the catheter will aid in reducing resistance, especially with constipated animals. Once the catheter has reached the lower intestine, saline solution is infused and retrieved several times and gentle massage of the colon may be applied to maximize return of diagnostic material. A swab and flotation may be performed on the retrieved sample. Parasite yield is much lower with this method than with a true fecal sample to analyze.

In the event of suspected or confirmed iatrogenic colonic or cloacal rupture, surgery is immediately indicated for primary repair of the defect and copious lavage of the coelom. Most cases of iatrogenic ruptures, unfortunately, go unnoticed until the animal presents with life-threatening coelomitis and sepsis.

Cloacal swabs for bacterial culture and sensitivity may be obtained in a manner similar to that performed in birds. Washing of the external vent is indicated to reduce contamination of the culturette upon insertion and sample retrieval.

Bandaging

Bandage application and wound care for skin defects are consistent with those of other companion animals with the exception that the healing process is prolonged. Except for deep or extensive wounds or those that may become contaminated, wounds on most lizards are best maintained open in a clean environment rather than bandaged. Bandages may be cumbersome to lizards or may be a source of rubbing or other behaviors that attempt to remove the bandage. Tape is contraindicated on all geckos or other lizards with fragile skin.

Bandage application may be indicated for tail autotomy and amputations as a temporary measure after surgery. Application of antibiotic ointments and gauze-packed syringe casings are ideal to allow hemorrhage control and prevent contamination. Typically these bandages are required for only a few days.

External coaptation of limbs is commonly performed as part of fracture management using materials and techniques applied for other companion animals. The same principles of stabilizing one joint above and below the fracture are followed. A potential splint for larger lizards is their own body. Under sedation, forelimbs are secured to the lateral chest wall, with care not to compress the chest cavity, especially in sedated animals. A similar application may be employed with the hindlimb to the tail. With this technique, however, proximal humeral and femoral fractures may not receive adequate reduction in motion of the proximal bone fragment, resulting in malalignment.

Spica splints are ideal for both forelimb and hindlimb unilateral or bilateral fracture management. Under sedation, the rigid splint for forelimb humeral fractures is incorporated into the soft bandage ventrally across the sternum, and in the hindlimb, the splint is applied dorsally across the dorsal pelvis. The soft support bandage of the hindlimb is wrapped in a figure-of-eight pattern incorporating both hindlimbs dorsally, creating abduction of both hindlimbs. A similar technique is applied to the forelimb soft bandage. This technique allows for the cloaca to remain free of bandage material and to reduce contamination of bandage material (Knafo and Karlin 2019). For more distal fractures of limbs, a modified Robert Jones bandage incorporating or encased by a plastic syringe casing and stirrups is ideal.

Carpal, tarsal, and digital fractures may be bandaged with soft bandage material. A ball bandage comprised of a cotton ball applied to the palmar or plantar aspect of the affected foot is wrapped by soft bandage (Knafo and Karlin 2019). For all bandage applications, lizards should be maintained on clean non-organic substrate such as paper or carpet, including those lizards requiring a higher humidity environment. Strict attention is given to cage and bandage sanitation and hygiene.

Assist Feeding

One of the most common signs of any disease state in lizards is anorexia. Assist feeding is employed when the normal feeding response is diminished or when the animal is physically incapable of normal prehension or swallowing of food or water.

The technique for assist feeding may also be applied to gastric oral medication administration and diagnostic gastric lavage. Some species of lizards may require sedation to access the oral cavity (*Uromastyx* spp., *Corucia zebrata*, and occasionally *Iguana* spp. and *Varanus* spp.). These species, especially *Uromastyx* and *Corucia*, are candidates for pharyngostomy tube placement when repeated assist feeding or oral medication is required.

Assist feeding of lizards is accomplished in several ways. Voluntary feeding for smaller lizards is applied when the patient's normal feeding response or mobility is compromised, but with a little enticement, the patient will readily prehend and swallow food. For large or dangerous lizards,

tongs or forceps are used to introduce food. Assist feeding is used for patients who can swallow but are otherwise reluctant to prehend prey items; the mouth may be gently opened and the food item placed into the mouth for the patient to swallow. Syringe feeding a prepared formula or homemade slurry is often easier than assist feeding prey items. Assist feeding is used for patients who are depressed and will not swallow or are incapable of chewing; food is provided by gastric or pharyngostomy feeding tube.

For insectivorous and carnivorous species that are fed only every other day or every few days in normal health, the normal feeding schedule may remain the same. It is important for all lizards not to overfeed them, especially if one is assisting in feeding normal dietary food items. Constipation or obstruction can result from overzealous feeding in these patients. For those species fed specially prepared gruels, either by mouth or through a feeding tube, daily feeding is recommended because it is likely that these diets are more rapidly digested and absorbed compared to the diet of normal health.

The procedures of tube assist feeding are similar to those applied for neonatal companion animals. The stomach of quadruped lizards is measured to the last few ribs. Anguiform lizards are treated as snakes for tube-feeding purposes. Rubber catheters or stainless-steel ball-tipped dosing needles are appropriate to use as feeding tubes. Because of the stresses imposed on the patient from restraint and opening the mouth by assist and assist feeding, feeding frequency is generally no more than once daily for these patients. Alternatively, placement of a pharyngostomy tube accommodates smaller volume multiple daily feedings (Figures 9.35 and 9.36).

Diets are based on identifying the patient as carnivorous (including juvenile omnivorous) or herbivorous (including adult omnivorous). The amount of feeding is a calculated daily energy need based on standard metabolic rate (SMR) measured in kcal/day. The formula is $SMR = 32 \times BW^{0.77}$ where BW = body weight in kilograms. Alert and relatively non-compromised patients receive 75% to 100% of daily energy needs in the first 24 to 48 hours. Weak or debilitated patients receive 40% to 75% of their daily energy needs in the first several days (Boyer and Scott 2019). The amount of feeding of the daily energy requirement is gradually increased to 100% as the patient's health and responsiveness improve. A crude calculation that can be used is to feed 1–2% of the patient's body weight every 12–24 hours depending on the species, their condition, and nutritional needs. Moreover, because the goal of assist feeding is to bring the patient back to voluntary feeding, the amount and frequency of assist feeding decreases or may abruptly stop pending the patient's recovery.

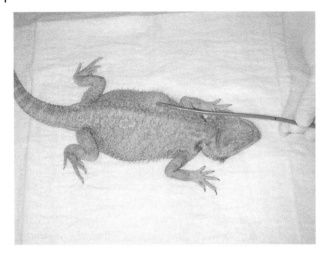

Figure 9.35 How to measure for the correct length of a feeding tube in a lizard. (Courtesy of Jody Nugent).

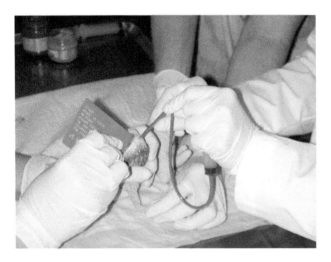

Figure 9.36 Assist feeding of a bearded dragon. (Courtesy of Jody Nugent).

A variety of enteral diets are available for both human and veterinary use. Good options for reptile patients include herbivore, omnivore, or carnivore diets made by Lafeber Company (Cornell, IL) or Oxbow Animal Health (Omaha, NE). The available energy in kcal/mL as well as protein, fat, carbohydrate, and fiber content, are available on the packaging.

Therapeutic Administration

Treatment of lizard patients with pharmaceuticals is performed in a manner consistent with that for mammals but with several exceptions. First, oral administration is not always the route of choice:

1. Oral access may be difficult or stressful for some patients receiving daily medications.

2. Gastrointestinal transit time and factors affecting absorption of medications vary among species.
3. Inexperience or reluctance of the client in administering oral medications may lead to unnecessary trauma to the patient or non-compliance by the owner. When properly counseled, however, most clients enjoy the opportunity to take an active role in restoring the health of their pets.

Examples of antibiotics commonly administered orally in lizards are enrofloxacin injectable and compounded suspensions (Baytril), metronidazole injectable and compounded suspensions, sulfadimethoxine (Albon), trimethoprim-sulfamethoxazole (Bactrim), and compounded tetracyclines. Additionally, many injectable antibiotics or ophthalmic preparations may be applied directly to oral mucous membranes rather than by injectable methods to achieve higher drug concentrations at the site of infection. The parasiticides fenbendazole (Panacur) and praziquantel (Droncit) and the antifungal agents terbinafine or voriconazole are administered PO. The application of antibiotics to drinking water or to food items for lizards is not recommended because of potential drug inactivity and the difficulty in accurate dosing.

Injections are performed using five methods. Subcutaneous (SC) and intramuscular (IM) techniques are most common. The intracoelomic (ICe) technique historically has been used for large volumes of fluids but this has fallen out of favor. Intravenous and intraosseous administrations are typically performed through an indwelling catheter, other than IV injections for sedation which are typically given through the ventral coccygeal vein as for venipuncture.

It is generally uncommon for clients to administer injectable medications to mammalian patients for routine infections. This practice is relatively common for reptile patients, but it must be approached with great attention to both the client's ability and the patient's cooperation. Considerations include:

1. What is the risk of injury to both the client and patient from the proposed procedure?
2. Is the client capable of adequately restraining the patient while administering the medication?
3. Is the client capable of determining if an undesirable side effect has occurred that prohibits further treatment?
4. Is there risk for abuse of the medication dispensed?

When dispensing injectable medication for the client to administer, adhere to the following:

1. Dispense the medication *premeasured* in syringes for each dose and *only* the amount for the specified number of doses. Administration should be only by the SC or IM route for home administration. If long-term treatment is required, dispense a portion of

the amount and only refill the medication with a recheck exam or consultation. Accurately and fully label drug name, concentration, route, frequency, and duration of administration with no abbreviations. Never dispense medications that are potentially dangerous to humans at the prescribed dose (large doses of aminoglycosides, chemotherapeutics, narcotics, etc.).

2. Describe, show, and allow the client to practice administration of the medication. Sterile saline may be used for a practice injection.
3. Instruct the client on the appropriate uncapping and capping of needles and handling of the sterile needle.
4. Counsel the client on potential side effects of the drug and potential side effects of administration. Describe "what can possibly go wrong" scenarios.
5. Encourage the client to give injections during business hours and call the office if there is a problem. If this is not possible, recommend they call upon opening the next business day, or have after-hours numbers available.
6. Have the client bring all medical waste products to the hospital or clinic for disposal.

Subcutaneous injections are made in the lateral scapular region. The skin is not drawn or lifted above the body wall as is common practice in mammals. The needle is advanced into the subcutaneous space, gentle aspiration is applied to check for incidental venous access, and the injection is administered. Serial injections are alternated between the left and right sides and among different locations within the region. Caution must be used in species with thin skin, and in *Chamaleo* spp., warn the owner the skin will temporarily discolor due to stimulation of chromatophores.

Intramuscular injections are administered in epaxial muscles or biceps or triceps muscles in large lizards. IM injections may not be possible in smaller lizards, but one must pay attention to volume of injection.

Intracoelomic injections are administered in the right lower quadrant of the abdomen slightly cranial dorsal to the rear leg (Perry and Mitchell 2019). Fluid therapy is the most common injection given intracoelomically, but this has fallen out of favor due to the inability to monitor absorption. A client should never be instructed to give an injection intracoelomically.

It is essential to understand not only the intended use of the medication but also potential undesired or side effects.

Side effects may be the result of a single administration, a series of administrations, a route of administration, or a cumulative dose. Individual variation as seen in mammals may also occur in reptiles. Side effects also involve the restraint or manipulation necessary to administer a particular drug. When considering the use of therapeutics, the old adage "do no harm" must be remembered.

Euthanasia

Euthanasia of captive lizards may be required for several reasons. The procedures for lizard euthanasia more closely resemble those of domestic laboratory animals than of dogs and cats. The relative inaccessibility of peripheral veins for injection, especially in small lizards, can make euthanasia more challenging. The client must be fully prepared for euthanasia techniques prior to performing the procedures, especially if they want to be present or take the remains home for burial. After euthanasia solution has been administered, it can take several hours for the heartbeat to stop due to prolonged electrical activity in the heart even after death. Death must be confirmed before the client can take the remains home, so often they must be prepared ahead of time they will need to leave their pet and pick up the next day.

Humane euthanasia in the veterinary hospital is best performed under heavy sedation with the dissociative agents ketamine or Telazol. Ketamine at a dose of 50–100 mg/kg IM, or Telazol at a dose of 25 mg/kg IM will assure adequate sedation but other options such as alfaxalone IM (as discussed in the "Anesthesia" section) can be used as well. Euthanasia solution as specified by the manufacturer for mammals is applied to lizards. If the ventral coccygeal vein is accessible and of appropriate size, this is typically the preferred site for injection. Injections may also be given intracardially with a sternal or lateral percutaneous approach to the heart. If the patient is dehydrated or severely debilitated and the cardiac approach is not possible, injection into the occipital sinus may be used. In small lizards where venous or cardiac access is impossible, intracoelomic injections may be given, aiming for the liver for faster absorption. In larger lizards, as long as the patient is completely anesthetized, euthanasia solution may also be given through the parietal eye into the brain.

References

Baines, F.M. and Cusack, L.M. (2019). Environmental lighting. In: *Mader's Reptile and Amphibian Medicine and Surgery*, 3rde (ed. S.J. Divers and S.J. Stahl), 131–139. St Louis: Elsevier.

Baker, B.B., Sladky, K.K., and Johnson, S.M. (2011). Evaluation of the analgesic effects of oral and subcutaneous tramadol administration in red-eared slider turtles. *J Am Vet Med Assoc* 238: 220–227.

Balsai, M. (1997). *General Care and Maintenance of Popular Monitors and Tegus*. Escondido: Advanced Vivarium Systems.

Banzato, T., Hellebuyck, T., Van Caelenberg, A. et al. (2013). A review of diagnostic imaging of snakes and lizards. *Vet Rec* 173: 43–49.

Barten, S.L. and Simpson, S. (2019). Lizard taxonomy, anatomy, and physiology. In: *Mader's Reptile and Amphibian Medicine and Surgery*, 3rde (ed. S.J. Divers and S.J. Stahl), 63–74. St Louis: Elsevier.

Bertelsen, M. and Sauer, C. (2011). Alfaxalone anaesthesia in the green iguana (*Iguana iguana*). *Vet Anaesth Analg* 38: 461–469.

Bogoslavsky, B. (2007). The use of ponazuril to treat coccidiosis in eight inland bearded dragons (*Pogona vitticeps*). *Proc ARAV* 8–9.

Boyer, T.H. and Scott, P.W. (2019). Nutrition. In: *Mader's Reptile and Mphibian Medicine and Surgery*, 3rde (ed. S.J. Divers and S.J. Stahl), 201–223. St Louis: Elsevier.

Boyer, T. (2019). Hypovitaminosis and hypervitaminosis A. In: *Mader's Reptile and Amphibian Medicine and Surgery*, 3rde (ed. S.J. Divers and S.J. Stahl), 1316–1317. St Louis: Elsevier.

Boyer, T.B., Garner, M.M., Reavill, D.R. et al. (2013). Common problems of leopard geckos (*Eublepharis macularius*). *Proc ARAV* 117–125.

Carman, E.N. et al. (2000). Photobiosynthetic opportunity and ability for UVB generated vitamin D synthesis in free-living house geckos (*Hemidactylus turcicus*) and Texas spiny lizards (*Sceloporus olivaceous*). *Copeia* 2000 (1): 245–250.

Chinnadurai, S.K., DeVoe, R., Koenig, A. et al. (2010). Comparison of an implantable telemetry device and an oscillometric monitor for measurement of blood pressure in anesthetized and unrestrained green iguanas (*Iguana iguana*). *Vet Anaesth Analg* 37: 434–439.

Cocilova, C.C., Flewelling, L.J., Granholm, A.A. et al. (2019). Intravenous lipid emulsion treatment reduces symptoms of brevetoxicosis in turtles (*Trachemys scripta*). *J Zoo Wildl Med* 50: 33–44.

da Silva, L.C.B.A., Sellera, F.P., Nascimento, C.L. et al. (2016). Spinal anesthesia in a green turtle (*Chelonia mydas*) for surgical removal of cutaneous fibropapillomatosis. *J Agri Vet Sci* 9: 83–86.

Deming, C., Greiner, E., and Uhl, E. (2009). Prevalence of Cryptosporidium infection and characteristics of oocyst shedding in a breeding colony of leopard geckos (*Eublepharis macularius*). *J Zoo Wildl Med* 39 (4): 600–607.

De Voe, R. (2019). Stomatitis. In: *Mader's Reptile and Amphibian Medicine and Surgery*, 3rde (ed. S.J. Divers and S.J. Stahl), 1345–1346. St Louis: Elsevier.

de Vosjoli, P. (1992). *The Green Iguana Manual*. Lakeside, CA: Advanced Vivarium Systems.

de Vosjoli, P. (1993). *The General Care and Maintenance of Prehensile-Tailed Skinks*. Lakeside, CA: Advanced Vivarium Systems.

de Vosjoli, P. (1995). *Basic Care of Uromastyx*. Santee, CA: Advanced Vivarium Systems.

de Vosjoli, P. (1997). *The Lizard Keeper's Handbook*. Santee, CA: Advanced Vivarium Systems.

de Vosjoli, P. and Ferguson, G. (ed.) (1995). *Care and Breeding of Panther, Jackson's, Veiled, and Parson's Chameleons*. Santee, CA: Advanced Vivarium Systems.

de Vosjoli, P. et al. (1997). *The Leopard Gecko Manual*. Mission Viejo, CA: Advanced Vivarium Systems.

de Vosjoli, P. et al. (2001). *The Bearded Dragon Manual*. Irvine, CA: Advanced Vivarium Systems.

Di Salvo, A., Giorgi, M., Catanzaro, A. et al. (2015). Pharmacokinetic profiles of meloxicam in turtles (*Trachemys scripta scripta*) after single oral, intracoelomic and intramuscular administrations. *J Vet Pharmacol Ther* 39: 102–105.

Divers, S.J. and Innis, C.J. (2019). Urology. In: *Mader's Reptile and Amphibian Medicine and Surgery*, 3rde (ed. S.J. Divers and S.J. Stahl), 624–649. St Louis: Elsevier.

Divers, S.J. (2019). Surgical equipment, instrumentation, and general principles. In: *Mader's Reptile and Amphibian Medicine and Surgery*, 3rde (ed. S.J. Divers and S.J. Stahl), 1014–1023. St Louis: Elsevier.

Divers, S.J., Papich, M., McBride, M. et al. (2010). Pharmacokinetics of meloxicam following intravenous and oral administration in green iguanas (*Iguana iguana*). *Am J Vet Res* 71: 1277–1283.

Eshar, D., Lapid, R., and Head, V. (2018). Transilluminated jugular blood sampling in the common chameleon (*Chamaeleo chamaeleon*). *J Herp Med Surg* 28: 19–22.

Ferguson, G. et al. (2005). Ultraviolet exposure and vitamin D synthesis in a sun-dwelling and a shade-dwelling species of anolis: are there adaptations for lower ultraviolet B and dietary vitamin D_3 availability in the shade? *Phys Biochem Zool* 78: 193–200.

Fink, D.M., Doss, G.A., Sladky, K.K., and Mans, C. (2018). Effect of injection site on dexmedetomidine-ketamine induced sedation in leopard geckos (Eublepharis macularius). *J Am Vet Med Assoc* 253: 1146–1150.

Gamble, K.C. (2008). Plasma fentanyl concentrations achieved after transdermal fentanyl patch application in prehensile-tailed skinks, *Corucia zebrata*. *J Herp Med Surg* 18: 81–85.

Gatson, B.J., Goe, A., Granone, T.D. et al. (2017). Intramuscular epinephrine results in reduced anesthetic recovery time in American alligatos (*Alligator mississippiensis*) undergoing isoflurane anesthesia. *J Zoo Wildl Med* 48: 55–61.

Giorgi, M., Salvadori, M., De Vito, V. et al. (2015). Pharmacokinetic/pharmacodynamics assessments of 10 mg/kg tramadol intramuscular injection in yellow-bellied slider turtles (*Trachemys scripta scripta*). *J Vet Pharmacol Ther* 38: 488–496.

Glaw, F. and Vences, M. (1994). *A Field Guide to the Amphibians and Reptiles of Madagascar*, 2nde. Bonn, Germany: Koenig.

Gobble, J. (2022). Oral fluralaner (Bravecto) use in the control of mites in 20 ball pythons (*Python regius*). *J Herp Med Surg* 32 (2): 111–112.

Goe, A., Shmalberg, J., Gatson, B.J. et al. (2016). Epinephrine or GV-26 electrical stimulation reduces inhalant anesthetic recovery time in common snapping turtles (*Chelydra serpentina*). *J Zoo Wildl Med* 47: 501–507.

Gould, A., Molitor, L., Rockwell, K. et al. (2018). Evaluating the physiologic effects of short duration Ultraviolet B exposure in leopard geckos (*Eublepharis macularius*). *J Herp Med Surg* 28: 34–39.

Greenacre, C.B., Schumacher, J.P., Talke, G. et al. (2006). Comparative antinociception of morphine, butorphanol, and buprenorphine versus saline in the green iguana, *Iguana iguana*, using electrostimulation. *J Herp Med Surg* 16: 88–92.

Hannon, D.E., Garner, M.M., and Reavill, D.R. (2011). Squamous cell carcinomas in inland bearded dragons (*Pogona vitticeps*). *J Herp Med Surg* 21: 101–106.

Heatley, J.J. and Russell, K.E. (2019). Hematology. In: *Mader's Reptile and Amphibian Medicine and Surgery*, 3rde (ed. S.J. Divers and S.J. Stahl), 301–319. St Louis: Elsevier.

Helfman, G.S. (1990). Mode selection and mode switching in foraging animals. *Adv Study Behav* 19: 249.

Holz, P., Barker, I.K., Burger, J.P. et al. (1997). The effect of the renal portal system on pharmacokinetic parameters in the red-eared slider (*Trachemys scripta elegans*). *J Zoo Wildl Med* 28: 386–393.

Jacobson, E.R. (2002). Chlamydiosis: an underreported disease of reptiles. In: *Proceedings of the North American Veterinary Conference (16)*. Gainesville, FL, 916–917.

Johnson-Delaney, C.A. and Gal, J. (2019). Zoonoses and public health. In: *Mader's Reptile and Amphibian Medicine and Surgery*, 3rde (ed. S.J. Divers and S.J. Stahl), 1359–1365. St Louis: Elsevier.

Juan-Sallés, C., Garner, M.M., Nordhausen, R.W. et al. (2014). Renal flagellate infections in reptiles: 29 cases. *J Zoo Wildl Med* 45: 100–109.

Kanui, T.I. and Hole, K. (1992). Morphine and pethidine antinociception in the crocodile. *J Vet Pharmacol Ther* 15: 101–103.

Kanui, T.I., Hole, K., and Miaron, J.O. (1990). Nociception in crocodiles - capsaicin instillation, formalin and hot plate tests. *Zool Sci* 7: 537–540.

Kharbush, R., Gutwillig, A., Hartzler, K. et al. (2017). Antinociceptive and respiratory effects following application of transdermal fentanyl patches and assessment of brain μ-opioid receptor mRNA expression in ball pythons. *Am J Vet Res* 78: 785–795.

Knafo, S.E. and Karlin, W.M. (2019). Orthopedic principles and external coaptation. In: *Mader's Reptile and Amphibian Medicine and Surgery*, 3rde (ed. S.J. Divers and S.J. Stahl), 1100–1103. St Louis: Elsevier.

Knotek, Z. and Divers, S. (2019). Pulmonology. In: *Mader's Reptile and Amphibian Medicine and Surgery*, 3rde (ed. S.J. Divers and S.J. Stahl), 786–804. St Louis: Elsevier.

Lai, O.R., Di Bello, A., Soloperto, S. et al. (2015). Pharmacokinetic behavior of meloxicam in loggerhead sea turtles (*Caretta caretta*) after intramuscular and intravenous administration. *J Wildl Dis* 51: 509–512.

Lewbart, G.A. and Lewbart, D.T. (2019). Laws and regulations – Americas. In: *Mader's reptile and amphibian medicine and surgery*, 3rde (ed. S.J. Divers and S.J. Stahl), 1457–1463. St Louis: Elsevier.

Mader DR. 2002. Ventral midline approach for the lizard coeliotomy. In: Proceedings of the North American Veterinary Conference (16). Gainesville, FL.

Mans, C., Sladky, K.K., and Schumacher, J. (2019). General Anesthesia. In: *Mader's Reptile and Amphibian Medicine and Surgery*, 3rde (ed. S.J. Divers and S.J. Stahl), 447–464. St Louis: Elsevier.

Mans, C., Lahner, L.L., Baker, B.B. et al. (2012). Antinociceptive efficacy of buprenorphine and hydromorphone in red-eared slider turtles (*Trachemys scripta elegans*). *J Zoo Wildl Med* 43: 662–665.

Mayer, J., Knoll, J., Wrubel, K.M. et al. (2011). Characterizing the hematologic and plasma chemistry profiles of captive crested geckos (*Rhacodactylus* [*Correlophus*] *ciliatus*). *J Herp Med Surg* 21: 68–75.

McArthur, S. and Machin, R.A. (2019). Cloacal prolapse. In: *Mader's Reptile and Amphibian Medicine and Surgery*, 3rde (ed. S.J. Divers and S.J. Stahl), 1090–1095. St Louis: Elsevier.

McKenzie, A., Li, T., and Doneley, B. (2022). A comparison of two techniques to identify the sex of the eastern blue-tongued skink (*Tiliqua scincoides scincoides*). *Aust Vet J* 100: 407–413.

McKeown, S. (1993). *The General Care and Maintenance of Day Geckos*. Lakeside, CA: Advanced Vivarium Systems.

Mitchell MA. 2009. Artificial lighting for reptiles: what we know and what you need to know. In: Proceedings of the North American Veterinary Conference (23). Gainesville, FL, pp. 1783–1785.

Norton, T.M., Cox, S., Nelson, S.E. Jr., et al. (2015). Pharmacokinetics of tramadol and o-desmethyltramadol in loggerhead sea turtles (*Caretta caretta*). *J Zoo Wildl Med* 46: 262–265.

Obst, F.J. et al. (1989). *The Completely Illustrated Atlas of Reptiles and Amphibians for the Terrarium*. Neptune City, NJ: TFH.

Olesen, M.G., Bertelsen, M.F., Perry, S.F. et al. (2008). Effects of preoperative administration of butorphanol or meloxicam on physiologic responses to surgery in ball pythons. *J Am Vet Med Assoc* 233: 1883–1889.

Pardo, M.A. and Divers, S.J. (2019). Catheter placement. In: *Mader's Reptile and Amphibian Medicine and Surgery*, 3rde (ed. S.J. Divers and S.J. Stahl), 422–429. St Louis: Elsevier.

Pare, J.A., Wellehan, J., Perry, S.M. et al. (2021). Onygenalean dermatomycoses (formerly yellow fungus disease, snake fungal disease) in reptiles. *J Herp Med Surg* 30: 198–209.

Parkinson, L.A. and Mans, C. (2018). Effects of furosemide administration to water-deprived inland bearded dragons (*Pogona vitticeps*). *Am J Vet Res* 79: 1204–1209.

Perrault, J.R., Barron, H.W., Malinowski, C.R. et al. (2021). Use of intravenous lipid emulsion therapy as a novel treatment for brevetoxicosis in sea turtles. *Sci Rep* 11: 24162.

Perry, S.M. and Mitchell, M.A. (2019). Routes of administration. In: *Mader's Reptile and Amphibian Medicine and Surgery*, 3rde (ed. S.J. Divers and S.J. Stahl), 1130–1139. St Louis: Elsevier.

Platt, S.R. (2019). Neurology. In: *Mader's Reptile and Amphibian Medicine and Surgery*, 3rde (ed. S.J. Divers and S.J. Stahl), 805–826. St. Louis: Elsevier.

Raiti, P. (2019). Endocrinology. In: *Mader's Reptile and Amphibian Medicine and Surgery*, 3rde (ed. S.J. Divers and S.J. Stahl), 835–849. St Louis: Elsevier.

Rivera, S., Divers, S.J., Knafo, S.E. et al. (2011). Sterilisation of hybrid Galapagos tortoises (*Geochelone nigra*) for island restoration. Part 2: phallectomy of males under intrathecal anaesthesia with lidocaine. *Vet Rec* 168: 79.

Rossi, J.V. (2019). General husbandry and management. In: *Mader's Reptile and Amphibian Medicine and Surgery*, 3rde (ed. S.J. Divers and S.J. Stahl), 109–130. St Louis: Elsevier.

Schumacher J. 2002. Critical and supportive care of reptiles. In: Proceedings of the North American Veterinary Conference (16). Gainesville, FL.

Schilliger, L.H., Morel, D., Bonwitt, J.H. et al. (2013). *Cheyletus eruditus* (taurrus): an effective candidate for the biological control of the snake mite (*Ophionyssus natricis*). *J Zoo Wildl Med* 44: 654–659.

Schilliger, L. and Girling, S. (2019). Cardiology. In: *Mader's Reptile and Amphibian Medicine and Surgery*, 3rde (ed. S.J. Divers and S.J. Stahl), 670–699. St Louis: Elsevier.

Silverman, S. and Janssen, D.L. (1996). Special techniques and procedures: diagnostic imaging. In: *Reptile Medicine and Surgery* (ed. D.R. Mader), 258–264. Philadelphia: W.B. Saunders Co.

Silverman, S., Sanchez-Migallon Guzman, D., Stern, J. et al. (2016). Standardization of the two-dimensional transcoelomic echocardiographic examination in the central bearded dragon (*Pogona vitticeps*). *J Vet Cardiol* 18: 168–179.

Sladky, K.K. and Mans, C. (2019). Analgesia. In: *Mader's Reptile and Amphibian Medicine and Surgery*, 3rde (ed. S.J. Divers and S.J. Stahl), 465–474. St Louis: Elsevier.

Sladky, K.K., Kinney, M.E., and Johnson, S.M. (2008). Analgesic efficacy of butorphanol and morphine in bearded dragons and corn snakes. *J Am Vet Med Assoc* 233: 267–273.

Sladky, K.K., Miletic, V., Paul-Murphy, J. et al. (2007). Analgesic efficacy and respiratory effects of butorphanol and morphine in turtles. *J Am Vet Med Assoc* 230: 1356–1362.

Stahl, S.J. and DeNardo, D.F. (2019). Theriogenology. In: *Mader's Reptile and Amphibian Medicine and Surgery*, 3rde (ed. S.J. Divers and S.J. Stahl), 849–893. St Louis: Elsevier.

Stahl SJ. 1999. Common medical problems of Old World chameleons. In: Proceedings of the North American Veterinary Conference (12). Gainesville, FL, pp. 814–817.

Tuttle, A.D., Papich, M., Lewbart, G.A. et al. (2006). Pharmacokinetics of ketoprofen in the green iguana (*Iguana iguana*) following single intravenous and intramuscular injections. *J Zoo Wildl Med* 37: 567–570.

Uney, K., Altan, F., Aboubakr, M. et al. (2016). Pharmacokinetics of meloxicam in red-eared slider turtles (*Trachemys scripta elegans*) after single intravenous and intramuscular injections. *Am J Vet Res* 77: 439–444.

Wambugu, S.N., Towett, P.K., Kiama, S.G. et al. (2010). Effects of opioids in the formalin test in the Speke's hinged tortoise (*Kinixy's spekii*). *J Vet Pharmacol Ther* 33: 347–351.

Wellehan, J.F.X. and Walden, H.D.S. (2019). Parasitology (including hemoparasites). In: *Mader's Reptile and Amphibian Medicine and Surgery*, 3rde (ed. S.J. Divers and S.J. Stahl), 281–300. St Louis: Elsevier.

Wilkinson, S.L. and Divers, S.J. (2020). Clinical management of reptile renal disease. *Vet Clin North Am Exot Anim Pract* 23: 151–169.

10

Snakes

Ryan Cheek

Introduction

Snakes are a diverse group of animals. They are found on every continent except for Antarctica, as far south as Tasmania and as far north as the Arctic Circle. They are found in the ocean and other bodies of water and at altitudes as high as 16,000 ft (about 5000 m). Snakes may be fossorial, terrestrial, arboreal, aquatic, or combinations thereof. They are found in biomes from the driest hottest deserts in the world to the most tropical rainforests around the equator. They range in all sizes, shapes, and colors. The largest species, *Python reticulatus* (reticulated python), can attain a length of nearly 30 ft (9 m) and weigh up to 400 pounds (180 kg), whereas the smallest snake, *Leptotyphlops carlae* (Barbados threadsnake) can attain a length of only 4 in. (10 cm). Snakes have adapted their body size and shape to accommodate their lifestyles and predation behaviors. Snakes can be described as large or small-bodied, and can even be described by the length of their tails. Some snakes, such as *Langaha madagascariensis* (Malagasy leaf-nosed snake), have elongated snouts that are a form of sexual dimorphism. The colors range from solid black in *Lampropeltis getula nigrita* (Mexican black kingsnake), to vibrant colors as seen in *Bitis parviocula* (Ethiopian mountain adder) or *Euprepiophis mandarinus* (Mandarin rat snake).

Taxonomically, snakes are in the order Squamata, along with the lizards. The order Squamata is further divided into three suborders: Lacertilia (lizards), Amphisbaenia (worm lizards), and Serpentes (snakes). Serpentes contains approximately 3,400 species in 500 genera and two infraorders: Scolecophidia, the blind and threadsnakes, contains 5 families and 15 genera; Alethinophidia contains the rest of the snake species and is comprised of 20 families and 9 subfamilies.

Keeping snakes in captivity has become increasingly popular over the years. It is estimated that there are 1.2 to 2.45 million snakes in approximately 555,000 to 846,000 households in the United States. Snakes represent 18% of the reptiles in captivity. With the increase in captive, specimens has come a greater demand for veterinarians and veterinary technicians who are educated in proper husbandry and treatment of reptiles. Annually, snake owners spend around $57.5 million on veterinary services and an additional $28.8 million on medications. The veterinary staff must be willing to keep up with current treatment protocols, as reptile medicine is ever-changing and still evolving. Beyond the medical aspect, it is important that the veterinary staff learn about natural history that includes where snakes live, the specific environmental conditions in which the species lives (including the microenvironment), and what and how they eat. The natural history is the single most important aspect of reptile medicine. Despite the importance of natural history, it is beyond the scope of this text. This text will focus on captive husbandry, comparative anatomy and physiology, diseases, and clinical skills.

Behavior

Snakes are solitary animals and should be housed separately unless attempting to breed. Some can exhibit territorial behaviors and be aggressive to other inhabitants. Signs of aggressive behavior toward other snakes include biting, constricting, and "head pinning." The head pinning is a courtship behavior as well. During breeding season, some of these behaviors are observed more often. If these signs of aggression are observed with snakes being housed together, they should be housed separately immediately. As with any animal, if snakes are fighting, care should be taken if interference is necessary. A person could be bitten while trying to separate the combating snakes. Using hooks or tongs is recommended when human interference is warranted.

Another downside with housing snakes together is that some species (i.e., king snakes) eat other snakes as part of their natural diet. For this reason, all king snakes should

Exotic Animal Medicine for the Veterinary Technician, Fourth Edition. Edited by Bonnie Ballard and Ryan Cheek.
© 2024 John Wiley & Sons, Inc. Published 2024 by John Wiley & Sons, Inc.
Companion Website: www.wiley.com/go/ballard/4e

be kept separate. Size or gender does not affect the snake's instinctive predatory behavior.

It is also important to know whether the snake is diurnal (active during day hours), crepuscular (active at dawn and dusk), or nocturnal (active during night hours). Knowing when the snake is the most active will aid in making several decisions, such as handling and ideal feeding times.

Anatomy and Physiology

Integument

As in mammals, the skin of snakes plays several crucial roles. The skin is the cellular protective barrier against the external environment. By being a protective barrier, it serves to protect the body from microbes and parasites, resists abrasions, and buffers the internal environment from the extremes of the external environment. The skin also holds other tissues and organs in place while being elastic enough to allow for respiration, movement, and growth. The skin also serves other roles such as physiologic regulation, sensory detection, respiration, and coloration.

The snake's skin consists of two main layers, the dermis and epidermis. The epidermis is covered completely by keratin. This layer of keratinous cells, stratum corneum, shields the living tissue below. The stratum germinativum, the innermost layer of the epidermis, divides continuously to replace the outer layer of dead keratinous cells. As the cells in the stratum germinativum are pushed outward, they slowly flatten, die, and keratinize to form the stratum corneum. The stratum corneum is composed of three layers, the Oberhautchen layer, the beta-keratin layer, and the alpha-keratin layer, from the surface inward, respectively.

The dermis consists of two layers, the stratum compactum and the stratum spongiosum. The stratum compactum is the innermost layer of the dermis and consists of densely knit connective tissue. The stratum spongiosum consists of connective tissue, blood vessels, glands, nerve endings, and other cellular structures.

Ecdysis, or shedding of the skin, is a normal occurrence throughout the snake's life. Young snakes will shed much more often and begin to have a longer resting period as they reach adult size. Because the top layer of snakeskin consists mostly of keratin, which is dead material, it is incapable of expanding during the snake's growth process. Therefore, it needs to be shed every so often. The cells of the upper stratum germinativum, the outer generation layer, begin to proliferate and differentiate. The germinative layer begins to divide producing new layers of cells. These new cells form the inner generation layer, which is the precursor to scales, or the outer generation layer, for the next ecdysis

cycle. At this stage the new epidermal layer is ready. The Oberhautchen then fills with lymph and enzymatic action produces a cleavage zone and the old epidermis is shed (Zug et al. 2001, p. 49).

Before a snake sheds, it secretes a lubricant underneath the outermost layer of skin. This is to assist with the shedding process. This lubricant is most noticeable in the snake's eyes. The eyes become opaque or blue in color due to this lubricant being secreted. Sometime after this optical opacity or dullness is noticed the snake will begin to shed its skin. It can take a week or two before the entire shedding process is over; shedding should be repeated at regular intervals. The snake may attempt to use any furnishings in the enclosure to assist in removing the dead skin. For this reason, one should make sure that all furnishings are not so abrasive as to cause injury to the snake. The snake may also attempt to soak in its water bowl to assist in shedding. Water softens the old skin and makes it easier to remove. If the humidity is too low, the snake may have problems shedding. A snake sheds its entire outer layer of skin all at once. All snakes, with the exception of large boids, should shed in one piece. If there are numerous pieces of the snake's shed skin or some still present on the snake, this is an abnormal shed. Snakes with abnormal shedding may need husbandry changes or may have ectoparasites and should be checked thoroughly. Age, nutrition, species, reproductive status, overall health, and hormonal balance also play a role in the frequency of ecdysis.

If some shedding is still present on the snake, soaking or spraying can be tried to assist in the removal of the skin. If skin is allowed to build up and not sloughed off naturally, infections can occur underneath the old skin.

While snakes are in shed, they should not be handled or fed. Their senses are dulled (eyes opaque) and because they feel vulnerable, they can also be very defensive. To avoid potential bites, handling is not recommended during this time. Also, it is unlikely the snake will eat, so feeding should not occur until after the snake has shed. If offering live prey items, feeding should not occur while the snake is in shed due to the higher potential for rodent bites.

Snakes are either entirely or partially covered by overlapping scales. The surface of each scale is composed of beta-keratin while the interscalar space, or sutures, is composed of alpha-keratin. This distribution of keratin gives a protective covering while allowing for flexibility and expansion. Certain species of colubrids and viperids are nearly scaleless. These species may only have labial and ventral scales. The remainder of the body is covered in a smooth keratinous epidermis. This anomaly is a recessive homozygous trait.

Snakes have paired scent glands at the base of their tails. These glands open at the outer edge of the cloaca. A large amount of semisolid, malodorous fluid is released for defensive behavior in some species and for courting behavior in other species.

Musculoskeletal System

Snakes possess a very complex cranial skeleton (Figure 10.1). Snakes have a cartilaginous anterior chondrocranium, the portion of the cranium that covers the brain (Zug et al. 2001, p. 52). This anterior portion of the chondrocranium consists of continuous internasal and interorbital septa and a pair of nasal conchae (Zug et al. 2001, p. 50). The chondrocranium calcifies between the eyes and ears and forms the basisphenoid. Further posteriorly, a pair of exoccipitals, the supraoccipital bones, and the basioccipital form just below and behind the brain. These occipital bones encircle the foramen magnum. The exoccipitals and the basioccipitals form a single occipital condyle and the articular surface of the skull and atlas.

The maxilla is loosely connected to the other cranial bones. The maxilla connects to a special process on the prefrontal bone. They are connected via a movable articulation. The maxilla is also loosely connected to the cranial bones by the ectopterygoid (Romer 1997, p. 126). The snout structures, the premaxilla, nasal, septomaxilla, and vomer, are movable as a separate series of bones from the maxilla and are also loosely connected to the cranial bones. This adaptation allows snakes to swallow large prey.

The mandible is highly specialized to allow for a large gape when swallowing large prey items (Romer 1997, p. 209). The mandible lacks a mandibular symphysis; an intramandibular hinge allows the mandible to flex in the middle, and an articulated streptostylic quadrate allows the mandible to move sideways (Figure 10.2).

The vertebral column in snakes is divided into the atlas and axis, 100–300 trunk or precloacal vertebrae, several cloacal vertebrae, and 10–120 caudal vertebrae (Zug et al. 2001, p. 57). Each precloacal vertebra has a rib attached. The zygapophyses are the intervertebral articular surfaces; each vertebra has a posterior and anterior pair. The anterior

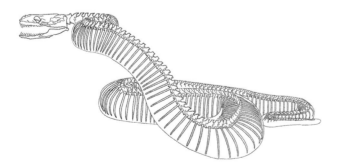

Figure 10.1 Snake skeletal anatomy. (Drawing by Scott Stark).

zygapophyses flare outward and upward while the posterior zygapophyses flare inward and downward. The angle of the zygapophyses gives reptiles their flexibility or rigidity. Snakes are able to have such great flexibility due to these articular surfaces being angled toward the horizontal plane.

The muscular system of snakes consists of several hundred multisegmental muscle chains composed of elongated and interconnecting segmental muscles and tendons. Movement is achieved through individual contraction patterns of the muscle chains. There are six types of locomotion divided into two classes (Pough et al. 2001, p. 272). Lateral undulation and slide-pushing have no static points of contact with the substrate. Rectilinear, concertina, sidewinding, and saltation do have static points with the substrate.

Lateral undulation is the most widely used method of locomotion in snakes. At fixed points in the snake's environment, force is generated by horizontal waves traveling down alternating sides of the body. These fixed points can be a rock, tree, or any other physical object that the snake comes in contact with. At each point, the body generates a force that pushes the body posterolaterally.

Slide-pushing is similar to lateral undulation but does not use fixed points in the physical environment. Slide-pushing involves very rapid alternating side body waves that generate sliding friction. This friction propels the snake forward.

Concertina locomotion is very slow and consumes large amounts of energy. This is a very complex system of locomotion. First, the anterior portion of the body will remain still while the posterior portion will draw up in a series of tight curves. The posterior end will then be stationary and the anterior end will extend forward. The sequence then repeats. Concertina locomotion is most effectively used on the ground where static friction is used to prevent rearward slippage.

Sidewinding is most commonly used on shifting soil such as mud or sand. Most snakes appear to have the ability to sidewind. The forces in sidewinding are directed vertically on the substrate. Sections of the body are alternately lifted, moved forward, and then set down. This produces a series of tracts that are parallel producing forward motion.

Saltation involves a very rapid straightening of the body from anterior to posterior lifting the entire body off the ground. This is used only by small species.

Rectilinear motion relies on the lateral muscles to work at the same time. The costocutaneous superior muscles pull the skin forward relative to the ribs. The ventral scales then anchor themselves to the ground. The costocutaneous inferior then pulls the ribs and with them the rest of the body forward relative to the stationary ventral scales. This form of locomotion is used by large-bodied snakes such as boids and vipers.

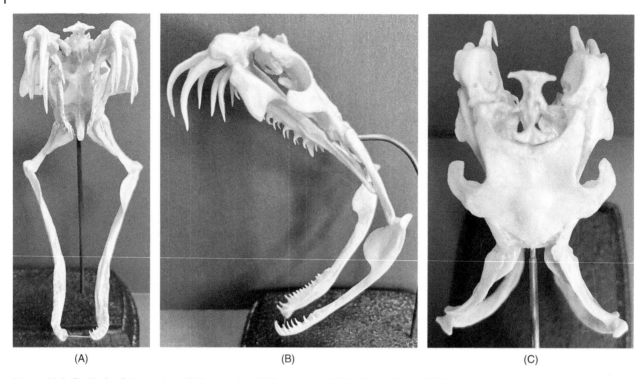

Figure 10.2 Skull of a Gaboon viper (*Bitis gabonica*) (A) Rostral view. (B) Left lateral view. (C) Dorsal view.

Cardiovascular System

The Heart

The hearts size, shape, structure, and position are all dependent on the species' anatomy, physiology, and behavior. Heart position has a direct correlation with arboreal, terrestrial, and aquatic habits (Vasse 1994, p. 75). Terrestrial species have a heart that is close to the head and have blood vessels in the distal portion of the body that dilate to receive extra blood. The heart of arboreal species is also located close to the head so that blood can more easily reach the brain when hanging vertically. Marine species have a heart that is found in the middle of the body so the pumping effort is minimal. Marine species do not have blood accumulation in the tail and the low blood pressure is compensated for by the external water pressure (Vasse 1994, p. 75). The heart consists of three chambers, right and left atria, and a single ventricle. The ventricle is further divided into the cavum arteriosum, cavum venosum, and cavum pulmonale. Even though the ventricle lacks a septum, the snake can still separate oxygenated and deoxygenated blood and can maintain different systemic and pulmonary pressures because the heart is functionally five-chambered (Pough et al. 2001, p. 206). There is a muscular ridge in the ventricle that separates the cavum pulmonale and the cavum venosum. The cavum arteriosum is located dorsal to the other two compartments and communicates with the cavum venosum through an intraventricular canal. There are two inflow routes—the right and left atria—and three outflow routes—the pulmonary artery, and the left and right aortic arches. The right atrium receives blood from the sinus venosus. The sinus venosus is a large chamber located on the dorsal surface of the atrium. It receives blood from four veins, the right and left precaval veins, the postcaval vein, and the left hepatic vein. The left atrium receives blood from the right and left pulmonary veins.

Blood flow through the heart starts when both atria contract. The atrioventricular valves open and allow blood to flow into the ventricle. When the atria contract, the valve between the right atria and the cavum venosum seals off the intraventricular canal allowing the oxygenated blood from the left atrium to flow into the cavum arteriosum, and the deoxygenated blood from the right atrium to flow into the cavum venosum and then to the cavum pulmonale. When the ventricle contracts, the blood pressure inside the heart increases. First, because resistance is lower in the pulmonary circuit, deoxygenated blood is expelled from the cavum pulmonale through the pulmonary artery. When the ventricle shortens, the muscular ridge that separates the cavum venosum and the cavum pulmonale comes into contact with the wall of the ventricle and closes off the passage between the two compartments. The atrioventricular valves are forced shut as the pressure inside the ventricle increases. When the atrioventricular valves are shut, the oxygenated blood from the cavum arteriosum is pushed through the intraventricular canal into the cavum

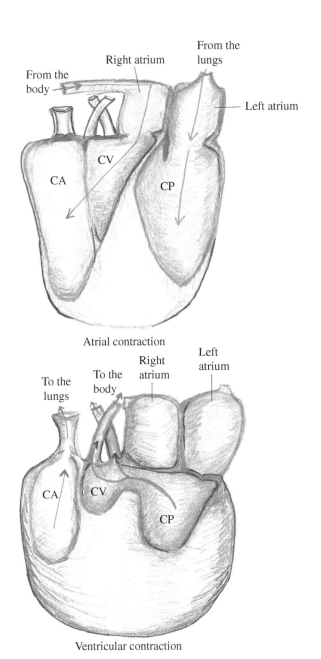

Figure 10.3 Cardiac cycle of non-crocodilian reptiles. CA: Cavum arteriosum, CV: Cavum venosum, CP: Cavum pulmonale (Drawing by Kara Caldwell).

venosum and out the left and right aortic arches. At this point, the pressure inside the cavum venosum is more than twice that in the cavum pulmonale (Figure 10.3).

Another remarkable ability that snakes, as well as other squamates and chelonians, have is the ability to perform intracardiac shunting. Intracardiac shunts are classified as left-to-right or right-to-left. In a right-to-left shunt, the deoxygenated blood that should normally be flowing out to the pulmonary circuit is expelled out to the systemic circuit via the aortic arches. This shunt increases the amount of circulating blood and decreases its oxygen content. Primarily, the right-to-left shunt is used to increase the body temperature and to bypass the lungs during breath-holding. The left-to-right shunt is used to help stabilize the oxygen content of the blood. The direction and degree of intracardiac shunting are dependent on the pressure differences between the pulmonary and systemic circuits and the washout of blood remaining in the cavum venosum.

The renal portal system exists in all fish, reptiles, and birds. The system collects blood from the caudal portion of the body and carries it to the kidneys. The blood is then filtered and returned to the heart via the postcaval vein. Blood that travels through the renal portal system only goes through the convoluted tubules and not the glomeruli (Holz 1999, p. 249).

The location of the heart, being so cranial, has two disadvantages. First, when a snake is holding its head down, blood flow to the tail will be compromised. Second, and most important, when the head is up or the entire body is in a vertical position, the blood from the tail has to travel all the way to the heart against gravity. The veins of snakes do not have valves to prevent backflow, so snakes have evolved three ways to ensure that the blood continues to flow toward the heart even while being vertical. First, contractions of the smooth muscles that line the vessels help push the blood toward the heart. Second, snakes will undulate or contract their skeletal muscles to massage the blood toward the heart. Third, the tight skin of arboreal species acts as an antigravity suit, further assisting the blood in traveling toward the heart (see Table 10.1).

The Lymphatic System

The lymphatic system in snakes, as well as all reptiles, is an elaborate drainage system. Microvessels collect lymph from all over the body. These microvessels merge into larger vessels that eventually empty into larger lymphatic trunk vessels and then into lymphatic sinuses. All three parts, the trunk, vessels, and sinuses, empty into veins. The lymph can be bidirectional but mostly flows toward the pericardial sinus and into the venous system. Reptiles have a pair of lymph hearts located in the pelvic region but do not possess lymph nodes.

Table 10.1 Approximate organ location in snakes.

First quarter	Trachea, esophagus, heart
Second quarter	Heart, liver, lung, stomach
Third quarter	Stomach, gallbladder, gonads, small intestine, pancreas, spleen, adrenal glands
Fourth quarter	Colon, kidneys, cloaca
Tail	Hemipenes, musk glands

Respiratory System

Snakes have an upper respiratory anatomy similar to mammals. Air enters and leaves the trachea through the glottis located in the back of the pharynx. The glottis and other cartilage form the larynx. The trachea of snakes has incomplete cartilaginous rings. The ventral portions of the rings are rigid and the dorsal portion is membranous.

Most snakes only have a single right lung and a small non-functioning left lung. The right lung is generally one-half or more of the snake's body length. In most species, the posterior one-third is an air sac, which can extend down to the cloaca in some aquatic species. Very few snakes have a right and left-functioning lung. In species that do have a functional left lung, such as boas and pythons, it is about 85% smaller than the right; however, variation exists between species. The right bronchus enters the lung and empties into a wall that is lined with faveoli. The faveoli are richly supplied with blood. Most of the gaseous exchange occurs in the faveoli (Zug et al. 2001, p. 173). Snakes that have only one functioning lung possess a tracheal lung. The tracheal lung is a vascular sac that contains many faveoli for gas exchange. The tracheal lung extends from the point where the tracheal rings are incomplete dorsally and posteriorly until it is touching the right lung. The air sac, or saccular lung, is not used for gas exchange but for air regulation.

All reptiles breathe using negative-pressure ventilation (Pough et al. 2001, p. 200). During inspiration, the intercostal muscles expand the ribs along the entire length of the body reducing the pressure inside the lungs to below atmospheric pressure and drawing in air. Then the intercostal muscles relax and the glottis closes, closing the respiratory tract. The snake then pauses for several seconds to several minutes before exhaling. Terrestrial and arboreal species normally have a period of apnea between respiratory cycles. When snakes are swallowing large prey, the ribs in the anterior portion of the body are unable to expand for proper inspiration. During ingestion of prey, the posterior ribs expand causing the saccular lung to inflate and deflate moving air through the respiratory system.

Nervous System

The central nervous system in snakes is organized the same as in all reptiles and similarly to that of mammals. The brain of snakes is divided into the forebrain and hindbrain. The forebrain contains the cerebral hemispheres, the thalamic segment, and the optic tectum and is further divided into the telencephalon, diencephalon, and mesencephalon. The cerebral hemispheres are pear-shaped and contain olfactory lobes that project anteriorly and end in olfactory bulbs (Zug et al. 2001, p. 61). The thalamic region is hidden by the cerebral lobes and the optic tectum; it is tube-shaped with a thick wall. The dorsal portion of the thalamic region has two dorsal projections: the anterior projection is the parietal body and the posterior projection, the epiphysis, is the pineal organ. The pineal organ is glandular in most snakes. The ventral portion contains the hypothalamus. The optic tectum is located on the dorsal part of the posterior portion of the forebrain and the ventral part contains the optic chiasma. The hindbrain contains the cerebellum and medulla and is also divided into the metencephalon and myelencephalon. Both are small in extant species of reptiles. Reptiles also have 12 pairs of cranial nerves.

The spinal cord runs the entire length of the vertebral column. Each vertebra contains a bilateral pair of spinal nerves, and each spinal nerve contains a sensory and motor root that fuse near their origin. The diameter of the spinal cord is uniform all the way down to the end.

Sense Organs

Cutaneous Sense Organs

Boids, pythonids, and viperids have specialized structures in the dermis and epidermis that contain heat receptors (Zug et al. 2001, p. 62). These pit organs sense infrared heat and are located in different locations in each taxon. In the boids, the pit organs are scattered on unmodified supralabial and infralabial scales. Boids have intra-epidermal and intradermal types. Pythonids have a series of pit organs in the labial scales. The heat receptors lie on the floor of each pit. In viperids, the pit organs are located bilaterally between the eyes and the nares. The opening of each pit is forward-facing and is overlapped by other receptors. The heat receptors are contained inside a membrane that stretches across the pit further enhancing its heat-seeking ability.

Ears

The ears of snakes have the same two functions as they do in mammals, hearing and balance. The middle ear in snakes is virtually non-existent (Platel 1994, p. 51). It is a very narrow cavity that does not contain a tympanic membrane but does contain one ossicle, the columella, that abuts the quadrate bone for transmission of vibrations. The inner ear of snakes is very similar to the inner ear of mammals. The utricle and saccule make up the semicircular canals that ensure balance. Vibrations are received in the inner ear via the columella and pass through the cochlear canal and onto the basilar papilla. Even with the absence of an outer ear and the virtual absence of a middle ear, snakes are adept at hearing (Platel 1994, p. 52). Since the columella senses vibrations from the quadrate bone that is located on the upper jaw, snakes will detect vibrations from the substrate on which their head rests (Funk 1996, p. 42). It is believed that arboreal snakes can detect aerial vibrations enabling them to catch avian prey in midflight.

Smell

It is difficult to determine the amount of olfactory sensation snakes have. Snakes have a large number of olfactory nerves, which leaves no doubt that snakes are macrosmatic animals. Their olfactory abilities do not work alone; they are closely associated with the vomeronasal sense as well as sight.

Vomeronasal Sense

The vomeronasal organ, or Jacobson's organ, plays a vital role in predation. It is connected to the oral cavity by the vomeronasal duct. The role of the vomeronasal organ is to detect non-aerial, non-volatile particulate odors. These odors are received by the chemoreceptors on the forked tongue. After picking up a scent, the snake then carries that scent to the vomeronasal organ. The sensory cells inside the vomeronasal organ react with certain molecules that then transfer the scent to the accessory olfactory bulbs, other encephalic centers, and the nucleus globosus. The vomeronasal organ is also used for interspecific interactions, and snakes can use the vomeronasal organ to sense a den for hibernating and for reproductive behaviors such as detecting pheromones.

Eyes

The eye anatomy of snakes is very different to that of other reptiles. Embryologically, the eyelids of snakes fuse to form a transparent spectacle (Zug et al. 2001, p. 64). This spectacle has an extensive vascular network that is optically transparent. The anterior layer of the spectacle is shed during each ecdysis cycle. The spectacle is separated from the cornea by an epithelial-lined subspectacular space. The globe of the eye is kept moist via secretions made by the harderian glands; snakes do not have lacrimal glands. The nasolacrimal ducts drain from the medial canthus to the roof of the oral cavity at the base of or just behind the vomeronasal organ. The globe has poorly developed rectus muscles and limited rotational muscles. Snakes lack the scleral ossicles and cartilage that lizards and chelonians have. Snakes possess a soft and pliable lens. They are able to focus using forward movement of the lens due to increased pressure of the vitreous applied by the ciliary muscle. The iris contains striated muscle making dilation and contraction of the pupil voluntary.

The retina, pupil shape, and lens color have gone through evolutionary changes to better fit the species' lifestyle (Platel 1994, p. 54). Diurnal species, most often, have a round pupil, yellow lens, and a retina made of all cones. Crepuscular species have a paler lens and the retina contains both rods and cones. Nocturnal species have a vertical slit-shaped pupil, a colorless lens, and a retina consisting mostly of rods with very few cones. But there are many exceptions to these generalized statements. For example, crepuscular or nocturnal pythons have a round pupil and a retina that contains a large quantity of both rods and cones.

Snakes have a very wide range of vision, from 125° to 135° for most species. They are also able to perceive depth and distance using binocular vision. The area that both eyes can see is between 30° and 45° (Platel 1994, p. 55).

Digestive System

The digestive system in snakes is a linear tract (Funk 1996, p. 40). It starts with the mouth that opens directly into the buccal cavity. The buccal cavity contains rows of teeth on the upper and lower jaws, the vomeronasal organs, the primary palate, the internal nares, and a highly specialized tongue. Aniliids, the false coral snakes, have developed a partial secondary palate. The morphology of the tongue is variable dependent on the feeding behavior of the snake. The buccal cavity contains many glands throughout the entire cavity. Multicellular glands are a component of the epithelial lining of the tongue. These glands produce and secrete mucus, which coats the prey making passage down the esophagus smooth. Snakes also have five types of salivary glands: labial, lingual, sublingual, palatine, and dental. Venom glands are modified salivary glands. The pharynx contains a muscular sphincter that controls the opening of the esophagus (Figure 10.4).

The esophagus is a muscular walled tube that connects the buccal cavity to the stomach. In snakes, the esophagus may be one-quarter to one-half of the body length. The stomach is a very large muscular tube that has the primary role of mechanical digestion and starting the chemical digestion process. Numerous glands in the stomach lining produce secretions to aid in digestion. The pyloric valve controls entry of the food bolus into the small intestine, which is a long, narrow, straight tube. The small intestine also has glands to help with the digestion process. At the junction with the large intestine, there is a marked difference in the size. The large intestine has a diameter several times that of the small intestine. Boids have a small

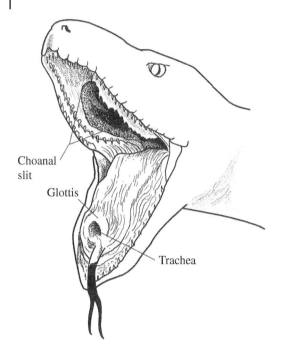

Figure 10.4 Oral cavity of a snake. (Drawing by Scott Stark).

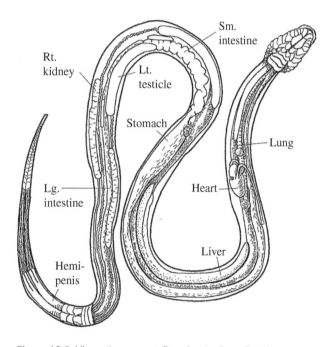

Figure 10.5 Visceral anatomy. (Drawing by Scott Stark).

cecum located at the proximal colon. The large intestine is the weakest and most thin-walled structure in the digestive tract. The large intestine ends at the anus and then leads to the dorsal portion of the cloaca, the coprodaeum (Figure 10.5).

The primary function of the liver in snakes is the same as in mammals. The liver produces bile that is stored in the gall bladder and then sent to the duodenum via the common bile duct. Bile aids in the digestion of fat. The liver is elongated and spindle-shaped. The pancreas produces digestive fluids into the duodenum. The pancreas is usually located in a triad with the spleen and gallbladder, although some species have a splenopancreas.

Since the feeding behavior of snakes is not all the same, different physiologic and morphologic changes occur with different feeding behaviors. Snakes that eat small, frequent meals tend to have a digestive system that is always in an active state. On the other hand, snakes that eat large, infrequent meals maintain their digestive system in an inactive state until a prey item has been ingested. When the prey is ingested, the gut begins to increase secretions of hydrochloric acid and digestive enzymes. Within one day, the small intestine will double in size and other organs in the digestive, respiratory, and circulatory systems will also gain in size. When the digestive tract is activated, the metabolic rate will increase as much as 44 times that of the resting metabolic rate. The energy needed to activate the intestinal tract must be received from stored reserves before the digestive process can begin for the new prey. Infrequent feeders usually maintain a metabolic rate half that of frequent feeders.

Urinary System

Snakes have a bilateral pair of lobulated and elongated kidneys. They are located in the dorsal caudal coelomic cavity. The right kidney is located cranial to the left kidney. The kidneys are metanephric in structure and have few nephrons and lack a loop of Henle and a renal pelvis (Divers 2000, p. 217). The ureters empty into the urodeum in the cloaca. Snakes do not have a urinary bladder.

Snakes excrete nitrogenous waste as uric acid. Uric acid is a purine, synthesized in several interlocking pathways, and is very insoluble in water. In the kidney tubule, urine stays dilute; water is reabsorbed when the urine reaches the cloaca, making the urine more concentrated, and some of the uric acid precipitates. The precipitation of uric acid reduces the concentration of the uric acid allowing more water to be reabsorbed. Again, this leads to more precipitation of uric acid. This process allows nitrogen to be excreted using very little water. The end product is a white or gray semisolid pasty material containing uric acid.

Endocrine and Exocrine Glands

Pituitary Gland

The pituitary gland is the so-called master gland of the body. It consists of two parts, the neurohypophysis and the adenohypophysis. The neurohypophysis produces hormones that stimulate the adenohypophysis or act directly on the target organs. The adenohypophysis releases six hormones: adrenocorticotropin, follicle-stimulating hormone, luteinizing hormone, prolactin, somatotropin, and thyrotropin.

Pineal Complex

The pineal complex consists of an epiphysis and a parapineal organ. They act as light receptors and are associated with cyclic activities such as circadian rhythms and seasonal cycles. As a gland, both organs release melatonin. All snakes have a pineal gland that lies on the brain but does not exit the skull as in some iguanids.

Thyroid Gland

The thyroid gland is located in the throat adjacent to the larynx and trachea and is nearly spherical. Snakes can have either a single or paired thyroid gland. The thyroid gland is responsible for accumulating iodine and producing and regulating hormones that control growth and development as well as ecdysis.

Parathyroid Gland

The parathyroid gland is located just cranial to the thyroid. The parathyroid gland functions as a blood calcium regulator.

Pancreas

The pancreas in snakes, like in mammals, functions as an endocrine and exocrine gland. As an exocrine gland, it secretes digestive enzymes, and as an endocrine gland, it secretes the hormone insulin via clusters of cells called the islets of Langerhans.

Gonads

The gonads produce the sex hormones. The function of the gonads is closely regulated by the brain and the pituitary. Hypothalamohypophyseal hormones and gonadotropins are produced by the brain and the pituitary, respectively, when the gonads are triggered by a hormonal response. Along with stimulating reproductive structures, the sex hormones also produce secondary sexual characteristics and provide a feedback mechanism to the hypothalamic–pituitary complex.

Adrenal Glands

The adrenal glands are a pair of bilateral glands located anterior to the kidneys. The adrenal glands have many functions. They produce adrenaline (epinephrine) and noradrenaline (norepinephrine), they affect sodium, potassium, and carbohydrate metabolism, and they affect the androgens and the reproductive process.

Reproductive Biology and Husbandry

Male Anatomy

All male snakes have right and left testicles and a pair of hemipenes. The testicles are ovoid masses of seminiferous tubules, interstitial cells, and blood vessels. They are located dorsomedially within the coelomic cavity between the pancreatic triad and the kidneys. The right testis is located just cranial to the left. Snakes do not have an epididymis. The hemipenes are located in the base of the tail and are held in place by a retractor muscle. Sperm is produced in the seminiferous tubules. During copulation, sperm travels to the hemipenis through the wolffian ducts. The sperm is able to enter the female by means of the sulcus spermaticus located on the outside of the hemipenis. During copulation, only one hemipenis is used. Many snakes, especially boids, have vestigial (pelvic) spurs. These spurs are used in copulation as stimulation and to help position the two cloacae together (Figure 10.6).

Female Anatomy

The paired ovaries are located similarly to the testes. Each consists of epithelial cells, connective tissue, nerves, blood vessels, and germinal cell beds encased in an elastic tunic. An inactive ovary is small and granular, whereas active ovaries are large, lobular sacs filled with spherical vitellogenic follicles. Snakes do not have a true uterus. The oviducts empty directly into the cloaca and have an albumin-secreting and shell-secreting function.

Sex Determination

Since snakes do not possess external genitalia, determining the sex can sometimes be challenging. There are

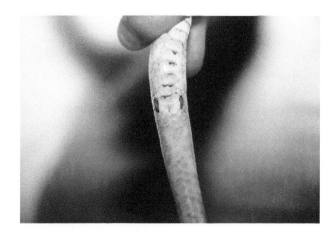

Figure 10.6 Large pelvic spurs.

several acceptable methods of sex determination, with various degrees of simplicity and accuracy. It is important to choose a method that best suits the particular snake. For a snake that is kept as a pet, it is best to stick with a more simple method of sex determination. Snakes kept for breeding should be sexed using the most accurate method for that species and size.

Secondary Sexual Characteristics

With the exception of the boids, most snakes do not show any secondary sexual characteristics. Male boids will sometimes have larger cloacal spurs than females. But only technicians who are very familiar with boids will be able to accurately determine the sex by using this method (see Figure 10.6). Another secondary sexual characteristic that can be used to determine the sex is a small bulge in the tail that indicates where the hemipenes are located. However, methods based on secondary sexual characteristics, although simple, are the least accurate.

Sexual Dimorphism

Sexual dimorphism occurs in most snakes. The most common form of sexual dimorphism is in size. Female snakes tend to be larger and have a shorter tail than males of the same species. This evolutionary adaptation allows the females to produce more and/or larger offspring, thereby increasing the chances of survival. The males have evolved to be shorter with a longer tail to accommodate the hemipenes and retractor muscles. The longer tail is beneficial during courtship, they can reach maturity at an earlier age, and have increased mobility. But, except in adult snakes, determining sex based on size and tail length may produce false results unless performed by the most experienced keepers.

Manual Eversion

A more accurate method of sex determination is manually everting the hemipenes. This method, often referred to as popping, is best used in juvenile snakes or snakes that are too small for other methods. For this process, firmly roll one thumb up the base of the tail starting distal and working proximal to the cloaca. If it is a male, the hemipenes will "pop" out. Care must be taken not to apply too much pressure or the hemipenes and the retractor muscles can be damaged. This method is unreliable in large snakes and some colubrids where manual eversion of the hemipenes is not possible.

Cloacal Probing

This is the preferred method of sex determination. It is very simple and accurate if done properly. The probe can

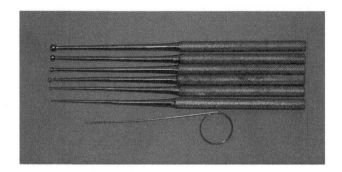

Figure 10.7 Commercial probe set used for sexing snakes.

be anything that is straight and has a blunt end. Commercial sex probes are available in sets of various diameters (Figure 10.7). Insert the lubricated probe into the cloaca and angle it caudally. Position the probe just lateral to the midline. Then gently slide the probe caudally into the base of the tail. If the snake is male, the probe will enter the inverted hemipenis and slide down several millimeters. If the snake is a female, the probe will either not be able to enter the tail base or will go only a couple of millimeters. Female snakes have blind diverticula that are smaller in diameter and shorter in depth than the hemipenes. A major cause of error in sexing is using a probe that is too small. A very small probe can enter the diverticula in females giving a false diagnosis. The technician must also be careful not to be forceful with the probe. The probe should slide smoothly with very little force needed. Generally, the distance the probe enters the base of the tail is measured in either millimeters or number of subcaudal scales. This number should be recorded in the file with the sex diagnosis (Figure 10.8).

Hydrostatic Eversion

Hydrostatic eversion is an accurate yet difficult method of sex determination. It involves injecting isotonic saline into the base of the tail just caudal to where the hemipenes would be located. Injection of the saline is continued until the hemipenes are everted or resistance is felt on the syringe. A possible danger of this procedure is injecting the saline into the hemipenes instead of caudally. For most snakes, anesthesia is required to perform this procedure. This method is accurate because the hemipenes are everted in males, and if the snake is female, the swelling around the cloaca allows for visualization of the oviductal papillae.

Other Methods of Sex Determination

Several other forms of sex determination are available. Imaging through ultrasonography is possible. However, the testes and ovaries can be mistaken for each other, and

Figure 10.8 Sex probing a snake. (A) Appropriate placement of probe prior to insertion. (B) Initial insertion of the probe. (C) Advancing the probe. (D) In males the probe advances farther than in females. (Drawings by Scott Stark).

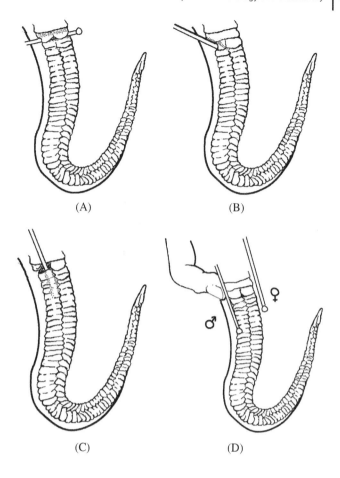

(A)   (B)

(C)   (D)

this method is best used to help determine the reproductive status of females. Direct visualization via laparoscopy is also an acceptable method, although it should be used as a last resort since other methods are available that have less risk associated with them.

Fertilization

Prior to egg production, fertilization occurs in the upper portion of the oviducts when the sperm and egg unite. In snakes, fertilization is usually delayed for a few hours to years after copulation. Sperm storage structures facilitate storage of sperm for long periods of time. This process of delayed fertilization permits females to mate with other males allowing multiple paternity among the offspring and giving a higher fecundity rate, although not all snakes practice this.

Parthenogenesis has been reported in several species of snakes. True parthenogenesis—asexual reproduction in an all-female species—is known to occur in one species of snake, *Ramphotyphlops braminus* (brahminy blind snake). More commonly facultative parthenogenesis occurs.

This occurs in species that are capable of sexual reproduction in the absence of males and has been observed in numerous species such as *Boa constrictor* (*boa constrictor*), *Epicrates maurus* (Columbian rainbow boa), *Agkistrodon contortrix* (copperhead), *Agkistrodon piscivorus* (cottonmouth), *Eunectes murinus* (green anaconda), and *Python bivittatus* (Burmese python).

Sexual Maturity

Sexual maturity in snakes is dependent on many factors; husbandry and nutrition are more important factors than age. Ultimately, it is the size of the snake that determines sexual maturity. Due to the large differences in care provided for captive snakes, the age of sexual maturity will consequently be different as well. With proper husbandry and nutrition, snakes will grow quickly and become sexually mature within their first or second year of life.

Follicle Maturation and the Fat Cycle

In the months before the female's reproductive cycle, she will begin to store fat (Ross et al. 1990, p. 60). This fat plays a major role in the reproductive cycle. Vitellogenesis, the production of yolk, will only occur if enough fat is stored. Also, at the end stages of gestation, snakes may not eat so the fat bodies are used for energy. The follicles mature within the ovaries, and when they are mature and palpable, some ova are released into the oviduct while other ova may be released before or after copulation. At this point, the snake will find a male and copulate and the female will become gravid. After the proper gestation period, the female will either lay eggs or give birth to live young. The female is now very thin and weak after using up all of her fat deposits during gestation and/or incubation. Until the fat stores have been replenished, she will not be able to stimulate follicular maturation. She then begins to eat and increases her fat bodies. After a couple to several months, the female snake is back to full weight and can begin the follicular maturation cycle again.

Courtship

It is important to know and observe signs of courtship so proper changes can be made. If communal cages are kept, insubordinate specimens should be separated from the courting pair. Temperature cycling patterns should be started before or at the first signs of copulation. Specimens should be removed or added if either of the specimens seen courting is inappropriate for breeding.

Many courtship behaviors are observed in snakes, and most behaviors are not species-specific. Four common courtship behaviors seen in many taxa are described here (Ross et al. 1990, p. 55).

1. The tactile chase behavior is characterized by the male pursuing the female in often jerky and erratic movements. The male may flick his tongue over the female's body and begin to crawl over her dorsum trying to align his body with hers. The female will continue to crawl away if unreceptive to the behavior.
2. In the tail search copulatory attempt the male will rotate his tail under the female's tail in an attempt to bring both cloacae together. A receptive female will then lift her tail or allow her tail to be lifted by the male. The male may use his spurs to stimulate the female to lift her tail.
3. Tactile alignment is characterized by the male aligning his tail with the female's, using his spurs as stimulation and to help align the cloacae.
4. Intromission and coitus occur when a female raises her tail and everts her cloaca to a male. The male will then align the two cloacae and copulation occurs. This behavior is also known as cloacal gaping.

Oviparous, Ovoviviparous, and Viviparous

Oviparous snakes are snakes that lay eggs that are protected by a hard shell. Around 70% of snakes are oviparous. Some of the more common oviparous species seen in a veterinary practice are king snakes and milk snakes (*Lampropeltis* spp.), rat and corn snakes (*Elaphe* spp.), and all pythons. Oviparous snakes will go to much trouble finding an appropriate place to lay their eggs. Some snakes will lay in a natural cavity, hollow stumps, or small mammals' burrows while others will dig their own burrow or make a nest. Most pythons will incubate their eggs by hugging them and increasing their own body heat through rhythmic contractions of their abdominal musculature. Oviposition occurs approximately 2–5 weeks after fertilization with embryos that are about 30% developed.

Research in squamates has shown that many species of lizards and snakes that give live birth do provide some maternal nutrition so the term viviparous, instead of ovoviviparous, is now used to describe snakes that give live birth. Viviparous snakes will incubate the eggs inside the oviducts until the eggs hatch. This process ensures proper humidity and temperature levels within the mother's thermoregulatory capabilities. In order for the snakes to be able to do this, their reproductive tract has evolved from a tract that was designed to house eggs for a short period of time (Blackburn & Stewart 2011). All viviparous snakes share a common oviparous ancestry and biological substrate. The formation of a placenta out of fetal membranes and the maternal oviduct enables these snakes to achieve successful reproduction. Within a given species and between taxa there are distinct differences in structural and functional attributes that reflect specialization for the individual snake's needs. Viviparous snakes often inhabit places where the ground is too cold to incubate eggs (Saint-Girons 1994, p. 99). However, viviparous species have a wide geographic and ecologic distribution and are not confined to cooler environments. There are viviparous representatives of arboreal, terrestrial, fossorial, and aquatic snakes from all biomes where snakes are found. However, viviparity brings many disadvantages. The gravid female moves very slowly, which makes her vulnerable to predation; she is only able to eat very small prey, which are hard to find at times; and she must focus more on thermoregulation. Viviparous snakes are born fully developed. Examples include boas, pit vipers, rattlesnakes, and garter snakes (*Thamnophis* spp.).

Egg Anatomy

After fertilization, the embryo begins to develop on the dorsal surface of the yolk. The yolk is then covered by the yolk sac and attached to the embryo by the yolk stalk at the umbilicus. Nourishment is provided by the yolk via the blood vessels of the yolk sac. The amnion is a fluid-filled sac that surrounds and protects the embryo. The allantois is a closed sac that collects waste products. The chorion is a membrane that surrounds and protects the embryo and yolk sac. Shell membranes cover these three membranes and provide gas exchange throughout the shell. Blood vessels in the shell membranes and the yolk stalk combine to form the umbilicus. As the egg passes through the oviducts, the shell and shell membranes are gradually applied by the shell glands.

Timing and Frequency of Reproduction

In most species, environmental factors trigger the breeding season. While other species will breed year-round, for temperate species the breeding season usually begins in spring after a hibernation period. Most equatorial species will breed year-round. There are exceptions to these rules. Some tropical boids reproduce in the cooler part of the year though temperatures may show greater diurnal changes than seasonal changes. Many species that live in areas where there is a rainy season, like the monsoons in Southeast Asia and India, time their reproductive cycle with the rainfall.

It is uncommon for a snake to reproduce more than once in a one year due to the lengthy gestation periods and the need to replenish fat deposits. The entire reproductive process, starting with follicle maturation and ending with the snake restored to full weight, could take several months to over a year depending on species. Viviparous species mostly breed once every two years or more.

Maternal Care

Very few snakes show any maternal care. Some pythons will coil around the eggs incubating them and protecting them from predators. Some viviparous species will show maternal care by helping the newborns out of the amniotic sac and consuming the infertile yolk sac. Maternal care with regards to teaching to acquire food, thermoregulation, or performance of other necessary life-sustaining activities is rarely observed in snakes.

Egg Incubation and Management

Artificial Incubation

It is recommended that eggs be artificially incubated only by experienced herpetoculturists. Many herpetoculturists artificially incubate eggs to increase the chance of hatching. In captivity, it is difficult for the female snake to keep the relative humidity high enough to incubate her own eggs. If the decision is made to artificially incubate the eggs, the herpetoculturist must be prepared well before the female lays the eggs; it is recommended that the incubator be ready several days in advance. The incubator should maintain a constant temperature and humidity that is ideal for the species being incubated. For most species, a temperature range of 86 to 91°F (30 to 32.5°C) is ideal. Eggs do not benefit from temperature variations so a constant temperature should be maintained. It is not critical to measure the relative humidity although a high relative humidity should be maintained. As long as condensation appears on the sides of the incubator, the humidity should be high enough.

When the female lays the eggs, the herpetoculturist should move quickly to remove them. Within a few hours after oviposition, the eggs will become adherent. It is preferable that the eggs be laid singly in the incubator so they can be properly monitored. Also, the conditions inside the enclosure may be inadequate for proper incubation, which can be detrimental to the eggs. Eggs can dehydrate within 48–72 hours. Gently remove the eggs and place them in the preheated incubator. The incubator should be checked several times a day for proper temperature and humidity and the eggs should be checked for viability.

Maternal Incubation

There are several reasons why maternal incubation should be performed. The eggs should be maternally incubated if the female is too large or aggressive to safely remove the eggs, if the female unexpectedly laid eggs and an incubator was not ready, or if normal incubation parameters are not known. The humidity in the cage should not fall below 75%. Because of the high humidity that must be maintained, the cage should be kept in a very clean environment with adequate circulation and a constant temperature inside the cage. The incubating female should not have to thermoregulate, which would require an excessive amount of energy that many incubating females do not have. The cage should be kept at 88°F (31°C) for most species of python. If maternal incubation was chosen due to the lack of experience of artificial incubation, extensive research on the natural history of the species should be done to determine the proper incubating temperature.

Incubator Design

Incubators can be commercially bought or one can easily be made. The basic requirements of an incubator are: the construction should prevent excessive heat and humidity loss; there must be a constant and reliable heat source; and there must be a thermostat to control the temperature. The actual design of the incubator can vary as long as the above three rules have been met.

When constructing an incubator, some general guidelines should be followed. The incubator should be uniformly heated. An easy way to accomplish this is by using heat tape that can be evenly positioned on the bottom of the incubator. Hot water can also be used. An inner container should be installed that is not resting on the bottom of the incubator. This will allow the heat to be evenly distributed throughout the entire incubator. The thermostat should be sensitive enough to control the temperature fluctuation within 1 degree, and the temperature should be monitored from the outside the incubator. To ensure adequate humidity, spray the incubator and eggs with water every two to three days. The water should be the same temperature as the incubator. The incubator should be lined with Styrofoam to maintain the desired temperature. The best substrates to use are vermiculite, sphagnum moss, potting soil, sand, shredded newspaper, pea gravel, and paper towels.

Determining Egg Viability

A viable clutch of eggs should be uniform in size, have a brilliant white color, and be pliable or elastic (Ross et al. 1990, p. 103). If an egg is smaller, discolored, hard, or rubbery, it usually is not fertilized. Some female snakes will reject an unfertilized egg from the clutch. If an egg does not adhere to the rest of the clutch, it should still be incubated until signs of egg death appear. Wrinkles or depressions at the time of oviposition are not signs of non-viability. A fertilized egg will not show significant change during the incubation period, whereas an unfertilized egg will quickly begin to show signs of decomposition.

It can sometimes be very difficult to determine the viability of an egg. If the viability is uncertain, the egg should be incubated until further signs appear. The rest of the clutch will not be in danger. The texture of an egg or irregular calcification should not be used as an indication of non-viability. Another method for determining egg viability is a technique called candling, which involves the use of a high-intensity light to transilluminate the egg. A viable egg should have a network of blood vessels and an embryo during the late stages of incubation. The absence of blood vessels indicates a non-viable egg.

Manual Pipping

Sometimes manual pipping is necessary for the embryo to live. An egg should be manually pipped only if most eggs in the clutch have hatched, no eggs have pipped by the estimated due date, or the due date is unknown. Manual pipping is a very delicate procedure that with time and practice can be a very effective method of saving a clutch. All that is needed to perform this technique is a pair of iris scissors and thumb forceps. Using the iris scissors, a small perforation is made in the shell. With the scissors pointing up toward the inner surface of the eggshell, a small incision is then made in the shell. At the site of the puncture, another small incision is made. This should make a "V" shaped incision. The wedge can be elevated using the thumb forceps and removed. If done properly, the shell membranes should all still be intact. During this process, one should avoid cutting large blood vessels—small vessels are impossible to avoid. The embryo should not be visible. With the thumb forceps, the shell membranes should be gently separated from the shell. One should start at the window that was made and begin working outward. More pieces of shell can be removed as the membrane is separated. When a large enough window has been made, the embryo can then be stimulated. To stimulate the embryo, prod it gently with a blunt tip instrument. If it is alive, the embryo will move freely in the egg. The embryo should be intermittently stimulated until the neonate has emerged from the shell. This process usually takes 12 to 24 hours.

Housing

When obtaining housing for a snake, a few things must be taken into consideration: (i) the size (length) of the snake to be housed; (ii) whether the snake is a terrestrial or an arboreal species; (iii) whether the housing is secure (escape proof); (iv) whether it has proper ventilation; (v) whether it allows for necessary cleaning/disinfecting; and (vi) whether proper heat sources can be provided (Figure 10.9).

Aquaria are certainly suitable and aesthetically pleasing enclosures for most species of snakes, but can be quite costly to obtain, especially when housing some of the larger species. Ideally the length of the enclosure should be no less than half of the length of the snake being housed. When housing arboreal species (e.g., green tree python), the enclosure should have more vertical space than horizontal to allow for placement of perches for the snake. If an aquarium is used, one needs to make sure that a lid can be secured on the tank appropriately. Lids that rest on top of the aquarium without any locking mechanisms are NOT appropriate for snakes as they are escape artists!! Also, if using an aquarium, the lid should allow proper ventilation (i.e., screen lids) if the aquarium itself does not have any ventilation holes (which most do not). One should make sure to choose a lid that does not present a potential fire hazard if using heat lamps above it. Plastic lids will melt.

Any aquaria with cracks should be avoided due to the potential for the glass to shatter resulting in injury to the animal. In short, aquaria can make wonderful enclosures and can be easily disinfected if the cost of obtaining an aquarium is not an issue.

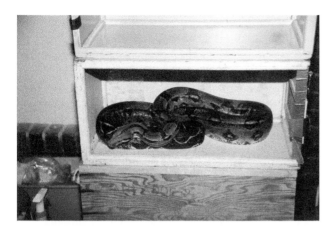

Figure 10.9 Inappropriate housing. The cage is too small and provides no source of heat or water.

Building an enclosure for a snake is usually the preferred method of housing. It is less expensive in most cases and allows for customizing according to the snake's needs. If one has the time and know-how, this is usually the best way to ensure the snake being housed has adequate room and the caging can be built using secure locking mechanisms. It can be enjoyable customizing an enclosure as long as a couple of guidelines are followed. Obviously, it would not be ideal to construct a cage solely of wood without any way to view the snake. Glass or Plexiglass should be included when constructing a wooden enclosure. Screen can be used on the sides or even the top of the enclosure to ensure proper ventilation. Without proper ventilation, bacteria can accumulate and it will become stagnant inside the enclosure. Incorporating screen into the top of the enclosure will allow proper lighting/heat fixtures to be fixed on top of the cage to allow illumination but not allow the snake to come into contact with it. Heat lamps should not be placed inside the enclosure where the snake can contact them due to the potential for burns. An enclosure should not be constructed solely of screen, however, as it can become too drafty. Pressure-treated wood should not be used for the construction. The wood used should be sanded and free of abrasive surfaces to prevent potential injury to the snake and treated/painted to allow regular cleaning without damaging the wood. Sealing/painting will also be necessary for cleaning purposes because of the possibility that feces and urates may soak into the porous wood. Priming and painting the inside of the enclosure white can assist you in spotting problems such as mites in the caging. The white paint reflects the lighting better as well.

Depending on one's preferred access to the inside of the cage, different locking mechanisms can be chosen. Everything from hinged doors with padlocks to sliding glass doors is suitable for securing the custom enclosure.

Commercially available enclosures specifically made for keeping reptiles can easily be acquired. Those designed specifically for snakes have consideration for the type of material, heating methods, accessing the snake, lighting, lifestyle, and aesthetic value. Enclosures are also made with the specific intention of housing venomous species or very large constrictors. Housing for venomous species should be made of a single piece construction, as with many molded high-density impact-resistant polyethylene cages. Large constrictors must be housed in a very secure cage with a front that allows for visualization, but also durable enough to withstand the snake pressing against it. Although these cages cost substantially more than building one yourself, they have many advantages that make them a good choice.

Substrate

Many different types of substrate are used in snake enclosures (Figure 10.10). There also is much debate on what is appropriate and what can be harmful. It is necessary to read as much as possible about the snake to obtain the maximum information about its natural habitat to better assist in making husbandry-related choices. Substrates can fall into two categories, naturalistic and simplistic.

Naturalistic substrates resemble the substrate that is found in the species' natural environment. Beyond aesthetic value, these substrates provide a means of enrichment for the snake being housed. They can also aid in the control of humidity and temperature. For example, wood chips tend to increase the humidity due to their ability to absorb moisture and also act as an insulator decreasing the effectiveness of under-tank heaters. Sand does not absorb moisture so tends to help keep the enclosure less humid and creates a great source of conductive and convective heat. However, the negative aspect is that any loose substrate ingested could potentially cause intestinal obstructions as well as stomatitis. The snake should not be fed in the enclosure and instead be placed inside a plastic box or other appropriate enclosure that does not contain naturalistic substrate to prevent the accidental ingestion of substrate. One needs to make sure the substrate is not being ingested, and if it is, the substrate should be changed to something more simplistic. Moist complex substrates will increase the chances of bacterial and fungal diseases since they can be difficult to clean and the hot, moist substrate is an ideal breeding ground for many species of bacteria and fungi.

Aspen shavings can be used for some snake species requiring an arid climate but should not be used for snakes requiring high humidity, for which there are more suitable substrates. One should make sure the aspen shavings have been treated through a "baking" process, which can help

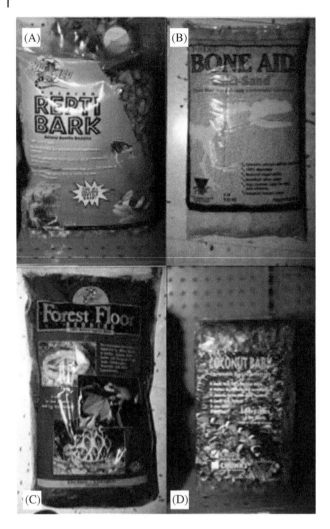

Figure 10.10 Various common commercially available substrates. (A) Repti Bark (fir bark). (B) Calcium carbonate granules. (C) Cypress mulch. (D) Ground coconut shell.

determines which type of sand to get if this is the substrate of choice.

Cypress mulch is another good substrate especially for species requiring higher humidity. It can make an enclosure look very natural, and it is relatively inexpensive. One needs to make sure that it is cypress mulch and not another type of mulch (i.e., eucalyptus) because these can be very aromatic and lead to respiratory problems. The mulch can be mixed with sphagnum moss if the goal is to make a natural appearing environment.

Potting soil should be used with caution. Most potting soils have fertilizers and other chemicals that could be toxic to snakes. If topsoil is used, one should make sure that it is organic and free of chemicals. Otherwise, topsoil can be a good substrate to use for snakes requiring high humidity because of its ability to retain moisture. This can be used for terrestrial and burrowing species.

Cedar/pine shavings are not recommended as substrate for any reptiles. The oils and natural aroma of these shavings can be toxic to snakes and can lead to respiratory disorders. Although some companies claim that they are great for snakes because they "repel mites and ticks," using any cedar or pine shavings should be avoided. Shavings can also lodge in the snake's oral cavity, which could cause stomatitis.

Aquarium gravel and corncob should not be used. Some gravel can be abrasive, and they can both cause impactions if ingested in large amounts.

Caution should be used if any tree limbs, substrate, or any other objects are collected from outside. They can contaminate the enclosure with parasites, molds/fungi, and so on. Sterilization can be attempted with these objects via boiling/baking or disinfecting with a diluted bleach solution to minimize contamination. Tree limbs taken from outside should not have any "sticky" substances such as sap on them.

Simplistic substrates are those that do not resemble anything seen in nature. They have the benefit of being easy to keep clean as the urates/feces is generally easily seen, and these substrates pose no risk of being ingested. However, they provide little enrichment to the snake and do little to help control heat and humidity. These substrates are recommended for sick or hospitalized patients, and those with external parasites. These are especially helpful during the treatment of mites.

Indoor/outdoor carpet is commonly used as substrate. It is aesthetically pleasing and does not present any immediate harm to the snake. It can be purchased by the yard at most local hardware stores. Routine cleaning and disinfecting will be more demanding than with other substrates because the carpet costs more and needs to be replaced frequently. When a snake defecates or passes urates, the carpet

to eliminate any parasites contained in the shavings, and ensure the shavings are free of toxic oils. Aspen shavings can also become lodged in the snake's mouth so as a precaution; the snake should not be fed on aspen shavings.

Sand is often used for desert species, and there are many contradicting statements regarding the use of sand in any reptile enclosure. However, it is the "natural" substrate of many desert species. While some people buy play sand at the hardware store to use, others buy sand sold at pet stores for reptile substrate. Some commercial brands of sand used as substrate for reptiles claim they are less likely to cause impactions than regular play sand if ingested due to their calcium content and fine grain. However, caution should still be used when feeding any reptile on a sand substrate; this not recommended, as already discussed. Also, consumption of large amounts of calcium can be just as harmful as calcium deficiency. Personal preference will absorb some of the matter and will need to be washed or replaced altogether. Otherwise, the carpet will become pungent and allow bacterial and/or fungal growth.

Newspaper is frequently used as substrate, especially when an individual keeps multiple snakes. Newspaper is plentiful, inexpensive, and easily obtained. It is absorbent and easily replaced when doing routine cleanings. It is especially good to use for animals in quarantine, and is the substrate best suited for feeding as the chances of it being ingested are not as great as with "loose" substrate. Although not as aesthetically pleasing as some forms of substrate, it is definitely easier to maintain. The ink from the paper can rub off onto the snake, but it will cause no harm as the ink is non-toxic.

Good judgment must be used when choosing an appropriate substrate. Knowing the geographic range of the particular snake housed and the benefits and risks of the substrates will aid in making husbandry decisions.

Heating and Lighting

Snakes are ectothermic, meaning they rely on their surroundings to regulate their body temperature. Unlike mammals, they are unable to do this on their own. Because of this, snakes kept in captivity require heating/lighting supplementation. Failure to maintain appropriate temperatures for the particular snake can lead to respiratory disorders, food regurgitation, anorexia due to lethargy, and even death (Table 10.2).

There are many species of snake kept in captivity today and sold commercially. Whether the snake is a desert-dwelling or tropical snake, it is necessary to maintain an enclosure that mimics its natural surroundings and climate zone. Ideally, snakes need a warm basking area to maintain good health and also a cooler area to retreat to in case they get too warm. To ensure that necessary temperatures are being met, thermometers must be purchased. These can be bought at most pet stores and have adhesives so they can be easily placed in the enclosure. Ideally, one thermometer should be affixed in the enclosure where the hottest temperature is achieved and one should also be affixed in the "cool zone." If the snake is a terrestrial species, the thermometer should be placed close to the bottom. With arboreal species, the thermometers should be placed near the areas where the snake can perch (Figure 10.11).

Heat rocks have been used in the reptile hobby for over 30 years. They have historically been known in the veterinary community as "death rocks" due to the large number of severe burns and subsequent deaths associated with their use. More recently, most of the heat rocks commercially available have a safety cut-off switch and an internal thermostat. Once the thermostat reaches a pre-set temperature,

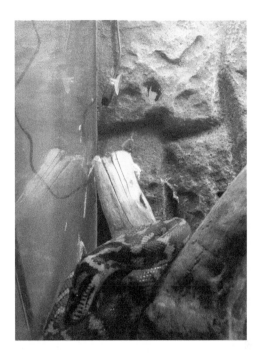

Figure 10.11 Probe for a thermometer and hygrometer located high in the cage of a *Morelia spilota variegata* (Irian Jaya carpet python).

the heating element cuts off. However, there are still many heat rocks sold commercially that do not have this safety feature. It is strongly advisable that only heat rocks with automatic cut-off switches be used. If the others are used, they should be buried in the substrate so that the snake does not have direct contact. It is also important to understand that the heat rock only provides conductive heat and should not be used as the sole source of heat as its action only works on objects directly touching it.

Heating tape, heating pads (often referred to as under-the-tank heaters), and heating cables are good sources of heat for snakes. These products are also sold commercially in the pet trade, and if used correctly are safer than heat rocks and can be used to help heat all or part of an enclosure. The pads and tape are often placed on the outside of the enclosure underneath the tank where the snake cannot make direct contact with the unit but benefits from the heat being emitted; these devices can also be placed on the sides of an enclosure. These heating mechanisms distribute the heat more evenly and in some cases cover the entire length of the enclosure. If a heating pad is used that has a temperature setting control, the setting should be kept on low. If the enclosure is made of thick wood or if there is a thick layer of substrate, one can adjust the setting of the pad to medium if the low setting is not producing enough heat to benefit the snake. The bottom of the enclosure should always be tested (via touch or thermometers) thoroughly to ensure it does not get too hot.

Table 10.2 Husbandry data for selected species of snake.

Common name	Scientific name	Average length[a]	Ambient temperature in Fahrenheit (day)[b]	Humidity (%)	Geographic range[c]
Boas					
Common boa	*Boa constrictor*	~6′–10′	80–85	50–70	Central America and South America
Brazilian rainbow boa	*Epicrates cenchria cenchria*	5′–7′	80–85	75–90	Brazil
Emerald tree boa	*Corallus caninus*	4′–6′	75–82	85–90	Amazon Basin
Rosy boa	*Lichanura trivirgata*	2′–3′	80–85	20–30	Southern CA, AZ, Mexico
Pythons					
Ball python	*Python requis*	3′–5′	80–85	60–65	Central Africa, West Africa, Borneo
Blood python	*Python curtus*	3′–6′	80–85	70–75	Borneo Islands, Malaysia, Sumatra
Burmese python	*Python molurus bivittatus*	12′–20′	80–85	70–80	SE Asia
Green tree python	*Morelia chondropython viridis*	4′–6′	75–85	85–90	Australia, New Guinea
Carpet python	*Morelia spilota*	6′–10′	80–85	60–70	Australia
Reticulated python	*Python reticulatus*	10′–25′	80–85	65–70	Thailand, Indonesia, Philippines (SE Asia)
African rock python	*Python sebae*	12′–20′	80–85	65–70	Africa
Colubrids					
Common king snakes	*Lampropeltis getula*	4′–5′	75–85	30–50	North and South America
Corn snakes	*Elaphe guttata*	4′–5′	75–85	50–60	Eastern United States, Midwest United States
Rat snake	*Elaphe obsoleta*	5′–7′	75–85	50–60	North America
Milk snake	*Lampropeltis triangulum*	2′–5′	75–85	50–60	North and South America
Gopher/bull/pine snake	*Pituophis* spp.	4′–7′	75–85	30–50	United States and Mexico
Garter/ribbon snakes	*Thamnophis* spp.	2′–4′	75–80	60–75	United States

a) Lengths refer to average adult lengths (in feet) not absolute min/max Lengths.
b) Temperatures given are average ambient temperatures; basking spots should be 5–10°F higher with a nighttime drop of 5–10°F.
c) AZ, Arizona; CA, California.

A high setting should never be used. One should not depend on the snake moving if the heating element gets too hot. Thermal burns are easily prevented if caution is used and regular checks are performed on the heating elements. If the pads do not have a temperature control setting or if using heat tape, the use of a thermostat is recommended. Heat tape has the advantage over heat pads in that it is cut to size and a single electrical source can be used to heat multiple cages, as in rack systems. Heat cables are relatively new to the trade. These come in sizes from 11 ft (3.5 m) and 15 watts up to 52 ft (16 m) and 150 W of power. The cables can be used inside the cage to add

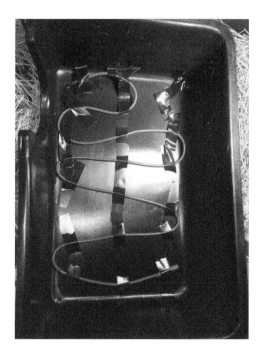

Figure 10.12 Heat cable used to heat a hide box. The heat cable maintains a temperature of 85°F. More or less heat cable could be used to increase or decrease the temperature.

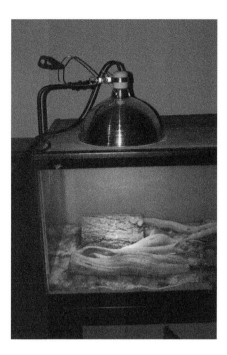

Figure 10.13 A light hood used to heat the cage of a *Heterodon nasicus* (western hognose). Note how the light is more than 12 in. from the snake and the snake has no access to the light.

conductive heat to cage furnishings such as branches; they can be used to heat hide boxes (Figure 10.12); or they can be taped to the underside of a tank to act like a heat pad. Multiple cages can be heated using these cables, and they are especially beneficial with rack systems.

Heat lamps are acceptable primary heat sources and also provide the snake with necessary day and night light cycles if actual lights are used. These can be used in conjunction with under-the-tank heaters for snakes requiring high temperatures. Clamp light fixtures are relatively inexpensive and can be purchased from local hardware stores, livestock supply stores, and pet stores (Figure 10.13). These can be placed on top of the enclosure (on a screen, not plastic or flammable material) or clamped to a surface allowing the light to be directed into the enclosure. Bulbs should be selected based on the snake's temperature needs and the design of the enclosure itself. Incandescent bulbs, ceramic heat emitters, or floodlamps can be used for heating purposes. Wattage of the bulb depends on the dimensions of the enclosure and the snake's temperature needs. In most cases, a 50–75-watt bulb is sufficient; if higher wattage is needed, one should reconsider the plan to heat the cage. Extremely high-wattage bulbs or bulbs used for food warming purposes should be used with extreme caution as these get extremely hot. The heat-emitting bulbs should be of sufficient distance from the snake so that burns do not occur; generally, 12–18 in. (30–45 cm) is acceptable. The snake should not have direct access to the bulbs. Burns can

be sustained from any heat source including bulbs if the snake is allowed direct access to them or if they are not placed at a safe distance from the snake being housed. The bulbs also cannot be allowed to get wet or be exposed to excessive humidity. By placing the lamp on one end of the enclosure, the snake is allowed a good basking area. One end of the enclosure should be free of any heat sources to provide a cooler zone to retreat to.

Another recent addition to the hobby is radiant heat panels (Figure 10.14). These come in several different sizes and are a very economical method of heating enclosures. These panels do not get warm to the touch, and most manufacturers claim to have a 50-year operational lifespan. The panels are most effective in a completely enclosed enclosure that has only a few vents for circulation. The panels must be connected to a thermostat or the enclosure will overheat.

When using lights, they should not be kept on all the time. Timers can be purchased that will control when the light switches on and off. This will assist in maintaining natural photoperiods or day/night cycles. Ideally, the snake should have around 12–13 hours a day of "daylight" followed by 11–12 hours of darkness to mimic "nighttime." The timers can be set to mimic the different seasonal day/night cycles by synchronizing them with the different day/night cycles that change slightly from season to season. Before deciding on a day/night cycle, one should always consider the species' natural history to make the best decision for the snake. For example, North American

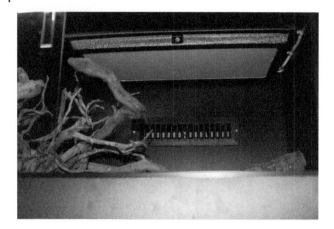

Figure 10.14 An 80-watt radiant heat panel used to heat a 12 ft (0.34 m³) cage to 83°F (28°C).

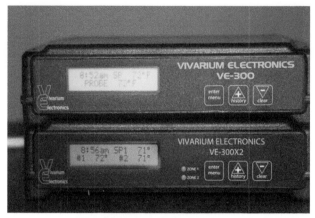

Figure 10.15 Thermostats used to control radiant heat panels in three different cages. The temperatures displayed are the nighttime temperatures.

species experience longer daylight hours in the summer than in winter. Therefore, daylight should be provided for approximately 13 hours in summer whereas in winter 11 hours of daylight is typical. The photoperiod is particularly important if breeding the snake is being considered. Some snakes are only receptive to breeding during certain seasons, so these seasonal changes must be recreated in captivity for successful breeding activity. However, if bulbs are the only source of heat being used, it may be necessary to purchase "night bulbs" to ensure the snake does not get too cool during the night hours. A slight drop in temperature at night is a natural occurrence but too much cooling can lead to illness. Night bulbs emit heat yet allow darkness. Red, blue, black light, ceramic bulbs or commercially available "night" bulbs can be purchased to achieve this. Reading the temperature gauges in the enclosure will assist you in making the appropriate decision on whether night bulbs will be necessary. Keeping the enclosure in a temperature-controlled room and away from drafty areas (i.e., windows) will aid in preventing drastic temperature changes at night when the heat lamps go off.

It is beneficial to wire the heating device (bulbs or pads) to a thermostat (Figure 10.15). This can assist in more accurately maintaining temperatures and decrease the chance of thermal burns. This is not to say that thermostats are always accurate or 100% dependable, but they add an extra level of protection. Frequent temperature checks should be performed when synchronizing thermostats. Several thermostats are available that can control multiple cages and provide an automatic night drop in temperature.

UV lighting or natural sunlight certainly can be beneficial to the snake, but their omission is not detrimental to the snake's overall health, unlike with diurnal lizards. It should be clear that there is no bulb available that can replace natural sunlight. During the warmer months,

if it is decided to keep a snake outside—which is not recommended—special precautions need to be taken. Glass or Plexiglass enclosures should not be used at all outside as they can get extremely hot with the direct sunlight and prove to be fatal to the snake. The inside of the enclosure can become hot, much like in a car with the windows rolled up and no air flow. With other enclosures used outside, there should always be a shaded area provided for the animal. They must be able to retreat to an area that is not receiving direct sunlight when they are finished basking, otherwise they will become overheated.

Water and Humidity

Depending on the geographic range the snake derives from, it may be necessary to supplement humidity as well as heat. Tropical species (e.g., emerald tree boas) need relatively high humidity and require some form of supplementation. In some cases, it may be necessary to make husbandry choices to prevent high humidity, as with desert species requiring arid environments.

Hygrometers (humidity gauges) can be purchased with thermometers and placed inside the enclosure to provide humidity readings. This will indicate when humidity needs to be increased or decreased to maintain ideal conditions.

High humidity can be maintained by misting the entire enclosure and even the snake. The mist should be fine and not extremely cold or hot water. It may be necessary to mist multiple times a day for tropical species. Some people even set up misting systems on timers to provide constant and consistent humidity.

One should remember that humidity is the presence of moisture in the atmosphere itself. If the enclosure does not allow humidity to stay contained, then it needs to be modified or a different enclosure should be used. Using enclosures made exclusively of screen for snakes requiring high humidity is not ideal due to the inability of the enclosure to retain moisture. Aquaria are good for maintaining humidity, but an appropriate lid needs to be made or purchased. However, one should ensure that the aquarium has some ventilation because the air and substrate can become stagnant. Typically, if water is added to supplement humidity (via misting, etc.), it should be evaporated at least within 24 hours. If it does not evaporate, then the enclosure is lacking appropriate ventilation. It may take some trial and error to get the humidity right. If one is obtaining tropical species requiring humid environments, an appropriate regime should be established before placing the snake in the enclosure. However, most species may not require any supplementation if appropriate enclosures and substrates are used.

A water supply is essential for all snakes, and this can assist in maintaining humidity as well. All snakes need an appropriately sized water container in the enclosure. Some enjoy soaking in the water prior to shedding, so the snake's size should be taken into consideration when choosing an appropriate bowl. Small ceramic bowls work well for smaller snakes (they cannot be tipped as easily as lightweight bowls), and plastic tubs work well for larger snakes. One needs to be careful not to overfill as the snake can cause large amounts of water to spill over when submerging. The water should be changed if it becomes soiled or stagnant. Regardless of contamination, it should be changed at least once a week. If the water container is placed over the heating element, (heating pad or tape) it will create some humidity and will evaporate quickly so the water levels should be watched closely. If the species requires low humidity, the water should not be placed near the heating elements.

Substrate can play a vital role in maintaining high humidity. Substrate materials such as topsoil, moss (sphagnum or peat), and mulch are great substrate choices for species requiring high humidity. They absorb and hold moisture well unless too much water is added. Regular mistings in conjunction with an appropriate substrate are keys in maintaining high humidity. Items such as newspaper, shavings, or rock gravel allow "pooling" and are not ideal for humid terrestrial environments.

Other Cage Furnishings

Hide boxes are easily constructed and really make a difference in the snake's overall demeanor. If the snake has a place to go where it feels secure, it will be less stressed in its captive environment. This has also been known to assist in the feeding response in some snakes (e.g., ball python). Hide boxes can be constructed from materials ranging from boxes, plastic pots, and Tupperware (not clear) to logs. They also may be purchased from reptile supply stores/dealers. No matter how elaborate or simple they are, hide boxes serve the same purpose and should be provided.

Tree branches or some sort of perching material should be provided with arboreal species. PVC pipe can be used for this purpose as well. The perch diameter should be no bigger than the largest diameter of the snake's body. One bigger than this will make perching difficult. One needs to make sure all perching materials are secured properly and free of abrasive surfaces.

Decorative rocks are nice additions to an enclosure but can also injure the snake if there are sharp edges. Snakes often use cage furnishings to assist them when shedding by rubbing against them. Anything with rough texture should not be placed in the enclosure.

Quarantine

All reptiles brought into a home or facility should undergo a quarantine period. This is especially necessary in environments where numerous reptiles are housed. Some reptile diseases can wipe out whole collections if proper quarantine procedures are not followed (e.g., inclusion body disease [IBD]).

A room should be set aside for quarantine purposes and should be absent of other animals, especially other reptiles. During the quarantine period, physical exams and fecal exams should be performed to check for internal/external parasites. Ideally, a fecal culture for salmonella should be performed as well. Salmonella is not only transmissible to other reptiles but also is zoonotic. The quarantine period should be no less than 30 days; however, 90 days may be more appropriate for some species, especially members of the Viperidae and Elapidae, due to the high incidence of paramyxovirus. Specimens with a history of contact with any viperid or elapid species should also be considered for 90-day quarantine, as all species of snakes are susceptible to the virus. Some facilities have even extended their quarantine period to 6 months for all reptiles. If the snake becomes ill the quarantine period should be extended, and continued until the snake is deemed healthy according to specific criteria established by the medical team; at which point, the quarantine period will start over for another 30 to 90 days.

Proper cleaning and disinfecting are very important during this time. The enclosures should be set up to meet the snake's individual requirements but also should allow for frequent cleaning. Newspaper is a good substrate to use for quarantined animals due to the ease of cleaning. It is easily changed and is cheap to replace. When the snake defecates or passes urates, the substrate should be changed completely. A dilute bleach solution, or other disinfectant that is appropriate to use with reptiles, should be used to clean surfaces in the enclosure. Ensure the enclosure is dry before replacing the snake. Gloves should be worn when cleaning soiled cages to prevent contamination. Any cage furnishings should be properly disinfected or replaced.

Nutrition

All snakes are carnivores that feed on whole prey items. Their digestive system is adapted to digest whole prey, and they "cast out" or defecate the parts of the prey that are not digested, such as fur. Eating whole carcasses provides them with added nutrients such as calcium from bone so that no further supplementation is needed. Feeding packaged meat and poultry products is not an appropriate, balanced diet for snakes. Feeding in this manner may be convenient for some, but it is not as nutritionally beneficial as whole prey items are. It should be remembered that just because a snake eats something readily does not mean it is nutritionally sound. It is the responsibility of the person who cares for the captive snake to make sure its nutritional needs are properly met. The health of the prey item is just as important as the type of prey item being fed. The prey item should be fed a nutritionally sound diet and be of a good body condition score with no signs of illness.

Although some commonly kept species feed on invertebrates in the wild, especially through their juvenile stages, most will readily feed using commercially bred mice and rats. What to feed the snake depends on multiple factors: (i) availability of prey item; (ii) natural diet; (iii) whether the snake was captive-bred or wild-caught; and (iv) size of the snake.

Prey Items

With the increase in popularity of keeping snakes in captivity, there is a larger and more diverse market for buying varieties of food items. At one point, the most accessible food items were "pet rodents" purchased from pet stores. Not only was this costly, but the pet rodent's nutritional needs were probably not as closely monitored as they are when sold as food items. It is essential that any prey item is fed a nutritionally sound diet. Prey items that have been starved, fed inappropriately, or otherwise neglected are going to be of little nutritional benefit to the snake that eats them. Just going through the motions of feeding the snake does not ensure nutritional requirements are being met.

Today, there are many companies that breed insects, rodents, rabbits, lizards, and many other prey items specifically for food to supply the exotic pet market, zoos, and aquaria. Every growth stage of rats and mice can be

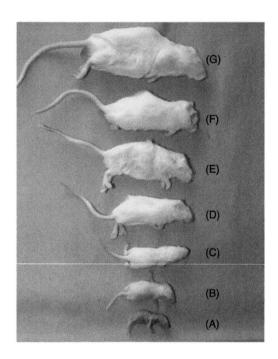

Figure 10.16 Comparison of common sizes of mice in relation to each other. (A) pinky, (B) fuzzy, (C) hopper, (D) weanling, (E) small adult, (F) large adult, (G) jumbo adult (Courtesy of Mice Direct).

purchased from these companies as well as various sizes and growth stages of other vertebrates. Commercially available snake food includes various growth stages of mice, rats, gerbils, rabbits, guinea pigs, and chickens (and other birds such as guinea chicks and quail). For smaller snakes (e.g., garter and ribbon snakes) that feed primarily on invertebrates, there are crickets, various worms, cockroaches, and even small fish available for feeding purposes. In some cases, other reptile and/or amphibian species, such as anoles or frogs, may be used to encourage finicky eaters to feed in captivity. However, most of the commonly kept species will feed on rodents. Table 10.3 describes some of the terms historically and currently used when specifying the stage of feeder rodents and rabbits, their age, and size (Figures 10.16 and 10.17). Due to the growing reptile hobby, many breeding facilities are increasing their stock to include many different names and sizes of mice and rats.

An appropriately sized meal consists of a prey item that is no larger than the widest part of the snake's body. Some people try to gauge prey size by the size of the snake's head. This can be deceiving because the snake's cranial skeletal anatomy allows for the expansion of the mandible, maxilla, and cranium to accommodate large prey items; therefore, it can feed on prey items that are much larger than its head. Gauging by the actual body itself will help to ensure the snake is being fed a large enough prey item and yet one that is not too big, which could cause discomfort for the snake and a large bulging appearance.

Table 10.3 Description, size, and age comparison of common rodent and rabbit prey items.

Common name	Description	Age	Length	Weight
Mice[a]				
XS pinkies	Have not formed a coat, still pink	1	0.5–1	1.5–2
Small pinkies		1–2	0.5–1	2–2.5
Large pinkies		3–4	0.5–1	2.5–3
Peach fuzzies	Fur is just visible	5–9	1–1.25	3–4.5
Fuzzies	Full coat, eyes not open	10–13	1.25–1.5	4.5–7
Hoppers	Eyes open, starting to eat on own	14–18	1.5–2	7–13
Weanlings	No longer nursing, but not adult size	21–25	2–2.5	13–18
Adults	Have reached sexual maturity	30–40	2.5–3	18–25
XL adults	Retired breeders, higher fat content	150–180	3–3.75	25+
Rats[a]				
Pinkies	Have not formed a coat, still pink	1–4	1.5–2	5–13
Fuzzies	Have developed a slight coat	10–13	2–2.5	13–20
Pups	Fuller coat, eyes not open yet	14–18	2.5–3.5	20–30
Weaned	No longer nursing, but not adult size	21–25	3.5–4.5	30–45
Small	Have not reached adult size yet	26–32	4.5–6	45–85
Medium		32–42	6–8	85–175
Large	Have reached sexual maturity	43–60	8–9	175–275
X large	Have reached full adult size	61–99	9–11	275–375
XX large	Retired breeders, higher fat content	100+	11–13	375–475
XXX large		100+	11–13	475+
Rabbits[b]				
X small	Weaned, but not adult size	20–30		0.5–1
Small		30–45		1–2
Medium		45–65		2–4
Large	Have reached adult size	65–100		4–6
X large	Have reached sexual maturity	100–179		6–8
XX large	Retired breeders, higher fat content	180+		8–10
XXX large		180+		11+

Data collected and averaged from Mice Direct and Rodent Pro.
a) Age is in days, length (inches) refers to body only, weight is in grams.
b) Age is in days, weight is in pounds.

Another benefit of using commercial rodent breeders is the ability to purchase rodents that are pre-killed and/or frozen. Some people find it disheartening and difficult to feed live rodents to snakes. In the wild, the snake will feed on live prey, but with the availability of pre-killed prey on the market, there is no need for this in captivity. Captive-bred specimens will readily feed on pre-killed or previously frozen prey items. Offering live prey to snakes causes unnecessary suffering to the rodent, and the snake might sustain rodent bites as a result. Significant rodent bites can cause many dermatologic problems; some even warrant systemic antibiotics and/or topical treatments of a dilute betadine or chlorhexidine solution. Scars from bite wounds are usually apparent in snakes that are offered live prey items.

Offering previously frozen prey rather than live prey has many other benefits. It is usually cheaper to buy them in this fashion and they may be purchased in bulk if freezer space is available. Another benefit is that a frozen rodent will certainly be less likely to introduce parasites to the snake and/or enclosure. Rodents are one of the main sources of parasitic contamination in captive snakes. If a frozen prey item had parasites (endoparasites or ectoparasites), the parasites will most likely be dead due to the freezing process. This is not to say, however, that it is acceptable to knowingly offer parasitized animals as food

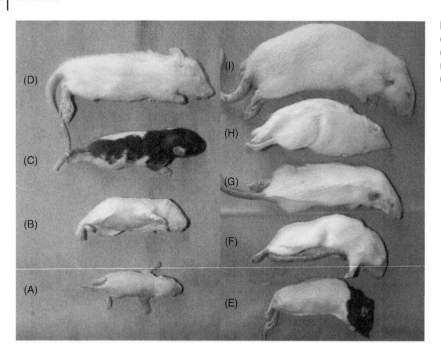

Figure 10.17 Comparison of common sizes of rats in relation to each other. (A) pinky, (B) fuzzy, (C) pup, (D) weanling, (E) small, (F) medium, (G) large, (H) jumbo, (I) colossal. (Courtesy of Mice Direct).

just because they were frozen. Buying snake food from a reputable company will assist in making sure the snake's nutritional needs are being met.

One should not attempt to feed a frozen rodent to the snake. It must first be thawed out. Putting it in a watertight plastic bag and submerging it in hot (not boiling) water is an easy way to do it. Some people even place the rodent on a warm surface (under a heat lamp, on a heat pad, etc.) to ensure the rodent is properly thawed. Microwaves are not an option for thawing rodents.

Feedings only need to occur about once a week to every 14 days for adult snakes due to their slow digestive process. For juveniles, it may be necessary to feed twice a week to ensure that proper nutritional requirements are being met during the growth phase. If a snake refuses one meal, do not panic. This happens occasionally, and the snake will not starve in one week's time. However, if several consecutive meals are skipped, then the snake's inappetence needs to be addressed. Snakes will often refuse food during the fall and winter months, despite strict environmental controls within the enclosure. It is also common for snakes to refuse food during reproductive cycles, when gravid, or when incubating eggs.

To avoid bites, some reptile hobbyists believe that snakes should not be fed inside their primary enclosure, especially when the only time the enclosure is opened is when the snake is being fed. This creates a feeding response and makes bites more likely to occur. Feeding outside the primary enclosure would be a safer practice and also could help to ensure that any loose substrate located inside the primary enclosure is not ingested during feeding.

Why Will My Snake Not Eat?

Anorexia in snakes is a common presenting complaint. In the absence of disease, there are many reasons why a snake will not eat. Following are some feeding guidelines and tips in case of snakes that are not eating.

Some snakes, such as boids and pit vipers, have heat-seeking pits that they rely on for locating their warm-blooded prey. These bilateral openings are located on the skin of the upper lip usually under the nares. If they confront a cold prey item (previously frozen), they are unlikely to show any interest. One should make sure that the prey item is warm before offering it to the snake, using the warming techniques described previously.

Besides warmth, motion also can trigger a snake to feed. Tongs should always be used when placing a pre-killed prey item into the enclosure. This is especially true when one entices the snake by moving the prey item around. Many snakebites occur during feedings and can be easily avoided if using tongs (not hands) when feeding and keeping a safe distance from the snake.

Wild-caught specimens are frequently reluctant to eat in captive environments, and there are several things to check for if one is not eating. It should be remembered that they have been taken from their natural habitat and placed in a cage. Not only that but in most cases, they are being offered prey they would never have encountered in their natural habitat. For example, a green tree python will feed primarily on birds, frogs, and occasional small mammals in its natural habitat. Once in captivity, it is offered white mice. This is an unnatural prey item as small mammals are not a large part of its natural diet. This is not to say that it will never accept commercially bred rodents in captivity, but adjusting to a new captive environment is tough. One should at least try to offer a natural diet initially. One can try feeding colored rodents rather than the typical white feeder rodents if the snake is reluctant to eat white rodents. Although more expensive than mice and rats, gerbils are another option to be used for prey. Gerbils look more like a natural source of prey than white rodents, and this sometimes helps with wild-caught snakes that are reluctant to eat. Wild-caught specimens will most likely be reluctant to take pre-killed prey initially because they are accustomed to live prey items. Attempting to feed pre-killed or frozen prey items to newly acquired wild-caught snakes will most likely be unsuccessful and will take time. Besides the moral issues with keeping wild-caught snakes, this is another reason why they should not be purchased.

Some people attempt to speed up the process of getting a wild-caught snake to accept commercially bred rodents by scenting them. This is achieved by taking the rodent and rubbing a natural prey item on it to leave a scent. This works mostly for hobbyists who keep multiple species of reptiles and amphibians. For example, if trying to feed a mouse to a snake that will mostly feed on lizards and frogs naturally, a person can rub the feeder rodent on a lizard or frog that is kept in their collection. This will leave the scent of that animal on the rodent, and possibly "trick" the snake into eating it. Others lacking a wide collection may keep a dead lizard or frog in the freezer. During each feeding, the scent item is thawed out, rubbed on the prey item, and then put back into the freezer.

Another common reason a snake may refuse food is inadequate provision of its environmental needs. If a snake is too cold or too hot, it will most likely refuse food. A snake needs to be within its preferred optimal temperature zone (POTZ) in order to properly digest food. Regurgitation occurs frequently in snakes kept too cold. If a snake is cold then it will spend most of its time in a heat-preserving posture and will not be interested in feeding. One should make sure all heat requirements are being met when dealing with a reluctant eater. Although humidity has less of an effect on feeding, extremes in either direction of the humidity spectrum can cause the snake to refuse food.

As a rule, when a snake refuses prey, one needs to make sure all husbandry requirements are being met properly. Even something as simple as the absence of a hide box (a secure place) will cause a snake to refuse prey.

If a snake is about to shed, it will most likely refuse food. Food items should not even be offered until the snake has fully shed to avoid excess stress.

Snakes that are ailing from respiratory disorders or other illnesses will most likely stop feeding as well. The onset of illness will affect their appetites just like any other animal.

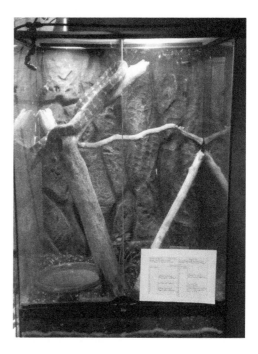

Figure 10.18 Cage of *Morelia spilota variegata* (Irian Jaya carpet python) with a cage card.

It is extremely important for the snake's owner to read as much literature as possible about their particular species of snake. Once again, knowing the natural geographic range of the snake will help in making husbandry decisions, which often lie at the root of many problems.

The use of a cage card is a very important and often overlooked aspect of keeping any reptile. Snakes are creatures of habit. They often will have a pattern of shedding, eating, and defecating. Knowing this pattern of their habits will aid the keeper in recognizing disease and reproductive cycles and will help them gauge when feedings should occur. Figures 10.18 and 10.19 show an example of a cage card and its placement on the cage. There are also computer applications designed to manage large collections of reptiles that will keep track of ecdysis cycles, feeding, weights, reproductive information, medical care, and many other aspects of husbandry practices (e.g., HerperPRO, Metzcal herp software, iHerp, ReptiStat).

Diseases and Clinical Conditions

Diseases Affecting the Reproductive Tract

Cloacal prolapse is a common problem seen in snakes. The prolapse can be the colon, hemipenes, uterus, or oviduct. It is usually caused by excessive straining or copulation. It is important to determine which organ has prolapsed before initiating treatment. The hemipenes are solid and

Month/Year: May 2013		ID: 1.0–325	Weight: 735 g
Species: *Morelia spilota variegata*		Common Name: Irian Jaya carpet python	
Food offered: XL mice and 2 week quail		Schedule: 1st & 2nd Sunday mouse/3rd Sunday quail	
Antivenom: Nonvenomous			
Day of Month		Day of Month	
1		17	
2		18	
3		19	Offered/ate quail
4		20	Changed water, under heat
5	Offered/ate mouse	21	
6	Changed water, under heat	22	
7		23	
8		24	In water all day
9	Heat light out-replaced	25	In water all day
10		26	Changed water, adj. humidity
11		27	Stool in water, changed water
12	Offered/ate mouse	28	Normal activity
13	Changes water, under heat	29	
14		30	
15		31	
16			

Figure 10.19 Example of a completed cage card for the specimen in Figure 10.18.

do not have a lumen, whereas the colon is smooth and has a lumen. Feces will normally be seen if the colon has prolapsed. The oviduct or shell gland will have longitudinal striations with a lumen, and prolapse of these will not have feces present.

Hemipenile prolapse, or paraphimosis, can be caused by several things. Infections with bacteria, fungi, or parasites, swelling secondary to forced probing, forced separation during copulation, constipation, or neurologic dysfunction in the hemipenes' retractor apparatus, cloacal vent, or anal sphincter muscles can all cause hemipenile prolapse. Treatment should start as soon as the diagnosis is made. The prolapsed hemipenis should be cleaned, lubed, and replaced. If replacement is unsuccessful or the hemipenis is necrotic, the hemipenis should be amputated. Since snakes have two hemipenes, their reproductive ability will not be affected.

A prolapsed colon is caused by excessive straining, usually from constipation. The tissue must be moistened and replaced. Most colon prolapses can be replaced through the cloaca, but occasionally surgery is required. When the tissue is replaced, it must also be inverted. If replaced properly a purse-string suture is not required. Since this condition is not the primary problem, both conditions must be treated.

Oviductal or shell gland prolapses are most commonly seen during normal oviposition or parturition. They are treated much the same as a colon prolapse. The prolapsed tissue must be kept moist and replaced through the cloaca. If a large segment of the oviduct is prolapsed or if the tissue is necrotic, resection is recommended.

Dystocia is another common reproductive disorder. There are two types of dystocia in reptiles, obstructive and non-obstructive (Lock 2000, p. 734). An obstructive dystocia is caused by an anatomic inability to deliver the eggs or live young or by a complication during oviposition. The anatomic defect may be fetal or maternal. Some common maternal anatomic defects that are seen in snakes include misshapen pelvis, oviductal stricture, non-oviductal masses, oviduct scarring from previous infection, or retained eggs or fetuses from previous pregnancy. Fetal defects include eggs that are too large or eggs that have adhered. Diagnosis is made through a physical exam, history, and radiographs or ultrasound. Treatment includes the surgical removal of the eggs or fetuses.

Non-obstructive dystocias are mostly caused by poor husbandry, infection, or poor physical condition (Lock 2000, p. 735). Improper temperature, humidity, diet, and nesting site can all cause a dystocia. Oviposition requires great strength, and most captive-raised snakes do not have the muscle mass that wild snakes have, which makes it very difficult for them to deliver eggs or live young. Treatments include massaging the eggs down, percutaneous ovocentesis, posterior pituitary hormones, and, as a last resort, surgery. When massaging, care must be taken not to trap a portion of the oviduct posterior to the egg or live young. If this happens, one should massage the egg or embryo back to its original position and start over (Ross et al. 1990, p. 79). Percutaneous ovocentesis can be performed in oviparous snakes. A needle is inserted into the egg through the ventrum and the contents are aspirated. It is important that the coelomic cavity is not contaminated with egg contents. The egg should pass naturally within 48 hours. Posterior pituitary hormones such as oxytocin can be used to assist with the oviposition. If all attempts have been made and the eggs or embryos are still retained, then surgery must be performed. Successful incubation of eggs after a dystocia is rare. Live fetuses have been raised after a salpingotomy, but it is uncommon. The prognosis for the female is good following a dystocia, and the future reproductive status is also good as long as there were no complications and at least one of the reproductive tracts was left intact. However, the female is more likely to retain eggs and live young in future breedings.

Disorders of the Integument

The most common disorder affecting the integument is dysecdysis, or difficulty in shedding. Causes of dysecdysis are numerous but are mostly associated with poor husbandry, including improper temperature or humidity, no shedding implements such as a rock or log, and malnutrition. Other causes of dysecdysis include systemic disorders, metabolic disorders, stress from excessive handling, loud noises, vibrations, overcrowding, or anything that limits the snake's movements. Treatment includes soaking the snake in tepid water for 1 to 8 hours a day and treating the underlying problem.

Increased ecdysis frequency can occur in snakes. Hyperthyroidism and dermatitis are the main causes of this condition. After a severe trauma, the natural function of healing is frequent ecdysis.

There are many clinical signs of dermatosis. Dysecdysis, abscesses, abrasions, blisters, bullae, discoloration, and nodules are all signs of a diseased integument. Abscesses are the most common dermatologic condition seen in captive reptiles. They are commonly caused by bites from prey or cage mates. Most abscesses are filled with a solid exudate. Treatment includes surgically removing the abscess and irrigating the area, and administering antibiotics pending a culture and sensitivity.

Bacterial dermatoses are also very common. The most common bacterial infection is caused by *Pseudomonas* spp. Other common bacterial pathogens include *Salmonella* spp., *Staphylococcus*, and *Streptococcus*, among others.

Fungal dermatoses are commonly seen in snakes that live in humid environments. Clinical signs of both fungal and bacterial infections include a brown to greenish–yellow discoloration, blisters, ulcers, nodules, crusts, and granulomas.

Vesicular dermatitis, popularly known as blister disease, is common in snakes kept in dirty, very humid enclosures. Fluid-filled blisters can appear all over the body. They are initially sterile, but as the condition continues, the fluid becomes cloudy and eventually results in bacteremia. Once bacteremia sets in, the prognosis is very poor.

Another bacterial infection caused by poor cage hygiene is ventral dermal necrosis (Lawton 1991, p. 254). Snakes kept in dirty enclosures can develop infections underneath their ventral scales. The signs include petechiation, ecchymosis, and eventual necrosis of the ventral scales. Fluid therapy is often needed due to the fluid loss from the damaged skin.

Contact dermatitis occurs when the snake is exposed to harsh chemicals such as pesticides, cleaning agents, and harsh aromatic compounds.

The diagnosis for all dermatoses includes a physical examination and history, culture (aerobic, anaerobic, and fungal), and cytology. Treatment usually involves topical or systemic antimicrobials and changes to the animal's husbandry and nutrition. During the treatment of any of these dermatoses, the snake should be housed on clean paper. The paper should be changed daily and also the cage should be disinfected daily until the condition has resolved.

Disorders of the Cardiovascular System

Cardiovascular disorders are uncommon in snakes. The clinical signs are non-specific, ranging from weight loss to a change in skin color. Nutritional disorders such as hypocalcemia, hypovitaminosis E, and hypercalcemia with hypervitaminosis D_3 have been associated with cardiovascular disease. Infectious diseases affecting the cardiovascular system are usually secondary to a systemic illness. There is potential for endocarditis with any Gram-negative bacterial pathogen. If bacterial sepsis is suspected, a blood culture should be taken. There have been reported cases of congestive heart failure associated with infectious disease and with cardiomyopathy.

Disorders of the Nervous System

Proliferative spinal osteopathy has been observed in all species of snakes commonly kept in captivity. This condition has not been observed in wild populations. The exact etiology is unclear, but there are several possible causes of this disorder. Trauma, unknown viral etiology, dietary deficiency, small enclosures, neoplasia, soft tissue bacterial infection, and septicemia have all been suspected or associated with proliferative spinal osteopathy (Fitzgerald & Knafo, 2019, p. 1343) It is suspected that a virus found in mice or a virus of snakes that is spread by mice may be a causative agent. Septicemia is suspected because bacteria are often cultured from the spinal lesions. An immune-mediated disease secondary to septicemia is also suspected. Finally, chronic trauma from excessive handling is thought to be a cause of this disease. Clinical signs include focal or multifocal swelling along the dorsum, pressure inducing a pain response, hyperreflexia cranial to the lesion, motor deficits, trembling, and spinal deformities. The diagnosis is made via clinical signs and radiographs. In the early stages of this disease, the snake is still able to function on its own. As the disease progresses, the snake will no longer be able to move, constrict, or swallow prey. Treatment includes blood and local aspirate cultures, antibiotics, anti-inflammatories, and surgical debridement. Intravenous administration of medications may need to be initiated since the areas affected may not be reached by other routes of administration. In some circumstances, medications may need to be implanted surgically. Treatment is often unsuccessful and requires months of care (Figure 10.20).

Organophosphate and carbamate toxicity have been reported in snakes. Treatment is similar to that of mammals. The snake should be given atropine and fluid therapy to maintain hydration and renal function. Its temperature should be decreased to slow conduction velocity of nerves to control seizures.

Disorders of the Respiratory Tract

The most common illnesses in snakes are respiratory infections, caused by bacterial, viral, fungal, or parasitic pathogens (Driggers 2000, p. 524). Bacterial pneumonia caused by Gram-negative pathogens is the most common respiratory illness. Viral infections are likely underdiagnosed due to the lack of diagnostic assays. Fungal infections are rare but have been reported. Common clinical signs of pneumonia include cyanosis, bubbles coming from the nares or glottis, wheezing or crackles

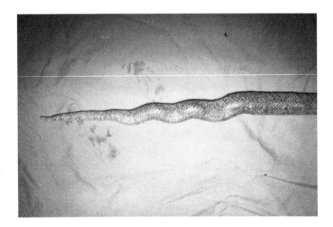

Figure 10.20 Suspected proliferative spinal osteopathy in the caudal region of this snake. Owners declined workup and the diagnosis could not be confirmed.

heard during auscultation, and petechiae of the oral cavity. Stomatitis is commonly seen in snakes with pneumonia (Driggers 2000, p. 524). The diagnostic plan should include culture and sensitivity, cytology, and radiographs. A transtracheal wash should be performed to obtain samples for culture and cytology. Antibiotics should be started and changed pending the results of the culture and sensitivity tests. Fluid therapy should be initiated with dehydrated snakes. The underlying cause of pneumonia in snakes is commonly husbandry-related. It is crucial to keep the snake within its POTZ and maintain proper humidity levels. Also, the cage needs to be kept clean at all times.

Other causes of respiratory disease include masses, trauma, aspiration of substrate, and dehydration. Dysecdysis can also compromise the respiratory tract causing disease (Driggers 2000, p. 528).

Disorders of the Urinary System

Unfortunately, early detection of renal dysfunction has not been reported in reptiles, although renal diseases are among the most common problems in older snakes.

Gout does occur, although not as common in snakes as in other groups of reptiles. Gout is the result of excessive protein metabolism or catabolism leading to uric acid production exceeding uric acid excretion. All diseases that lead to renal failure can cause gout (Miller 1998, p. 96). Gout is found in two forms. In the first form, urates are deposited on mesothelial surfaces. Urate deposits commonly occur on the pericardial sac, the peritoneum, the capsule of the liver, and within the parenchyma of the kidneys. In the other form of gout, urate deposits occur in joints, tendon sheaths, ligaments, and periosteum. Both forms of gout can occur simultaneously. Treatment for gout involves diuresis and changing to a low-purine diet. The prognosis is poor.

Bacterial nephritis is a common disease associated with the urinary system. It is often secondary to other bacterial infections or an immunosuppressive event (Miller 1998, p. 98). The primary cause should be detected and treated accordingly.

Disorders of the Eye

Retained spectacles are a common reason why snakes are brought into the veterinary clinic. Spectacles are retained when dysecdysis occurs. To remove the retained spectacle, place the snake in a very damp environment for 24 hours. Then wipe the eye with a gauze sponge or damp tissue. The retained spectacle will usually detach easily. If not, the snake should be kept in a warm, damp environment until the next ecdysis cycle and complete ecdysis occurs.

Surgical intervention should be a last resort. This is a delicate procedure and should be done carefully so the eye is not damaged. Sterile lubricant is applied to the eye and the spectacle is gently removed with forceps. If the old spectacle is still attached firmly, force should not be used to remove it. It may take several days of soaking and/or applying lubricant to fully remove the retained spectacle or any retained piece of shed.

Intraspectacular dermatitis will occur as a localized dermatitis or as part of a more generalized dermatitis. The majority of these cases are caused by retained spectacles. Often, enucleation is the treatment.

Pseudobuphthalmos is caused by obstruction of the nasolacrimal duct (Lawton 2019, p. 733). The obstruction is usually secondary to infectious stomatitis, a congenital obstruction, or parasites, or is idiopathic. Lacrimal fluid cannot drain from the eye due to the fluid being unable to overflow beyond the eyelid margin, which causes the distended subspectacular space. Long-term treatment involves surgically removing a 30° wedge of the ventral spectacle allowing for drainage, or conjunctivoralostomy.

Subspectacular abscesses are usually the result of an ascending infection in the oral cavity, a penetrating wound, or a systemic infection (Lawton 2019, p. 731). Treatment for these abscesses involves a wedge resection of the spectacle and flushing. The debris should be cultured and the snake should be started on appropriate antibiotics.

Disorders of the Digestive System

Infectious Stomatitis

Infectious stomatitis is a disease caused by poor husbandry and nutrition, stress, poor feeding techniques, or trauma. It is crucial that the snake be kept in its POTZ and proper humidity be maintained. When husbandry is deficient, the snake's immune system is weakened allowing opportunistic bacteria to reproduce. Stress from being in overcrowded cages, excessive handling, or loud noises can also weaken the immune system. Snakes that are fed live prey will commonly have small abrasions in their oral cavity that can lead to an infectious stomatitis. Finally, snakes that rub on the sides of the cage will have rostral abrasions that can lead to an infectious stomatitis (Figure 10.21).

Vomiting and Regurgitation

Vomiting can occur for many reasons. Stress can make a snake vomit. If disturbed after a meal, a snake may get nervous and vomit its meal. Also, feeding a prey item that is too large or is partially autolyzed, and keeping a snake below its POTZ are other common causes of vomiting. Parasitic infections, IBD, and bacterial infections can also cause vomiting in snakes. Regurgitation is usually

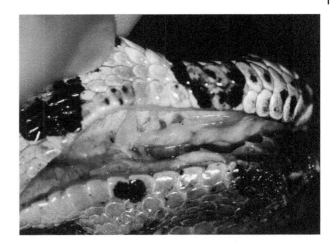

Figure 10.21 Infectious stomatitis.

associated with lesions in the esophagus, oral cavity, or pharynx.

Diagnosing Lumps and Bumps

Lumps and bumps are a common finding in snakes. These occur on the outside as well as on the inside. When a lump or bump is found on the surface of the snake a fine needle aspirate should be performed. Cytology, culture, and sensitivity should be performed on the sample. If the lump or bump is palpated in the coelomic cavity, a radiograph or ultrasound should be performed to determine the origin. A sample should be obtained and cytology performed. Causes of lumps and bumps in snakes range from parasites to abscesses to neoplasia. Once the diagnosis is made, treatment should begin accordingly.

Viral Diseases

The fer de lance paramyxovirus is the sole member of the genus *Ferlavirus*. Paramoxyvirus is mainly found in viperids but has been isolated in the families Boidae, Elapidae, Colubridae, and Crotalidae (Marschang 2019, p. 263). It is transmitted via secretions of the respiratory tract. Incubation is generally around 21 days but can exceed 90 days. Clinical signs are characterized by severe respiratory disease. Neurologic signs such as head tremors, excitement, star gazing, flaccid paralysis, or convulsions can also be seen. This disease may have a peracute presentation where the patient is found dead with no apparent clinical signs; an acute presentation where the patient rapidly progresses from first clinical sign to death in 1 to 3 days; or a more chronic form where clinical signs progress slowly for up to a year or more. A presumptive diagnosis of paramyxovirus should be considered when a pneumonia is unresponsive to antibiotics. Antemortem diagnosis can be made through virus isolation, RT-PCR testing, and hemagglutination inhibition assays. Tracheal washes are the preferred sample for testing, however oral and cloacal swabs may also provide a diagnostic sample. Titers reflect exposure, and a rising titer in paired samples is necessary for a diagnosis of active disease. A diagnosis can also be made by histologic examination of postmortem lung, liver, kidney, splenopancreas, and brain samples. There is no treatment for paramyxovirus, but supportive care and antibiotics to treat secondary bacterial infections should be in the treatment plan. The prognosis is grave. If an outbreak of paramyxovirus occurs in a collection, all sick snakes should immediately be quarantined and strict hygiene procedures must be followed. *Ferlavirus* infections have been observed in lizards and do not appear to be host-specific. Due to this, cross-contamination is possible and should be considered when housing a mixed species collection.

IBD is another serious viral infection that is only found in boids; however, a similar disease has been identified in colubrids and vipers. The etiologic agent of IBD is believed to be an arenavirus. The route of transmission is unknown, although it is suspected that arthropods, such as snake mites (*Ophionyssus natricis*), play a role. In boas, the most common first clinical sign is regurgitation, whereas in pythons the first clinical signs may be stomatitis and pneumonia. The disease progresses to severe neurologic signs such as head tremors, disorientation, flaccid muscle paralysis, and loss of the righting reflex. Secondary bacterial infections are common. Eventually, the snake will become anorectic and die. The disease progresses much more rapidly in pythons than boas. Documented cases of long-term survival in boas has been reported. Boas diagnosed with IBD should receive supportive care, however the prognosis is still poor (Origgi 2019, p. 1319). Table 10.4 Lists the various diagnostic testing to confirm IBD (Origgi 2019, p. 1319). Any molecular testing should be confirmed with histopathology or viral isolation. There are no treatments for IBD except supportive care and treating secondary bacterial infections. The snake will eventually die from this virus. Prevention of this disease involves strict quarantine procedures when introducing new snakes into an established collection. If confirmed carriers are identified in the collection, euthanasia is recommended to prevent more specimens from becoming infected with the virus.

Zoonotic Diseases

Snakes suffer from very few zoonotic diseases (Glynn et al. 2001, p. 9) (Table 10.5). There are two ways in which zoonotic diseases are transmitted. One is by direct contact

Table 10.4 Diagnostic tests for detecting IBD.

Test	Sample required[a]
RT-PCR (reverse transcription polymerase chain reaction)	Oral or cloacal swabs, whole blood, liver, or esophageal tonsilar biopsies
IHC (immunohisto-chemistry)	Liver, esophageal tonsils, pancreas, kidney, or brain biopsy
Cytological examination	Whole blood
Electron microscopy	Any affected tissues
Histopathology	Liver and esophageal tonsillar biopsies
Virus isolation	Any affected tissues

a) Consult your lab to determine what sample is needed and how to prepare the sample for testing and shipment.

Table 10.5 Common zoonotic diseases in reptiles.

Pathogen	Threat to humans	Mode of transmission
Salmonella spp.	Gastrointestinal	Fecal oral contact
Campylobacter spp.	Diarrhea and acute gastroenteritis	Fecal oral contact
Klebsiella spp.	Diarrhea and genitourinary infections	Direct contact
Enterobacter spp.	Diarrhea and genitourinary infections	Direct contact
Yersinia enterocolitica	Gastroenteritis and severe abdominal pain	Environmental contact
Pseudomonas spp.	Cutaneous, respiratory, and digestive	Ingestion, inhalation, or scratches or bites
Mycobacterium spp.	Cutaneous and subcutaneous nodule	Fecal oral contact, inhalation or oral or respiratory mucosa, or bites or scratches
Coxiella burnetii	Q-fever	Inhalation or direct contact

with the infected animal. The other is by indirect contact, which can be from contaminated feces, urine, secretions, blood, soil, fomites, and aerosols. Zoonotic diseases, for the most part, are easily avoided by following a few simple rules.

- One should not use the bathtub, sink, or shower as a place to soak a snake.
- One should not kiss a snake and hands should be washed after handling. A physician should be consulted if one is bitten by a snake and the area should be washed thoroughly.
- When cleaning a cage, one should wear the appropriate personal protective equipment such as gloves, respiratory protection, and possibly full facial protection.
- Finally, one should never clean any of the cage furnishings where human food is kept or prepared.

The most talked about zoonotic disease associated with reptiles is salmonellosis. It is believed that most reptiles carry *Salmonella* organisms in their intestinal tract and sporadically shed the organisms in their feces. An estimated 93,000 cases of reptile-associated human salmonellosis are diagnosed each year (Glynn et al. 2001, p. 9). All clients who either own a reptile or are considering owning a reptile for a pet should be educated about *Salmonella*. By simply following the guidelines outlined previously, salmonellosis is easily preventable.

Taking a History

Being able to take a complete history of the patient is the first crucial step in diagnosing and treating a sick snake. Such things as signalment, presenting complaint, husbandry and nutrition information, and any previous medical history are keys to proper diagnosis and treatment.

Signalment

Signalment includes the common and scientific names (e.g., ball python, *Python regius*), age, amount of time in owner's possession, whether it was captive-bred or wild-caught, and whether it is kept as a pet or as a breeder.

It is important that the common and scientific names of the snake are acquired when the appointment is made. With approximately 3,400 extant species of snake, it would be impossible for a single person to know the natural history, husbandry, and nutritional needs of every species. Therefore, it is important that the medical staff be prepared ahead of time to ensure that the owner meets the patient's proper husbandry and nutritional needs. Many species of snake have two or more common names, which can make identification very difficult. For example, most Americans refer to *Python regius* as a ball python, whereas most Europeans refer to *Python regius* as the royal python. By knowing the scientific name of the snake, proper identification can be made, and the appropriate information can be relayed to the owner.

Another key component to signalment is the age of the snake. If the actual age of the snake is unknown, then the amount of time that the owners have had possession of it is important information. The average lifespan of most captive snakes is relatively short. However, snakes are capable of living to a very geriatric age, with some species known to live more than 30 years. The reason for such short lifespans is mostly associated with poor husbandry.

It is important to know whether a captive snake has been wild-caught or captive-bred. Wild-caught snakes are those that have been taken from their natural habitats and sold through the pet trade. Unfortunately, this is a common occurrence in the reptile industry; however, the rate of importation has decreased with the popularity of captive breeding. Over the last seven years, the number of reptiles imported into the United States has decreased from 1.5 million to less than 600,000 annually. The majority of reptiles being imported are lizards and turtles. Wild-caught specimens typically have parasites (ticks, mites, and various internal parasites) and can take a long time to adjust to a captive environment, if they ever do. They also can have a host of other illnesses, such as respiratory infections, which become apparent while in captivity due to stress. Feeding wild-caught snakes can prove to be challenging due to their reluctance to eat in captivity. This reluctance is usually due to the difficulties that a wild-caught snake may have adjusting to a captive environment (especially if husbandry guidelines are not being followed) and the snake not being offered the natural diet it is accustomed to. For example, a snake such as *Candoia aspera* (viper boa), which feeds primarily on frogs in its natural environment, may not be receptive to the white lab mice that are sold commercially as snake feeders. This is not to say that it will never feed on mice in the future, but it will take some time to adjust and may require some "trickery."

Occasionally specimens called "captive hatched" will be available on the market. These snakes were "wild-caught" while still in the egg. The eggs were then taken into captivity and put into an incubator to hatch. Another term that may be used is "captive born" for viviparous snakes. Some snakes that are imported will be gravid and parturition then occurs in captivity. These snakes should be treated just as wild-caught ones since there is still much information that science does not know about the vertical transmission of many pathogens found in snakes. These snakes also retain their wild dietary instincts; however, they are generally easier to transition to a more convenient captive diet.

Captive-bred, or captive-born and bred, snakes are snakes that have been bred and raised in a captive environment. These are obviously better specimens due to their lack of exposure to the diseases and parasites found in wild-caught specimens. Captive-bred snakes also accept "commercially available" diets better (such as feeder rodents) when offered and are not as finicky about accepting pre-killed prey items, which is the recommended method of feeding. Although the temperament of a snake can never be guaranteed, captive-bred snakes tend to be more docile overall and can become more accustomed to handling.

For these reasons, it is important to know where the snake was bred and born. One should always recommend the purchase of captive-bred specimens to potential buyers to better ensure the snake's overall health. There are many reputable snake breeders to buy from who can provide a more reliable history for the snake. Often these specimens are less expensive than buying from pet retail stores. It is also important to know if the captive-bred snake has had any exposure to wild-caught specimens. Closed collections that observe strict quarantine guidelines are always recommended.

It also needs to be noted if the snake is kept as a pet or as a breeder. Snakes kept solely as pets usually do not need to be hibernated, so neither photoperiod nor nutritional requirements need to change throughout the year. Snakes kept for breeding do need nutritional and husbandry changes throughout the year. Temperate species should be hibernated, which takes several weeks of preparation. If hibernation is not done properly, the snake can become very sick and possibly die while hibernating. With regard to nutrition, many female snakes will not eat while gravid. The females will normally start eating again when the clutch is laid, the clutch hatches, or the live babies are born. Special nutritional needs must be met before the breeding season starts and when the snake starts eating again. Also, to ensure a successful breeding season, the photoperiod must be changed to simulate the natural photoperiod.

All snakes that are large enough should be sexed. It is a very simple procedure that should be included in the initial exam. For methods of sex determination, refer to Chapter 11 or the section of this chapter on "Sex Determination."

Presenting Complaint

The presenting complaint is the reason the owner brought the snake to be examined. Some common presenting complaints include wheezing, dysecdysis, anorexia, and lethargy. One should approach the presenting complaint as if one were examining a dog or cat. The owner should be asked when the problem started, were there any husbandry/nutritional changes, have the owners noticed any other problems, and so on. The medical staff is like a team of detectives who must gather as much evidence as possible to come up with a diagnosis and treatment plan. It is important to get as much information from the owners as possible.

Husbandry and Nutritional Information

The single leading cause of death in captive snakes is poor husbandry and/or nutrition. It is up to the veterinary technician to find out every detail of the husbandry practices and advise the owner if corrections need to be made. This part of the history will take 15 to 20 minutes. It is crucial to take time and record every detail. Following is a list of questions that the technicians should get answers to on the initial exam:

Caging:

- What are the dimensions of the cage?
- Where is the cage located?
- What is the cage made of?
- Is the cage designed for an arboreal or terrestrial species?
- What substrate is used?
- What cage furnishings are available (rocks, branches, hide box, etc.)?

Lighting:

- What is the day/night cycle?
- What light sources are available?

Heating:

- What is the day and night temperature range?
- What are the primary and secondary heat sources available?

Humidity:

- What is the humidity in the enclosure?
- What humidity devices and methods are used?

Nutrition/feeding/water:

- How is water offered (drip system, misting, bowl, etc.)?
- What food items are being offered and at what time of day are they offered?
- Is the snake fed live, frozen–thawed, or fresh-killed prey items?
- How is the prey offered (feeding tongs, set in the bottom of the cage, in a separate cage, etc.)?
- What is the feeding schedule?
- How are the prey items stored?
- Where were the prey items acquired?

Husbandry practices:

- How often is the cage cleaned and disinfected?
- What type of disinfectant is used?
- What is the ecdysis/defecation schedule?
- Are there other reptiles or other animals in the same air system?
- Are any of these animals sick or have any died within the past 3 months?
- Is proper quarantine performed on new and sick specimens? During subsequent exams on the same patient, the technician should ask about any changes to the husbandry or feeding since the last visit. It may be beneficial to ask specific questions about the husbandry and feeding instead of simply asking if anything has changed.

Previous Medical History

Any previous medical condition or diagnostic tests should be noted in the record. It is common for the client to perform their own fecal analysis for parasites and deworm according to their findings. The technician should inquire about their parasitology program and give advice as needed.

Preparing for the Physical Examination

The exam room must be prepared ahead of time to ensure a quick and complete physical exam. The exam room needs to be "snakeproof." The doors must be sealed so the snake cannot escape under the door, large drains in the sink should be covered, air vents should be covered with mesh to prevent the snake crawling in, and any other holes or cracks that the snake can access should be covered or sealed to prevent the snake from escaping or getting stuck. Appropriately sized sex probes with lubrication for sexing and an oral speculum (such as a spatula or credit card) for oral examination should be in the exam room. Restraining devices such as snake hooks, clear plastic restraining tubes, and capture tongs should be readily accessible for aggressive or venomous species. Large snakes could need two or more people for proper restraint. It may be necessary to have other technicians or assistants close by in the event that more help is needed. Other essential instruments that are needed for a physical exam are a good light source, ophthalmoscope, stethoscope, fecal collection system, and a magnifying glass to check for external parasites.

Transportation

When it becomes necessary to transport a snake, there are several ways to do it. The most common items used in transporting snakes are snake bags. These can be burlap sacks, pillowcases, laundry bags, or other linens, as long as they are made of a breathable fabric and can be secured. When using bags, the snake should be placed in the sack and a knot tied at the open end. One should remember that when transporting the snake in the bag, the bag should be grabbed above the knot, as a bite can still occur through a bag. Plastic tubs or clean paint buckets with lids can be used as well. This works well for larger species if a large enough bag cannot be obtained. One should ensure that the lid snaps down or can be secured properly in case the snake pushes on it. Breathing holes need to be cut in the plastic if tubs or buckets are used. One should make sure not to create abrasive or sharp edges that the snake could come into contact with when adding breathing holes in plastic containers.

Venomous snakes can easily be put into a bag using a snake hook and tongs. When tying the knot on the open end, use the snake hook to isolate the snake at the closed end of the bag to ensure they cannot access the handler's hand and bite through the bag (Figure 10.22). This method can also be used for aggressive non-venomous snakes. Venomous bagging systems have also been developed that allow for the snake to be bagged and then transferred safely into a container that provides more protection, such as a wooden box, plastic bucket, or plastic container. The container should give visibility of the snake so it can be safely removed. If the snake cannot be visualized, it should be left in the bag. When handling a venomous snake within a bag, tongs should be used (Figure 10.23). If the bag has to be grabbed without tongs, it should be grabbed above the knot. Venomous snakes should be transported in something more durable to safeguard against bites when at all possible.

Restraint

As stated previously, snakes can be very unpredictable and the handler should treat them as such to avoid being bitten.

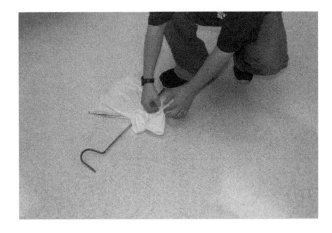

Figure 10.22 The snake hook is used to isolate the snake so that the handler can safely untie the bag from venomous or aggressive snakes.

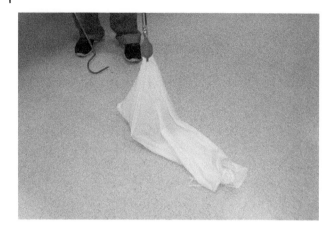

Figure 10.23 Tongs and a snake hook are used to remove venomous or aggressive snakes from a bag.

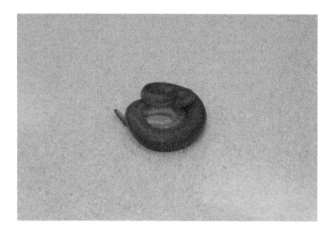

Figure 10.24 A Columbian rainbow boa (*Epicrates maurus*) in striking position. Notice the S-shaped posture.

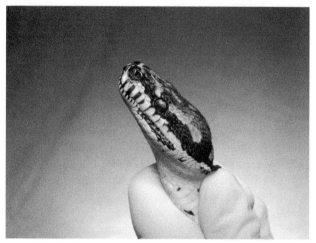

Figure 10.25 The head of the snake is secured to prevent injury to the snake or the restrainer. If this snake was aggressive, the hands should be held more cranially to prevent the snake from turning their head towards the handler's hands. Source: (Courtesy of Jody Nugent-Deal).

Even the most docile of snakes will bite if it feels threatened or cornered. One should watch for warning signs, such as hissing or an S-shaped striking posture before attempting to handle a snake (Figure 10.24).

Whether restraining or simply holding the snake, it is important to do so properly. If the snake is not held properly, not only can the handler get bitten, but also the snake can sustain injuries. The body should always be supported as much as possible. With larger snakes, it will take more than one person to hold and offer necessary support.

When manually restraining the snake, one should ensure that someone has control of the head. This should be the first part of the body to be restrained. The head should be held right at the base and without applying too much pressure around the neck area (Figure 10.25). Such pressure could obstruct the trachea causing a strangling effect and the snake to panic. The rest of the body can be held with a free hand or by assistants when handling large or aggressive snakes. The snake should have something that it can support itself on to feel more secure. It is important not to over-restrain the snake. Gripping tightly to the head will make even the most docile snake panic and become aggressive. The key is to secure the snake without causing undue stress. Do not place a snake (especially large snakes and/or constrictors) around your neck. This is commonly done and can be dangerous. If the snake feels threatened and insecure, it will begin to constrict around the neck. It is also recommended that there be one restrainer for each five-foot (1.5 m) section of the snake. This will give safe restraint for the snake and its restrainers and will also allow the snake to feel support throughout its entire body.

Different tools can be used to move snakes or assist in immobilization, including hooks, tubes, and tongs (Figure 10.26).

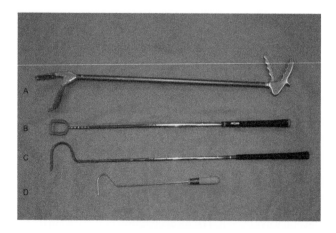

Figure 10.26 (A) Snake tong. (B) Pinning hook. (C) *Medium* snake hook. (D) Small snake hook.

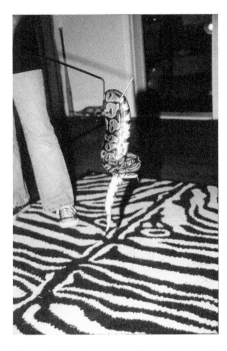

Figure 10.27 Proper use of a snake hook. Notice how the snake is able to balance on the hook.

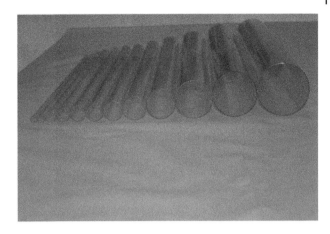

Figure 10.29 Set of plastic snake tubes. Sizes are available for all sizes of snakes.

Snake hooks allow a person to move a snake without having to touch the animal or get too close. This is advantageous when handling aggressive snakes. It can be used to get a snake out of an enclosure, as a guide, or as a pinning device. For example, to remove a snake from an enclosure, the hook is used to "hook" the snake one-third of the way down its body and then gently lift it (Figure 10.27). The hook can then be used to pin the head to take control of it but extreme caution must be used as any thrashing on the part of the snake can cause severe spinal cord injury. Only handlers experienced with the hook should use the pinning technique. A better option for pinning the snake is by using a pinning device (Figure 10.28). These devices have a thick rubber stretched between two pieces of metal. The rubber is tight enough to secure the head, and soft enough to prevent injuries. If the snake is hooked too close to the head or tail, the snake will usually slide right off. It may be necessary to use more than one hook for larger snakes. Snake hooks are also used when coercing a snake into a snake tube for physical exam or immobilization. Hooks can be purchased at most reptile supply shops.

Snake tubes are open-ended, clear, hard plastic or acrylic tubes that are used to hold a snake and view it safely during examination (Figure 10.29). The tube's diameter must be just large enough for the snake's head to fit into, but not allow the snake to turn around (Figure 10.30). One end of the tube should be aimed toward the snake's head and a snake hook used to entice the snake into the tube (Figure 10.31). Once one-third to one-half of the snake's body is in the tube, the handler should grasp the snake and the base of the tube so it cannot back out (Figure 10.32).

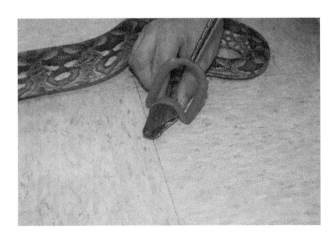

Figure 10.28 Pinning hook is placed at the base of the skull and the head is quickly secured.

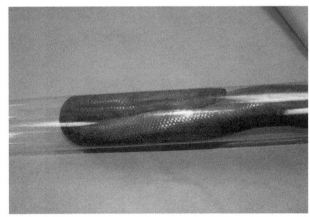

Figure 10.30 This tube is too large and poses a danger to the handler and to the snake.

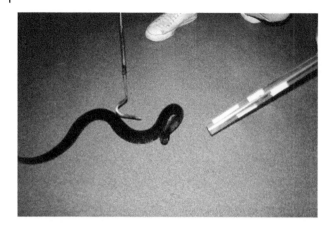

Figure 10.31 Using a hook to coax a snake into a plastic tube. Source: (Courtesy of Zoo Atlanta).

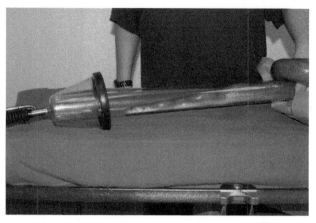

Figure 10.33 An anesthetic mask can be placed over the end of the snake tube to provide oxygen therapy or gas anesthesia.

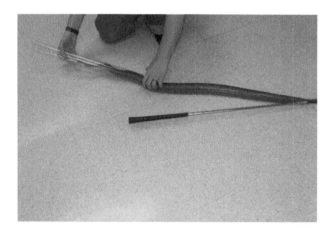

Figure 10.32 Once the snake is 1/3 in the tube, the handler should grasp the base to prevent further movement.

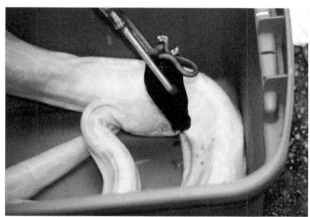

Figure 10.34 Feeding a python with tongs.

A face mask can be placed on the other end of the tube to administer gas anesthesia and immobilize the snake completely, if necessary (Figure 10.33). This is the safest way to manage aggressive snakes and venomous species. Most of these tubes are purchased from reptile supply stores or hardware stores (if appropriate materials are found) and come in various sizes.

Another method of capturing an aggressive non-venomous snake is to place a clear shield over its head. Once the shield is in place, the handler can grasp right behind its head taking control of it. A towel can also be used for similar purposes, but this is not recommended on very large and aggressive snakes. The towel is better suited for small to medium-sized non-venomous snakes.

Snake tongs can be used for many purposes. The most common use is for feeding (Figure 10.34). Offering food items via tongs is obviously safer than using one's hands to offer prey. Tongs allow the feeder to maintain some distance from the snake and the prey item. Tongs can also be

used to aid in the restraint of snakes or to move a small or medium-sized snake from one enclosure to another, which is especially helpful with handling venomous species. The tongs can also be used in conjunction with hooks. The hook is used to guide and control the head and the tongs are used to grasp the tail (Figure 10.35). Again, this technique is used mostly in small to medium-sized snakes. Despite their potential usefulness, tongs do have some caveats. Grabbing the snake with tongs can apply too much pressure and, depending on what part of the body is grasped, the snake can be injured. Snakes can also easily free themselves from tongs if not grasped properly. Tongs can be used to assist in handling the snake but not as a primary handling mechanism.

An undesirable method of restraint is to allow a snake to partially swallow prey. This will allow the handler time to take control of the head and the body before the snake can strike. However, often the snake will regurgitate the prey, making this technique undesirable.

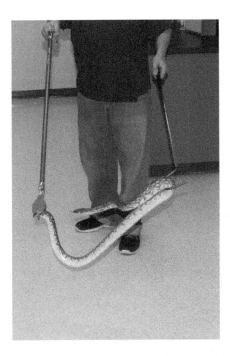

Figure 10.35 The tongs are used to control the tail and the hook is used to control the head.

To avoid bites, some reptile hobbyists believe that snakes should not be fed inside their primary enclosure, especially when the only time the enclosure is opened is when the snake is being fed. This creates a feeding response and makes bites more likely to occur. Feeding outside the primary enclosure would be a safer practice and also could help to ensure that any loose substrate located inside the primary enclosure is not ingested during feeding.

The Physical Exam

After a very thorough history has been taken and the exam room has been prepared, a complete physical exam should be performed. The physical exam should begin as soon as the owner brings the snake into the exam room. The snake should be observed as it moves around its environment. Body/muscle tone, proprioception, and mobility should be observed at this time. Any abnormalities should be noted. An accurate weight in grams or kilograms as well as the snout-to-vent length (SVL) should be measured to determine organ location and monitor growth in juvenile snakes. The cloacal temperature should be recorded to help determine the thermal environment in which the snake lives.

There are several approaches to performing a physical exam. Some clinicians prefer a head-to-tail evaluation while others have a specific order of body systems that are examined. It is important to follow the same routine with every physical exam so nothing is left out or overlooked.

Integument

The skin should be checked for parasites, thermal burns, trauma, skin tenting or ridges to assess hydration, dysecdysis, and bacterial or fungal infections. If ecdysis is currently in process, the stage of ecdysis should be recorded.

Respiratory System

The upper and lower airways should be auscultated for any crackles or increased respiratory sounds. Remember that most snakes only have a right lung, with the exception of the boids, which have a right lung and a small left lung. The nostrils should be clear of debris and any discharge. The glottis can easily be observed for proper function and for any inflammation. When the glottis opens during respiration, one should look down the trachea for any swelling, mucus, or foreign material.

Cardiovascular System

Auscultation of the snake's heart can sometimes prove to be difficult. It is crucial that the exam room be silent. Using a damp cloth or gauze sponge can help enhance the heart sounds. The heart is generally around one-quarter along the body from the snout. A heart rate should be obtained during auscultation. Peripheral pulses should be assessed via the use of a Doppler flow detector. The Doppler can be placed on the ventral tail vein or just cranial to the heart at the base of the glottis.

Neurologic Examination

Neurologic exams are very simple to perform on snakes. The exam starts with the initial presentation of the snake. One needs to watch for any jerking motions, absent or slow righting reflex, or the inability to strike at prey. The site of a spinal cord injury can be found by using the righting reflex. Snakes will right themselves up to the point of the injury. A hypodermic needle may be used to stimulate the panniculus reflex. A neurologically normal snake's skin will twitch up to the point of spinal injury. A cranial nerve exam should be performed if a neurologic disorder is suspected. Following are methods to use to examine the 12 cranial nerves in snakes.

CN I—A snake with a properly functioning olfactory nerve will recoil from the smell of noxious odors. Alcohol can be placed in front of the snake's nose to see if it reacts to the smell.

CN II—Since reptiles have an iris that is composed of skeletal muscle, the pupillary light reflex cannot be used to determine the function of the optic nerve. Carefully watch the eye movements of the snake to assess the function of the optic nerve.

CN III, CN IV, CN VI—This group of cranial nerves is extremely hard to assess in snakes. They are responsible for eye movement coordination.

CN V—Snakes with a malfunctioning trigeminal nerve will have abnormal jaw function and a loss of feeling around the face. They will not be able to thermoregulate or find prey.

CN VIII—The acoustic nerve is difficult to assess. Snakes may show signs of nystagmus, head tilt, rolling, and abnormal righting reflex.

CN IX, CN XI, CN XII—Dysphagia and abnormal tongue movements can be seen in a snake if one or more of these cranial nerves are damaged or malfunctioning.

CN VII and CN X—The facial and vagus nerves are impossible to assess in snakes.

Palpations

The entire length of the snake should be palpated for any abnormalities such as enlarged organs, internal masses, lumps, and bumps. In breeding females, eggs and pre-ovulatory follicles can be felt on palpation. Digital palpation of the cloaca can reveal several abnormalities and should be performed on all snakes that are large enough. An otoscope or endoscope can be used as well and may be necessary for smaller snakes.

Ophthalmic Exam

As discussed in the section on "Eyes," snakes have a transparent spectacle that covers the cornea. The eyes should be clear and smooth. Any retained sheds can easily be seen and removed. Any other abnormalities should be further examined with an ophthalmoscope.

Fecal Exam

All snakes presented for a physical exam should have a fecal examination performed. This exam should include a fecal centrifugation and two direct fecal smears, one prepared with a normal saline solution and the other prepared with a Lugol's iodine solution.

Oral Exam

Because most snakes become distressed during the oral exam, it is often best to perform the oral examination last. Gently open the mouth using an oral speculum. Determining the proper mucosal color can be difficult. Most species have a pale mucosa while others may have a more pink or bluish color. It is important to know the normal color for that species before the physical exam is performed. With all species, the oral cavity should be moist without any stringy or tenacious mucus. The clinician should look for

any caseous exudates, hemorrhage, and necrosis. Some parasites, such as *Kalicephalus* sp., may also be seen in the oral cavity.

Radiology

Positioning

As with all other animals, two views should be taken: a lateral and a dorsoventral (DV) view are most appropriate for snakes. Snakes should not be radiographed in the coiled position as this can distort internal organs and decrease detail (Figure 10.36). The snake should be stretched out over the cassette. If multiple films are required to image the region, the films should be labeled to match the region taken. There are several methods of doing this. The method used by this author is based on the number of films required to radiograph the snake. If four films are needed, the first film is labeled 1/4, the second film is labeled 2/4, and so on.

Restraint

With the exception of very sick snakes, most snakes will not be still enough to radiograph without proper restraint. For docile snakes, manually holding them on the table will be sufficient restraint for proper technique. For less docile snakes, placing them in clear plastic tubes will allow for proper positioning and technique. If this method is used, the kVp or mAs, depending on the technique chart used, may need to be slightly increased to compensate for the plastic. As a last resort, chemical restraint can be used: either injectable or inhalant anesthesia can be used. If injectable anesthesia is used, a short-acting drug or one that is reversible is preferred. Some injectable anesthetics can last for hours or even days in reptiles.

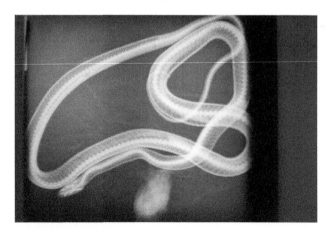

Figure 10.36 Snake radiographed inside of a bag. Notice the movement artifact and the many oblique angles.

Anesthesia

Anatomy and Physiology Considerations

The lungs of reptiles are very fragile. When performing intermittent positive pressure ventilation (IPPV) always stay under 20 cm H_2O to avoid pulmonary rupture (Bennett 1996, p. 30), and for routine ventilation, it is best to stay between 10 and 15 cm H_2O (Schumacher & Yelen 2006, p. 448). IPPV is required on all reptiles under anesthesia. IPPV can be accomplished through manual ventilation, but this method is labor-intensive and does not produce consistent rates and tidal volume. Small animal ventilators that are either pressure-driven or volume-driven are available and are ideal for reptilian anesthesia. The ventilator settings should be set at a rate of 4–6 breaths per minute, with a pressure not to exceed 12 cm H_2O, and an inspiratory time of 1–2 seconds (Mans et al. 2019, pg. 458). Ventilator settings should be adjusted to maintain an $ETCO_2$ between 10 and 25 mmHg. Since reptiles do not have a diaphragm, respiration is accomplished through other muscles throughout the thoracic and abdominal areas. Some of the muscles are paralyzed when the reptile reaches a surgical plane of anesthesia, making IPPV necessary. One should also keep in mind that many snakes can breathe hold and convert to anaerobic metabolism. Many species can live for hours without oxygen. This adaptation makes induction difficult to impossible in some species if inducing with inhalant anesthesia. It should also be important to understand that it is low oxygen concentration (PaO_2) that stimulates a reptile to breath. Hypoxemia will increase the respiratory rate, whereas hypercapnia generally has more effect on tidal volume.

Pre-anesthetic Examination and Considerations

Before placing a snake under anesthesia a very thorough physical examination should be performed. Also, a minimal amount of diagnostics, including a packed cell volume and total solids, should be recorded to help determine the health status of the snake. More diagnostics may be needed such as a biochemical profile, complete blood count, fecal analysis, radiographs, or cultures if infection is suspected. Any abnormalities on the physical examination or diagnostic testing should be treated or stabilized before the anesthetic episode. The snake should be fasted for 1 to 2 weeks for any elective procedures or non-emergency anesthetic procedures. Cardiopulmonary function can be compromised if a large prey is still being digested in the stomach.

Intravenous fluid therapy is needed for any debilitated snake or during long procedures (Bennett 1997, p. 32). If the snake is dehydrated, rehydration should occur before beginning the anesthetic episode. Any of the crystalloids are appropriate for use in reptiles (Lawton 2001, p. 788). There has been much debate over the use of any fluids containing lactate in reptiles. Lactate in reptiles builds to high levels after muscle fatigue and can only be metabolized by the liver. However, reptiles are able to handle a significant increase in lactate, and such lactate-containing fluids are fine to use in snakes. For dehydrated snakes, any balanced isotonic crystalloid can be used. If fluids are needed intraoperatively, an intravenous catheter must be placed in either the jugular vein or directly into the heart. The interoperative fluid rate should be 5–10 mL/kg/hour.

Pre-anesthetic Medications

Pre-anesthetics are not routinely used in all reptiles. Pre-anesthetic can be used to provide safer handling of larger snakes to facilitate smoother inductions for general anesthesia. They may also help decrease the amount of drugs needed for induction.

Anticholinergics

Anticholinergics such as atropine sulfate and glycopyrrolate for the most part are unnecessary as a pre-anesthetic medication. Glycopyrrolate has been shown to help prevent bradycardia; however, bradycardia is usually not a concern in reptile anesthesia.

Injectable Sedatives and Anesthetics

The use of injectable anesthetics and sedatives in reptiles has a very unpredictable effect. The same dose given to two individuals of the same species can yield completely different levels of sedation. Once the injection is given, the depth of anesthesia cannot be controlled. Since reptiles have a very slow metabolism, recovery can take from a couple of hours to a week with some anesthetics. Temperature can also have a drastic effect on the pharmacokinetic properties of the injected medication. Snakes kept below their POTZ can see a prolonged time to effect and intensity of clinical effect. Another factor that should be considered is location of injection for IM and SC routes. If giving injections in the caudal half of the body, it is possible that the drugs could pass through the liver prior to general circulation. It is advisable that all medications be administered in the cranial half of the body. Reptiles require a very high dose of narcotics to produce any sedative effects, hence narcotics are not recommended in reptiles for sedation as a sole agent; however, narcotics will produce analgesic effects.

Benzodiazepines are a common sedative for snakes. Midazolam and diazepam have both been used successfully to sedate snakes for restraint or minor procedures.

Midazolam is preferred over diazepam due to a shorter duration of action and onset of clinical effect. Benzodiazepines can be reversed using flumazenil. If reversing diazepam, flumazenil may need to be repeated due to the long duration of action of diazepam. Benzodiazpines can be combined with many other drugs, such as ketamine, narcotics, or α2-adrenergic agonists, to achieve the desired effect.

Ketamine is frequently used in snakes for sedation and induction and can also be used as a surgical anesthetic. Due to metabolic scaling, larger species require the lower end of the recommended dose (Bennett 1997, p. 34). When used alone, moderate to high doses of ketamine have been associated with increased heart rates, respiratory depression, hypertension, apnea, bradycardia, prolonged recovery times, and death (Bertelsen 2007). However, when ketamine is combined with benzodiazepines or α2-adrenergic agonists, better muscle relaxation and a reduction in required dose occur (Bertelsen 2007).

Alpha-2-adrenergic agonists are also commonly used to produce mild to heavy sedation as well as to provide some analgesic effects in snakes. Dexmedetomidine or medetomidine ([dex]medetomidine) has been used with great success in snakes. When given, it greatly reduces the amount of induction needed and also at higher doses gives enough sedation for quick procedures. (Dex)medetomidine is reversible with atipamezole. (Dex)medetomidine when given with ketamine shows better anesthetic effects than when given alone. Onset of clinical effects takes about 20 minutes when given as a sole agent. Dose-dependent cardiovascular effects as well as an initial period of hypertension and bradycardia may be seen. Due to the respiratory depression, supplemental oxygen therapy is recommended. (Dex)medetomidine can be reversed with atipamezole with a clinical effect taking around 20 minutes.

Telazol, a combination of tiletamine and zolazepam, is recommended as a tranquilizer or induction agent and not as the sole anesthetic. At a dose of 2–5 mg/kg, Telazol will sedate the snake enough for diagnostic procedures or for intubation. High doses of Telazol have been associated with prolonged recovery times (Schumacher & Yelen 2006).

Propofol is a very short-acting non-barbiturate that can be used as an induction agent or for short surgical or diagnostic procedures. The only disadvantage of propofol is that it must be given intravenously, which can be very difficult in some snakes. The advantages of propofol are that it produces very rapid induction and recovery times; it has minimal accumulation with repeated doses, and it produces very little hangover effect after recovery.

Recently, alfaxalone has gained popularity in veterinary medicine. It is a great sole agent or can be combined with other sedatives and narcotics to achieve sedation, induction, or maintenance anesthetic effects. Cardiovascular effects under alfaxalone are generally stable, the respiratory system however can see variable effects. Alfaxalone can be given SC, IM, or IV. Depending on the dose, if giving IM, several locations may need to be used due to the large volume of drug used.

Several neuromuscular blocking agents have been used in snakes. As these drugs do not produce unconsciousness or analgesia, the use of neuromuscular blockers should be limited to non-painful diagnostic procedures, or should be used in conjunction with analgesics and anesthetics. Since respiratory paralysis is likely, intubation with IPPV is necessary.

Inhalant Anesthetics

Inhalant anesthetics have become the standard of practice for reptiles. There are many advantages of inhalant anesthetics versus injectable anesthetics. First, the level of anesthesia is much more precisely controlled. Another big advantage is that the patient is intubated and receiving supplemental oxygen. Recovery from inhalant anesthetics is much quicker than with injectable anesthetics. Right-to-left intracardiac blood shunting can lead to increased induction times as well as a very rapid (and at times very unexpected) recovery. Usually, the patients are recovered in less than one hour after the anesthetic episode. A non-rebreathing system is recommended for patients weighing less than 5 kg and an oxygen flow rate of 300–500 mL/kg/min. Patients weighing more than 5 kg can use a rebreathing system at an oxygen flow rate of 1–2 L/min. IPPV is recommended in all anesthetized reptiles at a rate of four to eight breaths per minute.

Isoflurane is completely eliminated by the lungs so it causes no metabolic compromise, and can safely be used on debilitated or compromised patients. Induction is quick, taking 5 to 10 minutes, and recovery takes less than 30 minutes in most patients.

Sevoflurane gained popularity in the human and veterinary market because of its low blood–gas solubility. This allows for very fast induction and recovery times and improves the control of anesthetic depth. In humans, cardiovascular stability is better maintained with sevoflurane than with isoflurane. Sevoflurane is also completely eliminated by the lungs. Clinical experience shows that species and individuals respond differently to sevoflurane, with some being much more resistant than others.

Tracheal intubation is easy on snakes. The trachea sits at the base of their tongue and is easily visible when the mouth is open (Figures 10.37–10.40).

Analgesics

It was once believed that reptiles do not feel pain. Reptiles have the neurologic components, antinociceptive

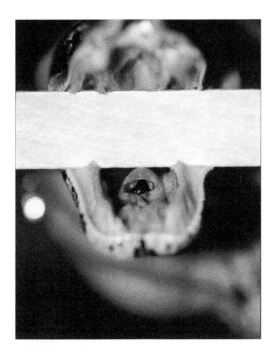

Figure 10.37 View of the glottis.

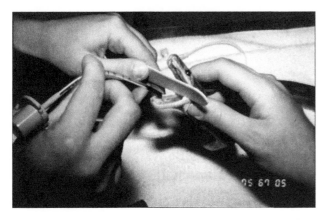

Figure 10.38 Endotracheal intubation of a snake. (Courtesy of Zoo Atlanta).

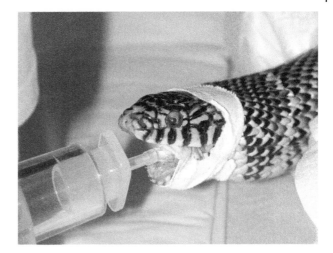

Figure 10.39 The endotracheal tube is secured with tape. (Courtesy of Jody Nugent-Deal).

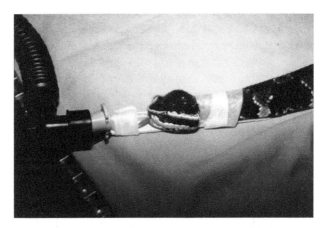

Figure 10.40 Longer endotracheal tubes can be secured with tape and a tongue depressor. (Courtesy of Zoo Atlanta).

mechanisms, and behavioral responses to pain that other animals have (Bradley 2001, p. 45). Reptiles can and do feel pain and therefore analgesics should be provided. Since pain is easier to prevent than treat, analgesics should be given before an anticipated painful procedure. Snakes also share many of the same signs of pain as domestic species. Commonly, snakes will show signs of avoidance of handling, withdrawal, restlessness, agitation, being easily startled, or anorexia when they are in pain. Some more obvious signs of pain are holding the body less coiled at the site of pain, stinting on palpation, and being tucked up and writhing in the affected area. Much like with anesthetics and sedatives, variable results occur with the use of analgesics between species, and it is essential that these

medications are administered into the cranial half of the body to avoid hepatic first-pass effect.

Opioids have been used extensively in snakes. μ-opioid receptor agonist have shown to provide the most evidence of pain management. Morphine, hydromorphone, methadone, and fentanyl have all been used successfully in snakes. Fentanyl patches can be applied and have shown to deliver a therapeutic plasma level as soon as 4 hours after administration and remain at therapeutic levels for 7 days (Darrow, et al. 2016). If signs of an overdose are seen, naloxone can be administered as a reversal. If the overdose is from transdermal fentanyl, the patch should be removed and the area cleaned with soap and water. Buprenorphine, a parial μ-opioid receptor agonist, has shown little efficacy in reptiles. Butorphanol should not be used as an analgesic in snakes.

Nonsteroidal anti-inflammatory drugs have seen limited uses in snakes. There is little data available on the efficacy of their usage in snakes. Multiple different injectable NSAIDs have been used for their analgesic effects and for their anti-inflammatory properties.

Recovery

Recovering patients should be placed in an environment that is quiet and within the species' POTZ. Close attention should be paid to the respirations since all anesthetics compromise the respiratory system. Also, observe the patient for any pain or discomfort and treat with analgesics accordingly. If the patient was receiving fluids during the procedure, the fluids should be continued until the patient is fully recovered.

Anesthetic Monitoring

The depth of anesthesia in snakes is very difficult to assess. As snakes become anesthetized, relaxation begins cranially and goes caudally, and this is reversed during recovery. One of the first reflexes a snake loses is the righting reflex. Other reflexes to check are the cloacal reflex and the tail pinch to help determine the depth of anesthesia. At a surgical plane, snakes should still have a tongue withdraw and will lose it if the snake is beyond the surgical plane. In a surgical plane of anesthesia, the snake should be apneic making the respiratory rate a factor in lighter planes or stages of anesthesia. As they get into deeper stages, the heart rate will begin to decrease.

Cardiovascular Monitoring

The cardiovascular system can be difficult to assess in an anesthetized snake. The heart rate is the only reliable measurement that is clinically available and that gives reliable readings. The Doppler flow device is the best tool in our arsenal for the measurement of the heart rate. The Doppler flow device should be placed directly over the heart. Capillary refill times and mucous membranes color as well as indirect blood pressure measurements are not reliable in snakes. Direct blood pressure measurement is reliable, but the clinical applications are limited. Although blood pressure measurement is not practical, it should be noted that reptiles under inhalant anesthetics are likely to be hypotensive.

Electrocardiogram (ECG) monitoring can be used to assess the electrical function of the heart. There is limited data published on ECG parameters in reptiles so the ECG is much more useful as a tool to assess trends. The ECG should look similar to a mammalian waveform with a P, QRS complex, and a T wave representing ventricular repolarization. In some patients, an SV wave will be seen before the P wave. The SV wave represents the depolarization of

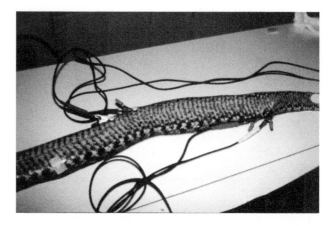

Figure 10.41 ECG lead placement on a snake. The head is to the right. (Courtesy of Zoo Atlanta).

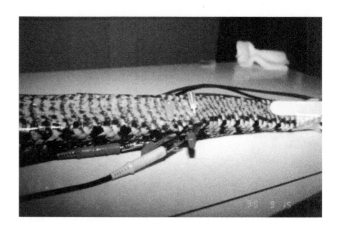

Figure 10.42 ECG lead placement close-up to show detail. (Courtesy of Zoo Atlanta).

the sinus venosus. The low amplitude of reptile patients will make interpretation difficult. The ECG lead should be placed two heart lengths cranial and caudal to the heart (Figures 10.41 and 10.42). An esophageal ECG can be used in patients who are large enough.

Respiratory Monitoring

Respiratory monitoring in snakes is also limited. Under a surgical plane of anesthesia, it is not likely that the patient will be breathing, however under lighter planes or stages, visual inspection of the rate and depth should be noted.

Pulse oximetry is useful in reptiles to monitor trends in arterial oxygen saturation. Pulse oximetry machines are calibrated to the mammalian oxygenhemoglobin dissociation curve and cannot be taken as an absolute number in reptiles. Pulse oximetry has only been verified in the green iguana (*Iguana iguana*) and it should only be used as a trend monitor. There are several factors that effect the efficacy of the readings. The snake respiratory and cardiac physiology and high levels of methemoglobin reported in reptiles will all effect the reading and therefore interpretation of the values reported. Reflectance pule oximeter probes can be used in the oral cavity, the esophagus, or cloaca.

Capnography is another tool we have that assesses ventilation. However, as discussed in other monitoring tools, there are some factors that must be considered. $ETCO_2$ has not been validated in reptiles. Reptiles also have the ability to have a right-to-left intracardiac blood shunting which will affect the interpretation of the results. Over time, the $ETCO_2$ reading may become significantly lower than the $PaCO_2$. Lastly, due to the small size of some of the patients, it is recommended to use an in-line capnography unit. The sidestream units may have inaccurate readings when dealing with very small tidal volumes.

Surgery

The basic principles of surgery are universal. Aseptic techniques should always be used. The patient should be prepared for surgery, induced with anesthesia, intubated, and placed on maintenance inhalant anesthesia. One should prepare the surgical site by an initial scrub with an approved surgical scrub such as chlorhexidine or betadine to remove any dirt or debris from the substrate. When the patient is stable under anesthesia, the patient can then be moved into the surgical suite. Once inside the surgical suite, all assistants should put on a cap and mask to maintain asepsis. The patient should be properly positioned and taped down to secure it to the table. Snakes can be positioned either in sternal, dorsal, or left or right recumbency. Once the patient is secured to the table, a sterile surgical scrub should be performed. The fluids used to prep the patient should be warmed to prevent cooling the patient. The patient should also be kept at their POTZ during the entire procedure and through recovery. This can be achieved by using a circulating hot water pad, forced air warmer, or hot water bottles.

Wound Healing

Wound healing has been studied extensively in snakes (Bennett & Lock 2000, p. 718). When a wound forms, proteinaceous fluid and fibrin fills the space to form a scab. A single layer of epithelial cells grows under the scab and then proliferates to restore the full thickness of the epithelium. Underneath this layer of epithelial cells, macrophages and heterophils move in to clean up any pathogens. Fibroblasts migrate to the area forming a fibrous scar. Heterophils are present until maturation has occurred. Ecdysis seems to help with the wound-healing

process (Bennett 1997, p. 38). It has also been observed that incisions having a cranial to caudal orientation heal faster than transverse incisions. Also maintaining the patient in the upper end of the species' POTZ promotes good wound healing (Bennett & Lock 2000, p. 719).

The incised skin of reptiles has a tendency to heal inverted. The skin should be closed using an everted suture pattern such as a mattress pattern. Skin staples can also be used for skin closure. The sutures should be removed in 4 to 6 weeks and preferably after the next ecdysis cycle.

Common Surgical Procedures

Celiotomies are routinely performed on snakes. The incision for a celiotomy should be made between the first two rows of scales dorsolateral to the large ventral scales (Bennett & Lock 2000, p. 721). This approach is performed to avoid the large mid-abdominal vein. A zigzag incision is made between the scales in the softer skin. Celiotomies are commonly performed for foreign body removal and exploratory surgery.

The most common surgery of the respiratory tract is removal of granulomas from the trachea. The approach is the same as for a celiotomy. The granuloma is found and removed. The two ends of the trachea are then anastomosed and the incision is closed. The snakes are usually back to breathing normally immediately.

Gastrointestinal surgeries are routinely done to repair abnormalities. These abnormalities may include foreign body removal or resection and anastomosis.

Surgery on the reproductive tract is usually not performed to prevent a reproductive problem (Lock 2000, p. 737). The most common female reproductive surgical procedures are for dystocia and ovariectomy or ovariosalpingohysterectomy. The last two procedures are performed to prevent another dystocia, to remove cysts or tumors, or to prevent another prolapse. The most common surgical procedure on the male reproductive tract is hemipenile amputation. The hemipenis may prolapse and become inflamed and non-retractable. Oftentimes the hemipenis can be replaced, but occasionally it will become necrotic and have to be amputated.

Parasitology

Diagnosing Parasites

Parasitic infections are relatively easy to diagnose. A fresh stool sample should be obtained being careful not to collect any urates. When an appointment is made for a snake, the client should be asked to bring in a fresh stool sample. The client can put the stool sample in a plastic sandwich bag and keep it in the refrigerator for up to 3 days. It is recommended that the stool sample be stored in a refrigerator that does not also store food for human consumption. A double or even triple-bag system can be used if the sample is stored with food for human consumption. If a fresh sample is not available, a colonic wash can be performed to obtain a sample. Two diagnostic tests should be performed: a centrifugation and a saline-prepared direct smear. The centrifuge will help diagnose protozoan cysts and nematode ova. The direct smear is used to diagnose moving or live parasites, mostly protozoans. The techniques used to perform these diagnostics are the same techniques used for diagnosing parasites in small animals. Some parasites, like *Cryptosporidium*, require specialized diagnostic testing.

Common Parasites of Snakes

External Parasites

Ticks

Ticks are common on wild-caught snakes, but can be very difficult to find, especially if the snake has dark skin, since they bury themselves under the scales to reach the skin and take their blood meal. Rarely do ticks occur in such high numbers on snakes as to cause anemia, but they can transmit blood parasites and viruses. All ticks should be removed with great care to remove all their mouthparts from the skin.

Mites

Ophionyssus natricis, the snake mite, is a common finding in pet snakes. The mites are small and appear red, gray, or black. The mite has four distinct life stages. The complete lifecycle of the snake mite can last up to 53 days in ideal situations; however, the nymphs can wait as long as a month, and possibly more, for a blood meal, extending the possible life cycle to 80 days or longer. The adults lay their eggs in dark, moist environments within the enclosure. After a 28–98-hour incubation, the eggs hatch into the free-living larval stage. The larvae stay within the hatching area for 18–47 hours, then molt into the parasitic protonymph stage, which can last 18–47 hours. After the skin hardens, they begin looking for a host, whereupon they crawl under the host's scales and begin taking a blood meal. The nymphs will crawl onto cage furnishings awaiting a host if one is not found easily. When they become engorged, they leave the host again and search out a warm, dark, moist environment where they molt into the non-parasitic deutonymph stage, which can last for 13–26 days. Finally, they molt again into adults, which again seek out a host and take a blood meal. Reproduction occurs at this stage, and the female can lay as many as 60–80 eggs after just a couple of feeds.

Snakes that are infected may spend long periods of time soaking in water or appear to rub or twist their bodies. Other common findings include dysecdysis, anemia, lethargy, anorexia, pruritus, and crusting dermatitis. Visualizing the mite is the only diagnostic method. If mites are suspected, a clean white paper towel or hand towel can be rubbed down the entire length of the snake's body. Often, the mites will detach onto the towel making for easier visualization. Treatment includes a combination of environmental control and drug therapy. The cage should be cleaned and disinfected. All substrate should be discarded, and any porous cage furnishings should be soaked in water and disinfected. The cage should be kept as simple as possible, resembling a quarantine cage setup. The snake should also be isolated from the rest of the population and strict infection control procedures should be initiated to prevent the spread of the mites. It is common to have large collections infested with mites, and this should be considered when deciding on treatment options. During treatment, the cage should be disinfected on a regular basis to kill those mites that are not on the snake. Insecticides may be indicated for heavy infestations. A number of products can be sprayed into the empty cage. Environmental control of this parasite disrupts the life cycle by killing the eggs, the larval stages, and the deutonymphs.

There are many products that can be used to treat the snake, and some of them can also be used to treat the environment. A brief description of the products and their uses follows.

Pyrethins and pyrethroids: There are numerous products on the market. After using any of these products, the snake should be rinsed off in warm water. Treatment should occur every 10–14 days, depending on the product, until no more mites are seen. Also, not all of these products are safe to spray directly onto the snake. Neonates, juveniles, and smaller snakes seem to be more sensitive to most of these chemicals. Some examples are as follows:
- Resmethrin II
- Permectin II: Dilute to 1% and use as a spray
- Pyrethrin: Dilute to 0.03% and use as a spray
- Permethrin: 0.5% spray

Fipronil: Frontline spay, and the many generic products, have been used to treat snake mites. The snake should be thoroughly sprayed, the excess fipronil should be wiped off with a damp gauze, and then washed off with water after 5 minutes.

Imidacloprid (100 g/L) plus Moxidectin (25 g/L): Spray the environment and the snake, wipe off the excess after a few mintues.

Ivermectin: Ivermectin has been commonly used to treat snake mites for many years. A topical spray is created by mixing 5 mg of 1% ivermectin in a quart (946 mL) of water. Ivermectin is not water soluble so the solution should be shaken vigorously before each application. Ivermectin can be repeated every 14 days until no mites are seen.

Alternative methods of mite control have been used by hobbyists with mixed results. One of the most common methods is soaking the snake in water. All stages of mites are unable to survive in extremely high humidity or in water. Soaking the snake will kill the life stages that are on the snake, effectively decreasing the population. However, the mites tend to crawl to the snake's head, which is not submerged. This treatment will not rid the environment of all mites, but it will significantly reduce the population, which would be beneficial in a severely debilitated patient. Since it helps depopulate the mites, it can serve as an adjunct to other environmental controls and drug therapies. It is important to understand that the treatment of mites must include environmental controls and drug therapies to be successful.

Recently, biological control methods have been used in the form of predatory mites. Currently, *Cheyletus eruditus* has been explored and is being sold as a treatment and preventive measure for snake mites. Studies by Schilling et al. (2013) have shown that these mites were able to significantly reduce the population of mites in the environment and on snakes with an active infestation. However, these mites did not completely rid the snakes of their parasitic mites. This new treatment should be considered as an aid to prevent mite infestations, and to help in the treatment of mites in addition to drug therapies and environmental controls.

Internal Parasites

Protozoa

Amoebiasis Of the many species of amoebae that are found in snakes, *Entamoeba invadens* is the most pathogenic (Wellehan & Walden, 2019, p. 288). This amoeba causes very high mortality and morbidity in snakes and is transmitted via the ingestion of infected reptile feces. This parasite has a direct life cycle leading to great difficulty in eradicating it from snakes. Clinical signs of amoebiasis are anorexia, dehydration, and wasting away. Later stages of the disease will show clinical signs of ulcerative gastritis and colitis. The organism can spread to other tissues causing renal and hepatic necrosis and abscesses. A diagnosis is made through a positive culture. Treatment of the disease includes a broad-spectrum antibiotic, amoebicide, and supportive care. The best way to prevent infections with this parasite is through strict infection control procedures and by maintaining a closed collection.

Coccidia Coccidiosis is a common finding in captive snakes. In wild snakes, coccidiosis is a self-limiting infection, but in captivity, coccidia can cause severe illness, and in young snakes or smaller species death may result. Coccidia have a direct life cycle, and most traditional treatments have led to inconsistent results. Sulfadimethoxine and trimethoprim-sulfamethoxazole, nutraceuticals, and probiotics have largely been found to be ineffective. Ponazuril has had some success in limited trials (Rockwell and Mitchell, 2019, p. 1165). Cage cleaning and strict hygiene protocols are the best way to prevent autoinfection and keeping the parasite load to a minimum.

Cryptosporidium serpentis is becoming a serious coccidial infection in snakes. The parasite is transmitted through fecal-oral contact, direct contact, or fomites. Once the oocyst is ingested, the sporozoite leaves the oocysts and penetrates the epithelial cells that line the stomach. Clinical signs of the disease include midbody swelling, weight loss, and regurgitation. *Cryptosporidium* oocysts can be shed by individuals with subclinical infection. Several cases of snakes shedding the oocysts for up to 20 years have been documented in individuals showing no clinical signs. The midbody swelling is a result of chronic gastric hypertrophy caused by the parasite.

Cryptosporidiosis is commonly diagnosed by visualization of oocysts on a microscopic exam. The oocysts can be detected in feces, mucus from a regurgitated meal, or from a gastric lavage, with the gastric lavage being the most sensitive. The sample can be prepared directly after centrifugation; however, this method is more sensitive if an immunofluorescent antibody stain (IFA) or acid-fast stain is used. The IFA is much more sensitive than the acid-fast stain. Merifluor is the IFA stain of choice. Merifluor will react to *Cryptosporidium parvum* so a false positive will occur if the snake ate a positive rodent. A dimethyl sulfoxide (DMSO) acid-fast exam can also be performed for proper diagnosis if the IFA is not available. Determination using the polymerase chain reaction (PCR) is also available. The concentration of oocysts increases postprandially, therefore it is recommended that the tests occur 3 days after feeding. Testing for serum antibody titers is also available to aid in the diagnosis of *Cryptosporidium*. After 6 weeks of infection, the snakes develop antibodies, but their presence indicates exposure but not necessarily active infection. A serum enzyme-linked immunosorbent assay (ELISA) test is available. Since it only represents exposure, this test should be performed in conjunction with other diagnostics. If both results are negative or positive, it can clarify the diagnosis. The ELISA test is unreliable due to the variable humoral response in infected individuals. Lastly, and most preferred, a gastric biopsy can be performed. Although more invasive, it can also help with making a prognosis because it will reveal the extent of gastric mucosal hyperplasia.

There are no safe and effective treatments for cryptosporidiosis. Trimethoprim sulfa, spiramycin, and paromomycin have been shown to reduce clinical signs and reduce or eliminate oocyte shedding. These drugs were given in conjunction with supportive care including fluids, high environmental temperatures, and tube feeding. Newer treatments such as hyperimmune bovine colostrum have shown promising results in reducing oocytes and clearing the patient of the parasite. Zoonotic potential has not been demonstrated with *Cryptosporidium serpentis*. *Cryptosporidium oocysts* are very stable in the environment and are not susceptible to many common commercial disinfectants.

Flagellated Protozoa There are many genera of flagellates found in snakes. Most are non-pathogenic although there is the potential for *Giardia* spp. to cause disease. Clinical signs include anorexia and weight loss. Metronidazole is the treatment of choice for flagellates.

Cestodes

The life cycle of cestodes involves many intermediate hosts. Snakes that are susceptible to cestode infections are those that are fed amphibians, fish, or crustaceans.

Nematodes

Several species of nematode affect snakes. The life cycle involves one or several intermediate hosts. Nematode infections are usually subclinical but signs can appear with severe infections. The only nematodes of great concern are the *Rhabdias* spp. and *Strongyloides* spp. *Rhabdias* spp. are known as lungworms in snakes because they migrate to the lungs. There are few clinical signs with minimal inflammatory response. In severe infections, the snake will show signs of dyspnea and mouth gaping. The diagnosis of lungworms can be made by discovering eggs and free-stage larvae in the oral secretions or in the feces.

Strongyles are nematodes that feed on the blood of the host. Clinical signs include anorexia, weight loss, hemorrhagic ulceration, and gastrointestinal obstruction. A fecal exam is performed for diagnosis. Treatment for all nematodes includes any of several anthelmintics and supportive care (Figure 10.43).

Blood Parasites

Extracellular and intracytoplasmic blood parasites are commonly seen in snakes. These rarely cause disease and are normally found on routine blood smears. Extreme cases can cause hemolytic anemia. If anemia is found, an antimalarial medication is indicated.

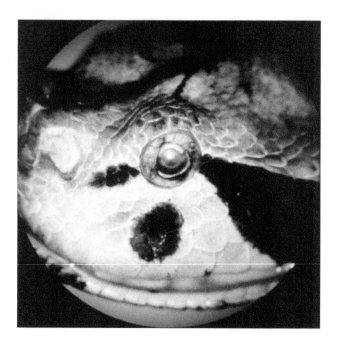

Figure 10.43 Ocular larva migrans in a snake (Courtesy of Zoo Atlanta).

Preventing Parasites

With parasites, like most other diseases, prevention is easier than cure. A few simple guidelines should be followed. The enclosures should be kept clean and disinfected often. New specimens should follow proper quarantine procedures. Do not feed wild prey items, and instead feed only thawed frozen prey to snakes. If live prey must be fed, start a breeding colony at home with a parasite-free male and female. Varying the prey offered can help to break any parasite life cycle.

Emergency and Critical Care

As more and more snakes are kept as pets, the need for proper emergency and critical care is increasing. The basics of emergency and critical care in snakes are the same as in any other animal. The patient is assessed, and diagnostics and treatments are quickly started. An emergency is defined as a sudden generally unexpected occurrence, or set of circumstances, demanding urgent action. Unfortunately, the need for urgent care is in the eyes of the owner and not trained medical professionals. Many owners wait for days to months to seek medical attention after first noticing a problem with their snake so that the initial problem turns into an emergency situation.

Phone Calls

Many owners will call the veterinary hospital seeking advice on their pet snake to determine if emergency medical treatment is necessary. Many problems with snakes that are reported after hours can wait until the morning when the regular veterinarian is available. Most diseases have been developing for weeks to months and initiating treatment can wait another several hours without detrimental effects to the patient. It is important that the technician screening the phone calls is familiar with snakes. For example, certain clinical signs that in dogs could be very serious are quite normal in a snake. A common non-emergency phone call is from an owner worried that his or her ball python (*Python regius*), or any other species, has not eaten in a week or sometimes in several months. Obviously, for a snake, this is not an emergency. Some of the more common emergencies that do need to be seen immediately are trauma, bite wounds, burns, hypothermia, hyperthermia, dyspnea, and cloacal prolapse. Common non-emergency clinical signs in snakes are lethargy, anorexia, dystocia, and constipation.

Initial Presentation and History

As soon as the patient comes into the veterinary hospital, a veterinary technician should make a quick assessment to determine the urgency of care. If the patient is stable, a thorough history should be obtained. If the patient is critical and needs immediate care, the patient should be taken to the attending veterinarian and a quick history should be obtained. This history should include such questions as:

- What is the ambient temperature in the enclosure?
- Is the snake eating and drinking normally?
- Do you feed live or dead prey?
- What heat sources are used?
- Has your snake been lethargic?
- Have you seen any coughing, wheezing, or nasal discharge?
- Has your snake regurgitated any food?
- Have there been any other medical problems in the past?

A more complete history can be obtained after the patient is stable and more time can be focused away from the patient. More questions may need to be asked pending the results of the physical examination.

Diagnostics

After the physical examination has been performed, the clinician will have a diagnostic plan. This may include a fecal analysis, biochemical profile, complete blood count, packed cell volume, total protein, or radiographs.

Treatment

After the diagnosis is made the treatment should begin. For dehydrated or severely ill snakes, fluid therapy should be initiated. Intravenous fluid therapy is preferable but other methods of fluid therapy will suffice. The fluids should be warmed to the preferred body temperature for the species being treated. The snake should be placed in a cage that is heated to the species' POTZ. Analgesics should be administered to patients who are in pain. Finally, other therapeutics should be started to treat the clinical signs and disease. Nutritional support should be started only after the patient is stable.

Emergency Conditions

Trauma

Trauma of any kind should be treated as an emergency. Bite wounds are common in snakes, and these normally occur from cage mates and live prey items left in the cage unattended (Figure 10.44). Lacerations are not so common in snakes, but they can be inflicted by exposed ends of wire mesh used on cages. Large snakes can easily break through glass cages, causing severe lacerations.

Bite wounds and lacerations are treated by either primary closure or secondary intention healing. If the wound is left open, antibiotic ointments rubbed on the wound work well as a barrier. Also, systemic antibiotics should be used on all bite wounds or lacerations. Analgesics should also be used.

Hypothermia

Occasionally snakes will escape from their enclosure and be found in a place that is excessively cold, causing their metabolism to slow or become virtually suspended. Frostbite may be seen on the tip of the snake's tail; if this is not necrotic, some pigment will be lost. Hypothermic snakes are unable to digest food and will often regurgitate prey. It is common to see respiratory disease several days to weeks after an episode of hypothermia. Snakes should be warmed up slowly over several hours and supportive care should be started.

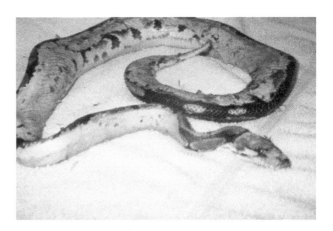

Figure 10.44 A snake suffering from trauma from a prey item (Courtesy of Dr. Sam Rivera).

Hyperthermia

Hyperthermia often occurs when the owner lets the snake outside in a glass or plastic enclosure in direct sunlight. Radiant heat quickly warms the snake and the animal is unable to move to a cooler environment. Treatment for hyperthermia includes subcutaneous or intracoelomic fluids and a quick, cool water bath to decrease the core body temperature.

Dyspnea

Snakes do not normally open-mouth breathe. If acute dyspnea occurs, the snake should be seen immediately. Dyspnea can be caused by several pathogens or disease processes but is most commonly associated with pneumonia.

Thermal Burns

Thermal burns are one of the most common emergencies seen in practice. Often, snakes will not show clinical signs of a burn for several days, making them difficult to treat. Thermal burns are most commonly caused by a malfunctioning heat source or improper use of a heat source. The two most common causes of thermal burns in snakes are hot rocks and heat lights, which snakes will coil around.

Burns are classified as superficial, partial, or full thickness. A superficial burn involves only the epidermis. The snake may appear to be in pain and have some discoloration on its scales. In severe superficial burns, some scales may be singed. Snakes with a superficial burn have a good prognosis. Antibiotic therapy should be initiated if any infection is noted. The snake should be housed in its POTZ and should heal by the next ecdysis. Little or no scarring is seen with superficial burns.

Partial-thickness burns involve complete destruction of the epidermis and extend into the underlying layers of skin. These burns appear red, ooze plasma, and will blister. Partial-thickness burns are also very painful and can take several months to completely heal. Analgesics should be administered immediately, the burn should be flushed thoroughly, and supportive care started. It is not uncommon for these patients to be in shock. After cleansing the burns, a burn cream, such as 1% silver sulfadiazine, should be applied and a sterile non-stick bandage should be placed when possible. Wet-to-dry bandages can also be used. The bandages should be replaced every day. The snake should be housed in a glass or Plexiglas container with no substrate until the wound is completely healed. The cage should also be disinfected daily. Antibiotics should be started to prevent infections, which are common in burn victims.

Full-thickness burns are characterized by a black eschar. They are not painful because all the nerves in the skin are destroyed. Full-thickness burns have a poor to grave prognosis and require very intensive treatment. The wound initially should be treated with a thorough cleansing, and fluid therapy administered to treat for shock. The burn should be debrided to promote healing, a bandage placed, and antibiotics started. Daily bandage changes and debridement are necessary for successful treatment. As the skin heals, the wound will become very painful. Analgesics should be started as soon as the patient feels pain. It can take months to a year for full granulation to occur. The owners must be told of the poor prognosis, long-term care, and financial expense of treating a full-thickness burn before treatment begins.

Critical Care Monitoring

The same principles apply to monitoring a critically ill snake as apply to monitoring a critically ill dog or cat. Neurologic, respiratory, and cardiovascular function all must be monitored and assessed.

The cardiovascular system is monitored by using a Doppler and ECG. A heart rate should be obtained from both the Doppler and ECG and recorded, and auscultation performed to monitor the respiratory system. The breath sounds should be clear without any wheezing or crackles, and a respiratory rate obtained and recorded. The patient is also observed for dyspnea, and a neurologic exam is performed daily. The snake should be housed in its POTZ.

Clinical Techniques

Administration of Medications

Intravenous (IV)

Intravenous injections can be given in the tail vein or directly into the heart. Use the same technique used for venipuncture to give the injection. Another option for IV injections is the palatine vein. This vein is located in the oral cavity and is best suited for very experienced phlebotomists due to its small size. The palatine vein should only be used in snakes with a healthy oral cavity and no signs of stomatitis.

Subcutaneous (SC)

Subcutaneous injections can easily be given when the snake is coiled and the skin folds become apparent. The needle should be placed between the scales on the lateral coelomic body wall, aspiration applied to the syringe to ensure a blood vessel has not been entered, and then the injection given. If the snake is not coiled, a small piece of skin can be lifted and the injection given.

Intramuscular (IM)

Intramuscular injections can be given in the epaxial and lateral muscle groups. The needle is placed between the scales, aspiration applied to the syringe to ensure a blood vessel has not been entered, and then the injection given.

Intracoelomic (ICe)

The snake should be restrained in dorsal or lateral recumbency. The needle is placed between scales in the lower quadrant of the coelomic cavity, taking care to be far enough caudal to avoid the lung. It is very important to aspirate back on the syringe before injecting. If any blood or other questionable fluid is aspirated, the needle should be removed and a new syringe and medication should be prepared. If giving ICe fluids, the fluids should be warmed to the snake's POTZ before administering.

Oral (PO)

Oral medications are very easy to give to snakes. The medication is drawn up into a syringe and then a red rubber catheter is attached to the end. To prevent it from passing into the trachea, the catheter should be too large to fit into the trachea. One should also open the mouth to ensure that the catheter has gone down the esophagus. After checking for correct placement, administration of the medication can begin. Using another syringe filled with water, the medication should be flushed down to ensure that no medicine is left in the catheter. This method can also be used to assist-fed snakes.

Venipuncture

Tail Vein

The snake can be placed in either dorsal or ventral recumbency (Figure 10.45). With the bevel of the needle facing cranially, the needle is inserted exactly on the midline at a 45° angle. While maintaining gentle suction, the needle is advanced until a flash of blood is seen. Occasionally the coccygeal vertebrae will be hit first and the flash of blood will be seen as the needle is withdrawn. The needle should be inserted caudal to the hemipenes and scent glands. With smaller snakes, a gentle suction and release may suffice to receive enough blood to perform diagnostic testing.

Cardiocentesis

Locate the heart by either manual palpation or by Doppler. One should apply pressure just caudal and cranial to the heart to stabilize it. After the heart has been stabilized, the needle is inserted at a 45–60° angle and advanced until a slight pop is felt indicating that the needle has entered the heart. One should then aspirate back until enough sample has been taken. Occasionally, pericardial fluid may be aspirated. If this happens, the needle should be withdrawn and the procedure started over with a fresh needle and syringe (Figures 10.46 and 10.47).

Palatine Vein

As stated previously, accessing the palatine vein is only recommended in a snake with a clean oral cavity and no signs of stomatitis. Moreover, this technique will only work

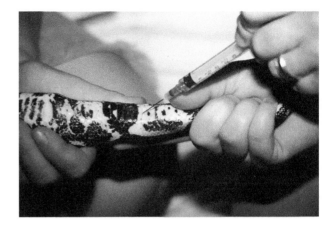

Figure 10.45 Venipuncture using the tail vein.

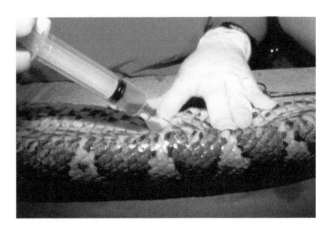

Figure 10.46 Cardiocentesis. The snake is placed dorsally on a table (Courtesy of Zoo Atlanta).

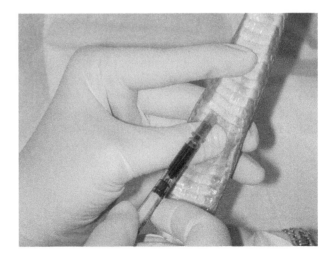

Figure 10.47 Cardiocentesis. The snake is held off of the table and the back is supported by the venipuncturist. (Courtesy of Jody Nugent-Deal).

on very docile or anesthetized snakes. One should restrain the snake with its mouth open. A 25–27-gauge needle is advanced into the vein; aspirate gently to prevent the vein from collapsing. Due to the risk of contamination from the saliva, this vein is best used only for IV injections, and as a last resort.

Intravenous Catheter Placement

The jugular vein is the preferred site for IV catheter placement. A cut-down incision is required for this procedure. The skin should be surgically prepped, and the incision made at the junction of the ventral scutes and lateral scales, just cranial to the heart by about four to seven scutes. It is necessary to bluntly dissect to expose the vein. Then the catheter is inserted until a flash is seen in the hub, whereupon the catheter is advanced into the vein. The skin is closed using sutures and with the catheter sutured to the skin. A bandage can be placed to keep the catheter site clean.

Other sites for IV access would include the heart and palatine vein. The palatine vein is only accessible while a patient is anesthetized and this route should not be used in venomous species due to the possibility of accidental envenomation. In an extreme emergency, a catheter can be placed in the heart for a short time. Employing the technique used for venipuncture. Once the catheter is placed, it should be secured with suture or tape.

Assist Feeding

One should properly restrain the snake with its mouth open. An appropriately sized prey item is grasped with large hemostats and copious lubrication is applied to the entire body of the prey. The prey is then inserted into the snake's mouth, gently forcing it down. Once the prey is completely inserted, one should milk the prey down the esophagus until it reaches the stomach. Care is taken that the prey does not scratch the esophagus with its incisors or claws. An easy way to prevent this is to trim the claws and teeth before assist feeding (Figure 10.48).

Ideally, snakes can also be assist fed by using the technique for giving oral medications. Liquefied whole prey or artificially prepared foods can be used. For neonates or smaller snakes, a device called a pinkie press can be used (Figure 10.49).

Tracheal and Lung Wash

Restrain the snake with its mouth open and pass a sterile red rubber catheter into the trachea; sedation is often needed. Once the catheter is in place, infuse sterile saline into the trachea and lung. Do not place more than 5 mL/kg

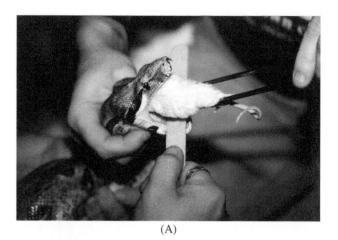

(A)

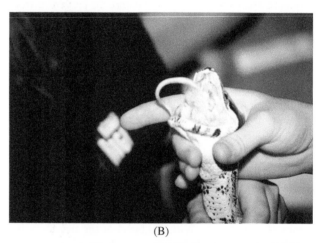

(B)

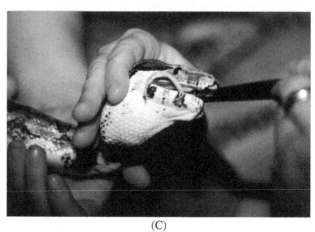

(C)

Figure 10.48 Assist feeding a snake. (A) The snake is properly restrained and a tongue depressor is used to open the mouth. The prey is then inserted into the oral cavity. (B) The prey is almost completely into the oral cavity. (C) Then the prey is gently pushed down the esophagus.

into the lung. After the sterile saline has been administered, aspirate as much of the saline as possible. The saline can be injected and aspirated as many times as needed to receive a proper amount of sample (Figure 10.50).

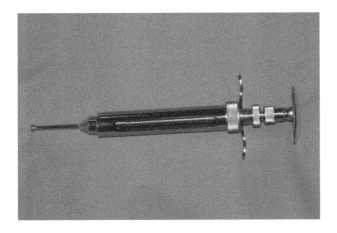

Figure 10.49 Pinkie press. Pinkies are inserted into the syringe and is then liquified by the compression of the syringe.

Colonic Wash and Enema

A well-lubricated red rubber catheter is inserted into the colon by entering the cloaca and aiming the catheter ventrally. Using a saline-filled syringe, begin flushing the saline into the colon and aspirating it back. This step should be repeated several times to get an adequate sample. This process also helps soften stools in constipated snakes. After aspiration, the sample can then be analyzed for parasites, cytology, and culture (Figure 10.51).

Venomous Snakes

It is not recommended to keep venomous snakes in private collections, especially by novice hobbyists. In some cases, it may be illegal to keep venomous snakes without proper permits. For this reason, it is rare that one would be brought into private practice for medical care. If this does occur, however, proper protocols need to be implemented. Whether a veterinary practice is even equipped for safe handling of venomous snakes needs to be addressed. At the very least, snake tongs, hooks, and tubes are needed for safer handling. Also, someone trained in handling venomous snakes is required. Although one can practice tubing and handling techniques on non-venomous snakes, there is obviously more risk involved in dealing with the venomous ones, and other people could be put at risk as well.

Most procedures on venomous snakes should be done while the snake is under anesthesia. This involves either tubing or placing the snake in an immobilization chamber. One should not attempt to manually restrain the head of a venomous snake. Those who milk snakes for venom have to do so but it is not a safe method of restraint. Some fangs are long enough to penetrate a hand while restraining the head.

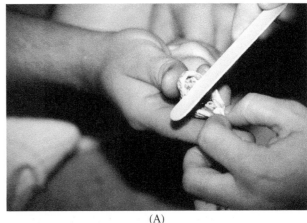

(A)

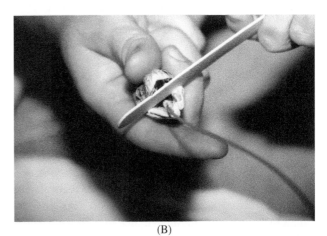

(B)

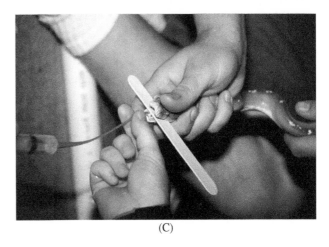

(C)

Figure 10.50 Tracheal wash. (A) With the snake properly restrained the mouth is opened. (B) A tongue depressor is used as a mouth gag, and the red rubber catheter is inserted into the trachea. (C) 0.9% sodium chloride is then gently flushed into the trachea and then aspirated back.

An envenomation protocol also needs to be in place at the facility. Most human hospitals only have antivenom for bites sustained by indigenous species. Imported species pose a greater risk to handlers due to the lack of accessible

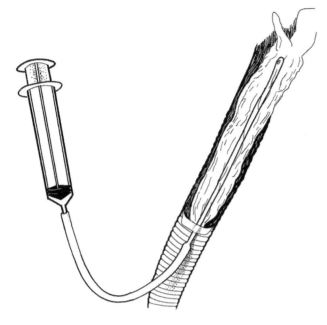

Figure 10.51 Colonic wash. The catheter should be inserted deep into the colon, especially if this procedure is done to relieve constipation. (Drawing by Scott Stark).

antivenom. Most facilities that handle venomous snakes keep the different types of antivenom in stock, not necessarily for self-administration should a bite occur, but to supply the nearest hospital if the hospital does not have any on hand. This is difficult though, due to both the expense involved and the lack of accessibility. Expiration dates on the antivenom have to be closely monitored as well.

One should establish secure lines of communication with local hospitals to see who is able to handle a venomous snakebite patient. Contacting the local poison control facility to establish a protocol would be helpful as well. Once again, these are all things that need to be addressed before venomous snakes are managed at the facility. Minutes count should a venomous snakebite occur, and one cannot afford to waste time calling hospitals to see if they can handle that particular bite. If this seems like too much of a hassle, then handling/treating venomous snakes should not be undertaken at all. Following are some basic guidelines that should be met if venomous species are seen:

- Never handle a venomous snake alone. Always have at a minimum two people.
- The snake should be handled in an enclosed room where, if the snake escapes, it cannot hide under or in anything.
- Never try handling the venomous snake without all of the appropriate equipment. If handling any of the spitting cobra species, wear full facial protection.
- The appointment should be scheduled at a time when no other clients and minimal staff will be on site. This will help eliminate possible exposures.

- The snake should be brought to the clinic inside a solid-sided, locked device such as a plastic or wooden box or plastic bucket. The owner of the snake should bring antivenom with them if the clinic does not have any. Enough antivenom to treat two people should be available.
- The snake should only be handled by trained individuals, even if anesthetized or inside a restraint tube.

Euthanasia

Unfortunately, not all patients can be saved. And although veterinary medicine has the privilege of being able to humanely euthanize animals suffering with terminal illnesses, euthanizing snakes can prove to be a difficult task. There are several humane methods of euthanasia that are acceptable in snakes.

One method starts with an injection of a sedative or anesthetic. If injectable anesthetics are not available, inhalant anesthesia can be used. Due to the ability of snakes to hold their breath for long periods of time, this can be a very lengthy process. After the snake is anesthetized or heavily sedated, a cardiac stick is performed and an overdose of a barbiturate is injected. In very small species or very dehydrated snakes, a cardiac stick can be difficult. In that case, a simple ICe injection of a barbiturate can be performed. It can take several minutes to several hours before the snake is finally deceased using this method. After the injection, the snake should be placed in a heated cage so that proper metabolism of the medication can occur.

The most difficult part of euthanizing snakes is determining death. There is no good answer to the question, is the snake deceased? An electrocardiograph, auscultation of the heart, or a Doppler can all be used to determine if the snake is deceased, but because reptile hearts can still beat for several hours postmortem, perhaps even once or twice per minute, these three tests can prove inaccurate. Many reptile clinicians have heard stories of the snake coming back to life 24 hours after the euthanasia. This can be easily avoided if the snake is left in the hospital overnight for observation.

Being a Responsible Snake Owner

As a part of the veterinary team, the technician is responsible for properly informing and educating clients of the needs of particular animals. It is also important to offer guidance when purchases are being considered. Knowing what is involved in snake care and having specific information about different species of snakes will aid in giving advice to those considering purchasing a snake as a pet.

Offering consultations to clients before purchases will help to eliminate a lot of the problems that arise after a snake is purchased. Snakes, in general, do not make good pets. This should be kept in mind when offering advice to potential buyers. Buying a snake that will reach lengths of 10 ft (3 m) or more is obviously not a choice that should be made by most people. These snakes often become neglected and the owners sometimes become fearful of them due to their size and sometimes their disposition, which may become aggressive.

More and more people are devising ways to get rid of their snakes when it is no longer convenient to own them. All too often these snakes are impulse buys that are thought of as disposable belongings. The most appalling of these occurrences is when people let them go in their backyards when they "don't want to deal with them anymore." Most captive specimens are not even indigenous to the country where their owners set them free. Not only will it most likely kill the animal, but it can upset the natural balance of that particular ecosystem. Some even choose to freeze the snake as their way of humanely euthanizing the animal so they will no longer be burdened. There is nothing humane about freezing a live animal. It is in fact a slow, painful death.

If it is decided that a snake is no longer wanted, then attempts should be made to place it in a home or facility that is ready and able to meet its needs. Mostly this occurs with the larger species of snakes. They can reach astounding lengths and girths and can be extremely dangerous—not to mention the size of the enclosure needed to properly house them. These are obviously not for novice keepers and should be discouraged when an inexperienced individual inquiries about obtaining one.

Another point to make about being a responsible snake owner is understanding that a lot of people fear them. Taking them out to public places to show them off is not doing the public any favors, especially not the snake. The snake may become scared by commotion, and its presence may cause alarm in people nearby. This is doing an injustice to the individual snake and to snakes in general. The public, as a whole, has a terrible phobia of snakes and forcing the issue by bringing snakes into public places only makes it worse. If owners want to display their snakes, they should offer educational exhibits and lectures. By displaying them in this way they can create a learning environment and the people have the choice whether to participate or not. A phobia (no matter how silly one thinks it is) is a phobia, and it is not something that can be changed forcibly.

References

Bennett RA. 1997. Reptilian surgery, parts 1 and 2. In: *Practical Exotic Animal Medicine* (ed KL Rosenthal). New Jersey: Veterinary Learning Systems.

Bennett RA. 1996. Anesthesia. In: *Reptile Medicine and Surgery* (ed DR Mader). Philadelphia: W.B. Saunders Co.

Bennett RA, Lock BA. 2000. Nonreproductive surgery in reptiles. In: *Veterinary Clinics of North America: Exotic Animal Practice*. Phildadelpia: W.B. Saunders Co.

Bertelsen MF. 2007. Squamates (snakes and lizards). In: *Zoo Animal & Wildlife Immobilization and Anesthesia* (eds G West, D Heard, N Caulkett). Iowa: Blackwell Publishing.

Blackburn DG, Stewart JR. 2011. Viviparity and placentation in snakes. In: *Reproductive Biology and Phylogeny of Snakes* (eds RD Aldrich, DM Sever) Enfield: Science Publishers.

Bradley T. 2001. Pain management considerations and pain-associated behaviors in reptiles and amphibians. In: Proceedings of the Association of Reptilian and Amphibian Veterinarians. Eastern State Vet Ass.

Darrow B, Myers G, KuKanich B, Sladky K. 2016. Fentanyl transdermal therapeutic system provides rapid systemic fenanyl absorption in two ball pythons (*Python regius*). *J Herpetol Med Surg* 26(3–4): 94–99.

Divers SJ. 2000. Reptilian renal and reproductive disease and diagnosis. In: *Laboratory Medicine: Avian and Exotic Pets* (ed AM Fudge). Philadelphia: W.B. Saunders Co.

Driggers T. 2000. Respiratory diseases, diagnostics, and therapy in snakes. In: *In the Veterinary Clinics of North America: Exotic Animal Medicine*. Philadelphia: W.B. Saunders Co.

Fitzgerald KT, Knafo SE. 2019. Spinal osteopathy. In: *Reptile Medicine and Surgery* (eds S Divers, S Stahl), 3rd edn. Missouri: Elsevier.

Funk RS. 1996. Snakes. In: *Reptile Medicine and Surgery* (ed DR Mader). Philadelphia: W.B. Saunders Co.

Glynn MK, et al. 2001. Knowledge and practices of California veterinarians concerning the human health threat of reptile-associated salmonellosis. *J Herpetol Med Surg* 11(2): 9–13.

Holz PH. 1999. The reptilian renal-portal system: influence on therapy. In: *Zoo and Wild Animal Medicine: Current Therapy* (eds ME Fowler, RE Miller), 4th edn. Philadelphia: W.B. Saunders Co.

Lawton MP. 2019. Ophthalmology. In: *Reptile medicine and surgery* (eds S Divers, S Stahl), 3rd edn. Missouri: Elsevier.

Lawton MP. 2001. Fluid therapy in reptiles. In: Proceedings of the North American Veterinary Conference. Eastern States Vet Ass.

Lawton MP. 1991. Lizards and snakes. In: *Manual of Exotic Pets* (eds PH Beymon et al.). Ames: Iowa State University Press.

Lock BA. 2000. Reproductive surgery in reptiles. In: *Veterinary Clinics of North America: Exotic Animal Practice.* Philadelphia: W.B. Saunders Co.

Mans C, Sladky K, Schumacher J. 2019. General anesthesia. In: *Reptile Medicine and Surgery* (eds S Divers, S Stahl), 3rd edn. Missouri: Elsevier.

Marschang RE. 2019. Virology. In: *Reptile Medicine and Surgery* (eds S Divers, S Stahl), 3rd edn. Missouri: Elsevier.

Miller HA. 1998. Urinary diseases of reptiles: pathophysiology and diagnosis. In: *Seminars in Avian and Exotic Pet Medicine* (ed AM Fudge). Philadelphia: W.B. Saunders Co.

Origgi F. 2019. Inclusion body disease. In: *Reptile Medicine and Surgery* (eds S Divers, S Stahl), 3rd edn. Missouri: Elsevier.

Platel R. 1994. Nervous system and sensory organs. In: *Snakes: A Natural History* (ed R Bauchot). New York: Sterling Publishing.

Pough FH, et al. 2001. *Herpetology.* 2d edn. New Jersey: Prentice-Hall Inc.

Rockwell K, Mitchell M. 2019. Antiparasitic therapy. In: *Reptile Medicine and Surgery* (eds S Divers, S Stahl), 3rd edn. Missouri: Elsevier.

Romer AS. 1997. *Osteology of the Reptiles.* Reprint. Malabar, FL: Krieger Publishing.

Ross RA, et al. 1990. *The Reproductive Husbandry of Pythons and Boas.* The Institute for Herpetological Research, Stanford, CA.

Saint-Girons H. 1994. Growth and reproduction. In: *Snakes: A Natural History* (ed Roland Bauchot). New York: Sterling Publishing.

Schilling LH, Morel D, Bonwitt JH, Marquis O. 2013. Cheyletus eruditus (tarrus): an effective candidate for the biological control of the snake mite (Ophionyssus natricis). *J Zoo Wildlife Med*; 44(3): 654–659.

Schumacher J, Yelen T. 2006. Anesthesia and analgesia. In: *Reptile Medicine and Surgery* (ed DR Mader), 2nd edn. Missouri: Saunders Elsevier.

Vasse Y. 1994. A cardiovascular system working against the forces of gravity. In: *Snakes: A Natural History* (ed R Bauchot). New York: Sterling Publishing.

Wellehan J, Walden H. 2019. Parasitology (including hemoparasites). In: *Reptile Medicine and Surgery* (eds S Divers, S Stahl), 3rd edn. Missouri: Elsevier.

Zug GR, et al. 2001. *Herpetology: An Introductory Biology of Amphibians and Reptiles*, 2nd edn. New York: Academic Press.

11

Chelonians

Sarah Camlic, Ryan Cheek, Pia Bartolini, and Samuel Rivera

Introduction

Chelonians belong to the class Reptilia, which is divided into four orders: Testudines (all chelonians), Crocodilia (crocodilians), Squamata (snakes and lizards), and Rhynchocephalia (tuatara). Chelonians are a group of animals that evolved into a shelled form millions of years ago. There are approximately 300 living species in the order Chelonia, with hundreds of species kept in captivity (Figures 11.1–11.3). Chelonians are divided into two suborders, the Cryptodira (hidden-necked) and Pleurodira (side-necked), referring to the way in which they withdraw their head and necks into their shell. Chelonians are extremely diverse, including the largest chelonian—the fully aquatic leatherback sea turtle (*Dermochelys coriacea*), the semi-aquatic and semi-infamous alligator snapping turtle (*Macrochelys temminckii*), popular pets such as the sulcata tortoise (*Centrochelys sulcata*) and the red-eared slider (*Trachemys scripta elegans*), and the largest terrestrial chelonian, the Galápagos tortoise (*Chelonoidis niger*).

Any discussion of chelonians requires first acknowledging the lack of standardized nomenclature: "turtle," "tortoise," and "terrapin" all have different meanings regionally, as well as in scientific versus common terminology. In the United States, "turtle" is most often used to reference any chelonian, but many use it to refer only to aquatic chelonians, sometimes with the exception of the terrestrial box turtles (*Terrapene* spp.) and wood turtles (*Glyptemys* and *Rhinoclemmys* spp.). "Tortoise" colloquially can refer to all terrestrial chelonians, or specifically to members of the Testudinidae family. To sum it up, some would say "all tortoises are turtles, but not all turtles are tortoises." Terrapins do not form a true taxonomic unit, and in the United States, the term is used infrequently by laypeople.

Elsewhere in the world, such as the United Kingdom, "turtle" is used to refer to marine species, and "terrapin" is

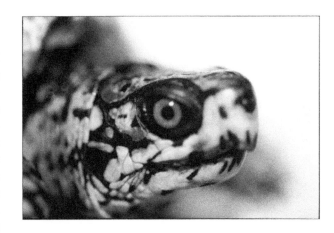

Figure 11.1 Male eastern box turtle (*Terrapene carolina carolina*) showing red eye.

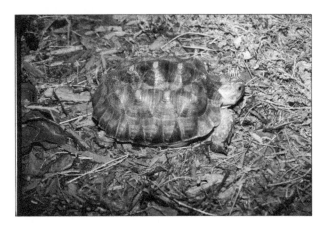

Figure 11.2 Sulcata tortoise (*Geochelone sulcata*).

used much more frequently to refer to a large group of semi-aquatic turtles found in fresh or brackish water. Because of the confusion in terminology, chelonians are often listed by their scientific name, which is uniform around the world.

As chelonians, and reptiles in general, become more popular as pets, it is important that veterinary staff have at

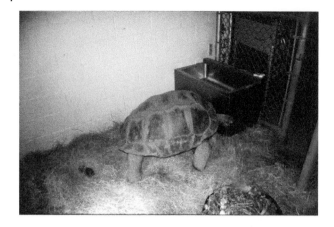

Figure 11.3 Aldabra tortoise (*Aldabrachelys gigantea*).

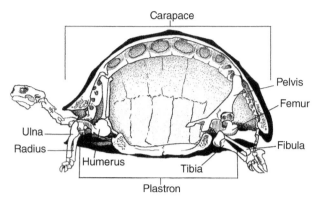

Figure 11.4 Skeletal anatomy. (Drawing by Scott Stark.)

least a basic understanding of how to care for these animals when they are injured or ill, and the ability to educate owners on proper wellness care. The goal of this chapter is to provide a basic understanding of chelonian anatomy, physiology, husbandry, common health problems, and basic clinical techniques.

Anatomy and Physiology

Musculoskeletal System

The most recognizable feature of chelonians is their shell, which is divided into two main parts. The dorsal portion of the shell is called the carapace, and the ventral portion the plastron; these two major components are connected by a bridge on either side extending from the plastron.

All species have 8 cervical and 10 thoracic vertebrae. The thoracic vertebrae, along with their expanded ribs, are fused to dermal bones to form the carapace. The ribs are single-headed, and the first and tenth ribs are significantly smaller than the others and often fused to their neighboring ribs.

The dermal bones along the dorsal midline are unpaired, and from cranial to caudal are the nuchal bone, the neural bones (usually eight), the suprapygal bone(s) (one or two), and the pygal bone. The neural bones are attached to the vertebrae. The costal bones are located on either side of the neural bones. The peripheral bones are located lateral to the costal bones and extend from the nuchal to the pygal bones on both sides of the carapace (Figure 11.4).

The bones of the plastron are less easily comparable to other animals, but investigations into their ontogeny suggest that the bones of the plastron are most likely homologous to the clavicles and gastralia (abdominal ribs) of other tetrapods, with the addition of the dermal bones unique to

chelonians. Chelonians show no embryological evidence of developing a sternum.

The plastron consists of eight paired bones and one unpaired bone. The unpaired entoplastral bone is on ventral midline and is surrounded by the epiplastral bones cranially and hyoplastral bones caudally. The hyoplastral bones are followed by the hypoplastral and xiphiplastral bones, consecutively. Some chelonians, most notably the accordingly named box turtle, have ligamentous hinges between plastral bones allowing them to close their shells partially or totally. In the box turtle, this hinge is located between the hyoplastral and hypoplastral bones. While in most chelonians, the margins of the scutes and plastral bones do not line up, in species with kinetic shells the margins correspond to allow the fully functional hinge.

Some species of chelonians have sexually dimorphic shells, with the males' being concave and the females' being more convex/steep to facilitate mounting; caution should be used in relying on this for sexing, especially in captive animals, as animals with improper husbandry may have abnormal shell morphology.

Chelonians have a triradiate pectoral girdle located deep to "inside" the carapace, consisting of the vertically oriented scapula with a more cranioventral prescapular process (acromion) and a caudoventrally oriented procoracoid. The acromion attaches to the plastron and the scapula attaches to the pleural bones and vertebrae by ligamentous and muscular connections. The pelvis is attached to the vertebral column by fibrous sacroiliac joints.

The bones of chelonians are overall homologous to those of other tetrapods, with the limb shape modified based on habitat, most drastically seen in sea turtles' flippers (Abdala et al., 2008).

The chelonian skull is unique among reptiles (and all living amniotes), in that it has no temporal fenestrae, which are openings in the skull that serve as muscular attachments. While species with no temporal fenestrae are classified as "anapsid," phylogenetic studies have provided evidence that chelonians are descended from diapsids and reverted to an anapsid-like state. The shape of the skull varies based on environment and feeding strategies of each species.

Integument

The portion of the chelonian epidermis on the limbs, head, neck, and tail is consistent with the general description of reptilian epidermis provided in Chapter 9. Terrestrial species often have very thickened areas of scales on the distal portions of their limbs that contribute to their defenses when their limbs are retracted into the shell.

The bones of the shell (detailed in the Section Musculoskeletal System) are covered with structures made of keratinized epithelium called scutes, with thin hinge regions between them. All scutes have names, which is useful for more exactly documenting lesion locations in written records. On the carapace, the scutes on the midline are unpaired; the most cranial is the nuchal scute (occasionally called the cervical scute), which is followed by five vertebral scutes. On either side of the vertebrals are a row of four costal scutes, and the scutes outlining the periphery are the marginal scutes. The plastron has six pairs of scutes, which from cranial to caudal are the gular, humeral, pectoral, abdominal, femoral, and anal scutes. The vast majority of chelonians follow this body plan, but there are some exceptions. Some have additional inframarginal scutes ventral to the marginal scutes, or additional axillary and/or inguinal scutes ventral to the limbs. Chelonians within the suborder Pleurodira will have an unpaired intergular scute between the gulars, while those in the other suborder, Cryptodira, do not.

Chelonians with softer shells, such as leatherback sea turtles (*Dermochelys coriacea*), pig-nosed turtles (*Carettochelys insculpta*), and those within the order Trionychidae "soft-shell turtles," have reduced ossification of the shell and do not have scutes.

Most terrestrial chelonians do not shed their scutes under normal conditions, and instead add new layers of epithelium to the base of the scute, forming visible rings of growth. The growth pattern of these scutes can show evidence of environmental/nutritional issues, which will be discussed in further detail later in this chapter. In aquatic turtles, during growth periods a lipid-rich layer of alpha-keratin forms from the hinge region toward the center of the scute and allows separation and shedding of the old corneus beta-keratin layer from the new one. There are some exceptions, such as the terrestrial box turtle (*Terrapene carolina*) which sheds scutes, and the freshwater American Blanding's turtle (*Emydoidea blandingii*), which does not shed them.

Cardiovascular System

As in squamates, chelonians have a three-chambered heart consisting of two atria and one semi-divided ventricle, from which the pulmonary artery and left and right aortic arches arise. Due to the anatomy of the ventricle, reptiles are capable of intracardiac shunting, which is important during phases of prolonged hypoxia or anoxia. This ability, along with the "dive reflex" and cardiac monitoring, are discussed in greater detail in the Anesthesia section. Like other reptiles, turtles have a renal portal circulation system, which functions to provide an alternate blood supply to the renal tubular cells and prevent ischemic necrosis when the arterial blood supply to the glomerulus is compromised (Holz 1999).

Chelonians have lymphatic vessels that are closely associated with their blood vessels; dilution of blood samples with lymph is a common occurrence.

Blood collection can be uniquely challenging in chelonians due to the presence of the shell. The jugular vein, which lies on the lateral aspect of the neck at the level of the tympanic scale, is ideal due to the decreased chance of lymph contamination and large volume able to be obtained but can be difficult or impossible to access without sedation.

The brachial vein/venous plexus, also called the ulnar vein, is the next most ideal location in terms of minimal lymph contamination; this site is located at the inner elbow ventral to the biceps brachii tendon. However, this location provides smaller volumes than the jugular, limiting its use to larger animals, and can still be difficult to access in awake chelonians.

The subcarapacial (located on dorsal midline caudal to the nuchal scute and dorsal to the cervical vertebrae) and dorsal coccygeal sinuses (on dorsal midline of the tail) are more accessible in awake patients who have retracted into their shells but have proximity to large lymphatics and the vertebral column, making lymph contamination a common occurrence and spinal trauma a more rare but certainly present risk.

More specific instructions on venipuncture, catheter placement, and routes of administration are discussed in the Clinical Techniques section later in this chapter.

Respiratory System

Chelonians breathe through paired nostrils located at the dorsocranial aspect of the premaxilla, which connect to internal nares (choanae) via the nasal sinus. The glottis is located at the base of the tongue. The trachea is relatively short and flexible to allow retraction of the head and is comprised of complete rings. It bifurcates into two mainstream bronchi that open into the paired lungs. The lungs are large, compartmentalized structures (multicameral) with a reticular surface containing bands of smooth muscle and connective tissue. The lungs are attached to the ventral aspect of the carapace and the viscera via connective tissue. As in all reptiles, turtles do not have a diaphragm. As chelonians do not have intercostal muscles and their ribs are rigidly fixed within the carapace, they cannot engage in costal ventilation like squamates. Instead, respiration is achieved by multiple opposing muscles whose contractions work to change the intracoelomic pressure, including the large serratus and transversus abdominus. Aquatic turtles can exchange oxygen through the mucosal surface of the oral cavity and cloaca. Soft-shelled turtles can exchange oxygen through their skin (Girgis 1961).

Chelonians, especially sea turtles, have a remarkable tolerance for low oxygen conditions and can breath-hold for extended periods of time (Trevizan-Baú et al. 2018; Lutcavage & Lutz 1991). The effects of chelonian's unique respiratory physiology on anesthesia and manual ventilation will be discussed later in this chapter.

Digestive System

Chelonians lack teeth and instead utilize their sharp beak to tear food. The tongue is short and unable to extend from the oral cavity, and in some aquatic species acts as an epiglottis by covering the tracheal opening (Fraher et al. 2010). Chelonian salivary glands do not produce digestive enzymes; these are secreted further along in the GI tract. In sea turtles, the oropharynx and esophagus have large caudally-facing conical papillae that help prevent retrograde movement of prey items such as jellyfish.

As in lizards, the alimentary tract consists of an esophagus, stomach, small and large intestine, and cloaca, which lie in the pleuroperitoneum (coelom) along with the other viscera. The esophagus lies along the left side of the neck. The stomach is in the left cranioventral aspect of the coelomic cavity encompassed by the left liver lobe. The small intestine has histologically discrete sections which can be grossly difficult to discern. The small intestine, cecum, and colon vary in size based on feeding strategy of each species, as does GI transit time. The GI tract empties into the coprodeum of the cloaca (Figure 11.5).

The liver and gallbladder are present in chelonians. The liver has two lobes (left and right) and has fossae for the heart, gallbladder, and stomach. The pancreas can be located near the spleen or in the mesentery along the duodenum and has both endocrine and exocrine glandular function.

Excretory System

Paired lobulated metanephric kidneys are located in the caudodorsal coelom. A renal portal system exists, with

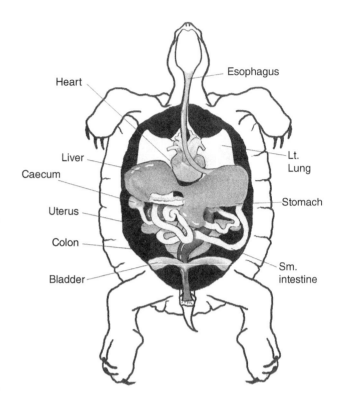

Figure 11.5 Visceral anatomy. (Drawing by Scott Stark.)

some anatomical variation among species; flow can be variable, allowing blood from the caudal body to bypass the kidneys. As in other reptiles, they lack a loop of Henle and are thus incapable of concentrating their urine above plasma tonicity. Nitrogenous waste excretion varies by species depending on habitat, with aquatic species tending to produce more urea and terrestrial species more uric acid. The ureters course caudoventrally into the urodeum of the cloaca, which has a cranioventral connection to the bilobed urinary bladder. Urine from the bladder can travel retrograde into the colon for reabsorption of water; terrestrial species in arid environments are known to store large volumes of urine within their bladders.

Animals will often void this stored urine when handled or otherwise stressed, and replacement of this fluid volume should be considered by the veterinary team, especially in any animals that are being imminently released back into the wild.

Reproductive System

Chelonians have paired testicles and ovaries that lie cranioventral and cranial, respectively, to their kidneys. All chelonians are oviparous, with the shell glands within the uterine portion of the oviduct forming the eggshell; the composition/rigidity of the shell is species-dependent.

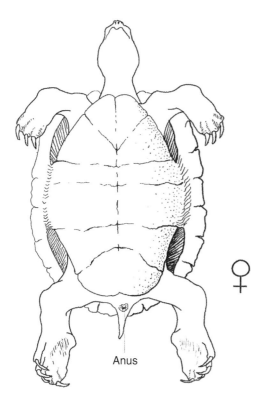

Figure 11.6 Female secondary sexual characteristics. (Drawing by Scott Stark.)

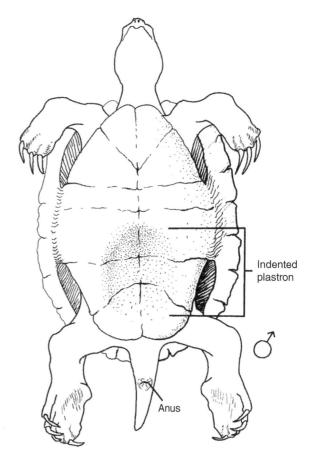

Figure 11.7 Male secondary sexual characteristics. (Drawing by Scott Stark.)

The oviducts and ductus deferentes empty into the proctodeum, the most caudal portion of the cloaca. The phallus is located on the ventral aspect of the proctodeum and has a central sulcus for semen delivery. It does not have urinary function, allowing amputation in the case of non-reducible and/or non-viable prolapse.

There is some sexual dimorphism among chelonians (Figures 11.6 and 11.7). Sexual size dimorphism is variable based on species and environment (Agha et al. 2018), and of course, captive individuals of varying ages and nutritional status should not be blindly compared regardless of the dimorphism of their wild counterparts. The male vent (cloacal opening) is usually located more caudally on the tail, past the shell margin. Male pond turtles (Family Emydidae) will often have more vibrant irises. In aquatic species, males will often have significantly longer nails on their forelimbs, but this can differ regionally even within species (Gibbons & Lovich 1990). As previously mentioned in the Musculoskeletal System section, males of some species have a concave plastron to allow mounting, and male tortoises also may have enlarged gular scutes for ramming the female during courtship; again, nutritional history should be considered when relying on skeletal traits for sex identification.

For many captive chelonians, owners are often unaware of their turtles' sex unless eggs are laid, or the phallus is prolapsed. Endoscopic sexing (coelioscopy and cloacoscopy) has become increasingly popular, especially with individuals or organizations that maintain breeding populations (Innis 2010; Stahl & DeNardo 2019).

Nervous System

The general arrangement of the chelonian nervous system is like the other amniotes: The central nervous system consists of a cerebrum, cerebellum, brainstem, and spinal cord, which as in other reptiles extends through the tail. The peripheral nervous system includes the 12 cranial nerves and many other peripheral nerves throughout the body.

While some reptiles can regenerate limbs and tails, chelonians are unique among amniotes in their ability to regain function after complete spinal cord transection, though function is usually limited compared to pre-injury (Rehermann et al. 2009).

Chelonians have also demonstrated "spinal walking" and "spinal swimming," reflexive movement patterns allowing hindlimb locomotion with severe spinal cord injury—this has been demonstrated in other amniotes including mammals (Stein 2018).

Sense Organs

Chelonians have moveable eyelids and a nictitating membrane; they lack a nasolacrimal duct.

Both lacrimal and Harderian glands are present in the adnexa. Scleral ossicles and cartilage are present in lizards. As in other reptiles, pupil dilation is under conscious control due to the presence of striated muscle in the iris. Chelonian eyes contain both rods and cones. The conus papillaris is a projection from the optic nerve that can be seen on fundic exam.

There is no external auditory meatus in chelonians; the tympanic membrane is covered by skin. Like most lizards, chelonians have a well-developed tympanic middle ear with a single ossicle, the columella, that connects to the tympanic membrane via the extracollumelar cartilage and expands into a cone shape at the oval window. While usually air-filled, in sea turtles varying amounts of fat are present within the middle ear. Chelonians have a bony otic capsule, and a narrow eustachian tube connecting the middle ear to the pharynx, features much more like mammals than other reptiles. There is evidence that chelonians are more sensitive to underwater sound than airborne sound (Christensen-Dalsgaard et al. 2012).

Chelonians have a well-developed olfactory system that likely plays a role in both feeding and social situations (Galeotti et al. 2007). It is thought that when chelonians exhibit "gular pumping" this is to aid in olfaction, not respiration (Druzisky & Brainerd 2001).

Husbandry and Nutrition

There are dozens of species of chelonia seen in the pet trade, and it is beyond the scope of this chapter to cover exact husbandry by species. A brief overview of the husbandry and nutritional requirements of aquatic, semi-aquatic, and terrestrial species will be given.

Aquatic and Semi-aquatic Species

Truly aquatic species of chelonian are only represented by the sea turtle species (*Dermochelys coriacea* and *Chelonidae* sp.), only coming out of the water for oviposition. Most other turtles are classified as semi-aquatic. How much of their daily life is in or out of the water is variable by species, and colloquially many are often appropriately referred to as aquatic. The use of the terms aquatic and semi-aquatic

are just as variable as the terms turtle and terrapin. For example, *Cuora* sp. and *Terrapene* sp. (Asian and North American box turtles) spend very little time in the water. They are mostly found wandering the land near water, yet can be found having an occasional snack in the water or sitting in shallow streams or ponds to get some water or relief from the hot sun. These species are typically considered terrestrial and their care will be discussed in the Tortoises and Terrestrial Turtles section below. On the other side, the pig-nosed turtle (*Carettochelys insculpta*) spends almost their entire life in the water, only occasionally coming out for thermoregulation or to scavenge some food on the banks of the rivers. Due to the differences in the natural history between species, the amount of water, depth of the water, and the amount of land will vary from species to species; however, the basic principles of husbandry for semi-aquatic species is the same for every species. This section will not discuss the captive husbandry or nutrition of sea turtles.

When considering setting up an enclosure of a semi-aquatic species, the first thing to consider is the overall size. There have been a few different methods of determining this. The Federation of British Herpetologists (2022) have suggested a minimum size of 8×4 plastron length (PL). The PL is the straight-line measurement of the plastron. This is generally a more accurate measurement from the straight carapace length (SCL) or carapace length (CL) which is the straight-line measurement from the most cranial aspect of the carapace to the most caudal aspect. The SCL or CL is not the distance over the dome of the carapace which makes this measurement more difficult to obtain. Once the PL is obtained, that measurement is multiplied by 8 to get the length and 4 to get the width. The height of the enclosure is determined by the species' need for water and land. For turtles that spend most of their time in the water, a minimum depth of water should be four times the carapace height. This will allow the turtle room to swim freely and stay submerged. This recommendation is easy as it gives actual floor and height measurements. Other references have suggested a minimum area of $4\,m^2$ for every $1\,m$ CL (Rossi 2019). This recommendation gives no specific calculation for water depth. More specific recommendations have been made that separate tortoise/semi-aquatic species to aquatic species as well as stating minimum versus ideal sizes. Those recommendations suggest for semi-aquatic species that the minimum size should be $0.2\,m^2/0.1\,m$ CL and an ideal size of $0.5\,m^2/0.1\,m$ CL. Aquatic species would need a minimum of $0.2\,m^3/0.1\,m$ CL and an ideal size of $0.5\,m^3/0.1\,m$ CL (Divers 1996). For these recommendations, an aquatic species would be one that rarely leaves the water. These last two recommendations do not give actual enclosure measurements so those have to be determined based on the square or cubic meters calculated. Regardless of the method used, these sizes are for a singly-housed turtle. About 20% should be added for each additional animal. See examples of these recommendations below:

For these examples, we will be using a turtle with a 0.2 m (8 in.) carapace or PL and a 0.07 m (3 in.) carapace height that is housed alone.

Example 1   8 × 4 PL and 4× carapace height

Cage dimensions should be 1.6 m long and 0.8 m wide with a water height of 0.28 m. This equals 1.28 m^2 or 0.36 m^3.

Example 2   4 m^2 for every 1 m CL

Cage size area of 0.8 m^2.

Example 3   semi-aquatic species: minimum size of 0.2 m^2/0.1 m CL and ideal size of 0.5 m^2/0.1 m CL

Minimum cage size area of 0.4 m^2
Recommended cage size area of 1.0 m^2

Example 4   aquatic species: minimum size of 0.2 m^3/0.1 m CL and ideal size of 0.5 m^3/0.1 m CL

Minimum cage size area of 0.4 m^3
Recommended cage size area of 1.0 m^3

Water quality is another factor that must be considered when caring for an aquatic or semi-aquatic species. Fortunately, chelonians do not breath through gills so ultraclean water is not needed. Many water quality issues associated with fish, such as the bacterial nitrification cycle, are not important with regards to turtles. However, turtles do produce more waste than fish and so it can be difficult to keep the water clean. Keeping the water clean involves preventing the water from getting dirty, having a good filtration system, and performing routine water changes. There is little that can be done to help keep the water clean. However, feeding in a separate enclosure will help. It is best to acclimate turtles when they are young to feed in a separate enclosure. Turtles can be quite messy eaters and will often defecate within a few minutes after a meal. Less food debris and feces will contribute to cleaner water and will help decrease the amount of water changes that is necessary. Most species can be housed in neutral pH water with no conditioners or additives. There are a few exceptions to this however. A few species live in brackish water, water having a salinity of 0.5–30 ppt. Species such as the Diamondback terrapin (*Malaclemys terrapin*) requires brackish water to thrive. For this species, 5 g of aquarium salt per liter (5 ppt) of water is needed. This amount could vary between species but is generally what is used for other species of brackish turtles. There are also a few species that have more specific pH requirements. These species are mostly represented in a group of South American species that live in a blackwater biotope (*Podocnemis erythrocephala, Hydromedusa tectifera,* and *Phyrnops* spp.). The water in this region is acidic, ranging from a pH of 4.5–6.5. Aquarium buffer systems are able to maintain this pH level.

Filtration systems designed for aquariums can be used in turtle enclosures, however, since turtles produce more waste than fish, a larger size filter will be needed than what is recommended for the size of the enclosure. For example, if the enclosure has 30 gallons of water, a filtration system for up to 50 gallons will not be sufficient. A filtration system that is rated for up to 100 gallons would be more practical. There are no published guidelines for how big of a filtration system that is needed. Trial and error will be the best judge for what size will be needed for each enclosure. Factors for the size of the filtration system would not only include what species and how many individuals are being housed in the enclosure, but also the temperature, substrate, and cage furnishings as this will also play a part. Biological and mechanical filtration units work well in turtle enclosures. If using biological filtration, dechlorinated water will need to be used as chlorine can kill the bacteria. External cannister filters are the best option for turtle enclosures. External cannister filters can provide excellent filtration as well as the option of adding sterilizing UV or ozone for disinfecting the water.

Periodic water changes will need to be done regardless of the filtration used. The frequency that water changes need to occur will depend on if the turtles are fed in the enclosure, the efficiency of the filtration system, temperature, and population density. When the water is changed, whole water changes are recommended. This can be made difficult based on the substrate used and any cage furnishings. Simple setups are easier to care for but may not provide the enrichment that the turtle needs.

Since turtles are ectothermic, environmental temperatures need to be maintained within the species preferred optimal temperature zone (POTZ) which includes water temperature as well. The water temperature can be maintained with a water heater designed for aquariums. Due to the larger filtration systems required, a larger water heater may also be needed. Water should be heated appropriately for the species housed, but most species can be kept between 24°C and 29°C (75–82°F). In each enclosure, there needs to be a place where the turtle can come out of the water and dry off and thermoregulate (Figure 11.8). At this site, a heat light should be placed to allow the animal a place to bask in the heat. If multiple turtles are housed together, multiple sites need to be placed to allow

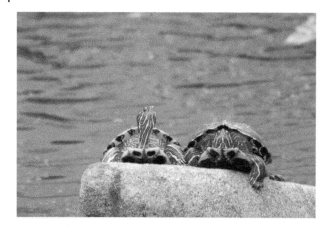

Figure 11.8 Sliders soaking up some morning sun.

each turtle a place to bask. It is common for a larger, or more dominant individual, to keep their cage mates from getting the benefits of basking. Lastly, the turtles need access to full-spectrum UV light. This can also be placed near the basking spot to allow for optimal exposure to the UV light. Certain species, such as matamatas (*Chelus fimbriata*) and pig-nosed turtles (*Carettochelys insculpta*) are almost exclusively aquatic and therefore do not need a dry basking spot, yet a heat light may still be indicated for these species.

The enclosure will need appropriate furnishings and substrate to allow for enrichment and normal functions of their daily lives. It is acceptable to have no substrate in the water portion of the enclosure. Turtles tend to eat the substrate, so it is good practice to not have any. However, many species like to burrow in sand and gravel, so for those species it is advisable to have something for them to burrow in. Any enclosure with an adult female (even in absence of males) needs to have a nesting area for oviposition. The nesting area should be four to five times larger than the female and twice as deep as the carapace length (Boyer & Boyer, 2019). The substrate within this nesting area should comprise a 50/50 mixture of moist sand and potting soil or peat moss. The nesting area should be a permanent fixture within the enclosure to help increase the likelihood of the turtle using it. This area can also double as the basking area. The enclosure should also have branches, rocks, and other items that closely resemble the species' natural environment. Turtles will often escape their enclosure. The water and land levels should be low enough so that the animal cannot escape. This is more of an issue with males as naturally, they tend to be more nomadic as they try to find a mate in neighboring ponds or streams (Figures 11.9 and 11.10).

Naturally, most chelonian species are solitary animals. However, most species will tolerate group housing. When introducing new animals, a strict quarantine period must

be observed, and the animal should only be released into the group once the animal has passed all post-quarantine testing. The group should be observed for any signs of aggression. Aggressive turtles will often times bite at the shell margins, tail, and neck of less dominant individuals. One may also see an individual not getting into the water. This is usually associated with a dominant individual who is not letting that individual come into the water. Group housing is only recommended for animals of the same size and species. Dominant turtles may also keep other individuals from basking or eating. Ensure that each animal in the group is growing. If one individual is large, and the rest are much smaller, the larger animal should be separated as it is preventing the others from getting the necessary food and heat. Species that should never be group housed include, but not limited to: softshell turtles (*Trionychidae*), common snapping turtle (*Chelydra serpentine*), alligator snapping turtle (*Macrochelys temminckii*), mud turtles (*Kinosternon* spp.), musk turtles (*Sternotheus* spp.), big-headed turtle (*Platysernon megacephalum*), Hamilton's pond turtle (*Geoclemys hamiltonii*).

Diets for feeding turtles should be composed primarily of a high-quality commercial fish-based aquatic turtle pellets. Other options that should make up the majority of the diet would be whole fish fed whole or chopped, and mice. Pinkies to adult mice can be fed whole or chopped but should be skinned to reduce the amount of indigestible keratin. The remaining diet, fed more as a treat, should consist of gut-loaded insects and other invertebrates. In species that are more omnivorous, dark leafy greens should be offered, especially as the turtle ages. Examples of species that undergo a shift in diet from primarily carnivorous to primarily herbivorous are mostly found in the Emydidae family of pond turtles and include *Chrysemys* spp. (painted turtles), *Graptemys* spp. (map turtles), *Pseudemys* spp. (cooters), and *Trachemys* spp. (sliders). Mineral blocks have no nutritional effect and should not be offered.

Tortoises and Terrestrial Turtles

Tortoises and terrestrial turtles only need enough water to soak in or to drink from depending on the species, but this does not make their husbandry requirements any easier. This group of chelonians come with their own unique challenges that will be discussed below.

The discussion first must start off with their size requirements. Tortoises need lots of space, and with some reaching sizes over 5 feet CL, this poses a serious commitment by the caretakers. As with the semi-aquatic and aquatic species, there have been some guidelines created to determine the size of the enclosure. The Federation of British Herpetologists (2022) maintain the same size

Figure 11.9 Aquatic habitat. (Drawing by Scott Stark.)

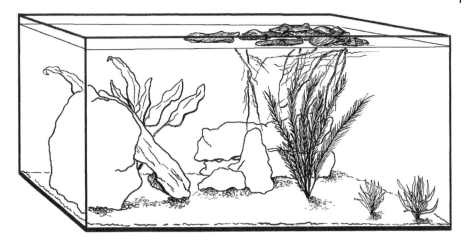

Figure 11.10 Semiaquatic habitat. (Drawing by Scott Stark.)

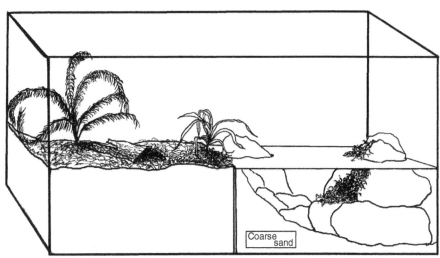

Coarse sand

recommendation of 8 × 4 PL. Other recommendations have stayed consistent with the formulas above; minimum floor area of 0.2 m²/0.1 m CL and recommended floor size of 0.5 m²/0.1 m CL. With these recommendations, even a modest-sized tortoise, like a red-footed tortoise (*Chelonoidis carbonarius*) with a carapace length of 30 cm (12 in.) would need a recommended area of 2 m × 0.75 m (79 in. × 30 in.). Also one needs to add at least 20% for each additional tortoise in the enclosure. Despite these recommendations, some species or individuals will still need a larger enclosure. Figure 11.11 houses a pair of Indian star tortoises (*Geochelone elegans*). The enclosure is 1.5 m² (16.47 ft²) which is above the recommended size of 1.2 m² (12.92 ft²) for the size and number of tortoises based on the 0.5 m²/0.1 m CL size recommendation. Notice how the tortoises have been demonstrating obsessive captive behaviors and not utilizing their floor space by circling the enclosure. This is evident by the lack of substrate at the periphery of the enclosure. These tortoises need a larger enclosure to help prevent the obsessive behaviors as well

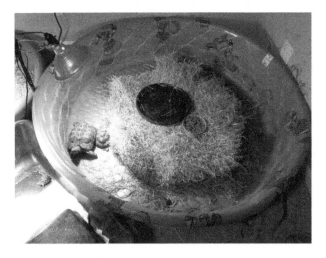

Figure 11.11 These tortoises are demonstrating behaviors that indicate a small and improperly designed enclosure.

as a better designed enclosure to help them utilize the rest of the space.

It is recommended that tortoises be housed outdoors as much as possible. This will allow them to get the appropriate lighting and space they need to thrive. Healthy tortoises can be placed outdoors when the temperature is above 18°C (65°F), and the mid-day temperature reaches 24°C (75°F) or above. There are some variations to these general temperature guidelines. Hatchlings and juvenile tortoises cannot tolerate temperatures below 21°C (70°F). Temperate species can tolerate temperatures slightly less than listed above, and tropical species do best in climates with less variability as they are not as tolerant of a wide temperature change throughout the day. Regardless of species, temperatures above 38°C (100°F) can become dangerous and a cool retreat should be provided during those times. The outdoor enclosure should contain a hide box as well as plenty of shade to allow the tortoises to escape from the hot sun. One common method to boost temperatures in an outdoor enclosure is to create a solarium. This can be accomplished with a ¼ in. safety glass leaned up against a solid structure at a 45° angle. The other end of the safety glass can be secured onto any structure that is raised up to a height that allows the individuals to access the solarium. Both ends of the solarium are left open to allow easy access as well as plenty of circulation. The solarium will be used primarily in the morning as the animals are waking up and seeking to warm up quickly, or during cooler days. It is also advisable to have a heated waterproof shelter in the enclosure. This is especially important for younger tortoises during cooler nights. When designing the rest of the enclosure one should consider the other needs of the species being housed. Grassland or desert species do not need much beyond plenty of grass and other species of plants to graze on. However, the enclosure should be designed so that they utilize the entire space. Hide boxes, solariums, and water sources should be placed strategically so that the animals do not just walk along the periphery of the enclosure. Tropical or forest species need a more elaborate design with plenty of plants that they can hide behind and that will also help with creating high humidity microclimates throughout the enclosure. All species need access to plenty of water with a water source large enough for them to soak in during hot days. The use of rocks, boulders, sticks, logs, and a varied topography will help ensure that the tortoises have plenty of objects to interact with to create an environment that is enriching to their lives (Figure 11.12).

Tortoises are notorious for their ability to escape from enclosures. Smaller or younger tortoises have the ability to climb small distances so the walls should be three times taller than the largest tortoise in the enclosure. The walls should be solid as any opening they can see through will just lead to an increased effort in that area to escape. Open fencing can also lead to injury as the tortoise could become entrapped in the fencing. If housing a species that burrows,

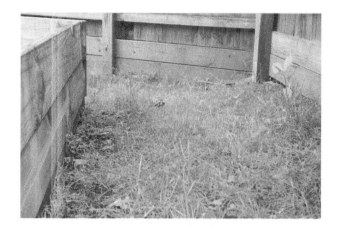

Figure 11.12 This outdoor enclosure provides plenty of grass and weeds for this juvenile Indian star tortoise (*Geochelone elegans*).

there needs to be a barrier placed underground to prevent the tortoise from escaping under the wall. For most species, this can be accomplished by burrowing hardware cloth several inches below the wall. However, if housing a larger species, such as sulcatas (*Centrochelys sulcate*), concrete bricks may need to be placed up to 2 feet underground to prevent escapes. Concrete bricks are always preferred over any type of metal wire. The metal wire in hardware cloth and chicken wire will eventually breakdown and will allow the tortoise to dig through easily, and these materials can also cause injury (Figure 11.13). Considerations for keeping the animals safe from predators and other nuisance animals should also be considered. Although tortoises are relatively free from natural predators, there are situations that occur. Canids, including domesticated dogs, will often times find tortoises to be a great chew toy, like a moving rawhide. Cats like to play with small tortoises, often times

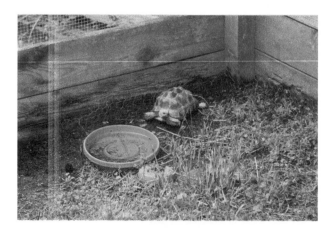

Figure 11.13 The exposed wire in this enclosure poses a danger to this tortoise. The tortoise could become entrapped in the wire.

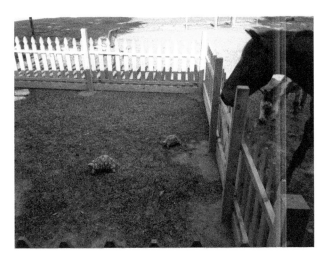

Figure 11.14 This horse found it fun to knock the tortoises over with his nose as they would walk by.

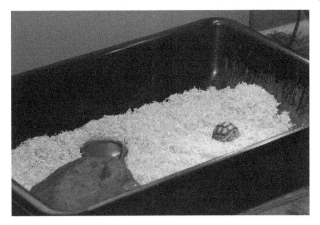

Figure 11.15 Indoor setup for a small tortoise.

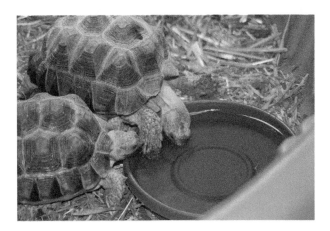

Figure 11.16 Two clutch mates that are housed together. Notice how the larger one is pushing the smaller one away from the water. These animals should be separated.

flipping them onto their backs as they swat at them. Occasionally falcons, hawks, or eagles will pick them up and usually drop them once they find that they will not be an easy meal. Depending on what potential predators are in the local area, a tall wall that cannot be climbed is the best defense. An electric wire system would also ward off any potential predators. Figure 11.14 shows a surprising predator.

When housing tortoises indoors during cooler times of the year, the same principles of enclosure design apply. They need a secure enclosure that will prevent escapes, it needs to be large enough for them to graze and be enriched, the enclosure needs to be designed so that they use the entire space, they have a private retreat, access full spectrum lighting and a basking light, and finally they need access to fresh clean water. They need a substrate that is appropriate for the species being housed. Desert and grassland species do well on alfalfa pellets, newspaper, indoor-outdoor carpeting, or cardboard. Forest or tropical species will need a substrate that is more humid such as soil, coconut coir, peat moss, bark, or a combination of these. This list is not all-inclusive; however, sand, gravel, cat litter, crushed corncob, and walnut shells should be avoided (Figure 11.15).

Group housing tortoises is also appropriate. Much like turtles, tortoises are generally solitary animals, but will tolerate being housed together. It is recommended to only house individuals together of the same species and of generally the same size. Watch for signs of aggression or dominance and separate those individuals. Dominant tortoises will keep others from basking under the heat lamp, will keep individuals out of hide or heat boxes, and will keep others from eating from a communal bowl. Aggressive individuals will commonly fight with others which may

end in tortoises being flipped over onto their backs. All of the individuals in the enclosure should grow at about the same rate, so if an individual is significantly larger than the rest, this could be a sign of dominance (Figure 11.16).

Tortoises are herbivorous species that tend to graze throughout the day eating dozens of different types of grasses and other plants throughout the year. This is impossible to replicate in the captive setting. Diet recommendations have changed significantly for tortoises over the past two decades. The overall diet should consist of <15% protein, 2–4% fat, and 25–30% fiber (Boyer & Scott, 2019). The current recommendations are that 80% of their diet should consist of a high-quality commercial pelleted diet (Table 11.1) and grass hays and the remaining 20% should consist of backyard weeds, spineless prickly pear cactus pads, dark leafy greens, flowers, and leaves. Table 11.2 highlights some examples from each of these categories. Fruits should not be fed as part of their normal diet; however, it can be given as treats. If a tortoise is refusing

Table 11.1 Basic nutritional composition of selected commercially available tortoise diets.

	Mazuri tortoise diet	Mazuri tortoise diet LS	Zoo med forest tortoise food	Zoo med grassland food	Fluker's tortoise diet	Exo terra soft pellets forest tortoise	Exo terra soft pellets European tortoise
Crude protein (min)	15.0%	12.0%	12.0%	8.5%	15.0%	13.0%	9.0%
Crude fat (min)	3.0%	4.0%	1.5%	1.9%	3.0%	2.0%	2.0%
Crude fiber (max)	18%	22%	23.0%	22.0%	18%	23.0%	26.0%
First ingredient	Soybean hulls	Timothy hay	Timothy hay	Whole wheat	Soybean hulls	Alfalfa meal	Alfalfa meal

Check current labels as recipes may change over time.

Table 11.2 A list of examples of nutritious food items for tortoises.

Backyard weeds	Dark leafy greens	Flowers	Leaves
Clover	Romaine lettuce	Roses	Mulberry tree
Burclovers	Bok choy	Nasturtiums	Grape
Purslane	Cabbage	Carnations	Banana
Spurges	Endives	Cactus flowers	Irish moss
Crabgrass	Collards	Chamomile	Coreopsis
Cheese weed	Mustard	Chrysanthemum	
Creeping wood sorrel	Escarole	Coreopsis	Geranium
Dandelions	Parsley	Geranium	Hibiscus
Bindweed	Turnip	Honeysuckle	Honeysuckle
Bittercress	Butter lettuce	Lavender	Lavender
Mustards			
Blessed thistle			
Butterfly bush			
Cat's ear			
Chickweed			
Chicory			
Evening primrose			
Wintercress			
Watercress			
St. John's wort			
Persimmon			
Kudzu			

to eat the commercial pellets and hay a few things can be done to entice them to eat these items. Recommendations include soaking the pellets and hay in water, mixing them in with things that they like, and avoiding feeding their absolute favorite foods as they will tend to eat those and not the pellets/hay. Persistence will pay off and they will eventually eat the pellets and hay. If feeding the above diet, supplemental calcium and multivitamin supplementation is not needed. The commercial diets are fortified with the proper amount of vitamins and minerals as well as

the supplemental fresh vegetables that are offered. If the tortoise is not eating commercial pellets, then each feeding should be dusted with calcium, and a multivitamin dusting a few times a month will be sufficient (Figure 11.17).

There have been some misconceptions regarding tortoise diets that have persisted in the reptile community (Boyer & Scott 2019). First, the concept that oxalate-containing greens should be avoided because they will bind to the calcium in the intestinal tract and decrease calcium absorption is sometimes heard. It is true that if a food

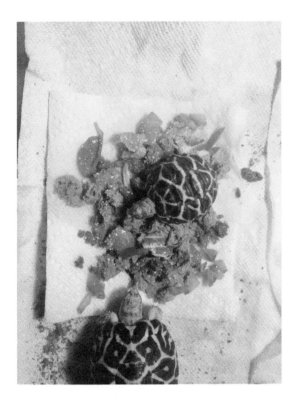

Figure 11.17 These baby tortoises are being weaned onto a commercial diet. The diet is moistened and mixed in with food that they like. A calcium supplement was dusted on top.

item is high in oxalate, it may not have any calcium that can be utilized by the body; however, one must consider the oxalate:calcium ratio to determine if the calcium will be utilized or not. Food items with an oxalate:Ca ratio of greater than 2 will not have any utilizable calcium and could bind to the calcium in other foods being eaten at the time. These food items include spinach and beet greens. However, there are many other food items that have an oxalate:Ca ratio below 2 indicating that the calcium will be utilized, and these food items will not affect the utilization of calcium in other foods being eaten at that time. Foods such as collards, Swiss chard, dandelions, kale, turnip greens, Brussels sprouts, and parsley are all low-oxalate foods. High-oxalate diets have also been accused of causing urocystoliths. Reptiles rarely form calcium oxalate stones, with only a couple of examples in the literature. Reptiles generally form urate stones. It is recommended to avoid feeding a large amount of high oxalate-containing foods; however, a small amount of the diet can contain these food items as they have other nutritional qualities to them. Another misconception is that food items from the Brassica family, which include cabbage, kale, mustard greens, broccoli, cauliflower, Brussels sprouts, and bok choy, can cause goiters. Goiters are very rare in tortoises with the few cases in the literature having no association with these food

items. These food items are perfectly safe in moderation as part of a balanced diet.

The last consideration with regards to creating a diet for tortoises is toxic plants. Fortunately, there have been very few cases of plant poisonings in tortoises. Numerous species of tortoises have natural diets that consist of plants that are toxic to other species. Tortoises tend to either avoid toxic plants or are resistant to their effects. There are a few plant species to avoid, however. These include rhododendrons, oleanders, chinaberry trees, tree tobacco, and toadstools.

Box turtles are opportunistic omnivores that tend to eat whatever they can get their mouth on. Younger box turtles are more carnivorous and tend to eat more vegetation as they age, but they stay omnivorous throughout their lifespan. In captivity, more than 50% of their diet should consist of a commercial box turtle or aquatic turtle pellets mixed with a live or pre-killed animal protein source. They should be fed a wide variety of invertebrates and can also be fed skinned chopped mice or pinky mice. The remainder of their diet should mostly consist of vegetables and a small portion consisting of fruits. The most important aspect of their diet is variety.

Common Disorders

Integument

"Shell rot" is a term used to describe superficial and deep pyodermas of the shell, most commonly in aquatic chelonians. Shell rot can be viral, bacterial, fungal, and/or algal and is usually initiated by trauma to the shell and/or underlying husbandry-related disease (Hoppmann & Barron 2007; White et al. 2011). The terms "wet" and "dry" shell rot are used to describe the appearance of the lesions and there have been associations made between gross appearance and causative agent (wet rot is more likely bacterial, dry is more likely fungal, etc.). However, appearance is not diagnostic by any means, and cytology and culture should be performed. Cases range from mild early forms, where only the scutes are affected and the lesions can generally be treated topically, to invasion of the underlying bone and/or septicemia that require systemic treatment—topical therapy such as chlorhexidine and/or other topical antibiotic preparations can be started empirically and based on cytology and patient stability systemic antibiotic or antifungal therapy may need to be started while culture results are pending.

Aquatic turtles need to be kept dry for at least 30–60 min after topical treatment. "Dry docking"—keeping the animal completely restricted from submerging—should be considered throughout treatment in mild cases and is required in cases with significant lesions; any animal that is dry-docked should have fluid therapy considered based on their systemic health and duration of treatment. Surgical debridement may be necessary in some cases.

Septicemic cutaneous ulcerative disease (SCUD) occurs when that spectrum of infections progresses to septicemia. It consists of the general sequelae of sepsis, including septic shock, coagulation disturbances, multi-organ dysfunction and failure, and eventually death. Outward signs, aside from the shell and skin changes, are likely nonspecific: severe lethargy to collapse, inappetence. Petechiation has been more highly correlated with septicemia in chelonians than in other reptiles (White et al. 2011). SCUD was previously attributed to specific bacteria (*Citrobacter freundii, Serratia* spp.) but is now recognized as a syndrome that can occur regardless of the infectious organism (Harkewicz 2001).

Burns are not quite as common as in squamates, but some owners will still utilize heating rocks or other inappropriate heat sources. Burns will appear as ulcerations and necrosis but can also progress to a more typical "shell rot" appearance as infection progresses.

Skeletal System

Traumatic injuries to the shell are relatively common, especially vehicular trauma in wild chelonians. In captive chelonians, dog bites to the shell and limbs are a common clinical presentation. In many cases, radiographs or computed tomography (CT scan) are necessary to determine the extent of the damage. Any fracture crossing the midline should be investigated for spinal cord trauma; as previously discussed spinal walking is possible, so ambulation does not rule out significant spinal cord trauma. The prognosis is grave/poor if the spinal cord is damaged.

Once the animal is relatively stable, the wounds must be cleaned, debrided, and flushed with sterile saline and diluted disinfectant (i.e., chlorhexidine or betadine). One must be careful when cleaning full-thickness fractures with exposed celomic cavity, especially since the lungs are closely associated with the carapace. As with significant injury in any species, pain management should also be provided—a fractured shell should be provided the same level of analgesia as would be given to any other animal with a fracture. Animals with full-thickness fractures, severe soft-tissue trauma, or predator bite wounds need systemic antibiotic treatment (Figure 11.18).

Superficial cracks on the shell can be repaired using sterile fiberglass cloth impregnated with polymerizing epoxy resin. Contact with the soft tissue should be avoided. Dental acrylic and other materials (surgical wire, zip-ties, etc.) can also be used (Figure 11.19). Full-thickness fractures where

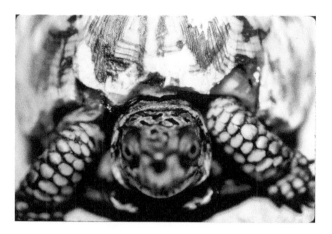

Figure 11.18 Traumatic injury to the shell. (Courtesy of Ryan Cheek, RVT.)

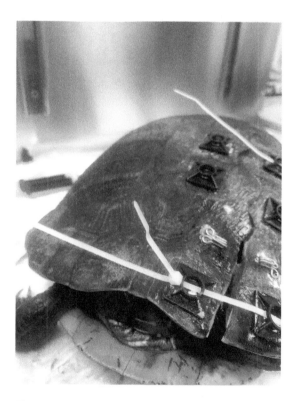

Figure 11.19 Repair of a traumatic injury to the shell. (Courtesy of Dr. Sarah Camlic.)

the celomic cavity has been exposed require surgical repair. In addition to shell repair, these animals require fluid and nutritional support and antibiotic therapy; fractured shells can take months to years to fully heal, and adequate supportive care and pain management are needed until the turtle is eating on its own and is free of infection. Aquatic patients often need to be dry-docked for the duration of the healing period, so daily fluid therapy may be necessary in addition to pain control and antibiotics. Placement of

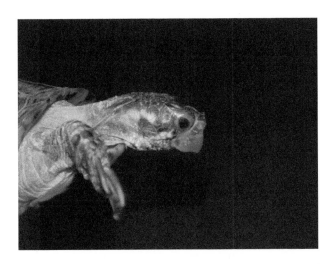

Figure 11.20 Overgrown beak. (Courtesy of Dr. Sam Rivera.)

an esophagostomy tube (detailed later in this chapter) at time of sedation/anesthesia is recommended for any individuals with major injuries where a long hospital stay and potential prolonged inappetence is predicted.

Some turtles will develop an overgrown beak in captivity. This has been associated with an inadequate diet. The overgrown beak needs to be trimmed on a regular basis. For the most part, this can be done without sedation with a dremel tool (Figure 11.20), though some animals will need sedation to adequately extend the head. The natural shape of the beak should be approximated as closely as possible, though this is sometimes not feasible with major deformities. As with avian beak trims, pulling up a photo of a wild individual from the same species to reference during the trim can be an excellent resource.

Shell deformities are also often found in captive animals due to inappropriate husbandry. Carapacial scute pyramiding (CSP), or "pyramiding," has specifically been linked to faster growth rates, which can be brought on by management choices such as not having an appropriate temperature drop at night and forgoing hibernation, and other factors including humidity and dietary protein have been implicated (Heinrich & Heinrich 2016; Ritz et al. 2012). Excessive calcium supplementation has not been shown to directly cause pyramiding, though improper dietary calcium balance can of course cause many orthopedic and systemic issues, to be expanded upon in the section on common nutritional disorders. Previous trauma can also cause warping of the shell during continued growth.

While the deformities themselves do not necessarily cause harm (though some may cause issues with ambulation, mounting, egg laying, etc.), they raise red flags about potential underlying systemic issues such as metabolic bone disease, immunocompromise, and other sequelae of poor husbandry. As with most issues of husbandry, factors

that most affect shell formation likely vary between species based on their natural diet and habitat, further highlighting how important it is to discuss species-specific husbandry with new owners.

Cardiovascular System

Few documented cases of cardiovascular disease in chelonians exist. Spirorchiid trematode infection has been documented in several aquatic turtle species and can cause endocarditis and arteritis; the flukes can affect several other body systems as well, both directly and secondary to thromboembolic disease (Schmidt & Reavill 2010). Congestive heart failure has been described in a spur-thighed tortoise (*Testudo graeca*) which temporarily responded to treatment with furosemide (Redrobe & Scudamore 2000), despite reptiles' lack of a loop of Henle. Methylated xanthines have also been shown to have diuretic effects in chelonians (Schilliger 2022).

ECG can be used in chelonians, though some adjustments may need to be made due to the presence of the shell (see Anesthesia section). Blood pressure can be measured in chelonians via either direct arterial means or via a cuff on the tail or limb if the patient is large enough; chelonians have a very low MAP, even compared to other reptiles, at approximately 15–40 mmHg (Schilliger 2022).

The heart cannot be distinguished on radiographs, so they are not useful as a screening tool for cardiomegaly.

Echocardiography is performed ideally through the cervical window, though trans-plastron echocardiography has been used successfully; normals exist for multiple chelonian species (March et al. 2020; Schilliger 2022).

Respiratory System

This is one of the most common presentations in clinical practice. Respiratory disease can range from upper airway disease, which can be infectious or allergic/inflammatory, to pneumonia. Infectious disease can be caused by bacteria, viruses, fungi, and certain parasites. Bacterial respiratory disease is most commonly caused by Gram-negative organisms and *Mycoplasma* (Studer & Di Girolamo 2021). There are many different viruses that have the potential to cause respiratory disease in chelonians, most notably herpesviruses and ranaviruses. Signs are not limited to the respiratory tract—encephalitis, papillomatosis, hepatitis, and other pathologies can all arise from these viruses—but conjunctivitis, rhinitis, stomatitis, and pneumonia are common, and disease can range from mild to fulminant (Okoh et al. 2021; Schmidt & Reavill 2010; Adamovicz et al. 2020). Ranavirus causes severe disease in chelonians and often leads to death via multi-organ failure; survival is rare but possible, and due to the existence of carrier states and reinfection, euthanasia should be considered in any previously positive animals even if they later test negative and is recommended if they are to have contact with any other susceptible animals (Adamovicz et al. 2020). Since clinical signs can be mild in survivors, testing for ranavirus should be strongly considered in any animals with upper respiratory signs and/or stomatitis, especially in managed collections.

Clinical signs of respiratory disease can include mucopurulent nasal discharge, oral discharge/foamy saliva, ocular discharge, abnormal respiratory noise (audibly and/or on auscultation), dyspnea (open mouth breathing, neck stretching, reluctance to swim), anorexia, weight loss, and lethargy; chronic disease can result in changes to the nares (Studer & Di Girolamo 2021) (Figure 11.21). Aquatic turtles may show abnormal buoyancy due to lung consolidation. Unfortunately, these signs are highly unlikely to point to one causative agent over another. Much like infectious respiratory disease complexes in other animals, chelonian respiratory disease will likely often be a combination of viral and bacterial pathogens, including opportunistic flora, brought on or exacerbated by stress and immunosuppression (transport, inappropriate husbandry, etc.).

Initial diagnosis of respiratory disease is based on clinical signs and imaging (radiographs and/or CT). Further modalities can be employed to attempt to reach a specific diagnosis, including bronchoscopy and bronchoalveolar lavage. Cytology, histopathology, culture and sensitivity, and PCR can be performed on retrieved samples.

Treatment includes appropriate antimicrobials (guided by diagnostics), heat support, fluid therapy, and nutritional support as indicated. Aquatic turtles with significant respiratory compromise should either have the depth of their water reduced and their docking space increased, or be dry-docked, as buoyancy issues and exercise intolerance can both lead to drowning.

Due to their lack of a diaphragm, reptiles cannot clear discharge in their lungs by coughing, so nebulization (saline and/or antimicrobial) and coupage can be helpful. Transcarapacial intrapulmonary catheter use has also been described for cases where systemic effects of drugs are a concern (Hernandez-Divers 2001).

Digestive System

While less common than in squamates, infectious and traumatic stomatitis can occur and are managed similarly. Chelonians with hypovitaminosis A can develop stomatitis in addition to the more classic signs of blepharoedema and aural abscessation. Testudinid herpesvirus (TeHV) can cause diphtheritic oral plaques in addition to other respiratory signs, and rarely neurologic signs (Okoh et al. 2021; Origgi 2012).

There is a wide range of diseases that affect the gastrointestinal tract of chelonians; the general approach to and differentials for gastrointestinal signs in chelonians is the same as in any other animal. The clinical signs of gastrointestinal disease are often nonspecific and include anorexia, vomiting/regurgitation, weight loss, lethargy, dehydration, and abnormal stool; GI tympany may be present in cases of obstruction, functional ileus, or volvulus, but may be difficult to identify due to the presence of the shell (Mans 2013).

Foreign bodies are relatively common and are often due to accidental ingestion of non-food material (rocks/gravel, etc.) while eating, though disorders such as pica can cause true dietary indiscretion. In aquatic species, floating debris is often mistakenly ingested—one of the more notable examples of this is sea turtles that mistake plastic bags for jellyfish. Fishing hooks and lines are also commonly ingested. The hook itself can become lodged in the oral cavity or remainder of the GI tract, and the line can act as a linear foreign body.

Physical examination and radiographs are the initial diagnostics for detection of foreign bodies. If radiographs do not show radiopaque foreign material and/or a definitive obstructive pattern, contrast radiography or advanced imaging may be needed. While ultrasound is limited by the shell, it has been used to directly identify foreign bodies and to identify intestinal plication from linear foreign bodies (Franchini et al. 2018); while this may or may not be feasible based on individual equipment and training, it would be reasonable for the average clinic to visualize and sample free coelomic fluid to assess for septic effusion. CT may be needed if other methods fail to identify a foreign body but clinical suspicion remains, or may be pursued

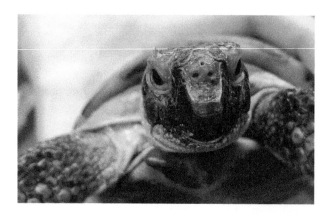

Figure 11.21 Erosions associated with the nares. (Courtesy of Sarah Camlic.)

even if a diagnosis is reached to determine a more precise location of the material within the GI tract and to aid in surgical planning.

If foreign material is found but is not obviously obstructive, medical management consisting of rehydration and lubricant laxatives can be attempted. It may take a prolonged period for objects to pass even with successful medical management due to chelonian GI transit time and the likelihood of concurrent function ileus; promotility agents such as metoclopramide and cisapride have been used with varying results in non-obstructive chelonian ileus and can be considered with caution. Bloodwork should be performed to assess for systemic consequences of the foreign body, and bloodwork and imaging should be reevaluated serially during any medical management. Both endoscopic and surgical techniques for foreign body removal have been described; the most appropriate modality will depend on a variety of factors including location, identity, and size of the foreign body.

Gastrointestinal parasitism is common and will be covered in depth in the "Parasitology" section.

Constipation is a common presenting complaint from owners across all species—while primary colonic/rectal disorders are certainly possible and should be investigated (especially if there is straining to defecate without production), general lack of defecation is frequently indicative of dehydration, ileus, anorexia, and/or other systemic disease.

Cloacal prolapse can involve the digestive, reproductive, and excretory systems and can have several causes including but not limited to enteritis, hypocalcemia, parasitism, obstructive dystocia, bladder stones, and neoplasia. As with any prolapse, during triage tissue damage should be assessed and the prolapsed tissue cleaned, lubricated, and if possible (usually only in cases of minor prolapse of cloacal tissue), replaced within the vent. Prolapse of any coelomic viscera is an emergency and will require anesthetized replacement. Prognosis is dependent on the degree of prolapse, the involved structures, underlying illness, and tissue viability.

Hepatobiliary disease can arise from the same variety of diseases that affect any organ system—infectious, nutritional, neoplastic, etc.—and can often have nonspecific signs such as anorexia and weight loss as the only outward indicators. Icterus and biliverdinuria may or may not be present, and bloodwork can be normal even in the face of severe disease (Mans 2013). Endoscopic evaluation and sample collection for histopathology/culture are frequently needed to achieve a diagnosis, which is also the case for many mammalian hepatopathies.

Excretory System

Renal disease is common in chelonians. As with many conditions, it can occur due to improper husbandry (inappropriate humidity/diet, lack of adequate water sources, oversupplementation of vitamin D), but there are many potential causes including but not limited to congenital disorders, toxic nephropathy, infectious nephritis, neoplasia, and age-related degeneration (Holz 2018). Signs are often nonspecific and can include lethargy, anorexia, and cachexia. As in companion mammals, a significant amount of renal function must be lost before blood values change. Increased uric acid level is more indicative than BUN and creatinine, though BUN may be of some use in the more ureotelic aquatic species (Holz 2018). Polyuria and polydipsia are reportedly uncommon. Animals are often in advanced renal failure by the time disease is identified, which carries a poor prognosis.

Underlying causes of renal disease should be investigated. Due to the absence of a loop of Henle, passage of urine through the cloaca, and reabsorption and secretion of metabolites within the rectum and bladder, urinalysis is of minimal use for assessment of renal function and urinary tract infection. While imaging can raise suspicion for renal disease, often endoscopic evaluation, biopsy, and culture are needed to find an underlying etiology.

Treatment includes addressing any underlying cause found, fluid therapy, and management of any secondary issues such as renal-secondary hyperparathyroidism or gout.

Gout is a condition that involves the deposition of urate crystals (tophi) in the visceral organs and/or joints. Gout can be caused by renal disease, dehydration, and/or high protein diets, as purines are metabolized into uric acid; clinical signs can include lethargy, anorexia, lameness, and swollen joints (Holz 2018). Diagnosis can be made by measuring serum/plasma uric acid levels, radiographs, and cytological evaluation of the material in the affected joints. The treatment involves the correction of the primary problem, but it is often unrewarding: medications and diet change can be employed to limit further deposition of crystals, but pre-existing crystals remain a source of discomfort, and advanced renal disease has limited treatment success. Pseudogout can also occur, which is deposition of calcium-based crystals.

Urolithiasis is also common in chelonians, especially tortoises in arid environments. Clinical signs often include straining/prolapse and hematuria, though many stones are found incidentally on radiographs (Keller et al. 2015). Common factors include dehydration, diet (vitamin under- or over-supplementation, high protein or oxalate content), and urinary tract infection.; stones are usually comprised of a combination of urate, calcium, and or phosphate and can be found in the cloaca or bladder (Keller et al. 2015; Holz 2018). Manual removal from the cloaca is possible; bladder stones necessitate cystotomy. Approaches through the plastron and prefemoral fossa have been described for cystotomy, endoscope assisted cystotomy is also an option in some cases (Divers 2019).

Reproductive System

Both preovulatory stasis and postovulatory stasis (dystocia) occur in chelonians (Stahl & DeNardo 2019). Preovulatory stasis occurs when follicles are neither ovulated nor resorbed, and cause disease by either ending up free in the coelom and causing a yolk coelomitis, becoming a nidus for infection, or by becoming a space-occupying lesion causing anorexia, dyspnea, etc. Dystocia can be caused by a variety of factors including but not limited to poor environmental conditions/metabolic disease (hypothermia, dehydration, abnormal shell formation or lack of reproductive tract motility due to hypocalcemia, etc.), infectious/inflammatory disease, and neoplasia. Clinical signs of all of these reproductive disorders can be nonspecific, including anorexia and lethargy, and with obstructive dystocia straining, bloody discharge from the cloaca, and prolapse can sometimes be seen.

Medical management of preovulatory stasis can be attempted and generally consists of providing appropriate nesting resources and providing hydration support and calcium supplementation if indicated (Stahl & DeNardo 2019). If medical management is unsuccessful, or if owners wish to avoid the high chance of the issue recurring in subsequent reproductive cycles, surgical intervention is indicated. Ovariectomy can also be offered at the first presentation to prevent possible decline.

The diagnosis of dystocia is based on diagnostic imaging or an obvious visible or palpable egg within the cloaca or any prolapsed tissue. Diagnosing dystocia in a clinically well turtle can be difficult, as they can retain eggs for prolonged periods of time past expected laying dates under normal circumstances (Gárriz et al. 2022). Presence of free coelomic fluid (which should be sampled if present) or bloodwork abnormalities such as a strong infectious/inflammatory leukogram or anemia are supportive of disease processes, but absence of bloodwork abnormalities does not preclude pathology. Bloodwork should be performed regardless of any suspected cases of dystocia to assess for common causes such as hypocalcemia. In nonobstructive dystocia, medical management in the form of calcium supplementation, fluid support, providing appropriate environmental parameters and nesting sites, and sometimes hormone and prostaglandin therapy

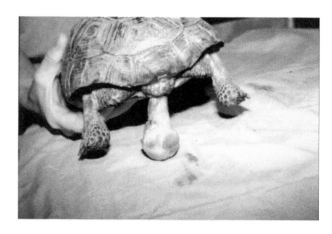

Figure 11.22 Phallus prolapse. (Courtesy of Zoo Atlanta.)

can be attempted (Stahl & DeNardo 2019). In obstructive dystocia and nonobstructive cases that have failed medical management, surgical intervention is warranted.

Eggs can sometimes be retrieved via cloacoscopy (Stahl & DeNardo 2019), and ovariectomy and ovariosalpingectomy can be performed via a prefemoral approach, both with and without laparoscopic assistance depending on animal size and surgeon preference (Innis 2010; Takami 2017; Hellebuyck & Vilanova 2022). Sometimes transplastron coeliotomy is necessary.

Cloacal, and sometimes oviductal, prolapse in females during parturition, and phallus prolapse in males during copulation can occur. Initial management is the same as for any prolapsed tissue (detailed in the Digestive System section above). Prolapse of the phallus is often caused by trauma, as the phallus swells and then cannot be retracted, but can also be caused by infection, cloacal impaction, myelopathy, and neoplasia. Severe cases often require amputation, which can be performed relatively easily as the phallus has no urinary function but does prevent reproduction (Figures 11.22 and 11.23).

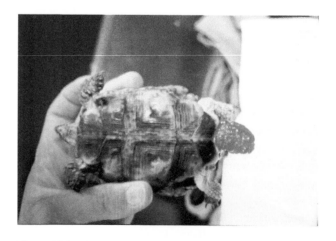

Figure 11.23 Cloacal prolapse. (Courtesy of Zoo Atlanta.)

Nervous System

There are few primary neurologic diseases discussed in the literature. Many of the more common "neurologic" presentations are secondary to other causes, such as seizures or paralysis after trauma, tremors and weakness from hypocalcemia, and hindlimb paresis from dystocia. Toxic causes of neurologic signs are discussed in the following section. If diagnosis is not apparent from history, examination, and screening bloodwork and radiographs, additional diagnostics including MRI, CSF evaluation, and infectious disease testing may need to be pursued.

There have been cases of chelonians exhibiting blindness and other neurologic abnormalities following hibernation, thought to be due to hypothermia-induced ischemic brain injury (Baron & Phalen 2018). As in any other animal, hyperthermia can lead to heat stroke, with CNS damage being one of the possible sequelae.

While testudinid herpesviruses (TeHV) more commonly causes respiratory signs, neurologic signs have been known to occur with TeHV-3, and mortality is often higher than with other TeHV; multiple serologic and molecular tests exist (though histopathology is often needed to confirm diagnosis) and some antivirals have been shown to be effective in treatment (Okoh et al. 2021).

Toxicity, Nutritional, and Miscellaneous Disorders

Hyperparathyroidism is a frequently encountered problem in reptiles. While primary hyperparathyroidism is rare, nutritional-secondary hyperparathyroidism (NSHP) and renal-secondary hyperparathyroidism (RSHP) are common (Rivera & Lock 2008). NSHP is caused by an improper calcium-to-phosphorus ratio in the diet and/or a vitamin D_3 deficiency. RSHP is caused by a drop in body calcium secondary to the accumulation of phosphorus and abnormal Vitamin D_3 metabolism as the kidneys fail. In response to low blood calcium levels, the parathyroid glands stimulate reabsorption of calcium from the skeleton. If enough decalcification occurs, animals develop clinically apparent "metabolic bone disease," also known as "fibrous osteodystrophy," in which the bones become obviously soft and potentially deformed on exam and radiolucent on imaging; animals will sometimes have multiple healed or active pathologic fractures apparent on physical examination or radiographs. While nutritional disease is sometimes reversible at this stage, any major deformities already present should be taken into consideration for ongoing quality of life. In the final stages of the disease, there is no longer enough total body calcium to maintain normocalcemia, and animals will present with clinical symptoms ranging from weakness, lethargy, and ileus to tremors, seizures, cardiac abnormalities, and sudden death. Prognosis at this stage is extremely guarded to grave. Treatment involves calcium supplementation, general supportive care, and review and correction of husbandry or treatment of the renal disease. Stabilization of end-stage disease is discussed in more depth in the Emergency and Critical Care section. This condition is generally accepted to be painful even when fractures are not present, so pain control should be provided.

Overgrowth or deformities of the beak can occur secondary to NSHP but can also be congenital or from previous trauma or infections (Mans 2013).

Vitamin A deficiency (hypovitaminosis A) is a common presentation in aquatic and terrestrial chelonians. It is caused by feeding a diet deficient in vitamin A. Clinical signs include conjunctivitis, blepharitis, nasal discharge, dyspnea, skin abnormalities, and aural abscesses. This condition is treated with parenteral vitamin A and diet correction.

The aural abscesses that develop with hypovitaminosis are thought to develop secondary to the squamous metaplasia that occurs within the middle ear. Organochlorine compounds have also been implicated as a cause of aural abscesses in wild box turtles (*Terrapene carolina carolina*), (Sleeman et al. 2008). Since reptile heterophils do not have the proteolytic activity necessary to make liquid pus, their abscesses consist of caseous pus, meaning surgical debridement is necessary as lancing alone will not drain the material as might be possible in mammalian abscesses. The tympanic membrane is incised, and the exudate removed, followed by debridement and lavage of the area. An antibiotic ointment may then be applied. The site is left open and treated daily. Pain management should be provided, and systemic antibiotics if indicated, until the wound heals by second intention. Culture and sensitivity should be strongly considered if systemic antibiotics are used. Radiographs and/or CT should be considered to screen for osteomyelitis.

Vitamin A toxicity (hypervitaminosis A) can also occur if there is excessive dietary supplementation or parenteral administration of vitamin A. It is much easier to cause over-supplementation with injectable means, so parenteral supplementation should be reached for first in only the most severe cases. Clinical signs include dry, flaky skin or sloughing of the skin with secondary bacterial infection. Treatment requires systemic antibiotics if secondary bacterial infection is present, and discontinuation of parenteral vitamin A or any source of over-supplementation.

Due to the presence of thiaminases in fish, which are not inactivated by freezing, frozen-thawed fish may be deficient in thiamine (vitamin B1); if these make up a large portion of an animal's diet, as may be the case in aquatic turtles, thiamine deficiency can occur, which generally presents as neurologic signs (Carmel & Johnson 2018). Supplementation should be provided to animals if their diet is primarily fish—supplements need to be stored properly and their expiration dates checked as thiamine degrades easily. Treatment consists of thiamine supplementation and supportive care.

Chelonians have a reportedly low incidence of neoplasia at around 10%; cutaneous squamous cell carcinoma is the most reported chelonian neoplasm, though many other tumor types have been described (Christman et al. 2017). Another neoplasm of note is viral fibropapillomatosis in green turtles (*Chelonia mydas*), likely caused by a herpesvirus (Jones et al. 2016). Biopsy is the diagnostic of choice for diagnosis of neoplasia, though cytology may be adequate depending on tumor type and location. While few reports of treatment of chelonian neoplasia exist (aside from a relatively significant body of information on treatment of fibropapillomas), many treatment modalities have been documented in chelonians and other reptiles with varying success (Christman et al. 2017).

Ivermectin has caused neurologic signs and death in multiple chelonian species, and as such avermectins should never be given in any chelonian by any route (Rockwell & Mitchell 2019).

Environmental toxins can present a problem in captive tortoises allowed to roam outside or fed gathered forage. Toxicities from oak leaves and ornamental plants have been described (Rotstein et al. 2003, Pizzi et al. 2005), and there are likely additional commonly kept plants that have the potential to cause significant toxicity. Husbandry evaluation should include a review of any plants present in the environment even if the owners have not witnessed the animal showing interest in them. There have been documented cases of lead toxicity causing digestive and neurologic signs in both aquatic and terrestrial species from ingestion of fishing weights and lead shot (Mitchell & Diaz-Figueroa 2005).

Many viruses can potentially affect chelonians. Herpesviruses and ranaviruses are covered in the respiratory system and nervous system portions of this section. Adenoviruses are another important emerging disease in chelonians. The adenoviruses detected in chelonians thus far are not members of the genus *Atadenovirus*, which is only genus that has been found to infect squamates. The adenoviruses in turtles also seem distinct from the other existing genera (though some atadenoviruses have been recently identified in chelonians) and a new genus "testadenovirus" has been proposed (Salzmann et al. 2021). Disease usually causes necrosis of the liver, bone marrow, and GI tract and has a poor prognosis (Marschang 2019).

Zoonoses

Most zoonotic diseases associated with keeping turtles involve bacterial pathogens. The most widely recognized disease is salmonellosis. *Salmonella* is a common bacteria flora of reptiles (Damborg et al. 2016). While the majority of human salmonella cases come from eating contaminated food, reptile-associated salmonellosis (RAS) is known to cause human disease (Sodagari et al. 2020; Bosch et al. 2016). The genus *Salmonella* contains many species with thousands of different serotypes. Many of these serotypes have been isolated from asymptomatic chelonians and have been associated with human salmonellosis; children, immunosuppressed individuals, and the elderly are at greater risk of contracting salmonellosis (Damborg et al. 2016). Symptoms in humans include abdominal pain, diarrhea, nausea, vomiting, and fever. In the 1960s and 70s, there were many human cases of salmonellosis linked to pet turtles as the source of infection; in 1975, laws were implemented banning the sale of baby turtles with a carapace length of 4 in (~10.2 cm) or less, as these animals were closely associated with cases of RAS in children (Bosch et al. 2016).

Many other bacteria of reptile origin including but not limited to *Aeromonas*, *Campylobacter*, and *Pseudomonas* have also been associated with illness in humans (De Luca et al. 2020; Goławska et al. 2019).

Reptiles can also be affected by several species of Mycobacteria that are known to cause disease in humans. *Mycobacterium* spp. can cause a variety of lesions across a number of organ systems in reptiles, ranging from asymptomatic infection to septic shock (Ebani et al. 2012).

The route of transmission for humans is through direct contact or inhalation of contaminated particulate matter; many of these species are widespread in the environment and infections often arise when there has been no contact with chelonians (Akram et al. 2022).

The hallmark of disease prevention and decreased risk of exposure to potential zoonoses is adequate hygiene. Owners should be made aware of the potential health hazard when keeping turtles as pets. Proper sanitation is essential to decrease the risk of exposure, as there is no effective or practical way to eliminate the bacteria from the intestinal flora of positive animals. The bacterial burden in the environment will greatly increase when the feces are allowed to build up in the enclosure, increasing the risk of transmission to humans. That is why it is so important to practice strict hygiene when keeping turtles or any other reptile. This goes for both the pet owner and the healthcare provider. When sick turtles are hospitalized, it is imperative that they be kept in a clean environment and handled carefully to prevent contamination of the hospital environment.

Parasitology

External Parasites

It is important to keep in mind that chelonians are also affected by ectoparasites. Ticks, leeches, mites, and myaisis can be found in chelonians (Wellehan & Walden 2019).

Amblyomma tuberculatam, known as the gopher tortoise tick, is an Ixodid tick that has the potential to infest chelonians. It can carry the *Anaplasma* species that is an emerging cause of anemia in tortoises.

Ivermectin is contraindicated in chelonians, as discussed in the section on toxicities. Cyfluthrin and permethrin were found to be the most effective and have the least side effects compared to other tested compounds when treating ticks in leopard tortoises (*Stigmochelys pardalis*) (Rockwell & Mitchell 2019).

Myiasis has been documented in chelonians, especially aquatic turtles. Eggs from myiatic fly species can be laid in existing wounds, and *Cistudinomyia cistudinis* is known to lay eggs on the healthy skin of box turtles (*Terrapene* spp.). Myiatic wounds need to be manually debrided of larvae and thoroughly cleaned. Topical nitenpyram can be used on the wounds as well as given orally or rectally. Antibiotics are generally recommended for extensive myiatic wounds.

Internal Parasites

Protozoans

Balantidium and *Nyctotherus* spp. are ciliates that are common within the gastrointestinal tract of chelonians. They are usually non-pathogenic but have the potential to cause disease.

As in other animals, coccidiosis is most frequently a gastrointestinal disease of young animals, though it can occur in any life stage and can have intestinal and extra-intestinal forms. Animals can be asymptomatic. *Cryptosporidium testudines* and *C. ducismarci* are the cryptosporidians most commonly found in tortoises. There are currently no known effective treatments for cryptosporidiosis in reptiles, though some medications have been shown to decrease clinical signs.

Identification of *Eimeria* spp. in fecal samples of asymptomatic animals generally does not indicate treatment.

Intranuclear coccidiosis of Testudines (TINC) is an emerging disease of chelonians that affects a wide range of species (Adamovicz et al. 2020). The coccidian parasite has an intranuclear developmental stage; cells of multiple organs can be affected. Clinical signs include rhinosinusitis, oronasal fistulae, lethargy, rapid weight loss, open mouth breathing, gastrointestinal signs, mucosal ulceration, and a swollen vent. Bloodwork changes can reflect a range of organ dysfunction. The degree and severity of clinical signs depend on species of the host, chronicity, and which organs are affected. The prognosis of animals showing signs associated with intranuclear coccidiosis is poor. Postmortem diagnosis is based on the histopathologic finding of intranuclear developing stages in multiple organs or by polymerase chain reaction (PCR) testing. Antemortem samples (cloacal/choanal/conjunctival swabs, nasal/cloacal biopsies) can be tested via PCR. Identification on fecal examination is difficult as the oocysts are very small and easily degraded. Treatment remains unrewarding; while ponazuril and toltrazuril have been initially effective in decreasing clinical signs the animals generally become chronically infected and die after a period of several months.

There are some flagellate species of note in chelonians. *Hexamita parvum* can either be an asymptomatic pathogen of the GI tract or cause severe and often fatal nephritis, generally in immunocompromised or juvenile animals (Holz 2018). *Hexamita* can sometimes be diagnosed on fecal or urinary samples, as a <8 μm fast-swimming binucleate flagellate without the disc seen in similar organisms such as *Giardia* (Wellehan & Walden 2019). Metronidazole may be effective for treatment, but studies are lacking.

Turtles can be subclinical carriers of pathogenic amoeba species. *Entamoeba invadens* is an example of an amoeba that causes low morbidity in turtles but can cause severe illness and death in snakes and lizards (Wellehan & Walden 2019). *E. invadens* trophozoites and cysts can sometimes be identified on fecal samples but can be confused with similar species. Amoebiasis in reptiles is generally treated with metronidazole.

Helminths

Trematodes

Spirorchiid trematodes are a family of flukes that cause cardiovascular disease in aquatic chelonians. Adults live in the major vessels and heart, eggs can obstruct the capillaries, and eggs can migrate into organs and cause granulomatous disease; clinical disease is caused by severe vasculitis, emboli of the organisms themselves, and ischemic organ injury (Wellehan & Walden 2019). Praziquantel may be used, but if there is a high number of organisms present the die-off can cause a fatal inflammatory response.

Nematodes

Nematoda is one of the largest and most diverse groups of parasites, and there are many organisms that have the potential to parasitize chelonians. The most significant nematode parasites of chelonians are within the orders Spirurida (spirurids) and Ascaridida (ascarids).

The spirurid genera *Spiroxys* and *Serpinema* can both be found in freshwater turtles; *Spiroxys* sp. can cause a severe granulomatous gastritis (Wellehan & Walden 2019). Eggs are smooth and larvated; eggs or larvae can be found on fecal exam.

Ascarid species have large, rough eggs and large three-lipped adults, who develop in the coelom and then travel to the GI tract when in their definitive hosts; *Krefftascaris, Sulcascaris, Anisakis, and Angusticaecum,* are genera that have been found to cause disease in chelonians (Wellehan & Walden 2019).

For large burdens of spirurids or ascarids, endoscopic removal of as much of the worm burden as possible is recommended prior to anthelminthic treatment due to the possibility of a fatal inflammatory response and/or gastrointestinal obstruction.

Topical emodepside/praziquantel has been used with varying efficacy in chelonian species (Mader routes of admin).

Cestodes

Cestodes are not usually pathogenic unless they are in an aberrant host. On fecal exam, eggs should contain an oncosphere with six hooks (Wellehan & Walden 2019).

Polystomatids are found in the conjunctiva, oral cavity, and cloaca/urinary tract of aquatic turtle hosts, and do not usually cause clinical disease.

Acanthocephalans

Acanthocephalans "thorny-headed worms" are large adults with a spiny proboscis that they use to burrow into the wall of the intestinal tract. Eggs are smooth and have multiple rings. A sedimentation procedure is usually necessary for identification of the eggs in fecal samples.

Traditional anthelminthics such as oxfendazole are used for treatment of nematodiasis, though acanthocephalans often do not respond as well as other nematode groups and may require surgical removal (Rockwell & Mitchell 2019). As previously discussed, avermectins are contraindicated in chelonians due to fatalities.

History, Restraint, and Physical Examination

History

A thorough history is one of the most important aspects of the clinical evaluation. Improper husbandry is often a major contributor to illness. A thorough husbandry investigation includes enclosure size and material, temperature, humidity, lighting, diet, type and route of supplementation, water quality/changes, cleaning procedures/products, conspecifics, and time outdoors. Reports of temperature and humidity levels should be followed by confirming if thermometers and hygrometers are present (rather than estimating based on their average home temperature) and where in the cage they are located. Owners should be asked how often the UVB lighting is changed, as UVB lights will stop emitting UVB rays long before they stop producing visible light, a fact that many owners are not aware of. If applicable, aquatic turtle owners should be asked if fish are fed live, fresh, or frozen-thawed. There are many other follow-up questions to general husbandry information that will come more easily with time and experience; it is highly recommended that a standardized husbandry form addressing these questions and the many other minutiae of reptile husbandry be used by the clinic and filled out by every owner and updated on a regular basis so that no details are forgotten.

While it is impossible for any individual to memorize the exact husbandry requirements of every chelonian species, let alone every exotic species they may come across, it is extremely important that both the clinicians and veterinary technicians have at least a basic understanding of terrestrial and aquatic husbandry, and a more in depth understanding of the requirements for any species they see very commonly. This serves to help find deficiencies that the owner can be educated on to prevent future illness, assess differentials for current illness, and instill confidence in owners that staff are familiar with the species under their care, especially with those clients who have extensive reptile experience.

One should always ask about current signs and any previous illness. Any change in appetite, behavior, weight, and defecation (consistency and frequency) should be recorded.

Hibernation season and reproductive activity should also be noted during the examination, as this can cause many changes in their behavior, physiology, and bloodwork. The origin of the animal (wild-caught vs. captive-bred, bought from a pet store vs. a private breeder) must be ascertained. Also inquire about other animals in the collection, whether there are other types of turtles and/or other reptiles in the household. Were any animals bought recently? Was the animal quarantined? All these questions will help to formulate a picture of the animal's environment and potential exposure to pathogens.

Restraint

The neck of many chelonians has an S-shaped curve that allows the animal to withdraw the head within the shell.

Up to a certain body size, the head can often be extended by applying gentle pressure with a thumb and index finger behind the mandibles. Once you have a hold behind the temporomandibular joints, apply gentle traction to overcome resistance being careful not to be too forceful. It is important to avoid dorsoventral pressure with your fingers as this can cause damage to the soft tissue of the neck and trachea. This technique is limited by the size, physical condition, and disposition of the animal; lack of retraction of the animal's appendages or minimal resistance to restraint is concerning for severe systemic illness. In many cases, the head can be grabbed by reaching from underneath, as animals will quickly withdraw when approached from the top. This quick withdrawal can cause the handler's fingers to be pinned between the shell and the appendages, which with larger species can cause significant damage to the handler—manual restraint should not be attempted in large animals unless they are significantly compromised.

The head of box turtles and other species with hinged shells can be harder to exteriorize, as they can move the cranial part of the plastron upward, making the shell an almost impenetrable fort. In this case a tongue depressor or smooth stainless-steel speculum can be utilized. Insert the tool between the carapace and plastron and apply gentle pressure downward. Once exposed, a limb can be grabbed, and one can attempt to restrain the head as described above.

Other approaches include holding the animal facing downward at a moderate angle, as they will often extend their head, or placing them in a small amount of warm water. Most individuals will attempt to get out of the water and when they do, you can attempt to restrain a limb or the head. If the first attempt at restraint fails, the animal should be placed in its holding container and tried later. Patience is a technician's best ally. In aquatic species with long nails, a towel can be used to wrap the animal and hold the legs within the shell, as the nails can inflict painful scratches on the handler. A towel can also be used to keep the head inside the shell of aggressive animals. Chelonians will also often urinate large volumes when picked up, which the handler should be prepared for. A reversible sedation protocol can be used to facilitate a physical exam and/or minor procedures if physical restraint is not successful or is unsafe. In apparently healthy animals, even if manual restraint is possible, sedation should still be considered for stressful procedures such as beak trims (Figure 11.24).

While the keratinized beak of any chelonian can inflict a serious bite, snapping turtles require special mention. Restraint of snapping turtles should only be performed by experienced individuals, as they have the capability of causing severe damage with their bites, and they can move very quickly and extend their necks a significant

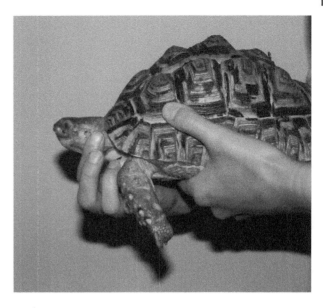

Figure 11.24 Proper restraint. (Courtesy of Ryan Cheek, RVT.)

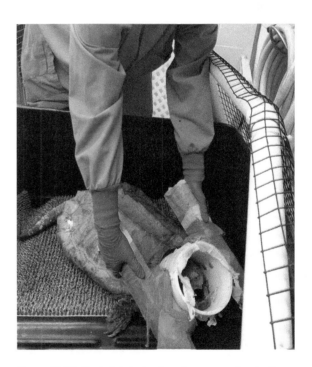

Figure 11.25 Restraint device for a large snapping turtle. (Courtesy of Dr. Sarah Camlic.)

distance in all directions. Restraint should be performed by grasping the very caudal part of the shell, or by using a purpose-made restraint device (Figure 11.25). In larger alligator snapping turtles, one hand can be used to grasp the nuchal scute as well for additional support—this should not be done in common snapping turtles as they have more retroflexion of their neck.

Physical Examination

The most important part of any physical examination is thoroughness and repeatability. A physical examination of any animal should be comprehensive and should be done in approximately the same way every time, so as not to miss anything. While it is tempting to address the most obvious injury or pathology first, a stepwise approach means not missing other more subtle changes that may affect possible differentials or decision-making.

The first part of any examination is the hands-off visual examination. While there may already be some changes due to stress from travel or a new environment, this will be the best chance at getting an accurate assessment of respiratory rate and effort, gait, and general demeanor. Buoyancy and intervals between surfacing should be assessed in aquatic animals.

Assess mentation—is the animal bright and alert, quiet, or worse? Levels of consciousness are often used incorrectly or interchangeably but do have specific meanings that veterinary staff should be aware of and use correctly to accurately track mentation changes regardless of who is performing the assessment. Dull/depressed/lethargic are some of the more subjective terms; while a perfect veterinary definition does not exist for each word, this author uses them to represent an animal that has a decreased level of energy and/or interaction while otherwise maintaining normal or near-normal responses to stimuli, and likely having some interest in the environment outside of direct stimulation. The next level is obtundation, which generally refers to having minimal to no interaction with the environment outside of direct stimulation, but still responding to non-noxious stimuli, though responses are usually slowed or inappropriate. The following level of consciousness is stupor/semi-coma, which means an animal that responds only to noxious and/or vigorous/repeated stimuli, and quickly returns to a state of non-responsiveness when the stimulus is removed. Coma is a state of complete non-responsiveness.

If an explanation for the mentation change is known, this should be noted as well—if an animal was just given an opioid and mentation decreased from a previous state of bright and alert, it would be more appropriate to use the term "narcotized" than "dull." Other assessments of mentation for animals exist, such as the Modified Glasgow Coma Scale, but these are difficult to apply to reptile patients due to the differences in examination parameters such as unreliable PLRs, etc.

Respiration should be very passive in reptilian patients; any obvious respiratory effort is a cause for concern. Normal respiratory rates in chelonians can be extremely low, sometimes less than once per minute in healthy animals.

Open-mouth breathing or any degree of orthopnea should be considered highly abnormal. Gular breathing, as discussed previously in this chapter, seems to be more associated with olfaction and has not been shown to be a sign of dyspnea. Any respiratory noise should be noted, as stridor or stertor can potentially help localize pathology to the upper respiratory tract. As in any animal without a diaphragm, respiratory signs can commonly occur secondary to space-occupying disease outside of the respiratory tract such as effusion or organomegaly. The lungs of chelonians can sometimes be auscultated by placing a wet hand towel between the carapace and the stethoscope to enhance the surface contact, or through the cervical inlet with the stethoscope directed upwards (Studer & Di Girolamo 2021).

Heart rate is most commonly measured via Doppler probe placed at the junction of the neck and forelimb. As chelonian heart rates can be quite slow, it is recommended to listen for at least 30 s if not a full minute to obtain the most accurate rate.

If possible, gait should be assessed—many chelonians will retreat into their shells in unfamiliar environments, so this may not be possible as part of the hands-off exam. A normal gait does not completely rule out orthopedic or neurologic abnormalities but can be an excellent screening indicator that most musculoskeletal and nervous system components are without significant damage, especially regarding polytrauma. As discussed previously, turtles can exhibit "spinal walking" even with spinal cord transection, but the gait they have in those situations is not a normal one.

General body condition and tone are important physical examination parameters. Is the animal well-muscled/conditioned and does it have a strong withdrawal into the shell? Animals should attempt to right themselves using their head and neck when placed in dorsal recumbency. Note: this is very stressful for the animal and does not necessarily have to be a part of a normal exam unless neurologic dysfunction is suspected.

While palpation may be slightly harder in chelonians than animals without a shell, one is generally able to get an assessment of body condition. Long bones and the shell should be palpated for any flexibility that might indicate metabolic bone disease, or for any evidence of current or healed fractures. In some species such as softshell turtles (Family Trionychidae) and pancake tortoises (*Malacochersus tornieri*) the shell is softer and more flexible, which should not be interpreted as pathology.

Normal appearance of the skin and shell varies slightly between species, especially when comparing terrestrial to aquatic animals, but there should be no extreme dryness/flaking, no dysecdysis, no discolored areas, and no erythema, ulceration/pitting, petechiae, wounds, masses, or other lesions. Loose scutes should not be pulled from the shell under normal shedding conditions, but any areas of concern can be gently investigated to see if there is any pathology underneath. The nails, nail beds, and rostrum should be evaluated for abrasions and other abnormalities.

Evaluate the head, eyes, nares, oral cavity, and tympanic membrane. Note any discharge, redness, swelling, plaques, abscessation, or other abnormalities. The mouth may not be able to be opened without gentle traction with a speculum or similar tool; chemical restraint may be necessary in larger animals (see Restraint section). The glottis and choanae should be carefully examined.

The vent should be examined for any prolapsed tissue, asymmetry, ulceration, masses, discharge, or other abnormalities. The cloaca should have tone and should contract when pinched. The tissue can be gently everted to look for any abnormalities of the mucosa.

While the presence of the shell limits palpation, the axillary and prefemoral fossae should be palpated for any eggs, bladder stones, masses, or effusion. The animal can be tilted to each side to allow coelomic viscera to fall closer to the fossae for palpation.

A weight should be obtained on every animal at every visit. Animals weighing greater than a kilogram can be measured using a regular scale; animals weighing less than a kilogram should be measured with a gram scale to ensure accuracy.

Radiology

Radiographs are an important diagnostic tool in the assessment of the musculoskeletal, respiratory, gastrointestinal, and reproductive systems. The dorsoventral (DV), craniocaudal (CC), and lateral views are recommended. For the lateral and CC views, a horizontal beam is desired. Tilting the turtle on its side is not recommended, as this will often cause distortion of the lungs, viscera, and reproductive organs (Figure 11.26).

The DV radiograph can often be easily taken by placing the animal on the table with no restraint; many will stay still long enough for image acquisition. If the animal does not stay still, placement into a plastic container is adequate for a DV view confirming a shelled egg or radiopaque urolith and may be useful for other views if being in a small container is enough to stop movement. Physical restraint also includes placement of a barrier such as a sandbag in front of the animal or elevating them by using a round container slightly smaller than the plastron or a similar item such as a yoga block. Make sure the legs cannot contact the platform, as they can then push off, causing movement

artifact and potential serious injury if they fall off the platform. The platform should also be stable enough that it does not fall with movement. Tape can also be used to secure the shell of smaller animals to the platform and can be used for restraint with other modalities (Figure 11.27). If this is not sufficient to stop movement, or retraction of the limbs and head is interfering with imaging, chemical restraint will be needed. If the lungs are being evaluated, retraction of the head and limbs into the shell can compress the lungs and lead to artifactual consolidation. Barnacles should be removed from marine turtles prior to imaging.

Computed tomography, or "CT scan," is a frequently utilized modality in chelonians. CT scans are becoming more common in small animal and exotic practices. The benefit of using CT versus a radiograph is that a CT scan produces a three-dimensional (3D) image while radiography produces a two-dimensional (2D) image. The 2D image has superimposition of structures, and therefore has a lower sensitivity in many cases compared to 3D CT images, especially with the presence of the radiopaque shell in chelonians. However, knowledge of the anatomy of the species is still imperative and having known normals is beneficial. There are exposure factors for both radiographs and CT scans, so radiation safety should be a consideration for both the staff and the patient.

There are different types of CT technology used in veterinary medicine. Older machines use axial imaging acquisition (multiple individual slices taken one at a time), which increases acquisition time, an important consideration in veterinary patients who may be sedated or anesthetized. Multidetector machines (MDCT) use helical continuous acquisition, which has a much shorter acquisition time. Cone-beam CT (CBCT) is a newer modality that utilizes a cone-shaped beam and requires only a single rotation for image acquisition; the machines can be compact and transportable and are becoming increasingly popular in veterinary medicine, especially for exotic animals.

Gastrointestinal and intravenous contrast have both been used in chelonians. Barium is used for gastrointestinal contrast and can be given orally (via gavage or esophagostomy tube) or cloacally depending on the purpose of the study. Iodinated contrast is used injectably. Information on these routes of administration and catheter placement is provided in the Clinical Techniques section.

Ultrasonography through multiple soft-tissue windows has been documented in desert tortoises (*Xerobates agassizii*) and was adequate for diagnosis of pericardial effusion and hepatic changes (Penninck et al. 1991). Ultrasonographic normals exist for red-eared sliders (*T. scripta elegans*) though not all organs could be visualized (Martorell et al. 2004). Soft-shelled species can be ultrasounded through the plastron.

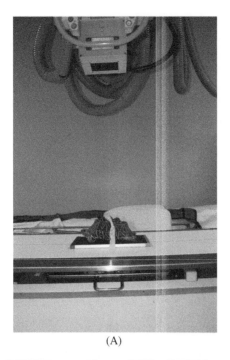

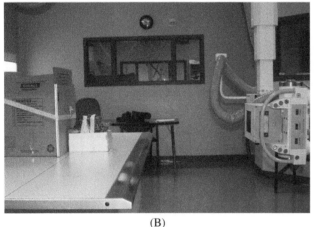
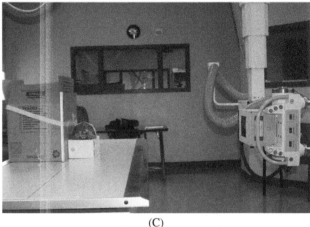

Figure 11.26 Restraint for radiographs. (A) Ventrodorsal view (B) Craniocaudal view (C) Lateral view. (Courtesy of Ryan Cheek, RVT.)

Anesthesia

Pre-anesthetic Considerations

The overall health of the patient should be established to assess anesthetic risk; a full physical examination (see above) and if possible, at least a minimum database of bloodwork should be obtained. During induction, anesthesia, and recovery, all reptiles should be kept at their POTZ, as deviations form this ideal temperature can affect the efficacy of injectable and inhalant agents and cause deviations of normal physiology, including intracardiac shunting. Electric heating pads should not be used as they put patients at risk for thermal burns; microwaved fluid bags should also be avoided as their temperature cannot be accurately regulated unlike recirculating water blankets.

Hydration status should be assessed using both physical examination and bloodwork parameters and fluid support provided if indicated peri-anesthetically. It was often said in the past that "reptile Ringer's" should be used for rehydration of reptiles and that lactated Ringer's should be avoided as reptiles have decreased clearance of lactate, but there has been evidence that lactate-buffered solutions do not cause appreciable negative effect in chelonians and can help correct the acidosis that critically ill chelonians often present with (Camacho et al. 2015). It has also been shown that lactated Ringer's does not appreciably increase lactate and that reptile Ringer's had negative effects when

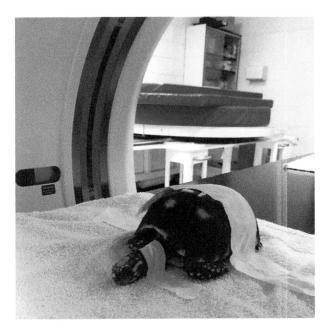

Figure 11.27 Taping to aid restraint for CT in a sedated patient. (Courtesy of Dr. Sarah Camlic.)

administered to bearded dragons (Parkinson & Mans 2020). While more research certainly still needs to be done in these areas across all reptile species, there exists no strong evidence that commercially available crystalloids, including those that are lactate-buffered, cannot be used in reptiles.

Anesthetic Agents and Induction

Chelonians can be anesthetized using inhalation agents via mask or chamber induction, but the presence of intracardiac shunting and the ability to breath-hold for prolonged periods of time, especially in aquatic species, makes this technique time-consuming for both induction and recovery. Because of this, inhalants are not recommended as a sole induction agent in chelonians. If gas induction is used, the uptake of the anesthetic agent can be increased by manipulating the limbs in and out, as this will enhance ventilation of the lungs.

The preferred method of inducing chelonians is to use a multimodal approach of parenteral drugs. The intramuscular and intravenous routes are frequently used for the administration of induction agents—access via these routes and others will be further discussed in the Clinical Techniques section. Practically, IM administration is often the first step in chelonian sedation/anesthesia due to the inherent difficulties in reliable IV access in awake chelonians.

A cotton tip applicator or tongue depressor can be used to gently move the tongue cranially while inserting the

endotracheal tube. External upward pressure on the soft tissue window between the mandibular bones can help expose the glottis. It is recommended to use a speculum to keep the mouth open and prevent the animal from biting the endotracheal tube. A piece of PVC pipe can be placed in the oral cavity during intubation to protect the person performing the intubation and can be secured in place to protect the ET tube during the procedure and recovery.

An uncuffed ET tube should be used due to chelonians' complete tracheal rings, and the tube should be inserted only a short distance, as the chelonian trachea bifurcates very cranially. Cole endotracheal tubes are very useful in reptiles as they prevent excessive advancement of the tube and help form a better seal.

The tube should be secured in place, generally taped to the beak/head. A rigid item such as a tongue depressor can be used to help keep the tube straight (Figure 11.28). As the shapes and sizes of chelonian skulls vary greatly, there is no one correct way to secure the ET tube and many creative approaches have been tried. As some would say: it's not stupid if it works.

Benzodiazepines

Midazolam can be given IM or IV at 0.5–2 mg/kg in chelonians. It has varying effects across chelonian species and is

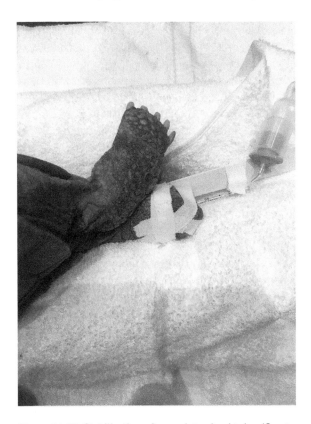

Figure 11.28 Stabilization of an endotracheal tube. (Courtesy of Dr. Sarah Camlic.)

often combined with other agents (Schnellbacher & Shepard 2019). Midazolam can be reversed by intramuscular or intravenous flumazenil; there are no pharmacokinetic studies of flumazenil in reptile but doses that have been described range from 0.01 to 0.3 mg/kg. It is sometimes recommended to give half of the flumazenil dose IM and half IV.

α-2 agonists

Dexmedetomidine and medetomidine alone and in combination with other agents have produced mild to deep sedation in various chelonian species and can be reversed with intramuscular atipamezole; intranasal administration in combination with ketamine has also been described in slider species (Schnellbacher & Shepard 2019). Dose-dependent cardiovascular depression occurs with these agents. While atipamezole is generally administered at an equal volume, it is important to note that some facilities use more concentrated formulations of α-2 agonists than are found in small animal practice, for which an equal volume of atipamezole will not suffice.

Opioids

Opioids are often part of anesthetic protocols, especially when the condition or procedure is considered painful. Morphine can be given via many parenteral routes and has been used intrathecally for regional analgesia (Schnellbacher & Shepard 2019). Butorphanol and tramadol have also been used in chelonians. Prolonged respiratory depression can occur with opioid administration in chelonians. Reversal with naloxone should be decided by weighing the level of respiratory compromise with the need for pain control/availability of other pain control agents. In the event of arrest or impending arrest, all reversal agents should be administered.

Dissociatives

Ketamine can be given IM or IV and should be paired with another agent, usually a benzodiazepine or opioid. Tiletamine is available in combination with the benzodiazepine zolazepam under various product names; efficacy and recovery can be unpredictable compared to ketamine combinations (Schnellbacher & Shepard 2019). Dissociatives have long been considered contraindicated in cases of known or suspected head trauma or other intracranial disease due to causing an increase in intracranial pressure; a recent preliminary systematic review of the human literature showed no obvious effects but was limited due to the quality of data available (Gregers et al. 2020). Until more definitive evidence is available in the human and veterinary worlds, it is still advisable to avoid these agents in these cases when possible. Due to the relatively quick onset of anesthesia from an IM injection, tiletamine-zolazepam is often used as the first part of multistep euthanasia protocols in captive and wild reptiles as well as for wildlife and shelter animals across species.

Propofol

Propofol is a hypnotic agent that has a rapid induction and recovery with minimal dysphoria and has been used in many chelonian species; limitations include that it is limited to IV or IO use, lacks analgesia, has significant respiratory depression, can cause hypotension if administered too rapidly, and is not reversible (Mans et al. 2019).

Alfaxalone

Alfaxalone is a neuroactive steroid that can be used as an IV induction agent or can be used IM for moderate to deep sedation; limitations include the lack of analgesia, dose-dependent respiratory and cardiovascular depression as with propofol, the relatively large volumes required for IM administration and associated expense, and hyperactivity during recovery (Schnellbacher & Shepard 2019). Previously alfaxalone lacked preservatives and the bottle had to be discarded shortly after opening, but a multidose formulation is now available.

Maintenance, Monitoring, and Recovery

Isoflurane and sevoflurane are the two inhalants currently most used in reptile anesthesia. Both produce dose-dependent cardiovascular depression, and there are minimal studies available investigating differences between the two in reptilian anesthesia (Mans et al. 2019).

While some degree of intracardiac shunting is possible in other reptile groups, chelonians, especially aquatic species, are notorious for having significant right-to-left shunting during anesthesia that can make achieving a surgical plane of anesthesia extremely difficult. Atropine at 1 mg/kg IV has been shown to eliminate intracardiac shunting in red-footed tortoises (*Chelonoidis carbonarius*) under isoflurane anesthesia by increasing pulmonary blood flow, lowering MAC, and providing a more stable anesthesia (Greunz et al. 2018).

Withdrawal reflexes/tone are generally reliable for monitoring anesthetic depth, and proceed in the following order: pectoral limbs, pelvic limbs and neck, righting reflex, tail and cloaca, and jaw tone (Mans et al. 2019). They should return in the reverse order. The palpebral reflexes are sometimes helpful but not always reliable for monitoring of anesthetic depth. An electrocardiogram (ECG) is ideal to monitor the cardiac function. The cranial ECG leads should ideally be placed on either side of the cervical region between the neck and forelimb, and the caudal leads either on the skin of the knees or caudal to the pelvic limbs (Schilliger 2022). In awake animals where that region cannot be accessed, there has been success in placing leads directly on the plastron (Kinoshita et al. 2022). Regular leads often do not adhere appropriately to reptilian skin; alligator clip leads attached to needles inserted through the skin often work very well. Reptile ECG has the same general components as mammalian ECG, though amplitudes are much lower. Other differences include a shorter PT interval and longer ST and QT intervals.

Doppler ultrasonography can be used to monitor the peripheral pulse in the limbs. A pulse oximeter with a reflectance probe can often be used to monitor oxygen saturation. Pulse oximetry is not validated in chelonians, but trends can be used for monitoring.

Neither Doppler nor ECG should be relied upon as indicators of life in reptiles. Pulseless electrical activity can occur as in any animal and may be hard to identify due to the normally low amplitude of the reptilian ECG. Reptiles often have cardiac contractions after death, so presence of a normal ECG or pulse does not rule out death.

End-tidal carbon dioxide ($ETCO_2$) can also be monitored during anesthesia; cardiac shunting can cause $ETCO_2$ values to underestimate $PaCO_2$, so the exact value is not as important as in mammalian anesthesia, though 10–25 mmHg is generally regarded as the ideal range. Trends can still be monitored, and abrupt changes should be investigated, as sudden drops can indicate either ET tube dislodgement/obstruction or decreased cardiac output such as in impending arrest.

All reptiles require intermittent positive pressure ventilation (IPPV) during anesthesia, either manually or via a mechanical ventilator. The ideal respiratory rate varies based on a variety of factors including species but is generally between 1 and 6 breaths per minute and should be titrated based on trends in $ETCO_2$ (Mans et al. 2019). PPV should not exceed 8 cm H_2O.

Arterial blood gas analysis, while ideal for respiratory monitoring during anesthesia in mammals, is difficult to obtain in chelonians (and reptiles in general), and mammalian normal cannot be extrapolated to reptiles due to the many significant physiological differences in their cardiovascular and respiratory systems outlined throughout this chapter.

While the mammalian respiratory stimulus is hypercapnia, the reptilian respiratory stimulus is hypoxemia. Because of this, it has historically been recommended that animals be taken off 100% oxygen as soon as possible during the recovery process, sometimes even slightly prior to the end of the procedure, and be manually ventilated with room air to prevent an extremely prolonged anesthetic recovery. However, recent studies have shown that this may not be the case, though as this was done in limited species and continued research is needed (Mans et al. 2019).

Epinephrine has been shown to decrease recovery times in common snapping turtles anesthetized with isoflurane (*Chelydra serpentina*) by increasing the tone of the systemic vasculature to counteract the shunting that occurs during apnea; the acupuncture point GV-26 was shown to have comparable effects (Mans et al. 2019).

Surgery

Some of the more common procedures performed in chelonians include shell fracture repair, amputations (often revision of traumatic amputations), ovariectomy/ovariosalpingectomy, cystotomy for urolith removal, and phallus amputation after prolapse. The shell of chelonians presents an obvious challenge for intracoelomic surgical procedures.

Transplastron coeliotomy is performed by cutting a rectangular window in the plastron with a surgical saw, with one side left partially attached to act as a hinge, preserving blood supply to the flap. After surgery, the cut section is placed back and covered with some combination of epoxy, resin, bone cement, and/or fiberglass mesh. Similar techniques are used to repair traumatic shell fractures, with the addition of devices to relieve tension (screws and wires, plates, anchors and zip ties, etc.) as needed; the multitude of approaches to turtle shell repair is beyond the scope of this chapter. Healing in reptiles is much slower than in mammals, and healing of the shell in chelonians can take many months.

With the increasing availability of endoscopy, there is much less frequent need for plastronotomy. Celioscopy in chelonians is most commonly done from a prefemoral approach, though other approaches can be used depending on the procedure. Endoscopic or endoscope-assisted techniques have been developed for many procedures in chelonians including sexing, sterilization, cystotomy, and foreign body removal (Divers 2019). Endoscopy is also an extremely useful diagnostic modality and can be used for evaluation of the cloaca, oral cavity, upper GI tract, and respiratory tract in addition to the coelom.

Limb fractures can be repaired using similar techniques as for mammalian fractures—cerclage wire, plates, etc.—as appropriate based on fracture location/type and animal size (Knafo & Karlin 2019b). If metabolic bone disease is present, healing will be compromised. Limb amputations are performed with the same general principles in mammals. For small chelonians, a partial amputation can be appropriate if indicated; for larger chelonians, full

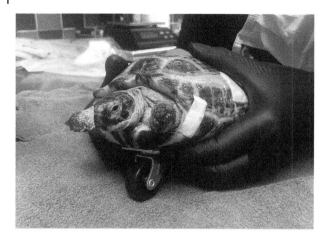

Figure 11.29 Fitting of a prosthetic to assist patient mobility. The pictured caster is too large, and a smaller prosthetic was obtained following the fitting. (Courtesy of Dr. Sarah Camlic.)

limb amputation is necessary to prevent ulceration of the remaining stump. Support structures such as a furniture caster (Figure 11.29) or a halved tennis ball can be secured to the plastron as prostheses (Knafo & Karlin 2019c).

Exact positioning varies depending on procedure, but preparation of the surgical site follows the same general rules as mammalian surgical prep. Adhesive plastic drapes are very useful for adhering to reptilian skin, especially for the chelonian shell.

Clinical Techniques

Venipuncture

The sites for blood collection in chelonians are the jugular, brachial, subcarapacial, tail (ventral and dorsal), and femoral veins, as well as the occipital sinus and the heart. Chelonians can prove challenging for blood collection. It is always a good idea to be familiar with multiple venipuncture sites. The supplies needed depend on the size of the animal. Prior to blood collection, slides, hematocrit tubes, small-volume (0.5 mL) heparinized tubes, alcohol swabs, needles, and syringes (0.5–3 mL) should be prepared. In patients smaller than 300 g, use a 25–27-gauge needle with a 0.5–1 mL syringe. In patients greater than 300 g, one can use a 22-gauge needle with a 3 mL syringe. Larger needles (20-gauge plus) can be used in turtles weighing over 5 kg (Figure 11.24). The venipuncture site should be cleaned well to prevent introduction of pathogens or debris into the animal, as well as to prevent inaccurate results (e.g., urates on the tail can cause a falsely elevated uric acid on bloodwork). Heparinized collection tubes are used—as with other non-mammals, EDTA will often lyse red blood cells.

Jugular vein

The jugular vein is relatively superficial and located dorsally on the neck in line with the tympanic scale. Blood can be collected from this location if the head can be exteriorized; sedation may be needed (see section on Restraint). The neck should be held in an extended position. In some patients, the vein can be visualized by applying digital pressure at the base of the neck; however, this is not always the case. Once the vein is located, the needle should be inserted at a 30° angle and negative pressure applied as the needle is advanced. The syringe will fill with blood as soon as the vein is entered. In some cases, the flow is slow. Once blood fills the hub of the needle, stop advancing and release suction on the plunger. Sometimes the vein will collapse. One should reapply gentle suction until the desired amount of blood is obtained (Figure 11.30).

Brachial vein

The animal should be placed in sternal recumbency. One should then gently pull either forelimb to expose the brachial-antebrachial joint. The brachial vein is located deep in the triceps tendon. This tendon can be palpated on the caudal aspect of the extended leg. The needle should be inserted perpendicular to the skin, in the groove located ventral to the distal end of the tendon. Once the skin is entered, negative pressure should be applied and the needle advanced. Redirecting the needle may be needed to find the vein (Figure 11.31).

Subcarapacial venous sinus/vein

This site is located ventral to the carapace along the dorsal midline. The animal should be restrained in sternal recumbency with the front end elevated at a 45° angle. With one hand, the head should be held inside the carapace. With the index finger of the other hand, the first vertebra that

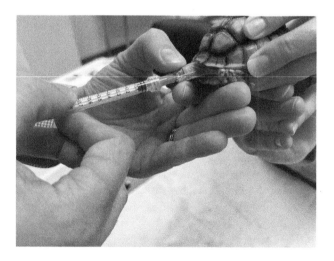

Figure 11.30 Jugular venipuncture.

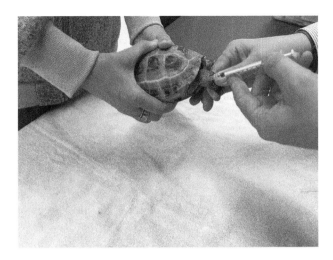

Figure 11.31 Brachial venipuncture.

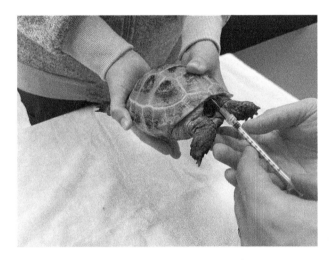

Figure 11.32 Subcarapacial venous sinus/vein venipuncture.

is fused to the carapace along the dorsal midline should be palpated. The needle is inserted in the midline position and slowly directed to the space between the carapace and the vertebrae. Negative pressure should be applied as the needle is advanced (Figure 11.32).

Dorsal coccygeal venous sinus/vein

The animal should be restrained in sternal recumbency. The tail should be held as straight as possible, and the needle inserted on the dorsal midline of the tail. One should insert the needle at a 30–45° angle, proximally near the junction between the tail and the caudal margin of the carapace. The needle is then advanced until the vertebral bodies are encountered. Negative pressure should be applied, and the needle moved gently out (1–2 mm) until blood flows.

Less common sites

For the ventral tail vein, the animal is restrained vertically with the plastron facing the phlebotomist or in dorsal recumbency. One should keep in mind that placing the animal in dorsal recumbency is stressful, therefore, this should be done for the shortest amount of time possible. The tail should be extended and held as straight as possible. One should then insert the needle in the ventral midline, distal to the vent. Remember that the further distally one goes, the smaller the diameter of the vein. The needle is then inserted at a 60° angle with the hub directed cranially, and the needle is advanced until the vertebral body is hit. Negative pressure should then be applied while gently moving the needle out (1–2 mm) until blood flows. This site is generally not productive as only a small volume can be obtained. Larger turtles in good physical condition can hold the tail close to the body making the tail very difficult to exteriorize.

For accessing the femoral vein, the animal should be restrained in sternal recumbency. The femoral vein courses through the femoral triangle, which is located at the most proximal and medial aspect of the hindlimb. With one hand, the hind leg should be extended, and the other hand should be used to withdraw the blood sample. This, like many of the other techniques, is a blind stick. The needle should be inserted at a 45° angle and suction applied as the needle is advanced. Repositioning the needle should be minimized as damage can be done to nerves and other vessels located in this area (Figure 11.33).

For the occipital venous sinus, the animal should be restrained in vertical recumbency with the carapace facing the phlebotomist or in sternal recumbency, and the head extended and gently ventroflexed. The sinus is located on the dorsal midline where the cervical vertebrae meet the skull; an obvious divot should be appreciated when this

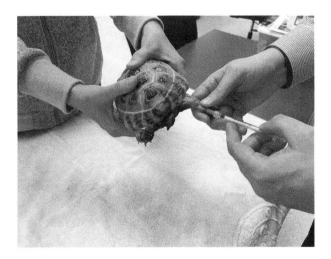

Figure 11.33 Femoral venipuncture.

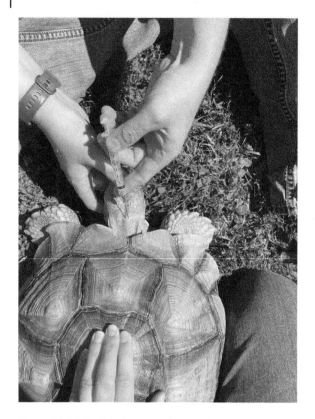

Figure 11.34 Occipital venous sinus venipuncture.

area is palpated. The needle should be inserted at a 60° angle. Negative pressure should be applied once the skin is penetrated as the needle is advanced. Sometimes the needle can be repositioned to either side of the midline as the sinus can extend laterally (Figure 11.34).

While techniques have been described for cardiac sampling, they are highly invasive and often fatal and are not recommended in clinical practice.

Intravenous and Intraosseous Catheter Placement

The jugular vein is the preferred site for intravenous (IV) catheter placement in chelonians; catheterization is often reserved for anesthetized animals or patients that are very critical, as patients that are relatively stable can sometimes make it difficult to access and maintain the catheter site (Figure 11.35). The procedure for IV catheter placement in a jugular vein is as follows (steps 2 and 3 may or may not be needed depending on animal size/skin thickness):

(1) Sterilely prepare the area of the jugular vein in the anesthetized patient.
(2) Make a full-thickness incision on the skin.
(3) Identify the jugular vein using blunt dissection.
(4) Apply pressure at the thoracic inlet to distend the vessel; insert an IV catheter of adequate size according

to the size of the animal—even if a full dissection is not performed, tenting the skin above the vessel and "pre-poking" with a needle is advisable due to the tough nature of reptilian skin.
(5) Place a butterfly tape over the catheter and cap and suture to the skin. Place a light wrap over the catheter if it is to be maintained in an awake patient.

Placement of an extension set can often help maintain access even if the patient withdraws their head, though withdrawal may cause the jugular catheter to occlude. The extension set can be secured to the carapace, making sure this is enough extra length to account for movement of the neck without putting tension on the catheter. A soft "donut" collar made of rolled stockinette and tape or similar materials can be placed at the base of the neck to prevent full retraction.

Central venous catheters "central lines" have been used successfully in chelonians and can potentially be maintained for up to 4 months or longer, if properly cared for (Pardo & Divers 2016). They are strongly recommended in the case of critically ill animals that will need intravenous medication and serial blood sampling. Commercially available central venous catheter kits can be used and placed via the jugular vein using sterile technique according to the enclosed instructions (modified Seldinger technique). ECG monitoring is recommended to assess for any arrhythmias if the catheter is inadvertently advanced too far. The catheter should be introduced to the level of the cranial aspect of the pectoral scutes—premeasure from the approximate point of insertion on the neck, with the neck extended. The catheter site should be covered with Tegaderm™ or a similar product. The ports can be secured to the shell, again making sure to allow for movement of the neck. Placement (cranial to the heart) needs to be confirmed with radiographs. Unless the animal is extremely compromised, sedation or anesthesia are recommended. Central venous catheters should be frequently cleaned and monitored for loss of patency or signs of infection as in a mammalian central line, and if any are seen the catheter should be removed.

The intraosseous (IO) route is not used as frequently in chelonians as it is in other reptiles due to their comparatively easier intravenous access but is available when needed (Figure 11.36). Sites include the distal femur or humerus and the bridge or gular plastron—the limb sites were shown to have better efficacy than the shell sites in one study in tortoises (Young et al. 2012). A spinal needle is ideal, but a needle with a smaller needle inside to serve as a stylet can be used. The size of the needle is dependent on the animal and the site.

The area should be thoroughly cleaned and sterilely prepared. While grasping the femur or humerus both

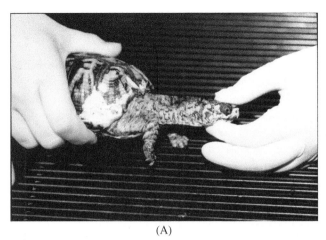

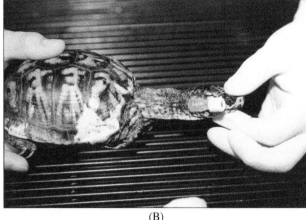

(A)
(B)

Figure 11.35 Jugular catheter placement. (A) Proper restraint for jugular catheterization. (B) Placement of jugular catheter. (Courtesy of Ryan Cheek, RVT.)

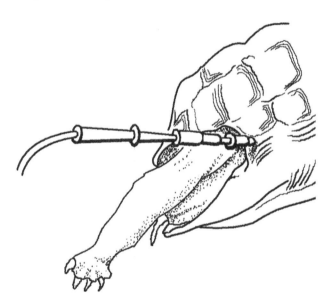

Figure 11.36 Intraosseous catheter (Drawing by Scott Stark.)

to provide stabilization and approximate the angle at which the needle needs to be introduced to stay within the medullary canal, the needle should be introduced to the distal aspect of the bone and advanced proximally using gentle pressure and twisting motions. Care should be taken that the stabilizing hand is not placed where it can be injured if the needle is inadvertently advanced back out of the bone more proximally. While the intravenous catheter techniques described above are easily extrapolated from mammals, it is recommended that, if possible, it is ideal to have IO catheter placement demonstrated by an individual with experience placing them rather than attempting alone the first time. Placement should be confirmed with orthogonal radiographs.

Therapeutic Administration

Intramuscular route

Many agents, including but not limited to antimicrobials, anesthetics, and calcium/vitamin supplementation, can be given intramuscularly (IM). The skin should be cleaned thoroughly before any injection. Intramuscular injections are ideally given in the triceps or pectoral muscles but can be given in the muscles of the hindlimbs as well. Due to the existence of the renal portal system, medications injected in the caudal half of the body may be filtered by the kidneys before entering the general circulation; drugs that are nephrotoxic or have significant first-pass elimination by the kidneys would therefore need to be given in the cranial half of the body. While some studies have shown differences in drug effects based on intravenous administration sites (Di Giuseppe et al. 2018), it remains best practice to give medications in the front half of the body, if possible. Staff safety should not be compromised in an effort to try to achieve cranial administration in the case of dangerous animals such as snapping turtles.

Subcutaneous route

Subcutaneous (SC/SQ) injections can be given under the skin of the axillary and prefemoral fossa. Absorption of medications and fluids administered subcutaneously is variable in reptiles (Perry & Mitchell 2019); this route is generally used for fluids more than for medications. The skin should be cleaned thoroughly before any injection. As reptile skin can be less elastic than mammalian, a slight twisting movement of the needle, as it is withdrawn, may help prevent leakage.

As with any animal, drugs with a very high or low pH should not be given by IM or SQ injection, and hyperosmotic fluids should not be given subcutaneously.

While recommendations do not exist for all drugs in reptile species, if a product is known to have adverse effects when given by these routes in mammals, the same can likely be extrapolated to reptiles.

Intravenous/intraosseous route

See the previous section for intravenous (IV) and intraosseous (IO) catheter placement instructions. The subcarapacial venous sinus has been used commonly to give fluids and medications. However, studies have shown that injections at this site can extravasate into the vertebral canal (Quesada et al. 2010; Rockwell et al. 2022) and respiratory tract (Rockwell et al. 2022); extravasation into the respiratory tract occurred in only one species of the three studied, likely due to species differences in how cranially the lungs extend. Advantages of this route include the ability for bolus or continuous administration of fluids and medications as needed, and the ability to give fluids with higher concentrations of dextrose if needed.

Intracoelomic route

The intracoelomic route (ICo/ICe) is used mostly for the administration of fluids, especially in sea turtles. While this route is used successfully, it carries a risk of injection of fluids into the respiratory tract or lacerating viscera. For this reason, other routes for fluid administration should be prioritized over intracoelomic if possible. Restrain the animal in lateral recumbency as this will cause the viscera and reproductive organs to shift away from the injection site. The needle should be inserted parallel to the plastron and directed cranially in the ventral aspect of the prefemoral fossa. When injecting fluids into the celomic cavity, keep in mind that the needle does not have to be inserted very deep. This route should not be used if there is any question of the integrity of the respiratory tract, such as with carapacial fractures.

Epicoelomic route

The epicoelomic route is useful for fluid administration in chelonians, especially if they are withdrawn into their shell or of a size that limits other administration methods. Restrain the turtle in sternal recumbency. The needle should be inserted into the potential space located dorsal to the plastron and ventral to the pectoral muscles, with the needle oriented parallel to the plastron. Discontinue administration if there is resistance to injection.

Oral route

The oral route (PO) is a good choice for fluid administration in mildly dehydrated animals and is also used for nutritional support and administration of enteral medications. The supplies needed are round-tip stainless steel gavage needles or red rubber catheters, speculums, and syringes of various sizes. Many sick turtles are anorexic, and nutritional support is essential for a full recovery. The most challenging part in many cases is opening the mouth. Some turtles will open their mouths when restrained—one can take advantage of this and insert a speculum quickly. If this fails, the mouth must be pried open. The upper beak in chelonians hangs slightly over the lower beak. A blunt tool can be inserted under the upper beak and inserted in the mouth, taking care not to cause damage to the beak. Once in the oral cavity, the tool should be twisted. Once the mouth is opened, the speculum can be inserted—materials like soft rubber are recommended to decrease the likelihood of damage to the beak. Food or medications being given into the oral cavity should be limited to small volumes and given slowly to avoid aspiration—administration via a stomach tube (gavage) is generally recommended to prevent complications. If medications or food are being gavage fed, the tube should be passed along the dorsal aspect of the oral cavity and into the esophagus while maintaining visualization of the glottis; the tube can then be advanced a pre-measured distance to the stomach (hold the head fully extended and measure the distance from the mouth to the pectoral scutes). The tube should be primed with the food or liquid medication ahead of time. The contents should be administered slowly while watching the oral cavity, and administration stopped if any reflux into the oral cavity is seen.

Refeeding should be started at most with a quarter of the calculated daily requirement (less if anorexia has been prolonged) and should be broken up into smaller feedings throughout the day if necessary; starting with a volume of 5 mL/kg per administration which is recommended to decrease the chance of regurgitation (Boyer & Scott 2019). Make sure to account for any volume of fluid used to flush the feeding tube, as this may be significant in smaller animals. If long-term medication or feeding is required, an esophagostomy tube "E-tube" should be placed.

Esophagostomy tube placement, maintenance, and use are essentially the same as in mammals, with the exception that the tube is generally secured to the carapace in chelonians, making sure to leave slack for neck movement. The tube should be premeasured to the pectoral scutes with neck extended as in gavage administration. Placement should always be verified with radiographs prior to use.

Cloacal route

Fluids and deworming medications can be administered via the cloaca. A lubricated red rubber catheter or gavage needle can be placed in the cloaca and the desired medication delivered. It is recommended to hold the turtle at an angle, with the cloaca elevated above the turtle's head to improve the absorption rate (Bonner 2000).

Topical route

A variety of topical medications have been used for wound care, and there are some topical acaricides that have been used in chelonians (see Parasitology section). Topical medications should be fully dry before aquatic chelonians are allowed to return to the water.

Nebulization

One of the most common problems seen in clinical practice is respiratory disease. Nebulization is a relatively stress-free method to deliver medications into the respiratory system. Turtles have lower respiratory rates than mammals and birds, therefore the nebulization time must be extended, generally for at least 1 h. Nebulization is generally performed by placing the animal in an enclosed chamber and ensuring that the chamber adequately fills with visible mist.

Miscellaneous Clinical Techniques

Wound care

Due to slow healing times and the need to leave wounds open to heal by second intention in reptiles, wound care can be a prolonged process. Placement of traditional bandages is limited by chelonians' unique anatomy, so tie-over bandages are often used on soft tissue wounds. Vacuum-assisted closure (VAC) has also been used successfully in chelonians. While purpose-made materials exist for VAC, alternatives that are more commonly available such as red rubber catheters, Tegaderm, and plastic wrap have been used successfully (Marin & Norton 2019) (Figure 11.37). It is important to monitor that a good seal is being maintained and discontinue VAC if the seal is lost, as loss of negative pressure can promote bacterial growth. Prolonged dry-docking in aquatic chelonians during wound management can lead to dehydration and inappetence. A technique has been described in which a plastic specimen cup with the bottom portion removed was epoxied around a wound, forming a waterproof shield for the wound, which could be accessed via removal of the cup lid as needed, allowing the animal to enter the water during recovery (Sypniewski et al. 2016). If wounds are limited to the carapace, animals can be maintained in shallow water, and if waterproof dressings can be successfully applied, full submersion may be possible without compromising wound healing (Patson et al. 2022). Watertight seals will be much easier to achieve in shell wounds than soft tissue wounds. Otherwise, fluid therapy is usually necessary throughout treatment, and placement of an esophagostomy tube should be considered.

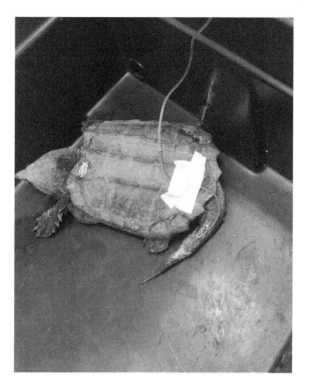

Figure 11.37 Improvised vacuum-assisted closure for traumatic wounds in an alligator snapping turtle (*Macrochelys temminckii*). (Courtesy of Dr. Sarah Camlic.)

Shell fractures are discussed previously in the Surgery section, but associated wounds can be treated similarly to soft tissue wounds, being careful to not instill any products into full-thickness shell fractures. Traditional external coaptation of limb fractures is limited due to the presence of the shell, but the shell itself can be used to immobilize the fractured limb by reducing the limb into the fossa and using tape or bandaging material to prevent extension (Knafo & Karlin 2019a). Alignment should be checked via radiographs afterward.

Fecal examination

It is important to collect a fresh fecal sample. Dry feces are not recommended as many protozoan organisms die as the feces dry out. The client should be advised to collect the feces at home, place the sample in multiple sealable plastic bags, and keep it refrigerated. Reiterate to the client the dangers of keeping reptile feces where food for human consumption is stored. If the sample is to be kept refrigerated, extreme hygiene is important to prevent cross-contamination. The sample can be refrigerated overnight, but longer refrigeration is not recommended. The fecal exams must be done using fecal material and not urates. If a fresh sample is not available, a colonic wash can be performed to obtain a sample.

Direct fecal exam: Using a small wooden stick, place a small amount of feces on a microscope slide. Place a cover slip on top and examine immediately; the longer the sample sits the more likely motile protozoans will die. Do not use the swab end of a cotton tip applicator as the cotton can absorb a substantial amount of your sample. You can stain the sample by adding one drop of Lugol's solution. It is ideal to prepare two direct smears, one stained and one unstained, as the Lugol's solution will kill motile protozoans.

Fecal flotation: The flotation technique is done in the same manner as that for small animals. For selected organisms, specialty flotation techniques may be needed (see Parasitology section).

Cloacal and colonic wash and enema

Colonic wash is performed when a sample for fecal examination has not been produced, and enemas can be used in cases of constipation. The techniques are the same as detailed in Chapter 9.

Respiratory tract sampling

Nasal flushes can be performed for both therapeutic (dislodgement of foreign material or accumulated secretions) and diagnostic purposes (Studer & Di Girolamo 2021). A catheter of appropriate size with needle removed is introduced into the nares and saline is flushed, taking care to either place something absorbent in the oral cavity or tilt the head downward to prevent aspiration of the fluid as it exits the choana. Since the nasal passages are not sterile environments results should be interpreted with caution.

Tracheal wash or bronchoalveolar lavage can be performed to assess for respiratory pathogens. The animal is anesthetized and intubated (see Anesthesia section) and a sterile catheter is advanced through the lumen of the sterile ET tube to the midcoelom—the tube should not be forced if resistance is met. Sterile saline is infused at 5 mL/kg; the saline can be aspirated and flushed multiple times and the patient can be rocked side to side or coupaged to increase the chance of obtaining a diagnostic sample (Knotek & Divers 2019).

Emergency and Critical Care

While many emergent reptile presentations are due to long-standing issues in husbandry and have poor to grave prognoses, this is not always the case, and any critically ill reptile that presents should be treated with the same level of care as a mammalian patient.

History and physical examination are exceedingly important in any emergency presentation and are detailed in the "History, Restraint, and Physical Examination" section earlier in this chapter. While a full history may not always be able to be obtained immediately, at least a brief triage history of inciting events should be obtained, and if available a second person can go obtain a more thorough history while the primary clinician works on stabilization. Many clinics have an option for the owner to approve a stabilization estimate, in which certain diagnostics and therapeutics up to a certain cost are detailed on a sheet that the owner can consent to prior to a full conversation with the clinician. This can be helpful to quickly rule in or out metabolic causes (hypocalcemia, hypoglycemia, etc.) in cases such as tremors/seizures, stupor, and similar presentations so that treatment is not delayed. Packed cell volume/total solids (PCV/TS), blood glucose, and blood lactate are commonly available triage diagnostics, and point-of-care blood gas machines that often include ionized calcium and osmolarity are also available in some clinics. Care should be taken when interpreting results as reptilian normals can be extremely different from mammalian normals (if normals for the species exist) and can also vary significantly by species and other environmental factors (Studer & Di Girolamo 2021).

Any major bleeding that is present on presentation should be addressed, and owners should be asked to estimate how much was lost at home—while owners may not be able to provide a volume amount, prompting them to describe blood spots based on the size of coins can sometimes provide a more accurate estimate.

A Prolapsed tissue should be addressed promptly (see the section on the digestive system within "Common Disorders"). Any open wounds should be covered with a non-adherent dressing if possible and pain medication should be provided for obvious major trauma. If obvious infection or major tissue compromise are found, or known bite wounds are present, samples for culture should be obtained and broad-spectrum antimicrobial therapy initiated (Norton et al. 2019). There is an argument to be made for starting antimicrobials when petechiation is present due to the previously discussed high correlation with sepsis in chelonians.

A Focused Assessment with Sonograph for Trauma (FAST) scan can be employed as part of initial assessment to look for free coelomic fluid—a FAST scan should be serially re-evaluated during rehydration in the event fluid begins to accumulate. Fluid should be sampled to direct differentials and therapy if enough is present and accessible.

As discussed in the section on pre-anesthetic consideration, the same principles that apply to mammals can likely be extrapolated to reptiles regarding fluid selection. Crystalloids should be used for rehydration and as a first step in volume resuscitation unless a specific indication for another fluid is present such as severe anemia or severe hypoproteinemia. PCV/TS is a valuable tool for assessing hydration status, as are physical examination and history. As many dehydrated reptiles have become dehydrated very chronically, care should be taken to not replace the deficit too quickly, with a goal of 48–72 h to avoid life-threatening cerebral edema as with chronic hypernatremia and similar conditions in mammals. If immediate volume resuscitation is needed, custom fluids may be required. In critically ill animals, IV access is the first choice for fluid resuscitation and drug administration; while IV access can be challenging in reptiles as previously discussed, severely compromised chelonians may be relatively easier to obtain jugular access in as they are less likely to be able to strongly withdraw into their shell.

Use of synthetic colloids has not been thoroughly investigated in reptiles, but a variety of adverse effects have been reported in mammals. While there is no correct answer due to the lack of research available, it might be beneficial to attempt resuscitation with blood products rather than colloids.

Chelonians tend to tolerate very low hematocrit levels (Brown 2022), but there are certainly cases where blood transfusion would be indicated, especially in the case of acute severe hemorrhage. The field of reptile transfusion medicine is young, but there have been several reports of successful transfusions, including xenotransfusions, in reptiles (Petritz & Son 2019), and several successful unpublished transfusions have occurred. Transfusion reactions have been reported, so a crossmatch should be performed if possible. Blood can be obtained from a healthy donor at 1% bodyweight (1 mL/100 g) into an anticoagulated syringe and line and administered through a filter.

While it is important to warm ill reptiles to their POTZ to bring their metabolism back to a more normal state, it may be beneficial to delay warming if the animal is thought to be hypovolemic as vasodilation from warming without fluid resuscitation could potentially lead to cardiovascular collapse—risks/benefits of this should be evaluated on a case-by-case basis. Warmed intravenous fluids (using a temperature-controlled fluid warmer) can be considered to concurrently provide volume support and thermal support.

Anemia and hyperlactatemia, including change in lactate over time, were found to be significant indicators of mortality in a variety of wild chelonian species (Gregory et al. 2022). A study in Eastern box turtles (*Terrapene carolina carolina*) presenting for trauma also found lactate to be a prognostic indicator. This study also developed a triage score that was correlated with acute and long-term mortality (Tucker-Retter & Lewbart 2022).

For wildlife, it is important to check if the animal is a protected species as there can be specific regulations regarding care and euthanasia of some species. It is prudent to check if deceased females have eggs present, especially in threatened or endangered species.

While every patient should be evaluated individually, euthanasia should be strongly considered in trauma patients in the following cases (Norton et al. 2019):

- Spinal or skull fractures
- Loss of >30% of the shell
- Internal injuries or evisceration, especially with obvious compromise of organs; bubbling from wound or fracture sites indicates some degree of respiratory tract involvement.

There is limited research on cardiopulmonary resuscitation (CPR) in reptiles. As previously discussed, reptiles have significantly higher tolerance to hypoxic and anoxic conditions, and anecdotally return of spontaneous circulation (ROSC) has been achieved after far longer periods of arrest than in mammals (Martinez-Jimenez & Hernandez-Divers 2007). Direct cardiac compression in chelonians is not possible due to the presence of the shell, but anecdotally pumping of the front legs has been performed in chelonian CPR. CPR should be performed in accordance with small mammal guidelines. Because drug doses differ, it is recommended that all hospitalized patients have a precalculated emergency drug sheet that is species-specific placed on their enclosure.

Euthanasia

In the veterinary community, there remains significant apprehension regarding euthanasia of chelonians—the propensity to leave euthanized animals out overnight, to draw a line around their body to ensure there is no movement when the cadaver is left to its own devices, etc. are common across clinics. It is believed that this reflects a general unfamiliarity with reptile physiology and approved methods of euthanasia, combined with a fear of causing undue suffering if the animal is not fully dead. The wish to prevent pain is admirable, but a thorough grasp of chelonian physiology and euthanasia should grant confidence and preclude the need for chelonian chalk outlines.

Confirmation of death is not straightforward in reptiles. Some of the signs that help confirm death include lack of response to painful stimuli, absence of a corneal reflex, rigor mortis, and absence of a heartbeat. However, in reptiles, the heart can continue to beat after death, and other spontaneous movement of the body can also persist. Because of this, euthanasia of reptiles should be a multistep process (Nevarez 2019; AVMA 2020).

The first step is IM or IV (SQ may be considered but usually at least IM injection is feasible) injectable anesthesia. As previously discussed dissociatives such as ketamine combinations or tiletamine-zolazepam are an excellent choice for IM injection, and propofol or alfaxalone can be used if there is IV access. Once unresponsive to painful stimuli, an injectable euthanasia agent such as pentobarbital or potassium chloride should be given (IV, IO, IC, or ICe). This should always be followed with a physical euthanasia method such as decapitation or pithing.

Owners may wish to be present for the euthanasia process. A frank discussion of the process and the need for physical methods in reptiles should be had with them. Owners will often still wish to be present for at least part of the process. Many veterinary practices have found that a good compromise is that owners may choose to be present for the IM sedation (or their animal is brought back to them immediately after IM injection) but not present for the euthanasia itself.

References

Abdala V, Manzano AS, Herrel A. 2008. The distal forelimb musculature in aquatic and terrestrial turtles: phylogeny or environmental constraints? *J Anat* 213(2): 159–172.

Adamovicz L, Allender MC, Gibbons PM. 2020. Emerging infectious diseases of chelonians: an update. *Vet Clin North Am Exot Anim Pract* 23(2): 263–283.

Agha M, Ennen JR, et al. 2018. Macroecological patterns of sexual size dimorphism in turtles of the world. *J Evol Biol* 31: 336–345.

Akram SM, Rathish B, Saleh D. 2022. Mycobacterium chelonae. In: *StatPearls [Internet]*. Treasure Island, FL: StatPearls Publishing.

AVMA. 2020. *AVMA Guidelines for the Euthanasia of Animals*. pp. 92–94.

Baron H, Phalen DN. 2018. Diseases of the nervous system. In: *Reptile Medicine and Surgery in Clinical Practice* (eds B Doneley, D Monks, R Johnson, B Carmel), pp. 331–344. Hoboken: John Wiley & Sons Ltd.

Bonner BB. 2000. Chelonian therapeutics. *Vet Clin North Am Exot Anim Pract* 3(7): 257–332.

Bosch S, Tauxe R, Behravesh CB. 2016. Turtle-associated salmonellosis, United States, 2006–2014. *Emerg Infect Dis* 22(7): 1149–1155.

Boyer TH, Boyer DM. 2019. Tortoises, freshwater turtles, and terrapins. In: *Mader's Reptile and Amphibian Medicine and Surgery* (eds SJ Divers, SJ Stahl), pp. 168–179. St. Louis: Elsevier.

Boyer TH, Scott PW. 2019. Nutritional therapy. In: *Mader's Reptile and Amphibian Medicine and Surgery* (eds SJ Divers, SJ Stahl), pp. 1173–1176. St. Louis: Elsevier.

Brown S. 2022. Providing critical care to sick tortoises. *In Practice* 44(4): 193–256.

Camacho M, Quintana M, et al. 2015. Acid-base and plasma biochemical changes using crystalloid fluids in stranded juvenile loggerhead sea turtles (*Caretta caretta*). *PLoS One* 10(7): e0132217.

Carmel B, Johnson R. 2018. Nutritional and metabolic diseases. In: *Reptile Medicine and Surgery in Clinical Practice* (eds B Doneley, D Monks, R Johnson, B Carmel), pp. 185–195.

Christensen-Dalsgaard J, Brandt C, et al. 2012. Specialization for underwater hearing by the tympanic middle ear of the turtle, *Trachemys scripta elegans*. *Proc R Soc B* 279: 2816–2824.

Christman J, Devau M, et al. 2017. Oncology of reptiles: diseases, diagnosis, and treatment. *Vet Clin North Am Exot Anim Pract* 20(1): 87–110.

Damborg P, Broens EM, et al. 2016. Bacterial zoonoses transmitted by household pets: state-of-the-art and future perspectives for targeted research and policy actions. *J Comp Pathol* 155(1): S27–S40.

De Luca C, Iraola G, et al. 2020. Occurrence and diversity of *Campylobacter* species in captive chelonians. *Vet Microbiol* 241: 108567.

Di Giuseppe M, Faraci L, et al. 2018. Preliminary survey on influence of renal portal system during propofol anesthesia in yellow-bellied turtle (*Trachemys scripta scripta*). *J Vet Med Allied Sci* 2(1): 12–15.

Divers S. 1996. Basic reptile husbandry, history taking, and clinical examination. *In Practice* 18(2): 51–65.

Divers SJ. 2019. Endoscope-assisted and endoscopic surgery. In: *Mader's Reptile and Amphibian Medicine and Surgery* (eds SJ Divers, SJ Stahl), pp. 1071–1076. St. Louis: Elsevier.

Druzisky KA, Brainerd EL. 2001. Buccal oscillation and lung ventilation in a semi-aquatic turtle, *Platysternon megacephalum*. *Zoology* 104(2): 143–152.

Ebani VV, Fratini F, et al. 2012. Isolation and identification of mycobacteria from captive reptiles. *Res Vet Sci* 93: 1136–1138.

Federation of British Herpetologists. 2022. *Recommended Minimum Enclosure Sizes for Reptiles*.

Fraher J, Davenport J, et al. 2010. Opening and closing mechanisms of the leatherback sea turtle larynx: a crucial role for the tongue. *J Exp Biol* 213(24): 4137–4145.

Franchini D, Valastro C, et al. 2018. Ultrasonographic detection of ingested fishing lines in loggerheads (*Caretta caretta*). *J Wildl Dis* 54(4): 68.

Galeotti P, Sacchi R, Rosa DP, Fasola M. 2007. Olfactory discrimination of species, sex, and sexual maturity by the Hermann's tortoise *Testudo hermanni*. *Copeia* 2007(4): 980–985.

Gárriz A, Williamson SE, et al. 2022. Transcriptomic analysis of preovipositional embryonic arrest in a nonsquamate reptile (*Chelonia mydas*). *Mol Ecol* 31(16): 4319–4331.

Gibbons JW, Lovich JE. 1990. Sexual dimorphism in turtles with emphasis on the slider turtle (*Trachemys scripta*). *Herpetol Monogr* 4: 1–29.

Girgis S. 1961. Aquatic respiration in the common Nile turtle, *Trionyx triunguis*. *Comp Biochem Physiol* 3: 206.

Goławska O, Zając M, et al. 2019. Complex bacterial flora of imported pet tortoises deceased during quarantine: another zoonotic threat? *Comp Immunol Microbiol Infect Dis* 65: 154–159.

Gregers MCT, Mikkelsen S, Lindvig KP, Brøchner AC. 2020. Ketamine as an anesthetic for patients with acute brain injury: a systematic review. *Neurocrit Care* 33(1): 273–282.

Gregory TM, Hubbard C, et al. 2022. Evaluation of prognostic indicators for injured turtles presenting to a wildlife clinic. *J Zoo Wildl Med* 53(1): 209–213.

Greunz EM, Williams C, et al. 2018. Elimination of intracardiac shunting provides stable gas anesthesia in tortoises. *Sci Rep* 8: 17124.

Harkewicz KA. 2001. Dermatology of reptiles: a clinical approach to diagnosis and treatment. *Vet Clin North Am Exot Anim* 4(2): 441–461.

Heinrich ML, Heinrich KK. 2016. Effect of supplemental heat in captive African leopard tortoises (*Stigmochelys pardalis*) and spurred tortoises (*Centrochelys sulcata*) on growth rate and carapacial scute pyramiding. *J Exot Pet Med* 25(1): 18–25.

Hellebuyck T, Vilanova FS. 2022. The use of prefemoral endoscope-assisted surgery and transplastron coeliotomy in chelonian reproductive disorders. *Animals* 12(23): 3439.

Hernandez-Divers SJ. 2001. Pulmonary candidiasis caused by *Candida albicans* in a Greek tortoise (*Testudo graeca*) and treatment with intrapulmonary amphotericin B. *J Zoo Wildl Med* 32(3): 352–359.

Holz PH. 1999. The reptilian renal portal system—a review. *Bull Assoc Reptil Amphi Vet* 9(1): 4.

Holz PH. 2018. Diseases of the urinary tract. In: *Reptile Medicine and Surgery in Clinical Practice* (eds B Doneley, D Monks, R Johnson, B Carmel), pp. 323–330. Hoboken: John Wiley & Sons Ltd.

Hoppmann E, Barron HW. 2007. Dermatology in reptiles. *J Exot Pet Med* 16(4): 210–224.

Innis CJ. 2010. Endoscopy and endosurgery of the chelonian reproductive tract. *Vet Clin North Am Exot Anim Pract* 13(2): 243–254.

Jones K, Ariel E, Burgess G, Read M. 2016. A review of fibropapillomatosis in green turtles (*Chelonia mydas*). *Vet J* 212: 48–57.

Keller KA, Hawkins MG, et al. 2015. Diagnosis and treatment of urolithiasis in client-owned chelonians: 40 cases (1987–2012). *J Am Vet Med Assoc* 247(6): 650–658.

Kinoshita C, Saito A, et al. 2022. A non-invasive heart rate measurement method is improved by placing the electrodes on the ventral side rather than the dorsal in loggerhead turtles. *Front Physiol* 13: 811947.

Knafo SE, Karlin WM. 2019a. Orthopedic principles and external coaptation. In: *Mader's Reptile and Amphibian Medicine and Surgery* (eds SJ Divers, SJ Stahl), pp. 1100–1103. St. Louis: Elsevier.

Knafo SE, Karlin WM. 2019b. Fracture fixation and arthrodesis. In: *Mader's Reptile and Amphibian Medicine and Surgery* (eds SJ Divers, SJ Stahl), pp. 1104–1108. St. Louis: Elsevier.

Knafo SE, Karlin WM. 2019c. Limb amputation. In: *Mader's Reptile and Amphibian Medicine and Surgery* (eds SJ Divers, SJ Stahl), pp. 1111–1112. St. Louis: Elsevier.

Knotek Z, Divers SJ. 2019. Pulmonology. In: *Mader's Reptile and Amphibian Medicine and Surgery* (eds SJ Divers, SJ Stahl), pp. 786–804. St. Louis: Elsevier.

Lutcavage ME, Lutz PL. 1991. Voluntary diving metabolism and ventilation in the loggerhead sea turtle. *J Exp Mar Biol Ecol* 147: 287–296.

Mans C. 2013. Clinical update on diagnosis and management of disorders of the digestive system of reptiles. *J Exot Pet Med* 22(2): 141–162.

Mans C, Sladky KK, Schumacher J. 2019. General anesthesia. In: *Mader's Reptile and Amphibian Medicine and Surgery* (eds SJ Divers, SJ Stahl), pp. 447–464. St. Louis: Elsevier.

March DT, Marshall K, et al. 2020. The use of echocardiography as a health assessment tool in green sea turtles (*Chelonia mydas*). *Aust Vet J* 99(1–2): 46–54.

Marin ML, Norton TM. 2019. Wound management. In: *Mader's Reptile and Amphibian Medicine and Surgery* (eds SJ Divers, SJ Stahl), pp. 1225–1231. St. Louis: Elsevier.

Martinez-Jimenez D, Hernandez-Divers SJ. 2007. Emergency care of reptiles. *Vet Clin North Am Exot Anim Pract* 10(2): 557–585.

Marschang RE. 2019. Virology. In: *Mader's Reptile and Amphibian Medicine and Surgery* (eds SJ Divers, SJ Stahl), pp. 247–269. St. Louis: Elsevier.

Martorell J, Espada Y, Ruiz de Gopegui R. 2004. Normal echoanatomy of the red-eared slider terrapin (*Trachemys scripta elegans*). *Vet Rec* 155(14): 417–420.

Mitchell MA, Diaz-Figueroa O. 2005. Clinical reptile gastroenterology. *Vet Clin North Am Exot Anim Pract* 8(2): 277–298.

Nevarez JG. 2019. Euthanasia. In: *Mader's Reptile and Amphibian Medicine and Surgery* (eds SJ Divers, SJ Stahl), pp. 437–440. St. Louis: Elsevier.

Norton TM, Fleming GJ, Meyer J. 2019. Shell surgery and repair. In: *Mader's Reptile and Amphibian Medicine and Surgery* (eds SJ Divers, SJ Stahl), pp. 1116–1126. St. Louis: Elsevier.

Okoh GR, Horwood PF, Whitmore D, Ariel E. 2021. Herpesviruses in reptiles. *Front Vet Sci* 8. doi: 10.3389/fvets.2021.642894.

Origgi FC. 2012. Testudinid herpesviruses: a review. *J Herpetol Med Surg* 22(1–2): 42–54.

Pardo MA, Divers S. 2016. Jugular central venous catheter placement through a modified seldinger technique for long-term venous access in chelonians. *J Zoo Wildlife Med* 47(1), 286–290.

Parkinson LA, Mans C. 2020. Evaluation of subcutaneously administered electrolyte solutions in experimentally dehydrated inland bearded dragons (*Pogona vitticeps*). *Am J Vet Res* 81(5):437–441.

Patson CN, Lemlet EM, Mans C. 2022. Outcome of common snapping turtles (*Chelydra serpentina*) treated for acute traumatic partial carapace avulsion: 12 cases (2014–2021). *J Exot Pet Med* 43: 4–10.

Penninck DG, Stewart JS, Paul-Murphy J, Pion P. 1991. Ultrasonography of the California desert tortoise (*Xerobates agassizii*). *Vet Rad* 32(3): 98–151.

Perry SM, Mitchell MA. 2019. Routes of administration. In: *Mader's Reptile and Amphibian Medicine and Surgery* (eds SJ Divers, SJ Stahl), pp. 1130–1138. St. Louis: Elsevier.

Petritz OA, Son TT. 2019. Emergency and critical care. In: *Mader's Reptile and Amphibian Medicine and Surgery* (eds SJ Divers, SJ Stahl), pp. 967–976. St. Louis: Elsevier.

Pizzi R, Goodman G, et al. 2005. *Pieris japonica* intoxication in an African spurred tortoise (*Geochelone sulcata*). *Vet Rec* 156: 487–488.

Quesada RJ, Aitken-Palmer C, Conley K, Heard DJ. 2010. Accidental submeningeal injection of propofol in gopher tortoises (*Gopherus polyphemus*). *Vet Rec* 167(13): 464–500.

Redrobe SP, Scudamore CL. 2000. Ultrasonographic diagnosis of pericardial effusion and atrial dilation in a spur-thighed tortoise (*Testudo graeca*). *Vet Rec* 146(7): 183.

Rehermann MI, Marichal N, Russo RE, Trujillo-Cenóz O. 2009. Neural reconnection in the transected spinal cord of the freshwater turtle *Trachemys dorbigni*. *J Comp Neurol* 515(2): 197–214.

Ritz J, Clauss M, Streich WJ, Hatt J. 2012. Variation in growth and potentially associated health status in Hermann's and spur-thighed tortoise (*Testudo hermanii* and *Testudo graeca*). *Zoo Biol* 31: 705–717.

Rivera S, Lock B. 2008. The reptilian thyroid and parathyroid glands. *Vet Clin North Am Exot Anim Pract* 11(1): 163–175.

Rockwell K, Mitchell MA. 2019. Antiparasitic therapy. In: *Mader's Reptile and Amphibian Medicine and Surgery* (eds SJ Divers, SJ Stahl), pp. 1111–1112. St. Louis: Elsevier.

Rockwell K, Rademacher N, Osborn ML, Nevarez JG. 2022. Extravasation of contrast media after subcarapacial vessel injection in three chelonian species. *J Zoo Wildl Med* 53(2): 402–411.

Rossi JV. 2019. General husbandry and management. In: *Mader's Reptile and Amphibian Medicine and Surgery* (eds SJ Divers, SJ Stahl), pp. 109–130. St. Louis: Elsevier.

Rotstein DS, Lewbart GA, et al. 2003. Suspected oak, *Quercus*, toxicity in an African spurred tortoise, *Sulcata*. *J Herpetol Med Surg* 13(3): 20–21.

Salzmann E, Müller E, Marschang RE. 2021. Detection of testadenoviruses and atadenoviruses in tortoises and turtles in Europe. *J Zoo Wildl Med* 52(1): 223–231.

Schilliger L. 2022. Heart diseases in reptiles: diagnosis and therapy. *Vet Clin North Am Exot Anim Pract* 25(2): 383–407.

Schmidt RE, Reavill DR. 2010. Cardiopulmonary disease in reptiles. In: Proceedings of the Association of Reptilian and Amphibian Veterinarians Conference. pp. 90–98.

Schnellbacher RW, Shepard M. 2019. Sedation. In: *Mader's Reptile and Amphibian Medicine and Surgery* (eds SJ Divers, SJ Stahl), pp. 441–446. St. Louis: Elsevier.

Sleeman JM, Brown J, et al. 2008. Relationships among aural abscesses, organochlorine compounds, and vitamin a in free-ranging Eastern box turtles (*Terrapene carolina carolina*). *J Wildl Dis* 44(4): 922–929.

Sodagari HR, Habib I, et al. 2020. A review of the public health challenges of *Salmonella* and turtles. *Vet Sci* 7(2): 56.

Stahl SJ, DeNardo DF. 2019. Theriogenology. In: *Mader's Reptile and Amphibian Medicine and Surgery* (eds SJ Divers, SJ Stahl), pp. 849–893. St. Louis: Elsevier.

Stein PSG. 2018. Central pattern generators in the turtle spinal cord: selection among the forms of motor behaviors. *J Neurophysiol* 119: 422–440.

Studer K, Di Girolamo N. 2021. Respiratory disorders in chelonians. *Vet Clin North Am Exot Anim Pract* 24(2): 341–367.

Sypniewski LA, Hahn A, et al. 2016. Novel shell wound care in the aquatic turtle. *J Exot Pet Med* 25(2): 110–114.

Takami Y. 2017. Single-incision, prefemoral bilateral oophorosalpingectomy without coelioscopy in an Indian star tortoise (*Geochelone elegans*) with follicular stasis. *J Vet Med Sci* 79(10): 1675–1677.

Trevizan-Baú P, Abe AS, Klein W. 2018. Effects of environmental hypoxia and hypercarbia on ventilation and gas exchange in Testudines. *PeerJ*. doi: 10.7717/peerj.5137.

Tucker-Retter EK, Lewbart GA. 2022. Corticosterone, lactate, and injury severity as short-term and long-term prognostic indicators in Eastern box turtles (*Terrapene carolina carolina*) with traumatic injuries admitted to a wildlife rehabilitation clinic *J Herpetol Med Surg* 32(4).

Wellehan JFX, Walden HDS. 2019. Parasitology (including hemoparasites). In: *Mader's Reptile and Amphibian Medicine and Surgery* (eds SJ Divers, SJ Stahl), pp. 281–300. St. Louis: Elsevier.

White SD, Bourdeau P, et al. 2011. Reptiles with dermatological lesions: a retrospective study of 301 cases at two university veterinary teaching hospitals (1992–2008). *Vet Dermatol* 22(2): 150–161.

Young BD, Stegeman N, Norby B, Heatley JJ. 2012. Comparison of intraosseous and peripheral venous fluid dynamics in the desert tortoise (*Gopherus agassizii*). *J Zoo Wildl Med* 43(1): 59–66.

12

Herpetoculture and Reproduction
David Martinez-Jimenez

Introduction

In 2021, the US spent $123.6 billion on their pets, of that, $34.3 billion were spent on vet care and product sales. This is a $33.1 billion increase from 2018 and an indication that this is a growing market (APPA). According to the 2021–2022, APPA National Pet Owners Survey, 70% of US households own a pet which represents about 90.5 million homes. The reptile pet industry is a growing field with an estimated 13.4 million pet reptiles in 2007/2008 (APPA 2007/2008). This has gone from 4.8 million households in the United States to more than 5.7 million households (APPA 2021/2022).

In the United States, the reptile industry has been shifting over the past 20 years toward domestic captive breeding. Through selective breeding of uniquely colored patterns (morphs and/or phases), captive breeding is becoming a viable profession (The Modern US Reptile Industry). In 2009, 11.3 million live reptiles were exported from the United States while only 900,000 were imported. (United States Fish and Wildlife Service, Law Enforcement Management Information System ("LEMIS") data.)

Proper management and husbandry remain the major obstacles to maintaining a healthy reptile collection. Veterinary care is still one of the largest expenses for reptile owners and the 2010 APPA Survey reported $475.5 million spent on non-surgical veterinary care for owned reptiles each year (APPA 2010). As a breeding collection, the veterinarian and veterinary technician need to pay attention to the health of the entire collection and not just of the individual.

The importance of neonatal care and reptile breeding has a growing significance in the management of these captive reptile collections. Proper captive population management is essential to decrease inbreeding and disease spread. Reptile rarities through selective breeding in the form of morphs can have important health and ethical implications.

The purpose of this chapter is to cover the fundamentals for a healthy reptile collection, and the principles behind captive breeding.

Basic Principles for Breeding and Care

Stock Selection

Despite the increase in reptile pet ownership, reptile importation remains about the same. This can be explained by the increase in captive-bred reptiles (HSUS 2001). Unfortunately, this trade continues as captive breeding has not yet been mastered for all species of reptiles such as chameleons (HSUS 2001) (Table 12.1).

Careful selection of breeding stock is very important to meet future goals and prevent genetic problems. There are three types of breeding stock: captive-bred (animal is born by crossing two animals that were maintained and bred under human care), captive-hatched (animal was born in human care but breeding parents were wild born), and wild-caught (animal came from the wild).

Captive-bred is by far the best stock. It allows a more sustainable way of nourishing the pet market, decreases the chances of introducing foreign diseases, and promotes the breeding of more suitable traits like non-aggressiveness and tolerance to captivity.

Table 12.1 Species of reptiles by taxa. About 8734 species of reptiles are divided up as follows:

Amphisbaenia (amphisbaenians)	168 species
Sauria (lizards)	5079 species
Serpentes (snakes)	3149 species
Chelonia (turtles and tortoises)	313 species
Crocodylia (crocodiles)	23 species
Rhynchocephalia (tuataras)	2 species

Exotic Animal Medicine for the Veterinary Technician, Fourth Edition. Edited by Bonnie Ballard and Ryan Cheek.
© 2024 John Wiley & Sons, Inc. Published 2024 by John Wiley & Sons, Inc.
Companion Website: www.wiley.com/go/ballard/4e

Understanding Genetics

The careful planning and maintenance of the breeding stock has important implications in the management of the collection as well as the end result through the breeding of desirable morphs. Morphs transformed the reptile industry between the 80's and the 90's. The discovery of rare and colorful wild snakes (albinos) led to an increased demand for these unusual colors by the mid-90s.

As a goal, it is important to decide what type of genetics are best to be kept within the breeding stock. This would help in planning for possible new and desirable morphs as well as maintaining some genetic materials in case of a come-back of past valuable morphs. To understand this genetic diversity within the breeding stock, for example, just within the ball python species, there are currently over 100+ morphs (Clarke 2021). Because of this, breeding would also require a basic understanding of genetics.

This genetic blueprint is coded within the chromosomes. Chromosomes are structured into genes and a gene might control a particular phenotype. A phenotype is the observable characteristic controlled by the gene. To complicate things further, multiple genes can also work together to control a given phenotype and multiple phenotypes may be controlled by a single gene (in this case, these gene variations are referred to as alleles). Because chromosomes exist in pairs, genes do too. Homozygous means that both chromosomes of the pair possess the same allele while heterozygous means that only one chromosome carries the allele. The alterations on this blueprint are referred as mutations, which are the genetic basis of the various colors and pattern morphs in reptiles. There are dominant mutations when only one chromosome of the pair must have the mutation and recessive when both chromosomes must have the mutation in order for this phenotype to be observed (e.g., albinism).

There is a variation of dominance that is referred to as incomplete dominance. In this case, an individual that is heterozygous for the allele will have one mutant phenotype, while an animal that is homozygous for that allele will have a different phenotype. This is an example of the fire and pastel ball python morphs. Heterozygous pastel morphs have a lightened coloration, while homozygous pastel pythons have an even lighter coloration. In the case of the heterozygous fire morph, there is a reduction in brown pigments as well as a pattern reduction but the homozygous (generally referred as "super fire") have a leucistic phenotype (similar to albinos except they lack the pink eyes).

Another important term is co-dominance. This is when two different alleles cause phenotype changes in the same animal. In this case, the mutation is not recessive and is expressed in both heterozygous and homozygous states. An easy way to explain this would be to imagine an allele responsible for red-scale pigmentation and an allele responsible for blue-scale pigmentation. In this example, an individual having both red and blue alleles would likely have a purple phenotype.

This is important because it would allow the breeder to have input on the results of this breeding. For example, when breeding a homozygous albino male to a heterozygous albino female, 50% of the offspring will be homozygous albino and 50% will be heterozygous albino. Because the albinism mutation is recessive, heterozygous individuals will appear to be normal and those albinos would be homozygous.

Physical Examination and Sexing

Every incoming reptile should have a complete physical examination. This would include an examination of the cloaca. This is where copulation takes place and therefore it is directly involved during reproduction.

Sex determination is part of this physical examination. Properly sexed individuals would prevent the waste of time and energy as well as the monetary loss from failing to breed during the breeding season.

There are different ways of sexing reptiles but none of them is applicable for all reptile species. Methods of sex determination in reptiles are the following:

- Sexual dimorphism
- Probing
- Manual eversion of hemipenes or popping
- Hydrostatic eversion of hemipenes
- Digital palpation (crocodilians)
- Plasma testosterone
- Morphometric measurements
- DNA sexing (karyotyping)
- Ultrasonography
- Coelioscopy/laparoscopy

Sexual Dimorphism

Sexual dimorphism is the difference in appearance between males and females of the same species. This is usually apparent in some species of chelonians (turtles and tortoises) and saurians (lizards). Sexual dimorphism is generally apparent in adults but can be very difficult to determine sub-adults and juveniles. General guidelines for the identification of chelonian males are a longer tail with a cloacal opening beyond the rear carapacial shell margin, and a plastral concavity (Figure 12.1). Some other species-specific characteristics are long front limb

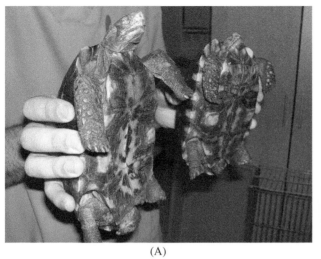

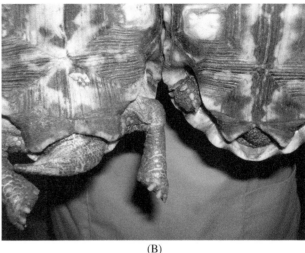

(A)   (B)

Figure 12.1 Sexual dimorphisim in a chelonian species, Red-footed tortoise (*Geochelone carbonaria*). (A) Plastral concavity is more pronounced in male chelonians than females to facilitate mating. (B) Male chelonians commonly have longer tails with the cloacal opening beyond the rear carapacial shell margin. (Courtesy of David Perpiñan LV, MSc, Veterinary Talent, Badalona, Spain.)

toenails in slider turtles (*Pseudemys* spp., *Trachemys scripta*), painted turtles (*Chrysemys picta*), and map turtles (*Graptemys* spp.); a red iris in the male Eastern box turtles (*Terrapene carolina carolina*); and more prominent mental glands, gular scutes, and body size in male desert tortoises (*Gopherus agassizii*). The female leopard tortoise (*Geochelone pardalis*) has larger toenails in the rear legs than in the male, and the female map turtles and diamondback terrapins are significantly larger than the males.

Although many lizard species are monomorphic, male lizards have a pair of hemipenes located at the base of the tail. In mature iguanids, geckos, and varanids, a paired bulge from these hemipenes may identify the individual as a male. Some lizards, especially agamids, geckos, and iguanids, also have pores on their ventral thighs (femoral pores) or on the ventral procloacal skin (precloacal pores). These pores are relatively larger in adult males than in females (Figure 12.2). Male monitors have a bone structure in their hemipenes termed the hemibaculum. The *Varanus* species reported to have hemibacula are *acantharus*, *beccarii*, *caudolineatus*, *eremius*, *giganteus*, *gilleni*, *gouldii*, *indicus*, *karlschmidti*, *komodoensis*, *olivaceus*, *panoptes*, *salvadorii*, *storii*, *tristis*, and *varius*. In these species, the use of radiography would make apparent the presence of the hemibacula (Funk 2002). Other dimorphism among lizards is based on ornamentation, such as the three large rostral horns in male Jackson's chameleon (*Chamaeleo jacksonii*), or more robust appearance (especially of the head) in males such as iguanas and Gila monsters (*Heloderma suspectum*).

Sexual dimorphism among snakes is very rare. Among boid snakes, the spurs, located just lateral to the vent, are

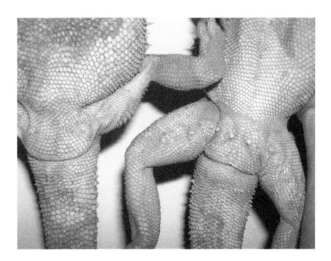

Figure 12.2 Sexual dimorphism in a lizard species, Bearded dragon (*Pogona vitticeps*). The male is on the right and female on the left. Femoral pores and tail bulge from the hemipenes are obvious in the male. (Courtesy of David Perpiñan LV, MSc, Veterinary Talent, Badalona, Spain.)

larger in males than in females. These spurs are used for tactile stimulation of the female during courtship. The spur size is highly reliable in the case of the rosy boa (*Charina trivirgata*) and the sand boas (*Eryx* spp.).

Probing

Probing is a technique in which a lubricated blunt-tipped probe is used for sexing. Only water- or saline-based lubricants should be used because some other lubricants may be spermicidal. This technique is only valid for the Squamata (lizards and snakes); however, probing is not reliable in most lizard species (Stahl & DeNardo 2019). Males are those individuals in which the sexing probe goes farther down into the tail as the sexing probe enters the hemipenial pocket. The depth of the hemipenial sac varies among species. In females, probing results in the total inability or limited ability to insert the probe into the tail base. This is the result of probing a pair of blind diverticula, and female lizards may have a tiny homologous structure called hemiclitori. Common species in which these diverticula are well developed, thus creating difficulty in sexing by this method, include the monitors (*Varanus* spp.) and the blood python (*Python curtus*).

Manual Eversion of Hemipenes (Popping)

Popping, or manual eversion of the hemipenes, is a common method for determining the sex of neonatal colubrid snakes. This is accomplished by firmly rolling one's thumb proximally up the tail base toward the cloaca. In females, the oviductal papillae can sometimes be identified as two small reddish openings located laterally in the cloaca.

Hydrostatic Eversion of Hemipenes

Hydrostatic eversion of hemipenes involves injecting isotonic saline solution (as much as 100 mL) into the tail just distal to where the hemipenes are located. If the technique is performed correctly, the hydrostatic pressure created by the saline solution causes the hemipenes to evert (Figure 12.3). This also causes swelling of the tissue surrounding the cloaca, and may partially evert the cloaca through the vent. For larger species such as boids, monitors, iguanas, and Gila monsters, anesthesia may be required as the retractor penis muscle can counteract the hydrostatic pressure created therefore preventing eversion of the hemipenes.

Digital Palpation

Digital palpation is the preferred method for crocodilian species. This involves palpating the ventral aspect of the cloaca for the presence of a penis in the otherwise smooth-walled cloaca.

Plasma Testosterone

Plasma testosterone concentration has been used for sexing chelonian juveniles, with or without the use of follicle-stimulating hormone (FSH) stimulation test (Lance et al. 1992; Owens et al. 1978; Rostal et al. 1994). Males typically have higher levels than females. However, this test also has limitations because older females may

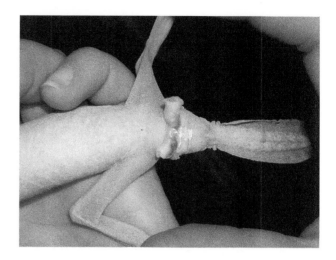

Figure 12.3 Everted hemipenes in a Lineated leaf-tailed gecko (*Uroplatus lineautus*). (Courtesy of David Perpiñan LV, MSc Veterinary Talent, Badalona, Spain.)

normally have elevated testosterone levels; moreover, prolonged handling of both sexes has been reported to elevate testosterone levels (Innis & Boyer 2002; Rostal et al. 1994).

Morphometrics

Morphometrics is the use of body measurements to determine sex. However, this is not a reliable way to differentiate males and females as there are many exceptions among species. It is more common for males to be larger than females in lizards. Female turtles are generally larger in body size than males. However, this may be different in tortoises. For example, the male desert tortoise (*Gopherus agassizii*) is larger than the female.

DNA Sexing

Karyotyping is the use of DNA to determine gender. It can be used for both temperature-dependent sex determination (TSD) species and non-TSD species (Demas et al. 1990; Innis & Boyer 2002). Although this technique is feasible, it has received little attention.

Ultrasonography and Laparoscopy

Ultrasonography may be useful in determining males and females by identification of ovaries, follicles, or eggs in the celomic cavity of females; and testes or hemipenes in the case of the males (Figure 12.4). Laparoscopy has also been used for sexing. This is a surgical procedure in which an endoscope is guided through the celom to directly visualize the testis or ovarian tissue (Figure 12.5). The advantage is that it permits visual evaluation of the reproductive tract and detection of possible abnormalities.

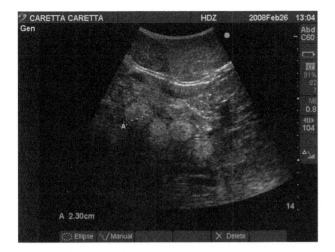

Figure 12.4 Coelomic cavity ultrasound in a gravid female. Note the presence of the follicles (increased round echogenicity) as they lack the more mineralized eggshell. (Courtesy of David Perpiñan LV, MSc, Veterinary Talent, Badalona, Spain.)

Record Keeping and Size of the Collection

Record keeping is very important for proper care not only of the individual's health but of the overall health of the collection. This also allows an insight into the results of the collection itself such as natality, mortality, and breeding. The minimum data to be recorded would include feeding details, shedding dates, medical problems or concerns, weight, fecal and urine elimination, and reproductive activity. During breeding, temperature and humidity cycling, results following introduction (e.g., fighting, mounting, and copulation), results of breeding (successful pairs, number of animals born, mortality, reproductive-related problems, and genetic outcomes in the form of morphs) should be documented.

Quarantine

Quarantine is the isolation of animals and persons to prevent the spread of infectious diseases. This is the most important step in preventive medicine. The recommended quarantine period for reptiles is about 3 months, but up to 6 months for snakes because of the risk of ophidian paramyxovirus. Quarantine should be carried out in an off-site location. When this is not possible, a separate room that does not exchange air with other facilities would be adequate. It is also ideal to have two isolation areas, one for new arrivals and one for those animals of the collection that become sick.

New arrivals in quarantine should be examined at the beginning of the quarantine for evidence of external parasites (e.g., snake mites, *Ophionyssus natricis*) and signs of illness. Body weight, ecdysis (normal skin shedding), behavior, feeding, and urination/defecation should be monitored throughout the quarantine period and recorded appropriately. Accurate record-keeping is vital for the assessment of the collection's health and disease identification.

Quarantined animals should be handled last, after attending to the established collection animals. Cages, furniture, and bowls should be identified properly so they do not leave the quarantine area and are not exchanged among quarantine animals. The quarantine area should have foot baths, foot pump water faucets, and soap dispensers to prevent cross-contamination. Furthermore, individual cage accessories (bowls, hide boxes, etc.) should be minimal and should not be cleaned together with accessories from other cages. In order to minimize the exchange of pathogens between quarantine cages, cages should be maintained so as to facilitate cleaning and disinfection (e.g., disposable paper towels as substrate). Common disinfectants

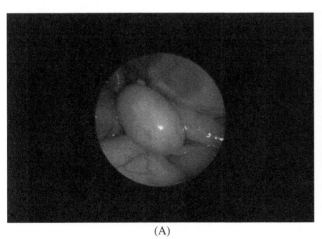
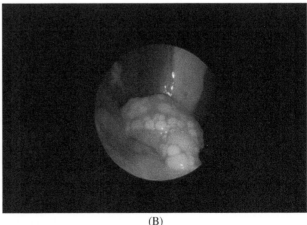

(A)   (B)

Figure 12.5 Endoscopic visualization of (A) a testis in a male green iguana (*Iguana iguana*) and (B) an ovary in a young female Hermann's tortoise (*Testudo hermanni*). (Courtesy of Xavier Valls Badia LV, Xavivallsvet.com, Barcelona, Spain.)

used are household bleach (sodium hypochlorite) at 1:30 concentration (1 part of bleach per 30 parts of water, in other words 30 mL per liter of water or ½ cup per gallon), 5% ammonia solution (which is effective against coccidia and cryptosporidia), and quaternary ammonium against common reptile pathogens at 1:200 to 1:400 for reptile cages and bowls. Other substances commonly used are listed in Table 12.2.

Quarantine is managed according to the "all-in-and-all-out" principle. Once a group of reptiles has started quarantine, those individuals remain as a group and no other reptiles enter the quarantine section or area until the quarantine is over. The introduction of new reptiles entails beginning the quarantine period all over again.

Ideally, three negative fecal tests for gastrointestinal parasites and protozoa are required. Each fecal test is performed 3–4 weeks apart. Once parasitism is diagnosed, appropriate treatment is started immediately. Those parasites with direct life cycles (e.g., coccidia) are particularly difficult to eliminate, requiring a regular screening and deworming schedule. Complete blood analysis should be performed at the beginning and end of the quarantine period. In the case of healthy animals, this establishes normal baseline values for future reference in the collection. More specific diagnostics can be performed during this period in an attempt to detect some of the most infectious diseases and isolate seropositive from seronegative individuals (Stahl 2001). See Table 12.3. Individuals who become sick should be isolated, and any casualty or euthanasia must have a complete necropsy and tissue sampling for histopathology. A detailed necropsy allows proper sampling and special testing for infectious diseases.

Pest control is important not only at quarantine, but also for the collection in itself. Arthropods (insects) can facilitate spread of infectious disease between exhibits, cages, and collections.

Collection Management and Housing

Managing Large Collections

Managing large collections of reptiles requires a thorough understanding of each species (natural history, husbandry requirements, etc.), an understanding of reptile zoonoses, regulations (local, national, and international), and preventive medicine. Preventive medicine includes individual identification, sanitation and disinfection, nutrition, physical examination and quarantine, parasite and disease surveillance, necropsy, and pest control.

In order to maintain a large collection of animals, a population management plan is required. In other words, the following questions should be asked:

- What is the size of the animal collection?
- How many different species will there be?
- What is the purpose of the collection (private hobby, captive breeding for commercial purposes, education, zoological, etc.)?
- How does one manage the surplus of animals?
- How is the genetic pool of the collection monitored?

Once the purpose of the collection is established, then one can focus on fulfilling the collection's specific requirements in order to successfully manage it.

Record keeping is fundamental. Data may include feeding details, waste output (fecal/urate), sheddings, weight, reproduction details (number of offspring), and any medical condition. Reproductive data should include temperature and humidity cycling, light cycles, monitoring of time of introduction, courtship behavior, and mating. In order to maximize offspring and avoid reproduction-related problems such as dystocia, gravid females should be monitored throughout the gestation time and oviposition (egg-laying). Once the oviposition occurs, it is very important to document the number of live offspring, stillborns, and slugs for viviparous species, and the number of healthy-looking eggs, abnormal eggs, and slugs in the case of oviparous species.

It is important to maintain a proper identification system for the collection so that there is a system of documenting mortality, percentage of viable offspring, compatible breeding pairs, and so forth. For larger collections of animals, a visual (physical pattern, carapace marking, etc.) and a permanent system (e.g., microchip) would be ideal. Proper microchip placement in reptiles is summarized in Table 12.4.

Reproducing reptiles in captivity can be complex. Husbandry is very important as they rely entirely on their environment to reproduce successfully. A period of cool temperature is necessary for most species to initiate reproductive behavior. Seasonal cooling is usually referred to as hibernation or brumation (Figure 12.6); in any case, this is very complex and species-specific. For this reason, the author strongly recommends extensive literature research on the species before attempting breeding. Another important factor for reproduction is space availability, which can affect proper copulation and egg deposition. Unfit reptiles are more prone to egg retention or dystocia (Figure 12.7). Another common cause of dystocia is improper laying conditions such as lack of a nesting box.

Sanitation and disinfection require a routine schedule. Properly done, it requires a written protocol of cleaning and disinfecting agents used, as well as when and how to use them. Disinfectants can only be used after removal of organic matter and cleaning.

Nutrition should be based on the species maintained. Diet can be complex and almost impossible to reproduce

Table 12.2 Characteristics of disinfectants

Type	Strength	Effectiveness	Advantage/Disadvantage	Contact time
Chlorine (e.g., Sodium hypochlorite)	2–10%	Fungi, bacteria, alga, enveloped and non-enveloped viruses. Good against tuberculosis microorganisms and mycoplasma. Not effective against spores	Corrosive, irritant to mucous membranes, eyes, and skin in high concentration. Germicidal activity decreases in high water pH (ideally between 6 and 8), and when temperature is below 65°F. Inactivation in presence of organic material and some soaps	Several minutes for maximal efficacy (10 min)
Iodophors (e.g., betadine)	10–100%	Fungi, bacteria, and enveloped and non-enveloped viruses. Good activity against tuberculosis organisms and mycoplasma. Poor sporocidal activity but better than chlorine products	Inactivated by presence of organic debris and alcohol. Stains skin, fabric and porous material	1–5 min depending on the concentration
Biguanides (e.g., chlorhexidine)	90 mL/gal	Fair bactericidal (most Gram-positive and few Gram-negative), viricidal against enveloped viruses, sporocidal and low to moderate fungicidal activity. Good activity against tuberculosis organisms and mycoplasma	Not an irritant. Maintains effectiveness in presence of organic matter or alcohol, but affected by alkaline pH (precipitation of the active ingredients)	5–10 min
Alcohol (e.g., ethyl alcohol or isopropyl alcohol)	Full strength	Strong bactericidal (both Gram-positive and negative), slight fungicidal, and viricidal (effective against enveloped viruses). Not effective against bacterial spores and non-enveloped viruses	Long contact time and inactivated by organic matter. Tissue irritant but non corrosive. Poses a fire hazard	20 min
Oxidizing agents (e.g., hydrogen peroxide)	Full strength	Great for anaerobic bacteria, but not viricidal. Tissue irritant. Blended and/or stabilized peroxides can be used for disinfection of equipment surfaces. Stabilized peroxides may be blended with iodophors or quaternary ammonia. Some products are effective against a much broader range of pathogens including both enveloped and non-enveloped viruses, vegetative bacteria, fungi, and bacterial spores. Examples include: Hyperox, VirkonS	Inactivated by organic matter. Not effective against bacterial or fungal spores	1–10 min

Table 12.2 (Continued)

Type	Strength	Effectiveness	Advantage/Disadvantage	Contact time
Phenol-based compounds (e.g., Lysol, synPhenol-3)	Full strength	Fair bactericidal (especially gram-positive bacteria) and viricidal (enveloped viruses). No effective against non-enveloped viruses or spores. Fungicidal.	No inactivated by presence of organic matter, skin irritation if prolonged exposure and corrosive to skin, toxic to cats and reptiles	10 min
Ammonia Quaternary ammonium compounds (e.g., Roccal, Parvosol, etc.)	5% 1:200–1:400	Coccidia and *Cryptosporidia* Good bactericidal, moderate fungicidal activity, and poor viricidal (effective against enveloped viruses). Poor activity against non-enveloped viruses and no effective against fungi and bacterial spores. Good activity against tuberculosis microorganisms and fair activity against mycoplasma	Inactivated by organic matter and soaps, and poor activity in hard waters. Low toxicity but prolonged contact can be irritating	10 min
Aldehydes (e.g., glutaraldehyde)	Full strength	Bactericidal, viricidal, fungicidal and sporocidal. Effective against tuberculosis organisms and *Chlamydophila* spp.	Effective in the presence of moderate organic matter. Corrosive, toxic, and irritant to the eye, skin, and respiratory tract	20 min

what would be encountered in the wild. Vitamin and mineral supplements are usually required. Generally, neonates and youngsters require supplementation on a daily basis or every other day and adults require it about once a week. Palatability and composition of invertebrates vary considerably with stage and species. Certain species of wild insects may contain pollutants and can potentially be toxic (e.g., lightning bugs). Commercial pellet diets are available in the market; however, the animals' nutritional requirements are not completely known and such diets should not be used as the only food source.

Reptiles should be examined biannually or annually depending on age and reproductive stage. The implementation of physical examinations, quarantine, and necropsy aids disease surveillance within the collection. Early detection of an infectious and metabolic disease would permit prompt correction and lower morbidity and mortality.

Pest control has important implications for personal safety as well as prevention of disease spread within the collection. Possible pest species should be carefully identified and a control plan instituted. Whatever system is implemented, it has to be safe for the species in the collection. The quality of the program has to be carefully monitored and recorded. For example, rodent traps should be inspected regularly and the number of animals trapped monitored for control purposes. An increase in the number of rodents trapped may simply correlate with a change in the management such as waste disposal.

Managing Large Collections of Dangerous Species

Dangerous reptiles are those that can inflict serious injuries from a bite (e.g., crocodile), strangulation (e.g., large boids), or venom (e.g., rattlesnake). The same principles discussed already for keeping a large reptile collection apply for dangerous species. However, these species require further safety precautions such as proper caging and, in most cases, a legal permit. In cases where multiple persons are

Table 12.3 Common infectious diseases

Disease	Species	Clinical signs	Diagnostic test
Snakes			
Inclusions body disease or IBD (Arenavirus)	Boas, pythons	Regurgitation, head tremors, ataxia, and incoordination	Histopaholoyg biopsy, CBC/blood smear, PCR from lung/tracheal wash, whole blood, cloacal or oral swabs
Ophidian paramyxovirus or OPMV (Ferlavirus)	Viperids, less common in boas, pythons, and colubrids	Anorexia, regurgitation, head tremors, "star gazing," and respiratory difficulty	Blood titers (HI), histopathology and PCR from lung/tracheal washes, whole blood, cloacal swabs or oral swabs, HI and ELISA
Sunshine virus	Pythons, boas	Respiratory disease, stomatitis, regurgitation and dermatitis	PCR from oral and cloacal swabs, blood and tissues
Nidovirus	Pythons	Excess salivation, open mouth breathing, pneumonia, anorexia, and death	PCR test of respiratory secretions, choanal swabs, or lung tissue
Snake fungal disease (*Ophydiomyces ophidiocola*)	All snakes	Pustules, scabs, swelling, dysecdysis, ulcers, and cloudy eyes	Fungal culture, histopathology, and PCR
Helminth parasites	All snakes	Gastrointestinal disease	Fecal examination
Arthropods (e.g., *Ophionyssus natricis* or snake mites)	All snakes	Anemia, anorexia, anemia, weakness, vector to other diseases	Visual examination
Cryptosporidiosis (*Cryptosporidium sp.*)	Boas, pythons, colubrids	Thickened of the gastric mucosa (swelling may appear the middle of the body) and regurgitation	Acid-fast staining feces or stomach wash, IFA, ELISA, histopathology stomach
Amoebiasis (*Entameoba invadens*)	All snakes	Anorexia, bloody diarrhea, rectal prolapse, and acute death	Cysts in eosin-stained feces, PCR, and immunochemistry
Chelonians			
Bunyavirus (TBD) or turtle fraservirus 1	Turtles	Weakness, lethargy, swollen, closed or sunken eyelids, discharge from the nose or eyes, and splotchy red discoloration on softshells	PCR, histopathology
Adenovirus	Turtles and tortoises	Nasal and ocular discharge, mucosal ulcers and palatine erosions	Oral and cloacal swab PCR
Herpesvirus	Tortoises	Respiratory disease	ELISA/serum neutralization
Ranavirus	Turtles and tortoises	Lethargy, anorexia, dyspnea, nasal discharge, conjunctivitis, oral ulcerations, severe subcutaneous cervical edema, ulcerative stomatitis, and "red-neck disease"	Oral and cloacal swab PCR , whole blood and ELISA
Iridovirus	Turtles and tortoises	Respiratory disease with palpebral edema, ocular and nasal discharge, and stomatitis	PCR
Mycoplasma (*Mycoplasma agassizii*)	Tortoises	Respiratory disease	ELISA/culture/PCR

Table 12.3 (Continued)

Disease	Species	Clinical signs	Diagnostic test
Dermatomycosis (*Endomyces testavorans*)	Turtles	Ulcerative shell lesions, scute defects, and pliable scutes	PCR, culture, histophatology
Testudinade intranuclear coccidia (TINC)	Turtles and tortoises	Severe lethargy, rapid weight loss, weakness, gasping respiration, conjunctivitis, nasal discharge, oronasal fistulas and swollen erythematous vents with ulceration	Histopathology and conjunctival-choanal-cloacal swab PCR
Amoebiasis	Tortoises	Anorexia, listlessness, and diarrhea	Histopathology
Cryptosporidium	Turtles and tortoises	GI disease and dead	Acid-fast staining feces, IFA, ELISA, EM, PCR histopathology stomach
Lizards			
Adenovirus	Bearded dragons, blue-tongued skinks	Neurological disease and GI disease in bearded and respiratory in skinks	Liver biopsy, necropsy, histopathology, PCR oral-cloacal swab
Nidovirus	Skinks	Respiratory disease	Conjunctival-tracheal-oral swab PCR, histopathology
Iridovirus	Bearded dragons	Lethargy and poor doing, intracytoplasmic inclusions bodies in erythrocytes	Whole blood, PCR, histopathology
Yellow fungal disease (*Nannizziopsis* spp.)	Lizards and crocodiles	Swelling, ulceration, crusting, and deep necrosis of the skin	Skin swab PCR, histopathology
Microsporidium (*Encephalitozoon* spp.)	Bearded dragon	Lethargy, anorexia, granulomatous lesions affecting internal organs	Oral-cloacal swab PCR, histopathology
Cryptosporidium spp.	Leopard geckos, gila monsters, chameleons	Severe enteritis, diarrhea, and cachexia	Acid-fast staining (feces), biopsy/histopathology, IFA
Isospora amphiboluri	Bearded dragons	From asymptomatic or cause anorexia, lethargy and diarrhea	Fecal testing
Arthropods	All lizards	Anemia, anorexia, anemia, weakness, vector to other diseases	Visual examination
Bacterial dermatitis (*Devrisea agamarum* and *Chrysosporium guarro*)	Mainly family Agamidae (genera Pogona, Uromastyx, Agama)	Dermatitis and/or septicemia	Culture
Crocodilians			
Chlamydia	Various crocodilian species	Fibrinopurulent blepharoconjunctivitis and hepatitis	Culture, PCR, and histopathology
Mycoplasma	Various crocodilian species	Lethargy, weakness, anorexia, white ocular discharge, polyarthritis, paresis, edema (facial, periocular, cervical, limbs)	ELISA, histopathology
Poxvirus	Various crocodilian species	Skin lesions	PCR, histopathology
WNV	Various crocodilian species	Ranging from sudden death to neurological disease (swimming in circles, head tilt, muscle tremors, weakness), lethargy, and anorexia	PCR and viral culture

ELISA, enzyme-linked immunoassay; EM, electron microscopy; HI, hemoagglutination inhibition assay; IFA, immunofluorescence assay; PCR, polymerase chain reaction.

Table 12.4 Sites for microchip placement in reptiles

Animal	Suggestive site
Chelonians (turtles and tortoises)	Subcutaneously in left hindleg or intramuscularly in thin and small species
Sauria (lizards)	Left quadriceps muscle or subcutaneously in that area. In very small species, subcutaneously on the left side of the body
Ophidia (snakes)	Subcutaneously on the left side of the neck area at about twice the length of the head
Crocodilians	Cranial to nuchal cluster

Source: Based on guidelines of the British Veterinary Zoological Society.

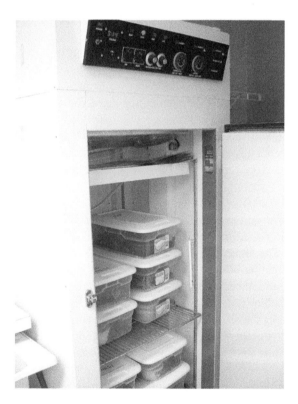

Figure 12.6 A temperature-and humidity-controlled hibernaculum allowing normal reptile hibernation or brumation. (Courtesy of David Perpiñan LV, MSc, Veterinary Talent, Badalona, Spain.)

handling dangerous species, a written emergency protocol is fundamental. The appropriate protocol would address every danger in the case of injury or escape, minimizing the likelihood of mortality or permanent disability. Every protocol must be specific for the type and number of dangerous reptiles in the collection, and in the case of certain venomous species, maintenance of antivenom may

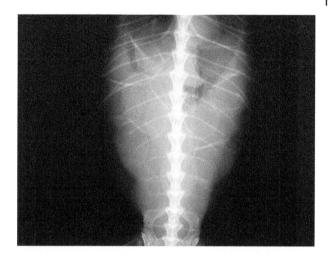

Figure 12.7 Egg retention (dystocia) in a green iguana (*Iguana iguana*). Notice the distended abdomen full of calcified eggs. (Courtesy of David Perpiñan LV, MSc Veterinary Talent, Badalona, Spain.)

be required. The American Zoo and Aquarium Association and the American Association of Poison Control Centers list the amount and location of available antivenoms for most venomous species. In any case, it is strongly advisable to notify the local hospital about the ownership of venomous species so that medical staff are prepared in the case of a venomous animal bite.

Dangerous species require proper labeling, and their handling is restricted to appropriately trained people. Access is restricted by the use of a lock, and the cages are properly secured at all times. This is especially important in the case of venomous species. Venomous reptiles are coded as 1 or 2 depending on their potential to inflict life-threatening injury. Code 1 animals are those capable of causing death, long-term illness, or permanent disability, while code 2 animals are unlikely to cause severe or long-lasting effects.

In the event of injury and escape, the victim would be responsible for securing the area first and then seeking medical care. A first-aid kit should be available and personnel should be trained in providing first-aid care.

A capture plan should also be part of the protocol, including immediate measures to secure the area, a contact list of people responsible to respond to an escape, equipment necessary for safe capture and handling, and so forth. If the animal cannot be safely captured, humane killing may be indicated.

Nutrition

Nutrition plays an important role in reproduction. Properly nourished and healthy individuals would be more likely to breed successfully. Therefore, diet history, feeding regimen, and nutritional supplementation should be carefully evaluated during the off-breeding season (Stahl 2001). During the off-season, reptiles should be fed heavily to condition them for breeding. This is especially important in reptiles as many of them would not eat during breeding and gestation. Weight and size playsan important role in reproductive maturity, therefore both the veterinarian and breeder should be familiar (Stahl 2001).

Feeding the Neonate

Hatchlings usually begin feeding within 1 to 14 days of leaving the egg, and most neonatal snakes do not eat until their first shed at about 1 to 3 weeks after hatching (Mader 2006). Feeding appropriately is critical for their proper growth and development. The yolk will provide nutrients for the first few days but proper food type and size is fundamental thereafter. A thorough understanding of the dietary requirements of the species is essential. Some species prey on particular species that are not commercially available, so "scenting" is required to train the neonate to eat alternate food items. This is accomplished by rubbing the alternate food (e.g., rodent) with the proper food item (e.g., fish or frog). Herbivorous reptiles can be offered a mix of fresh vegetables. Vegetables should be presented finely chopped to the appropriate size. Insectivorous and carnivorous reptiles can be offered insects such as crickets, mealworms, grubs, wingless fruit flies, termites, slugs, small fish (guppies or comets), pinky mice, small lizards (anoles or geckos), small frogs (toads can be toxic), chick legs, hatchling quails, and mouse parts. In any case, the offered food item should never be larger than the width between the reptile's eyes, or otherwise, it will potentially be too large to be ingested.

The nutritive value of the diet should be enhanced with commercially available vitamin and mineral supplements, and this is especially important for herbivores and insectivorous species. There are two basic methods for vitamin/mineral enhancement: dusting and gut loading. Dusting entails sprinkling the supplement over the food item. This technique may decrease the palatability of the food item so careful monitoring is required to assure that the food is completely eaten. In the case of insects, if these are not ingested immediately the insects can self-groom and remove these powders thereby decreasing the supplement available for the reptile. Alternatively, enriched media can be offered to the insects for a few days before they are fed to the reptiles. This is called gut loading.

In cases of anorexia, assisted feeding may be required. This can be accomplished by the use of an appropriately sized stomach tube to deliver the food into the stomach.

Commercially available foods or purees of appropriate food items (rodent parts, eggs, vegetables, etc.) can be used. Assisted feeding is provided by forceful placement of the food into the reptile's mouth; this can potentially damage the back of the mouth (oropharynx) and esophagus and is stressful. Snakes can be stimulated to eat by using a technique called "slap feeding," by gently tapping the snake's nose with the food item. This tends to initiate a reflex in the snake to strike and grasp the food item (Mader 2006).

Breeding Management

Reproductive Behavior

The development of secondary sexual characteristics coupled with courtship behavior is an indication that sexual maturity is approaching (Innis & Boyer 2002). Sexual maturity is dependent upon the reptile's size and not its chronological age (Taylor & Denardo 2005). In captivity, reptiles reach sexual maturity at a younger age than their wild counterparts. For instance, captive leopard tortoises (*Geochelone pardalis*) may reproduce successfully in 4 to 6 years whereas their wild-born counterparts do not reach sexual maturity for 15 years (Innis & Boyer 2002). As a rough generality in captive species, snakes usually mature in 2 to 3 years, small lizards in 1 to 2 years, large lizards in 3 to 4 years, and chelonians usually in 5 to 7 years (Denardo 2006).

In most reptile studies to date, high plasma levels of testosterone and corticosterone coincide with the mating period. The female's estradiol level increases at the onset of the mating season, ultimately declining at the onset of the nesting season. Progesterone levels are high close to ovulation and the beginning of the nesting season, and finally decrease during the nesting season (Schramm et al. 1999). Therefore, monitoring the reproductive cycle is possible via plasma chemistry and hormone assays (Innis & Boyer 2002).

The most common stimulus to reproduction in reptiles is a change in temperature. Other factors are photoperiod and food availability. The reproductive cycle in chelonians is linked to the temperature and humidity determined by their natural habitats. For temperate species, reproductive activity is restricted to the warmer months of the year when the day length is longer. In general, females will ovulate and be fertilized in the spring, nest in the late spring and summer, and begin folliculogenesis for the following year's eggs in late summer and fall. An exception to this is tropical boids (boas and pythons), which tend to breed during the cooler period (Denardo 2006). In tropical climates, the reproductive cycle follows the rainfall patterns, as temperature and day length fluctuations are minimal (Innis & Boyer 2002).

Light plays also an important role in sexual behavior. Behavioral studies have proven the importance of full-spectrum lighting (UVA, UVB, and visible light; 280–700 nm) and its role not only in motion perception and foraging but also in intersexual recognition.

Courtship and Mating Behavior

In most species, some degree of courtship behavior is noted. Courtship may last from minutes to hours, and it may even resume on subsequent days. Most terrestrial tortoises, such as the Mediterranean tortoises (*Testudo* spp.), display a lunging behavior toward the females, battering the anterior edge of their carapace against the female. The male red-footed tortoise (*Geochelone carbonaria*) may stand in front of the female with his stretched neck low to the ground, moving it rhythmically side to side while uttering low-pitched grunting sounds. In some North American aquatic species (e.g., red-eared slider, *Trachemys scripta*), males will fibrillate the elongated nails of their forelimbs near the female's face (Innis & Boyer 2002).

Copulation is a short event only lasting for several minutes. Many chelonians and lizards display biting behavior as the male mounts the female from behind (Innis & Boyer 2002). In snakes, the male of the colubrid neck-banded snake (*Scaphiodontophis annulatus*) grabs, holds, and bites the female during copulation as part of the mating behavior (Sasa & Curtis 2006).

During copulation, one hemipenis is everted into the female's cloaca in the case of snakes and lizards (Figure 12.8A–C). In the case of chelonians and crocodilians, a single penis arising from the floor of the cloaca is everted. In both cases, the sperm flows through a single groove called the seminal groove, or sulcus spermaticus, from the vas deferens down the penis or hemipenis and down to the anterior portions of the female's cloaca. The spermatozoa travel upward through the oviduct where fertilization occurs. In some species, such as iguanids, sperm storage allows the female to lay subsequent clutches (Funk 2002).

Reproduction Without Mating

Amphigonia retardata, or sperm storage, has been described in turtles and snakes. This adaptation allows a female to produce several clutches from a single mating in one season, but also to reproduce in subsequent seasons. The viability of the stored sperm is not indefinite and varies with the species, ranging from several months to up to 6 years (Mader 2006).

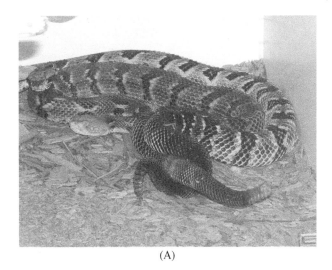

(A)

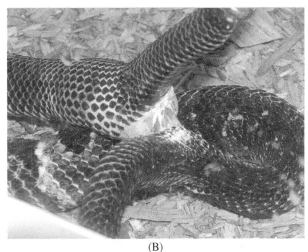

(B)

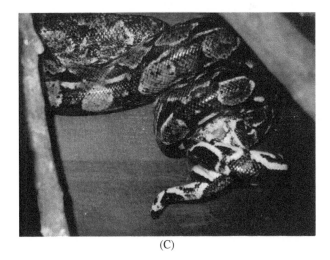

(C)

Figure 12.8 (A) Snake copulation and (B) copulation in timber rattlesnake (*Crotalus horridus*). (Courtesy of B W Smith (Animal South LLC).) (C) copulation of common bao constrictor (*Boa constrictor*). (Courtesy of Susana Ringenbach MVZ, Fauna Silvestre, Merida, Mexico.)

Table 12.5 Reptile families in which parthenogenesis has been described

Family Gekkonidae (Geckoes)	5 species
Family Agamidae (Agamids)	1 species
Family Chamaelonidae (Chameleons)	1 species
Family Xantusiidae (Night lizards)	1 species
Family Lacertidae (Lacertids)	5 species (e.g., Genus *Darevskia*)
Family Teiidae (Whiptails and tegus)	15 species (e.g., Genus *Cnemidophorus*)
Family Typhlopidae (Blind snakes)	1 species

Another strategy to reproduce without mating is parthenogenesis. In this case, the female becomes gravid in the absence of a male and produces only female offspring (Mader 2006). Interestingly, genetic polymorphism is present to some extent despite the lack of genetic recombination. In true parthenogenetic species, such as the Caucasian rock lizard (*Darevskia unisexualis*), studies have shown that mutations can make a significant contribution to population variability (Badaeva et al. 2008). Parthenogenesis has been reported in more than 30 species of lizards and in some snakes. Some common examples include members of the genera *Cnemidophorus* (whiptails), *Darevskia* (rock lizards), *Hemidactylus* (geckos), Komodo dragon (*Varanus komodoensis*), and snakes such as *Ramphotyphlops braminus* (blind snake) (Table 12.5).

Vitellogenesis is the major step of follicle maturation with the accumulation of yolk. Estrogen triggers the liver to convert lipid from the body's fat stores to vitellogenin, which will be selectively absorbed by the follicles. Calcium also accumulates in the yolk during this stage so that the yolk will act as the main calcium reservoir for the embryo. Furthermore, a significant amount of calcium is drawn from the eggshell in oviparous species. The mature ovum is 10-fold to 100-fold larger than its previtellogenic size. In the oviduct, the ovum becomes an egg when albumin and a shell are added for oviparous species. In the case of viviparous species, placentation takes place instead. This maternal-embryonic relationship varies among viviparous species, with the most extreme example being some skinks (*Mabuya* spp.) in which the mother contributes more than 99% of the neonatal mass through a chorioallantoic placenta (Denardo 2006).

Clutch Dynamics

The frequency with which reptiles reproduce is dependent on the species, environmental conditions, and the health status of the specific individual. Reproduction has detrimental effects for the mother, and female reptiles will cease feeding during the latter stages of pregnancy. The length of time during which feeding is reduced varies, but it is much shorter in oviparous (weeks) than in viviparous (months) species. This limited amount of energy allocated to reproduction has direct effects on offspring and clutch size. Invariably, the amount of energy is extraordinary, especially in snakes where more than 40% of the female's body mass can be allocated to reproduction (Denardo 2006).

Clutch size is extremely variable in reptiles. For oviparous species, it ranges from a single egg in the case of anoles (*Anolis* spp.) and pancake tortoise (*Malocochersus tornieri*) to 200 in the green seaturtle (*Chelonia mydas*). In viviparous species, the numbers may be slightly lower, with a range from one in the case of shingleback skinks (*Trachysaurus rugosus*) to 92 in the gartersnake (*Thamnophis radix*) (Denardo 2006).

Many oviparous species have the ability to produce more than one clutch per year. This is more common among chelonian and lizards than snakes. Due to the restraints of viviparity, viviparous reptiles are limited to a single clutch per year.

Oviparous, Ovoviviparous, or Viviparous; and Parthenogenesis

The oviduct's function in lizards and snakes is fertilization, sperm storage, egg transport, eggshell deposition, maintenance of the early embryo, and expulsion of the egg or fetus. In viviparous species, the oviduct also contributes to the placenta, which is responsible for gas exchange and nutrient provision to the fetus (Blackburn 1998).

For a long time, three modes of reptile reproduction have been recognized: oviparous, ovoviviparous, and viviparous. The term ovoviviparity (ovovivipary) was applied to those species in which the young are born alive but there was no placental connection between the mother and the offspring. However, more recent investigations have demonstrated some nutrient transfer and therefore the term ovovivipary may be inappropriate (Funk 2002).

Thus, the term oviparity refers to the condition of laying fertilized eggs and viviparity refers to the condition of giving birth to live offspring regardless of how nutrient exchange may have occurred between the mother

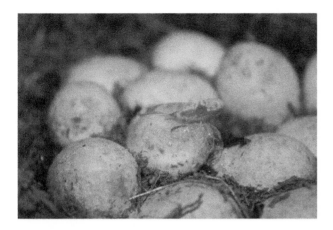

Figure 12.9 Amelanistic corn snake (*Pantherophis* guttatus) hatching. The head is upside down. (Courtesy of Olivia Barron.)

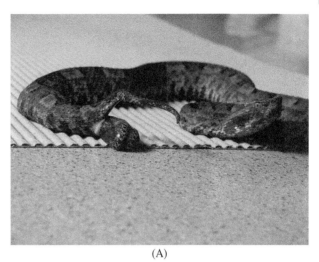

(A)

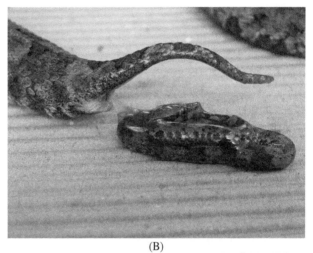

(B)

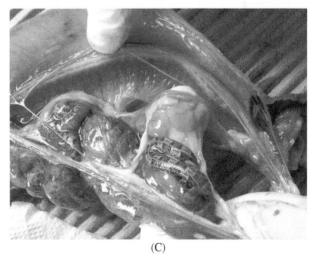

(C)

Figure 12.10 Viviparity in a rainforest hognose viper (*Porthidium nasutum*). (A) Hognose viper is giving birth; (B) offspring surrounded by the plancenta membrane (C) necropsy of a rainforest hognose viper in which several fetuses are contained within a plancenta membrane within the oviduct. (Courtesy of Alejandro Ramirez (Student of Veterinary Medicine and Supervisor of the group in Ophidism-Scorpionism University of Antioquia, Colombia.)

and the offspring. An example of oviparity can be seen in Figure 12.9. Chelonian and crocodilian species are oviparous, while 20% of squamates (some lizard and snake lineages) are viviparous (Benirschke 2007; Funk 2002) (Table 12.6).

Although viviparity has a clear advantage over oviparity, there are several disadvantages that are worth mentioning. Sustaining the fetuses over an extended period of time will limit the female to a single clutch per year. Bearing the offspring also has detrimental effects on the female as viviparous females cease feeding during the latter stages (Denardo 2006) (Figure 12.10A–C). However, viviparous reptiles have the advantage to regulate incubation temperature and enhance fitness of the offspring. For this reason, a phylogenetic transition from oviparity to viviparity has occurred in cold climates (Webb et al. 2006).

Parthenogenesis or asexual reproduction has been reported in more than 30 species of lizards and some snakes (Stahl and Denardo 2019).

Egg Incubation Versus Maternal Incubation

A number of factors determine the length of gestation such as season, ambient temperature, housing, and food supply among others (Mader 2006). Parental care in reptiles is minimal, with few exceptions among crocodilians and pythons. Female pythons are known to brood their eggs during incubation by coiling around the eggs until hatching. Periodic rhythmic contractions of the mother's abdominal musculature is capable of maintaining a mean body temperature of 7.3°C above the mean ambient surface temperature (Mader 2006).

Table 12.6 Oviparity and viviparity of commonly kept reptiles

Oviparous
All crocodilians
All chelonians
Most lizards
  All monitors (*Varanus* spp.)
  Most iguanids
    Iguanas (*Iguana* spp.)
    Water Dragons (*Physignathus* spp.)
  All geckos
  Most chameleons
    Veiled Chameleon (*Chamaeleo calyptratus*)
    Panther Chameleon (*Chamaeleo pardalis*)
Some snakes
  All pythons
  Most colubrids
    Kingsnakes and Milksnakes (*Lampropelis* spp.)
    Ratsnakes and Cornsnakes (*Elaphe* spp.)
Viviparous
Some lizards
  Some skinks
    Blue-tongued skinks (*Tiliqua* spp.)
    Shingle-backed skink (*Trachysaurus rugosus*)
    Prehensile-tailed skink (*Corucia zebrata*)
Some chameleons
  Jackson's Chameleon (*Chamaeleo jacksonii*)
Some snakes
Most boas (excepting *Charina reinhardti*, *Eryx jayakari*)
  Most vipers
    All rattlesnakes (*Crotalus* spp.)
  Some colubrids
Gatersnakes (*Thamnophis* spp.)

Source: Adapted from Denardo (2006).

Egg Incubation Methods

Viable eggs are usually firm, dry, and chalky white. Soft-shelled or pliable eggs occur in all snakes, most lizards, and some chelonians, whilst the eggs of crocodilians, many chelonians, and some lizards are hard-shelled and therefore rigid (Figure 12.11).

Artificial incubation is relatively simple. Incubators can be easily designed and maintained by fulfilling three basic requirements: proper regulation of temperature and humidity; even distribution of heat; and a reliable thermostat to control temperature. Although insulation prevents the loss of heat and humidity, some degree of ventilation should be permitted (e.g., small holes on the lid of the egg chamber). A study on sea turtle eggs showed that

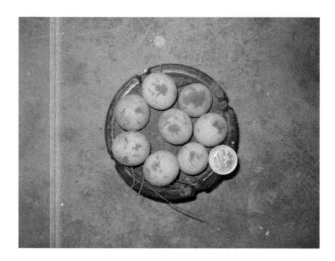

Figure 12.11 Hard-shelled eggs of the Mediterranean spur-thighed tortoise (*Testudo graeca*). (Courtesy of Jose Luis Crespo Picazo LV, Valencia, Spain.)

poor ventilation increases incubation time and reduces survival of embryos (Funk 2002). Commercial incubators are available for reptiles, and even chick incubators can be used with minor modifications such as stopping the movement of the egg trays. Most incubators are designed on a double-chamber principle so that the eggs are located inside a box, and this box is inside the larger incubator chamber. A Styrofoam cooler can be used as a cheaper alternative for the containment chamber of the nest box. Plastic storage boxes can be used as a nest or inside box. The lid should fit tightly so that the air humidity approaches saturation. The moistened substrate material is filled halfway, and then water is added appropriately so that it is only slightly damp. Heat is provided by heating coils, strips, and pads, and a thermostat assures that the temperature stays constant within the inner chamber, with the set-up based on the species' eggs. As long as the three main principles of reptile egg incubation are fulfilled, any container with controlled heat, humidity, and ventilation may be suitable (Figure 12.12).

The eggs should be placed in the incubator in the same orientation as they were laid. A pencil mark on top of the egg may help maintain the orientation when the egg is moved. Soft-shelled eggs are then half-buried within the moist substrate and separated from each other by a small distance. In the case of hard-shelled eggs, these may be placed in a small depression in the substrate. Maintaining a certain distance between the eggs prevents the spread of disease among the eggs. Where two or more eggs are strongly adhered to each other, they will have to be half-buried together; attempting to separate them may lead to permanent damage (Figure 12.13A–C).

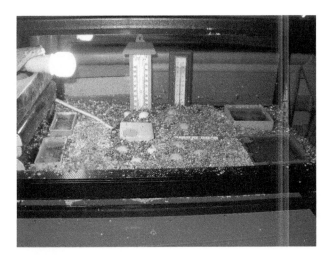

Figure 12.12 A hand-made incubator can be easily designed by creating an environment of controlled temperature and humidity, even distribution of heat and some degree of ventilation. (Courtesy of Jose Luis Crespo Picazo LV Valencia, Spain.)

Incubation requirements for most reptilian eggs are similar. Very important factors to remember in reptile reproduction are ambient temperature, humidity, and substrate.

Temperature

The ambient incubation temperature directly affects the length of incubation and, in some species, gender determination (Table 12.7). There are two types of sex determination systems: genotypic sex determination (GSD) determined by the sex chromosomes, and temperature-dependent sex determination system (TSD), in which temperature affects sex determination (Delmas et al. 2008; Wibbels et al. 1991). The relevance of TSD over GSD is still unknown but may be related to environmental fitness (Warner & Shine 2008). However, sex determination is very complex in reptiles, and both systems can even be present in a single species. For example, sex determination in the montane scincid lizard (*Bassiana duperreyi*) is regulated genetically by sex chromosomes but temperature can override chromosomal sex generating phenotypically male offspring from XX eggs in cool nests (Radder et al. 2008). TSD occurs in all studied crocodilians and tuataras, is very common in chelonians, less frequent in lizards, and unknown in snakes (Delmas et al. 2008). Although TSD has evolved in several lineages of lizards, there is less information on these than other reptile taxa. The time in which TSD occurs is called the thermosensitive period and is about the middle one-third of embryonic development (Delmas et al. 2008; Wibbels et al. 1991). TSD may be also evident in viviparous lizards, in which sex ratios fluctuate with thermal conditions. In the spotted

skink, (*Niveoscincus ocellatus*) there is a higher proportion of male offspring in colder years (Wapstra et al. 2009). There are two distinct patterns of TSD. In pattern I, there is a single transition zone at which eggs incubated below this temperature zone result predominantly in males, and those above the temperature zone hatch predominantly as females. Pattern II has two transition zones, with males predominating at the intermediate zone and females at both extremes. Pattern I occurs chiefly in turtles in which the adult females are larger than the adult males, while pattern II is primarily present in species in which females are smaller than males or in non-dimorphic species (no difference between males and females). Some *Sternotherus* and *Chelydra* spp. are exceptions in that a constant incubation temperature within the transition zone yields 100% males (Eti 2008).

Incubation length is usually reduced by high temperatures, but this increases the risk of congenital defects (Denardo 2006). Furthermore, abnormally high or low temperatures will affect the health of the hatchlings (Mader 2006). In general, incubation temperature ranges from 26°C to 32°C (80–90°F) (Denardo 2006).

Gestation periods vary. The eggs of most snakes and small lizards hatch in 45 to 70 days, whereas eggs from larger lizards such as iguanas and monitor lizards can take 90 to 130 days. Gestation lengths vary not only among species, but also within the same species and within the same clutch. For example, the incubation time of the leopard tortoise (*Geochelone pardalis*) can range from 250 to 540 days and show 30 to 40 days variation within the same clutch (Denardo 2006).

Substrate

Commonly used incubation substrates include perlite, vermiculite, potting soil, sand, sphagnum moss, and shredded paper. There is also commercially available substrate for reptile incubators based on a pre-prepared mixture of the already mentioned substrates. Perlite and vermiculite are preferred by many hobbyists as they are very light, absorbent, siliceous materials that naturally resist molding. In any case, the purpose of the substrate is to provide a medium that will retain water and maintain humidity within the egg container while preventing excessive fungal growth.

Humidity

The amount of water added to the substrate varies but should be enough to create clumping of the media without dripping of water. Water will be required throughout the incubation period and therefore more may need to be

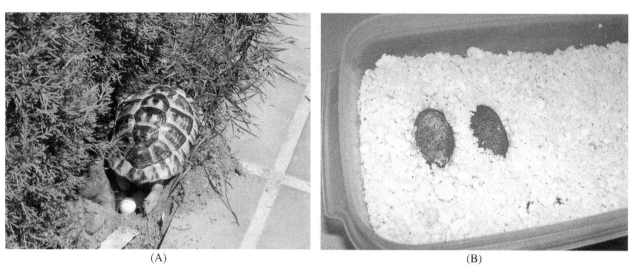

(A)   (B)

Figure 12.13 After egg deposition, the eggs are removed and placed into the incubator chamber. (A) Egg laying of a Mediterranean spur-thighed tortoise (*Testudo graeca*). (Courtesy of Jose Luis Crespo Picazo LV, Valencia, Spain.) (B) The egg chamber would contain the half-buried eggs set into the moistened substrate and separated from each other by a small distance. Maintenance of a certain distance between the eggs would prevent the spread of disease processes among the eggs. (Courtesy of David Perpiñan LV MSc, Veterinary Talent, Badalona, Spain.)

added. Dampened sphagnum moss can be used to cover the eggs to help prevent desiccation; however, it will prevent or make more difficult visual checking of the viability of the eggs.

It is advisable to weigh the incubation box and its eggs periodically so that water can be added to keep the box at its original weight. If water needs to be added, water should be at the same temperature as the incubator.

Caring for the Newborn

Reptilian neonates are born precocious. In other words, they are fully independent and capable of survival from birth. Adult reptiles rarely provide any care for their offspring. Parental care can be defined as the parental actions after oviposition or parturition that may increase the offspring's chances of survival (Funk 2002). Parental care has been documented in at least 100 species of reptiles, but it is limited and non-essential for survival of the offspring (Denardo 2006). Among lizards, there are a few examples of maternal care, but this is basic and limited to nesting care against predators in the case of some skinks. Nest guarding has also been documented in chelonians (e.g., Burmese mountain tortoise, *Manouria emys*), snakes (e.g., king cobra, *Ophiophagus hannah*, and cobras, *Naja* spp.), and virtually all species of crocodilians. In the case of the skink *Eumeces obsoletus*, the female assists during hatching and subsequently licks the hatchlings' cloacas, as well as supplying them with food until about the 10th day (Mader 2006). As a part of nest guarding, crocodilians

assist the neonates in emerging from the nest and guard them after hatching. Rattlesnakes will remain with their offspring until the neonates' first shed (Denardo 2006).

In captivity, neonate care can be divided into three categories: environmental conditions, space, and proper food. The care provided to newborns is minimal and merely a scaled-down version of the care for adults. Hatching can take from 1 to 4 days. In the case of chelonians, the neonate's shell begins to unfold facilitating yolk absorption. Absorption of the yolk sac may take several days after hatching so neonates should be kept in a clean and moist environment. In general, hatchlings are maintained at or near the incubation temperature, and many breeders leave them in the incubator for the first few days. A plastic container with clean, moist paper towels is also commonly used for the first few days. Once the yolk sac is fully absorbed and the umbilicus sealed, the neonates can be transferred to a cage with other substrate. Neonates are very prone to dehydration, and thus humidity should be close to 100%. After the neonates leave the incubator, their environmental temperature range should be close to that of the adults but with slightly higher humidity. Higher humidity can be easily accomplished by using moistened paper towels and a humidity box. A humidity box is a confined box containing moistened paper towels with a small opening that allows the youngsters to get in and out easily. Being such a confined and closed space, this allows a relative humidity of almost 100% as long as the substrate is replaced on a daily basis. Other more naturalistic substrates can be used as the youngsters grow

Table 12.7 Patterns of temperature sex determination in reptiles

Sauria (Lizards)	
Family Geckonidae	
African fat-tailed gecko (*Hemitheconyx caudicinctus*)	Pattern II
26–29°C (78.8–84.2°F) results in females	
30–32°C (86–89.6°F) results in males	
34–35°C (93.2–95°F) results in females	
Japanese gecko (*Gekko japonicus*)	Pattern I
Females at higher temperatures, males at lower temperature	
Leopard gecko (*Eublepharis macularius*)	Pattern I
26.7–29.4°C results in 90% females	
>32.2°C results in 90% males	
Rainbow lizard (*Agama agama*)	Pattern I
26–27°C (78.8–80.6°F) results in females	
29°C (84.2°F) results in males	
Jacky dragon (*Amphibolurus muricatus*)	Pattern I
Chelonians (Turtles and tortoises)	
Males are generally produced at lower temperatures and mostly females at higher	
Some Bataguridae	Pattern I
Carettochelydae	Pattern I
Cheloniidae	Pattern I
Dermochelydae	Pattern I
Emydidae	Pattern I
Testudinidae	Pattern I
Pelomedusidae	Pattern II
Kinosternidae	Pattern II
Macroclemys temminckii (Chelydridae)	Pattern II
Few Bataguridae	
All Crocodilians	Pattern II

but paper is generally the preferred option because it is cheap and easily cleaned.

Aggression is very common among neonatal lizards and snakes as part of a survival instinct. Providing enough space is therefore fundamental for them to thrive and minimize stress. If aggression is obvious, the hatchlings should be separated. Separating the clutch into smaller groups will not only decrease aggression but also helps monitor the health status of the group (weekly weight monitoring) and their appetite.

Medical Problems Arising from Reproduction

Diagnosing Egg Problems

In order to diagnose egg problems, it is important to understand the basic differences among reptilian eggs. The eggshell in snakes and most lizards is leathery and soft; however, the egg of chelonians, crocodilians, and geckos has a hard calcareous shell. Both soft-shelled and hard-shelled eggs have three internal membranes (the amnion, chorion, and allantois) that retard outward water diffusion and allow embryonic respiration. Even the hard-shelled eggs will take water from the environment to some extent and swell in size during embryonic development. All the nutrients come from the yolk and the white, and any remaining yolk in the egg will be incorporated into the hatchling's celomic cavity (Mader 2006).

Death of the egg can occur when the environmental conditions for egg development are not fulfilled. Incorrect humidity (high or low), temperature (high or low), and improper ventilation are very common problems that can cause egg death. Other potential causes are excessive handling or trauma. In any case, it may be difficult to determine the cause of embryonic death. Reptiles from temperate zones can withstand temperature variations better than tropical species. For instance, the embryos of the tropical green iguana (*Iguana iguana*) fail to develop at temperatures varying more than 2°C from the optimum 30°C (86°F) (Funk 2002).

Health assessment of the eggs is based on daily monitoring for color and texture changes. A collapsed egg is a sign of dehydration but not necessarily egg death. Marked changes in color or texture, or fungal growth are usually signs of a non-viable egg, either an egg that has died or a non-fertile egg (Table 12.8).

Two diagnostic ways to assess the health of an egg are "candling" and ultrasonography for non-calcified eggs (most squamates). A high-intensity light source (e.g., transilluminator) placed in direct contact with the side of the egg in a dark room can reveal a developing vascular pattern in a viable egg as the embryo grows or a homogeneous, diffuse, yellow-white luminescence in a dead egg. Ultrasonography must be used carefully as the ultrasound gel can potentially damage the eggs due to clogging of the pores used for gaseous exchange. Ultrasonography of the

Table 12.8 Common signs encountered during egg incubation, treatment, and prevention

Problem	Signs	Treatment	Prevention
Diapause	Fails to develop	Correction of environmental conditions	Some eggs enter diapause and resume growth after proper environmental conditions
Egg death	Fails to develop	Proper environmental conditions	Proper environmental conditions, proper monitoring and design of incubator
	Infertile egg	Not treatment	Sex determination of individuals, correct level of maturity, and proper pairing
	Fungal growth	Clean fungus gently with cotton tip	Avoid excessive humidity and contact between eggs
Trauma	Depression or deformity	No treatment	Mark egg's orientation with a pencil and avoid trauma or excessive handling
Dessication	Egg shrinkage	Rehydrate with warm spring water	Proper monitoring of humidity and temperature
Fungal growth	Mold on egg surface	Remove growth with a cotton tip, and sprinkle antifungal powder (e.g., athlete's foot powder)	Prevent excessive humidity and avoid contact between eggs. Remove any death egg
Slugs	Waxy yellow deformed and shrink eggs	No treatment	Discarded unfertilized ova. It may imply an underlying issue with the female. Seek veterinary attention

developing embryo requires a high-frequency ultrasound transducer (7.5–10 MHz) to properly assess development (Mader 2006). In any case, ultrasonography is a valid means not only to distinguish the general stages of follicle and egg development but also to predict birth—this can be reasonably predicted by monitoring the loss of yolk, with birth occurring about a week after yolk is no longer detectable (Denardo 2006).

Genetic Related Diseases

Genetically derived health problems have been reported. Because concerns regarding quality of life, organizations like the International Herpetological Society (IHS) have actively banned their sales in their shows. In any case, there is no entity regulating reptile breeding and ultimately this falls within the hands of the breeder and health providers. It is suggested that genetic mutations that reduce pigmentation often show signs of developmental and neurological abnormalities, including deafness, hereditary megacolon, reduced vision, and poor coordination. When these mutations are homozygously present, severe or even lethal developmental abnormalities are observed (Fox 2020).

IHS Banned Morphs:
Lemon Frost Leopard Gecko (Figures 12.14A–D).
Incomplete dominant inheritance. This mutation produces white body coloration with bright white/grey eyes, a brightened yellow and orange areas on their bodies, and a pattern that wraps to their underbellies. It also causes skin tumors (iridophoroma) with potential metastasis in homozygous individuals (Guo et al. 2021).

Enigma Leopard Geckos (Figures 12.15A and B).
Dominant inheritance. The enigma mutation affects neurological function causing dysfunction of coordination and cognition. Unfortunately, this is a late-onset neurological disease making it difficult for breeders to know which of their individuals are affected. Symptoms vary from mild (stargazing, head tilting, occasional circling, and abnormal behavior) to severe (inability to catch food, seizures, constant circling, and death rolls).

Super Motley Boa
The Motley mutation causes an increased black pigmentation resulting in a completely black or brown boa. The homologous form of the mutation is expressed when the boa has two homologous alleles of the mutated gene. This is referred to as the "super" form. The super or homologous

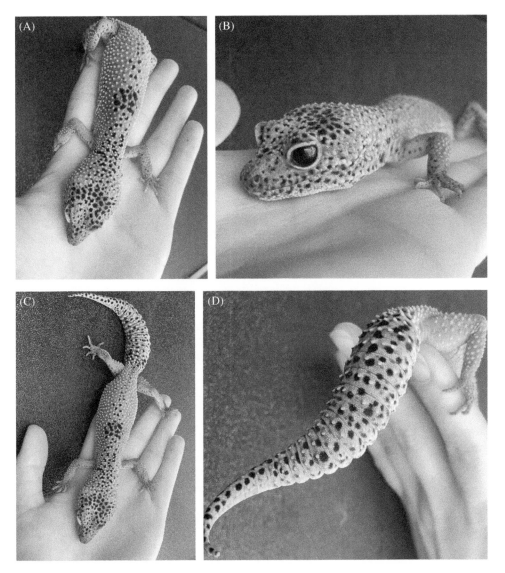

Figure 12.14 (A) Lemon Frost Leopard Gecko. (B) Head of the Lemon Frost Gecko. (C) Body view from above. (D) Tail view (Courtesy of Jessica Fennen.)

dominant form of this mutation is lethal within the first two years due to underdeveloped muscles.

Spider or Spider Webbed Ball Python

Incomplete dominant inheritance. The homozygous form of this gene is lethal (generally referred as super Spider). Also, this Spider gene, even when combined with any other number of mutations, causes neurological signs. This is generally referred to in the hobby as "wobbles" because of the head tremors. Signs are more obvious when the animals get excited or stressed, the wobble can range from very minor to extreme with some spiders struggling to even feed themselves. The gene is still very common in the hobby trade (Figures 12.16 and 12.17).

Jaguar Carpet Python

Incomplete dominant inheritance of the Coastal carpet python (*Morelia mcdowelli*). The resulting phenotype is characterized by a reduced pattern and an increase in yellow pigment. The mutation is linked to neurological signs of head wobbling, spinning, tremors, erratic movement, and head jerking (Fox 2020). The homozygous Jaguar (Super Jaguar) seems to have a lethal gene and these snakes do not live more than a few days.

There are genetically derived health problems that can also affect their musculoskeletal system. Some examples are the caramel albino ball python and the super cinnamon ball python (Figure 12.18A and B). In bearded dragons, breeding visual translucent with translucent can result

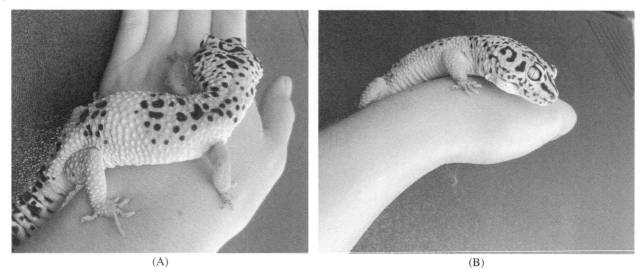

(A)   (B)

Figure 12.15 (A) Enigma Leopard Gecko. (B) Front view of an Enigma Leopard Gecko.(Courtesy of Jessica Fennen.)

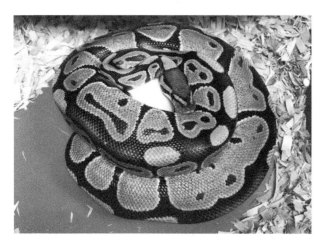

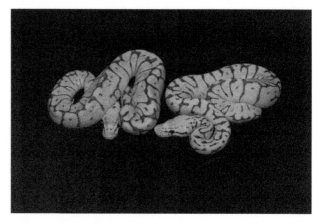

Figure 12.16 Normal morph ball python, it is also referred to as "wild-type" or "classic." (Courtesy of Tim Bailey.)

Figure 12.17 KillerBee which is a Super Pastel Spider (Courtesy of Tim Bailey.)

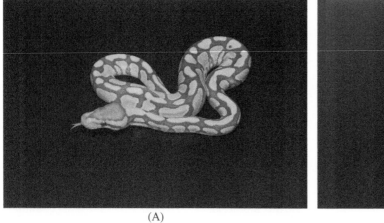

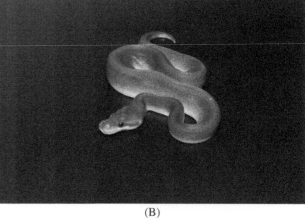

(A)   (B)

Figure 12.18 (A) Caramel Albino (B) Super Cinnamon ball python. (Courtesy of Tim Bailey.)

in bearded dragons with kinked backs, deformed limbs, neurological problems, and failure to thrive. An attempt to cover all available morphs and health-related problems would be outside the scope of this chapter.

Common Reproductive Diseases

Bites or trauma due to seasonal aggression, courting, or mating.

Phallus or hemipenes prolapse. About 35% of all cloacal prolapses involve the male reproductive organ. This is generally due to trauma with subsequent inflammation preventing retraction followed by infection and necrosis.

Oviductal prolapse. It is generally seen during dystocia or as a consequence of other reproductive-related issues like salpingitis, oviduct rupture/tear, abnormally shaped or sized ova, ectopic ova. and follicular stasis.

Follicular stasis. It occurs when mature follicles develop but do not ovulate or resorb, becoming static.

Egg yolk coelomitis. Inflammatory response in coelom due to the leakage of yolk material due to complications associated with pre-ovulatory stasis.

Dystocia. The inability of giving birth, either term eggs or fetuses. Dystocias can be divided into obstructive and non-obstructive.

Scent gland adenitis (snakes). This is an inflammation/impaction of the scent gland in snakes.

References

APPA. 2007/2008. *APPA's 2007/2008 National Pet Owners Survey.* American Pet Products Association.

APPA. 2010. *APPA's 2010 National Pet Owners Survey.* American Pet Products Association.

APPA. 2021/2022. *APPA's 2021/2022 National Pet Owners Survey.* American Pet Products Association.

Badaeva T, Malysheva D, et al. 2008. Genetic variation and de novo mutations in the parthenogenetic Caucasian rock lizard *Darevskia unisexualis. PLoS One* 3(7): e2730.

Benirschke K. 2007. Jackson's chameleon *Chamaeleon jacksonii xantholophus.* In: *Comparative Placentation* (ed K. Benirschke). Ithaca, NY: International Veterinary Information Service.

Blackburn D. 1998. Structure, function, and evolution of the oviducts of squamate reptiles, with special reference to viviparity and placentation. *J Exp Zool* 282(4–5): 560–617.

Clarke E. 2021. Ball python wizardry: basic medicine and husbandry, *VWX Conference in Orlando, Florida (5 June 2021).*

Delmas V, Prevot-Julliard A-C, et al. 2008. A mechanistic model of temperature-dependent sex determination in a chelonian: the European pond turtle. *Funct Ecol* 22(1): 84–93.

Demas S, Duronslet M, et al. 1990. Sex-specific DNA in reptiles with temperature dependent sex determination. *J Exp Zool* 253:319–324.

Denardo D. 2006. Reproductive biology. In: *Reptile Medicine and Surgery* (ed D Mader), pp. 376–390. St Louis, MI: Saunders Elsevier.

Fox B. 2020. *Hypopigmentation as the Cause for the Neulogical Disorder "Spider Wobble" in Python Regius. College Essay.* Columbus State Community College.

Funk R. 2002. Lizard reproductive medicine and surgery. *Vet Clin Exot Anim* 5(3): 579–613.

Guo L, Bloom J, et al. 2021. Genetics of white color and iridophoroma in "Lemon Frost" leopard geckos. *PLoS Genet* 17(6): 1–19.

HSUS. 2001. *The Trade in Live Reptiles: Imports to the United States.* Washington, DC: Humane Society of the United States.

Innis C, Boyer T. 2002. Chelonian reproductive disorders. *Vet Clin Exot Anim* 5(3): 555–578.

Lance V, Valenzuela N, et al. 1992. A hormonal method to determine the sex of hatchling giant river turtles, *Podocnemis expansa*: application to endangered species research. *Amer Zool* 32: 16A.

Mader D. 2006. Perinatology. In: *Reptile Medicine and Surgery* (ed D. Mader), pp. 365–375. St Louis, MI: Saunders Elsevier.

Owens D, Hendrickson J, et al. 1978. A technique for determining sex of immature *Chelonia mydas* using radioimmunoassay. *Herpetologica* 34: 270–273.

Radder R, Quinn A, et al. 2008. Genetic evidence for co-occurrence of chromosomal and thermal sex-determining systems in a lizard. *Biol Lett* 4(2): 176–178.

Rostal D, Grumbles J, et al. 1994. Non-lethal sexing techniques for hatchling and immature desert tortoises (*Gopherus agassizii*). *Herp Mono* 8: 83–87.

Sasa M, Curtis S. 2006. Field observation of mating behavior in the neckbanded snake *Scaphiodontophis annulatus* (Serpentes: Colubridae). *Rev Biol Trop* 54(2): 647–650.

Schramm B, Casares M, et al. 1999. Steroid levels and reproductive cycle of the Galapagos tortoise, *Geochelone nigra*, living under seminatural conditions on Santa Cruz Island (Galapagos). *Gen Comp Endocrinol* 114(1): 108–120.

Stahl S. 2001. Reptile reproduction medicine. *Semin Avian Exotic Pet Med* 10(3): 140–150.

Stahl S, Denardo D. 2019. Theriogenology. In: *Mader's Reptile and Amphibian Medicine and Surgery* 3rd edn (ed. S Divers and S Stahl), pp. 849–893. St Louis, MI: Saunders Elsevier.

Taylor E, Denardo D. 2005. Sexual size dimorphism and growth plasticity in snakes: an experiment on the Western Diamond-backed Rattlesnake (*Crotalus atrox*). *J Exp Zool A Comp Exp Biol* 303(7): 598–607.

Wapstra E, Uller T, et al. 2009. Climate effects on offspring sex ratio in a viviparous lizard. *J Anim Ecol* 78: 84–90.

Warner D, Shine R. 2008. The adaptive significance of temperature-dependent sex determination in a reptile. *Nature* 451: 566–568.

Webb J, Shine R, et al. 2006. The adaptive significance of reptilian viviparity in the tropics: testing maternal manipulation hypothesis. *Evolution* 60(1): 115–160.

Wibbels T, Bull J, et al. 1991. Chronology and morphology of temperature dependent sex determination. *J Exp Zool* 260: 371–381.

13

Infectious Diseases of Reptiles
Pia Bartolini

Introduction

There are over 11,730 species of reptiles currently known in the world (http://www.reptile-database.org). Emerging diseases also continue to be on the rise from improved modular and diagnostics techniques with many of these pathogens being detected by polymerase-chain reaction (PCR). Next-generation sequencing (NGS) techniques have had a rapid increase in the described viruses and other pathogens in captive and wild vertebrates (Hotaling et al. 2021, O'Dea et al. 2016, Tetzlaff et al. 2017). The development of these diagnostic tools has become essential for exotic veterinary medicine. Despite many advancements, there can be cases that are not straightforward in infectious disease epidemiology. These can be due to complex factors such as host relationships, viruses/pathogens, environment, and other co-infections in the animal. Pathogens may also have a healthy carrier state or be asymptomatic compounding the epidemiological effect with "Typhoid Mary" as an example. Using a multimodal approach with clinical signs, patient history, and evidence-based diagnostics and validated testing when available for diagnosis and treatment plans is essential (Mitchell & Perry 2017). It is imperative not to misinterpret diagnostics such as culture and sensitivity or molecular diagnostic test results because many of these organisms may be nonpathogenic in reptilian species. Normal bacterial flora can cause illness when a patient is immune-suppressed or otherwise debilitated by a pathogen causing a secondary infection. There have also been multiple reports of co-infections which show the complexity of viral infections in various herpetofauna (Keller et al. 2017, Racz et al. 2021, Rostad et al. 2019).

With the increasing number of reptile species entering into the pet hobby trade the technician can use comparative medicine when there is a lack of information about a given species. The best model to use typically is the closest phylogenetically relative from which data is available (Wellehan 2014). Treatment, drugs, and drug doses are commonly extrapolated with many of the species not having pharmacokinetic (PK) data available. Over the last decade, there has been an increase in the utilization of technicians in educating clients not only on the advancements of reptile husbandry, quarantine, biosecurity, but also the need for disease surveillance and infectious disease testing. An initial database ideally should be obtained for every patient including a full physical examination, complete blood count, plasma biochemistry, fecal evaluation, (direct, float, and acid-fast stain) and radiographs or computerized tomography (CT) scan. As veterinary clinics add advanced modalities such as CT-scans, they can be utilized for the baseline of the patient which could possibly identify a subclinical disease in non-domestic patients that commonly hide their illness. It is paramount that technicians understand differential diagnoses of the presenting complaint of the patient, thus helping to ask appropriate questions while taking the patient's history and initial database. To further the technician's knowledge base, a recommended resource for a comprehensive overview is the second edition Infectious Diseases and Pathology of Reptiles: A Color Atlas and Text by Jacobson E (Boca Raton, FL, USA: CRC Press; 2021) as well as the third edition of Mader's Reptile Medicine and Surgery by Divers and Stahl (St. Louis, MO, USA: Elsevier; 2019). The Association of Reptile and Amphibian Veterinarians' Infectious Disease Committee puts together a quarterly list of reptile infectious disease publications in peer-reviewed literature, entitled "Infectious Diseases of Reptiles and Amphibians: Peer-Reviewed Publications." These lists are published in the Journal of Herpetological Medicine & Surgery and are a valuable resource for technicians and veterinarians.

Exotic Animal Medicine for the Veterinary Technician, Fourth Edition. Edited by Bonnie Ballard and Ryan Cheek.
© 2024 John Wiley & Sons, Inc. Published 2024 by John Wiley & Sons, Inc.
Companion Website: www.wiley.com/go/ballard/4e

Biosecurity and Quarantine

Technicians are commonly the first and last person the client engages with at the veterinary clinic. Therefore, technicians have a vital role in ensuring clients are educated on all aspects of reptile care, including biosecurity, infectious disease testing, and quarantine of new incoming animals. Quarantine is defined as a length of time the new incoming animal is kept isolated from the existing pets in the household. This is important for observing behavior, testing for infectious diseases, and allowing time for the new animal to acclimate to their new environment to reduce stress. Most importantly, the quarantine period may protect the established population in the household from an infectious disease carried by the incoming animal. The length of time and how to isolate new animals will be determined on a case-by-case basis; however, an arbitrary 30 up to 90-day quarantine is commonly used. A few factors to consider include where the origin of the animal was, the age, species, and was the animal captive born or wild-caught as this could shorten or length the time of quarantine with unknown history needing longer quarantine times. It is also important that other animals in the home have been tested for infectious diseases, and that they have not also been exposed to unknown animals prior to introducing a new pet into an existing collection. This includes exposure to other animals at pet shops, reptile expos, and other homes. Inadvertently exposing an established reptile collection to an infectious agent can be devastating to the health of the established collection with both emotional and financial costs. It has been well-documented that the stress of transport and exposure to novel infectious agents in new environments may cause the new incoming animal to be more susceptible to these agents and can increase the likelihood to shed the infectious agents. The area where the animal is isolated for quarantine should be separate from the main collection, and cared for ideally on separate days from the main collection with separate tools and husbandry items or after the main collection is cared for. An "All In" protocol as described in the American Animal Health Association (AAHA) isolation sample protocol for entering and exiting an isolation area can be adapted (https://www.aaha.org).

1. Before entering the isolation area, remove outerwear (e.g., laboratory coat) and any equipment (e.g., watch, cell phone) and leave outside the isolation area.
2. Gather any necessary supplies and medications before putting on personal protective equipment (PPE).
   a. PPE can be as simple as an old scrub top, t-shirt or jacket and a pair of slip-on shoes.
3. Perform hand hygiene and then put on a quarantine top, gloves and changing shoes before entering the isolation room.
4. Clean and disinfect any equipment used while caring for the animal.
5. Before leaving the isolation area, remove PPE; remove shoes last when stepping out of the isolation room and avoid touching the outer surface of the shoes. Avoid contact with external portions of the door when exiting the isolation room.
6. Perform hand hygiene and then disinfect any surfaces (e.g., doorknobs) that may have accidentally been contaminated when the room was exited. Wash hands again before leaving the anteroom.

Sample Collection, Diagnostic Testing, and Shipping

Technicians have a crucial role in collecting and shipping diagnostic samples to the appropriate laboratories. The technician's role is to assist in ensuring that the sample that is collected is the correct one for the diagnostic test, it is stored appropriately in the appropriate media, and that the sample is labeled appropriately (patient name, identification number, date, species, and sampling site). Depending on the disease in question or health surveillance risk analysis, different sample types and testing are required. Understanding the methods of the diagnostic test is imperative for a good clinical approach. Microbial infections should be cultured with sensitivity but understanding that some bacteria can by normal or some bacteria such as mycobacterium and mycoplasma do not culture well. Therefore, a PCR which amplifies specific DNA/RNA may be a better diagnostic test. The sample collected should be adequate without any contamination. A fresh tissue biopsy sample can also be used for culture and in conjunction with a PCR. A benefit with PCR is that sequencing can be performed to confirm specific pathogens which can assist in clinical treatment approaches. Since PCR is highly sensitive and contamination or degradation of samples is a significant concern, care needs to be taken with sample collection and transport. Laboratories may have different shipping and sample preservation requests so contact the specific laboratory prior to shipping. Other modalities can be used with formalin-fixed tissue biopsies such as histopathology, immunohistochemistry, and in situ hybridization. Additionally, some samples can be collected for a quick in-house diagnostic test such as cytology, complete blood count, plasma biochemistry, and fecal evaluation. Some of these modalities can be done microscopically in-house with the use of special stains to assist in ruling in or out diseases while the patient is still at the clinic. Cytological evaluation of Gram stains can characterize bacteria and morphology into Gram-positive or Gram-negative bacteria which can also assist with antibiotic selection prior to receiving the final sensitivity results from the laboratory (Eatwell 2007). Wright–Giemsa and lactophenol cotton blue are used to characterize yeasts and fungal hyphae. Other stains such as Acid-fast stains are used to identify Acid-fast staining bacteria like mycobacterial infections, Nocardia, and some parasitic infections, such as Cryptosporidium. In addition, several factors can affect results from types of immune responses in reptile patients including reproductive status, age, seasonal variation, endogenous cortisol levels, and exogenous administration of corticosteroids affecting the clinical pathology. The technician should understand that there are two major approaches to testing for infectious agents not only in reptiles but for all patients. One is by looking at the patient's acquired immune response to an agent and the second is the presence of an infectious agent. Then the acquired immunity can be additionally specified to a test that can evaluate an antibody production against the specific pathogen to assess a humoral immune response. Some examples of tests that look at humoral response are enzyme-linked immunosorbent assays (ELISA), hemagglutination inhibition (HI), virus neutralization, and agarose gel immunodiffusion. Importantly, technicians should understand that humoral immunity is only part of the acquired immune response, and what it means to have a positive humoral immunity but negative PCR. Another diagnostic modality is electron microscopy (EM) which obtains a high-resolution image of biological specimens giving detailed structures of tissues, cells, organisms, viruses, etc. EM uses a variety of ancillary techniques such as immuno-labeling and negative staining to identify species pathogens (Jacobson & Garner 2021).

All these diagnostic tests are tools to look for the presence of the infectious agent or evaluate the health of the patient. The knowledge of the pathobiology of the infectious agent is needed to determine the appropriate sampling, testing modality, and treatment plan. When the veterinarian is interpreting test results, the evidence of an infectious agent or an immune response does not mean that the agent is pathogenic and causing disease. Likewise, the absence of the agent may not mean that it is not occurring due to false negatives of testing. Some pathogens may show clinical disease only after a viremia has occurred, and the agent is no longer present for identification. During the initial examination, the patient needs a clinical assessment of any underlying factors that can contribute to the reptile's medical condition. Also with treatment of underlying disease, thermal support, and improved husbandry largely influences clinical improvement and recovery in herpetofauna. The poikilothermic patient's immune response, metabolism of drugs, and hydration support are thermally dependent (Kurath & Adams 2011). Reptilian patients that

are ambulatory can be provided a thermal gradient that is appropriate for the species; noted that some species may need to be cooled. For patients who are non-ambulatory, a temperature selection should be based on the species and clinical need. Technicians need to be aware of the husbandry of common species that are seen in their clinic and resources for uncommon species. As with any patient seen at the clinic, stabilization may include hydration support, nutritional support, analgesics if indicated, and a reduction of exposure to any environmental stressors. A routine minimum database should be collected with advanced diagnostics if indicated to confirm a clinical diagnosis. Careful selection of antimicrobial or antiparasitic medications is warranted after diagnostic samples have been collected to reduce antibiotic/antiparasitic resistance or complicating factors of diagnostic test results. Also, inappropriate administration of antibiotics, antiparasitic, or antifungal medications can cause significant side effects to the patient (Eatwell 2007).

With regard to diagnostic sample shipping, there may be the potential for hefty fines if shipping is done incorrectly. Samples may be considered hazardous goods, thus requiring specific shipping parameters. Prior to shipping contact the shipping company (USPS, UPS, FedEX, DHL, etc.) via phone call or website for additional information and guidelines. The IATA Dangerous Goods Regulations (DGR) manual is a standard recognized by airlines as the global reference for shipping dangerous goods by air. Shipping requirements can change therefore an up-to-date protocol is necessary. If shipping liquid, it should be in a secure primary receptacle such as a vial or specimen cup and can be further secured with parafilm. It can then be placed inside a secondary receptacle such as a sealed plastic bag or Whirl-pac with absorbable material such as paper towels added. Ensure that the sample can withstand shipping conditions and arrive at the laboratory without damage, such as in a cardboard and/or styrofoam box Similarly, dry samples and swabs should be shipped within a secondary receptacle to ensure they arrive at the laboratory without damage, such as in a sterile vial (Figures 13.1-13.8).

Veterinary diagnostic samples are subject to the country's Postal Service regulations. Check with the diagnostic laboratory for specific shipping requests and possibly pre-addressed mailers prior to submission (https://about.usps.com).

FedEx and UPS have similar shipping guidelines with examples below. The IATA regulations require that shipments containing Biological Substances, Category B are triple packaged according to Packing Instruction 650. Refer to the Dangerous Goods Regulations, Packing Instruction 650 for more information regarding marking, labeling, and packing requirements (https://www.fedex.com).

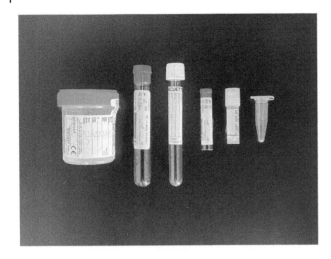

Figure 13.1 An example of primary containers for liquid or a secondary container for a swab sample.

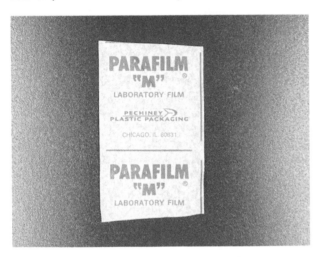

Figure 13.2 An example of Parafilm to seal a primary container with a liquid sample.

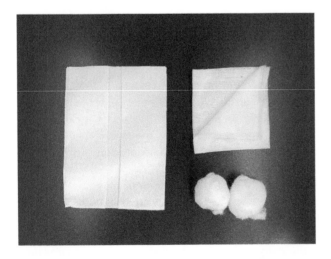

Figure 13.3 An example of absorbable material to place inside the secondary container for a liquid sample.

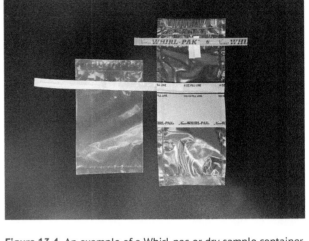

Figure 13.4 An example of a Whirl-pac or dry sample container.

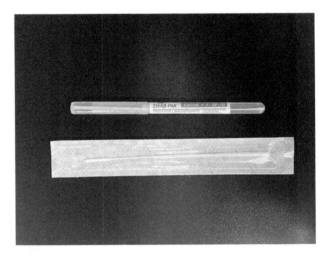

Figure 13.5 An example of a sterile swab for PCR testing.

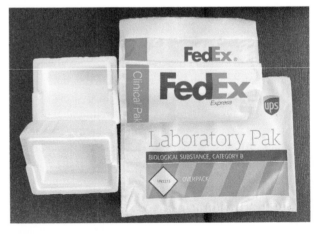

Figure 13.6 An example of a soft clinical package supplied by a shipping company with a styrofoam box.

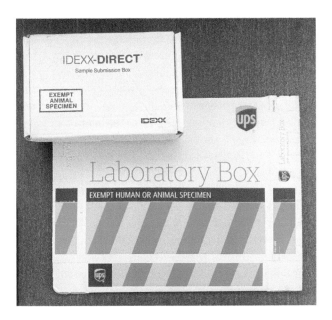

Figure 13.7 An example of a cardboard clinical package supplied by a shipping company.

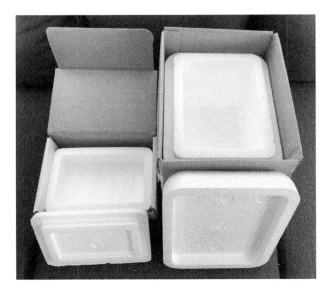

Figure 13.8 An example of a cardboard box with accompanying styrofoam box.

Infectious Diseases

Bacterial

Mycoplasma (URTD)

Disease/Definition: Mycoplasma is a genus of bacteria that lacks a cell wall and is also referred to as a "soft skin" bacteria in the class Mollicutes. Also known as upper respiratory tract disease (URTD) (Jacobson et al. 2014, Jacobson & Garner 2021).

Symptoms/Clinical Signs: Presentation can depend on the species and tissues affected. Non-specific complaints of malaise (anorexia, lethargy, decreased activity) mild and non-specific upper and lower respiratory signs, ocular discharge, palpebral edema, increased oral discharge, redness of gums or stomatitis, wheezing and increased respiratory effort, open mouth breathing or "coughing," weight loss, dehydration and/or dysecdysis, change in behavior. Other clinical signs include arthritis, otitis, and granulomas (Jacobson et al. 2014, Jacobson & Garner 2021, Racz et al. 2021).

Epidemiology: Most *Mycoplasma spp.* are more common than significantly causing disease but likely with co-infections. No sex or age predilection is known but juvenile or immunocompromised animals are more susceptible (Jacobson et al. 2014, Jacobson & Garner 2021, Racz et al. 2021).

Etiology/Pathophysiology: Commonly associated with hyperplasia and lymphoplasmacytic inflammation (Jacobson & Garner 2021, Marschang et al. 2016, Penner et al. 1997).

Differential Diagnosis: Respiratory and granulomatous disease differentials include bacterial (chlamydia), viral (herpesvirus, ranavirus, adenovirus, reovirus, paramyxovirus, picoronavirus) parasitic (intranuclear coccidiosis), fungal, trauma (nasal or tracheal foreign body), neoplasia, or cardiac disease (Divers & Stahl 2019, Jacobson & Garner 2021).

Initial Database: Full physical examination, complete blood count, plasma biochemistry, fecal evaluation (direct, float, and acid-fast stain), and radiographs or CT scan as a baseline. A leukocytosis may be present.

Advanced/Confirmatory Testing: Since *Mycoplasma* sp. are highly susceptible to desiccation during transport, PCR, EM, or ELISA serology are the best to confirm. Serum or heparinized plasma separated into a sterile plastic tube can be submitted for ELISA. Tissue biopsy, oral/nasal swab or nasal wash can be submitted for PCR (Jacobson et al. 2014, Racz et al. 2021).

Treatment: Macrolides and tetracyclines are currently the best therapeutic choice with any husbandry deficiencies corrected. Eradication of *Mycoplasma* may be difficult with patients being chronic asymptomatic carriers (Eatwell 2007, Hedley et al. 2021).

Pearls/Considerations/Tech Tip: Upper respiratory tract disease "URTD" is the common name in tortoises commonly seen without pneumonia. Speciation is important to evaluate *Mycoplasma* species because not all species have been shown to cause disease. There are two species of *Mycoplasma* that are a pathogenic and causative agent of URTD in chelonians. They are *Mycoplasma agassizii* and *Mycoplasma testudineum* (Jacobson et al. 2014).

Prevention: Maintaining a closed group of animals with a known negative status with proper husbandry, quarantine, and strict biosecurity. Introduction of new animals only after above-mentioned quarantine and infectious disease screening (Divers & Stahl 2019).

Chlamydia (Neochlamydia, Parachlamydia, and Simkania)

Disease/Definition: Chlamydia is a unique, obligate intracellular, gram-negative bacterial pathogen that can cause an acute or chronic bacterial infection in reptiles. Chlamydia can cause granulomatous lesions in internal organs, proliferative pneumonia, necrotizing enteritis, myocarditis, hepatitis, conjunctivitis, or be asymptomatic. They are in the genera Chlamydiae, including *Chlamydophila, Neochlamydia, Parachlamydia,* and *Simkania* (Divers & Stahl 2019, Jacobson & Garner 2021, Mitchell 2011, Mitura et al. 2017, Racz et al. 2021).

Symptoms/Clinical Signs: Presentation can depend on the species and tissues affected. Non-specific complaints of malaise (anorexia, lethargy, and decreased activity), mild and non-specific respiratory signs, regurgitation and weight loss, dehydration, and/or dysecdysis (Divers & Stahl 2019, Jacobson & Garner 2021).

Epidemiology: Commonly seen in emerald tree boas (*Corallus caninus*). No sex or age predilection is known but juvenile or immunocompromised animals are more susceptible (Divers & Stahl 2019, Inchuai et al. 2021).

Etiology/Pathophysiology: Most commonly seen is *Chlamydophila pneumoniae* and should be speciated because of differences in both ecology and zoonotic risk with different *Chlamydia* species (Divers & Stahl 2019, Jacobson & Garner 2021).

Differential Diagnosis: Respiratory and granulomatous disease differentials include bacterial (mycoplasma), viral (herpesvirus, ranavirus, adenovirus, reovirus, paramyxovirus, and picoronavirus) parasitic (intranuclear coccidiosis), fungal, trauma (nasal or tracheal foreign body), neoplasia, or cardiac disease (Divers & Stahl 2019, Jacobson & Garner 2021).

Initial Database: Full physical examination, complete blood count, plasma biochemistry, fecal evaluation (direct, float, and acid-fast stain), and radiographs or CT-scan as a baseline.

Advanced/Confirmatory Testing: Direct impression smears and cytologic staining can be done in-house, choanal or upper esophageal swabs can be submitted for PCR (it is preferred), immunohistochemistry with monoclonal antibodies against chlamydial lipopolysaccharide (LPS). Biopsies of granulomatous disease should be examined with a Machiavello stain or by immunohistochemistry (Divers & Stahl 2019, Jacobson & Garner 2021).

Treatment: Tetracyclines and azalides are currently the best therapeutic choice with husbandry deficiencies corrected. PK data is available in azithromycin in royal/ball pythons (*Python regius*), rat snakes (*Elaphe obsoleta*), green iguanas (*Iguana iguana*), corn snakes (*Elaphe gutatta gutatta*), carpet pythons (*Moreilia spilota*), red-eared terrapins (*Trachemys scripta elegans*), Hermann's tortoises (*Testudo hermanni*) and Greek tortoises (*Testudo graeca*) (Eatwell 2007, Hedley et al. 2021, Jacobson & Garner 2021).

Pearls/Considerations/Tech Tip: *Chlamydophila pneumoniae* is zoonotic and a significant concern and should be discussed with the client. Two novel chlamydial species have been described: *Chlamydia serpentis* and *Chlamydia poikilothermis*. Co-infections with other pathogens like Mycoplasma, serpentovirus, etc. can likely occur, however, clinical relevance still needs to be studied (Racz et al. 2021, Taylor-Brown et al. 2015).

Prevention: Maintaining a closed group of animals with a known negative status with proper husbandry, quarantine, and strict biosecurity. Introduction of new animals only after above-mentioned quarantine and infectious disease screening (Divers & Stahl 2019).

Devriesea agamarum

Disease/Definition: A newly discovered species of bacteria, a Gram-positive, short 1–2 μm rod that appears in pairs or short chains. In the phylum Actinobacteria that has been associated with severe hyperkeratotic dermatitis, cheilitis, and potential septicemia in Uromastyx species and agamid species (Hellebuyck et al. 2009a,b, Jacobson & Garner 2021).

Symptoms/Clinical Signs: Presentation can depend on the species and tissues affected. Non-specific complaints of malaise (anorexia, lethargy, decreased activity), mild and non-specific dermatitis, chronic proliferative dermatitis, cheylitis (chapped lips), ulcerative lesions, peri-cloacal dermatitis, septicemia, and chronic subcutaneous abscesses (Hellebuyck et al. 2009a,b).

Epidemiology: Common cause of dermatitis and septicemia in lizards (*Uromastyx spp.*) and can affect asymptomatically other lizard species especially the bearded dragon (*Pogona vitticeps*) with *D. agamarum* as it is part of the normal mouth flora (Hellebuyck et al. 2009a,b, Schmidt-Ukaj et al. 2014).

Etiology/Pathophysiology: Healthy carriers in captive colonies can be a significant health concern and can become a chronic problem. No sex predilection is known but juvenile or immunocompromised animals are more susceptible.

Differential Diagnosis: Dermatitis differentials include bacterial dermatitis, viral-causing cutaneous lesions (Poxvirus, Herpesvirus), parasitic (scale mites, cutaneous larva migrans) fungal dermatopathies ("CANV" *nannizziopsis*, *Mucor spp.*, *Penicillium spp.*, *Candida spp.*), trauma-induced dermatopathies (thermal burns), or neoplasia (Divers & Stahl 2019, Jacobson & Garner 2021).

Initial Database: Full physical examination, complete blood count, plasma biochemistry, fecal evaluation (direct, float and acid-fast stain) and radiographs or CT-scan as a baseline.

Advanced/Confirmatory Testing: PCR is preferred by histopathology or by microbiological evaluation. Biopsies of dermatological lesions should be examined by histopathology. Swabs can be submitted for microbiological examination with antibiotic sensitivity. Crusty skin/ecdysis or skin scrape/swabs can be submitted for PCR (Divers & Stahl 2019, Hellebuyck et al. 2009a,b).

Treatment: A study of an intramuscular injection of ceftiofur at 5 mg/kg q24h eliminated *D. agamarum* with clinical recovery. Surgical debridement may also be required with analgesia. Supportive treatment for bacterial overgrowth, analgesia, and wound care with husbandry deficiencies corrected (Eatwell 2007, Hedley et al. 2021, Hellebuyck et al. 2009a,b).

Pearls/Considerations/Tech Tip: Seen in dry desert species such as *Uromastyx spp.*, some tropical species like *Basiliscus spp.*, *Physignathus spp.* (water dragons) *Eublepharis spp.* (leopard geckos), *Furcifer spp.* (chameleons) and others. Asymptomatic carriers can occur. It has been reported that enrofloxacin did not eliminate *D. agamarum* (Hellebuyck et al. 2021).

Prevention: Maintaining a closed group of animals with a known negative status with proper husbandry, quarantine, and strict biosecurity. Introduction of new animals only after above-mentioned quarantine and infectious disease screening (Divers & Stahl 2019).

Enterococcus lacertideformus

Disease/Definition: Novel species of *enterococci* that causes multi-systemic disease and seems to be invariably fatal. More common *Enterococcus spp.* are in the order Lactobacillales and are chain-forming Gram-positive cocci (Agius 2021).

Symptoms/Clinical Signs: Presentation can depend on the species and tissues affected. Non-specific complaints of malaise (anorexia, lethargy, decreased activity), mild and non-specific facial swelling, lethargy, and death (Agius 2021).

Epidemiology: Has been seen in four species of captive lizards: Carolina anole (*Anolis carolinensis*), Cape girdled lizard (*Cordylus cordylus*), Balkan green lizard (*Lacerta trilineata*), and European green lizard (*Lacerta viridis*), Common house gecko (*Hemidactylus frenatus*), and in invasive brown anoles (*Anolis sagrei*) in Florida, USA.

No age or sex predilection is known but likely juvenile or immunocompromised animals are more susceptible (Agius 2021, Ossiboff et al. 2020, Rose et al. 2017).

Etiology/Pathophysiology: Known to have hardened cell walls, osmotic and antibiotic resistance cause an infection of *Enterococcus* difficult to treat. With *E. lacertideformus* large colonies replace the bone and the soft tissues in the head of the infected animal which compresses and replaces the normal parenchyma of the infected tissues. Interestingly, the biofilm that *E. lacertideformus* is surrounded by appears to cover the host animal's immune system. This in turn causes a limited inflammatory response in the host (Agius et al. 2021).

Differential Diagnosis: Differentials for facial swelling include bacterial dermatitis, viral-causing cutaneous lesions (Poxvirus, Herpesvirus), parasitic (cutaneous larva migrans) fungal dermatopathies, trauma-induced dermatopathies (subcutaneous emphysema), or neoplasia (Divers & Stahl 2019).

Initial Database: Full physical examination, complete blood count, plasma biochemistry, fecal evaluation, (direct, float, and acid-fast stain) and radiographs or CT-scan as a baseline.

Advanced/Confirmatory Testing: Microscopically, chains of bacterial cocci are surrounded by a thick biofilm-like matrix (Agius 2021).

Treatment: PK study of enrofloxacin showed that it likely achieved sufficient plasma concentrations therefore enrofloxacin and amoxicillin-clavulanic acid were possible treatment options. Also supportive treatment for secondary bacterial overgrowth, analgesia, and wound care with husbandry deficiencies corrected (Agius 2021, Eatwell 2007, Hedley et al. 2021).

Pearls/Considerations/Tech Tip: Seen in wild invasive brown anoles and wild species of geckos in Southeast Asia and should be on the list of differentials facial swelling of newly imported animals based on exiting and importing ports (Agius 2021, Ossiboff et al. 2020).

Prevention: Maintaining a closed group of animals with a known negative status with proper husbandry, quarantine, and strict biosecurity. Introduction of new animals only after above-mentioned quarantine and infectious disease screening (Divers & Stahl 2019).

Austwickia chelonae

Disease/Definition: *Austwickia* (formerly *Dermatophilus*) *chelonae*, a Gram-positive filamentous Actinobacteria in the Dermatophilaceae family causing fatal granulomatous disease in diverse captive reptile species but unknown presence in wild or free-ranging populations (Divers & Stahl 2019, Jacobson & Garner 2021, Jiang et al. 2019, Rostad et al. 2019).

Symptoms/Clinical Signs: Dermatophilosis from *A. chelonae* has distinctive granulomas that appear like wart-like growths or boils with these lesions being up to 1 cm wide in larger chelonian specimens (Divers & Stahl 2019, Jacobson & Garner 2021).

Epidemiology: Commonly seen in tortoises, lizard species such as bearded dragon (*P. vitticeps*), crocodile lizard (*Shinisaurus crocodilurus*) but can be seen in any reptile species. No sex predilection is known but juvenile or immunocompromised animals are more susceptible (Divers & Stahl 2019, Jacobson & Garner 2021, Liguori et al. 2022).

Etiology/Pathophysiology: *A. chelonae* irritates the deep layers of skin tissue and causes an inflammatory growth reaction or a hypersensitivity reaction. The granulomas first appear as a bump and then usually grow into a larger yellowish boil where a scab can form as well. Infected chelonians typically have granulomas formed on the legs and jaw, and scabs on the nose (Divers & Stahl 2019, Jacobson & Garner 2021).

Differential Diagnosis: Dermatitis differentials include bacterial dermatitis, viral causing cutaneous lesions (Poxvirus, Herpesvirus), parasitic (scale mites, cutaneous larva migrans) fungal dermatopathies ("CANV" *nannizziopsis, Mucor spp., Penicillium spp., Candida spp.*), trauma-induced dermatopathies (thermal burns), or neoplasia. Granulomatous disease differentials include bacterial (*Mycobacterium spp., Chlamydia spp.*), viral, parasitic, fungal, trauma, or neoplasia (Divers & Stahl 2019, Jacobson & Garner 2021).

Initial Database: Full physical examination, complete blood count, plasma biochemistry, fecal evaluation (direct, float, and acid-fast stain), and radiographs or CT-scan as a baseline.

Advanced/Confirmatory Testing: Biopsies of dermatological lesions should be examined by histopathology. Crusty skin/ecdysis or skin scrape/swabs can be submitted for PCR. Notify laboratory that *A. chelonae* is suspected due to growing faster at 27°C than 37°C (Tamukai et al. 2016).

Treatment: Antibiotic sensitivity was shown in one study to cephalothin, minocycline and ampicillin, but not to kanamycin, gentamicin, streptomycin, and clarithromycin, suggesting a possible treatment for the infected crocodile lizards with husbandry deficiencies corrected. However, surgical resection of the nodules as early as possible was recommended. Supportive treatment for secondary bacterial overgrowth, analgesia, and wound care with husbandry deficiencies corrected (Divers & Stahl 2019, Eatwell 2007, Hedley et al. 2021).

Pearls/Considerations/Tech Tip: Co-infections with Ranavirus has been seen Inland Bearded Dragons (*P. vitticeps*). Also referred to as "Rain Rot" in the reptile community (Tamukai et al. 2016).

Prevention: Maintaining a closed group of animals with a known negative status with proper husbandry, quarantine, and strict biosecurity. Introduction of new animals only after above-mentioned quarantine and infectious disease screening (Divers & Stahl 2019).

Fungal

Ophidiomyces ("Snake Fungal Disease")

Disease/Definition: *Ophidomcyes ophiodiicola* is a fungus in the Onygenaceae family causing crusting dermatitis commonly around the head and lips of snakes. Commonly referred to as snake fungal disease "SFD" which can be a broad term for any fungal lesion and formerly, *Chrysosporium ophiodiicola*. Similar fungal isolates formerly grouped under the appellation "*Chrysosporium* anamorph of *Nannizziopsis vriesii* (CANV) complex" led to major taxonomic revisions and *Nannizziopsis* now includes nine species within reptiles and human hosts. Then *Ophidiomyces*, with a single species *Ophidiomyces ophiodiicola* (Divers & Stahl 2019, Jacobson & Garner 2021).

Symptoms/Clinical Signs: Range from a mild dermatitis with hyperkeratosis, scab/crusting of skin (commonly around face), deep granulomatous dermatitis, facial swelling that progresses to dermatitis, subcutaneous nodules, abnormal behavior (restlessness), open-mouth breathing (occluded nares), premature shedding of the skin and corneal opacities (Divers & Stahl 2019, Jacobson & Garner 2021).

Epidemiology: Mycosis can affect a wide range of reptilian species. The presence of fungus is normal on skin and environment. Pathogenic mycosis can be spread between individuals by direct contact, environmental transmission, and cross-contamination. No sex or age predilection is known but juvenile or immunocompromised animals can be more susceptible (Divers & Stahl 2019).

Etiology/Pathophysiology: Infection occurs when the arthroconidia colonizes dead stratum corneum at the surface of the skin where the hyphae proliferates the deeper dermis (Jacobson & Garner 2021, Picquet et al. 2018).

Differential Diagnosis: Differentials include bacterial, viral, parasitic (ectoparasite/mites), trauma-induced dermatopathy, inappropriate husbandry (i.e., severe dehydration, thermal burns), other fungal dermatopathies ("CANV" *nannizziopsis, Mucor spp., Penicillium spp., Candida spp.*) or neoplasia (Divers & Stahl 2019).

Initial Database: Full physical examination, complete blood count, plasma biochemistry, fecal evaluation, (direct, float, and acid-fast stain) and radiographs or CT-scan as a baseline.

Advanced/Confirmatory Testing: Biopsies of dermatological lesions should be examined by histopathology particularly if diagnostic arthroconidia are present. Biopsy preferred but crusty skin/ecdysis or skin scrape/swabs can be submitted for PCR (Jacobson & Garner 2021, Picquet et al. 2018).

Treatment: Surgical debridement, antifungals, supportive treatment for secondary bacterial overgrowth, analgesia, and wound care with husbandry deficiencies corrected. Terbinafine nebulized ± systemic antifungals such as itraconazole and voriconazole with care taken to not cause toxicity (Divers & Stahl 2019, Kane et al. 2017).

Pearls/Considerations/Tech Tip: Commonly seen in vipers and colubids. 70% ethanol or bleach are effective disinfectants on clean nonporous surfaces. SFD is often misdiagnosed (*Chrysosporium anamorph Nannizziopsis vriessii* (CANV) complex). Snakes often exhibit abnormal feeding behaviors, inappropriately thermoregulating, and hyperthermia. Lesions around the face and mouth may interfere with vision and feeding ability. Species with heat-sensing ability may also be affected, although this effect has not been fully researched. In early signs of the disease, scale discoloration and facial swelling should be evaluated along with narrowing of the nares or secondary jaw misalignment. Grossly, the lesions appear to resolve after a shed but re-initiation of the disease can occur with previously infected scales appearing abnormal or scarred after a shed. Death can occur in severe cases of ophidiomycosis (Anderson et al. 2021). Multiple biopsies should be taken to submit for histopathology and save frozen for additional testing such as PCR (Divers & Stahl 2019, Jacobson & Garner 2021, Picquet et al. 2018).

Prevention: Maintaining a closed group of animals with a known negative status with proper husbandry, quarantine, and strict biosecurity. Introduction of new animals only after above-mentioned quarantine and infectious disease screening (Divers & Stahl 2019).

Paranannizziopsis ("CANV," "White Spot Disease")

Disease/Definition: *Paranannizziopsis* is a fungus in the Onygenaceae family causing crusting dermatitis with a high mortality rate that affects species of snakes, lizards, and tuataras (Cnossen 2021, Divers & Stahl 2019, Jacobson & Garner 2021, Paré & Sigler 2016).

Symptoms/Clinical signs: Range from a mild dermatitis, small pale yellow/white skin lesions on head and dorsum, subcutaneous nodules, crusting hyperkeratosis, scab/crusting of skin (commonly around face), deep granulomatous dermatitis, facial swelling that progresses to dermatitis, abnormal behavior (restlessness), open-mouth breathing (occluded nares), premature ecdysis, osmotic imbalances in aquatic species, and death (Divers & Stahl 2019, Jacobson & Garner 2021, Paré & Sigler 2016).

Epidemiology: Mycosis can affect a wide range of reptilian species. Presence of fungus is normal on skin and environment. Pathogenic mycosis can be spread between individuals by direct contact, environmental transmission, and cross-contamination (Divers & Stahl 2019, Jacobson & Garner 2021).

Etiology/Pathophysiology: Infection occurs when the arthroconidia colonizes dead stratum corneum at the surface of the skin where the hyphae proliferates the deeper dermis (Paré & Sigler 2016).

Differential Diagnosis: Differentials include bacterial (*D. agamarium* or *A. chelonae*), viral (ranavirus), parasitic (ectoparasite/mites), trauma-induced dermatopathy, inappropriate husbandry (i.e., severe dehydration, thermal burns), other fungal dermatopathies ("CANV" *nannizziopsis, Mucor spp., Penicillium spp., Candida spp.*), or neoplasia (Divers & Stahl 2019).

Initial Database: Full physical examination, complete blood count, plasma biochemistry, fecal evaluation (direct, float, and acid-fast stain), and radiographs or CT-scan as a baseline.

Advanced/Confirmatory Testing: Biopsies of dermatological lesions should be examined by histopathology. Biopsy preferred but crusty skin/ecdysis or skin scrape/swabs can be submitted for PCR (Divers & Stahl 2019, Jacobson & Garner 2021, Paré & Sigler 2016).

Treatment: Surgical debridement, antifungal, supportive treatment for secondary bacterial overgrowth, analgesia, and wound care with husbandry deficiencies corrected. Terbinafine nebulized ± systemic antifungals such as itraconazole and voriconazole with care taken to not cause toxicity. Itraconazole is ineffective to *P. australasiensis* in bearded dragons with husbandry deficiencies corrected (Paré & Sigler 2016).

Pearls/Considerations/Tech Tip: Commonly seen in aquatic snakes and can be misidentified as "CANV" in bearded dragons in Australia, however, more research is needed. Death can occur in severe cases of mycosis. Multiple biopsies should be taken to submit for histopathology and save frozen for additional testing such as PCR (Bertelsen et al. 2005, Divers & Stahl 2019, Paré & Sigler 2016).

Prevention: Maintaining a closed group of animals with a known negative status with proper husbandry, quarantine, and strict biosecurity. Introduction of new animals only after above-mentioned quarantine and infectious disease screening (Divers & Stahl 2019).

Nannizziopsis ("CANV," "Yellow Fungus Disease")

Disease/Definition: *Nannizziopsi guarroi* (formerly *Chrysosporium guarroi*) in the Onygenaceae family causing necrotizing crusting dermatitis with a high mortality rate that commonly affects lizards but can affect other squamata species. The main causal agent of "Yellow Fungus Disease" in captive bearded dragons (*P. vitticeps*) (Cabañes et al. 2014, Divers & Stahl 2019, Jacobson & Garner 2021, Paré & Sigler 2016).

Symptoms/Clinical Signs: Range from a mild dermatitis with skin lesions that can be anywhere on the body but typically are on the head but can affect limbs, pericloacal, and tail area. Subcutaneous nodules, crusting hyperkeratosis, scab/crusting of skin (commonly around face), deep granulomatous dermatitis, facial swelling that progresses to dermatitis, abnormal behavior (restlessness), open-mouth breathing (occluded nares), premature ecdysis, and death (Divers & Stahl 2019, Jacobson & Garner 2021, Paré & Sigler 2016).

Epidemiology: Mycosis can affect a wide range of reptilian species. Presence of fungus is normal on skin and environment. Pathogenic mycosis can be spread between individuals by direct contact, environmental transmission, and cross-contamination (Divers & Stahl 2019, Jacobson & Garner 2021, Paré & Sigler 2016).

Etiology/Pathophysiology: Infection occurs when the arthroconidia colonizes dead stratum corneum at the surface of the skin where the hyphae proliferates the deeper dermis (Divers & Stahl 2019, Paré & Sigler 2016).

Differential Diagnosis: Differentials include bacterial (*D. agamarium* or *A. chelonae*), viral (ranavirus), parasitic (ectoparasite/mites), trauma-induced dermatopathy, inappropriate husbandry (i.e., severe dehydration, thermal burns), other fungal dermatopathies (*Paranannizziopsis spp.*, *Mucor spp.*, *Penicillium spp.*, *Candida spp.*) or neoplasia (Divers & Stahl 2019, Paré & Sigler 2016).

Initial Database: Full physical examination, complete blood count, plasma biochemistry, fecal evaluation (direct, float, and acid-fast stain), and radiographs or CT-scan as a baseline.

Advanced/Confirmatory Testing: Biopsies of dermatological lesions should be examined by histopathology. Biopsy preferred but crusty skin/ecdysis or skin scrape/swabs can be submitted for PCR (Divers & Stahl 2019, Jacobson & Garner 2021, Paré & Sigler 2016).

Treatment: Surgical debridement, antifungals, supportive treatment for secondary bacterial overgrowth, analgesia, and wound care with husbandry deficiencies corrected. Terbinafine nebulized ± systemic antifungals such as itraconazole and voriconazole with care taken to not cause toxicity (Divers & Stahl 2019, Gentry et al. 2021, McEntire et al. 2022, Paré & Sigler 2016).

Pearls/Considerations/Tech Tip: Commonly called by reptile hobbyists "Yellow Fungus Disease" previously misidentified term as CANV and shouldn't be used which has caused confusion in both the academic and the private sector. The term nannizziomycosis should be used.

Itraconazole toxicosis can be seen in bearded dragons. Co-infections with *D. agamarum* and *N. guarroi* have been seen in bearded dragons. Death can occur in severe cases of mycosis. Multiple biopsies should be taken to submit for histopathology and save frozen for additional testing such as PCR (Divers & Stahl 2019, Jacobson & Garner 2021).

Prevention: Maintaining a closed group of animals with a known negative status with proper husbandry, quarantine, and strict biosecurity. Introduction of new animals only after above-mentioned quarantine and infectious disease screening (Divers & Stahl 2019).

Parasitic

Intranuclear coccidiosis ("TINC")

Disease/Definition: Tortoise intranuclear coccidiosis (TINC) is an emerging disease affecting chelonians (Divers & Stahl 2019, Hofmannová et al. 2019, Jacobson & Garner 2021, Wellehan et al. 2022).

Symptoms/Clinical signs: Range from mild to severe rhinosinusitis, ocular discharge, nasal discharge, oronasal fistula, lethargy, anorexia, rapid weight loss, open-mouth breathing, diarrhea, swollen vent, and death. The severity of clinical signs depend on chronicity and which organs are affected. Most patients who present with clinical disease have a grave prognosis (Divers & Stahl 2019, Hofmannová et al. 2019, Wellehan et al. 2022).

Epidemiology: Has been detected in radiated tortoises (*Astrochelys radiata*), leopard tortoises (*Stigmochelys pardalis*), red-footed tortoises (*Chelonoidis carbonaria*), Eastern box turtle (*Terrapene carolina*), and other chelonian species. No sex or age predilection is known but juvenile or immunocompromised animals can be more susceptible (Divers & Stahl 2019, Jacobson & Garner 2021, Wellehan et al. 2022).

Etiology/Pathophysiology: Infecting the epithelial cells causing lymphoplasmocytic epithelial hyperplasia with a mixed inflammation and necrosis of the tissue. Coccidian oocyte has an intranuclear developmental stage found in multiple organ systems including GI tract, liver, kidney, spleen, and upper respiratory tract. Complete details of its life cycle are unknown and additional research is needed (Divers & Stahl 2019, Jacobson & Garner 2021, Wellehan et al. 2022).

Differential Diagnosis: Differentials include bacterial (*Mycoplasma spp., Mycobacterium spp.*), viral (herpesvirus, ranavirus, adenovirus, reovirus, paramyxovirus), parasitic, fungal, trauma (nasal foreign body), inappropriate husbandry (i.e., thermal burns, nutritional deficits), or neoplasia (tracheal chondromas) (Divers & Stahl 2019, Jacobson & Garner 2021).

Initial Database: Full physical examination, complete blood count, plasma biochemistry, fecal evaluation, (direct, float, and acid-fast stain) and radiographs or CT-scan as a baseline.

Advanced/Confirmatory Testing: Choanal/cloacal/conjunctival swabs can be submitted for PCR. Postmortem diagnosis is based on histopathologic findings of the intranuclear developing stages in multiple organs or by PCR testing (Divers & Stahl 2019, Jacobson & Garner 2021, Wellehan et al. 2022).

Treatment: Anecdotal evidence of treatment of asymptomatic positive animals with Ponazuril may halt progression of the disease with husbandry deficiencies corrected. The prognosis of animals showing signs associated with intranuclear coccidiosis is poor (Divers & Stahl 2019, Wellehan et al. 2022).

Pearls/Considerations/Tech Tip: Co-infections can occur however, bacterial or fungal stomatitis is rare in chelonians (Divers & Stahl 2019, Wellehan et al. 2022).

Prevention: Maintaining a closed group of animals with a known negative status with proper husbandry, quarantine, and strict biosecurity. Introduction of new animals only after above-mentioned quarantine and infectious disease screening (Divers & Stahl 2019).

Cryptosporidium

Disease/Definition: Cryptosporidium is in the phylum Apicomplexa and is a unicellular organism. The Apicomplexa also includes genera like Coccidia species such as Eimeria and Toxoplasma. There are many species of Cryptosporidium that can affect a wide range of hosts (Divers & Stahl 2019, Jacobson & Garner 2021).

Symptoms/Clinical Signs: Range from intermittent regurgitation, anorexia, weight loss, diarrhea, lethargy, stunted growth, maldigestion, mid-body swelling, and death (Bogan 2019, Divers & Stahl 2019, Jacobson & Garner 2021).

Epidemiology: Has been detected in a wide range of reptilian species including chelonians but is more commonly seen in colubrid snakes and lizard species. *Cryptosporidium serpentis* is commonly seen in snakes and affects the stomach whereas *Cryptosporidium varanii/saurophilum* is seen in lizards and affects the small intestinal tract. Has a fecal-oral transmission and has been shown to shed intermittently. No sex or age predilection is known but juvenile or immunocompromised animals can be more susceptible with most at risk being overcrowding or poor husbandry (Bogan 2019, Divers & Stahl 2019, Jacobson & Garner 2021, Koehler et al. 2020).

Etiology/Pathophysiology: Clinically mid-body swelling is attributed to massive gastric mucosal hypertrophy which eventually narrows the gastric lumen, causing chronic regurgitation. Once ingested excystation occurs where the sporozoites invade the targeted mucosal cells, then it begins with multiple rounds of merogony, differentiating into the trophozoite stage, then releasing merozoites before entering gametogony. These merozoites can reinfect the host cell and reproduce asexually via schizogony. Oocytes can persist in the environment for long periods of time (Bogan 2019, Divers & Stahl 2019, Jacobson & Garner 2021, Koehler et al. 2020).

Differential Diagnosis: Differentials for GI symptoms include bacterial (*Chlamydophia spp.*, *Salmonella spp.*, bacterial dysbiosis), viral (adenovirus/atadenovirus), other parasites (Amoebiasis, Nematodiasis, *Cryptosporidium spp.*, *Giardia spp.*), fungal, trauma (GI foreign body/obstruction), inappropriate husbandry (i.e., nutritional deficits, low temperature, inappropriate prey size), organ system dysfunction (renal/hepatic disease), or neoplasia (Divers & Stahl 2019, Jacobson & Garner 2021).

Initial Database: Full physical examination, complete blood count, plasma biochemistry, fecal evaluation, (direct, float, and acid-fast stain) and radiographs or CT-scan as a baseline.

Advanced/Confirmatory Testing: Microscopic examination of feces, gastric wash, or impression smear of regurgitated items with an acid-fast stain. Gastric biopsies examined by histopathology and PCR. Species-specific PCR needed to differentiate the *Cryptosporidium* species (Bogan 2019, Divers & Stahl 2019, Jacobson & Garner 2021, Koehler et al. 2020).

Treatment: No treatments have been completely successful, however, reports of effective treatment with oral paromomycin. Reported that nitazoxanide has not been effective. Other antibiotics have been used such as azithromycin or sulfadiazine and trimethoprim in combination with any husbandry deficiencies being corrected. Historically hyperimmune anti-*C. parvum* bovine colostrum has been used (Bogan et al. 2021, Bogan et al. 2022, Divers & Stahl 2019, Eatwell 2007, Hedley et al. 2021, Jacobson & Garner 2021).

Pearls/Considerations/Tech Tip: *C. serpentis* is commonly seen in colubrids. *C. serpentis* can cause severe and life-threatening gastric disease. One account of *C. serpentis* reported in the gallbladder of a corn snake (*Pantherophis guttata guttata*). Extremely hardy in the environment and most disinfectants are not effective. Disinfectant needs to be a high concentration of hydrogen peroxide, ammonia, or moist high temperature. PCR needs to be specific to identify the *Cryptosporidium* species since *C. muris* is a pass-through from rodent-eating reptiles which doesn't cause disease. Co-infection with an orthoreovirus has been detected in a snake (Bogan et al. 2021, Bogan et al. 2022, Divers & Stahl 2019, Jacobson & Garner 2021).

Prevention: Maintaining a closed group of animals with a known negative status with proper husbandry, quarantine, and strict biosecurity. Introduction of new animals only after above-mentioned quarantine and infectious disease screening (Divers & Stahl 2019).

Isospora amphibolurus

Disease/Definition: Coccidia are a single-celled spore-forming obligate intracellular protozoan parasite belonging to the phylum Apicomplexa, in the genera *Eimeria spp.* and *Isospora spp. Isospora amphibolurus* has been primarily detected as a gastrointestinal (GI) parasite in bearded dragons (*P. vitticeps*) (Divers & Stahl 2019, Jacobson & Garner 2021).

Symptoms/Clinical Signs: Range from subclinical to weight loss, weakness, lethargy, diarrhea, head tilt, and neurological symptoms due to hepatoencephalopathy from hepatocellular necrosis, and death (Divers & Stahl 2019).

Epidemiology: Common parasite of inland bearded dragons (*P. vitticeps*). Coccidians are intracellular parasites with oocytes sporulating within the gastrointestinal tract and/or liver. Damage to intestinal or hepatic cells can cause malabsorption or dysfunction. They have an in-direct life cycle with a fecal-oral transmission route. Secondly, co-infections of bacteria or viruses are common in bearded dragons. No sex or age predilection is known but juvenile or immuno-compromised animals can be more susceptible with most at risk being overcrowding or poor husbandry (Divers & Stahl 2019, McAllister et al. 1995, Walden & Mitchell 2021).

Etiology/Pathophysiology: There are signs of adverse synergistic co-infections with adenovirus that may increase morbidity and mortality. The pre-patent period from exposure to shedding the parasite in feces is 15–22 days with most shedding seen between 17 and 20 days post infection. Oocysts are spherical to slightly subspherical, smooth with bilayered walls. Oocysts have been measured at 22.7–25.4 μm in diameter with the oocyst wall measured at 1.1–1.4 μm. *I. amphiboluri* appears to have a typical life cycle for enteric coccidians with a homoxenous life cycle. Once ingested excystation occurs in the duodenum where the sporozoites invade the local mucosal cells, begin merogony (schizogony), and then release merozoites with multiple rounds of merogony before entering gametogony (Jacobson & Garner 2021, Walden & Mitchell 2021).

Differential Diagnosis: Differentials for GI symptoms include bacterial (*Mycobacterium spp.*, *Salmonella spp.*, bacterial dysbiosis), viral (adenovirus/atadenovirus), other parasites (Amoebiasis, Nematodiasis, *Cryptosporidium spp., Giardia spp.*), fungal, trauma (GI foreign body), inappropriate husbandry (i.e., nutritional deficits), organ system dysfunction (renal/hepatic disease), or neoplasia (Divers & Stahl 2019).

Initial Database: Full physical examination, complete blood count, plasma biochemistry, fecal evaluation (direct, float and acid-fast stain) and radiographs or CT-scan as a baseline. Fecal direct smear and flotation of intestinal contents should yield *Isospora* sp.

Advanced/Confirmatory Testing: Fecal evaluation followed by PCR for identification or histopathology (Divers & Stahl 2019, Jacobson & Garner 2021).

Treatment: Oral ponazuril with husbandry deficiencies corrected (Walden & Mitchell 2021).

Pearls/Considerations/Tech Tip: Reported to be a widespread parasite in commercially bred inland bearded dragons (*Pogona vitticeps*) with up to 15% mortality in young lizards. Co-infections with adenovirus are likely (Kim et al. 2002).

Prevention: Maintaining a closed group of animals with a known negative status with proper husbandry, quarantine, and strict biosecurity. Introduction of new animals only after above-mentioned quarantine and infectious disease screening (Divers & Stahl 2019).

Pentastomids

Disease/Definition: Pentastomids are endoparasites that mature primarily in the respiratory system of carnivorous reptiles. They are in the subphylum Crustacea of the Arthropoda phylum with two orders: Cephalobaenida and Porocephalida (Divers & Stahl 2019, Jacobson & Garner 2021, Paré 2008).

Symptoms/Clinical Signs: Range from subclinical to non-specific signs such as mild respiratory signs, anorexia, lethargy, oral/nasal discharge, open mouth breathing, excessive basking, and death (Divers & Stahl 2019, Jacobson & Garner 2021, Mendoza-Roldan et al. 2020, Paré 2008).

Epidemiology: Porocephalida has a greater zoonotic risk than Cephalobaenida. *Porocephalus crotali* has been detected in the USA affecting many native species including Eastern indigo snakes (*Drymarchon couperi*), vipers and has been detrimental to small vipers such as dusty pygmy rattlesnakes (*Sistrurus miliarius*) in the Southeast. *Kiricephalus coarctatus* is more commonly seen in North American colubrids. No sex or age predilection is known but juvenile or immunocompromised animals can be more susceptible (Divers & Stahl 2019, Jacobson & Garner 2021, Mendoza-Roldan et al. 2020, Paré 2008).

Etiology/Pathophysiology: They have an indirect life cycle that can involve one or more intermediate hosts. Adult worms are typically found in the lungs. On microscopic examination they have the presence of four hooks surrounding their mouth, which attach to respiratory tissue to feed on the host's blood. Pentastomid infections can often be asymptomatic, however adult and larval pentastomids can cause severe pathology resulting in the death of their intermediate and definitive hosts by obstruction of the host's airways and/or a secondary bacterial and/or fungal infection. Ova are coughed up, then swallowed and/or also passed in the feces (Divers & Stahl 2019, Jacobson & Garner 2021, Mendoza-Roldan et al. 2020, Paré 2008).

Differential Diagnosis: Differentials for respiratory symptoms include bacterial pneumonia (*Mycoplasma spp., Chlamydia spp.*), tongue sheath abscess, intraoral mass, stomatitis, viral (paramyxovirus, ferlavirus, nidovirus/serpentovirus, reovirus, herpesvirus), other parasites, fungal pneumonia, trauma (nasal occlusion, tracheal obstruction), inappropriate husbandry (i.e., dysecdysis, exposure to respiratory toxins, high ammonia within enclosure), pulmonary neoplasia (Divers & Stahl 2019, Jacobson & Garner 2021).

Initial Database: Full physical examination, complete blood count, plasma biochemistry, fecal evaluation, (direct, float, and acid-fast stain) and radiographs or CT-scan as a baseline.

Advanced/Confirmatory Testing: Fecal evaluation, wet mount of pulmonary wash, visualization on radiographs of adult worms, direct endoscopic visualization of the adult worm in the lungs, and PCR (Divers & Stahl 2019, Jacobson & Garner 2021, Mendoza-Roldan et al. 2020, Paré 2008).

Treatment: Some reports of ivermectin but can be toxic to some species, surgical removal of the adult worm from the lung is the best treatment, possibly antibiotics for secondary bacterial infections with husbandry deficiencies corrected (Divers & Stahl 2019, Eatwell 2007, Hedley et al. 2021, Jacobson & Garner 2021, Mendoza-Roldan et al. 2020, Paré 2008).

Pearls/Considerations/Tech Tip: ZOONOTIC, reptiles act as definitive hosts for most of the pentastome species. In North America, pentastomiasis can be fatal to dogs from eating infected snakes with *Porocephalus crotali* (Ayinmode et al. 2010).

Prevention: Maintaining a closed group of animals with a known negative status with proper husbandry, quarantine, and strict biosecurity. Introduction of new animals only after above-mentioned quarantine and infectious disease screening (Divers & Stahl 2019).

Viral

Adenoviruses/Atadenovirus (AdV, "Wasting Disease," "Star-Gazing Disease")

Disease/Definition: Adenoviruses (AdV) are a DNA, non-enveloped, double-stranded virus 70–90 nm. They are highly resistant in the environment, referred to as atadenovirus and in the private sector called "wasting disease" or "star-gazing disease" (Divers & Stahl 2019, Jacobson & Garner 2021, Marschang 2011).

Symptoms/Clinical Signs: Range from asymptomatic/subclinical, a failure to thrive, anorexia, weight loss, lethargy, diarrhea, green feces, or urates. A secondary parasitic or bacterial infection that persists. Neurologic deficiencies from hind leg weakness, abnormal postures, head tilt, opisthotonus, circling, to sudden death (Divers & Stahl 2019, Jacobson & Garner 2021, Marschang 2011).

Epidemiology: Bearded dragons (*Pogona vitticeps*) are most affected but has been seen boa constrictors (*Boa constrictor*), rosy boas (*Lichanura trivirgata*), royal/ball pythons (*Python regius*), corn snakes (*Pantherophis guttatus*), Jackson's chameleons (*Trioceros jacksonii*), savannah monitors (*Varanus exanthematicus*) and a leopard tortoise (*Geochelone pardalis*). Transmission can be from direct contact or ingestion of virus and can be vertically from mother to offspring. Healthy carriers may not show any clinical signs. The duration of viral shedding is not completely known. No sex or age predilection is known but juvenile or immunocompromised animals can be more susceptible with most at risk being overcrowding or poor husbandry (Divers & Stahl 2019, Farkas et al. 2002, Jacobson & Garner 2021, Marschang 2011).

Etiology/Pathophysiology: AdV has been known to spread to the liver, kidneys, brain, and bone marrow in reptiles. AdV primarily causes intranuclear inclusion bodies that distend the nucleus of the affected tissue (Divers & Stahl 2019, Jacobson & Garner 2021, Marschang 2011).

Differential Diagnosis: Differentials for GI symptoms include bacterial (*Mycobacterium spp., Salmonella spp., Chlamydia spp.*, TINC, bacterial dysbiosis), other viruses (Arenaviruses "IBD," herpesvirus, reovirus), parasites (Amoebiasis, Nematodiasis, Coccidiosis, *Cryptosporidium spp., Giardia spp.*), fungal, trauma (GI foreign body, stomatitis), inappropriate husbandry (i.e., nutritional deficits, inappropriate temperatures, nutritional secondary hyperparathyroidism, toxicity, stress), organ system dysfunction (renal/hepatic disease, vestibular), or neoplasia (Divers & Stahl 2019, Jacobson & Garner 2021).

Differentials for neurologic symptoms include bacterial (meningitis, encephalitis), other viruses (Arenaviruses "IBD," paramyxovirus), parasites (protozoal encephalitis, helminth migration, mites), fungal, head or spinal trauma, inappropriate husbandry (i.e., nutritional deficits, thiamine deficiency, hypocalcemia, hypoglycemia, nutritional secondary hyperparathyroidism, hyperthermia, toxicity), organ system dysfunction (renal/hepatic disease), or neoplasia (xanthomas) (Divers & Stahl 2019).

Initial Database: Full physical examination, complete blood count, plasma biochemistry, fecal evaluation, (direct, float, and acid-fast stain) and radiographs or CT-scan as a baseline.

Advanced/Confirmatory Testing: Feces or oral swabs but cloacal swabs are preferred and can be submitted for PCR. Postmortem diagnosis is based on histopathologic findings or by PCR testing (Divers & Stahl 2019, Jacobson & Garner 2021, Marschang 2011).

Treatment: Nutritional and thermal support, fluid therapy, treatment for secondary bacterial overgrowth, hepatic support, ±analgesia (NSAIDs), with husbandry deficiencies corrected. No current antiviral treatment for *Adenovirus* exists and euthanasia should be considered depending on patient prognosis and clinical signs. Some reports of antiviral (cidofovir) medications have been used with some success (Divers & Stahl 2019, Jacobson & Garner 2021, Marschang 2011).

Pearls/Considerations/Tech Tip: Very commonly seen in bearded dragons (*Pogona vitticeps*) with additional co-infections. Positive animals can recover but should be kept apart from negative animals. Co-infections have been documented with reovirus (Divers & Stahl 2019, Jacobson et al. 1996, Marschang 2011, Romanowski et al. 2001).

Prevention: Maintaining a closed group of animals with a known negative status with proper husbandry, quarantine, and strict biosecurity. Introduction of new animals only after above-mentioned quarantine and infectious disease screening (Divers & Stahl 2019).

Ferlaviruses (FDLV)

Disease/Definition: Ferlavirus is a negative-strand, enveloped RNA virus in the *Paramyxoviridae* family. Ferlavirus was named after being discovered in fer-de-lance pit vipers, also called (FDLV) (Divers & Stahl 2019, Jacobson & Garner 2021, Marschang 2011).

Symptoms/Clinical Signs: Range from subclinical to neurorespiratory, malaise (anorexia, lethargy, decreased activity) mild and non-specific respiratory signs, increased oral discharge, redness of gums or free blood in oral cavity, hemorrhagic pneumonia, wheezing and increased respiratory effort, open mouth breathing or "coughing," changes in behavior, abnormal posture, opisthotonus, regurgitation, head tremors, dermatological sign in chelonians, and sudden death (Divers & Stahl 2019, Jacobson & Garner 2021, Marschang 2011).

Epidemiology: FDLV can be seen in colubrid, boids, pythons, and venomous snakes. However, mostly seen in snakes but there are rare reports in chelonians, monitors, caiman lizards (*Dracaena guianensis*), and a flat-head knob-scaled lizard (*Xenosaurus platyceps*). Transmission can be from direct contact and/or ingestion of virus. Currently, there are no reports of vertical transmission but there is evidence for vertical transmission of other paramyxovirus viruses. Healthy carriers may not show any clinical signs. The duration of incubation and viral shedding is not completely known. No sex or age predilection is known but juvenile or immunocompromised animals can be more susceptible with most at risk being overcrowding or poor husbandry (Divers & Stahl 2019, Jacobson & Garner 2021, Marschang 2011, Pees et al. 2019).

Etiology/Pathophysiology: FDLV commonly affects the respiratory tract of reptiles causing proliferative interstitial or caseous pneumonia that can have debris filling the respiratory tract including the trachea, lungs, and air sacs. Other organs can be affected causing pancreatic hyperplasia or necrosis, and lesions in the brain. Hemagglutination inhibition assays can be done for antibody titers, but the results should be interpreted cautiously (Divers & Stahl 2019, Jacobson & Garner 2021, Marschang 2011).

Differential Diagnosis: Differentials for respiratory symptoms include bacterial pneumonia (*Mycoplasma spp., Chlamydia spp.*), tongue sheath abscess, intraoral mass, stomatitis, viral (paramyxovirus, nidovirus/serpentovirus, reovirus, herpesvirus, sunshinevirus), parasites (TINC, pentastomiasis), fungal pneumonia, trauma (nasal occlusion, tracheal obstruction), inappropriate husbandry (i.e., dysecdysis, exposure to respiratory toxins, high ammonia within enclosure), pulmonary neoplasia (Divers & Stahl 2019).

Differentials for neurologic symptoms include bacterial (meningitis, encephalitis), other viruses (Arenaviruses "IBD," paramyxovirus), parasites (protozoal encephalitis, helminth migration, mites), fungal, head or spinal trauma, inappropriate husbandry (i.e., nutritional deficits, thiamine deficiency, hypocalcemia, hypoglycemia, nutritional secondary hyperparathyroidism, hyperthermia, and toxicity), organ system dysfunction (renal/hepatic disease), or neoplasia (xanthomas) (Divers & Stahl 2019).

Initial Database: Full physical examination, complete blood count, plasma biochemistry, fecal evaluation (direct, float, and acid-fast stain), and radiographs or CT-scan as a baseline.

Advanced/Confirmatory Testing: Oral, cloacal swabs but preferred tracheal washes for RT-PCR testing, hemagglutination inhibition test (HI), and postmortem diagnosis is based on histopathologic findings or by PCR testing (Divers & Stahl 2019, Jacobson & Garner 2021, Marschang 2011).

Treatment: Nutritional and thermal support, fluid therapy, treatment for secondary bacterial pneumonia, ±analgesia, ±anti-inflammatories (NSAIDs), with husbandry deficiencies corrected. No current antiviral treatment for *Ferlavirus* and euthanasia can be considered depending on patient prognosis (Divers & Stahl 2019, Jacobson & Garner 2021, Marschang 2011).

Pearls/Considerations/Tech Tip: Typically has an acute onset and has been seen in North, South America, and

Europe (Divers & Stahl 2019, Jacobson & Garner 2021, Marschang 2011).

Prevention: Maintaining a closed group of animals with a known negative status with proper husbandry, quarantine, and strict biosecurity. Introduction of new animals only after above-mentioned quarantine and infectious disease screening (Divers & Stahl 2019).

Herpesviruses (HVs)

Disease/Definition: Herpesviruses (HVs) are a double-stranded DNA, enveloped virus measuring 120–200 nm in the subfamily of *Alphaherpesvirinae* (Divers & Stahl 2019, Jacobson & Garner 2021, Marschang 2014).

Symptoms/Clinical signs: Range from subclinical/asymptomatic to respiratory symptoms, nasal discharge, upper respiratory disease, anorexia, stomatitis, necrotizing stomatitis, mucocutaneous lesion(s), lethargy, peracute hepatitis, enteritis, and sudden death (Divers & Stahl 2019, Jacobson & Garner 2021, Marschang 2014).

Epidemiology: Seen in snakes, lizards, chelonians, and crocodilians. HVs have co-evolved along with reptiles and have been characterized in the subfamily *Alphaherpesvirinae*. Some HVs can cause proliferative lesions that may progress to neoplasia. Transmission can be from direct contact and/or ingestion of virus. Currently, there are no reports of vertical transmission but there is evidence for vertical transmission. Healthy carriers may not show any clinical signs. The duration of incubation and viral shedding is not completely known. No sex or age predilection is known but juvenile or immunocompromised animals can be more susceptible with most at risk being overcrowding or poor husbandry (Bicknese et al. 2010, Okoh et al. 2021, Sim et al. 2015, Wellehan & Johnson 2005, Wellehan et al. 2005).

Etiology/Pathophysiology: HVs have been one of the more studied viruses in reptiles with many of the herpesvirus' co-evolving with the reptile host. They can cause a latent infection and persist for the lifetime of the host. HVs replicate in the host cell nucleus causing proliferative mucocutaneous lesions that may progress to neoplasia. Death may occur before an inflammatory response may be seen in peracute disease. HVs can affect multiple organ systems and cause disease and lesions to organs such as the liver, spleen, pancreas, kidneys, lungs, nose, mouth, choana, tongue, and trachea (Divers & Stahl 2019, Jacobson & Garner 2021, Marschang 2014).

Differential Diagnosis: Differentials for respiratory symptoms include bacterial pneumonia (*Mycoplasma spp., Chlamydia spp.*), oral/nasal abscess, intraoral mass, stomatitis, other viral disease (iridovirus, reovirus, ranavirus paramyxovirus, nidovirus/serpentovirus, sunshinevirus), parasites (TINC, pentastomiasis)), fungal pneumonia,

trauma (nasal occlusion, tracheal obstruction), inappropriate husbandry (i.e., dysecdysis, exposure to respiratory toxins, high ammonia within enclosure), pulmonary neoplasia (Divers & Stahl 2019).

Initial Database: Full physical examination, complete blood count, plasma biochemistry, fecal evaluation (direct, float, and acid-fast stain), and radiographs or CT-scan as a baseline.

Advanced/Confirmatory Testing: Cloacal/choanal/conjunctival swabs or biopsies can be submitted for PCR. Postmortem diagnosis is based on histopathologic findings of the organs or by PCR testing (Divers & Stahl 2019, Jacobson & Garner 2021, Marschang 2014).

Treatment: There is no 100% effective antiviral treatment for *Herpesvirus,* however, there have been cases and published studies with limited data of success with acyclovir, lactoferrin, eprociclovir, ganciclovir, and Lysine. Although the complete effects are uncertain, Lysine may inhibit replication in HVs. Treatment includes nutritional and thermal support, fluid therapy, treatment for secondary bacterial pneumonia, liver support medications, ±analgesia, and anti-inflammatories (NSAIDs), with husbandry deficiencies corrected. Euthanasia can be considered depending on patient prognosis, but some species or individuals can survive with HVs without clinical signs (Allender et al. 2013, Eatwell 2007, Gandar et al. 2019, Marschang et al. 2021).

Pearls/Considerations/Tech Tip: Typically seen in chelonians with respiratory symptoms. Co-infections with organisms like *Mycoplasma* spp. are also documented. Latent period and be quiescent for the remainder of the animal's life, or until sufficiently stressed for the virus to reappear as clinical disease (Divers & Stahl 2019, Jacobson & Garner 2021, Marschang 2014).

Prevention: Maintaining a closed group of animals with a known negative status with proper husbandry, quarantine, and strict biosecurity. Introduction of new animals only after above-mentioned quarantine and infectious disease screening (Divers & Stahl 2019).

Iridoviruses ([IIV, Ranavirus [Rv], Erythrocytic Virus [ENV])

Disease/Definition: The family of *iridoviruses* (IIV) are double-stranded DNA, enveloped viruses measuring 120–300 nm which includes: *Ranavirus* (Rv), erythrocytic virus (ENV) and IIV. Also has been referred to as Toddia or Pirhemocyton. Belonging to a group of large DNA viruses called nucleo-cytoplasmic large DNA viruses (NCLDV) (Divers & Stahl 2019, Jacobson & Garner 2021, Marschang 2014).

Symptoms/Clinical Signs: Range from subclinical/asymptomatic to respiratory symptoms, nasal discharge, upper respiratory disease, anorexia, lethargy, swollen eyelids, buoyancy issues in aquatic species, anemia, stomatitis, oral lesion(s), necrotizing stomatitis, mucocutaneous lesion(s) on feet, hepatitis, enteritis, and sudden death (Divers & Stahl 2019, Jacobson & Garner 2021, Marschang 2014).

Epidemiology: Rv has been seen in reptiles including box turtles (*Terrapene carolina carolina*), flat-tail gecko (*Uroplatus fimbriatus*), four-horned chameleon (*Chamaeleo quadricornis*), and green pythons (*Morelia viridis*). Transmission can be from direct contact, ingestion of virus, or contact of water exposed to infected animals. Vertical transmission is suspected however, it remains unknown. The duration of incubation and viral shedding is not completely known. Large mixed animal collections may be at a higher risk of transmission. Invertebrates could be a potential vector for transmission of IIV in insectivorous reptiles. No sex or age predilection is known but juvenile or immunocompromised animals can be more susceptible with most at risk being overcrowding or poor husbandry (DeVoe et al. 2004, Divers & Stahl 2019, Hyatt et al. 2002, Jacobson & Garner 2021, Johnson et al. 2008, Marschang et al. 2002, Marschang 2014).

Etiology/Pathophysiology: Histological lesions of necrotizing and ulcerative stomatitis, esophagitis, conjunctivitis, tracheitis, splenitis, gastritis, enteritis, hepatitis, with vasculitis and/or thrombosis can occur. The kidney, liver and spleen are commonly seen with necrosis of the hematopoietic tissue, basophilic intracytoplasmic inclusions can be seen within the epithelial cells of the oral mucosa, esophagus, stomach, and trachea or within endothelial cells, macrophages, hepatocytes, and hematopoietic cells on rare occasions (Divers & Stahl 2019, Jacobson & Garner 2021, Marschang 2014).

Differential Diagnosis: Differentials for respiratory symptoms include bacterial pneumonia (*Mycoplasma spp.*, *Chlamydia spp.*), oral/nasal abscess, intraoral mass, stomatitis, other viral disease (herpesvirus, reovirus, ranavirus paramyxovirus, nidovirus/serpentovirus, sunshinevirus), parasites (TINC, pentastomiasis), fungal pneumonia, trauma (nasal occlusion, tracheal obstruction), inappropriate husbandry (i.e., dysecdysis, exposure to respiratory toxins, high ammonia within enclosure), pulmonary neoplasia (Divers & Stahl 2019).

Initial Database: Full physical examination, complete blood count, plasma biochemistry, fecal evaluation, (direct, float, and acid-fast stain) and radiographs or CT-scan as a baseline.

Advanced/Confirmatory Testing: CBC can show anemia. Oral, choanal, swabs, or biopsies can be submitted for PCR. Postmortem diagnosis is based on histopathologic findings of the organs or by PCR testing or EM (Divers & Stahl 2019, Jacobson & Garner 2021, Marschang 2014, Marschang and Müller 2021).

Treatment: Includes nutritional support and thermal support, fluid therapy, treatment for secondary bacterial pneumonia, ±analgesia, ±anti-inflammatories (NSAIDs), with husbandry deficiencies corrected. Antiviral treatment for Rv is limited and euthanasia should be considered depending on patient prognosis and clinical signs (Divers & Stahl 2019, Jacobson & Garner 2021, Marschang et al. 2021).

Pearls/Considerations/Tech Tip: Commonly seen in box turtles (*Terrapene spp.*), chelonians, and is more commonly seen in the spring. More resistant to the environment than other enveloped viruses. IIV can also be isolated from the prey animals of reptiles, for example, commercially grown crickets fed to lizards, and could be an incidental passthrough if tested, clinical signs and sequenced from PCR (Divers & Stahl 2019, Jacobson & Garner 2021, Marschang 2014).

Prevention: Maintaining a closed group of animals with a known negative status with proper husbandry, quarantine, and strict biosecurity. Introduction of new animals only after above-mentioned quarantine and infectious disease screening (Divers & Stahl 2019).

Paramyxoviruses (PMVs, OPMV)

Disease/Definition: Paramyxoviruses (PMVs) are enveloped, negative single-stranded RNA viruses measuring 150–300 nm. Also known to cause measles and distemper in mammals. Can be misclassified as *ferlaviruses* and *sunshinevirus* (Divers & Stahl 2019, Hyndman et al. 2013, Jacobson & Garner 2021, Marschang 2014).

Symptoms/Clinical signs: Range from subclinical to neurorespiratory, malaise (anorexia, lethargy, decreased activity) mild and non-specific respiratory signs, increased oral discharge, redness of gums or free blood in oral cavity, hemorrhagic pneumonia, wheezing and increased respiratory effort, open mouth breathing or "coughing," change in behavior, abnormal posture, opisthotonus, encephalitis, regurgitation, head tremors, and sudden death (Divers & Stahl 2019, Jacobson & Garner 2021, Kurath et al. 2004, Marschang 2014).

Epidemiology: PMVs are transmitted by both fecal and oral routes and have been seen in colubrid, boids, pythons, and elapids. Mostly seen in snakes but in rare reports in chelonians, monitors, caiman lizards, and a flat-head knob-scaled lizard. Transmission from oral or respiratory secretions and direct contact. Currently, there are no reports of vertical transmission but there is evidence for vertical transmission of other paramyxoviruses viruses like *sunshinevirus*. Healthy carriers may not show any clinical signs. The duration of viral incubation and shedding is not completely known. No sex or age predilection is known but juvenile or immunocompromised animals can be more susceptible with most at risk being overcrowding or poor husbandry (Divers & Stahl 2019, Jacobson & Garner 2021, Marschang 2014, Pees et al. 2010).

Etiology/Pathophysiology: PMVs commonly affect the respiratory tract of reptiles causing proliferative interstitial or caseous pneumonia that can have debris filling the respiratory tract including the trachea, lungs, and air sacs. Genotypes A, B, C have been sequenced with genotype B causing the most pathology in the lungs. Pancreatic hyperplasia or necrosis, lesions in the brain, and other organs can also be affected. HI assays for antibody titers can be done, but the results should be interpreted cautiously. Histologically lesions of paramyxoviruses can resemble reoviruses. Intracytoplasmic inclusions may be seen in small numbers but are not always present (Divers & Stahl 2019, Jacobson & Garner 2021, Marschang 2014).

Differential Diagnosis: Differentials for respiratory symptoms include bacterial pneumonia (*Mycoplasma spp., Chlamydia spp.*), tongue sheath abscess, intraoral mass, stomatitis, viral (ferlavirus, nidovirus/serpentovirus, reovirus, herpesvirus, sunshinevirus), other parasites, fungal pneumonia, trauma (nasal occlusion, tracheal obstruction), inappropriate husbandry (i.e., dysecdysis, exposure to respiratory toxins, and high ammonia within enclosure), pulmonary neoplasia (Divers & Stahl 2019).

Differentials for neurologic symptoms include bacterial (meningitis, encephalitis), other viruses (Arenaviruses "IBD," ferlavirus, sunshinevirus), parasites (protozoal encephalitis, helminth migration, mites), fungal, head or spinal trauma, inappropriate husbandry (i.e., nutritional deficits, thiamine deficiency, hypocalcemia, hypoglycemia, nutritional secondary hyperparathyroidism, hyperthermia, toxicity), organ system dysfunction (renal/hepatic disease), or neoplasia (xanthomas) (Divers & Stahl 2019).

Initial Database: Full physical examination, complete blood count, plasma biochemistry, fecal evaluation, (direct, float, and acid-fast stain) and radiographs or CT-scan as a baseline.

Advanced/Confirmatory Testing: Oral/cloacal swabs but preferred tracheal washes for RT-PCR testing, hemagglutination inhibition test (HI), and gross pathology/histopathology (Divers & Stahl 2019, Jacobson & Garner 2021, Marschang 2014).

Treatment: Nutritional and thermal support, fluid therapy, treatment for secondary bacterial overgrowth, ±analgesia, anti-inflammatories (NSAIDs), with husbandry deficiencies corrected. No current antiviral treatment for *Paramyxovirus* and euthanasia should be considered depending on patient prognosis and clinical signs (Divers & Stahl 2019, Eatwell 2007, Jacobson & Garner 2021, Marschang 2014).

Pearls/Considerations/Tech Tip: There is evidence that if the patient survives an OPMV infection and then seroconverts, a subsequent immunity could be built. Therefore, a positive serological test with a negative PCR should be evaluated with clinical signs and patient history. (Divers & Stahl 2019, Jacobson & Garner 2021, Marschang 2014). Co-infection can also occur as seen in a corn snake (*Pantherophis guttatus*) (Abbas et al. 2011).

Prevention: Maintaining a closed group of animals with a known negative status with proper husbandry, quarantine, and strict biosecurity. Introduction of new animals only after above-mentioned quarantine and infectious disease screening (Divers & Stahl 2019).

Serpentoviruses (Nidovirus, "Python RI")

Disease/Definition: Nidoviruses are enveloped, positive-stranded RNA viruses in the *Coronaviridae* family, containing the largest known RNA genomes. Coronaviruses are typically known to target not only the epithelial cells of the respiratory tract but also gastrointestinal tract (Divers & Stahl 2019, Jacobson & Garner 2021, Marschang 2014).

Symptoms/Clinical Signs: Ranges from asymptomatic/subclinical to upper and lower respiratory signs, malaise (anorexia, lethargy, decreased activity) mild and nonspecific respiratory signs, increased oral discharge, redness of gums or stomatitis, wheezing and increased respiratory effort, open mouth breathing or "coughing," weight loss, dehydration and/or dysecdysis, change in behavior and sudden death (Divers & Stahl 2019, Hoon-Hanks et al. 2019, Jacobson & Garner 2021, Marschang 2014).

Epidemiology: Since its description in 2014, reptile *nidovirales* (now reclassified in snakes as *serpentoviruses*) have become a primary differential of respiratory disease in pythons in North America, Europe, and Taiwan. Serpentoviruses are a major infectious threat to captive snake collections, as they spread rapidly and can be associated with high morbidity and mortality. Incubation, shedding patterns and transmission are currently not completely known, likely similar to other coronaviruses by oral or respiratory secretions and/or direct contact. Possibly healthy carriers may not show any clinical signs but still be infectious. Nidovirus has been detected in the boidae family such as Indian rock pythons (*Python molurus*), royal/ball pythons (*Python regius*), green tree pythons (*Morelia viridis*), carpet pythons (*Morelia spilota spp.*), other *Morelia spp.*, blood pythons (*Python brongersmai, P. curtis, P. breitensteini*), *Boa constrictor*, *Colubridae spp.*, *Homalopsidae spp.* (water/mud snakes) along with other nonpublished species. Nidovirus has also been detected in chelonian species: Bellinger River snapping turtle (*Myuchelys georgesi*), lizard species including veiled chameleon (*Chamaeleo calyptratus*) shingleback skink (*Tiliqua rugosa*). No sex or age predilection is known but juvenile or immunocompromised animals can be more susceptible with most at risk being overcrowding or poor husbandry (Dervas et al. 2020, Divers & Stahl 2019, Hoon-Hanks et al. 2019, Hoon-Hanks et al. 2020, Jacobson 2021, Leineweber 2023, Marschang 2014, Martinez 2019, Zhang et al. 2018).

Etiology/Pathophysiology: Commonly affecting the upper and lower respiratory tract of reptiles causing proliferative interstitial and/or caseous pneumonia. Mucoid or caseous debris can fill the respiratory tract, nasal cavity trachea, lungs, and air sacs. Histologically, multifocal extensive respiratory epithelial necrosis, hyperplastic of the respiratory and squamous epithelium with heterophils, lymphocytes, plasma cells, and macrophages. A fibrinonecrotic rhinitis, stomatitis, diffuse chronic tracheitis has also been reported. Nidovirus/serpentovirus-associated proliferative disease with epithelial hyperplasia in the nasal cavity, trachea, and lung, as well as mucus and inflammatory cells filling the faveolar space is often reported. Also, individual reports of encephalitis, conjunctivitis, pancreatic necrosis, nephritis, nephrosis, salpingitis, hepatic lipidosis, and multifocal dermatitis that may or may not be nidovirus/serpentovirus associated (Divers & Stahl 2019, Hoon-Hanks et al. 2019, Jacobson & Garner 2021, Marschang 2014).

Differential Diagnosis: Differentials for respiratory symptoms include bacterial pneumonia (*Mycoplasma spp.*, *Chlamydia spp.*), tongue sheath abscess, intraoral mass, stomatitis, viral (paramyxovirus, ferlavirus, reovirus, herpesvirus, and sunshinevirus), other parasites, fungal pneumonia, trauma (nasal occlusion, tracheal obstruction), inappropriate husbandry (i.e., dysecdysis, exposure to respiratory toxins, high ammonia within enclosure), pulmonary neoplasia (Divers & Stahl 2019).

Initial Database: Full physical examination, complete blood count, plasma biochemistry, fecal evaluation (direct, float, and acid-fast stain), and radiographs or CT-scan as a baseline.

Advanced/Confirmatory Testing: Choanal/upper esophageal swabs, pulmonary wash or biopsies can be submitted for PCR. Postmortem diagnosis is based on histopathologic findings of the organs or by PCR testing (Divers & Stahl 2019, Jacobson & Garner 2021, Marschang 2014).

Treatment: Currently, there is no antiviral treatment, but supportive care and treatment includes nutritional and thermal support, fluid therapy, treatment for secondary bacterial overgrowth, ±immune support medications, anti-inflammatories (NSAIDs), with husbandry deficiencies corrected. Euthanasia can be considered depending on patient prognosis but many species but there are reports

of subclinical or asymptomatic snakes living with serpentovirus for years (Eatwell 2007, Divers & Stahl 2019, Hedley et al. 2021, Jacobson & Garner 2021, Marschang 2014).

Pearls/Considerations/Tech Tip: Commonly seen in respiratory infection in royal/ball pythons (*Python regius*), carpet and green tree pythons (*Morelia spp.*), Burmese pythons (*Python bivittatus*), blood pythons (*Python spp.*), and has been seen in chameleons, skinks and aquatic turtles. Typically seen as a wax and waning RI that is nonresponsive to antibiotic treatment but can also present as an acute RI. There are reports that it is more common in the winter. This proliferative pneumonia has recently been called nidovirus-associated proliferative disease (NPD) (Divers & Stahl 2019, Jacobson & Garner 2021, Li et al. 2020, Marschang 2014, Parrish et al. 2021).

Prevention: Maintaining a closed group of animals with a known negative status with proper husbandry, quarantine, and strict biosecurity. Introduction of new animals only after above-mentioned quarantine and infectious disease screening (Divers & Stahl 2019).

Sunshineviruses (SunCV, Sunshine Coast Virus)

Disease/Definition: Sunshinevirus (SunCV) is a negative single-stranded RNA virus in the Order *Mononegavirales*, newly created family *Sunviridae*. Previously described in the *Paramyxoviridae* family. Named from the location it was first described; Sunshine Coast, Australia in 2012 then classified to its own Family in 2016 (Divers & Stahl 2019, Jacobson & Garner 2021, Marschang 2014).

Symptoms/Clinical signs: Range from asymptomatic/subclinical to neurorespiratory, malaise (anorexia, lethargy, decreased activity) mild and non-specific respiratory signs, increased oral discharge, redness of gums or stomatitis, wheezing and increased respiratory effort, open mouth breathing or "coughing," weight loss, dehydration and/or dysecdysis, dermatitis, change in behavior, and sudden death (Divers & Stahl 2019, Jacobson & Garner 2021, Marschang 2014).

Epidemiology: First described in Australia in black-headed pythons (*Aspidites melanocephalus*), woma pythons (*Aspidites ramsayi*), spotted pythons (*Antaresia maculosa*), carpet pythons (*Morelia spp.*), one report on a royal/ball python (*Python regius*) in Germany, in *Boa constrictor* in Thailand, and unpublished reports in North America. Incubation and shedding patterns have been seen over several months but are not completely known. Likely similar to other paramyxoviruses transmission by oral, respiratory, and cloacal secretions and/or direct contact. SunCV has been isolated from whole blood which may lead to a possible ectoparasitic component and a report of vertical transmission in one species. Possibly vertical transmission however, all infected embryos were dead and may be self-limiting. No sex or age predilection is known but juvenile or immunocompromised animals can be more susceptible with most at risk being overcrowding or poor husbandry (Divers & Stahl 2019, Hyndman et al. 2012a,b, Hyndman & Johnson 2015, Jacobson & Garner 2021, Marschang 2014).

Etiology/Pathophysiology: SunCVs commonly affect the brain and histologically most lesions are seen within the hindbrain white matter appearing as spongiosis and gliosis, neuronal chromatolysis, and neuronal necrosis. Necrotic cell debris with low numbers of gitter cells, primarily located in the meninges and surrounding parenchymal of the blood vessels. Bronchointerstitial pneumonia can be seen causing diffuse or extensive pulmonary consolidation and hyperplasia of the respiratory tract including the trachea, lungs, and air sacs. Histologically lesions of SunCV can resemble paramyxoviruses (Divers & Stahl 2019, Hyndman et al. 2012a,b, Hyndman & Johnson 2015, Jacobson & Garner 2021, Marschang 2014).

Differential Diagnosis: Differentials for respiratory symptoms include bacterial pneumonia (*Mycoplasma spp., Chlamydia spp.*), tongue sheath abscess, intraoral mass, stomatitis, viral (paramyxovirus, ferlavirus, nidovirus/serpentovirus, reovirus, herpesvirus), parasites (TINC, pentastomiasis), fungal pneumonia, trauma (nasal occlusion, tracheal obstruction), inappropriate husbandry (i.e., dysecdysis, exposure to respiratory toxins, high ammonia within enclosure), pulmonary neoplasia (Divers & Stahl 2019).

Differentials for neurologic symptoms include bacterial (meningitis, encephalitis), other viruses (Arenaviruses "IBD," paramyxovirus), parasites (protozoal encephalitis, helminth migration, mites), fungal, head or spinal trauma, inappropriate husbandry (i.e., nutritional deficits, thiamine deficiency, hypocalcemia, hypoglycemia, nutritional secondary hyperparathyroidism, hyperthermia, toxicity), organ system dysfunction (renal/hepatic disease), or neoplasia (xanthomas) (Divers & Stahl 2019).

Initial Database: Full physical examination, complete blood count, plasma biochemistry, fecal evaluation (direct, float, and acid-fast stain), and radiographs or CT-scan as a baseline.

Advanced/Confirmatory Testing: Oral, choanal, swabs, or biopsies can be submitted for PCR. Postmortem diagnosis is based on histopathologic findings of the organs or by PCR testing or EM (Divers & Stahl 2019, Hyndman et al. 2012a,b, Hyndman & Johnson 2015, Jacobson & Garner 2021, Marschang 2014).

Treatment: Currently, there is no antiviral treatment for SunCV, but supportive care and treatment includes nutritional and thermal support, fluid therapy, treatment for secondary bacterial overgrowth, ±immune

support medications, anti-inflammatories (NSAIDs), with husbandry deficiencies corrected. Euthanasia can be considered depending on patient prognosis (Divers & Stahl 2019, Eatwell 2007, Jacobson & Garner 2021, Marschang 2014).

Pearls/Considerations/Tech Tip: Possibly SunCV will be an emerging neurorespiratory disease in captive snakes in North America (Divers & Stahl 2019, Hyndman et al. 2012a,b, Hyndman & Johnson 2015, Jacobson & Garner 2021, Marschang 2014).

Prevention: Maintaining a closed group of animals with a known negative status with proper husbandry, quarantine, and strict biosecurity. Introduction of new animals only after above-mentioned quarantine and infectious disease screening (Divers & Stahl 2019).

Reoviruses (Orthroreovirus)

Disease/Definition: Reoviruses are a non-enveloped RNA viruses that are 70–85 nm, icosahedral shaped, in the genus *Orthoreovirus* (Divers & Stahl 2019, Jacobson & Garner 2021, Marschang 2014).

Symptoms/Clinical Signs: Range from asymptomatic/subclinical to neurorespiratory, malaise (anorexia, lethargy, decreased activity) mild and non-specific respiratory signs, increased oral discharge, redness of gums or free blood in oral cavity, hemorrhagic pneumonia, wheezing, and increased respiratory effort, open mouth breathing or "coughing," change in behavior, abnormal posture, opisthotonus, encephalitis, regurgitation, enteritis, hepatitis, head tremors, and sudden death (Divers & Stahl 2019, Jacobson & Garner 2021, Marschang 2014).

Epidemiology: Reovirus has been seen in many species of reptiles including snakes, lizards, chelonians, and is very stable in the environment. However, more commonly in snakes including royal/ball pythons (*Python regius*), emerald tree boa (*Corallus caninus*), *Boa constrictor*, rough green snakes (*Opheodrys aestivus*), black ratsnake (*Elaphe obsolete*), corn snakes (*Pantherophis guttatus*), leopard geckos (*Eublepharis macularius*), associated with papillomas in the green lizard (*Lacerta viridis*), and in Europe spur-thighed tortoises (*Testudo graeca*) (Ahne et al. 1987). Incubation and shedding patterns are currently not completely known, but transmission is by fecal-oral or respiratory secretions and/or direct contact. No sex or age predilection is known but juvenile or immunocompromised animals can be more susceptible with most at risk being overcrowding or poor husbandry (Divers & Stahl 2019, Jacobson & Garner 2021, Kugler et al. 2016, Lamirande et al. 1999, Marschang et al. 2002, Marschang 2014).

Etiology/Pathophysiology: Reoviruses affect multiple organ systems including the kidney, liver, spleen, respiratory tract, and brain. In snakes, it causes neurologic signs, pneumonia, tracheitis, and fatal proliferative interstitial pneumonia. Rhinitis, stomatitis, and pharyngitis in chelonians. In one case epithelial necrosis of the tongue was associated with reoviral infection in a tortoise. Similar lesions to herpesviruses, iridoviruses, and picornaviruses in chelonians. Lizards like snakes have respiratory signs of pneumonia. Diagnosis is challenging due to the histologic lesions resembling paramyxoviruses with no inclusions (Divers & Stahl 2019, Jacobson & Garner 2021, Marschang 2014).

Differential Diagnosis: Differentials for respiratory symptoms include bacterial pneumonia (*Mycoplasma spp., Chlamydia spp.*), tongue sheath abscess, intraoral mass, stomatitis, viral (paramyxovirus, ferlavirus, nidovirus/serpentovirus, herpesvirus), parasites (TINC, pentastomiasis), fungal pneumonia, trauma (nasal occlusion, tracheal obstruction), inappropriate husbandry (i.e., dysecdysis, exposure to respiratory toxins, high ammonia within enclosure), pulmonary neoplasia (Divers & Stahl 2019).

Differentials for neurologic symptoms include bacterial (meningitis, encephalitis), other viruses (Arenaviruses "IBD," paramyxovirus), parasites (protozoal encephalitis, helminth migration, mites), fungal, head or spinal trauma, inappropriate husbandry (i.e. nutritional deficits, thiamine deficiency, hypocalcemia, hypoglycemia, nutritional secondary hyperparathyroidism, hyperthermia, toxicity), organ system dysfunction (renal/hepatic disease), or neoplasia (xanthomas) (Divers & Stahl 2019).

Initial Database: Full physical examination, complete blood count, plasma biochemistry, fecal evaluation, (direct, float, and acid-fast stain) and radiographs or CT-scan as a baseline.

Advanced/Confirmatory Testing: Oral, choanal, swabs, or biopsies can be submitted for PCR. Postmortem diagnosis is based on histopathologic findings of the organs or by PCR testing or EM (Divers & Stahl 2019, Jacobson & Garner 2021, Marschang 2014).

Treatment: Currently, there is no antiviral treatment, but supportive care and treatment includes nutritional and thermal support, fluid therapy, treatment for secondary bacterial overgrowth, ±immune support medications, anti-inflammatories (NSAIDs), with husbandry deficiencies corrected. Euthanasia can be considered depending on patient prognosis (Divers & Stahl 2019, Jacobson & Garner 2021, Marschang 2014).

Pearls/Considerations/Tech Tip: Secondary infections are common from immune suppression. Co-infections with reovirus and adenoviruses have been documented. Similar presentation in snakes as paramyxovirus, ferlavirus, nidovirus/serpentovirus with proliferative pneumonia (Divers & Stahl 2019, Jacobson & Garner 2021, Marschang 2014).

Prevention: Maintaining a closed group of animals with a known negative status with proper husbandry, quarantine, and strict biosecurity. Introduction of new animals only after above-mentioned quarantine and infectious disease screening (Divers & Stahl 2019).

Reptarenaviruses ("IBD" or "BIBD")

Disease/Definition: *Reptarenaviruses* is a bisegmented negative-sense RNA virus. Arenaviruses have recently been separated into two genera *Mammarenavirus* and *Reptarenavirus* including the virus causing boid inclusion body disease (BIBD) or also known as just inclusion body disease (IBD). First thought to be a Reovirus in 1993, then later an Arenavirus in 2013 to current classification as a Reptarenavirus in 2016 (Divers & Stahl 2019, Jacobson & Garner 2021, Marschang 2014).

Symptoms/Clinical Signs: Range from asymptomatic/subclinical to neurorespiratory, malaise (anorexia, lethargy, decreased activity) mild and non-specific respiratory signs, increased oral discharge, wheezing and increased respiratory effort, open mouth breathing or "coughing," regurgitation, lymphoproliferative disorders, round cell tumors, change in behavior, abnormal posture, opisthotonus, torticollis, encephalitis, head tremors, flaccid paralysis, and sudden death (Divers & Stahl 2019, Jacobson & Garner 2021, Marschang 2014).

Epidemiology: Primarily seen in *Henophilia* species of boas, pythons, and related families. Seen in green anaconda (*Eunectes murinus*), yellow anaconda (*Eunectes notaeus*), rainbow boa (*Epicrates cenchria*), Haitian boa (*Epicrates striatus*), Madagascar tree boa (*Sanzinia madagascariensis*), annulated boa (*Corallus annulatus*), Indian rock python (*Python molurus*), reticulated python (*Python reticulatus*), royal/ball python (*Python regius*) and carpet python (*Morelia spilota spp.*). Similar inclusions seen in palm vipers (*Bothriechis marchi*) and eastern kingsnakes (*Lampropeltis getula*) but virus cause is unknown. Transmission can be from direct contact or ingestion of virus and has been seen to be vertically from mother to offspring in *Boa constrictor*. Healthy carriers may not show any clinical signs. The duration of viral shedding is not completely known. No sex or age predilection is known but juvenile or immunocompromised animals can be more susceptible with most at risk being overcrowding or poor husbandry (Divers & Stahl 2019, Jacobson & Garner 2021, Keller et al. 2017, Marschang 2014, Raymond et al. 2001, Simard et al. 2020).

Etiology/Pathophysiology: *Reptarenaviruses* are characterized by intracytoplasmic inclusion of epithelial cells of affected organs and neurons. Other clinical signs and diseases that are associated with "IBD" and/or "BIBD" include pneumonia, lymphoproliferative disorders, leukemia, and undifferentiated cutaneous sarcomas (Divers & Stahl 2019, Jacobson & Garner 2021, Marschang 2014).

Differential Diagnosis: Differentials for neurologic symptoms include bacterial (meningitis, encephalitis), other viruses (paramyxovirus), parasites (protozoal encephalitis, helminth migration, mites), fungal, head or spinal trauma, inappropriate husbandry (i.e., nutritional deficits, thiamine deficiency, hypocalcemia, hypoglycemia, nutritional secondary hyperparathyroidism, hyperthermia, toxicity), organ system dysfunction (renal/hepatic disease), or neoplasia (xanthomas) (Divers & Stahl 2019).

Initial Database: Full physical examination, complete blood count, plasma biochemistry, fecal evaluation (direct, float, and acid-fast stain), and radiographs or CT-scan as a baseline.

Advanced/Confirmatory Testing: Whole body, oral/choanal swabs, or biopsies can be submitted for PCR. Postmortem diagnosis is based on histopathologic findings of the organs or by PCR testing or EM (Divers & Stahl 2019, Jacobson & Garner 2021, Marschang 2014).

Treatment: Currently, there is no current antiviral treatment for *Reptarenavirus* but supportive care and treatment includes nutritional and thermal support, fluid therapy, treatment for secondary bacterial overgrowth, ±immune support medications, anti-inflammatories (NSAIDs), with husbandry deficiencies corrected. Euthanasia should be considered depending on patient prognosis (Divers & Stahl 2019, Eatwell 2007, Jacobson & Garner 2021, Marschang 2014).

Pearls/Considerations/Tech Tip: Can have co-infection with other viruses. Originally seen primarily in Burmese pythons (*Python bivittatus*) but now more commonly seen in *Boa constrictors*. Data denotes that asymptomatic snakes have positive over a couple years. Snake mites (*Ophionyssus natricis*) may also play a role as a vector (Divers & Stahl 2019, Hepojoki et al. 2015, Jacobson & Garner 2021, Marschang 2014).

Prevention: Maintaining a closed group of animals with a known negative status with proper husbandry, quarantine, and strict biosecurity. Introduction of new animals only after above-mentioned quarantine and infectious disease screening (Divers & Stahl 2019).

References

https://www.aaha.org/aaha-guidelines/infection-control-configuration/protocols/entering-and-exiting-isolation-area2/

https://amphibiaweb.org/amphibian/speciesnums.html#:~:text=There%20are%20three%20orders%20of,salamanders%2C%20and%20215%20are%20caecilians.http://www.reptile-database.org/db-info/SpeciesStat.html#:~:text=Species%20Numbers%20(as%20of%20March%202022)&text=Note%20that%20currently%201046%20reptile%20species%20have%20a%20total%20of%202%2C442%20subspecies.

Abbas MD, Marschang RE, Schmidt V, Kasper A, Papp T. 2011. A unique novel reptilian paramyxovirus, four atadenovirus types and a reovirus identified in a concurrent infection of a corn snake (Pantherophis guttatus) collection in Germany. *Vet Microbiol* 150(1–2): 70–79.

Agius JE, Phalen DN, Rose K, Eden JS. 2021. Genomic insights into the pathogenicity of a novel biofilm-forming Enterococcus sp. bacteria (Enterococcus lacertideformus) identified in reptiles. *Front Microb* 12: 635208.

Agius J. 2021. *Combating a Novel Pathogen Threatening Critically Endangered Reptiles in a Biodiversity Hotspot* (Doctoral Dissertation). University of Sydney.

Ahne W, Thomsen I, Winton J. 1987. Isolation of a reovirus from the snake, *Python regius. Arch Virol* 94(1): 135–139.

Allender MC, Mitchell MA, Yarborough J, Cox S. 2013. Pharmacokinetics of a single oral dose of acyclovir and valacyclovir in North American box turtles (*Terrapene* sp.). *J Vet Pharmacol Ther* 36(2): 205–208.

Anderson KB, Steeil JC, Neiffer DL, Evans M, Peters A, Allender MC, Cartoceti AN. 2021. Retrospective review of ophidiomycosis (ophidiomyces ophiodiicola) at the smithsonian's national zoological park (1983–2017). *J Zoo Wildlife Med* 52(3): 997–1002.

Ayinmode AB, Adedokun AO, Aina A, Taiwo V. 2010. The zoonotic implications of pentastomiasis in the royal python (*Python regius*). *Ghana Med J* 44(3).

Bertelsen MF, Crawshaw GJ, Sigler L, Smith DA. 2005. Fatal cutaneous mycosis in tentacled snakes (*Erpeton tentaculatum*) caused by the *Chrysosporium anamorph* of *Nannizziopsis vriesii. J Zoo Wildlife Med* 36(1): 82–87.

Bicknese EJ, Childress AL, Wellehan JFX. 2010. A novel herpesvirus of the proposed genus Chelonivirus from an asymptomatic bowsprit tortoise (*Chersina angulata*). *J Zoo Wildlife Med* 353–358.

Bogan JE. 2019. Gastric cryptosporidiosis in snakes, a review. *J Herpetol Med Surg*, 29(3–4): 71–86.

Bogan JE, Hoffman M, Dickerson F, Mitchell MA, Garner MM, Childress A, Wellehan JF. 2021. Evaluation of paromomycin treatment for *Cryptosporidium serpentis* infection in eastern indigo snakes (*Drymarchon couperi*). *J Herpetol Med Surg* 31(4): 307–314.

Bogan Jr, JE, Hoffman M, Mitchell MA, Garner MM, Childress A, Wellehan JF. 2022. Evaluation of the drug combination Nitazoxanide, azithromycin, and rifabutin as a treatment for *Cryptosporidium serpentis* infection in Eastern Indigo snakes (*Drymarchon couperi*). *J Herpetol Med Surg* 32(4): 291–295.

Cabañes FJ, Sutton DA, Guarro J. 2014. Chrysosporium-related fungi and reptiles: a fatal attraction. *PLoS Pathog* 10: e1004367. doi: 10.1371/journal.ppat.1004367.

Cnossen A. 2021. *Dermatomycosis in Squamate Reptiles* (Doctoral dissertation). Ghent University.

Dervas E, Hepojoki J, Smura T, Prähauser B, Windbichler K, Blümich S, Ramis A, Hetzel U, Kipar A. 2020. Serpentoviruses: more than respiratory pathogens. *J Virol* 94(18): e00649-20.

DeVoe R, Geissler K, Elmore S, Rotstein D, Lewbart G, Guy J. 2004. Ranavirus-associated morbidity and mortality in a group of captive eastern box turtles (*Terrapene carolina carolina*). *J Zoo Wildlife Med* 35(4): 534–543.

Divers S, Stahl S. 2019. *Mader's Reptile and Amphibian Medicine and Surgery*, 3rd edn. St. Louis, MO: Elsevier

Eatwell K. 2007. Antibiotic therapy in reptiles. *J Herpetol Med Surg* 17(2): 42–49.

Farkas SL, Benkő M, Élő P, Ursu K, Dán Á, Ahne W, Harrach B. 2002. Genomic and phylogenetic analyses of an adenovirus isolated from a corn snake (*Elaphe guttata*) imply a common origin with members of the proposed new genus Atadenovirus. *J Gen Virol* 83(10): 2403–2410.

Gandar F, Marlier D, Vanderplasschen A. 2019. In vitro and in vivo assessment of eprociclovir as antiviral treatment against testudinid herpesvirus 3 in Hermann's tortoise (*Testudo hermanni*). *Res Vet Sci* 124: 20–3. doi: 10.1016/j.rvsc.2019.02.001

Gentry SL, Lorch JM, Lankton JS, Pringle A. 2021. Koch's postulates: confirming *Nannizziopsis guarroi* as the cause of yellow fungal disease in *Pogona vitticeps*. *Mycologia* 113(6): 1253–1263.

Hedley J, Whitehead ML, Munns C, Pellett S, Abou-Zahr T, Calvo Carrasco D, Wissink-Argilaga N. 2021. Antibiotic stewardship for reptiles. *J Small Anim Pract*, 62: 829–839.

Hellebuyck T, Couck L, Ducatelle R, Van den Broeck W, Marschang RE. 2021. Cheilitis associated with a novel herpesvirus in two panther chameleons (*Furcifer pardalis*). *J Comp Pathol* 182: 58–66.

Hellebuyck T, Martel A, Chiers K, Haesebrouck F, Pasmans F. 2009a. *Devriesea agamarum* causes dermatitis in bearded dragons (*Pogona vitticeps*). *Vet Microbiol* 134(3–4): 267–271.

Hellebuyck T, Pasmans F, Haesebrouck F, Martel A. 2009b. Designing a successful antimicrobial treatment against *Devriesea agamarum* infections in lizards. *Vet Microbiol* 139(1–2): 189–92. doi: 10.1016/j.vetmic.2009.05.003. Epub 2009 May 19. PMID: 19497687.

Hepojoki J, Salmenpera P, Sironen T, et al. 2015. Arenavirus coinfections are common in snakes with boid inclusion body disease. *J Virol* 89: 8657–8660.

Hoon-Hanks LL, Stöhr AC, Anderson AJ, Evans DE, Nevarez JG, Díaz RE, ..., Stenglein MD. 2020. Serpentovirus (nidovirus) and orthoreovirus coinfection in captive veiled chameleons (*Chamaeleo calyptratus*) with respiratory disease. *Viruses* 12(11): 1329.

Hoon-Hanks LL, Ossiboff RJ, Bartolini P, Fogelson SB, Perry SM, Stöhr AC, Stenglein MD. 2019. Longitudinal and cross-sectional sampling of serpentovirus (nidovirus) infection in captive snakes reveals high prevalence, persistent infection, and increased mortality in pythons and divergent serpentovirus infection in boas and colubrids. *Front Vet Sci* 6: 338.

Hofmannová L, Kvičerová J, Bízková K, Modrý D. 2019. Intranuclear coccidiosis in tortoises—discovery of its causative agent and transmission. *Eur J Protistol* 67: 71–76.

Hotaling S, Kelley JL, Frandsen PB. 2021. Toward a genome sequence for every animal: where are we now? *Proc Natl Acad Sci USA* 118: e2109019118.

Hyatt AD, Williamson M, Coupar BEH, et al. 2002. First identification of a Ranavirus from green pythons (*Chondropython viridis*). *J Wildl Dis* 38(2): 239–52.

Hyndman TH, Johnson RS. 2015. Evidence for the vertical transmission of Sunshine virus. *Vet Microbiol* 175(2–4): 179–184.

Hyndman TH, Shilton CM, Marschang RE. 2013. Paramyxoviruses in reptiles: a review. *Vet Microbiol* 165(3–4): 200–213.

Hyndman TH, Shilton CM, Doneley RJ, Nicholls PK. 2012a. Sunshine virus in Australian pythons. *Vet Microbiol* 161(1–2): 77–87.

Hyndman TH, Marschang RE, Wellehan Jr, JF, Nicholls PK. 2012b. Isolation and molecular identification of Sunshine virus, a novel paramyxovirus found in Australian snakes. *Infect Genet Evol* 12(7): 1436–1446.

Inchuai R, Weerakun S, Nguyen HN, Sukon P. 2021. Global prevalence of chlamydial infections in reptiles: a systematic review and meta-analysis. *Vector-Borne Zoonotic Dis* 21(1): 32–39.

Jacobson ER, Garner MM (eds). 2021. *Infectious Diseases and Pathology of Reptiles: Color Atlas and Text, Diseases and Pathology of Reptiles*, Volume 1. CRC Press.

Jacobson ER, Brown MB, Wendland LD, Brown DR, Klein PA, Christopher MM, Berry KH. 2014. Mycoplasmosis and upper respiratory tract disease of tortoises: a review and update. *Vet J (London, England : 1997)* 201(3): 257–264.

Jacobson ER, Kopit W, Kennedy FA, Funk RS. 1996. Coinfection of a bearded dragon, *Pogona vitticeps*, with adenovirus-and dependovirus-like viruses. *Vet Pathol* 33(3): 343–346.

Jiang H, Zhang X, Li L, Ma J, He N, Liu H, Han R, Li H, Wu Z, Chen J. 2019. Identification of *Austwickia chelonae* as cause of cutaneous granuloma in endangered crocodile lizards using metataxonomics. *PeerJ* 7: e6574. doi: 10.7717/peerj.6574. PMID: 30886772; PMCID: PMC6420803.

Johnson AJ, Pessier AP, Wellehan JF, Childress A, Norton TM, Stedman NL, ..., Jacobson ER. 2008. Ranavirus infection of free-ranging and captive box turtles and tortoises in the United States. *J Wildlife Dis* 44(4): 851–863.

Kane LP, Allender MC, Archer G, et al. 2017. Pharmacokinetics of nebulized and subcutaneously implanted terbinafine in cottonmouths (*Agkistrodon piscivorus*). *J Vet Pharmacol Therap* 40: 575–579.

Keller S, Hetzel U, Sironen T, Korzyukov Y, Vapalahti O, Kipar A, Hepojoki J. 2017. Co-infecting reptarenaviruses can be vertically transmitted in boa constrictor. *PLoS Pathog* 13(1): e1006179.

Kim DY, Mitchell MA, Bauer RW, Poston R, Cho D-Y. 2002. An outbreak of adenoviral infection in inland bearded dragons (*Pogona vitticeps*) coinfected with dependovirus and coccidial protozoa (*Isospora* sp.). *J Vet Diagn Invest* 14(4): 332–334. doi: 10.1177/104063870201400411.

Koehler AV, Scheelings TF, Gasser RB. 2020. *Cryptosporidium cf. avium* in an inland-bearded dragon (*Pogona vitticeps*)–a case report and review of the literature. *Int J Parasitol Parasites Wildl* 13: 150–159.

Kugler R, Marschang RE, Ihász K, Lengyel G, Jakab F, Bányai K, Farkas SL. 2016. Whole genome characterization of a chelonian orthoreovirus strain identifies significant genetic diversity and may classify reptile orthoreoviruses into distinct species. *Virus Res* 215: 94–98.

Kurath G, Adams A. 2011. Foreword: pathogens and immune responses of fish and reptiles. *Vet Res* 42(1): 1–1.

Kurath G, Batts WN, Ahne W, Winton JR. 2004. Complete genome sequence of Fer-de-Lance virus reveals a novel gene in reptilian paramyxoviruses. *J Virol* 78(4): 2045–2056.

Lamirande EW, Nichols DK, Owens JW, Gaskin JM, Jacobson ER. 1999. Isolation and experimental transmission of a reovirus pathogenic in ratsnakes (*Elaphe* species). *Virus Res* 63: 135–141. doi: 10.1016/S0168-1702(99)00067-2.

Leineweber C, Marschang RE. 2023. Detection of nidoviruses in samples collected from captive snakes in Europe between 2016 and 2021. *Vet Rec* e2588.

Li WT, Lee MS, Tseng YC, Yang NY. 2020. A case report of reptile-associated nidovirus (serpentovirus) in a ball python (*Python regius*) in Taiwan. *J Vet Med Sci* 82(6): 788–792.

Liguori BL, Ossiboff RJ, Stacy NI, Graham EA, Oliveira LJ, Childress AL, ..., Wellehan JF. 2022. Austwickia chelonae in a wild gopher tortoise (*Gopherus polyphemus*) and evidence of positive selection on the diphtheria-like toxin gene. *J Wildlife Dis* 58(1): 1–7.

Marschang RE, Salzmann E, Pees M. 2021. Diagnostics of infectious respiratory pathogens in reptiles. *Vet Clin Exotic Anim Pract* 24(2): 369–395.

Marschang RE, Müller E. 2021. Effects of the antivirals lysine and lactoferrin on testudinid herpesviruses and a ranavirus in cell culture. *J Herpetol Med Surg* 31(2): 151–158.

Marschang RE, Heckers KO, Dietz J, Kolesnik E. 2016. Detection of a *Mycoplasma* sp. in a *Python* (*Morelia spilota*) with stomatitis. *J Herpetol Med Surg* 26(3–4): 90–93.

Marschang RE. 2014. Clinical virology. *Curr Ther Rep Med Surgery* 32–52.

Marschang RE. 2011. Viruses infecting reptiles. *Viruses* 3(11): 2087–2126.

Marschang RE, Becher P, Braun S. 2002. Isolation of iridoviruses from three different lizard species. In: Proceedings of the Association of Reptilian and Amphibian Veterinarians, pp. 99–100. Reno.

Martinez J. 2019. *Associations Between Gastrointestinal Parasites and Nidovirus Infection in Western Australian Shingleback Lizards* (Tiliqua rugosa) (Doctoral dissertation). Murdoch University.

McAllister CT, Upton SJ, Jacobson ER, Kopit W. 1995. A description of *Isospora amphiboluri* (Apicomplexa: Eimeriidae) from the Inland Bearded Dragon, *Pogona vitticeps* (Sauria: Agamidae). *J Parasitol* 81(2): 281–284. doi: 10.2307/3283934.

McEntire MS, Reinhart JM, Cox SK, Keller KA. 2022. Single-dose pharmacokinetics of orally administered terbinafine in bearded dragons (*Pogona vitticeps*) and the antifungal susceptibility patterns of *Nannizziopsis guarroi*. *Am J Vet Res* 83(3): 256–263.

Mendoza-Roldan JA, Modry D, Otranto D. 2020. Zoonotic parasites of reptiles: a crawling threat. *Trends Parasitol* 36(8): 677–687.

Mitchell MA, Perry SM. 2017. Evidence-based advances in reptile medicine. *Vet Clin Exotic Anim Pract* 20(3): 857–870.

Mitchell MA. 2011. Zoonotic diseases associated with reptiles and amphibians: an update. *Vet Clin Exotic Anim Pract* 14(3): 439–456.

Mitura A, Niemczuk K, Zaręba K, Zając M, Laroucau K, Szymańska-Czerwińska M. 2017. Free-living and captive turtles and tortoises as carriers of new *Chlamydia spp.PLoS One* 12(9): e0185407.

O'Dea MA, Jackson B, Jackson C, Xavier P, Warren K. 2016. Discovery and partial genomic characterisation of a novel nidovirus associated with respiratory disease in wild shingleback lizards (*Tiliqua rugosa*). *PLoS One* 11: e0165209. doi:10.1371/journal.pone.0165209.

Okoh GSR, Horwood PF, Whitmore D, Ariel E. 2021. Herpesviruses in reptiles. *Front Vet Sci* 8: 642894.

Ossiboff RJ, Caudill M, Childress A, Guzman-Vargas V, Enge KM, Shender L. 2020. Systemic Enterococcosis in brown anoles (*Anolis sagrei*) in Florida. In: *Paper presented at the Sixth Annual Wildlife and Aquatic Veterinary Disease Laboratory PALOOZA*. Gainesville, FL.

Paré JA, Sigler L. 2016. An overview of reptile fungal pathogens in the genera Nannizziopsis, Paranannizziopsis, and Ophidiomyces. *J Herpetol Med Surg* 26(1–2): 46–53.

Paré JA. 2008. An overview of pentastomiasis in reptiles and other vertebrates. *J Exot Pet Med* 17(4): 285–294.

Parrish K, Kirkland PD, Skerratt LF, Ariel E. 2021. Nidoviruses in reptiles: a review. *Front Vet Sci* 8: 733404.

Pees M, Schmidt V, Papp T, Gellért Á, Abbas M, Starck JM, ..., Marschang RE. 2019. Three genetically distinct ferlaviruses have varying effects on infected corn snakes (*Pantherophis guttatus*). *PLoS One* 14(6): e0217164.

Pees M, Schmidt V, Marschang RE, Heckers KO, Krautwald-Junghanns ME. 2010. Prevalence of viral infections in captive collections of boid snakes in Germany. *Vet Rec* 166(14): 422–425.

Penner JD, Jacobson ER, Brown DR, Adams HP, Besch-Williford CL. 1997. A novel *Mycoplasma* sp. associated with proliferative tracheitis and pneumonia in a *Burmese python* (*Python molurus bivittatus*). *J Comp Pathol* 117(3): 283–288.

Picquet P, Heckers KO, Kolesnik E, Heusinger A, Marschang RE. 2018. Detection of Ophidiomyces ophiodiicola in two captive Bocourt water snakes (*Subsessor bocourti*) and one captive Pueblan milk snake (*Lampropeltis triangulum campbelli*). *J Zoo Wildlife Med* 49(1): 219–222.

Racz K, Salzmann E, Müller E, Marschang RE. 2021. Detection of mycoplasma and chlamydia in pythons with and without serpentovirus infection. *J Zoo Wildlife Med*, 52(4): 1167–1174.

Raymond JT, Garner MM, Nordhausen RW, Jacobson ER. 2001. A disease resembling inclusion body disease of boid snakes in captive palm vipers (*Bothriechis marchi*). *J Vet Diagn Investig* 13(1): 82–86. doi: 10.1177/1040638701 01300118

Romanowski EG, Yates KA, Gordon YJ. 2001. Antiviral prophylaxis with twice daily topical cidofovir protects against challenge in the adenovirus type 5/New Zealand rabbit ocular model. *Antiviral Res* 52(3): 275–280.

Rose K, Agius J, Hall J, Thompson P, Eden J-S, Srivastava M, et al. 2017. Emergent multisystemic *Enterococcus* infection threatens endangered Christmas Island reptile populations. *PLoS One* 12: e0181240. doi: 10.1371/journal.pone.0181240.

Rostad SJ, Brandão J, Ramachandran A, Chien RC, Confer AW. 2019. Austwickiosis in captive African spurred tortoises (Geochelone sulcata) co-infected with *Cryptosporidium ducismarci*. *J Comp Pathol* 173: 1–7.

Sim RR, et al. 2015. Identification of a novel herpesvirus in captive Eastern box turtles (*Terrapene carolina carolina*). *Vet Microbiol* 175(2–4): 218–223.

Simard J, Marschang RE, Leineweber C, Hellebuyck T. 2020. Prevalence of inclusion body disease and associated comorbidity in captive collections of boid and pythonid snakes in Belgium. *PLoS One* 15(3): e0229667.

Schmidt-Ukaj S, Loncaric I, Klang A, Spergser J, Häbich A-C, Knotek Z. 2014. Infection with *Devriesea agamarum* and *Chrysosporium guarroi* in an inland bearded dragon (*Pogona vitticeps*). *Vet Dermatol* 25: 555–e97.

Tamukai K, Tokiwa T, Kobayashi H, Une Y. 2016. Ranavirus in an outbreak of dermatophilosis in captive inland bearded dragons (*Pogona vitticeps*). *Vet Dermatol* 27(2): 99–e28.

Taylor-Brown A, Rüegg S, Polkinghorne A, Borel N. 2015. Characterisation of Chlamydia pneumoniae and other novel chlamydial infections in captive snakes. *Vet Microbiol* 178(1–2): 88–93.

Tetzlaff SJ, Ravesi MJ, Allender MC, Carter ET, Degregorio BA, Josimovich JM, et al. 2017. Snake fungal disease affects behavior of free-ranging massasauga rattlesnakes (*Sistrurus catenatus*). *Herpetol Conserv Biol* 12 624–634.

Walden M, Mitchell MA. 2021. Pathogenesis of *Isospora amphiboluri* in bearded dragons (*Pogona vitticeps*). *Animals* 11(2): 438.

Wellehan JF, Jacobson E, Stilwell J, Gibbons PM, Garner MM, Rosenoff E, ..., Boyer TH. 2022. Testudine intranuclear coccidiosis (TINC). *J Herpetol Med Surg* 32(2): 144–154.

Wellehan Jr, JFX. 2014. Clinical aspects of evolution in reptile medicine. *Curr Ther Reptile Med Surg* 20.

Wellehan JFX, et al. 2005. Varanid herpesvirus 1: a novel herpesvirus associated with proliferative stomatitis in green tree monitors (*Varanus prasinus*). *Vet Microbiol* 105(2): 83–92.

Wellehan JF, Johnson AJ. 2005. Reptile virology. *Vet Clin Exot Anim Pract* 8(1): 27–52.

Zhang J, Finlaison DS, Frost MJ, Gestier S, Gu X, Hall J, ..., Kirkland PD. 2018. Identification of a novel nidovirus as a potential cause of large scale mortalities in the endangered Bellinger river snapping turtle (*Myuchelys georgesi*). *PLoS One* 13(10): e0205209.

Section V

Amphibians and Aquatic Animals

14

Amphibians
Brad Wilson

Introduction, Taxonomy, and Natural History

A more complete understanding of amphibian natural history and physiology has led to tremendous improvement in providing husbandry and medical care for captive amphibians. The advent of captive amphibian conservation programs is the primary driving force of this better understanding. These programs have provided large colonies of animals for study and research of both physiologic and infectious disorders which field studies and pet industry clinical cases would not facilitate. This research knowledge has translated well to the clinical setting of the captive amphibian pet industry. Though much variation between species regarding physiology, nutrition, and disease susceptibility prevents a generalization approach to husbandry and medical care of all amphibians; the exotic animal clinician and technician now can approach a myriad of captive animal disorders to gain both valid results and to expect treatment success.

Taxonomy

The biological saying "ontogeny recapitulates phylogeny" is most appropriately applied to the natural history of amphibians. The life cycle of the amphibian from egg to adult (ontogeny) is the abridged version of the monumental evolutionary adaptations of amphibians (phylogeny) that enabled the vertebrates to leave water and colonize the land 350 million years ago (Wright 2001e; Goin et al. 1978). Modern amphibians comprise approximately 8000 (AmphibiaWeb 2021) species that are classified into three orders based on anatomic characteristics. The orders are listed with the modern accepted nomenclature followed by commonly used traditional nomenclature in parentheses: the caecilians, Gymnophiona (Apoda); the sirens, salamanders, and newts, Caudata (Meantes and Urodela); and the frogs and toads, Anura (Salientia). See Table 14.1 for species commonly kept in captivity.

Amphibians of the order Gymnophiona, Caecilians, are uncommonly kept as pets and even less commonly observed clinically. Originating in the eastern and western tropics, caecilians may be terrestrial (yellow-striped caecilian, *Ichthyophis kohtaoensis*) or totally aquatic (*Typhlonectes compressicauda*) as adults. To many, caecilians resemble snakes or oversized earthworms. All known species are limbless with greatly reduced eyes. Some species are oviparous (egg-laying) and some are viviparous (live-bearing). All known species are carnivorous and consume various arthropods, annelids, or gastropods. Because of their secretive nature, it is likely that many species remain undiscovered. Longevity of captive caecilians is reported at 9 years (Goin et al. 1978).

The order Caudata, tailed amphibians, consists of salamanders, newts, sirens, and amphiumas. Sirens were once classified in a separate order, Meantes (Trachystomata). The majority of species inhabit North America, with one species in Africa and no species in Australia or Antarctica (Goin et al. 1978, Duellman & Trueb 1994). Many species of all sub-orders are maintained as pets, though few are commercially available. Few species venture far from water or moist environs and most species require water for some portion of reproduction or development. Some species are fully aquatic, some facultatively aquatic, some terrestrial, and some American newts (*Notophthalmus viridescens*) are aquatic as larvae, terrestrial as juveniles, and aquatic again as adults. Salamanders are carnivorous as both larvae and adults and consume various arthropods, gastropods, arachnids, annelids, crustaceans, and other vertebrates including mammals. The longevity of salamanders is known to be up to 55 years for the Japanese giant salamander (*Adrias japonicus*) (Goin et al. 1978). Generally, larger species have a longer lifespan than smaller species (Figures 14.1 and 14.2).

Table 14.1 Amphibians commonly kept in captivity.

Common name/ species name	Origin	Habitat	Size (cm)[a]	T/H[b]	Repro[c]	Feed[d]	Care[e]	Handling concerns[f]
Gymnophiona								
Yellow-striped, *Ichthyophis kohtoaensis*[g,h]	SE Asia	Fossorial, tropical	50	25/mod	Oviparous	an,ar	Mod; large	Docile, sturdy; escape
Aquatic caecilian, *Typhlonectes* spp.[g,h]	S America	Aquatic, tropical	to 50	25	Viviparous	an,ar	Easy; medium	Docile, sturdy; escape
Caudata Cryptobranchidae (Giant salamanders)								
Hellbender, *Crypto-branchus alleganiensis*[g]	N America	Aquatic, temperate	to 75	15	Oviparous	cr,ar,v	Diff+; large+#	Occas. aggressive, sturdy
Sirenidae (Sirens)								
Greater siren, *Siren lacertina*[g]	e N America	Aquatic, temperate	80	20	Oviparous	ar,cr,v	Mod; large+	Occas. aggressive, sturdy
Amphiumidae (Amphiumas)								
Amphiuma, *Amphiuma means*[g]	e N America	Aquatic, temperate	to 100	20	Oviparous	ar,cr,v	Mod; large+	Aggressive, sturdy
Proteidae (Neotenic salamanders)								
Mudpuppy, *Necturus maculosus*[g]	e N America	Aquatic, temperate	40	15	Oviparous	ar,cr,v,g	Diff; large#	Docile, sturdy
Ambystomatidae (Mole salamanders)								
Axolotl, *Ambystoma mexicanum*[g]	C America	Aquatic, tropical	20	20	Oviparous	ar,cr,v	Easy; medium	Aggressive, sturdy
Tiger salamander, *Ambystoma tigrinum*[g]	N America	Terrestrial, fossorial	25	22/mod	Oviparous	ar,an,v	Easy; small	Aggressive, sturdy
Waterdog, *Ambystoma tigrinum*[i]	N America	Temporary aquatic; terrestrial	20	20	n/a	an,ar,cr,v	Easy; small	Aggressive, sturdy
Plethodontidae (Lungless salamanders)								
Arboreal salamander, *Aniedes lugubris*[j,k]	w N America	Terr/arbor, temperate forest	10	14–17/mod	Oviparous	ar	Mod; small	Occas. aggressive, sturdy
Palm salamander, *Bolitoglossa* spp.[h]	C,S America	Terr/arbor, tropical forest	8–14	14–20/high	Oviparous	t,ar	Diff+; medium	Docile, fragile
Ensatina, *Ensatina* spp.[j,k]	w N America	Terrestrial, temperate forest	7	14–17/mod	Oviparous	ar	Mod; small	Docile, sturdy
Red salamanders, *Pseudotriton* spp.[k]	N America	Semiaquatic, streams, forests	15	20/mod	Oviparous	an,ar mod; small	Docile, sturdy	

Table 14.1 (Continued)

Common name/ species name	Origin	Habitat	Size (cm)[a]	T/H[b]	Repro[c]	Feed[d]	Care[e]	Handling concerns[f]
Anura Pipidae (Clawed frogs)								
Dwarf frog, *Hymenochirus curtipes*[h,l]	Africa	Aquatic, tropical	4	25	Oviparous	an,ar	Easy; small	Docile, sturdy
Surinam toad, *Pipa pipa*[h,l]	S America	Aquatic, tropical	20	25	Oviparous	v,an,ar	Mod; large+	Docile, sturdy
African clawed frog, *Xenopus laevis*[h,l]	Africa	Aquatic, tropical	12	25	Oviparous	v,an,ar	Easy; medium	Docile, sturdy
Pelobatidae (Spadefoot toads)								
Asian leaf frogs, *Megophrys* spp.[h]	SE Asia	Terrestrial, tropical	to 15	20–22/mod	Oviparous	ar,v	Mod; medium	Docile, sturdy
Bufonidae (True toads)								
Harlequin toads, *Atelopus* spp.[i]	C,S America	Terrestrial, montane tropical	to 5	15–20/high	Oviparous	ar,t	Diff+; medium	Docile, fragile
American toad, *Bufo americanus*[h]	N America	Terrestrial, temperate	to 10	20/low	Oviparous	ar,g,v	Easy; medium	Docile, sturdy
Marine toad, *Bufo marinus*[h]	C,S America	Terrestrial, temp/ tropical	23	22/low	Oviparous	ar,g,v	Easy; large	Occas. aggressive, sturdy
Asian tree toads, *Pedostibes* spp.[h]	SE Asia	Terrestrial, tropical	to 10	25–27/high	Oviparous	t	Diff; large	Docile, fragile to sturdy
Microhylidae (Narrow mouth toads)								
Tomato frogs, *Dyscophus* spp.[h,l]	Madagascar	Semiaquatic, tropical	to 10	25/mod	Oviparous	ar	Easy; medium	Docile, sturdy
Malaysian toad, *Kaloula pulchra*[h,l]	SE Asia	Terrestrial/ fossorial, tropical	7	25/high	Oviparous	ar,t	Easy; medium	Docile, sturdy
Dendrobatidae (Poison dart frogs)								
Dendrobates, Phyllobates, *Epipedobates* spp.[h,m]	C,S America	Terrestrial, tropical	1.5–5	22–30/high	Oviparous	ar,t	Easy to diff; varies	Occas. aggressive— see below
Hylidae (Tree frogs)								
Red-eyed treefrog, *Agalychnis callidryas*[n]	C America	Arboreal, tropical	7	25/high	Oviparous	ar	Easy; medium	Docile, sturdy
Green treefrog, *Hyla cinerea*[h]	N America	Arboreal, temperate	6	25/mod	Oviparous	ar	Easy; medium	Docile, sturdy
Monkey frogs, *Phyllomedusa* spp.[n]	C, S America	Arboreal, tropical	to 10	25/low to mod	Oviparous	ar	Mod; med to lg	Docile, sturdy
White's treefrog, *Litoria caerulea*[g,n]	Australia	Arboreal, desert/forest	10	25/low to mod	Oviparous	ar	Easy; medium	Docile, sturdy

(continued)

Table 14.1 (Continued)

Common name/ species name	Origin	Habitat	Size (cm)[a]	T/H[b]	Repro[c]	Feed[d]	Care[e]	Handling concerns[f]
Ranidae (*True frogs*)								
Mantellas, *Mantella* spp.[h]	Madagascar	Terrestrial, tropical	3	18–22/high	Oviparous	ar,t	Easy; small+	Docile, fragile to sturdy
American bullfrog, *Rana catesbeiana*[h]	N America	Semiaquatic, temperate	to 20	22/mod	Oviparous	v,ar	Easy; large+	Aggressive, sturdy
African pyxie frog, *Pyxicephalus adspersus*[h]	Africa	Semiaquatic, temperate	to 20	25/mod	Oviparous	v,ar	Easy; large+	Aggressive, sturdy
Eyelash frog, *Ceratobatrachus guentheri*[h]	Solomon Islands	Terrestrial, tropical	8	25/mod	Oviparous	ar	Mod; medium	Docile, sturdy
Leptodactylidae (*Tropical frogs*)								
Surinam horned frog, *Ceratophrys cornuta*[h]	S America	Terrestrial, tropical	20	25/mod	Oviparous	v,ar	Diff; medium	Aggressive, sturdy
Ornate horned frog, *Ceratophrys ornata*[h]	S America	Terrestrial, tropical	12	25/mod	Oviparous	v,ar	Easy; medium	Aggressive, sturdy

a) Average maximum adult size.
b) Average day temperature/relative humidity for adults of species or typical of genus in captivity.
c) Oviparous (ovi-), egg laying; viviparous (vivi-), live birth.
d) Diet of the adult amphibian *in nature* listed in order of importance for each species: *an*, annelids; *ar*, arthropods; *cr*, crustaceans; *g*, gastropods; *t*, termites and ants; *v*, vertebrates. Many animals will adapt to domestically raised food items.
e) Difficulty for captive maintenance of wild-caught and some captive-born animals. (Generally, captive-born animals adapt well with proper conditions.) Second value is minimum terrarium size. *Easy*, adapts well to terrarium; *moderate*, specialized feeding, temperature, housing required; *difficult*, only most experienced keepers; *difficult+*, should only be attempted by zoological parks. *Small*, 10 gallon terrarium; *medium*, 15–20 gallon terrarium; *large*, 30 gallon terrarium; *large+*, 55 gallon or specially constructed; *#*, may require chilled water.
f) Typical response of patient to handling (all animals will resist handling): *Docile*, will not attempt to bite, no special defenses. All caecilians may escape; terrarium must be well sealed. *Occasionally aggressive*, may attempt to bite, but generally will not cause injury to handler. Can bite and seriously damage or kill cage mates. Avoid skin or direct/indirect mucous membrane contact with wild-caught dart frogs and all marine toads. *Aggressive*, species that will routinely bite as defense (Amphiuma) or conditioned feeding response (mole salamanders) or will attempt to eat any cage mates (frogs, mole salamanders). Amphiumas, pyxie frogs, and horned frogs must be approached and handled with caution; bites from adult animals may cut skin and may be painful. *Fragile*, amphibians that may be easily stressed, damaged, or killed by handling. *Sturdy*, amphibians that are not likely damaged from responsible handling.
g) Wright (2001g, 3–14).
h) Obst et al. (1988).
i) Lotters (1996).
j) Stebbins (1985).
k) Petranka (1998).
l) Mattison (1987).
m) Walls (1994).
n) de Vosjoli (1996).

The order Anura, tailless amphibians, consists of frogs and toads. This order represents the great majority of all species of modern amphibians and the majority of captive amphibians. A great number of species are available in the pet trade as captive-born animals (Figures 14.3 and 14.4).

Frogs are to amphibians as lizards are to reptiles. Frogs have managed to adapt and to populate many terrestrial, arboreal, and aquatic (and even several flying or gliding) habitats on Earth. Adaptation and specialization of skin, diet, and reproductive strategy have all made this expansion

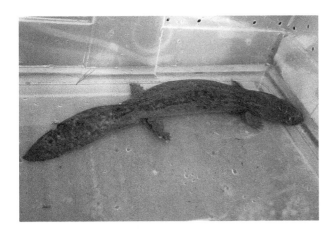

Figure 14.1 Eastern Hellbender (*Cryptobranchus alleganiensis alleganiensis*). (Courtesy of Sandy Skeba, LVMT.)

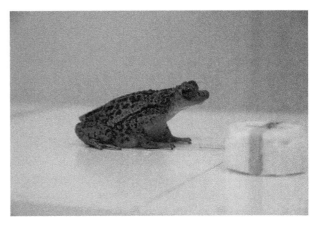

Figure 14.3 Puerto Rican Crested Toad (*Peltophryne lemur*), a critically endangered species found only in Puerto Rico and the Virgin Islands. (Courtesy of Sandy Skeba, LVMT.)

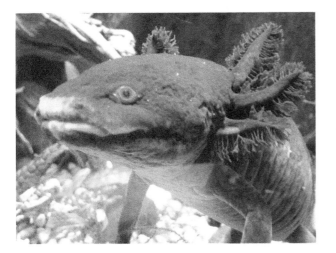

Figure 14.2 Axolotl or Mexican Salamander (*Ambystoma mexicanum*), a neotenic species of salamander (meaning it retains juvenile characteristics throughout its adult life). (Courtesy of Sandy Skeba, LVMT.)

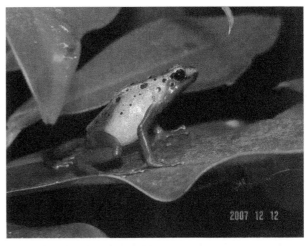

Figure 14.4 *Dendrobates tinctorius*, a common dart frog kept as a pet. (Courtesy of Dr. Sam Rivera.)

possible. Several species of frogs are totally aquatic and several are adapted to estivate in the driest deserts for months or years. All adult frogs are carnivorous and the majority of their larvae, tadpoles, are herbivorous. Some tadpoles are omnivorous and some are carnivorous. Adult frogs feed on many insects, crustaceans, annelids, and other vertebrates, and some species are specialized to feed primarily on other frogs (*Ceratophrys* spp., *Hemiphractus* spp.). The known longevity for some species is up to 36 years (Goin et al. 1978).

Amphibians begin development as fertilized eggs, and with most species, the eggs hatch into free-swimming gilled larvae, and then the larvae metamorphose into adults. The post-hatching larvae depend upon a moist environment such as water, inside a gelatinous terrestrial egg (some species undergo direct development and metamorphose

to adults inside the eggs), inside a brooding adaptation of the parent (Gastrotheca cornuta and Pipa pipa), or inside a uterus-like oviduct (some amphibians are live-bearing or viviparous). Not all amphibian larvae require standing water to complete development. Similarly, all adult amphibians do not depend on standing water to reproduce, though traditionally most amphibians do return to water both to mate and to disperse eggs. Some amphibians are entirely aquatic and cannot survive out of water for any extended periods of time, whereas others inhabit deserts or may estivate for extended period (years) with no exogenous water. Completely aquatic amphibians are represented in all three families. Some salamanders are neotenic (Figure 14.2), in which metamorphosis to the typical adult form never occurs yet the larvae develop gonads internally and the larvae are capable of reproduction.

Though most numerous in temperate to tropical environments, amphibians are distributed worldwide. Frogs are found among nearly every habitat on Earth except the open ocean and Antarctica. Particularly interesting among the frogs is their colonization of harsh deserts. Adaptation for desert environments is most widespread among the frogs of Australia as seen in both terrestrial (*Arenophryne rotunda*) (Mattison 1987) and arboreal (*Litoria* spp.) species and among the South African terrestrial species (*Breviceps* spp.). Several South American species (*Atelopus* spp.) are adapted to cool elevations well over 10,000 feet (Lotters 1996) and some species of North American frogs (*Rana sylvatica*) are known to freeze solid during hibernation and then thaw following winter to resume normal physiology (Duellman & Trueb 1994, Mattison 1987, Stebbins 1985).

The veterinary technician should be familiar with herpetological scientific nomenclature and common terminology. It is not uncommon that scientific order, family, or group names of both plants and animals may be modified for use in general conversation or popular and scientific publications. For instance, when speaking of the three orders of amphibians, frogs, and toads (Anura) are commonly called anurans. Salamanders (Caudata) are called caudates. In the salamanders and frogs, the family names are commonly modified when discussing several of the larger families: the mole salamanders (Ambystomatidae) are ambystomatids, the lungless salamanders (Plethodontidae) are plethodontids, the poison dart frogs (Dendrobatidae) are dendrobatids, the tree frogs (Hylidae) are hylids, the true toads (Bufonidae) are bufonids, and so on.

A great deal of this chapter focuses on frogs. This is due to the fact that frogs are, by far, the most popular and widespread amphibian group in the pet industry. Much of the medicine, anesthesia, and surgery techniques applied to frogs are extrapolated to all amphibians. The general discussion of amphibian medicine focuses on metamorphosed juvenile and adult amphibians with a separate general discussion of larvae. The husbandry and disorders of larvae can differ significantly from the adults of some species.

Anatomy and Physiology

General anatomy is similar across all three orders of amphibians and is discussed as applies to all amphibians. Anatomical specializations and clinically significant differences in anatomy are described for the three orders. Physiology varies tremendously, even among genera and species of the same order, and clinically significant differences are noted in the following discussion.

Integument

The evolutionary development of amphibian skin is one of the greatest adaptations that enabled vertebrates to leave the water and exist on land. The epidermal layer of amphibian skin is shed routinely (ecdysis) in a manner consistent with that of lizards and snakes. Ecdysis may occur piecemeal or entirely, and some caecilians, frogs, and salamanders consume the shed skin—a process called keratophagy or dermatophagy. The dermis layers of skin serve a respiratory function and are highly vascularized. Some caecilians possess small scales that are embedded in the skin (Goin et al. 1978, Duellman & Trueb 1994).

The respiratory function of amphibian skin is particularly important for larvae, adult caecilians, most adult salamanders, and many frogs. Several species of amphibians and one family of salamanders (Plethodontidae) have absent or greatly reduced lungs and rely on cutaneous respiration for the majority of oxygen and carbon dioxide exchange. The hellbenders (*Cryptobranchus* spp.) and giant Asian salamanders (*Adrias* spp.), both of which are aquatic, have well-developed lateral skin folds which increase surface area for cutaneous gas exchange. An interesting behavior exhibited by *Cryptobranchus* spp. is a rocking motion in which the salamander sways the body from side to side in slow-moving or poorly oxygenated water, presumably to "ventilate" the skin (Duellman & Trueb 1994, Petranka 1998).

The amphibian epidermis is rich with glands. Some epidermal glands produce secretions that moisten the skin to facilitate cutaneous respiration and some frogs (*Phyllomedusa* spp.) secrete waxy substances that protect against dehydration and dessication (Wright 2001b). Poison glands are present in all salamanders and frogs. These are most notable among the poison dart frogs (Dendrobatidae) of Central and South America and toads worldwide. Of all amphibians, the skin secretions of *Phyllobates terribilis*, the golden dart frog of Colombia, are the most toxic (Walls 1994). The Chaco Indians of Columbia use skin secretions of three species of *Phyllobates* to coat blow darts used to hunt monkeys, hence the common family name of these frogs. Of the 170 species of Dendrodatidae, only *P. terribilis* is considered lethal to man from simply touching the toxin. Interestingly, wild-caught dart frogs of all species fed domestic diets in captivity and frogs born in captivity lose the majority of their skin toxins (Daly et al. 1994).

Several species of toads and salamanders possess large parotid glands dorsally on the head, just caudal to the skull. These glands are elliptical and commonly the site of profuse toxin excretion. Skin toxins from many frogs and toads are dangerous to domestic animals such as dogs and cats. The author has observed a 20-kg Labrador Retriever suffer violent vomiting, diarrhea, and convulsions following the accidental ingestion of a Cuban treefrog (*Osteopilus septentrionalis*). Anecdotal reports exist of deaths in dogs and cats following exposure to or ingestion of toxic secretions of marine toads (*Bufo marinus*). In general, all terrestrial frogs and toads should be considered potentially dangerous to dogs and cats. Other captive amphibians that should be considered toxic include the European salamander (*Salamandra salamandra*), the American newt (*Notophthalmus viridescens*), and some mole salamanders (*Ambystoma* spp.).

Many of the more toxic amphibians exhibit aposematic coloration and are conspicuous or active by day. Animals that exhibit aposematic or warning colors rely on a learned response of the potential predator to avoid interaction with the particular animal or suffer distasteful or noxious stimuli. Some of the commonly observed aposematically colored amphibians include the European salamander (*Salamandra salamandra*), the red eft phase of the American newt (*Notophthalmus viridescens*), red salamanders (*Pseudotriton* spp.), some poison dart frogs (Dendrobatidae), some harlequin frogs (*Atelopus* spp.), the golden mantella (*Mantella aurantiaca*), and the semi-aquatic fire-bellied toads (*Bombina* spp.). As with some insects and snakes, mimicry in coloration occurs in several "non-toxic" species that co-occur with more toxic species.

Several species of frogs possess unique skin adaptations for raising young. The aquatic female Surinam toad (*Pipa pipa*) carries eggs on her back over several months during which time the eggs invaginate into the skin and undergo direct development into juvenile frogs. Upon hatching the juvenile frogs swim out of the holes in the skin, ending parental care. Another female South American frog, the marsupial frog (*Gastrotheca* spp.), possesses a pouch on the dorsum in which eggs hatch into tadpoles (or undergo direct development in some species) and are then released into a suitable aquatic habitat.

Skeletal System

The skeleton of amphibians is comprised of both an endoskeleton and exoskeleton that is ossified. Exoskeleton

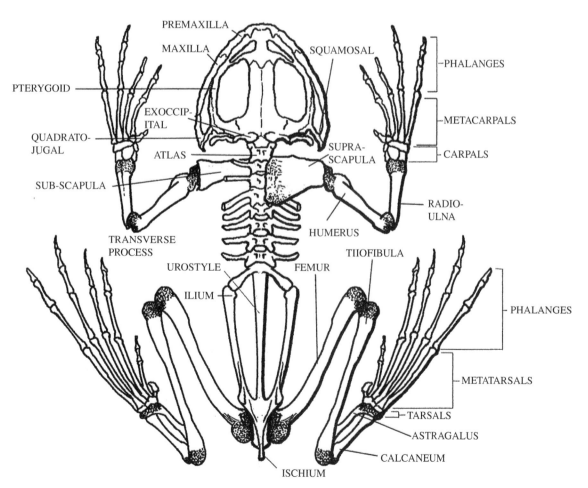

Figure 14.5 Skeletal anatomy of a frog. (Drawing by Scott Stark.)

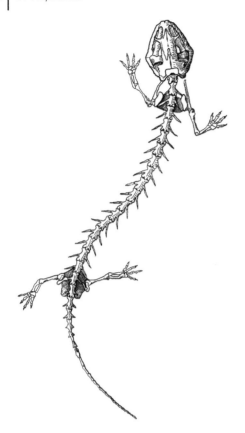

Figure 14.6 Salamander skeletal anatomy. (Drawing by Scott Stark.)

is bone formed in the dermis that fuses with underlying endoskeleton and is most notable in the skull of amphibians, particularly in frogs and toads. The amphibian skeletal system has three functions: protection, locomotion, and support for terrestrial existence. A major adaptation for locomotion on land is the development of pelvic and pectoral girdles. These are absent in caecilians, but well-developed in most salamanders and all frogs. Great variation of the appendicular skeleton exists among species of frogs and toads. In most frogs and some salamanders, the hyoid bones are modified to eject the tongue for prehension of prey (Figures 14.5 and 14.6).

Digestive System

All adult amphibians are carnivorous and have a digestive tract similar to that of higher carnivorous vertebrates and similar among the three orders of amphibians. The oral cavity of salamanders and frogs is spacious and generally designed for capturing and swallowing whole prey items. A fleshy tongue is present in most species. Aquatic salamanders have a primary fish-like tongue and aquatic frogs (Pipidae) have no tongue (Goin et al. 1978). Amphibian

teeth are replaced through life when lost (Goin et al. 1978, Duellman & Trueb 1994).

Prehension of prey may occur by one of several modalities in amphibians: suction, hellbender (*Cryptobranchus* spp.) and Surinam toad (*Pipa pipa*); ambush or direct pounce and capture, mole salamanders (*Ambystoma* spp.) and toads (*Bufo* spp.); luring and capture, horned frogs (*Ceratophrys* spp.); foraging and prehension with tongue, palm salamanders (*Bolitoglossa* spp.) and dart frogs (*Dendrobates* spp.); and scavenging, *Amphiuma* spp., *Siren* spp., and aquatic caecilians (*Typhlonectes* spp.) (Helfman 1990).

The esophagus, stomach, small intestine, and large intestine are similar to those of higher vertebrates. The cloaca is homologous to that of reptiles. The pancreas and gall bladder are present and aid in digestion. The liver serves to convert ammonia into nitrogenous waste products, primarily urea. In at least one frog species, the Australian gastric-brooding frogs, *Rheobatrachus* spp., the female ingests the fertilized eggs into the stomach where the eggs hatch into tadpoles and then metamorphose into juvenile frogs. During the brooding period, all digestive secretions are stopped in these species (Duellman & Trueb 1994) (Figure 14.7).

Respiratory System

Amphibians exhibit four modalities of respiration: branchial, buccopharyngeal, cutaneous, and pulmonic (Wright 2001c). Adult salamanders use the four modes of respiration; adult caecilians and frogs do not use the branchial mode. In most amphibians, the left and right

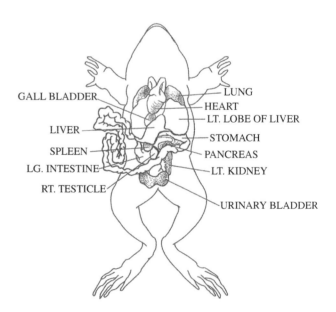

GALL BLADDER

LIVER

SPLEEN

LG. INTESTINE

RT. TESTICLE

LUNG

HEART

LT. LOBE OF LIVER

STOMACH

PANCREAS

LT. KIDNEY

URINARY BLADDER

Figure 14.7 Visceral anatomy of a frog. (Drawing by Scott Stark.)

lungs are of equal size. Some caecilians have a greatly reduced or absent left lung, as observed in snakes.

Branchial or gill respiration is present in free-swimming larvae of all amphibians and in neotenic or aquatic salamanders. Those species with external gills may exhibit varying degrees of gill development dependent upon environmental conditions such as dissolved oxygen. In more stagnant oxygen-deprived environments, the gills are larger to increase oxygen-absorbing surface area. In well-oxygenated water, the gills are typically smaller. Some aquatic species (Sirenidae, Proteidae, and Pipidae) may rely more on buccopharyngeal and pulmonic respiration by gulping air when oxygen content is critically low. Cutaneous respiration is discussed in the Integument section.

Buccopharyngeal respiration is primarily driven by air gulping in aquatic species and gular or buccal pumping in terrestrial species. Atmospheric air is pulled in through the nostrils to the nasopharynx and oral cavity by negative pressure during buccal expansion and then driven out by the collapse of the gular skin. Oxygen exchange occurs through the thin-walled buccopharyngeal capillaries. This pumping action also drives both inspiratory and expiratory pulmonic respiration in terrestrial amphibians. Buccopharyngeal gas exchange in amphibians is analogous to that of some freshwater air-gulping fishes such as the electric eel (*Electrophorus electricus*) and the lungfishes (*Protopterus* spp. and *Lepidosiren* spp.).

All terrestrial amphibians, except salamanders of Plethodontidae, which do not have lungs, use pulmonic respiration. Amphibian lungs are sac-like, with alveoli most well-developed in the Anurans. The lungs of some aquatic amphibians serve as hydrostatic or buoyancy organs in addition to the respiratory function (Wright 2001c).

Vocalization is best developed in frogs but is also observed in caecilians and salamanders of various species. Frogs are the only order of amphibians in which anatomic vocal structures are well developed and in which vocalization is known to serve as communication for mating, territorial defense, and escape from predators (Duellman & Trueb 1994). Vocalization is unique for every species and is also present in aquatic species. Males are the most vocal of the sexes, but females of some species have "distress calls" which are used when escaping predators or "release calls" to signal males when the female is unreceptive during opportunistic breeding congregations.

Excretory System

The kidney of amphibians is mesonephric and empties into the urinary bladder. The urinary bladder of some amphibians may be bilobate. As in reptiles, urine is collected by the Wolffian duct (mesonephric duct in amphibians, metanephric duct in reptiles) and then routed to the cloaca and not the urinary bladder. Urine passes retrograde from the cloaca into the urinary bladder (Goin et al. 1978).

Nitrogenous wastes of primarily aquatic amphibians are excreted as ammonia, whereas many terrestrial amphibians secrete urinary wastes as urea or uric acid. This conversion of ammonia to urea and uric acid conserves water for terrestrial amphibians and reduces the toxicity of ammonia in the blood. Frogs of the genus *Phyllomedusa* are uricotelic, being able to convert urea to uric acid for excretion (Wright 2001c).

Reproductive System

Amphibians have paired internal gonads that are hormonally regulated. Collecting ducts (oviducts in female) transport gametes to the cloaca where they are expelled from the body. Viviparous species are present in all three orders and the larvae undergo metamorphosis in the oviduct of the female and are born as fully functional juveniles. Fat bodies are located adjacent to the gonads of all amphibians and are presumed to provide nutrient stores for developing gametes. These bodies enlarge during non-breeding season and are greatly diminished at the end of breeding season.

The testes of frogs are a collection of seminiferous tubules connected to the mesonephric ducts by collecting ducts. Frogs exhibit the greatest organizational structure of seminiferous tubules among the amphibians. The testes (and ovaries) enlarge dramatically in response to breeding season. Copulation is observed in all caecilians but only one species of frog, and fertilization is internal in these species. Fertilization for all other frogs is external. Interestingly, fertilization for all but two families of salamanders (Hynobiidae and Cryptobranchidae) is internal with no copulation. Male salamanders secrete a jellylike substance in the cloaca that encases the sperm, the spermatophore, and expel this structure during breeding. The female salamander collects the spermatophore in the cloaca and fertilization occurs internally. Fertilization is internal in only a few frogs.

The amphibian ovaries are located in proximity to the kidneys as seen in higher vertebrates. Following ovulation ova are contained within a thin membrane, the ovisac, which ruptures and releases eggs into the coelom. Eggs are funneled into the ostium of the oviduct by cilia lining the coelomic mesentery and then passed to the cloaca to be expelled into the environment. The lining of the oviduct of viviparous caecilians is consumed by developing larvae as nourishment during development. In oviparous species, the oviducts serve to store or hold eggs until spawning occurs. In salamanders, a diverticulum of the dorsal wall of the cloaca forms the spermatheca, which stores collected sperm to fertilize eggs upon spawning.

Amphibians, especially frogs, exhibit tremendous adaptation in parental care of developing eggs and larvae. These adaptions are discussed throughout various sections in this chapter.

Cardiovascular System

The cardiovascular system is comprised of a three-chambered heart, arteries, veins, and lymphatics. The heart of *Siren intermedia* and *Necturus maculosus* contains an interventricular septum, making a four-chambered heart (Goin et al. 1978). As with reptiles, oxygenated and deoxygenated blood mixes minimally in the common ventricle.

The three orders of amphibians exhibit great variation in the development of aortic arch vasculature. A prominent ventral abdominal vein is present in amphibians as in reptiles. This is the vein of choice for blood collection in large frogs or toads. In salamanders not capable of tail autotomy (release of the tail when stressed), blood can be sampled from the ventral tail vein as described for snakes and lizards. Many frogs can also be sampled from the ventral lingual plexus in the mouth (see Techniques).

Lymphatics and lymphatic circulation are well-developed in amphibians. All blood cells and proteins except erythrocytes are found in amphibian lymph. Lymph hearts that beat synchronously and independently of the cardia control lymph circulation. Diagnostic samples may be retrieved from lymph sacs, which are found in various locations of the body. Most notable of these are paired lymphatic sacs in the skin dorsal and caudal to the pelvis in frogs.

Amphibian blood and tissue fluids have a lower osmolality (200–250 mOsm) than mammals (300 mOsm) (Wright 2001c). Thus, isotonic fluids used for mammals are hypertonic to amphibians and result in dehydration of the amphibian patient with long-term exposure. Mammalian saline is 0.9% NaCl. A 0.6% NaCl solution is most appropriate for use with amphibians.

Nervous System

The amphibian nervous system is modified from that of fish with the enlargement of the cerebral hemispheres and the development of more complex neural networks in the spinal cord for the innervation of pectoral and pelvic limbs. A withdrawal response is observed in amphibians as a result of trauma such as damage to limbs and toes.

Sense Organs

Amphibian eyes, though not as highly adapted as those of reptiles for complete terrestrial existence, are greatly modified from the eyes of most fish. Movable eyelids and lacrimal glands to moisten the eye are among the most notable adaptations. The eyelids are not present in amphibian larvae, most aquatic amphibians, and the neotenic axolotl. A third eyelid or nictitating membrane is present in many terrestrial frogs. It is similar to the same membrane of dogs and cats and its closure is passive, being achieved by contraction of the retractor bulbi muscle followed by withdrawal of the eye into the eye socket. A portion of the levator bulbi muscle actively controls retraction of the third eyelid back to its resting position.

The amphibian auditory system, while anatomically and physiologically interesting, has relatively little clinical significance. Jacobson's organ, the vomeronasal organ, is present in amphibians, but is much less developed than in snakes and lizards. This sense organ is suspected to function in food recognition and in plethodontid salamanders (and possibly other genera) is thought to function for pheromone detection during courtship and mating.

Husbandry

A basic understanding of the life history requirements of the amphibian species in question (or extrapolated from a closely related species) is needed to gain a thorough history and develop a diagnostic and treatment plan for amphibians. Even among different related species of amphibians, however, there may be dramatic diversity of environmental needs within a single genus. These differences are particularly evident among the genera of Dendrobatidae (*Dendrobates*, *Ameerga*, *Ranitomeya*, *Excitobates*, *Phyllobates*, *Epipedobates*) and the genera *Atelopus* and *Mantella*. The Dendrobatids are a diverse and geographically widespread group occurring from sea level to 2,600 m elevation; some species are terrestrial, some are entirely arboreal; some are 1.5 cm as adults, and some are more than 5 cm (Walls 1994). Similarly, the Atelopids have species groups that are termed highland (2,600–4,500 m) or lowland (<1,000 m) (Lotters 1996). If a highland species is maintained as a lowland species or vice-versa, the frog will fail to thrive and typically perish within days. Similar though less extreme environmental diversity is seen among *Mantella* spp.

Many of the natural history-related criteria for evaluating lizards (see Chapter 9) apply to amphibians. The following list highlights the more pertinent information with which the technician and clinician should be familiar for a given species:

1. Origin of the captive patient: Is the patient captive-born or wild-caught? For the more common species in captivity, know which of these are more likely caught in the wild or propagated in captivity.
2. Preferred microhabitat: Is the patient fossorial, terrestrial, arboreal, aquatic, or semi-aquatic? What is the preferred air and/or water temperature of the patient? What is the preferred humidity of the patient?
3. Behavior: At what time of day is the patient active in normal health? Does the patient exhibit seasonal behavioral patterns such as hibernation? Does the patient exhibit certain defensive postures or behaviors when stressed or threatened?
4. Diet: What is the patient's preferred food in nature and what food items is it known to consume in captivity? What is the preferred size of food item? Is the patient an aggressive feeder that may attack or consume cage mates? At what time of day or night does the patient feed in its habitat? What is the normal feeding behavior of the species in question?
5. Anatomy and physiology: What is the anatomy of the normal healthy patient, including size or coloration differences between sexes of a given species? Are certain physical characteristics seasonally variable? Is the patient potentially toxic to cage mates?

The diversity of species' environmental adaptations necessitates this knowledge of amphibians even more than among the lizards, snakes, tortoises, and terrapins. Unfortunately, the majority of amphibian diseases progress rapidly or have a narrow window of treatment, making the speed of diagnosis and treatment critical.

The greatest progress in successfully maintaining amphibians in captivity, particularly with the frogs, may be attributed to an understanding of the captive environment for each species. As with many reptiles, success with captive maintenance and breeding of amphibians has improved dramatically in the last 10–15 years through the research and experimentation of zookeepers and private hobbyists.

Enclosures and Environment

The four basic generalized amphibian cage designs are arboreal, terrestrial, semi-aquatic, and aquatic. On occasion, a mix of these designs is appropriate for some animals and each design may be slightly modified to house a particular species. With each of these habitats, there may be dramatic variation between species with regard to temperature and humidity in any given environment. With many species in their permanent enclosure, effort should be made to somewhat reproduce the natural environment to reduce stress and increase adaptability. Once again, having

fundamental natural history knowledge of the patient is essential.

The health of the captive amphibian may be directly proportional to the "health" of the terrarium. Certain characteristics apply to all amphibian enclosures. These include security from escape; visual and noise security; refuges for hiding; substrate; and the environmental parameters of lighting, temperature, humidity, ventilation, and water quality.

Security to prevent escape is of primary importance. The most elaborate climate-controlled naturalistic enclosure is of no help to the dried-out carcass of an amphibian on the floor of a room. The evolutionary development of legs has greatly improved the ability for escape by amphibians when compared to fish; some of the most escape-prone amphibians, however, are the legless caecilians and the sirens and amphiumas, both of which have reduced limbs. Many fish enthusiasts can attest to similar escapes with eels, ropefish, lung-fish, and other anguiform fish species. Though many aquatic and semi-aquatic amphibians perish in the dry environment of a climate-controlled room, some, if they find suitable moist habitat elsewhere in the room, can survive quite well outside their intended enclosure. Barnett et al. (2001) mention the placement of "moist oases" along the walls of such rooms to prevent dessication in case an escape occurs. These may be plastic containers lined with moistened moss and an adequate opening for entry.

Visual, noise, and vibration security is essential for many species. With the exception of the most dominant or aggressive species (*Ceratophrys* spp., *Pyxicephalus* spp., large *Bufo* spp., large Ranidae spp., some *Ambystoma* spp., *Amphiuma* spp.), many amphibians rely on camouflage or escape as the first defense. Thus, when threatened, many frogs attempt to escape by jumping. Most enclosures are not of adequate size to prevent collision with the cage walls and the collisions may stimulate further escape behavior. Similar evasion may be seen with some salamanders and many aquatic amphibians, though salamanders typically seek retreats or subterranean refuge. Physical trauma, however, may not be as significant as the stress created and the resultant maladaptation to a captive environment without adequate cover.

Visual security is provided by both internal and external cage design. Painting the external surfaces of the terrarium or applying other external visual barriers is helpful to prevent incessant escape attempts through the cage walls and to reduce sudden visual stimulation from movements outside the enclosure. Certain cage ornaments, accessories, and artificial or live plants are applied inside the cage for refuge and visual security. Clean plastic pots, sections of PVC pipe, the bases of plastic soda bottles, cork bark, sticks or logs, and rocks are all valuable as refuges. Though less natural, the benefit of plastic refuges is that they are easily cleaned or sterilized for reuse. Cork bark may be autoclaved (if an autoclave is available), though it is not recommended to use certain detergents, ammonia, or bleach on any natural or porous cage accessories for amphibians. Soaking organic items in clean, fresh water for several hours may be required to remove cleaning agent residues. Dried hardwood leaves are an excellent renewable refuge for salamanders and smaller frogs. It is also possible to clean these items with diluted bleach solution prior to use.

Understanding the behavior of a species in nature is helpful to proper cage design. Many arboreal frogs, for example, will not use substrate-interfaced or many horizontally oriented refuges but instead require vertically suspended flat leaves (*Agalychnis* spp., *Hyla* spp.) or horizontal branches (*Phyllomedusa* spp.) for resting. Similarly, terrestrial salamanders typically do not benefit from vertically spacious, heavily planted terrariums, though the terrestrial cover provided by such plantings may be beneficial for reducing ground lighting. Larger terrestrial amphibians such as marine toads and mole salamanders seem particularly fond of artificial refuges in a terrarium and regularly return to these areas when inactive. Aquatic caudates such as *Cryptobranchus* spp. and *Necturus* spp. occur in fast-moving coldwater streams and require large rocks, logs, or other submerged refuges to escape the currents. Often these animals also forage for food in these microhabitats because many food items similarly use the refuges to avoid strong currents.

Certain plants provide ideal refuges for some caudates and anurans. Bromeliads are an ideal tropical enclosure plant for smaller hylids, some dendrobatids, and the tropical *Bolitoglossa* spp. Some bromeliads, however, may have sharp defensive spines that can prove perilous to many amphibians and their owners. Many smaller aroids (peace lilies, *Spathiphyllum* spp.) are ideal for treefrogs. (Gagliardo, personal communication). Large terrestrial amphibians are best maintained in terrariums that are sparsely planted or contain large sturdy plants. Marine toads, horned frogs, tiger salamanders, and large ranids are quite capable of trampling and eventually killing all but the sturdiest plants in a terrarium. In similar fashion, larger aquatic amphibians (all aquatics except dwarf aquatic frogs and newts) uproot or damage planted aquatic terrariums in a matter of minutes to hours, though these species typically benefit from copious floating or suspended aquatic vegetation.

Plants for the terrarium are selected based on utility and aesthetic quality. Consideration must be given to the possibility of introduction of harmful pesticides, fertilizers, detergents, and potential pathogens. All plants, regardless of their origin, should be cleaned of all soil and thoroughly washed before planting. Furthermore, plants from one established amphibian enclosure should never be moved to another amphibian enclosure to reduce the risk of parasite or other disease transmission to uninfected or otherwise unexposed animals. This must be strictly observed for plants originating from any enclosures containing wild-caught amphibians. Avoid using plants that originate in regions where there are known frog populations inhabiting or contacting the plants.

Basic requirements of an ideal soil-type substrate are a slowly degradable, well-drained, well-aerated, slightly moisture-retentive soil that is free of pesticides, fertilizers, or other potentially toxic chemicals. These soils, though all organic, contain many non-traditional components which include horticultural grade charcoal, orchid bark, tree fern or palm trunk fiber, milled sphagnum, and some peat. Generally, this substrate is adapted from epiphytic orchid or tropical pitcher plant (*Nepenthes* spp.) soil mixes that are designed to be well-drained and aerated (Gagliardo, personal communication). The author has maintained several larger well-planted terrariums of dart frogs with these soil mixes for more than years with no soil changing. This soil type is best used for dart frogs, harlequin toads, mantellas, hylids, and other arboreal species requiring a well-planted enclosure.

The major benefit derived from this soil type is for the maintenance of plants in the enclosure. An invariable outcome of most peat-based or ready-made houseplant soil mixes in terrariums is rapid decomposition, compaction, and inadequate aeration. As this process progresses, the roots of plants die and the plants fail to thrive. Eventually, the health of the entire terrarium deteriorates and animals fail to thrive. The bark/charcoal/peat mix requires a longer time period (2–3 years) for decomposition and rarely, if ever, compacts in the terrarium. A disadvantage to the "*Nepenthes* mix," however, is that it cannot be used for burrowing species of amphibians. The bark, charcoal, and tree fern are all potentially abrasive to amphibian skin. This does not appear to create a problem for most small (<5 cm) terrestrial frogs or toads but can be irritating to larger frogs and some salamanders.

Another soil suitable for substrate is composted leaf litter that is free of fertilizers, pesticides, or other chemicals. This is particularly useful for salamanders and burrowing frogs. Commercially available topsoil preparations must be used with caution because they may contain chemical additives.

Proper lighting of a terrarium raises many questions regarding the light needs of amphibians. Generally, the specific requirements of ultraviolet light (particularly UV-B required for the synthesis of vitamin D_3) are unknown for amphibians (Barnett 1996). Histopathology studies of several Panamanian amphibians (*Gastrotheca cornuta*, *Hemiphractus fasciatus*) indicate that nutritional secondary hyperparathyroid disease occurs in these species (personal observation). Addition of UV-B radiation and feeding a calcium-enriched diet has demonstrated reduction of clinical signs of nutritional secondary hyperparathyroidism (NSHP) in captive-born *Gastrotheca cornuta*. Certainly, questions arise regarding the requirements of nocturnal, fossorial, or fully aquatic amphibians. For terrariums containing live plants, attempts are made to simulate natural sunlight so that the plants will thrive. The incidental effects of this lighting scheme on amphibians may be beneficial. As with most terrestrial vertebrates some light is required for vision and photoperiodic behavior.

The amphibian owner should attempt to recreate the lighting scheme of the amphibian in nature. In general, most terrestrial salamanders and nocturnal frogs do not require bright lighting and may avoid it altogether. A natural method to reduce lighting on the cage floor is a well-planted terrarium with full spectrum lighting. It is not unusual for some nocturnal hylids to rest on leaves or branches that are exposed to full sun during some part of the day (White's tree-frog, *Litoria caerulea*; green treefrog, *Hyla cinerea*). Therefore, suitable basking sites should be provided for these species. Light fixtures are suitably placed above the enclosure, preferably within 46 cm (18 inches) of the cage floor (Barnett et al. 2001). It is important to note that ultraviolet radiation does not penetrate plastic and glass; thus, any lids that may shield the light should be replaced with screen. Unfortunately, screen also diffuses the penetration of UV radiation into an enclosure (author, personal observation). Also, when a full aquarium hood is used as lid and light source for the enclosure, a tight fit is essential to prevent escape of the inhabitants.

Commercially available full-spectrum lights for terrariums are available as fluorescent tube, coiled compact fluorescent, mercury vapor, and compact halogen. Most, if not all, of the incandescent lights available for aquariums and terrariums do not produce adequate UV-B radiation despite packaging claims. Additionally, because most incandescent bulbs produce copious heat, they should be used with caution for amphibian enclosures. Many brands of full-spectrum lights are available for both plants and animals, each with their own claims of benefits. To date, coiled compact fluorescent, mercury vapor, and compact halogen lights are the best producers of UV-B radiation. Baines et al. (2016) have published some general guidelines for common captive species.

Temperature, humidity, and ventilation for the terrarium are all interrelated and their control and management often dictate cage design more than any other environmental parameter. As many fish hobbyists can attest, the larger the aquarium the easier it is to manage temperature. The same is true for terrariums. This is particularly true for humidity and ventilation. Surprising to many, amphibians as a group inhabit a wide variety of climates from the equator to the Arctic Circle. Caecilians and salamanders are somewhat less adapted to extreme climates than frogs are. Thus, discussion of the more extreme temperature and humidity requirements primarily pertain to certain species of anurans. Some species of amphibians require seasonal cooling to stimulate ovulation and spermatogenesis for breeding. Knowledge of the specific patient's natural history with regard to environmental parameters is essential.

Enclosure temperature for many amphibian patients is controlled by room temperature. The great majority of amphibians can adapt to normal household room temperature of 25°C to 30°C (75°F to 85°F), though there are some exceptions. Most highland tropical frogs (*Atelopus* spp. and some *Mantella* spp.) as well as most North American salamanders fail to thrive for extended periods at temperatures above 21–24°C (70–75°F) (Lotters 1996, Obst et al. 1988). The Pacific giant salamander (*Dicamptodon ensatus*), the hellbender (*Cryptobranchus alleganiensis*), and the mudpuppy (*Necturus maculosus*) may all require refrigerated water or air conditioning throughout the year. Aquatic species such as the Surinam toad (*Pipa pipa*) and the African dwarf frog (*Hymenochirus* spp.) require heated water with protected submersible aquarium heaters.

Supplemental heating of the terrestrial amphibian enclosure is generally not required, though some species of frogs and toads benefit from basking lights or heat sources such as incandescent lights or ceramic heaters. These species include some toads, monkey, frogs (*Phyllomedusa* spp.), and White's treefrogs (*Litoria* spp.). Most diurnal frogs (Dendrobatids, Atelopids, Mantellids) typically do not require basking areas in the terrarium. Behaviorally, however, many diurnal species may be observed "basking" or exposing themselves to shafts of sunlight in the forest. Additionally, some nocturnal species may spend their daytime resting period directly exposed to sunlight (*Phyllomedusa* spp., *Litoria* spp.). One should avoid heating enclosures with hot rocks or heating elements with which amphibians can make direct contact to prevent dessication and thermal burns.

Enclosure humidity and ventilation are somewhat inversely proportional. Though other factors such as temperature and amount of water in the enclosure contribute to humidity, ventilation has the greatest and most rapid effect on increasing or decreasing humidity. Ideally, the amphibian enclosure should be well-ventilated with appropriate humidity. A partial or full-screen terrarium lid or cover is ideal for allowing evaporation and creating ventilation. Partially occluding the screen lid increases or decreases ventilation and inversely raises or lowers humidity. For large or tall terrariums, small ventilation holes may be drilled in the cage wall and covered with screen to allow ventilation of the otherwise stagnant lower reaches of the enclosure. A small fan may be placed outside the roof of the enclosure to create cross ventilation from these lower air intake ports.

Most terrestrial amphibians benefit from a humidity gradient in the terrarium. This gradient is created by shelters in the terrarium, additional ventilation to portions of the terrarium, and with basking sites as described with lighting. Small depressions, pools, or streams of water may be created in the terrarium with pond liner or plant watering trays. For small frogs, particularly for dendrobatids and mantellids, it is imperative that even the smallest water reservoir have multiple escape routes. Many small frogs are incapable of swimming and will drown in even one centimeter of water. Many salamanders are capable of semiaquatic life and generally can withstand submersion for longer periods. Placement of limbs, plants, raised gravel, or other cage accessories within or around the water ensures the ability for escape. Similarly, the sides of water enclosures for terrestrial amphibians should have tapered ramps in all directions for small amphibians to escape the water.

Moving water in the enclosure is also helpful to increase both humidity and to a lesser extent ventilation. Small waterfalls, humidifiers, or vaporizers may be used for this purpose. Transfer of vaporized air is achieved by connecting an appropriate size PVC pipe from the vaporizer outflow into the enclosure at the desired location. Connecting the vaporizer to an automatic timer is helpful to create several periodic mistings per day. The misting effect in the terrarium can be quite dramatic. Humidifiers and vaporizers must be cleaned weekly to prevent the growth of potential pathogenic organisms in the water reservoir. Soaking with a dilute bleach solution (1 fl oz or 30 mL in 1 qt or 946 mL water) for 15 min and then thorough rinsing is sufficient for disinfecting (Barnett et al. 2001).

Water for the amphibian enclosure should be free of potential pathogens and all treatment chemicals. Aged tap water (allowed to ventilate in a container for 24 h) in many cases is the best water for the terrarium (Barnett et al. 2001). Alternatively, carbon-filtered water may be used, though this water treatment may result in developmental abnormalities of tadpoles. Water moving in the terrarium over soil, gravel, or charcoal will generally be filtered biologically. Water that is stationary in containers should be changed as often as possible. Many terrestrial amphibians defecate in these water bowls and bacterial or fungal growth in these containers may be rapid. Cleaning the water bowls in a dilute bleach solution as described for vaporizer reservoirs is recommended at least weekly.

Enclosure Design

The Terrestrial Enclosure

By employing the general principles of security and environmental parameters, design of the amphibian enclosure, based on the species, is relatively straight-forward and dictated by practicality. With the exception of temporary housing or quarantine, the smallest recommended amphibian enclosure is a 10-gallon aquarium. Though there is no maximum size limit of a terrarium, access for cleaning, visualization, and environmental control must all be considered (Figure 14.8A and B).

An appropriate substrate is most important for establishing a well-balanced naturalistic arboreal, terrestrial, or semi-aquatic terrarium, and the soil composition is quite variable depending upon the species of amphibians and plants contained within. The type of soil or gravel, however, is only one part of establishing a suitable amphibian substrate. Proper design of the cage floor-substrate interface is crucial for maintaining a long-lasting planted or naturalistic terrarium. Ideally, the soil mix should be elevated above the cage floor to allow for water and airflow through the soil and the development of a moisture gradient within the soil and terrarium.

Elevation of the soil above the cage floor is achieved by one of several methods. Wright (2001e) uses a standard cage design at National Aquarium in Baltimore (NAIB) by creating a raised platform or false floor of overhead fluorescent light panels (egg crate) cut to fit the tank floor and then raised 2 cm above the true cage floor by pilings cut from PVC pipe (Barnett et al. 2001). This false floor is then overlaid with window screen or horticultural shade cloth and then covered by 1–2 cm of gravel and then the sheet moss directly above the gravel. In one corner of the enclosure, a 2.5-cm diameter clear plastic tube is placed vertically through the false floor extending to just below the roof of the cage. This tube allows siphoning off the cage floor with a separate smaller siphon tube passed to the bottom of the cage. An optional but highly recommended bulkhead and spigot may be placed through a drilled hole in the cage floor to allow drainage thereby eliminating the need for the siphon tube.

The author has used a modified version of this design developed by Ron Gagliardo at the Atlanta Botanical Garden with great success. The egg crate false floor is typically inexpensive, but when using standard fish aquariums, prefabricated under-gravel filters (the economy models) are made to fit the size of the tank and come complete

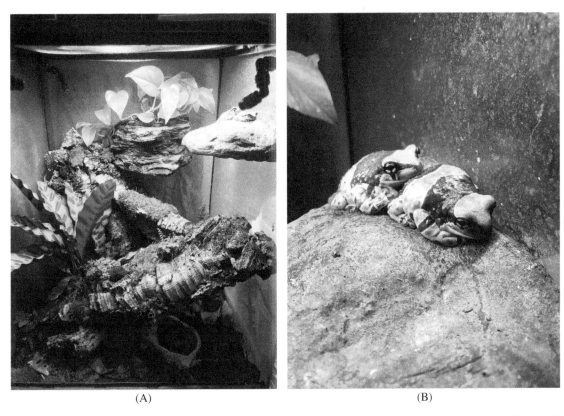

Figure 14.8 (A) Typical housing for a tropical species of amphibian. (B) In this case, it is housing Amazon milk frogs (*Trachycephalus resinifictrix*) (Courtesy of Dr. Stacey Wilkinson.)

with siphon tubes. One or more of these siphon tubes may be used as access for siphon drainage of the cage floor. Additionally, an alternative to the use of aquarium gravel between the filter plate and the soil is to use washed large or medium horticultural grade charcoal that is commonly available for orchids or other special planting mixes. The benefits of the charcoal are lighter weight (especially for large enclosures) and the gradual filtration of organic and inorganic compounds from the water and soil. The benefit of gravel is the large surface area for biologic filtration that likely also occurs with the charcoal. Charcoal has been used as both an enclosure base layer and as a component of custom mixed terrarium soils by the Atlanta Botanical Garden for many years with no known adverse effects on various species of frogs.

For a planted terrarium a soil depth of at least 5 cm is recommended. Over time some settling of the soil will occur. Plants are added bare root (no soil on the roots) to the soil mix and lightly watered to settle the surrounding soil. Generally, plants smaller than the eventual desired size are planted and allowed to grow in the terrarium. Plants in an amphibian terrarium should never be fertilized. Theoretically, soil decomposition, animal feces, and microbes provide all the nutrients necessary for the growth of terrarium plants. It is common that many suitable plants soon outgrow the enclosure and require routine trimming.

For many conservation assurance populations, the false bottom of the cage may remain bare to facilitate washing and removal of organic waste on a routine basis. This is particularly important to reduce the risk of reinfection by lungworms (Rhabdias spp.) and various other intestinal parasites.

The water level of the terrestrial terrarium is maintained to achieve desired humidity and fill pools or streams contained within. Plumbing for water accessories may be achieved through drilled holes or siphon tubes through the lid of the terrarium. Water pumps, moving part mechanical devices, and electrical cords should never be inside the terrarium proper. These may be routed through sealed conduits or contained outside the terrarium entirely. Similarly, outflow siphon hoses must be fully protected from cage inhabitants and preferably are located beneath the false floor of the enclosure.

The Aquatic Enclosure

The aquatic enclosure for many obligate aquatic or facultative aquatic amphibians is somewhat similar to the basic tropical fish or goldfish aquarium. Large aquatic amphibians such as *Amphiuma* spp., large sirens, and *Cryptobranchus* spp. are best housed in a 55-gallon or larger aquarium. *Cryptobranchus* and *Necturus* spp. both require chilled water with very high filtration. These animals should not be kept in captivity without properly providing for exact water quality conditions. One requirement for aquatic amphibians is sufficient access to the water surface to breathe air. Because a majority of aquatic amphibians are relatively large and somewhat active, all refuges and ornaments must be secure in their placement. Aquarium heaters (if required) should be contained within a shroud such as PVC or other durable plastic into which numerous holes or slits are drilled to allow water movement over the element and proper heat dissipation. This is to prevent the accidental breaking of glass or ceramic heating elements. The lid must be tight fitting and preferably latched to prevent escape. With a swimming start, many larger aquatic amphibians are capable of opening lids to a standard aquarium hood.

Some form of water flow is desired for most aquatic amphibians, though frogs such as *Pipa* spp., *Xenopus* spp., and *Hymenochirus* spp. adapt well to still water. Cleanliness of the terrarium is essential and necessitates some type of filtration system. Under-gravel filtration as provided for a fish aquarium is ideal for most aquatic amphibians. Those species requiring high water flow typically require a canister filter or other high-flow rate external water pump and/or filter. Most temperate aquatic amphibians require no supplemental heating and adapt well to room temperatures during the entire year. Tropical species are likely to require some supplemental heating if room temperatures fall below 72–75°F.

Amphibian-Environment Interaction

Several common problems can be avoided in captive amphibians with a practical approach to cage design. First, the substrate and cage accessories should be appropriate so they do not physically injure the animal. This includes even "natural" elements such as plants. Sharp spines on certain bromeliads or other plants can be lethal to frogs. Certain plants are toxic to amphibians. The toxicity is not necessarily from direct contact but occurs secondary to ingestion by food items such as crickets or other insects. This is mostly a concern with the introduction of field-collected insects. For example, some plant-sucking insects such as aphids can feed on toxic plants (such as milkweeds, *Asclepias* spp.) and not become distasteful to the smaller amphibians. In the case of milkweeds, the toxicity usually results in death of the animal.

Substrate ingestion is a major problem for captive amphibians. The substrate should be either too large to ingest or small enough that ingested particles are passed through the digestive tract. This may require modifying the substrate in a particular enclosure as the amphibian pet grows.

Almost paradoxically, water in the terrestrial enclosure can result in fatalities of some amphibians. Small terrestrial frogs (mantellids, dendrobatids, and atelopids) are incapable of swimming or will exhaust very easily in water. If a water enclosure is located in the corner of a terrestrial terrarium with no escape possibility against the glass, death of some cage inhabitants from drowning is a certainty. To adequately maintain these species in captivity, standing water is optional or can be provided in the form of a petri dish or other shallow container. Unfortunately, to successfully breed both *Mantella* and *Atelopus* spp., some form of moving or standing water is usually required in the enclosure.

One can assume that any opening to the outside of the cage will be used for escape. The lid or covering for the enclosure must be tight-fitting or completely sealed. Even strictly terrestrial frogs are capable of limited climbing and jumping to reach the top of the cage. Some salamanders are also capable of climbing glass or plastic.

Amphibian–Amphibian Interaction

A common question of many amphibian enthusiasts is "Can different species be housed together?" The safe answer to the question is "No." Nevertheless, with experience and thorough knowledge of the species in question, many species that co-occur in nature may be housed communally with proper cage design.

The ultimate rule of housing multiple species (or even the same species from different sources) is that wild-caught individuals from different sources should never, ever be housed together. Clinically, amphibians (particularly frogs) appear to be more commonly parasitized than reptiles, even among captive-born individuals. Exposure of naive animals to certain parasites or bacteria and fungi can result in disaster for an entire collection. An emerging disease concern for terrestrial amphibian owners is the chytrid (Chytridiomycosis) fungus. This pathogenic fungus is suspected to be at least one of the causes of worldwide mortality among wild populations of amphibians, and it has been identified as widespread and easily transmitted among captive amphibians (see Common Disorders) (Berger et al. 1998, Daszak et al. 2000, Morell 1999).

Aside from contagious disease is the question of compatibility. For the average amphibian owner, large frogs and salamanders (*Ceratophrys*, *Pyxicephalus*, large *Rana*, large *Bufo*, and *Ambystoma*) are best housed singly in an enclosure. All large amphibians are typically conditioned to feed on anything that is small enough to fit in their mouth. Ambystomatids in captivity are particularly conditioned to bite anything that touches the flanks, even animals larger than they are. The author has witnessed numerous leg amputations and lacerations of frogs and other salamanders that were temporarily housed with a tiger salamander of equal size. Frogs such as *Ceratobatrachus guentheri*, *Ceratophrys*, *Hemiphractus*, *Megophrys*, and *Pyxicephalus* spp. prey on other frog species and other vertebrates as a substantial part of their diet and therefore are generally unsuited for cohabitation with any other amphibians.

Toxicity between different species of amphibians is also a concern, even among the same family of frogs. Many anecdotal reports exist and the author has witnessed that other amphibians (and other *Rana* spp.) enclosed with wood frogs (*Rana sylvatica*) die rapidly, leaving only the wood frogs alive (Duellman & Trueb 1994, Mattison 1987). The exact nature of this suspected toxicity is not fully known. It is possible that similar toxicity exists between different species of wild-collected dart frogs, though there is no observed toxicity among captive individuals.

Quarantine

The role of quarantine for new amphibians in a collection cannot be overemphasized. Segregation of new arrivals is most important for those animals that will be introduced into multi-species displays. The quarantine procedure for amphibians, however, is more designed to protect the individual animal from occult disease that may manifest itself sometime after arrival into the new enclosure (Pessier & Mendelson 2014).

The quarantine enclosure is quite basic. A 10-gallon glass aquarium or plastic sweater box with ventilation holes is ideal for quarantine of most terrestrial amphibians. Larger aquatic amphibians should be maintained in an appropriately sized enclosure. For terrestrial amphibians, the cage substrate should be non-bleached paper towel and possibly a hide box or other disposable cage ornament to provide security. The quarantine enclosure should be located in a low-traffic area of the room where the inhabitants may be monitored for activity from a distance. If necessary, the sides of the enclosure may be painted or covered with paper to provide visual security. If possible, a feeding station should be provided in the form of a petri dish or shallow dish so that the feeding response can be monitored. Arboreal frogs and salamanders can be quarantined similarly with the addition of horizontal branches

for perching. If forced to remain on the cage floor, arboreal frogs may become stressed and fail to acclimate.

A fundamental purpose of quarantine is the collection of fecal material for analysis. This should be performed as soon as the first sample is available. Subsequent fecal samples should be examined every three to five days, depending on availability, and then rechecked every 2 weeks following a negative or "clean" sample. A final recheck 2 months after a negative sample is also advised (Wright & Whitaker 2001c).

The quarantine period should be at least thirty days following a negative fecal sample for apparently healthy individuals (Wright & Whitaker 2001c). Wild-collected amphibians, despite the status of fecal testing, should be quarantined for sixty days. Under no circumstances should wild-collected amphibians be introduced into an enclosure with any other animals. Despite antiparasiticide, antibiotic, and antifungal treatment it is possible for these individuals to carry undetected infectious diseases and later transmit them to other naive animals.

It is not uncommon to prophylactically treat new amphibian arrivals for gastrointestinal parasites and some cutaneous fungi. Though this practice is no substitute for fecal examination, it can be effective in eliminating or reducing the burden of some infectious diseases. Unfortunately, there is a risk of adverse side effects with this practice. The author has observed the death of long-term captive imported frogs following deworming with fenbendazole at recommended doses. The animals were four green and black poison dart frogs, *Dendrobates auratus*, which were confirmed infected with various nematodes including great numbers of lungworms, *Rhabdias* spp. None of the animals had exhibited clinical disease and were breeding in captivity. Following a single oral treatment with fenbendazole at 100 mg/kg two of the four frogs immediately stopped eating and subsequently died within 5 days. A third stopped feeding and then resumed feeding and survived. The fourth frog was not adversely affected. Both surviving frogs continued to shed *Rhabdias* spp. larvae in the feces following treatment, yet the number of larvae were reduced. The author has not observed this phenomenon in other similarly infected *Dendrobates* spp. or *Mantella* spp.

A common prophylactic antiparasite regimen includes administering fenbendazole orally at 100 mg/kg followed by ivermectin topically at 0.2 mg/kg (Wright & Whitaker 2001c). Repeating the treatment in 3 weeks is recommended, along with rechecking a fecal sample prior to treatment. The author has observed that ivermectin treatment may be fatal is some species including Central American glass frogs (Centrolenidae) and the lemur leaf frog (*Hylomantis lemur*). The frog deaths were observed in frogs that were infected with *Rhabdias* spp. Ongoing research and personal observations on the treatment of *Rhabdias* spp. infections in multiple Central American amphibian species indicates that a complete "cure" or elimination of *Rhabidias* spp. infection may not be possible in captive amphibians.

Record keeping of feeding and treatments is essential. The client should record all observations of activity, feeding response, food items consumed, and other pertinent behavior. Weekly weights are also beneficial for healthy individuals when this can be performed accurately and in a stress-free manner.

Nutrition

If the nutritional needs for amphibians were as simple as tossing a few crickets into the enclosure from time to time, they would all be more popular pets. Instead, the nutritional maintenance for many captive amphibians is as labor intensive (or more so) as that of insectivorous lizards, and the nutritional demands of amphibians are more a consequence of the animals being such generalists rather than being specialists on one food item. The variety of food items consumed in the wild likely results in a tremendously varied vitamin, mineral, amino acid, and fatty acid intake that is not duplicated with captive diets. Very little scientific data exists regarding the exact diet and its nutritional composition of amphibians in the wild. Unfortunately, much is learned about the proper or improper nutrition of amphibians through histopathology.

There is great variability in the feeding preferences of different life stages of metamorphosed amphibians, and this variability has been observed in those animals that have been successfully bred over several generations. For instance, froglets of the golden mantella (*Mantella aurantiaca*) are no more than 8 mm in length at metamorphosis. To a frog this small, even the smallest of domestic fruit flies is too large to eat. These froglets must be raised for several weeks on small insects called springtails (order Collembola) until they may be fed small fruitflies. Adult mantellas, however, are quite ravenous and will eat crickets that are nearly 20% of their body size.

The feeding method of amphibians is also somewhat important when selecting food items. All frogs should be considered food gulpers; after capturing the prey item, it is swallowed whole with little to no chewing. In contrast, large salamanders and especially aquatic amphibians (Necturus, Amphiuma, Siren, and *Cryptobranchus spp.*) all exhibit some chewing motions when feeding. This is especially observed in sirens and amphiumas that may repeatedly move food items in and out of the mouth while crushing them. Choosing appropriate food items, or more importantly, avoiding improper food items for certain species, is important.

Another important point to remember regarding most terrestrial amphibians is that they are sight feeders. Generally moving food is preferred over stationary food. Some larger frogs, toads, and salamanders may be conditioned to feed on stationary pre-killed or frozen and thawed food items, but this is more the exception than the rule. Thus, when approaching the dilemma of a non-feeding amphibian, always consider the type and size of food offered.

Perhaps the most important consideration when feeding amphibians is the timing of feeding. The client must be fully informed of the feeding habits of the species in question. Nearly all terrestrial salamanders and many tree frogs are nocturnal and will only feed at night. Many of the larger nocturnal frogs and toads, being opportunists, will feed any time in captivity. The tiger salamander, *Ambystoma tigrinum*, though nocturnal in its native habitat, will readily adapt to daylight feeding. Night feeding may make the monitoring of food consumption difficult with some amphibians. For newly established pets, encourage the client to observe the feeding habits with a flashlight or red light illumination if necessary.

To compensate for the known vitamin and mineral imbalances in food items and for suspected deficiencies in amino acids, many hobbyists apply several commercially available vitamin/mineral powders (called dusting) to the food items prior to feeding. The process of dusting food items is discussed in Nutrition section of the chapter on lizards. Additionally, food products specifically for the prey items to consume are designed to enrich the prey item prior to feeding to the amphibian pet. This process is called "gut-loading."

Based on known dietary disorders, several basic provisions must be made for captive amphibians. Calcium and phosphorous (Ca:P) should be provided in a ratio of 1:1 to 2:1 to prevent several nutritional diseases (Wright 2001d, Wright & Whitaker 2001a, Donoghue & Langenberg 1996). Additionally, vitamin D_3 is supplemented in the diet or produced endogenously by the amphibian when exposed to the appropriate quality and quantity of ultraviolet light. A ratio that is too low in calcium or too high in phosphorous may result in NSHP. A ratio too high in calcium or vitamin D_3 may contribute to hypervitaminosis D and secondary renal failure (Wright & Whitaker 2001b). Powdered supplements are available from Rep-Cal (Los Gatos, CA; www.repcal.com) and Nekton (Clearwater, FL; www.nekton.de). Additionally, feeding insects or small mammals high in fat content is highly suspected of causing cholesterol and fat deposits on the cornea known as lipid keratopathy.

Neonatal and young amphibians appear to be most affected by NSHP because of increased calcium demand by growing bones. The frequency for calcium supplementation of these animals is increased compared to that of adults. Neonatal or young, growing amphibians may receive calcium and vitamin D_3 supplementation twice weekly when fed daily and most adult amphibians should receive calcium-supplemented food items once weekly or less often. Larger amphibians fed whole animal vertebrate diets such as thawed frozen rats or mice likely do not require supplemental calcium in the diet.

Aquatic or semi-aquatic amphibians fed diets comprised solely of fish may develop a thiamine (vitamin B_1) deficiency (Wright & Whitaker 2001b, Donoghue & Langenberg 1996). This disorder is the result of high levels of thiaminase in the food items that inactivates dietary and endogenously produced thiamine in the amphibian. Several susceptible species include aquatic salamanders, aquatic caecilians, horned frogs (*Ceratophrys* spp.), African bullfrogs (*Pyxicephalus* spp.), and other semi-aquatic frogs.

Food Items

Most clients who maintain breeding colonies or large colonies of amphibians are required to raise their own food items because the expense of purchasing food items can be excessive. The simplest factor dictating the feeding of captive amphibians is the size of the animal and the size of the food item. The standard diet for most larger salamanders and frogs is crickets and the diet of choice for smaller amphibians is fruit flies. Some wild-collected insects such as termites may be available seasonally or throughout the year in warmer climates.

Domestic or gray crickets (*Acheta domestica*) of various sizes are the standard diet for most medium to large terrestrial amphibians. Crickets are commercially available in sizes ranging from 1/16 inch (pinheads) in length to 1 inch (adults) from pet shops and mail order from a variety of sources. The Ca:P for crickets is 0.2:2.6 (Donoghue & Langenberg 1996). Periodic dusting of crickets with calcium and vitamin D_3 powders is recommended for all amphibians.

A variety of specialized cricket diets are available to enrich crickets with nutrients. The efficacy of these products is debatable. Generations of frogs that have been fed crickets raised on fresh vegetables and fruits such as squash, greens, and oranges have reproduced and lived for five or more years with no apparent health abnormalities to themselves or offspring.

Another cultured food item for medium to large amphibians is mealworms. The mealworm is actually larvae of the beetle, *Tenebrio molitor*, which may be cultured easily in one of several different grain meals supplemented with cut pieces of apple or vegetable for moisture. Because the adult beetles are required to reproduce for new mealworms, a tight-fitting, ventilated lid is required to maintain the culture. Mealworms are generally a poor food choice for amphibians because of the hard exoskeleton. Though the softer-bodied, newly molted larvae are acceptable, the author has witnessed the unexplained deaths of several frogs and lizards following the feeding of mealworms. Necropsy on several lizards has revealed peritoneal abscessation that was attributed to gastrointestinal perforation from the hard body parts or possibly chewing of the larvae. Because mealworms do not provide an improved Ca:P ratio (0.1:1.2) (Donoghue & Langenberg 1996) as compared to crickets, their use as a primary food item for most amphibians is not recommended. Finke (2002) provides an exceptional reference on the nutritional value of various insects raised commercially for captive animals.

Similarly, most beetles and other large insects with hard exoskeletons are not a good food source for amphibians. An exception might be made for large frogs and especially toads, which may be observed to nearly consume their weight in beetles while feeding in habitats during summer months. Large terrestrial salamanders and aquatic amphiumas and sirens are generally capable of crushing these insects following capture and therefore may adequately digest them and have minimal risk of gastrointestinal injury.

The flour beetle, *Trilobium* spp., which is a relative of the larger *Tenebrio* spp., is a smaller beetle that can safely be fed to small frogs. These beetles are approximately 5 mm in length as adults with comparable small larvae. They are raised and harvested similar to *Tenebrio* spp., though the adult beetle is fed as commonly as the larvae.

Wingless or flightless fruit flies are the standard diet for smaller frogs and salamanders, particularly for poison dart frogs, mantellas, harlequin frogs, and neonatal amphibians. Two species of flies, *Drosophila melanogaster* (the small vestigial or wingless fruit fly) and *Drosophila hydei* (the larger flightless fruit fly), are commercially available. Fruit flies are easily cultured by the client and may be the sole food source for many captive amphibians. They are cultured in reusable canning jars or disposable plastic cups, both of which are sealed with a permeable (but escape-proof) ventilated lid. Fruit fly growing media is available from Carolina Biological Supply Co. (Burlington, NC; www.carolina.com) or can be made from instant potato flakes, brewer's yeast, and a mold inhibitor. Fruit flies are typically dusted with powdered supplements as with crickets.

Another small food item that is relished by nearly all amphibians is the termite. In warmer climates, such as the southeastern U.S. coastal plain, termites can be collected any time of year. There are methods of "culturing" termites in the wild that involve burying coffee cans punctured with drain holes in the ground and filling them with rolled cardboard. Unfortunately, the risk of infestation to homes and other wooden structures is great, so this practice should not be recommended to clients. Nevertheless, wild-collected termites do not appear to cause harm to captive amphibians, and certain nutrients not otherwise available to these animals may be provided. Similarly, parasites or other toxins ingested by the termites could put captive animals at risk for disease.

An important but often overlooked food item for small frogs is springtails or leafhoppers of the insect order Collembola. These very small (<1 mm) white to gray insects that are commonly seen in most terrariums containing soil. They feed on detritus and decaying plant material and can be easily cultured to feed neonatal or very small frogs and salamanders. A plastic container such as a margarine container or plastic shoebox filled with approximately 1–2 inches of potting soil is ideal. The soil is slightly moistened and a few pinches of fish food flakes are sprinkled on the surface of the soil. The springtails may be introduced from a decaying leaf from outdoors or from a previously existing culture. A method for easily removing the springtails is to place a small block (10 cm × 5 cm × cm) of horticultural tree fern fiber on the soil surface, then remove and gently tap the block to remove springtails when feeding is desired.

The only acceptable vertebrate food sources for captive amphibians are fish and thawed frozen pink mice or rats. Large frogs, toads, and salamanders with conditioned feeding responses usually accept these items when offered by forceps, or in the case of fish when offered in a shallow dish. These larger amphibians generally accept other vertebrate prey such as other amphibians, reptiles, large beetles, and large insects such as grasshoppers and locusts. The client should carefully consider the health risk to the amphibian before feeding such items. The risk of parasitism with endoparasites or bacterial or fungal infections is great. Of paramount concern must be the Chytridiomycosis fungus when offering any amphibians. This disease is extremely serious for amphibians and should be viewed on the level of the immunodeficiency viruses that affect cats and humans when considering prevention.

Aquatic amphibians consume a wide variety of food items. Earthworms and fish are the standard diets with other arthropods and some frozen foods are occasionally accepted. Ideally, the food should be cultured or purchased as cultured rather than collected from the wild. This reduces the risk of introducing infectious diseases into the enclosure.

Certain amphibians, particularly several frog species, are specialists in their feeding choices and may be difficult to feed in captivity. The bizarre casque-headed tree frogs, *Hemiphractus* spp., of South America and several species of horned frogs, *Ceratophrys* spp., are known frog-eating specialists (Mattison 1987, Obst et al. 1988). It may be necessary to feed live frogs to these species while trying to train them to eat various invertebrate or vertebrate prey items. Another finicky large frog (8–10 cm) is the climbing toad, *Pedostibes hosei*, of southeast Asia. This frog is known to specialize in ants and termites and may not accept crickets or other large invertebrates in captivity (Obst et al. 1988). This frog may be transitioned to a cricket-only diet by feeding smaller size crickets or beetles. Among aquatic amphibians the hellbenders, *Cryptobranchus* spp., as adults typically feed only on crayfish and must be coaxed to accept other aquatic food items if captive.

Finally, many clients may be misinformed regarding the feeding of manufactured pelleted diets. It is unreasonable to expect any terrestrial amphibians to eat non-moving prepared foods. It is more likely, though not common, that aquatic amphibians will readily accept these diets. Salamanders and newts, more than frogs, will adapt to these diets, but they are rarely substitutes for live foods. Clients should be informed about this fact prior to purchasing amphibian pets. For some, the cost of live foods or the time to culture them may not meet their expectations for proper maintenance of amphibian pets. One exception of note is the fact that marine toads (*Bufo marinus*) have been observed and videotaped eating dry dog food from outdoor food bowls in south Florida. So, one can never underestimate the resourcefulness of these animals when it comes to adaptation.

Common Disorders

The great majority if not nearly all health disorders of captive amphibians are preventable with appropriate husbandry, nutrition, and biosecurity. The clinician and technician will soon learn that treatment failure for many disorders is common due to the protracted nature of the disease prior to presentation for diagnosis and treatment. Therefore, a thorough understanding of natural history and appropriate captive conditions is paramount for providing education to the keeper to reduce incidence of disease.

The captive environment presents a multitude of challenges for the amphibian keeper to maintain optimal health of frogs and salamanders. Many, if not most, health abnormalities in amphibians require a quick response if not immediate treatment to prevent death of the individual or population. It is important for the keeper to recognize the initial and often more subtle signs of disease in an individual animal and then determine if the disorder is infectious or non-infectious. This determination will dictate a course of action needed for management of just a single individual or entire captive population. It is also important to realize that the manifestations of some non-infectious processes (poor water quality, toxins, and food contamination) may resemble the pathophysiology of infectious disease. This fact further complicates the epidemiologic approach to multiple diseased animal scenarios with captive amphibian populations. Additionally, not all infectious diseases among amphibians are contagious.

Unfortunately, many clinical signs or manifestations of disease in captive amphibians are similar which prohibits an exact diagnosis based on clinical signs alone. Despite a thorough history and pre-mortem laboratory testing, exact diagnosis may escape all testing except necropsy and histopathology. For this reason, it is common to establish a "working diagnosis" and recommend treatment on the most logical or practical suspected disorder. Response to therapy can be just as valuable diagnostically as any clinical test.

Determining a course of treatment may be based not only on observed clinical signs and laboratory testing, but also on clinical experience with the collection or specific species, known tendencies of a particular species, or even rationalizing which of a given set of disease possibilities is most likely. Successful treatment may result as much from recognizing when no treatment is indicated as opposed to choosing the most appropriate pharmaceutical.

Treatment of the diseased amphibian commonly requires the manipulation or correction of abnormal environmental parameters that may have contributed to alterations in physiology or behavior that is the underlying cause of disease. Treatment of some infectious diseases, however, may be enhanced or augmented by the alteration of typical environmental parameters outside the range of the animal's optimal captive environment. This treatment synergy requires an understanding of baseline environmental conditions for the animal prior to onset of the disease in question. Therefore, routine monitoring of a captive population as well as observation and understanding of "normal" anatomy, physiology, and behavior for each species in the collection are all an essential aspect of collection management. It is essential to understand that for some species "normal" parameters in captivity may be different than "normal" parameter in the native habitat.

For many diseases in captive amphibians, successful treatment is measured by a return to the typical physiologic or behavioral state by the individual or by the survival of the majority of affected animals under treatment. For survival assurance conservation collections, success is measured as survival plus a return to the captive breeding population. For these animals, it is essential to consider future reproductive success of the individual animal as its primary value to the collection. Determining treatment for survival assurance colonies may be more based on health of the population rather than health of the individual.

Though it is rare that a clinical sign or observed abnormality is pathognomonic, an observant keeper may quickly recognize the presentation of a few disorders. Successful management of some diseases is predicated on quick recognition and initiation of treatment. A clinical signs approach to categorize potential diseases is often helpful for the trained observer to begin the diagnostic and treatment processes.

Anorexia

Anorexia is defined as a loss of appetite or inability to eat. Both of these circumstances may apply to the disorder of anorexia in captive amphibians. This disorder may occur acutely or develop and progress chronically and is a disorder that is fully reliant on the observations of a trained keeper familiar with the living collection. In order to diagnose a non-feeding amphibian, the keeper must have observed the affected animal(s) feeding routinely at some point. Both acute and chronic anorexia may be attributed to virtually any infectious or non-infectious disease.

One cause of acute anorexia common to larger amphibian species is gastrointestinal obstruction caused by non-edible material and typically affects a single animal or very few individuals in a collection at one time. Most commonly this is a result of accidental ingestion of substrate. In the pet trade captive amphibians that are particularly prone to this problem are horned frogs, toads (various genera and species), and larger salamanders such as ambystomatids. Ingestion of the foreign body is usually the result of an instinctual or reflex feeding response in which the foreign material is either repeatedly ingested (sand or soil) or in which a larger object is not recognized and swallowed with (or instead of) the prey item. Unfortunately, many substrate materials may be unrecognized by the captive amphibian as foreign material, or the captive animal is housed so that it is forced to be in contact with a substrate while feeding. Examples may include a treefrog that must feed on ground-dwelling insects in captivity, but in its native habitat would never be in contact with the ground to feed or a horned frog that is housed on pebbles or gravel but in its native habitat would only live in leaf litter, soil, and water.

The gastrointestinal foreign body is diagnosed by trained keepers or veterinary staff by a combination of thorough history, physical exam, palpation, and possibly radiographs. Single foreign bodies of the stomach only, may be safely corrected by sedation of the animal and simple retrieval through the oral cavity. Foreign material in the lower gastrointestinal tract may require surgical correction. Constipation (impaction of the colon or large intestine with feces) may also occur as a cause for inappetence.

If a gastrointestinal foreign body is not suspected, then investigation of all other infectious and non-infectious diseases must begin. The list of possible disorders is reduced by good observations and records of the animal(s) involved and familiarity with the collection. When multiple animals within an enclosure are simultaneously affected, infectious diseases must be considered as the top (though not exclusive) potential diagnosis. It is not uncommon for non-infectious nutritional diseases to affect groups of animals within a short time period. Simultaneous occurrence of nutritional disease, however, is quite uncommon as these disorders appear to have variable rates of onset and manifestation among individuals.

Weight Loss

Weight loss is another vague clinical abnormality that is commonly observed in captive amphibians and is not specific to any given disorder. It may be observed concurrent with nearly every clinical disorder that affects captive amphibians. Though it may be intuitively associated as a consequence of anorexia, this is not always the case. Similar to anorexia, weight loss is most commonly diagnosed by the routine observations of a trained keeper familiar with the animals under their care. Typically, weight loss is a sign of chronic disease and therefore once diagnosed must be considered a potentially life-threatening abnormality as the animal may have been diseased for some time.

Several of the more common causes of weight loss in captivity include inappropriate feeding or underfeeding, competition with cage mates, parasitism, other infectious disease, NSHP, and old age. Because parasitism is the one disease that may be definitively diagnosed by clinical testing in amphibians, it must be ruled out in every case of weight loss. Even if competition with cagemates is suspected, it is possible that the stress caused by this competition may allow for immunosuppression and subsequent parasite proliferation in the individual. If parasites are absent, then diagnosis of the underlying disorder relies on clinical history and observation. Weight loss of multiple animals in an enclosure as opposed to just a single animal may suggest infectious or nutritional disease.

The first and most important step toward mitigating and diagnosing weight loss is to isolate the affected animal in a suitable enclosure where feeding may be observed and feces may be collected. If the patient fails to eat, then assist feeding may be required during treatment for the suspected underlying disorder. This process must be performed or supervised by a trained amphibian keeper as serious damage to the animal may result from improper technique.

Activity or Behavior Disturbance

Though this category of abnormal clinical appearance is not a disease itself, it is nevertheless a very important abnormality that may require immediate attention. Typically, any amphibian that deviates from its normal daily or nightly routine as a pattern of behavior change is diseased or stressed. Diagnosis, intervention, and mitigation of the underlying cause of the behavior disturbance must be a priority for the affected animal(s).

Typical behavior disturbances include nocturnal animals becoming active in the daytime or vice-versa; constant activity in an otherwise sedentary animal or vice-versa; failure to perch, rest, or sleep in typical location; spastic hopping or jumping; persistent or progressive color change; repeated or constant rubbing of the skin or "scratching;" repeated gaping or "yawning;" or other deviations from the typical observed patterns of behavior.

Many deviations in behavior reflect another underlying disorder that could become life-threatening. Because there is moderate risk for infectious disease if any of these clinical changes are observed, the affected animal(s) should be isolated and observed.

Dysecdysis or Excessive Skin Shedding

Many amphibians routinely shed their skin and may be observed to do so at the beginning of their daily or nightly activity period. This routine physiologic event should not be mistaken as a disorder by observers unfamiliar with the animal's typical behavior. Rarely is excessive skin shedding observed as the only clinical abnormality in a diseased animal. Commonly, this clinical sign is observed in conjunction with activity or a behavioral disturbance, inactivity, refusal to feed, or weight loss among other abnormalities.

Because many frogs shed and eat their skin, the excessive skin shedding may not be observed, but on occasion, an excessive amount of skin may be observed retained in the mouth as the animal is not feeding normally and still ingesting skin sheds that it cannot swallow. For highly aquatic species, layers of shed skin may be observed floating in water or loosely attached to the animal's body. In many cases, excessive skin shedding is a single animal disorder in an enclosure.

In all cases of increased skin shedding, the risk for chytridiomycosis due to *Batrachochytrium dendrobatidis* or *B. salamandrivorans* must be assessed and ruled out. Most excessive skin shedding is a result of irritation to all or a portion of the skin. Potential etiologies include inappropriate water quality, infectious disease, and physical or chemical irritation not associated with water. It is essential as a first step to determine if water is a direct or indirect cause of the observed problems. Elevated ammonia levels and/or sudden alterations to water pH are most commonly implicated with water quality problems in aquatic or semi-aquatic environments. Because many institutions with captive amphibians may use amphibian water misting bottles that are very similar to cleaning agents, it is essential that these containers are clearly labeled or stored in separate locations. Once water quality and environmental irritants can be ruled out, infectious diseases including bacterial, fungal, and parasitic diseases should be investigated.

The best first response to address excessive shedding despite the underlying cause is to separate the affected animal(s) to a clean environment with clean, fresh water. The initial use of a clear plastic container will facilitate examination of all surfaces of the animal without handling which could further damage the skin. The presence of skin lesions or red discoloration of the skin does not always indicate active infectious disease but is suggestive that opportunistic bacterial infection will develop. Therefore, treatment with appropriate topical antibacterial agents is indicated. Suitable treatments may include antibiotics applied topically on the lesion(s), injected, or applied as a bath. For most amphibians, all of these applications will result in both focal reduction of bacteria as well as systemic treatment facilitated by direct absorption into the blood or lymphatic systems through the skin.

It is important to understand that this is a disorder that may commonly result in rapid death of individual animals and several causes have the potential to become infectious to other animals in the enclosure. In some cases, by the time clinical signs have developed there may be no treatment options to correct the affected animals and humane euthanasia must be considered. Management focus then moves to prevention of disease in other animals within the enclosure.

Dehydration

Clinical dehydration is a diagnosis that is suspected given a narrow range of clinical abnormalities and history. Dehydration is most commonly encountered in newly acquired animals or in animals that have been shipped over long distances and introduced into a new enclosure.

Understanding normal behavior of the species in question may be essential to recognizing this condition. Because many frog species absorb water from the environment through their skin, animals that maintain increased contact with moist areas of the enclosure or are seen pressing their ventral surfaces against the substrate for prolonged time should be suspected of dehydration. Another more subtle clinical sign is the sudden loss of "stickiness" to the tongue. This is most easily observed among poison dart frogs and toads. If an animal is observed attempting to prehend food items and cannot seem to pull small insects into the mouth, dehydration may be suspected.

It is important to note that the lack of stickiness to the tongue is reported as a common sign of hypovitaminosis A in several toad species. This condition is reported as "Short Tongue Syndrome." In the case of dehydration, this change is a relatively sudden onset as opposed to gradual onset in long-term captive animals with Hypovitaminosis A and would likely develop after an animal has been shipped or coupled with the pressing behavior described above.

Treatment is relatively straightforward by increasing enclosure moisture and humidity. Typically rehydration is gradual and may require one or more days for the affected animal to return to normal. Because prolonged dehydration may result in prolonged inability to feed, it may lead to a cascade of negative physiologic changes that cannot be easily reversed. Maintaining routine observation of animals within the collection and their enclosures is the best method for prevention.

Seizures/Paralysis/Weakness

Seizures and Paralysis are somewhat ill-defined and vague clinical signs that are not pathognomonic for any particular disease. Seizures may occasionally appear suddenly, though more commonly they are preceded by alteration of normal physiology or behavior over one or more days, usually characterized by weakness or inactivity. Classically, seizures are manifested as uncontrolled stretching or extension of the hind limbs commonly followed by apparent paralysis. The recognition and response to this disorder is best handled by trained amphibian conservation staff as a thorough understanding of history is required to recognize the abnormal behavior and to discern potential causes of paralysis. Several of the more common causes of seizures and paralysis in captive amphibians are NSHP, septicemia, dehydration, other nutritional disorders, and toxicity (water quality or chemically induced).

Weakness, however, has a much broader list of possible etiologies which include many environmental or husbandry factors. These particularly may include non-optimal temperature and humidity. When determining a cause for weakness, it is important to discern between an inactive frog and a truly weak frog. The truly weak frog (unable to hop, non-responsive) is an emergency condition and without intervention, the affected animal will die. The inactive frog, capable of normal activity when stimulated, is rarely an emergency, though determination and mitigation of the underlying cause of inactivity should be investigated. In some species, inactivity may be caused by intra or interspecific cage mate aggression.

Cloacal Prolapse

Cloacal prolapse is a condition in which internal organs or tissues are everted through the vent. These organs may include one or more of the cloaca, colon, oviduct, and urinary bladder. This condition should always be considered a potential emergency. There are a variety of potential etiologies for prolapse of internal organs ranging from trauma to intestinal parasitism to nutritional disorders. Determining the cause of the prolapse is not necessary when providing first aid. Cloacal prolapse is most commonly a single-animal disease. When multiple animals are affected (particularly multiple animals of a young age class), nutritional disorders such as NSHP or gastrointestinal parasites may be implicated. Treefrogs and other arboreal frog species seem to be more affected than terrestrial species.

Initial therapy consists of isolating the affected animal in a clean humid environment (Figure 14.9). The primary concern is maintaining the integrity of the fragile prolapsed tissues. The affected animal should be maintained initially on moist paper towels as a substrate in a completely enclosed high-humidity environment. Any soil or fecal debris should be gently washed or cleaned with fresh isotonic solution. In the event that immediate veterinary attention is not available, a sugar solution (commonly 50% dextrose) may be applied once or twice to the prolapsed tissues after cleaning. This hypertonic solution is applied in an attempt to reduce swelling (commonly caused by edema) to facilitate replacement of the tissues into the body as soon as possible. Replacement of prolapsed tissue should only be attempted by a well-trained, experienced keeper or under the direct supervision of a veterinarian. It may be necessary for the trained veterinary staff to aspirate fluid from distended prolapsed tissues to minimize tissue trauma and to facilitate replacement.

In the event that 50% dextrose is not available, a suitable substitute is to mix table sugar with water. Mix ½ teaspoon of table sugar (sucrose, not a sugar substitute) in 14.0 mL water. This solution then may be applied directly to the swollen prolapsed tissues.

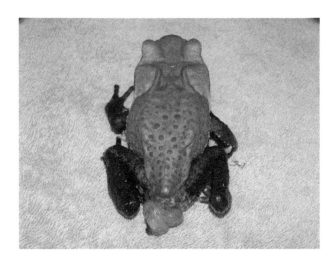

Figure 14.9 Cloacal prolapse in a Smooth-Sided Toad. This is a common presentation. (Courtesy of Dr. Sam Rivera.)

Gastrointestinal Foreign Body Obstruction

A rather common though avoidable non-infectious disease in amphibians is foreign body obstruction. Typically the result of inappropriate substrate or feeding practices, this problem often goes unnoticed for some time. The primary presenting complaint is anorexia or occasionally regurgitation. Gravel, soil particles, or rarely an invertebrate exoskeleton may cause obstruction. Diagnosis may be presumptive based on history and husbandry practices or definitive with abdominal palpation and radiographic study.

The degree of obstruction, size of patient, and nature of the foreign body dictate treatment. For organic foreign materials, oral laxatives such as psyllium and mineral oil may aid in passage of the obstruction. For larger amphibians, surgery may be indicated. Larger gastric foreign bodies may be easily removed with forceps via the oral cavity and through the esophagus while the patient is sedated.

Trauma and Cutaneous Injury

Physical injuries are among the most easily recognized disorders in captive amphibians. Recognition of trauma, however, is dependent upon a complete understanding of normal anatomy of the species in question. Generally, traumatic injuries affect only one animal within a collection; rarely are multiple animals affected at one time. Two common classes of trauma are injuries to the skin (lacerations and ulcerations) and fractures and luxations to bones and joints respectively. There are many potential etiologies of skin trauma which may include both infectious and non-infectious disease. Fractures may be the result of forceful trauma (lid closure to limbs) or the consequence of dietary/lighting disorders (NSHP).

Initial therapy for fracture management should include isolating the affected animal into a small enclosure to prevent further activity which may exacerbate the observed abnormality. Once isolation is achieved, then further evaluation will be initiated to determine potential underlying causes of the injury and potential treatments to correct the disorder. Except in very rare circumstances, external coaptation or fracture fixation is not a practical treatment for captive amphibians.

Though fractures may initially appear to be a more significant health problem, skin injuries are by far the most serious threat to survival of the captive amphibian. Any damage to the skin of the amphibian may allow entrance of environmental or other potentially infectious organisms into the bloodstream. This condition is known as septicemia. It is likely that septicemia is ultimately the leading cause of death among captive amphibians.

The common etiology of skin trauma is a result of escape attempts through clear plastic lids, screens, glass enclosures, or inter- or intra-species aggression. During transport, prevention of abrasions may be accomplished with opaque transport containers and packing of the amphibian with moss or another soft substrate to reduce movement within the container. In the permanent captive enclosure, prevention of skin trauma may also result from the provision of adequate visual security and environmental enrichment.

Traumatic injuries to limbs are commonly similar to rostral abrasions. Trauma may occur secondary to accidents with enclosure lids closing on legs or bite wounds from cage mates with some species. These wounds typically require aggressive antibiotic therapy initially rather than just observation. If severe trauma to underlying bone is suspected, amputation is recommended early in treatment to prevent the development of systemic disease (Figures 14.10–14.13).

Though bacterial culture and sensitivity is a hallmark of infectious wound management of mammals, this diagnostic test has limited value in the initial management of amphibian skin disease. Many gram-negative potentially infectious bacteria inhabit the surface of the amphibian skin and as a result, many of the active cutaneous and septicemia infections of amphibians are a result of these opportunistic organisms. A more practical initial test is the impression smear of the affected lesion. Multiple impression contacts with a microscopic slide may be collected from the lesion, then stained to evaluate for the presence of bacteria, fungi, or protozoa.

The two goals of treatment for traumatic injuries with amphibians is facilitation of repair of the primary wound and prevention of septicemia as a consequence of the wound. Wound repair is most commonly achieved by second intention of the non-infected wound. Upon the

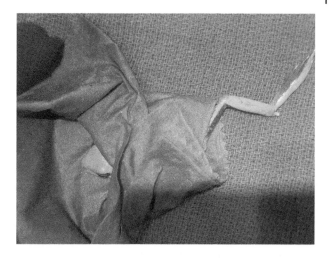

Figure 14.10 A frog with a rear limb fracture. (Courtesy of Susan Coy, CVT.)

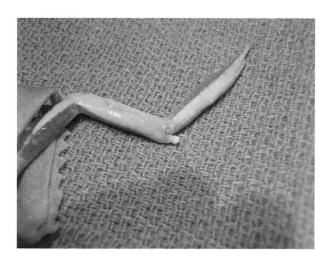

Figure 14.11 A close-up view of the frog's injury. (Courtesy of Susan Coy, CVT.)

initial observation of skin trauma, initiate treatment with one of several topical antibacterial medications. Preferred choices for treatment include Baytril Otic Solution (Bayer); Gentamicin, Tobramycin, Neomycin, or Terramycin. Ophthalmic solutions or ointments; or for initial treatment (first aid) only, Neosporin or other topical antibacterial ointments. If lesions are restricted only to the eyes, then ophthalmic solutions or ointment are required; Baytril Otic Solution should not be applied directly to the eye.

Active lesions associated with erosive dermatitis or osteomyelitis require aggressive diagnostic and therapeutic intervention. Bacterial culture and sensitivity, and cytology if possible, from an impression smear or tissue sample in formalin may be collected to confirm diagnosis. In addition to topical therapy, systemic antibiotics are indicated. Enrofloxacin at a dose of 5–10 mg/kg TO every

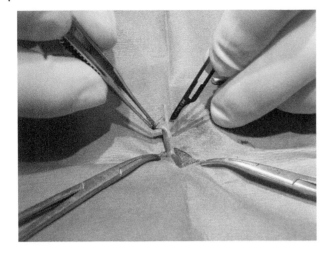

Figure 14.12 Amputation of the distal rear limb. (Courtesy of Susan Coy, CVT.)

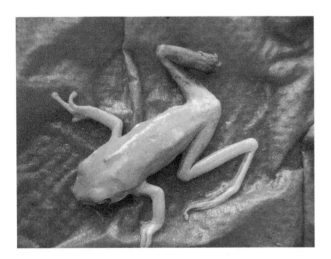

Figure 14.13 The frog after the amputation. (Courtesy of Susan Coy, CVT.)

24 h for 7 days (Taylor 2001) is recommended pending culture results. The client must be vigilant of the patient with regard to healing of these lesions. Amphibians with substantial rostral abrasions should be maintained in a quarantine enclosure for cleanliness and observation.

Infectious Skin Diseases: Bacterial Dermatitis

Primary bacterial and fungal skin infections (non-trauma origin) are common in amphibians and may present as discolorations, erythema, erosions, and ulcerations. Bacterial dermatitis may be difficult to diagnose on visual inspection alone. Many infections are the result of immunosuppression from a number of factors including improper husbandry, inadequate diet, or the stress of shipping. The resultant infectious agent may arise from the patient's environment, normal skin flora, or from an apparently unaffected cage mate. Some infections are contagious and the result of improper quarantine procedures when introducing new animals or a result of improper biosecurity practices with water or equipment.

Definitive diagnosis of these diseases is achieved with histopathology, but this is an impractical method for diagnosis in the living patient. As explained with traumatic diseases, bacterial culture and sensitivity rarely assist in the development of the immediate treatment plan. Commonly, by the time test results are available the patient has either recovered with treatment or is deceased. Culture and sensitivity, however, is an essential aspect of population management or herd health and is of particular importance when performing a necropsy. Because the bacterially infected amphibian is commonly septicemic, correlation of bacterial populations among both skin and internal organs is helpful when addressing population declines that are suspected to be secondary to bacterial origin.

The most practical and quick method for diagnosis is the impression smear (see Techniques). Impression smears of active lesions are generally effective to differentiate bacterial, fungal, protozoal, or mixed infections on the skin or deeper tissues. A modification of the impression smear is to evaluate stained specimens of shed skin from the amphibian patient. Many amphibians with dermatitis will shed skin more rapidly. When placed in a container of shallow physiologic saline (0.6%) or Amphibian Ringer's solution, these shed pieces of skin may be gently retrieved, mounted on a slide, stained, and then evaluated microscopically either wet or dry (see Table 14.2). This method is particularly effective for screening for *Batrachochytrium dendrobatidis* infection in frogs.

Amphibian Ringer's solution recipe

Distilled water: 1 L
NaCl: 6.6 g
KCl: 0.15 g
$CaCl_2$: 0.15 g
$NaHCO_3$: 0.2 g

It should be noted, however, that two of the most lethal dermal diseases of captive management, *Batrachocytrium dendrobatidis* and *B. salamandrivorans* (chytridiomycosis,

Table 14.2 Making 0.6% NaCl using common sized fluid bags of 0.9% NaCl.

0.9% NaCl Bag Size	Volume of 0.9% NaCl	Volume of sterile water[a]
1000 ml	667 ml	333 ml
500 ml	333 ml	167 ml
250 ml	167 ml	83 ml
100 ml	67 ml	33 ml

a) Remove equal amount of 0.9% NaCl from bag b before adding sterile water.

"chytrid," or "Bd/Bsal") are rarely diagnosed from an impression smear and is difficult to diagnose with other methods of skin cytology. Success in diagnosis of Bd via cytology is (1) directly proportional to the experience of the clinician or diagnostician and (2) the infection level of the patient. Therefore, when available, Bd PCR testing is necessary to achieve a diagnosis or more importantly to eliminate the possibility of Bd as a background disease in the population.

Physical examination alone is rarely of assistance in determining the cause of dermatitis in the living or deceased amphibian. None of the known bacterial or fungal dermatitides have pathognomonic signs and the clinician must refrain from making assumptions regarding an exact diagnosis based on visual inspection. What may be assumed, however, is that any amphibian with dermal disease has a poor prognosis for survival without immediate medical intervention.

Initial treatment and management of suspected infectious dermatitis in the amphibian patient in the absence of a positive Bd test result is systemic antibiotics, meticulous husbandry management of the hospital enclosure, and reduction of stress for the patient. The patient(s) must be isolated. This practice is helpful for several reasons: (1) The patient may be more closely evaluated for improvement or decline in health; (2) in many cases, treatment may be applied in the isolation enclosure without handling the patient; (3) the risk for horizontal transmission of contagious disease is reduced. Reduction of disease transmission is absolutely essential as many dermatitides in amphibians originate from multiple pathogens, some of which may be viral or fungal (Bd) both of which are typically highly contagious. Placing the affected individual in isolation also heightens the awareness of contagious infectious disease among caregivers thus improving biosecurity practices in the facility.

The compromised patient must first be housed in an enclosure and environment that meets the known optimal environmental parameters for that species in captivity (temperature, humidity, and ventilation). Because the functionality of the skin to maintain hydration in the dermatitis-compromised patient is reduced, opportunity to maintain adequate hydration must be provided daily. For the severely compromised patient, daily soaks in isotonic solutions (0.6% NaCl or Amphibian Ringer's solution) for 15–30 min are necessary. The patient must be supervised as weak patients may be unable to maintain the nostrils above the water line and drowning is possible.

For suspected bacterial dermatitis or septicemia, systemic antibiotics are administered as injections, applied topically, or applied as baths and are initiated immediately. enrofloxacin at 10 mg/kg daily or chloramphenicol (injectable) are reliable first choices for treatment.

Treatment for 7–10 days pending clinical improvement is required.

Infectious Skin Diseases: Chytridiomycosis

Batrachocytrium dentrobatidis is the causative organism for the disease chytridiomycosis in frogs and salamanders and is commonly referenced as chytrid or Bd. The recently described disease, *Batracochytrium salamandrivorans*, is an emerging disease from Europe and appears to be specific to salamanders (Martel et al. 2013). Current diagnostics and therapy for the disease Bd will be discussed.

Bd is a fungal pathogen of the epidermis of amphibians (Longcore et al. 1999). Bd is highly contagious and has been linked to multiple population declines in wild and captive amphibians. It is a pathogen that may be present in captive collections at very low levels and cause sporadic deaths. Certain species of amphibians may have innate resistance or tolerance to Bd and be considered immune carriers including the American bullfrog and African clawed frog. It is theorized that one or both of these species may be partially responsible for the worldwide introduction and spread of this disease among amphibians (Fisher & Garner 2007). Because of species variation in the sensitivity to Bd, no assumptions about the presence or absence of this disease may be made in a captive setting.

The most sensitive and specific test for Bd in amphibians is qPCR. It must be noted that sample collection technique, sample handling, sample storage, shipping conditions, maintenance of equipment, cleanliness of the lab, and proficiency of laboratory staff all influence test results both positive and negative. When test results are in doubt, duplication of testing may be required. Also, low-level Bd-positive animals may yield a negative test. Therefore, a structured disease surveillance program with designed retesting of individuals is essential to establish assurance of the absence of Bd.

Because chytridiomycosis is the single most lethal threat to a large number of species of captive amphibians, disease management plans designed to control the introduction and spread of Bd effectively mitigate nearly all other infectious disease threats to captive amphibians. The infective sporozoites of Bd live and are motile in water, therefore control of the movement of water is essential within a captive amphibian population to reduce the infectivity of the disease. It is unknown if Bd may move or be transmitted dry or in a resting state. There are no effective tests for Bd in the natural environment. Quarantine and testing of all new individual animals in a collection is essential. If new animals originate from other captive collections or wild populations where Bd is suspected known to exist, each animal should be treated despite the known testing status.

The current best practices treatment is a 10-minute bath of 0.005% itraconazole repeated once daily for 10 days. This treatment is designed for non-post-metamorphic amphibians only and has demonstrated toxicity for some larval amphibians. This is an updated dosage from the previously reported 0.01% solutions (Taylor 2001) and takes into account observed clinical effectiveness of a lower concentration and takes into account certain species sensitivities to the drug. Immediately following each treatment, the amphibian must be returned to a disinfected enclosure with all enclosure structures disinfected and any organic materials replaced. If returned to the original pre-treatment enclosure, the amphibian patients risk reinfection from possible low-level Bd contamination, and treatment failure will result. For chytridiomycosis-diseased individuals, there is increased risk for secondary bacterial infection and concomitant antibiotic therapy may be required.

Chief among clinically effective alternatives to itraconazole therapy is use of the antibiotic chloramphenicol in a bath at concentration of 0.002% (Young et al. 2014). This therapeutic regimen may be applied when itraconazole is unavailable and has been clinically effective for safely treating tadpoles.

Miscellaneous Skin Diseases

Ectoparasites are uncommon among amphibians and are clinically most prevalent among toads. Treatment consists of physical removal of the parasite or ivermectin at 0.4 mg/kg PO or TO given once weekly for at least 4 weeks (Poynton & Whitaker 2001). Some amphibian species have shown sensitivity to higher doses of ivermectin (2 mg/kg) (Poynton & Whitaker 2001, Klingenberg 1993). The author is reluctant to use ivermectin for any amphibians given the apparent multiple species sensitivity to the drug.

Ranavirus infections are documented to cause skin lesions in adult amphibians (Miller et al. 2011). These infections cannot be differentiated from any other skin disease based on clinical signs alone. Tadpoles appear highly sensitive to this disease, and it is responsible for mass mortalities in amphibians. Testing for ranavirus is achieved by PCR testing of the living or deceased patient or histopathology of the deceased patient. There is no known treatment for ranavirus infections in amphibians.

Saprolegniasis caused by one or more water molds of the genus *Saprolegnia* is reported as a cause of population decline in amphibians (Fernández-Benéitez et al. 2008). This disease has been reported in multiple species from the Pacific northwestern United States.

Nutritional Disorders: Nutritional Secondary Hyperparathyroidism

NSHP (previously referred to as metabolic bone disease, or MBD) is the leading diagnosed nutritional disorder of captive amphibians. NSHP is an artifact of the captive environment and is not documented from wild-collected animals. It is a disease requiring prevention as recovery from the clinical state of NSHP is rarely successful.

Current research (Tapley et al. 2015, Michaels et al. 2015) supports the theory that calcium and/or vitamin D3 is physiologically required for the appropriate growth and development of post-metamorphic anurans and that a deficiency in these nutrients will lead to NSHP. The control of dietary absorption, distribution, storage, and resorption of calcium in the presence of vitamin D3 in mammalian vertebrates is well documented (DeLuca 2004, Giustina & Bilezikian 2018). Nevertheless, it is unknown if comparable physiologic processes control calcium metabolism among different species or families of amphibians.

Skeletal developmental abnormalities, seizure-like manifestations, reduced vigor, and mortality have been observed in multiple species of young and growing, captive-born amphibians in multiple institutions (Griffith, Wilson, Baitchman, Pessier, Gratwicke, pers. obs. and comm., 2006–2014). These developmental problems were believed to be the result of abnormal calcium metabolism based on histopathology. Nutritional secondary hyperparathyroid disease was further suspected when the modification of captive animals' diets and lighting resulted in a reduction in clinical signs (Griffith, Wilson, Gagliardo, pers. obs. and comm., 2008–2012). However, there have been few controlled studies to determine the exact causes of suspected NSHP.

In many terrestrial vertebrates, vitamin D3 is synthesized in the skin in response to exposure to UV-B radiation. Metabolites of vitamin D3 then facilitate calcium absorption in the gut. Calcium metabolism is then regulated by both bone and kidneys for absorption and storage or excretion. Hormones from the parathyroid gland drive this regulation. Calcium in the vertebrate body is required for physiologic neurologic and muscular functions primarily by means of facilitating neurotransmitter release of nerves and regulating action potential in heart muscle. Additionally, in many mammals (including humans) Vitamin D3 may be sourced dietarily making UV-B exposure unnecessary for physiologic gut absorption of calcium.

Although a variation in calcium and vitamin D physiology is not known among closely related species of amphibians, this variation has been documented between two species of lizards within the same genus, *Anolis lineatropis* and sagrei. Ferguson et al. (2013) concluded that *A sagrei* may facultatively utilize dietary vitamin D3 whereas *A lineatropis* obligately requires UV-B exposure to synthesize Vitamin D3. This finding suggests that dietary vitamin D3 absorption or bioavailability may differ even among species of the same genus in reptiles making oral supplementation ineffective for some species. Several researchers have made similar observations of species variation in Vitamin D3 metabolism (Browne et al. 2009) and there is suspicion that the mechanism of calcium and vitamin D3 metabolism cannot be generalized among all amphibian species (Ferguson et al. 2005, Michaels et al. 2014, van Zijll Langhout et al. 2017).

The question of whether captive amphibians require UV-B radiation to synthesize Vitamin D3 is inconclusive. Both field and clinical observations are highly suggestive that UV-B exposure is required for some species including many species which are considered nocturnal. Van Ziill et al. did observe basking behavior in the nocturnal species *Pelobates fuscus* in a captive environment with permanent UV-B radiation access. Field observations further support penetration of UV-B radiation of at least 1–2 uW/cm^2 even in highly shaded locations (Griffith, Wilson, Gagliardo, pers. obs. and comm., 2006) indicating that incidental UV-B exposure may occur in resting animals that do not necessarily behaviorally seek natural UV-B exposure. It is probable that we cannot generalize either a dietary or UV-B source for vitamin D3 metabolism among all amphibian species.

It is standard practice in many captive breeding conservation programs to provide some level of daily exposure to UV-B radiation to amphibians. This practice has been documented to greatly reduce the incidence of clinical signs and histopathologically diagnosed NSHP and greatly increase survival of captive-born offspring to maturity. It is necessary, however, to provide a UV-B exposure gradient in any enclosure so that the individual animal has an ability behaviorally to avoid or reduce UV-B exposure. Increased heat commonly associated with many commercially available UV-B bulbs must be controlled.

Supplemental calcium via dusting with commercially available calcium supplements (Michaels et al. 2014) or gut-loading of feeder insects (Livingston et al. 2014) is considered a standard for providing adequate calcium for captive insectivorous amphibians and reptiles. The author (Wilson et al. 2019) demonstrated that cohorts of newly metamorphosed captive-born Evergreen toads (*Incilius coniferus*) developed clinical and radiographic signs of NSHP if denied dusted supplemental calcium when fed an exclusive cricket diet. Those groups provided calcium-dusted crickets did not exhibit signs of NSHP nor radiographic evidence of bone density loss (see Figure 14.14). To prevent NSHP in amphibians, gut loading and/or calcium dusting is recommended particularly for young growing animals.

Clinical signs of chronic low calcium levels from any cause in amphibians may include anorexia, depression, inactivity, weakness, paralysis, seizures, remodeling of bones, bloating, and cloacal prolapse. It is common to observe an acute onset of clinical signs with NSHP despite the fact that the underlying disease is most commonly chronic. Once therapy is initiated, recovery from the abnormal clinical state and resolution of clinical signs is commonly prolonged requiring weeks or months. Bone deformities resultant from NSHP in amphibians are permanent and the treatment plan should be reflective of this understanding and the patient's value to the collection. The prognosis for full recovery with observed clinical signs is poor.

Diagnosis of NSHP is presumptive based on age of the animal, nutritional history, and clinical signs. Blood testing for ionized calcium is impractical because of the small size of most patients. Non-invasive radiographs may be helpful, but an understanding of normal bone density for the species in question is required to make an accurate assessment.

Treatment of NSHP in amphibians is supportive. Calcium gluconate at a dose of 100 mg/kg PO, SQ, or ICe (Wright & Whitaker 2001b) and dietary correction is essential. Oral vitamin D3 is recommended to enhance the absorption of calcium from the gastrointestinal tract (Wright & Whitaker 2001b, Donoghue & Langenberg 1996). Patients with neurologic disease secondary to NSHP may require calcium gluconate 10% at 100 mg/kg ICe every four to six hours until signs resolve.

Nutritional Disorders: Hypovitaminosis A

Though NSHP may be the most commonly observed nutritional disease in amphibians, hypovitaminosis A may be the most underdiagnosed. Hypovitaminosis A is a common disease of captive amphibians (Pessier et al. 2002). This disease progresses in amphibians similar to that observed in reptiles with the hallmark histopathologic change of squamous metaplasia. Multiple organ systems may be affected and clinical signs may vary widely. Wright (2009) recommends vitamin A treatment for any clinically ill captive amphibian for which there is no clear diagnosis or clinical sign of disease. It is very likely that a myriad of health abnormalities and reproductive failures in captive amphibians are secondary to hypovitaminosis A.

Prevention of hypovitaminosis A is paramount as recovery of an individual or captive population of animals suspected of this disorder is challenging. Vitamin A enters the body dietarily primarily as pro-vitamin A carotenoids.

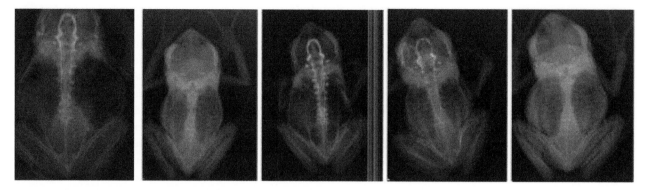

Figure 14.14 Radiographs of young Evergreen Toads, *Incilius coniferus* illustrating lack of bone mineralization. From L to R, images 2 and 5 are 6-month post-metamorphic cohorts denied supplemental calcium and fed only crickets.

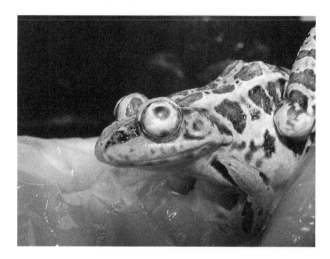

Figure 14.15 Lipid keratopathy in a Pickerel frog. This is a common presentation. (Courtesy of Dr. Sam Rivera.)

Three primary metabolites vitamin A (retinol, retinal, retinoic acid) are created and stored in the vertebrate body with retinol a cofactor in cell metabolism, retinal the chemical basis of vision, and retinoic acid modulating gene activation, gamete production, and embryo differentiation. The condition of hypovitaminosis A is the result of chronic total body depletion of these metabolites and full recovery may take months to a year with treatment. An overview of multiple health benefits of dietary carotenoid supplementation in the red-eye treefrog, *Agalychnis callidryas*, should serve as a model for dietary management of most captive insectivorous amphibians (Ogilvy et al. 2012). Richard Preziosi (pers. comm.) has further noted that gut-loading feeder insects with natural carotenoid-rich vegetables and fruits are as effective as commercially available vitamin supplements to achieve results in preventing hypovitaminosis A.

Historically treatment consisted of Aquasol A (retinol) 1 IU vitamin A/g body weight once daily for 2 weeks or until clinical signs resolve (Wright 2009). Because this medication is considered unavailable, compounded products have been applied, but inconsistency of formulation has been observed (E.V. Valdes, pers. comm.). Therefore, sourcing compounded retinol medications from reputable compounding pharmacies with high-level quality control is essential. The technician and veterinarian should also note that different from carotenoids, active metabolites of vitamin A have very narrow margins of safety and must be dosed accurately.

Nutritional Disorders: Lipid Keratopathy

Corneal lipidosis may be commonly confused with infectious or traumatic inflammatory disease and typically slowly progresses to eventually involve the cornea of one or both eyes. The author has observed this disorder clinically in primarily large treefrogs (*Litoria caerulea, Gastrotheca cornuta, Triprion spinosus*) which consume large insect (typically crickets) prey or occasionally pink mice in the pet industry. To date, this disorder is considered irreversible (Figure 14.15). Treatment is supportive and should be directed at reduction of dietary fat or cholesterol by altering prey item selection and reducing frequency of feeding (Wright 2009).

Nutritional Disorders: Spindly Leg Syndrome

A mysterious disease of newly metamorphosed frogs is called spindly leg disease or syndrome (SLS). With this abnormality tadpoles develop normal or nearly normal hind legs, yet the forelimbs either fail to erupt from the skin or are extremely thin and weak, almost as if there were only skin and bone with no muscle. This syndrome has been reported extensively among dendrobatid frogs. This high rate of occurrence may be due to the fact that these frogs are bred in captivity in such great numbers and therefore the chance for occurrence is greater. Frogs that metamorphose and leave the water usually fail to eat and die within days. SLS normally affects multiple metamorphic individuals in a single clutch and rarely is a single animal occurrence. SLS is a disease that must be prevented as there is no treatment for affected individuals with this disease process.

The potential causes for this syndrome are diet of the tadpole or parents, improper environmental conditions (water quality, temperature, lighting, etc.), genetics, toxins, and possibly chytridiomycosis. Camperio Ciani et al. (2018) demonstrated that water quality of the tadpoles may play a leading role in SLS development in the harlequin toad, *Atelopus glyphus*. Based on strong anecdotal evidence in poison dart frogs (Dendrobatidae) vitamin A levels of the female is suspected as a contributing factor. Several reputable U.S. and European dart frog breeders have observed that without a resting period away from breeding for several months, offspring of long-term breeding females would begin to manifest SLS and that the same females, once rested, would produce normal-limbed offspring. This suggests a possible etiology of total body reduction in vitamin A stores for this class of amphibians. A hypovitaminosis-derived cause for SLS is further supported by the molecular role of retinoic acid in embryonic limb bud development and differentiation in amphibians, birds, and mammals (Niaze 1996; Stratford et al. 1996; Power et al. 2000). There is no treatment for affected individuals with this disease process.

Parasitism

Intestinal parasitism is clinically widespread among terrestrial amphibians and somewhat less common among arboreal species. Amphibians are infected with a wide variety of protozoa and metazoan parasites. It is common that routine fecal exams of amphibians reveal these organisms in otherwise healthy patients. Some protozoans may not be pathogenic and may not require treatment. Some protozoan and many metazoan (nematodes, trematodes, and cestodes) parasites may inhabit amphibian tissues and remain in "balance" with the host with a competent immune system.

The onset of stress and subsequent immunosuppression that results from transport, poor diet, or inappropriate husbandry can rapidly lead to accelerated reproduction, migration, and infestation of these parasites. Similarly, the direct life cycle of many parasites only compounds the reinfection rate when the patient is subject to confinement in a terrarium. This is the likely cause for the apparent higher clinical prevalence of these parasites in terrestrial rather than arboreal species because there is greater likelihood for contact with the infective oocysts or larvae.

Intestinal parasites are best treated when diagnosed. Nevertheless, the client must be educated regarding the potential side effects of treatment. More commonly there is greater risk of death or debilitation from the host's immune response to sudden parasite death than from side effects of appropriately dosed medications. For very valuable animals, treatment of apparently healthy animals should be carefully weighed against the potential loss of the patient. When groups of animals are to be medicated, treatment of a few animals in the group is preferable to medicating the entire group at once.

The most important factor in breaking the life cycle of direct parasites is maintenance of the patient in an immaculately clean, well-maintained enclosure. Removal of all feces immediately after passage is imperative. Feeding of the patient should only be performed in an enclosure with no fecal contamination because food items may browse on contaminated surfaces and reinfect the host. Prophylactic treatment for intestinal parasites is discussed in the Quarantine section of Husbandry.

Protozoan parasites present both a diagnostic and treatment challenge. For suspected pathogenic *Trichomonas* spp. and *Entamoeba* spp. infections, metronidazole is indicated. Dose ranges for adults vary from 10 mg/kg PO every 24 h for seven to ten days for *Trichomonas* to 100 mg/kg PO every 14 days for *Entamoeba* (Poynton & Whitaker 2001). Metronidazole baths at 250 mg to 500 mg/L fresh water for 6–8 h once weekly are indicated for larval amphibians (Poynton & Whitaker 2001).

Coccidiosis is not uncommon in amphibians, yet its diagnosis is complicated by the fact that oocysts are intermittently shed in the feces. Thus, repeated fecal exams over protracted periods are required in some cases for definitive diagnosis. As seen in mammals, coccidiosis is primarily a clinical disease of the very young, very old, or immunosuppressed animal. Nevertheless, treatment is indicated upon diagnosis and consists of trimethoprim-sulfamethoxazole at 15 mg/kg PO daily for fourteen days (Poynton & Whitaker 2001). The dosage of TMS in exotic animals is based on the combined concentration of both the trimethoprim and sulfa medications.

Trematodes and cestodes have indirect life cycles in amphibians and interruption of the vector for reinfection is essential for treatment. Treatment consists of praziquantel at 8–14 mg/kg PO every 14 days for three or more treatments (Poynton & Whitaker 2001).

Nematodes are treated as described for lungworms (*Rhabdias* spp.) in the section on Respiratory System and Quarantine for prophylactic treatment. It may be difficult to specifically diagnose each species of nematode parasite on fecal exam, though the treatment for each is similar.

Parasites are not limited to the digestive tract in amphibians. A common respiratory pathogen is the lungworm (*Rhabdias* spp.). Though this nematode is diagnosed with moderate frequency among terrestrial frogs, clinical disease associated with the organism is infrequent. It is likely that the migration of larvae through host tissues and secondary invasion of bacteria with or without septicemia contributes greatly to debilitation of the patient.

Rhabdias spp. infection is diagnosed by demonstrating larvae on direct fecal examination or flotation or by cytology of a tracheal wash. Patients exhibiting apparent respiratory distress in association with *Rhabdias* spp. infection is best treated with anthelminthics concurrent with antibiotics such as enrofloxacin for secondary bacterial infections. Those patients that exhibit no active clinical disease are treated only with anthelminthics such as fenbendazole 100 mg/kg PO every 14 days for three treatments or ivermectin at 0.2–0.4 mg/kg PO or TO at the same rate of administration (Poynton & Whitaker 2001). The combination anthelminthic Drontal-plus (Bayer) contains praziquantel, fenbantel, and pyrantel. Drontal-plus can be compounded to a suspension of 2.27 mg/mL dosed at 5 mg/kg po q 14 days (Gagliardo et al. 2008). Because the life cycle of this infection (as well as other amphibian nematodal infections) is direct, isolation and strict hygiene are essential to reducing parasite burdens.

References to the use of ivermectin as a topical treatment for amphibian parasites are published (Panayotova-Pencheva 2016). The author advises great caution with amphibian treatments as there appears to be a great discrepancy of safety among species with the smallest amphibians being particularly susceptible to sudden death. Use of ivermectin is advised based on prior experience or well-documented published experiences with any given species.

Bloating

Bloating or body distention is one of the most nebulous clinical signs of disease and likely the most difficult to diagnose the underlying cause in the captive amphibian. As with excessive skin shedding, the underlying cause may be initiated by inflammation in the body. In addition to the inflammation caused by inappropriate water quality or infectious disease, mechanical obstruction of lymphatics, neoplasia, cardiovascular failure, renal failure, trauma, respiratory disease, and medication side effects are all potential causes for bloating. Unfortunately, many of the typical underlying causes of the imbalance result in permanent alteration of physiology or a cascade of physiologic changes from which the individual animal may never return to normal function or appearance.

The first step in determining a potential cause for bloating is to determine what exactly is causing the distention. The two types of distention are air and water. Though much less common, air distention may be a normal physiologic or behavioral defense tactic by some frogs. Generally, this state is not persistent and resolves once the initial threat is mitigated. Rupture of the lung or air sac may result in intracoelomic free air which the body cannot quickly eliminate. Though rare, this cause for bloating may carry the most favorable prognosis as treatment involves aspirating the free air and then allowing time for the tissue rupture to reseal. Determination of a cause of the air sac rupture must be made and appropriate treatment initiated.

Fluid is much more common than air for causing body distention in amphibians. There is no one cause of fluid distention that should be considered likely or common and each possibility must be systematically assessed when establishing a working diagnosis. When associated with profound weakness or non-responsiveness an infectious vasculitis (inflammation of lymphatic or cardiovascular system) should be suspected and appropriate antibacterial treatment should be initiated. Most animals with these clinical signs progress to death within hours and many do not survive even with appropriate therapy.

Fluid distention may be compartmentalized in one of several areas in the living amphibian. The first and possibly most common location is within the coelomic (body) cavity. Next is between the skin and body wall and this compartmentalization of fluid is most commonly associated with abnormality of the lymphatic system. Lastly, more localized distention may be caused by edema in which the fluid may be between fascial planes or between cells in the affected animal. Edema is more commonly associated with localized trauma or acute localized infection and may progress to a more widespread distention in time.

Despite the cause and location of fluid accumulation within the body of the living amphibian, there are very few treatable conditions from which the animal may be recovered to a normal physiologic state. Of these causes, infectious diseases caused by fungus or bacteria are the most likely scenarios in which medical treatment will be successful. The most common non-infectious cause is poor or inappropriate water quality. Recent histopathologic evaluation of bloated frogs has identified one potential associated disorder as a form of polycystic kidney disease (Pessier et al. 2014).

Water quality must always be ruled out as a cause for bloating in amphibians and should be highly suspected when multiple animals that are housed together or sourced with the same water become bloated. Though rarely diagnosed as a sole cause for bloating in clinical situations, some of the causes for bloating secondary to poor water quality are (1) sudden use of hypotonic water (such as distilled water) for housing amphibians, (2) sudden elevations of nitrogenous waste including especially ammonia and nitrites, (3) sudden elevations in pH.

It is typically not necessary or recommended to reduce bloating immediately in amphibians. Commonly, aggressive practices of "deflating" the affected animal by aspirating fluid or placing animals in hypertonic solutions are very detrimental to health. Removing a portion of retained fluid for diagnostic purposes is generally desired, but sudden removal of fluid may deplete the animal of osmotic proteins and other dissolved minerals or electrolytes. Soaking the animal in hypertonic solution typically does not directly "draw out" fluid retained in body cavities, but instead dehydrates the skin and cardiovascular fluids that likely will further physiologically compromise the animal.

The best initial treatment of the bloated patient is placement in a slightly drier than typical enclosure with isotonic fluids. Commonly a slightly moistened paper towel and hide box with good ventilation is adequate. If poor water quality is diagnosed as the most likely cause of the bloating, then this therapy and time may be all that is required for the animal to recover. If water quality is likely not the cause for the bloating, then a review of biosecurity and chytrid status of the patient are required. If the patient is further compromised by lethargy, inactivity, weakness, or skin irritation/ulceration then systemic antibiotic therapy must be initiated. Testing for chytrid infection must be concurrent with this treatment. If chytrid infection is known to be present within the collection, then initiating chytrid treatment is suggested.

The author has observed repeated seasonal fluid distention with one tropical toad species, *Incilius coniferus*, in a captive setting. Males appeared more affected, yet otherwise maintained normal health in all other aspects. There is suspicion that the natural history of this species in the wild may require seasonal dry periods and maintenance of these individuals in continual moist enclosures may lead to physiologic water retention. Extended periods of drying the animals has resulted in resolution of the fluid retention without any additional medical treatment.

For frogs that recover, a diagnosis of the initial cause is often not achieved. For those that are deceased, histopathology may assist in achieving a diagnosis, but commonly the exact cause of bloating may not be determined with just one specimen. These diagnoses are most commonly achieved over time with histopathologic study of a population of animals from the same or similar habitats.

Toxicity

Amphibians are quite sensitive to environmental contamination from both naturally occurring and synthetic toxins. These include ammonia, nitrites, nitrates, excessive salts, chlorine, organophosphates, pyrethrins and pyrethroids, and many solvents used in glues and sealants. It is imperative that any cleaning compounds used to disinfect enclosures or enclosure accessories be thoroughly rinsed, soaked, and dried prior to reintroduction into the enclosure. Diana et al. (2001) report toxicosis among dendrobatid frogs within enclosures that were misted by a newly constructed system composed of PVC pipes. Organic solvents from the pipe cement were found to be the cause of toxicosis. Similar attention must be observed with aquarium glass sealants.

Zoonoses

Amphibians are known to carry several bacteria which are potentially pathogenic to man and other animals. Though not infectious, certain amphibian toxins are potentially dangerous to man and domestic animals.

Bacteria such as *Listeria monocytogenes*, *Salmonella* spp., and *Yersinia enterocolitica* are all reported as isolated from the feces or digestive tracts of some amphibians (Taylor 2001). There is no link to clinical disease in man from these bacteria arising from amphibians. Care and common sense, however, must be exercised when handling amphibians regarding zoonotic potential. Human carelessness is often a contributing factor to zoonoses when related to exotic animals.

It is the responsibility of the veterinary clinician and technician to educate the client regarding proper handling of the amphibian pet to reduce the risk of potential exposure. The following are several guidelines that should be followed:

1. Do not handle amphibians unless absolutely necessary. Most (if not all) amphibians show no apparent health or quality of life benefit from human contact. In fact, stress may be increased as well as tissue trauma that may lead to an increased incidence of disease in the animal.
2. Never handle or clean amphibians, amphibian foods or food containers, or amphibian enclosures near a human food preparation area or human sanitation area such as a kitchen sink, kitchen table or countertop, bathroom sink, or bathtub.
3. Never allow children to handle amphibians without direct adult supervision and make sure that hands are washed immediately after handling.
4. Do not allow amphibians to remain loose or uncontained in a building intended for human occupation, sanitation, or food preparation.

Unfortunately, the above suggestions may seem to be common sense, but the breakthroughs in common sense are always reported in the popular press by relatively uneducated media professionals, implicating exotic animals in zoonotic disease. Without the responsible education of pet owners, there is a great risk of continued legislation prohibiting private possession of these animals.

Larval Amphibians

Tadpoles and larval salamanders face a variety of disorders that, for the most part, are never diagnosed or treated. Under controlled conditions with captive breeding the incidence of disease is relatively low, yet many may be susceptible to disease when stressed with substandard environmental conditions. There is tremendous variability in natural and cultural conditions of larval amphibians and some species demand exacting environmental parameters, while others are adapted to what might be considered nearly unsurvivable conditions.

For practical purposes, all larval caecilians and salamanders are carnivorous. Some caecilians are viviparous and consume oviductal secretions while developing in the adult female and are then born as juveniles. For salamanders, carnivory leads to cannibalism in crowded conditions, particularly as metamorphosis approaches. It is possible that the survival strategy of some communal pond-breeding salamanders depends on this strategy for a few animals to survive. In contrast, most frog larvae, tadpoles, are herbivorous. There are, however, a few notable exceptions. Though not commonly bred by hobbyists in captivity, horned frogs (*Ceratophrys* spp. and some other Leptodactylidae) have carnivorous, or more reputedly cannibalistic, tadpoles. Successful rearing of these tadpoles and larvae of other carnivorous species necessitates isolation into individual enclosures for each larva.

The most critical husbandry issue for larval amphibians is water quality. Understanding the natural history and reproductive strategy for a particular species is important for proper care of the tadpoles. Most dart frogs, for example, lay eggs out of water on leaves, in leaf axils, or on flat surfaces near the ground. After hatching, the tadpoles are then transferred to a suitable water area that is generally a small plant with water supplied only from rain. For these species in captivity, elaborate filtration and moving or constantly filtered water is not essential for survival and metamorphosis. Aged tap water or spring water changed periodically generally yields success.

Species that lay eggs above streams or have tadpoles that inhabit moving water usually require some water oxygenation or filtration for survival. Some of these species, such as many larger Central and South American hylids, feed on particulates suspended in the water and require the water movement to supply a constant source of food. Many of these species rapidly perish if maintained in still or stagnant water.

Feeding of larval amphibians, particularly tadpoles, is not difficult in most cases. An exceptional food for larval herbivorous dendrobatids is spirulina powder (Earthrise Co., Petaluma, CA) which is available from most health food stores. The author has raised many generations of various species of dendrobatids and *Mantella* spp. tadpoles on this diet with absolutely no developmental abnormalities. Overfeeding must be avoided, however. Water quality deteriorates rapidly without filtration and death is rapid. Many dendrobatids and possibly other frog species give parental care to tadpoles in the form of "feeder eggs." Information on these species is available in many hobbyist texts.

Larval salamanders can be problematic in that many species in early development require live foods. Daphnia, gammarus (fairy shrimp), and other small crustaceans must be cultured or made readily available. Wild collection of these food items is not recommended, because this is commonly a source for infection with the trematode *Gyrodactylus spp.*, the body fluke. These microscopic parasites can be rapidly fatal to larvae and may be the inciting cause of cutaneous ulcers in adults. Treatment may be accomplished with dilute salt or formaldehyde baths (1.5 mL of 10% formalin in 1-L water for 10 min) and survivability is good with early diagnosis. The amphibians undergoing treatment must be watched very closely and removed to freshwater at the first sign of distress in formalin. Dipping the infected animals into the treatment solution within a net is the most practical method for rapid removal.

Larval amphibians are subject to the same bacterial and fungal infections as adults. Treatment is with medicated baths rather than by individual dosing. Diagnosis of a specific infection is usually obtained by sacrificing one or more larvae from a group for bacteriologic or microscopic analysis.

History, Restraint and Physical Examination

History

A complete and accurate history of the amphibian patient may be the most important procedure in developing a diagnosis of disease (or health). Unfortunately, amphibian patients are commonly presented moribund or altered from the original onset of clinical signs, making it difficult to diagnose the underlying etiology based on physical exam. Similarly, the clinician may be presented with a deceased patient from a group of animals and a diagnosis may be required to develop a treatment plan for the remaining group of apparently healthy individuals. Additionally, when gaining new clients who own amphibians (and reptiles), much time is spent in phone conversations with clients who are reluctant to bring the patient into the clinic. Though there is little substitute for a physical exam of the patient, there is even less substitute for not having patience with a potential first time client.

The first step in obtaining an accurate history is identification of the correct scientific name of the patient to at least the genus (and preferably to species) level. It may be difficult to obtain natural history information based on common or colloquial names. Identification to the subspecies level (many salamanders) or the variety level (many Dendrobatidae) is not important for developing a history and diagnosis.

Establish the origin of the patient; is it captive-born or wild-caught and imported? This information is particularly important for amphibians because the likelihood of acclimation to a captive environment and the potential pathogens in wild-caught animals must be considered. The client may not know this history, particularly if the animal was purchased at a pet store or reptile and amphibian trade show or swap meet. One characteristic of captive-born amphibians includes juvenile age or relatively young animals when obtained by the client. Imported animals are usually adults because they are more frequently captured in the wild and more likely to survive shipping. Today certain species of frogs are almost exclusively captive-born. Many salamanders and most caecilians are wild-caught.

A particularly important question of the client is the medical history of the patient; has the patient been treated at home prior to or following the client's possession of the patient? Has the patient received treatment from another veterinarian? Home treatment of exotic pets, particularly reptiles and amphibians, is common. Occasionally results are favorable with home treatment, but more commonly the clinical condition fails to respond or deteriorates.

All husbandry parameters should be fully investigated. Descriptions of the enclosure, substrate, accessories, cage mates, feeding schedule, and environmental conditions of both the enclosure and the room housing the enclosure are important. When multiple individuals or species of amphibians are housed together, the client should be questioned regarding the health of these animals as well as any quarantine procedures that were performed.

The exact nutrition (which food items are consumed) of the captive amphibian is generally not as much of a clinical concern as whether or not the patient is actually eating.

With respect to food items offered, particularly insects, it is important to learn the size of insect that is fed and the timing of the feedings. Also, ask the client if the patient is observed to actually eat the food items or if the food simply disappears from the cage. Many times insects may escape or hide beneath cage ornaments, leading the client to believe that the insects were consumed. This is particularly true of nocturnal amphibians. Question the client regarding food supplements such as vitamin/mineral powders and frequency of application. For aquatic amphibians, it is important to know the exact food items offered (live or processed). Many captive amphibians refuse prepared diets such as pellets initially and must be fed live food.

Restraint

The primary consideration when restraining an amphibian is stress on the patient and the potential health consequences of handling. The patient should be touched or restrained only when absolutely necessary. All diagnostic tests or treatments should be prepared prior to handling to consolidate procedures into the fewest episodes of physical manipulation of the patient. Consideration must also be given to the safety of the handler. Some species are capable of producing toxic skin secretions that are irritating and noxious, but rarely lethal to humans.

The following species when known to be wild-collected should be handled with extreme caution: golden poison frog (*Phyllobates terribilis*), black-legged poison frog (*Phyllobates bicolor*), Colorado River toad (*Incilius alvarius*), and marine toad (*Rhinella marina*). It is unlikely that either of the poison frogs listed will ever be seen in practice as wild-caught individuals because they are relatively inaccessible for collection and exportation from Colombia, and both species are now widely available as captive-born juveniles and adults. Captive-born dart frogs have greatly reduced skin toxins and are generally not toxic to humans (Daly et al. 1994). Nevertheless, an imported *Phyllobates terribilis* should be considered lethal to humans. The toxins of *P. bicolor* are only 1/50 the strength of *P. terribilis*, yet a wild-caught frog should be considered dangerous (Walls 1994).

The toads of the family Bufonidae are a concern not as much for their degree of toxicity, which is significant, but for the manner in which the toxin may be secreted. Both species are capable of ejecting copious amounts of toxin from the parotid glands. Reports exist of this toxin spraying six feet or more from the animal (Wright & Whitaker 2001d). Entry of the toxin into an unprotected eye can be serious, not just from the standpoint of direct physical irritation, but also from absorption and systemic effects. All larger Bufonids and all wild-caught dart frogs are best handled with powder-free latex gloves. Additionally, protective eyewear is recommended when handling or manipulating larger toad species.

When possible, amphibians are best observed in a clear enclosure such as a plastic shoebox, deli cup, plastic bag, or other small enclosure. Handling of all amphibians is performed with a powder-free exam glove that has been cleaned, rinsed, or moistened with distilled water. Small frogs are best restrained with the hind legs extended and held securely between the thumb and index finger. This frees the head, body, and front legs for examination or treatment, yet adequately prevents jumping or escape attempts. Larger frogs and toads may require support from two hands to the body between the front and hind legs. Medium to large salamanders are restrained with a delicate grip of the fist, allowing the head to protrude between thumb and index finger and the tail exiting at the little finger. As in lizards, tail autotomy is possible for many species of salamanders. Most adult anguiform amphibians (caecilians, amphiumas, and sirens) are nearly impossible to restrain manually and are best examined in an aquarium or chemically restrained (see Anesthesia).

Physical Examination

As with all exotic animals, the most important physical observations of the patient are made without handling. With the exception of some frogs and in contrast to most turtles, lizards, and snakes, the posture of amphibians is not as significant in revealing clinical disease. This is due to the fact that many species are nocturnal and cryptic, preferring to remain inactive or burrowed during the day. Species in which posture is generally significant are the dendrobatids, atelopids, mantellids, perching hylids such as *Phyllomedusa* spp., and most newts. Activity of the patient may be significant for some species. During a daytime examination, all of the previously mentioned species (with the exception of hylids) should be bright, alert, and responsive. In contrast, nocturnal species such as hylids, some toads, ranids, and salamanders are generally inactive. A common indication of poor health in hylids, typically nocturnal, is activity during daylight hours. Red-eyed treefrogs, for example, generally rest on the sides of the enclosure with eyelids shut in daylight. Aquatic amphibians, though generally nocturnal, are generally active in the enclosure on presentation. Exceptions may include some aquatic or large semiaquatic frogs that, by nature, typically are not very active foragers and prefer to wait and ambush prey.

Observing the feeding response of diurnally active amphibians is a practical method to assess overall health. A failure to respond to the proper food item is generally a sign of illness or stress. Nocturnal or shy animals, however, rarely feed upon observation in daylight hours.

With a basic understanding of normal anatomy and body condition of the species in question, the visual exam should first focus on body condition. Is the patient normal weight, underweight, overweight, or bloated? It is important to remember that some frogs will inflate with air as a defense mechanism and may appear bloated, but suffer from no abnormal physiology. Air inflation is not a physiologic adaptation of salamanders and caecilians. As with other animals, emaciation does not occur in hours or days, but in weeks or months. Even the smallest frogs have distinct muscle groups that reveal weight loss. Poison dart frogs, for example, exhibit emaciation particularly on the back, scapulas, and pelvis.

Observe the cloaca for prolapse. This abnormality may remain unnoticed by the client. Also, observe a fresh stool sample. For most terrestrial amphibians, the feces are ejected as a pellet and should be somewhat moist and dark brown in color. Abnormalities in color and consistency may be significant. A microscopic fecal exam is essential for all captive-born and imported amphibians.

Abnormalities in respiratory effort can be difficult to detect in terrestrial amphibians. Normal respiration is driven primarily by buccal or gular pumping rather than by diaphragmatic or intercostal muscle contraction. There is rarely a noticeable variation in this rhythmic pumping motion, even in diseased animals. Bubbling from the mouth or nostrils in terrestrial amphibians, however, is abnormal and a possible clinical sign of respiratory disease.

Abnormality of the integument is one of the more common abnormal physical findings and a common presenting complaint for diseased amphibians. Understanding the natural history and normal characteristics of the integument for a given species is essential. Most toads, terrestrial newts, and some tree frogs have relatively dry skin. Many larger tree frogs such as *Phyllomedusa* spp. and *Litoria* spp. can produce waxy secretions to prevent dessication. Amphibians slough skin, ecdysis, throughout their lives, and this process should not be confused with disease. Coloration varies widely, particularly in frogs, and with many this coloration is bilaterally symmetrical. Even cryptic amphibians exhibit some color and pattern symmetry; therefore, observe closely for abnormalities in symmetry of color, texture, and morphology. Amphibians typically do not exhibit color-changing ability as seen in some lizards, though variation will occur from day to night in many hylids. Ulcers, erosions, plaques, and crusts are not normal. Newly acquired or recently imported frogs are susceptible to rostral abrasions that may rapidly progress into necrotizing ulcerations.

Most salamanders and terrestrial frogs have closable eyelids and frogs possess a nictitating membrane that is semitransparent. When awake and alert the amphibian eye should have eyelids open and clear corneas. Iris coloration is variable among amphibians but is always bilaterally symmetrical. As with mammals, unilateral ocular changes are most suggestive of trauma or focal disease and bilateral ophthalmic abnormalities are more suggestive of systemic disease. Iris vasculature may be apparent in the normal amphibian eye. There is great variation in pupil structure from circular to horizontally and vertically elliptic. An ophthalmoscope illuminator or slit lamp is helpful for examination of the eye. Commonly used mammalian mydriatics such as atropine and proparacaine are not effective in dilating the amphibian eye. Wright (2001b) recommends the combination of D-tubocurarine and benzalkonium chloride applied topically for mydriasis (Whitaker 2001).

An oral exam requires physical or chemical restraint in most species. Some species of frog, *Ceratophrys* and *Hemiphractus* spp., are known to gape as a defensive tactic, making oral examination possible without restraint on occasion. Similarly, some larger terrestrial salamanders (*Ambystoma* spp., *Dicamptodon* spp.), particularly those maintained long-term in captivity, may exhibit a conditioned feeding response and can be coaxed into biting a soft speculum to examine the mouth. Though it is not recommended as normal practice, these animals, when routinely hand-fed, will bite fingers waved in front of the face. It is unlikely that any injury will result to a human from the bite of an ambystomatid salamander. Large frogs (*Ceratophrys*, *Pyxicephalus*) and large aquatic salamanders (*Amphiuma*, Siren, *Cryptobranchus*) are capable of painful bites to humans. These species generally require chemical restraint for both physical restraint and oral examination.

The clinician and technician should be aware that mandibular bones of many small amphibians are easily fractured with improper or forceful techniques to open the mouth. When properly restrained, the mouth of many smaller amphibians may be opened with a variety of apparatus such as plastic cards, laminated paper, coverslips, and small rubber spatulas. Nearly all amphibians will resist the oral exam if not sedated. Observe for uniformity and symmetry in shape and coloration of the oral mucosa and the tongue. Occasionally parasites such as flukes and leeches may be observed attached to the oral mucosa (Figure 14.16A and B).

Palpation is easily accomplished for larger amphibians but should generally be avoided in smaller species to prevent iatrogenic trauma. Internal organs of the smallest species may be evaluated by transillumination of the patient through a clear plastic container. This process is ineffective for large or dark-pigmented patients. The heart, liver, spleen, gonads, and some vasculature may be observed in this manner. Palpation of larger species may reveal abnormalities such as foreign bodies and calculi, though normal structures may be difficult to assess or identify.

The heartbeat may be visible as pulsations of the skin in the region of the xiphoid on the ventral thorax in some amphibians. Similarly, in some frogs, pulsation of the lymphatic hearts is occasionally observed lateral to the urostyle. Cardiac auscultation is possible in larger amphibians, though the clinical significance of this procedure during wellness exams is questionable.

Radiology

As with reptiles, radiology is valuable in the diagnosis of some amphibian diseases. This imaging is particularly useful for the diagnosis of skeletal disorders, urinary tract calculi, tissue mineralization, pulmonary disease, gastrointestinal foreign bodies, and other gastrointestinal disease with the aid of contrast materials. Unless an abnormality is present, it is generally not possible to clearly differentiate coelomic cavity structures radiographically in amphibians.

Techniques for radiographic exposure are similar to those described for reptiles. Because of the small size of most amphibians, a table-top exposure with detail cassettes yields the best quality image. Generally, an exposure setting consistent with the lowest mammalian extremity setting is sufficient, though with smaller patients overexposure is still possible. For technician safety, the use of a collimator to achieve the smallest exposure field is essential. With this technique, multiple exposures are possible on a single cassette.

Restraint of the amphibian patient during radiology is a hands-off affair. Many frogs will sit briefly directly on the cassette for exposure. For those who are reluctant to remain still, placement of the patient in a plastic bag facilitates restraint and manipulation for proper exposure (Stetter 2001a). When possible, a lateral and dorsoventral exposure should be made of every patient imaged. This typically requires the movement of the radiographic beam into a horizontal beam projection as the patient sits on the tabletop or platform (Figures 14.17–14.19).

Contrast studies are easily performed in amphibians. Barium sulfate is the contrast medium of choice and is given orally via a rubber catheter or feeding tube. The dosage varies greatly based on the size of amphibian. A range of 10–15 mL/kg PO is generally sufficient, though the technician should approximate the volume of the calculated dose to the patient's body size and adjust accordingly.

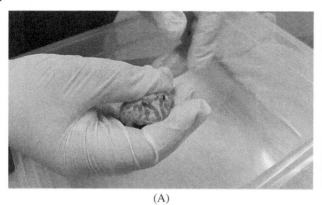

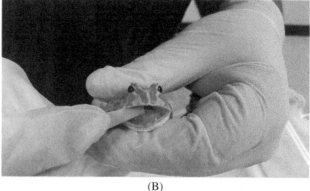

(A)

(B)

Figure 14.16 (A) Physical examination of an albino pacman frog (*Ceratophrys cranwelli*). (B) Oral exam. The blue object is the fingernail pick that comes with surgical scrub brushes. It works great as an atraumatic mouth opener for amphibians and reptiles. (Courtesy of Dr. Stacey Wilkinson.)

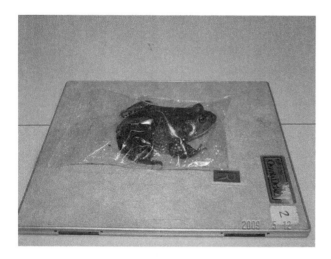

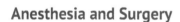

Figure 14.17 A plastic bag used for temporary restraint of a bullfrog (*Rana* catesbeiana) for radiographs. (Courtesy of Dr. Sam Rivera.)

Percloacal barium administration is also performed for suspected colonic foreign bodies, strictures, or other disease. Great care must be used when manipulating catheters with these tissues to prevent iatrogenic trauma.

Ultrasound can also be used to diagnose disease in amphibians. It is particularly useful in evaluating celomic structures (Figure 14.20).

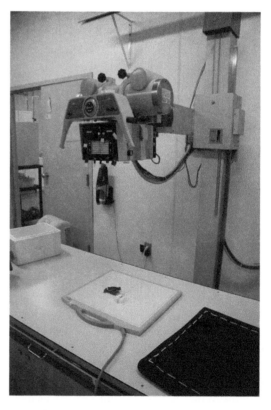

Figure 14.18 Radiograph being taken of a Puerto Rican Crested Toad. (Courtesy of Sandy Skeba, LVMT.)

Anesthesia and Surgery

Anesthesia

Anesthesia for amphibians is useful for physical examination of aggressive or reluctantly restrained patients, certain diagnostic and therapeutic procedures, and surgery. Reports exist for the use of injectable anesthetics in amphibians, though current consensus regards these medications as impractical and ineffective for safe chemical restraint. The anesthetic of choice for amphibians is tricaine methanesulfonate (Syncaine: Syndel USA, Ferndale, WA; formerly: MS-222/tricaine-S/FINQUEL,) (Wright 2001f). It is a white crystalline powder that may be mixed with water to anesthetize fish and amphibians. Amphibians are immersed in a bath of tricaine methanesulfonate until anesthesia is achieved and then maintained

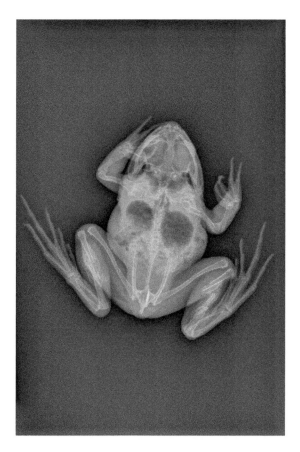

Figure 14.19 Radiograph of a bullfrog (*Rana catesbeiana*. Note the bilateral tibiofibular healing fractures). (Courtesy of Dr. Sam Rivera.)

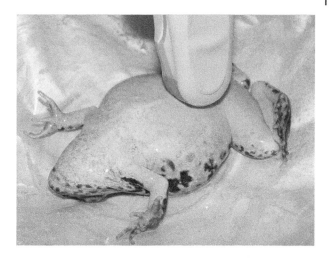

Figure 14.20 Coelomic ultrasound in an anesthetized Pickeral frog. (Courtesy of Dr. Sam Rivera.)

in fresh water for the particular procedure to be performed. For longer procedures, the patient may be immersed in a 50% dilution of the original induction solution or intubated and maintained on isoflurane.

Preparation of tricaine solution is described in the package insert with product. Because tricaine is quite acidic, the solution must be buffered to a pH of 7–7.4, which is the physiologic range of amphibian tissue. This is accomplished with either sodium biphosphate (Na_2HPO_4) or sodium bicarbonate (Na_2CO_3). Tricaine is not stable in water when exposed to light. Therefore, unless multiple anesthesia episodes are planned, they should be mixed only in the quantity desired for a single anesthetic episode. Generally, a 1-L solution is adequate. All dissolved tricaine should be discarded after use and not reused for other patients.

Standard instructions for mixing tricaine can be somewhat confusing. A simplistic, safe, and effective method is to mix equal parts by volume of tricaine and baking soda into the desired solution for anesthesia. The author commonly uses ½ teaspoon tricaine (equivalent of 1 g) plus ½ teaspoon baking soda into 1 L 0.6% NaCl as the standard

anesthetic bath for most adult terrestrial amphibians. This solution is used directly and there is no stock solution to add to more confusion. About 0.6% NaCl solution may be easily mixed in the clinic by diluting a 1L bag of 0.9% NaCl which is isotonic for most amphibians as opposed to distilled water. Loss of the righting reflex and lack of voluntary movement is an indication of adequate induction. Loss of the withdrawal or deep pain reflex indicates surgical anesthesia.

The patient is then transferred out of the induction chamber onto a treatment pan or receptacle and maintained in clean fresh distilled water or a 50% dilution of tricaine (0.05%) for the duration of the procedure (Wright 2001f). The patient's nostrils and mouth must be maintained above the water level to prevent aspiration. At this time, for longer surgical procedures, large amphibians may be intubated and maintained on oxygen (with or without isoflurane) with intermittent positive pressure ventilation (IPPV). Continued exposure to the 0.05% tricaine bath maintains adequate anesthesia in the absence of isoflurane.

The patient should be monitored for heartbeat throughout the anesthetic procedure. Respiration is reduced or nearly absent and oxygenation of the tricaine bath with oxygen is recommended to enhance oxygen absorption through the skin. The patient is recovered from tricaine anesthesia in clean 0.9% NaCl water, making sure that the nostrils and mouth are not underwater to prevent aspiration. The recovery period may range from thirty to sixty minutes.

An additional anesthetic protocol is the topical application of liquid isoflurane. A mixture of 3 cc liquid isoflurane with 1.5 cc water and 3.5 cc KY-Jelly is made in a 10-cc syringe and shaken. The resulting liquid is then applied to the back of the patient at a dose of 0.025–0.035 cc/g body weight. The lower dose is applied to frogs and salamanders and the higher dose is for toads. The patient is induced in a sealed container over 5–15 min. Following induction, the remaining gel is wiped from the skin and anesthesia will last for 45–80 min. Though effective, the author finds that isoflurane is quite irritating to the skin of most amphibians and does not recommend its use unless absolutely necessary.

Surgery

Though surgical procedures on amphibians are not routine, several pathologic conditions may require surgical treatment. Celiotomy, mass removal, and limb amputation are the most commonly performed procedures (Figure 14.21). Other procedures include enucleation and orthopedic surgery. All invasive surgical procedures are performed with general anesthesia using tricaine or isoflurane. Pre- and post-surgical administration of antibiotics are recommended for invasive procedures.

The amphibian skin is prepped using 0.2% chlorhexidine (Wright 2001f) or 0.2% chloroxylenol diluted to 0.75% with water. Isopropyl alcohol and iodine compounds are potentially toxic to amphibians and should be avoided. The surgical prep should have as long a contact time as possible prior to surgery, preferably ten minutes. The surgical site should be moistened with saline prior to draping and surgery. Depending on the procedure, draping may not be performed. For celiotomy, sterile clear plastic drape is applied. Peripheral to the plastic drape a sterile cloth drape may be used to maintain a sterile field for surgical instruments.

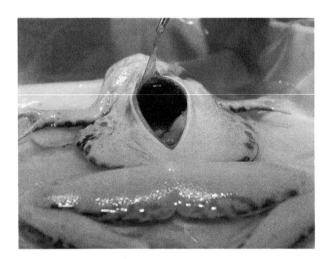

Figure 14.21 Coelotomy to remove a mass in a Pickeral frog. (Courtesy of Dr. Sam Rivera.)

As with lizards, a paramedian ventral midline incision is recommended to avoid the large ventral abdominal vein that lies on the ventral serosal surface of the coelomic cavity. Closure of surgical incisions is accomplished with non-absorbable monofilament sutures of appropriate size.

Techniques

Venipuncture

Blood collection in amphibians can be a challenge, yet in some species, with proper technique and anatomical knowledge, the task is routine. Prior to sampling the skin should be prepped with diluted 2% chlorhexidine or 2% chloroxylenol at a 1:40 dilution (Wright 2001f). Alcohol should not be used because of irritation and dessication to the patient. Sampling from salamanders is performed from the ventral tail vein as described for snakes and lizards. A 1-cc or smaller syringe with a 25- or 27-gauge needle is ideal for most amphibians and the sample is preserved in lithium heparin.

Phlebotomy in frogs and toads is performed from a variety of locations. In larger frogs and toads, the ventral abdominal vein is the best choice for both quality and quantity of the blood sample. Sampling from this vein is performed in the same manner as described for lizards (Figures 14.22–14.24). Because the lymphatic system of amphibians courses parallel to the blood vessels, it is not uncommon to collect lymphatic fluids with peripheral blood. Other sites of blood collection that are generally accessible in large frogs include the femoral vein and the lingual vein located on the ventral surface of the tongue. The volume of blood collected should be no more than 1% of the patient's body weight or 0.5% from a debilitated patient (Wright 2001f).

Celiocentesis

This technique is performed to analyze fluid retained in the coelomic cavity of amphibians. It may be both diagnostic and therapeutic. Fluid may accumulate in the coelom secondary to cardiac, renal, hepatic, or other osmotic imbalances. Similar to phlebotomy, a 25- or 27-gauge needle on a 1- to 3-cc syringe is ideal. The sample site is prepped with a 1:40 dilution of 2% chlorhexidine or chloroxylenol. The preferred collection site is from the mid-lateral flank or mid-ventral coelomic cavity. The syringe should fill with fluid on gentle aspiration and forceful aspiration should be avoided to prevent damage to delicate internal organs. Fluid may be smeared immediately or submitted in lithium heparin for cellular and chemical analysis.

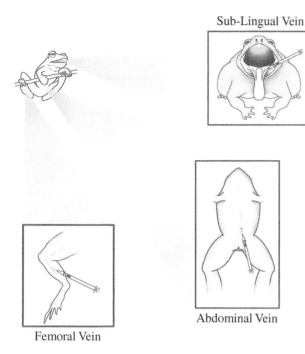

Sub-Lingual Vein

Abdominal Vein

Femoral Vein

Figure 14.22 Venipuncture sites in a frog. (Drawing by Scott Stark.)

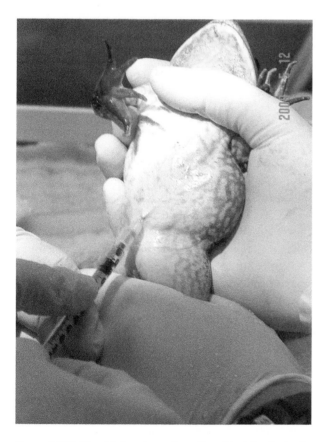

Figure 14.23 Blood being drawn from the mid-abdominal vein of a bullfrog. (Courtesy of Dr. Sam Rivera.)

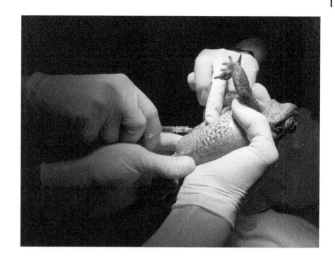

Figure 14.24 Blood draw in a Marine toad (*Rhinella marina*). (Courtesy of Sandy Skeba, LVMT.)

Fecal Examination

A fecal exam is one diagnostic test that can be performed in all terrestrial amphibians and nearly all aquatic amphibians with relative ease. Collection of feces is facilitated particularly well during quarantine. The amphibian is maintained on paper towel in a clean cage such as a plastic shoebox or storage container that is adequately ventilated and a sample is collected.

The sample should be examined directly in 0.9% saline and by fecal floatation with standard commercially available fecal flotation solutions. Common parasite ova include nematodes, trematodes, coccidia, various protozoans, and lungworm larvae (see Parasitology).

Cloacal Wash

Cloacal wash is performed in larger amphibians (>5 cm) to collect fecal material for microscopic analysis when a fresh stool sample is unavailable for analysis. A lubricated semi-rigid plastic or rubber catheter attached to a 1-mL syringe is gently inserted into the cloaca and isotonic saline (0.6%) is infused from and retrieved into the syringe. The fluid volume may be between 0.5 and 1 mL and not all fluid will be retrieved. A portion of the sample is then viewed with a microscope for pathogens. For smaller amphibians, (<5 cm) cloacal wash is generally too traumatic to attempt. Examination of fecal samples is recommended for these species.

Transtracheal Wash

The techniques for tracheal wash are identical to those in other terrestrial vertebrates. The patient must be anesthetized (see Anesthesia and Surgery) and delicate handling of the tissues and apparatus must be performed. A sterile tomcat or small gauge mammalian intravenous catheter may be inserted into the glottis on the floor of the mouth. Depending on patient size, 0.25–0.5 cc sterile isotonic (0.6%) saline is infused and gently retrieved.

The sample may then be smeared and stained for microscopic analysis.

Skin Scrape and Impression Smear

These processes are designed to identify fungal, bacterial, and protozoal elements to the skin or wounds on the skin. An impression smear is performed when tissue is damaged or ulcerated and a scraping will only create further trauma. Shed skins are particularly helpful for microscopic analysis and may be fixed in formalin for histopathologic staining to identify certain bacterial and fungal pathogens. A skin scraping is performed with the edge of a coverslip and wet mount examination.

Assist Feeding

Assist feeding is required for amphibians who are diseased and unable or unwilling to voluntarily feed. It is important that the owner understand that this procedure may be stressful on the patient and debilitated patients may not survive repeated handling; nevertheless, this may also be a lifesaving procedure designed to return the patient to a normal feeding response. Wright and Whitaker (2001d) list the standard metabolic rates (SMR) for caecilians, salamanders, and frogs at temperatures ranging from 5°C to 25°C and they recommend that caloric intake for diseased animals should exceed the SMR by 50% on a daily basis.

An ideal feeding formula for amphibians is Oxbow Critical Care Carnivore (Oxbow Animal Health, Omaha, NE). This liquid product is easy to administer through a small to medium bore feeding tube and provides nutrients and calories evenly in suspension. The patient's normal food items are provided daily under observation to assess for a return to normal feeding. Assist feedings are not made daily to reduce handling. Instead, the calculated daily dose may be multiplied by the number of days between feedings (three, five, etc.), and the total dose for those days is administered at one time.

The feeding procedure is accomplished in a manner similar to that of reptiles. A red rubber catheter, intravenous catheter, tomcat catheter, or ball-tipped feeding needle is passed into the stomach and the food preparation is infused. The technician should be aware that the stomach of most amphibians (especially frogs) is relatively proximal in the coelom; thus, passage of the tube no more than one-third to one-half of the patient's body length (excluding the tail) is recommended.

An alternative to Carnivore Care is a mashed or ground mixture of invertebrates such as fruit flies or crickets administered in the same manner. The author has had great success with anorectic dart frogs using this technique on an every 72 h basis. Several patients have required 2 weeks or more of assist feeding before feeding voluntarily.

Therapeutic Administration

Amphibians present fewer problems than one may expect with medications. The semipermeable skin enables the clinician to apply some medications topically (TO) for systemic absorption, a technique not applicable to reptiles. Additionally, medicated baths may be used to treat both cutaneous and systemic diseases. Oral (PO) administration is possible and standard for some medications such as deworming agents and antibiotics. Finally, injections may be given intramuscularly (IM) or intracoelomically (ICe) in large amphibians or subcutaneously (SC) in frogs and some salamanders. Intravenous (IV) administration is rare and difficult at best in all but the largest amphibians. Physical restraint of the patient is required for all but the topical route of therapeutic administration.

The application of injectable medications in a topical manner is very practical for amphibians with permeable skin. This method likely results in lower percutaneous absorption rates in toads or in species that produce a waxy skin coating. Antibiotics such as enrofloxacin and ivermectin have been applied topically with great success for various bacterial and parasitic diseases. Baths with medications such as gentamicin, nitrofurazone, itraconazole, sulfamethazine, metronidazole, and other medications have shown success and safety in combating various diseases.

Oral administration is possible in nearly all sizes of amphibians and is the preferred route of treatment when possible, to achieve maximum systemic absorption. This route is contraindicated in those species that are refractory to handling or physical manipulation. Metal feeding tubes or rubber catheters are used in large animals and microliter pipettes are used for small patients. Dilution of the commercially available preparations or compounding of medications is required for smaller amphibians. Dosing for most oral medications is daily or less often depending on the drug.

Injections are possible in amphibians but carry moderate risk of trauma to muscles or internal organs and may result in chemical trauma or excessive pain and disability at the injection site. Many injectable medications applied orally in amphibians show good systemic absorption. This is particularly true of enrofloxacin which may be otherwise irritating to amphibian skin and may cause skin irritation, discoloration, or sloughing from topical administration or injection. The intracoelomic route is preferred for fluid administration in critically ill or dehydrated amphibians. The method of injection is similar to that of celiocentesis.

A considerable benefit to choosing the topical route for medicating the patient is allowing the client to treat at home for non-critical cases. All other routes of administration require hospitalization or repeated visits to the clinic for treatment by the technician or clinician. Medications should be dispensed in individual syringes with the appropriate amount for each dose drawn up and ready to apply. This negates the possibility of inappropriate dosing by the client. The client should return the used syringes for disposal at the end of the treatment period to allow both a recheck of the patient and to assess compliance of therapeutic administration.

An important fact regarding amphibian disease is that pharmaceuticals are not required to treat or cure every disease. It cannot be overemphasized that diseases resulting from improper husbandry comprise a substantial percentage of presenting complaints with amphibians and reptiles. The number one consideration when choosing pharmaceuticals for disease management is side effects. Though it may be difficult for the client to appreciate that environmental manipulation alone can correct improper health, it is even more difficult to understand further debilitation caused by unnecessary treatment.

Euthanasia

Invariably treatments fail to gain a response or patients are too debilitated to withstand treatment and the client elects euthanasia. Amphibians and reptiles can pose some problems with euthanasia in that the heart may continue to beat for some time after neurologic incapacitation or death has occurred.

Reducing patient suffering and pain and client discomfort with the euthanasia process may be difficult. If possible, the patient may be sedated with one of several anesthetic agents prior to administering euthanasia injections. Ketamine at a dose of 100 mg/kg IM or telazol (tiletamine–zolazepam) at a dose of 10 mg/kg IM (Wright 2001f) is sufficient to achieve sedation for euthanasia. The clinician and technician should understand that both of these injections are likely to cause pain and discomfort to the patient at the injection site. Alternatively, tricaine (Syncaine) may be used as a pre-euthanasia sedative or if overdosed as a euthanasia solution (Wright & Whitaker 2001b).

Administration of a barbiturate euthanasia solution such as pentobarbital at a dose of 100 mg/kg intracardiac (if possible) results in instant death. Alternatively, the injection may be given intracoelomically or intracranially through the foramen magnum, though cardiac death may be delayed.

If histopathology is required of the patient, then minimizing trauma to vital organs is essential. In this case, an overdose of tricaine given intracoelomically or immersion of the sedated patient in 20% ethanol will result in death (Wright & Whitaker 2001d). Most importantly, clients should be informed of the euthanasia alternatives and fully understand the procedure to be performed if they wish to be present during the euthanasia process.

References

AmphibiaWeb. 2021. *Amphibian species by the numbers* amphibiaweb.org/amphibian/speciesnums.html.

Baines M, Dale J, Garrick D, Gill I, Goetz M, Skelton T, Swatman M. 2016. How much UVB does my reptile need? The UV-Tool, a guide to the selection of UV lighting for reptiles and amphibians in captivity. *J Zoo Aquarium Res* 4(1): 42–63.

Barnett SL. 1996. The husbandry of poison-dart frogs (Family Dendrobatidae). *Proc Assoc Amph Rept Vet* 1–6.

Barnett SL, et al. 2001. Amphibian husbandry and housing. In: *Amphibian Medicine and Captive Husbandry* (eds KM Wright, BR Whitaker). Malabar, FL: Krieger Publishing Co.

Berger L, et al. 1998. Chytridiomycosis causes amphibian mortality associated with population declines in the rain forests of Australia and Central America. *Proc Natl Acad Sci USA* 95: 9031–9036.

Browne RK, Verschooren E, Antwis RE, Vercaammen F. 2009. UV-B, vitamin D3, and amphibian health and behaviour. *Ark Sci Res* Retrieved from http://www.amphibianark.org/research/Amphibian-UV-B-and-vitamin-D3.pdf.

Camperio Ciani JF, Guerrel J, Baitchman E, Diaz R, Evans M, Ibáñez R, et al. 2018. The relationship between spindly leg syndrome incidence and water composition, overfeeding, and diet in newly metamorphosed harlequin frogs (*Atelopus* spp.). *PLoS One* 13(10).

Daly JW, et al. 1994. Dietary source for skin alkaloids of poison frogs (Dendrobatidae)? *J Chem Ecol* 20(4): 943–98.

Daszak P, et al. 2000. Emerging infectious diseases of wildlife—threats to biodiversity and human health. *Am Assoc Adv Sci* 287: 443–449.

DeLuca HF. 2004. Overview of general physiologic features and functions of vitamin D. *Am J Clin Nutr* 80(6 Suppl): 1689S–1696S.

de Vosjoli P. 1996. *Care and Breeding of Popular Tree Frogs.* Santee, CA: Advanced Vivarium Systems, Inc.

Diana SG, et al. 2001. Clinical toxicology. In: *Amphibian Medicine and Captive Husbandry* (eds KM Wright, BR Whitaker). Malabar, FL: Krieger Publishing Co.

Donoghue S, Langenberg J. 1996. Special topics: nutrition. In: *Reptile Medicine and Surgery* (ed DR Mader). Philadelphia: W.B. Saunders Co.

Duellman WE, Trueb L. 1994. *Biology of Amphibians.* Baltimore: Johns Hopkins University Press.

Ferguson GW, Gehrmann WH, Karsten KB, Landwer AJ, Carman EN, Chen TC, Holick MF. 2005. Ultraviolet exposure and vitamin D synthesis in a sun-dwelling and a shade-dwelling species of Anolis: are there adaptations for lower ultraviolet B and dietary vitamin D3 availability in the shade? *Physiol Biochem Zool* 78(2): 193–200.

Ferguson GW, Kingeter AJ, Gehrmann WH. 2013. Ultraviolet light exposure and response to dietary vitamin D3 in two Jamaican Anoles. *J Herpetol* 47(4): 524–529.

Fernández-Benéitez M, et al. 2008. *Saprolegnia diclina*: another species responsible for the emergent disease 'Saprolegnia infections' in amphibians. *Fed Eur Microbiol Soc.*

Finke MD. 2002. Complete nutrient composition of commercially raised invertebrates used as food for insectivores. *Zoo Biol* 21: 269–285.

Fisher A, Garner T. 2007. The relationship between the emergence of Batrachochytrium dendrobatidis, the international trade in amphibians and introduced amphibian species. *Fungal Biol Rev.* 21: 2–9.

Gagliardo R. *Atlanta Botanical Garden.* Personal communication.

Gagliardo R, Crump P, Griffiths E, Mendelson JR III, Ross H, Zippel KC. 2008. The principles of rapid response for amphibian conservation using the programmes in Panama as an example. *Int Zoo Yearbook* 42: 125–135.

Giustina A, Bilezikian JP. 2018. *Vitamin D in Clinical Medicine.* Basel: Karger.

Goin CJ, Goin OB, Zug GR. 1978. *Introduction to Herpetology,* 3rd edn. New York: W.H. Freeman and Co.

Helfman GS. 1990. Mode selection and mode switching in foraging animals. *Adv Study Behav* 19: 249.

Klingenberg RJ. 1993. *Understanding Reptile Parasites.* Lakeside, CA: Advanced Vivarium Systems.

Longcore J, et al. 1999. *Batrachochytrium dendrobatidis* gen. et sp. nov., a chytrid pathogenic to amphibians. *Mycologia* 91: 219–227.

Lotters S. 1996. *The Neotropical Toad Genus Atelopus.* Koln, Germany: M. Vences and F. Glaw Verlags GbR.

Martel A, et al. 2013. *Batrachochytrium salamandrivorans* sp. nov. causes lethal chytridiomycosis in amphibians. *Proc Natl Acad Sci USA* 110: 15325–15329.

Mattison C. 1987. *Frogs and Toads of the World.* New York: Facts on File Publications.

Michaels CJ, Antwis RE, Preziosi RF. 2015. Impacts of UVB provision and dietary calcium content on serum vitamin D3, growth rates, skeletal structure and coloration in captive oriental fire-bellied toads (*Bombina orientalis*). *J Anim Physiol Anim Nutr* 99(2): 391–403.

Michaels CJ, Antwis R, Preziosi RF. 2014 Manipulation of the calcium content of insectivore diets through supplemental dusting. *J Zoo Aquarium Res* 2(3): 77–81.

Miller D, et al. 2011. Ecopathology of ranaviruses infecting amphibians. *Viruses* 3: 2351–2373.

Morell V. 1999. Are pathogens felling frogs? *Science* 284: 728–731.

Niaze IA. 1996. Background to work on retinoids and amphibian limb regeneration: studies on anuran tadpoles—a retrospect. *J Biosci* 21(3): 273–297.

Obst FJ, et al. 1988. *The Completely Illustrated Atlas of Reptiles and Amphibians for the Terrarium.* Neptune City, NJ: TFH.

Ogilvy V, Preziosi R, Fidgett A. 2012 A brighter future for frogs? The influence of carotenoids on the health, development and reproductive success of the red-eye tree frog. *Anim Conserv* 15(5): 480–488.

Panayotova-Pencheva M. 2016. Experience in the ivermectin treatment of internal parasites in zoo and captive wild animals: a review. *Der Zoo Garten* 85(5): 280–308.

Pessier AP, et al. 2014. Causes of mortality in anuran amphibians from an ex situ survival assurance colony in Panama. *Zoo Biol* 33: 516–526.

Pessier AP, Mendelson JR (eds). 2014. *A Manual for Control of Infectious Diseases in Amphibian Survival Assurance Colonies and Reintroduction Programs.* Apple Valley, MN: IUCN/SSC Conservation Breeding Specialist Group.

Pessier AP, Roberts DR, Linn M, et al. 2002. "Short tongue syndrome," lingual squamous Metaplasia and suspected hypovitaminosis A in captive Wyoming toads. *Proc Assoc Rep Amphibian Vet* 151–153.

Petranka JW. 1998. *Salamanders of the United States and Canada.* Washington, DC: Smithsonian Institution Press.

Power S, Lancman J, Smith S. 2000. Retinoic acid is essential for shh/hoxd signaling during rat limb outgrowth but not for limb initiation. *Dev Dyn* 216(4): 469–480.

Poynton SL, Whitaker BR. 2001. Protozoa and metazoa infecting amphibians. In: *Amphibian Medicine and Captive Husbandry* (eds KM Wright, BR Whitaker). Malabar, FL: Krieger Publishing Co.

Livingston S, Lavin SR, Sullivan K, Attard L, Valdes EV. 2014. Challenges with effective nutrient supplementation for amphibians: a review of cricket studies. *Zoo Biol* 33: 565–576.

Stebbins RC. 1985. *Peterson Field Guide to Western Reptiles and Amphibians*. Boston: Houghton Mifflin Co.

Stetter MD. 2001a. Diagnostic imaging of amphibians. In: *Amphibian Medicine and Captive Husbandry* (eds KM Wright, BR Whitaker). Malabar, FL: Krieger Publishing Co.

Stratford T, Horton C, Maden M. 1996. Retinoic acid is required for the initiation of outgrowth in the chick limb bud. *Curr Biol* 6(9): 1124–1133

Tapley B, Rendle M, Baines FM, Goetz M, Bradfield KS, Rood D, Lopez J, Garcia G, Routh A. 2015. Meeting ultraviolet b radiation requirements of amphibians in captivity: a case study with mountain chicken frogs (Leptodactylus fallax) and general recommendations for pre-release health screening. *Zoo Biol* 34(1): 46–52.

Taylor SK. 2001. Mycoses. In: *Amphibian Medicine and Captive Husbandry* (eds KM Wright, BR Whitaker). Malabar, FL: Krieger Publishing Co.

van Zijll Langhout M, Struijk R, Konning T, van Zuilen D, Horvath K, van Bolhuis H, Maarschalkerweerd R, Verstappen F. 2017. Evaluation of bone mineralization by computed tomography in wild and captive European common spadefoots (Pelobates fuscus), in relation to exposure to ultraviolet b radiation and dietary supplements. *J Zoo Wildl Med* 48(3): 748–756.

Walls JG. 1994. *Jewels of the Rain Forest—Poison Dart Frogs of the World*. Neptune City, NJ: TFH Publications.

Whitaker BR. 2001. The amphibian eye. In: *Amphibian Medicine and Captive Husbandry* (eds KM Wright, BR Whitaker). Malabar, FL: Krieger Publishing Co.

Wilson B, Myers C, Yin Y. 2019. *Supplemental Dietary Calcium Essential for Growth, Bone Mineralization, and Survival of Post-Metamorphic Evergreen Toads (Incilius coniferus) in Captivity*. Atlanta Botanical Garden Unpublished Research.

Wright KM. 2001b. Anatomy for the clinician. In: *Amphibian Medicine and Captive Husbandry* (eds KM Wright, BR Whitaker). Malabar, FL: Krieger Publishing Co.

Wright KM. 2001c. Applied physiology. In: *Amphibian Medicine and Captive Husbandry* (eds KM Wright, BR Whitaker). Malabar, FL: Krieger Publishing Co.

Wright KM. 2001d. Diets for captive amphibians. In: *Amphibian Medicine and Captive Husbandry* (eds KM Wright, BR Whitaker). Malabar, FL: Krieger Publishing Co.

Wright KM. 2001e. Evolution of the amphibia. In: *Amphibian Medicine and Captive Husbandry* (eds KM Wright, BR Whitaker). Malabar, FL: Krieger Publishing Co.

Wright KM. 2001f. Surgical techniques. In: *Amphibian Medicine and Captive Husbandry* (eds KM Wright, BR Whitaker). Malabar, FL: Krieger Publishing Co.

Wright KM. 2001g. Taxonomy of amphibians kept in captivity. In: *Amphibian Medicine and Captive Husbandry* (eds KM Wright, BR Whitaker). Malabar, FL: Krieger Publishing Co. pp. 3–14.

Wright KM, Whitaker BR. 2001a. Nutritional disorders. In: *Amphibian Medicine and Captive Husbandry* (eds KM Wright, BR Whitaker). Malabar, FL: Krieger Publishing Co.

Wright KM, Whitaker BR. 2001b. Pharmacotherapeutics. In: *Amphibian Medicine and Captive Husbandry* (eds KM Wright, BR Whitaker). Malabar, FL: Krieger Publishing Co.

Wright KM, Whitaker BR. 2001c. Quarantine. In: *Amphibian Medicine and Captive Husbandry* (eds KM Wright, BR Whitaker). Malabar, FL: Krieger Publishing Co.

Wright KM, Whitaker BR. 2001d. Restraint techniques and euthanasia. In: *Amphibian Medicine and Captive Husbandry* (eds KM Wright, BR Whitaker). Malabar, FL: Krieger Publishing Co.

Wright KM. 2009. Three things you must know to see amphibians. *Proc North Am Vet Conf* 23: 1822–1825. (Gainesville, FL).

Young S, Speare R, Berger L, Skerratt L. 2014. Chloramphenicol with fluid and electrolyte therapy cures terminally ill green tree frogs (*Litoria caerulea*) with chytridiomycosis. *J Zoo Wildl Med* 43: 330–337.

15

Fish
Sandy Skeba and Bonnie Ballard

Natural History

Fish are a member of the Phylum Chordata. They are mostly ectothermic, meaning they derive their body temperature from their ambient environment. A typical fish lives in water, obtains oxygen with gills, and usually has scales and lays eggs, although there are exceptions to these rules. About half of the living species of all vertebrates in the world are fish. Fish can be found in nearly every aquatic environment, from freshwater caves, to Antarctic depths, to warm, tropical reefs. Fish are an important source of food, but in this chapter, we will investigate the medical care of fish kept as pets in home aquaria.

Fish originated about 530 million years ago during the Cambrian Explosion when vertebrates first began to appear and diversify (Nelson 2006). The first fish were jawless and were strictly filter feeders. One of the earliest known fish, *Haikouichthys*, may also be the ancestor of all vertebrates. Its unique (for the time) anatomy included a notochord (the precursor to a spinal column), rudimentary vertebrae, and a defined head and tail. The next important step in fish evolution was the development of the jaw. The jaw formed from the gill arches (the bony part of the gill). Fish with jaws were able to ingest larger items and could exploit many more diverse ecological niches. With jaws, fish could pursue active prey animals (rather than just filtering microscopic zooplankton), and most developed more streamlined body shapes and efficient swimming methods. Fish could become much larger, such as the armor-plated Dunkleosteus, which grew to over seven meters (23 feet) long and was considered one of the first apex predators. During the Devonian Era, or "Age of the Fishes," jawed fishes became so successful that all but a few of the jawless species became extinct. It was during this time that the transitional labyrinthodont fish, the precursor to the amphibians, appeared. But fish are more than just a stepping stone to the amphibians. They are highly evolved to be masters of their watery environment. They come in many forms, have the ability to eat a huge variety of foods, and have populated almost every body of water. Fish are the most common vertebrate, with approximately 31,000 species alive today (Weber 2011). In comparison, the next most common vertebrates are birds, with a mere 8,600 species (Romer and Parsons 1985).

Fish can be divided into three classes; the Agnatha (jawless fishes including hagfish and lampreys), the Chondrichthyes (cartilaginous fish, including sharks, rays, and skates), and the Osteichthyes (bony fish). The overwhelming majority of aquarium fish are from the class Osteichthyes (Nelson 2006). There are many orders of fish within this class, but a few orders comprise most of the aquarium fish popular today:

- **Anguilliformes** (eels)
- **Cypriniformes** (carps and goldfish)
- **Characiformes** (tetras, headstanders, piranhas)
- **Siluriformes** (catfish)
- **Cyprinodontiformes** (killifish and guppies)
- **Atheriniformes** (rainbowfish)
- **Beryciformes** (squirrelfish, soldierfish)
- **Gasterosteiformes** (pipefish, seahorses)
- **Scorpaeniformes** (scorpionfish, lionfish)
- **Perciformes** (cichlids, darters, perches, angelfish, butterfish, gouramies, gobies)
- **Tetraodontiformes** (triggerfish, boxfish, puffers).

Fish can also be divided into two broad types: freshwater fish and saltwater fish, although some species (such as the salmon) spend part of their lives in one habitat before switching to the other (Nelson 2006). There are also fish that utilize moderately saline environments called brackish water species (such as anglerfish and killifish). Brackish, freshwater, and saltwater fish are all kept in home aquariums.

Exotic Animal Medicine for the Veterinary Technician, Fourth Edition. Edited by Bonnie Ballard and Ryan Cheek.
© 2024 John Wiley & Sons, Inc. Published 2024 by John Wiley & Sons, Inc.
Companion Website: www.wiley.com/go/ballard/4e

History

The earliest aquariums date back to the Roman Empire. Early Romans kept local freshwater fish in marble tubs for enjoyment, rather than eating. In the mid-1300s, the Chinese popularized the keeping of goldfish in porcelain bowls. During the 1800s, aquarium keeping began to take off as a hobby among Europeans, and many great strides were made in the science of keeping fish alive in artificial habitats. Around 1908 the first air pump (initially water-powered) was invented, and this is credited as a pivotal moment in the development of home aquaria. The later addition of the reliable availability of electricity enabled aquaria to be heated, filtered, and aerated. Initially, people kept native fish or goldfish. But this changed after methods were developed to keep fish alive during overseas trips, such as using a bicycle pump to aerate fish in barrels. The addition of exotic species greatly added to the popularity of the hobby (Brunner 2003).

Anatomy and Physiology

The definition of "fish" is an exclusionary one; that is, a vertebrate that lives in the water and is not a mammal, reptile, or amphibian. Therefore, the group is comprised of many different evolutionary lines (Nelson 2006). Many diverse types of fish exist. The characteristics of those found most commonly in home aquaria will be discussed.

Basic Body Shapes

As previously noted, fish come from many evolutionary lines, and each species is a product of its environment. The universal shape thought of when one mentions "fish" is the torpedo-shaped, streamlined one, flattened laterally. However, there are as many fish shapes as there are environments that fish are found in. Algae eaters, such as the *Plecostomus*, are flattened dorso-ventrally, with a ventrally placed mouth and stiff side fins, ideal for grazing under and around algae-covered rocks. Flatfishes, such as flounder, have one of the most extreme body arrangements. When hatched, they resemble a "typical" fish. But as they grow, they begin to flatten, laterally, and one eye migrates over to one side to join the other. The result is a pancake-like fish, perfectly adapted to hiding on or under the sandy bottom of its aquatic home. On the other end of the scale, seahorses and pipefishes exhibit bizarre, upright shapes, designed to fit in among quiet reef systems, providing good camouflage among the corals and sea fans.

Integumentary System

The skin of most bony and cartilaginous fishes is covered by scales. Scales vary tremendously in size, shape, and structure, ranging from rigid armor plates in fishes such as seahorses and boxfishes, to microscopic or absent in fishes such as eels and anglerfishes. The morphology of a scale can often be used to identify the species of fish it came from. Fish scales are mesodermal in origin (Stoskopf 1993). The same genes responsible for scale development in fish are also involved in tooth and hair development in mammals. This distinguishes fish scales from reptile scales, which are derived from epidermal origins. Scales have many functions, including protection (from the elements and predators) and streamlining for swimming. This outer barrier is further enhanced by a layer of mucus covering the scales. Fish mucus, or slime, has antibiotic properties and is constantly being renewed (Andrews 2003). This sloughs off debris and discourages external parasites. Fish mucus production increases in times of stress, whether it be environmental or illness. Transport also is a stressor. There are artificial slime preparations, such as Stress-coat™, (Mars Fishcare, Chalfont, PA, 18914) that can be added to the water to soothe and replenish the natural slime layer. Beneath the scales lies the dermis and epidermis. Altogether, fish skin, mucus, and scales are the first line of defense against illness (Andrews 2003).

Bony fish, or teleosts (the most common type of aquarium fish), have leptoid scales. As they grow, they add concentric layers. Leptoid scales overlap each other smoothly, in a head-to-toe direction, which reduces drag as the fish swims through the water and provides great flexibility. There are two types of leptoid scales. Cycloid scales have smooth outer edges and are found in fish such as goldfish and salmon. Ctenoid scales have a toothed or spiny outer edge, causing a rough feel to the scale. Fish with ctenoid scales include cichlids and perches, and many saltwater fish. Both types of scales can be found on some fish. For example, some species of flatfish (flounders) can have ctenoid scales on the eyed (up) side, and cycloid scales on the blind (down) side (Stoskopf 1993).

Cartilaginous (Chondrichthyes) fish, such as sharks and rays, have placoid scales. This type of scale is also known as dermal denticles, so called because they are structurally similar to teeth. These scales are tiny but very rough. The texture of placoid scales reduces drag through the water, making sharks more efficient and quieter swimmers than bony fishes.

Fins

All fish have fins. The primary purpose of fins is to assist with the fish's motion through the water, although some species also use their fins for internal fertilization (guppies), crawling (mudskippers), and protection (venomous lionfishes). Fins consist of soft and/or bony rays projecting from the body, usually covered with skin to join each ray together. The skin adhering to these rays ranges from almost transparent to thick and fleshy, depending on the type of fish (Williams et al. 2013). Each fin or set of fins has a different function in moving the fish, and some fish have lost various fins during evolution. See Figure 15.1. The main fins are:

- Dorsal fin—runs along the dorsal spine for varying lengths according to the type of fish. The dorsal fin of most fish is used for stabilization during swimming. Some fish, such as male guppies, use their dorsal fin for courtship and can raise and lower them voluntarily. The dorsal fin, though single, can be separated in some species into two sections running down the back of the fish.
- Pectoral fins—paired set of fins that emerge from the ventral surface of the fish, just behind the gill openings. Pectoral fins are used during turning and stopping. Some fish, such as mudskippers, use modified pectoral fins for pulling themselves along ("walking") on damp land.
- Pelvic fins—paired set of fins located ventrally, behind the pectoral fins. They assist the fish in turning and stopping. In some fish, such as gobies, the pelvic fins are fused into a sucker, allowing the fish to fasten onto rocks.
- Anal fin—a single fin located on the ventral surface of the fish, just behind the anus in teleosts, and the cloaca in chondrichthyes. It is primarily a stabilizing fin. In male guppies, the anal fin has modified into a structure called the gonopodium, which is used to internally fertilize the female.
- Caudal fin—this is the "tail" fin, a single fin at the rear terminus of the fish. It is the only fish fin controlled by the skeleton of the fish (the spine). It is used for propulsion in most species.

Osmoregulation

Fish are immersed in their environment and are constantly battling the osmolality of the water they rely on for life. For a freshwater fish, its internal osmolality is higher than that of its surroundings, meaning that its molecules are constantly trying to pass from the area of higher concentration (the fish) to one of lower concentration (the fresh water). To combat this, freshwater fish have very efficient kidneys and excrete water rapidly. Internal salt loss is minimized by absorption from the kidneys before copious, dilute urine is excreted, and by absorption from the environment by chloride glands in the gills. Saltwater fish have the opposite

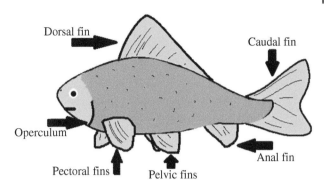

Figure 15.1 Fins of fish. (Courtesy of Sandy Skeba.)

problem; the tendency is for water to be lost from the fish's tissues into the saltier environment. Adaptations to prevent dehydration include drinking large quantities of water (but excreting small amounts of concentrated urine) and using chloride glands in the gills to actively excrete salt (Andrews 2003).

Senses

Water affects the way fish perceive the world. It absorbs light rapidly and increased particulate matter can further reduce visibility. Sound travels more quickly in water than in air. Water also contains many chemicals, so a fish must have excellent taste and smell to find food.

Sight

Like many animals, predatory fishes usually have better binocular vision (eyes located toward the front of the head), and prey fish have better peripheral vision (eyes on the sides of the head). Fish eyes are similar in structure to other vertebrate eyes, but the lens is almost spherical to allow both up-close and distant focus by moving the lens closer or further from the retina. Most fish have a fixed iris, with the exception of some sharks. There are also fish that have diminished or no visual capabilities due to their life in dark habitats, such as the ocean bottom and caves. Fish have limited vision above the water, due to the difference in light refraction. Most fish have good color vision (Helfman et al. 2009).

Sound

Sound travels in water as pressure waves. Fish are very sensitive to these waves. Internal ears are used to detect specific frequencies, and some species can use their swim bladder to amplify sounds. Fish also perceive sound through a unique lateral line system. The lateral line runs the length of the fish, laterally about mid-body. It consists of a series of tiny indentations filled with modified epithelial cells (called "hair" cells) which are extremely sensitive to motion in the water. The lateral line is especially tuned toward lower-frequency sounds and is designed to ignore background noise. It plays a large role in facilitating schooling behavior and in hunting prey. The number and placement of hair cells can vary greatly among species; some fish have them throughout the body, whereas others only on the head and lateral line (Helfman et al. 2009).

Taste/Smell

Fish have very well-developed chemical senses, and taste and smell are almost indistinguishable. They are able to sort out dissolved substances in the water pertaining to not just food, but potential mates, potential predators, and natal homes (such as salmon). Sharks can judge the distance to a certain smell by the timing of its arrival on each nostril, similar to how mammals judge distance by hearing. Chemoreceptors are concentrated in the nostrils and mouth, but in some species may be scattered around the head, or even the entire body.

Proprioception

As in mammals, the inner ear of fish is also used to register position, or "tilt," of the body. Fish fins are also thought to have analogous functions to mammalian limbs in determining orientation, by sending nerve messages as to velocity and bending of the rays of the fins (Williams et al. 2013).

Many bony fish also possess a swim bladder that allows them to regulate their buoyancy without movement. This is a thin-walled, gas-filled one or two-chambered sac inside the body cavity that runs ventrally just below the spine. Some fish have a connection between the swim bladder and the gastrointestinal (GI) tract and can increase air in the bladder chamber by gulping at the surface. Other species, lacking this connection, use a gas gland. The gas gland regulates the amount of air in the swim bladder. With the gas gland, the fish can increase or decrease the amount of air, and subsequently rise or lower itself in the water (Stoskopf 1993). The swim bladder also resonates sound well and is used in some fish to produce or amplify noises. The resonance of sound off of the swim bladder is what makes fish "visible" to fish-finding sonar systems.

Respiratory System

Although animals get energy from the food they eat, their bodies need oxygen to perform the necessary chemical reactions. Fish acquire oxygen through their gills. Fish respiration is very efficient, which is necessary because water contains only five parts per million (ppm) of oxygen, as opposed to approximately 210,000 ppm in the air (Mortimer 1956). Gills are highly vascular, filamentous tissues located bilaterally just behind the head. They are supported on bony arches, and protected by exterior, skin-covered bony flaps called opercula (singular, operculum). Gaseous exchange of oxygen and carbon dioxide is accomplished by simple osmotic pressure. Fish generate water flow over the gills by opening and closing their mouths, with the exception of most sharks, which need to be in motion to move water (and thus oxygen) over their gills. The fish opens its mouth to bring water in, then closes its mouth and opens the opercula to allow the water to flow out and over the gills (Stoskopf 1993). This motion is also known as "gilling."

Oxygen levels in home aquaria can be affected by several factors. One of the most important is temperature. Oxygen levels are inversely proportional to water temperature. That is, dissolved oxygen is lower in warmer temperatures, and increases as water temperature decreases. The second most important factor is surface area. Oxygen diffuses into water primarily though the interchange of the water's surface, and the air. Agitating or breaking up the water surface increases the amount of oxygen in the water. Bubblers placed under the water have some effect but are not the primary source of oxygen in a closed system (such as aquaria) (Andrews 2003).

Gill structure can be thought of as a branching tree and consists of the gill arch (trunk), gill filaments or primary lamellae (branches), and secondary lamellae (leaves). Oxygen exchange occurs in the secondary lamellae. The secondary lamellae are also the site of osmoregulation (as noted previously), plus they excrete waste products, such as ammonia, and salt in marine fish. Teleost fish (bony fish) typically have four gill arches, protected by one operculum on each side of the head. Cartilaginous fish, such as sharks, can have five to seven gill arches, and each arch is protected by its own operculum (Stoskopf 1993). Gills also have an anterior process called a "gill raker," on the leading edge of each gill arch. Originally, these structures kept large particles ingested in the water from hitting and damaging the gills, but as these particles are often nutritious, gill rakers evolved in use to trap food and direct it to the esophagus.

Some fish are able to extract oxygen in other ways. This enables them to survive in water with low oxygen content. Mudskippers can absorb oxygen through their skin, much as some amphibians do. Some catfish can absorb oxygen through their intestinal tract or swim bladders. Other fish, such as bettas and gouramis, have a specialized labyrinthine organ above the gills which can absorb oxygen (Stoskopf 1993). Fish with these capabilities typically live in small lakes or ponds that are subject to seasonal drying. Some of these fish are capable of surviving for months in what may be no more than damp mud.

Cardiovascular System

The cardiovascular system is a single closed loop that connects every part of the fish's body. Blood is the liquid tissue that flows within this system. Its primary functions are to deliver oxygen and nutrients to the body's cells and remove carbon dioxide and metabolic waste. Blood is a complex media consisting of cells, water, salts, and the materials being transported. As in mammals, a fish's most numerous blood cells are the oxygen-carrying red blood cells, which, unlike mammalian red blood cells, are nucleated. Thrombocytes are next in number and are the cells analogous to mammalian platelets. Unlike platelets, they are nucleated but play the same role in coagulation. White blood cells are the least numerous and have the same function in immune health as in mammals.

The heart is located just behind and below the gills. Fish have a primitive heart consisting of four chambers with only two valves. These chambers, unlike other vertebrate hearts, lie sequentially in a row or S-shape. The first chamber, in which low-oxygenated blood collects from the hepatic and cardinal veins, is the sinus venosus. From here, blood enters the atrium, where it travels into the much more muscular ventricle. The ventricle supplies the main pumping action of the heart. The final chamber is the bulbous arteriosis (teleost fish) or conus arteriosis (elasmobranchs). Multiple valves therein distribute the blood to the ventral aorta, where it passes through the gills and picks up oxygen. After leaving the gills, the blood flows through the dorsal aorta into the rest of the body (Romer & Parsons 1985).

Gastrointestinal System

The GI system of each type of fish is a reflection of its diet. Like mammals, carnivorous fish tend to have a straight, simple gut shorter than their body length, and herbivores more complex and longer than their body length. Carnivorous fish usually have sharp teeth for apprehending slippery prey items. These teeth reside in the premaxilla, maxilla, and mandible. Herbivorous fish may have thick, rough bony plates, set in the front of the esophagus, which begin the process of breaking down the food. Many species have a second set of jaws, known as the pharyngeal jaws, which are derived from bones in the throat. These bones are dermal and contain modifications based on diet. Fish that eat hard items such as shellfish can have crushing, molar-like teeth on the pharyngeal jaw, while others have pointed teeth that assist in prey capture. Notably, some fish such as moray eels can protrude their pharyngeal jaw to procure prey. When a fish ingests a meal, the esophagus delivers it to the stomach. The process of digestion begins, and nutrients begin to be absorbed as they pass into the intestinal tract. In many fish, notably trout, there are numerous outgrowths of the intestine called pyloric caeca. These increase the absorptive surface of the intestinal tract (Stoskopf 1993). As the food moves through the intestines, digestive enzymes from the liver and pancreas are added. Nutrients are absorbed into the bloodstream in the lower GI tract. Fish utilize nutrients—lipids (fats), proteins, carbohydrates, and minerals—as do other animals. Many of these nutrients, after bodily demands are met, are stored in the liver or as adipose (fat).

Urogenital System

The kidney functions to remove waste from the bloodstream in most animals, but in fish, it also has an osmoregulatory function. The kidney is divided into anterior and posterior segments. The anterior segment's primary function is to produce blood cells (fish have no bone marrow). The posterior kidney is the excretory organ and regulates osmolality. In saltwater fish, which tend to lose fluids in their environment, the kidney concentrates urine and returns liquid to the body. In freshwater fish the opposite happens; because they are constantly ingesting and absorbing water, their urine is copious and dilute (Andrews 2003). Cartilaginous fish such as sharks have a single excretory opening, known as a cloaca, which serves the kidneys, gonads, and intestinal tract. However, in most bony fishes, the three openings (though close together) are separate.

Reproduction is varied in fish. Male fish possess testes, and females, ovaries, although some species are able to change sex due to age or environmental conditions. Most fish perform external fertilization, where the female produces eggs in the environment, and the male excretes sperm and seminal fluid (also known as milt) over the eggs.

Some notable exceptions exist, such as sharks and rays. Males of these species have a set of intromittent organs called claspers, which are modified pelvic fins used to internally fertilize the female. Guppies also use modified fins for internal fertilization.

Most fish are egg layers or oviparous. Egg-producing fish exhibit varying degrees of parental care from total neglect, to protection from predators, to extremes such as mouth-brooding. Amazonian discus (*Symphysodon* spp.) is a popular variety of aquarium fish which tend to their eggs carefully, fanning water over them to keep them oxygenated and removing any dead or diseased eggs to protect the healthy ones. After hatching, the young feed from nutritious slime excreted by the skin of the parents, for up to four weeks.

Newly hatched fish are called larvae and are poorly developed until they absorb enough nutrients from their yolk sac to grow into juveniles, when they begin feeding on their own.

Some fish produce live young. Ovoviviparous fish, such as guppies, produce eggs but retain them internally. The larvae rely on the nutrients from the egg yolk sac to develop, and are expelled as well-formed, tiny fishes. Viviparous species, such as lemon sharks (*Negaprion brevirostris*), retain their eggs and nourish them from the body, using a placenta-like structure. Aquarists use the term livebearers to describe non-egg-laying species.

If fish are to be bred, the owner must research the reproductive strategies of the individual species and provide the appropriate setting. For example, guppies will produce fully formed, swimming young, but unless they are separated from the other tank inhabitants or given hiding places (such as grass mats), they will be quickly devoured.

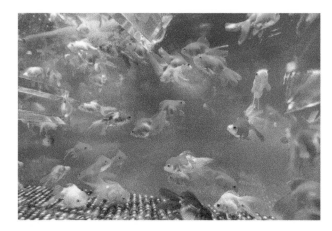

Figure 15.2 Various goldfish (*Carassius* sp.) for sale. (Courtesy of kazuend https://unsplash.com/.)

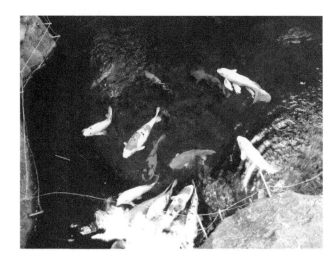

Figure 15.3 Koi (*Cyprinus* sp.) in a pond. (https://pixabay.com/images/search/aquarium%20fish.)

Husbandry

Aquarium fish can be divided into three broad categories:

Temperate freshwater fish—include the popular cyprinid species, goldfish (*Carassius auratus*), and koi (*Cyprinus carpio*). Both of these types of fish have been cultivated for centuries, and many coveted colors and varieties exist. Goldfish and koi, while separate species, have much the same requirements in temperature and space, and are often found together in home ponds. However, goldfish are much smaller, and unlike koi are often kept in home aquaria. There are over 30 varieties of ornamental goldfish available in the pet trade, and some of these sport bizarre mutations, such as a large bubble beneath each eye, excessive tissue growth over the head, and double-finned fish (Figure 15.2). Koi are available in many colors and scale patterns, and individuals with desired traits can be quite valuable. Koi will grow too large for most home aquaria and are best suited to life in an outside pond (Figures 15.3 and 15.4A and B). When kept together in a pond, goldfish and koi will readily interbreed and usually produce inferiorly colored hybrids. Other species of temperate freshwater fish include popular North American game fish such as sunfish, trout, and bass. While sunfish can be quite attractive, they are generally too aggressive for the home aquarium, and game fish require large, complex systems for life support.

Tropical freshwater fish—these are the most popular type of fish typically kept in the home aquarium and require warmer temperatures than temperate water fish. This necessitates the use of a heating system within the tank. These fish can further be grouped into community and aggressive species; it is common to see these designations

Figure 15.4 (A) A large koi pond on the back patio of a private residence. (B) Three of the koi in that pond are 34 years old, weigh 30–35 pounds and are 30–40 inches long. (Courtesy of Terry and Carol Mills.)

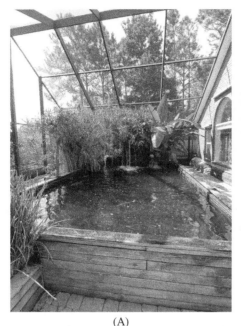

(A)

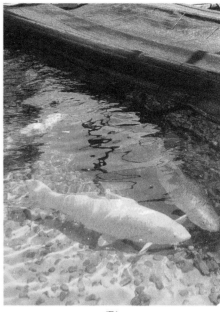

(B)

on the tanks used in a fish store. Amateur aquarists would do well to heed the advice of the pet store personnel when acquiring species with which they are unfamiliar.

Typical examples of these fish include:

Community—schooling or non-aggressive fish such as guppies and mollies (*Poecilia* spp.), tetras (Characiformes), angelfish (*Pterophyllum* spp.), gouramis (*Helostoma* spp.), swordtails (*Xiphophorus helleri*), rainbow fish (*Melanotaenia* spp.), and some cichlids (Cichlidae). Often a tank will also include a non-aggressive algae eater, such as a *Plecostomus* catfish (Figures 15.5–15.7). Fish that do well in a community but have more stringent water parameter requirements, such as discus, should be kept in a single-species tank.

Aggressive—Some cichlids (such as oscars, [*Astronotus ocellatus*], piranha (Serrasalmidae), snakeheads (Channidae), bettas ("Siamese fighting fish," *Betta splendens*), and tiger barbs (*Puntigrus tetrazona*) (Figures 15.8–15.10).

Some fish labeled "aggressive" will do fine when combined with fish of their own size; conversely, "community" fish may bully those much smaller than themselves.

Amateur aquarists should also investigate the possibility that a particular fish they are interested in could outgrow the aquarium they live in such as the fish in Figure 15.6 and the Ripsaw Catfish (*Oxydoras niger*) named Dudley who had to find a new home in a public aquarium (Figure 15.11). This catfish can grow to a length of 36 inches.

Tropical saltwater fish—saltwater systems are more demanding and complex to recreate than most freshwater systems, due to stringent salinity needs and the

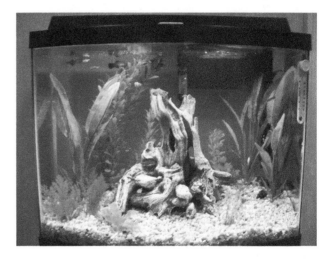

Figure 15.5 A 28-gallon freshwater community tropical fish tank with guppies (*Poecilia reticulata*) and red wagtail platys (*Xiphophorus masculatus*). (Courtesy of Dr. Bonnie Ballard.)

sensitivity of certain species to trace minerals such as copper (Figures 15.12 and 15.13). The popularity of saltwater fish is largely due to their brilliant colors and size. However, these fish come with a much higher price tag than typical freshwater fish which means that problems getting the tank established can be costly and heartbreaking. (See water quality section.)

Many saltwater aquarists also strive for the perfection of a reef tank, which incorporates not just fish, but hard and soft corals, tube worms, and colorful shrimps, clams, and crabs. As with tropical freshwater fish, specimens should be carefully selected based on their ability to "get along with"

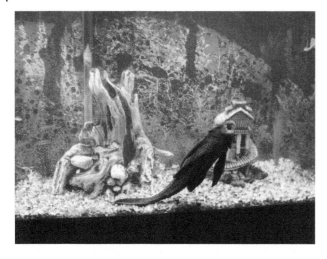

Figure 15.6 A 55-gallon freshwater community tropical fish tank with a large *Plecostomus* in the foreground. (Courtesy of Dr. Bonnie Ballard.)

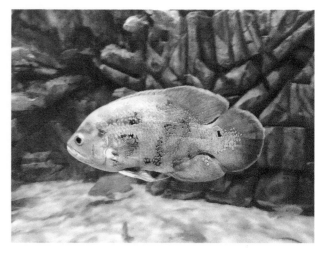

Figure 15.8 An Oscar (*Astronotus ocellatus*), a cichlid that can outgrow most home aquaria. (Courtesy of Amir Shahabi, https://unsplash.com/.)

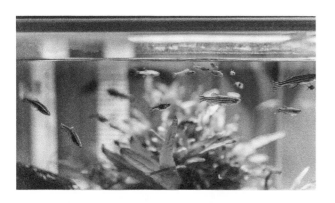

Figure 15.7 Freshwater community tank with zebra fish (*Brachydanio rerio*) and cloud fish (*Tanichthys albonubes*). (Courtesy of Jerry Wang https://unsplash.com/.)

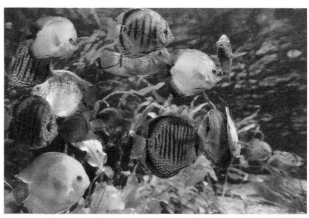

Figure 15.9 Captive bred discus (*Symphysodon*) in various colors. (Courtesy of Daniel Corneschi https://unsplash.com/.)

other members of the tank. Since a home aquarium is a closed system, fish that are being persecuted are unable to escape their aggressors. Tank "furniture," such as rocks and plants, may help by giving pursued fish a place to hide, but this may also ensure that some fish are hidden from view. If the persecution is severe enough, fish may starve due to being kept away from food (Figures 15.14–15.16).

Many types of freshwater fish are bred in captivity. Captive-bred fish usually are better acclimated to aquarium living, are free from the parasites and diseases carried by wild-caught fish, and are less expensive. All goldfish and koi are captive-bred. Many community-type fish are also, including most livebearers (guppies, mollies, and swordtails). Cichlids can be found that are captive-bred; however, part of the attraction of cichlid keeping is finding new and novel species, and many are still being brought into the pet trade from the wild.

Conversely, most saltwater fish are wild-caught. This makes keeping saltwater fish somewhat of a controversial hobby. Environmentalists fear that the saltwater fish trade not only decreases wild populations directly, but methods of catching wild saltwater fish are often injurious to the environment, such as using cyanide to temporarily stun desired fish but leaving other fish to die in the poisoned water. However, more and more saltwater fish are being bred in captivity. Most notable are the clownfish, made popular by the movie *Finding Nemo*.

Water Quality

Fish keeping involves many factors, but the number one defining aspect of good fish husbandry is proper water quality (Andrews 2003). Fish are vulnerable to changes in their environment, even more so than terrestrial animals.

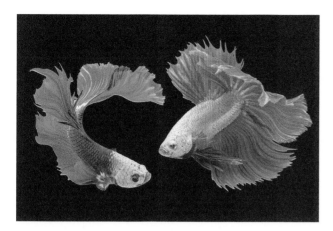

Figure 15.10 Two Siamese fighting fish (*Betta splendens*), a popular species for home aquaria however they must be housed singly. (Courtesy of Worachat Sodsri https://unsplash.com/.)

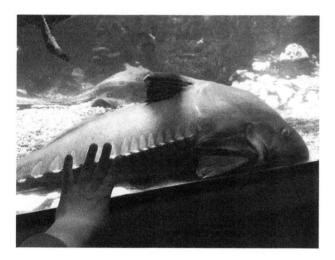

Figure 15.11 Dudley, a Ripsaw Catfish (*Oxydoras niger*) outgrew his aquarium and now has a home in a public aquarium.

As aquaria are invariably closed systems, it is up to the fish keeper to provide all of the water purification needs. In nature, water is purified by precipitation, filtering through sand and sediment, and inhabitant bacteria. Large masses of water dilute toxins and flowing water sweeps them away. Fish owners must be familiar with the nitrogen cycle, as it is the first defense in keeping the home aquarium livable.

Fish waste, dead plants, and uneaten food all contribute to ammonia in the fish tank. Ammonia is toxic to fish. *Nitrosomas* bacteria oxidize ammonia, breaking it down into nitrite. Nitrite is also toxic to fish, even in small amounts. The presence of another type of bacteria, *Nitrobacter*, is required to further reduce nitrite into nitrate. Fish are much more tolerant of nitrates in the water. Eventually, anaerobic bacteria turn nitrates into simple nitrogen gas (Figure 15.17). The more of each type

of bacteria present in the system, the more capacity there is to control toxic ammonia and nitrite levels. Nitrifying bacteria inhabit the filter, substrate, and walls of the fish tank or pond. Often, filters will contain numerous irregular objects, such as pumice, to provide even more surface area for the bacteria to grow. This process is called biological filtration (Andrews 2003).

Mechanical filtration uses various densities of filter material to remove particulate matter from the water. Filter pads containing carbon will also clarify the water. A good home aquarium system utilizes both methods of filtration. Fish kept in bowls, such as bettas and goldfish, may not require filtration if they receive substantial, timely water changes.

A common problem for the beginning hobbyist is New Tank Syndrome. The excited fish-owner-to-be buys a tank, decorates it, fills it with water, and immediately chooses a dozen fish to place into the new environment. Inevitably, there is an ammonia spike due to the new inhabitants, and because the tank is fresh and clean, there are no bacteria to degrade the toxic ammonia. One by one the fish succumb to the toxic conditions, with perhaps the exception of one or two hardy individuals. Discouraged, the owner puts the tank and all accessories up for sale and resolves never to try fish keeping again. The key here is patience; when a new tank is set up, only one or two small fish are introduced at first (preferably inexpensive ones, just in case). They produce waste, but in small amounts, so that the bacteria have time to increase in population. As time goes by, more fish can be added as the capacity for the nitrogen cycle grows (Figure 15.17). However, there is a limit for each tank as to how many fish can comfortably exist within it. A very general rule is an inch of fish per gallon of water, keeping in mind that fish will grow, and that substrate and tank "furniture" take up space that would be part of the water volume (Andrews 2003).

There are many water test kits available that an aquarist can use to check the levels of ammonia, nitrite, and nitrate in the aquarium. When waiting for a new tank to "cycle" (as the nitrogen cycle process is referred to), these levels should be tested daily. In established tanks, weekly testing should be sufficient (Andrews 2003).

Beyond the nitrogen cycle, there are many other factors to keeping fish healthy. As fish come from many different environments is the wild, each species has different parameters in which they will be comfortable when kept in an aquarium.

pH

The pH scale runs from 1 to 14 and represents the level of acid or alkaline in a substance. The lower the number, the more acidic the pH, and higher means more alkaline. A

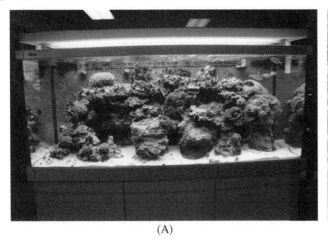

(A)

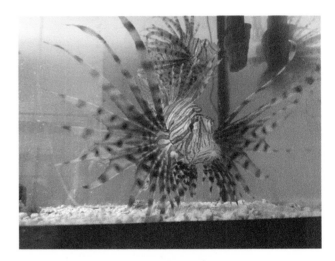

(B)

Figure 15.12 Saltwater tank A and B.

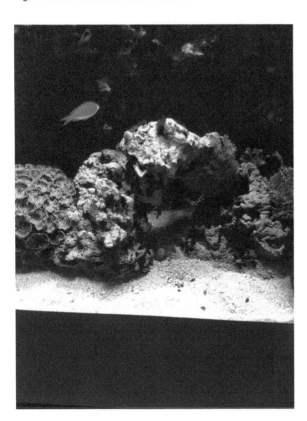

Figure 15.13 Blue damselfish (*Chrysiptera cyanea*) in a live coral tank.

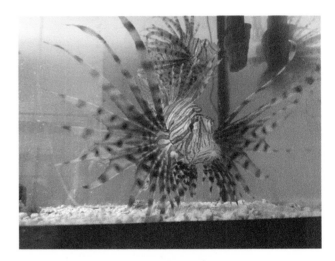

Figure 15.14 Lionfish (*Pterois antennata*).

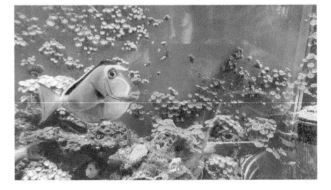

Figure 15.15 Naso tang (*Naso lituratus*). (Courtesy of Terry and Carol Mills.)

pH of 7 is considered neutral. The pH scale is logarithmic, with each step being ten times the previous. Therefore, a pH of 5 is 10 times more acidic than a pH of 6. Most organisms thrive when their environment is close to neutral. However, with both plants and animals, there are species that prefer their environment to be a little more acid or alkaline. In fishkeeping, most aquariums should be close to neutral. Notable exceptions are discus (which prefers a pH around 6.3) and saltwater fish (saltwater aquaria usually are more alkaline, with a pH between 8 and 9). The best course of action for each type of fish would be to investigate what the pH is in its natural environment and

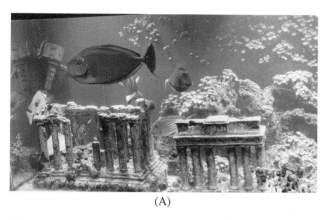
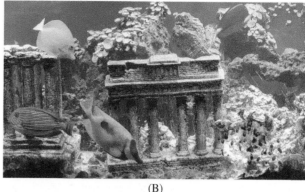

(A) (B)

Figure 15.16 (A) A 260-gallon saltwater tank that has numerous species of fish in a home. (B) These fish are approximately 22 years of age. (Courtesy of Terry and Carol Mills.)

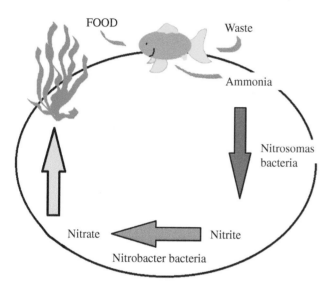

Figure 15.17 Nitrogen cycle. (Courtesy of Sandy Skeba.)

to group together fish that are comfortable in the same pH (Andrews 2003).

An increase in ammonia levels will decrease pH, making the water more acidic. Fish respiration also decreases pH. An aquarium system's buffering capacity is a direct measure of how well the water can deal with pH changes. In general, "hard" water with dissolved salts and minerals (such as calcium and magnesium) is better able to buffer against pH changes than "soft," or pure water (Andrews 2003). pH can be directly affected by adding different materials to the water. Aquarium peat will decrease water pH naturally. Coral rocks or shells will increase pH as their calcium carbonate dissolves. There are also commercial solutions available for adjusting pH levels to that which is most natural for the fish.

Oxygen

As stated in respiration, oxygen levels in the water are a direct consequence of the amount of surface area of the tank. Oxygen levels typically must be around 5 ppm to sustain life in an aquarium. Temperature is also a factor in oxygenation. Warm water has less ability to hold oxygen than cooler or cold water. Low oxygen levels will quickly kill fish, as with any other vertebrate, although some species have developed abilities to deal with low water oxygenation, such as gulping air from the surface, or respiring through the skin. Oxygen measuring kits are available, but it is not a typically monitored component, as it is usually easy to maintain adequate oxygenation in the home aquarium.

Temperature

As with pH, the temperature that fish are comfortable with is a direct reflection of what their environment would be in the wild. There are three main groups of aquarium fish in this regard: Cold freshwater species, such as goldfish and koi; warm freshwater species, such as cichlids and tetras, and warm saltwater species, which includes tropical reef fish (the most common kind of saltwater hobby aquaria). As with other parameters, investigate the preferred temperatures of each species, and keep only temperature-compatible fish in the same aquarium.

Heaters are available for every size of aquarium. Care must be taken to ensure electrical safety when using immersion heaters. Likewise, glass heating elements must be used with care, as leakage of chemicals into the tank from broken or cracked heaters can quickly kill fish.

Chlorine and Chloramine

Chlorine and chloramine are two substances commonly added to our municipal tap water for their disinfectant properties. However, both are toxic to aquarium fish. Sodium thiosulfate is a chemical that neutralizes both of these. However, chloramine also contains ammonia, and this must also be dealt with before adding to the tank

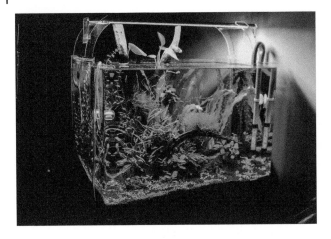

Figure 15.18 Freshwater aquarium with live plants. (Courtesy of Huy Phan https://unsplash.com/.)

(Andrews 2003). Water chlorine and chloramine removers are available at any pet store. Tap water should never be used directly to replace tank water without being first conditioned.

Salinity

Salinity refers to the amount of dissolved salts in the water. In general, freshwater aquaria contain less salts than saltwater systems. However, most freshwater tanks benefit from having some salts, which, along with minerals, increase the buffering capacity of the water. Most saltwater fish require a salinity of 31–36 g per liter. Brackish water salinity is between 3 and 10 g per liter. Salinity can also be measured by the specific gravity of the water. A specific gravity of 1.020–1.023 is ideal for most marine fish (Stoskopf 1993). Keep in mind that salinity in fish-keeping is more than just sodium chloride. Marine water is a complex mix of many salts and chemicals. Artificial seawater mixes are available that closely mimic the salt and mineral components of natural ocean water. In addition to sodium chloride, these mixes also contain potassium chloride, sodium bicarbonate, boric acid, and calcium and magnesium. These dry mixes are easy to use; just add water until the desired specific gravity is achieved. One should keep in mind that, due to evaporation, salinity will increase from water evaporation in a closed marine system, so the aquarium water itself must be monitored, and fresh (low-saline) water is used occasionally to replenish the tank. A marine fish keeper living near the ocean may use natural sea water for tank water changes, but pollution and variable water quality are negative factors to take into consideration.

Planted Tanks

An aquarium with a balance of healthy fish and lush, green plants is a delight to behold (Figure 15.18). Plants add oxygen to the water. Plants also provide hiding places for docile fish and break up the sight line between more aggressive fish. However, there are some drawbacks to keeping live plants in an aquarium. Plants provide environmental enrichment to fish, in the form of nibbling (or downright eating), to digging up, and displacement. These natural behaviors can quickly turn even the most enthusiastic fish keeper to using plastic plants. In addition, dying plant material adds to ammonia levels in the tank and can quickly clog filters. Plants also reverse-respire at night, when not practicing photosynthesis, and can draw oxygen out of the water. Plants removed from other fish-inhabited areas (such as a wild lake or pond) can be a source of fomites for fish disease or parasites. Planted tanks also have specific lighting needs, requiring the purchase of often expensive bulbs. Increasing the light in an aquarium can also lead to algae blooms. Again, the key is research into which types of plants are hardy enough to withstand the aquarium environment.

Feeding

Since fish come in so many diverse types, there are many different types of fish food available. When choosing food, remember to try to approximate the fish's natural diet. Therefore, a diet containing cornmeal as a primary ingredient would be inappropriate for a piscivorous (fish-eating) fish, but more suited to a herbivore (such as koi). Fish food comes in many different forms:

- Pelleted and flaked foods: Most people think of these when they envision fish food. Different variations of these foods are available for different types of fish. They are usually formulated as a whole, balanced diet. But many fish have more stringent needs, and alternating food items can be used as a form of environmental enrichment.
- Freeze-dried: Whole food items, such as krill or blood-worms, may be conveniently bought in a freeze-dried form. Freeze-dried foods are easy to use and store and make a good dietary enrichment item. Most freeze-dried foods are not nutritionally complete.
- Frozen foods: Prepared, complete diets can be frozen and stored until just before use. Commercial preparations are available, usually in small "breakaway" cubes. Some fish owners, especially marine aquarium keepers, prefer to make their own frozen diets by buying different types of fish, shrimp, vitamins, and minerals, and blending them according to recipes designed for each type of fish.

- Live food: Carnivorous fish are especially fascinating when they are chasing live food. Indeed, that is the appeal to most people when they purchase an aggressive carnivore, such as snakeheads or piranhas. Whole food items are usually a complete meal. However, when feeder fish such as goldfish or minnows are used, parasites may be transferred from them to the collection fish. Whole food items may not be completely consumed and will add to the ammonia burden of the tank. Also, the availability of prey items may be sporadic. A fish that is used to live food only may turn down less exciting meals, such as frozen or freeze-dried.

Quarantine

Quarantine is a very important part of maintaining a healthy tank to prevent a disease or parasitic outbreak, acclimating and acquiring baseline information of the new addition. It is in the best interest of the current residents to quarantine any new additions for 30–45 days or longer if needed. Depending upon the size of the fish, it will need the appropriate sized tank with separate water and filtration, ensuring excellent water quality. Avoid cross-contamination of any equipment used, such as nets, siphon hoses, buckets, or brushes, by having a set for both systems. Watch these animals very closely for the next several days for any signs of disease (see common disorders for fresh water or marine fish). Keep the quarantine holding system simple for ease of cleaning and stress reduction.

Some freshwater fish can tolerate a saltwater dip or a low salt bath (1–3 ppt or 3–5 ppt) for 21 days to help mitigate some potential diseases and inhibit *Chilodonella*. One should verify what fish can tolerate this before starting. Occasionally, it may be necessary to treat a bacterial disease with an antibiotic. It is best to work with a veterinarian who has fish experience to determine the appropriate treatment, and if there is a large mortality event examining some of those animals would be beneficial.

Some marine fish can tolerate fresh water dips. For those that do, it is advisable to provide a 1–3-minute dip to remove any potential diseases and parasites, less time if the animal is becoming stressed.

Keeping good records of water quality, water changes, feeding behaviors (food offered and eaten) and any treatments given is important; if there are any issues that occur, accurate records will help determine the problem/s.

Common Diseases of Aquarium Fish

Most problems found in aquarium fish can be directly related to water quality issues. Due to the necessary confinement of pet fish, they are unable to escape from inadequate conditions. High levels of ammonia or nitrite can cause fish to become sick, as can keeping them in less-than-ideal conditions for their particular species. Each fish type has certain parameters of water hardness, pH, oxygenation, and aquarium décor. A healthy fish can survive in imperfect conditions but will be more susceptible to illness. The first step in evaluating the sick fish patient is to obtain accurate water sample parameters. It should be kept in mind that many presenting complaints for ill fish are not diseases per se but are signs that can indicate more than one type of disease process.

Ammonia or Nitrite Poisoning

Signs of a fish sickened by poor water quality include clamped fins, listlessness, or gasping at the surface. Prolonged exposure may lead to ragged fins, hemorrhagic discolorations on the fins, or even death. Also, pond fish are susceptible to run-off from fertilizers or other chemicals applied to lawns, with similar resulting illnesses.

Hypoxia

Lack of oxygen in the water can cause discomfort, distress, or death of all but air-breathing species. Hypoxic fish gasp at surface of the water or gather at water inlets where oxygen levels are highest. Causes include overcrowding, poor water circulation, and algae crash (decomposition of dead algae uses up available oxygen in the water). Correction of the inciting problem is essential.

Fungal Infections

True fungal infections in fish are rare. *Aspergillus*, *Fusarium*, and *Candida* are all geneses of fungi that can systemically cause chronic health issues. However, it is quite common for an ill or injured fish to fall prey to opportunistic attack by water molds or fungi. An affected fish will present with cottony growths on the skin or gills. Usually, there is a history of poor water quality, decreased water temperature, or trauma, which allows the normally environmental fungi to colonize the fish. To confirm, a skin scraping should be performed on the affected area. Under microscopic exam, broad, non-septate fungal hyphae will be visible. *Saprolegnia* is the most common genus of water mold affecting fish (causing Saprolegniasis), but other fungi can cause the disease as well.

Dropsy

Dropsy is a broad term meaning swelling of the coelomic cavity. It can range from normal in some ornamental goldfish, to mild, to severe enough that the fish's scales protrude from its body, giving it a "pine cone" appearance. This condition can be a sign of many disease processes, including peritonitis (bacterial, parasitic, or viral), a mass or neoplasia, obesity, egg binding, or coelomic effusion. Radiographs and/or aspirate of the coelom can help diagnose the cause.

Egg Binding

When female fish ovulate, they wait for the right environmental conditions in which to lay their eggs. In captivity, there is often an absence of those conditions. While some fish can safely resorb unlaid eggs, others will retain them, causing digestive and/or buoyancy problems. In severe cases, unlaid eggs can even pile up year after year in the coelomic cavity. In these cases, inspissation occurs, and the only treatment is surgical removal.

Less often, egg binding can be secondary to another disease, such as a mass causing uterine blockage.

Color Change

Fish change color normally for many reasons, such as age or to indicate reproductive readiness. But when a fish becomes ill or stressed, maintaining normal pigment takes less precedence than maintaining other bodily functions. A fish with pale patches or dulled colors can be suffering from many types of illness. Red discoloration of the body or fins can indicate septicemia or toxic changes to the water.

Ragged Fins

A very common presenting complaint with many possible etiologies, fin damage can be caused by poor water quality, parasitism, trauma (tank mate aggression or rough objects in the water), or septicemia.

Ulcerations

Fish can develop raised, reddened ulcerated areas on the skin due to many problems, including trauma with secondary bacterial infection, ectoparasite attachment, or poor water quality.

Mycobacteriosis

A true illness, *Mycobacterium marinum* can affect fish despite excellent husbandry. This acid-fast bacterial rod causes granulomas to form within the body of the fish, although sometimes fish can be affected externally as well. Fish sickened by mycobacteriosis lose weight and become listless, and eventually succumb. Importantly, this is a zoonotic disease, called "Fish Handler's Syndrome."

People who place their hands in infected tanks develop small granulomas on their fingers. Fortunately, in healthy individuals, the disease is superficial due to the bacteria's inability to grow at human body temperature, which limits it to the extremities. A full course of the proper antibiotics is usually curative in humans. Due to zoonotic potential and difficulty in treatment, affected fish are usually culled. Sygnathids (pipefish and seahorses) are especially susceptible.

Lateral Line Disease/Hole-in-the-Head

Fish affected by this disease syndrome typically begin showing small erosions along the lateral line. These lesions progress until the skin around the lateral line and head becomes large, erosive lesions that can develop secondary bacterial infections. Flagellate protozoa have been associated with the lesions, but whether they are primary pathogens or opportunistic invaders is not known. Poor nutrition is also thought to be a factor.

Scoliosis

Fish, like any vertebrates, can suffer from deviation of the spine. Poor nutrition, trauma, or genetics can all cause scoliosis. There is no treatment. Affected fish may be able to live with the deformity if they are able to apprehend food. Due the possible genetic etiology, affected fish are usually culled.

Swim Bladder Disease

Since the swim bladder provides the fish with buoyancy control, a fish with Swim Bladder Disease usually presents floating upside down or unevenly. Multiple causes for this condition exist, such as trauma, septicemia, or gastric problems. Sometimes the condition is self-curing; otherwise, the affected fish can live with the condition as long as it is able to procure food. Goldfish, especially heavy-bodied ornamental varieties, are quite prone to this disease.

Gas Bubble Disease

Although Gas Bubble Disease, like Swim Bladder Disease, can affect a fish's buoyancy, the etiology is usually different. When the water becomes supersaturated with gases (usually oxygen but sometimes nitrogen), the gas can force itself into the tissues of the fish. Affected fish show clear bubbles in the fins, under the surface of the skin, and within the eyes. Causes of gas supersaturation include malfunctioning pumps, a sudden influx of oxygen-rich water, and rapidly heating cool, oxygen-rich water (which releases the dissolved gas). Severe events can even cause death from bursting of blood vessels within the body. Correcting the inciting event usually corrects the problem; however, large, visible pockets of gas can be safely aspirated with a needle and syringe to provide instant relief.

Exophthalmos

Although bulging eyes are a desired characteristic in some fancy goldfish, sudden onset in other species is not normal. Causes for exophthalmos include increased intraocular pressure (as in Gas Bubble Disease), mass or tumor (especially if unilateral), and septicemia.

Lymphocystis

Another true disease (rather than just a sign), lymphocystis is caused by Lymphocystivirus, an iridovirus. It is the most common viral infection in both salt and freshwater fish. Affected fish start out with a white dusting on the skin, which progresses to neoplastic-like masses. Although disfiguring, the disease is self-limiting, and recovered fish are thought to have some immunity thereafter. Diagnosis is based on a skin scraping of the lesions, which, when microscopically examined, reveal greatly enlarged dermal fibroblasts. Control includes isolating affected fish, decreasing stress, and prophylactic antibiotics to ward off secondary bacterial infections.

Parasitology

Wild fish are usually infested with parasites, but it is presumed that they live in balance with their parasitic load. A healthy fish can harbor some parasites without noticeable ill health effects. However, captive-bred fish can be sickened by a wide range of parasites and can succumb to their infestations due to exacerbation of parasitic disease by various conditions such as overcrowding, unfavorable water conditions, and improper nutrition (Stoskopf 1993). Parasites that take advantage and overwhelm an already sickened host are known as opportunistic parasites.

Unlike most domestic pets, it is more usual for a fish to be debilitated by ectoparasites rather than by endoparasites. The methods used for detection of ectoparasites, the gill clip and the skin scrape, are described under diagnostics and are two of the most commonly performed procedures in aquarium fish medicine. Endoparasites in fish also occur, but it can be difficult to obtain a fecal sample from an aquatic organism such as a fish. Endoparasites are often diagnosed at necropsy, and the other inhabitants of the tank can be

presumed to have the discovered parasite, also. The tank can then be treated as a "herd-health" situation.

Parasites can be difficult to treat. The best course of action is to have an effective quarantine system to avoid introducing parasites into the tank or pond in the first place. Treatments for ectoparasites commonly are referred to as "baths" (prolonged exposure to a low level of the treatment agent in the water) or "dips" (quick immersion, up to 15 min, in a higher concentration solution of the treatment agent).

Parasites in fish come from many different types, but often the symptoms exhibited by a fish infested with ectoparasites are similar (Andrews 2003).

- Reddened or raised scales
- Rapid opercular movement (gilling/respiration) or gulping air at the surface of the water
- Increase in mucus production
- Rapid, darting movements, often sideways ("flashing" to show the side and belly)
- Listlessness, such as lying still on the bottom or floating in the corner of the tank
- Scratching against objects in the tank
- Frayed fins, or clamped fins against the body
- Discolorations on the scales, such as white or black spots

Treatment of parasites varies, of course, with the target organism, but in general freshwater fish can be dipped briefly into a saltwater bath, which will eliminate many parasites adapted to living strictly on freshwater species, and vice versa for saltwater fish. There are many over-the-counter treatments, often proprietary, that are offered by different aquaculture companies. These can be very effective as long as the directions are followed carefully. Below, some of the more common parasites, and their basic treatments, are discussed.

Flagellates

Flagellates are microscopic, single-celled protozoa with one or more whiplike organelles used for locomotion. Most flagellates have a simple life cycle, where reproduction is by cell division. Many flagellates have the ability to change into a cyst form, which is better able to survive inhospitable conditions in the environment. The cyst form is infective but no longer motile. Typical flagellate parasites of fish include:

Hexamita and *Spironucleus* flagellates can affect fish both externally (skin and gills) and internally (intestine and muscle tissue). They cause a disease known in the aquarium world as Hole-in-the-Head. These parasites can be found in low numbers in healthy fish, but when the fish is debilitated by poor environmental conditions or diet, they lose the immune ability to keep parasite numbers in check. *Hexamita* burrows into sensory pits in the skin, causing erosion and decay, eventually showing up as rutted, mucoid lesions on the skin of the fish. Secondary bacterial infections are not uncommon. Treatment is usually metronidazole, in bath form, or in the feed if the fish is still eating. These flagellates measure approximately 10 × 6 μm (Noga 2010).

Ichthyobodo, previously known as Costia, and *Chilodonella* are two other opportunistic flagellates that can be present in low numbers in a healthy aquarium without causing harm. These protozoa cause "slime disease" when they overgrow on their fish host. Increased mucus production occurs, especially around the gills, and death can be rapid due to suffocation. The excessive mucus production is due to irritation as the parasites feed off of skin cells. Both these parasites can be treated with formalin. *Chilodonella* measures between 30–80 and 20–60 μm. *Icthyobodo* is one of the smaller flagellates, measuring 6–8 μm (Noga 2010).

Piscinoodinium, also known simply as *Oodinium*, is a dinoflagellate that causes "velvet disease." These protozoa have a more complex life cycle, with a free-swimming form that seeks out a host, and a cyst form that lodges under the skin of the fish and feeds off the epithelial tissue. Infected fish often exhibit what appears to be gold dust on the scales. This is caused by large numbers of the attached parasites. This parasite can also be found on the gills. Copper is the preferred method of treatment but must not be used in tanks with denizens sensitive to copper, such as most invertebrates. Salt baths may also be effective. *Oodinium* measures 40–100 μm (Noga 2010). *Amyloodinium* is a similar organism that causes a disease in saltwater fish called "Marine Velvet." It can be found in the gills, skin, and fins.

Ciliates

Ciliate protozoa are single-celled organisms with hair-like projections called cilia, which are used for locomotion. Cilia are similar to flagella but are usually shorter and more numerous. Ciliate protozoa are generally larger than flagellates. Ciliates reproduce by cell fission.

Ichthyophthirius multifiliis, also known as "Ich," is probably the most common parasitic infestation seen in the home aquarium. Known as "white spot," "ich," or "ick," this disease is particularly difficult to eradicate once established in a habitat, in part due to its life cycle (Figure 15.19). The infective form is the trophozoite stage, which encysts in the skin and gills of the host and feeds on the tissues. When finished, it falls off and forms the reproductive tomont stage, which adheres to objects in the environment. A single tomont can divide up to 10 times, producing mobile theronts, which seek out new

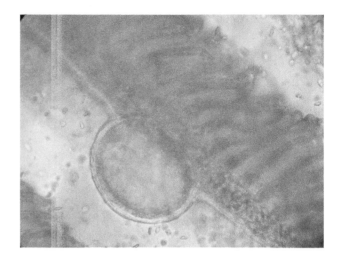

Figure 15.19 *Ich* in a gill.

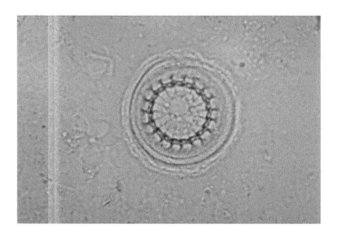

Figure 15.20 *Tricodina.*

hosts. Treatment includes increasing the environmental temperature to speed up the life cycle and treating the entire tank with increased salt levels or malachite green. *Ichthyophthirius* trophozoites exhibit a wide range of sizes, anywhere from 30 to 1000 μm (Noga 2010). *Cryptocaryon irritans,* known as "Marine Ich," is found on the skin and fins of saltwater fish. The organism looks similar to the freshwater counterpart, but the large horseshoe-shaped macronucleus is not as defined.

Trichodina is considered by many to be the most beautiful ciliate parasite of fish (Figure 15.20). This large (50–100 μm) disc-shaped protozoa has several rings of cilia that not only provide locomotion but also suction for clinging to the host. Most trichodinids are not direct parasites but use the fish as a base from which to feed on bacteria and detritus. Described as looking like a "flying saucer" or "scrubbing bubbles," this organism can cause extreme damage to gills and skin due to the presence of a denticle ring, which provides secure adhesion to fish tissue.

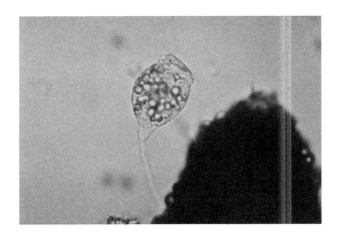

Figure 15.21 *Epistylus.*

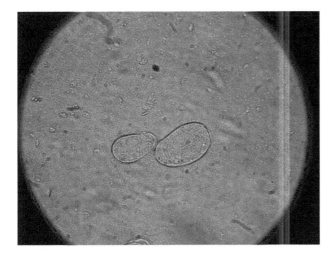

Figure 15.22 *Brooklynella.*

Formalin baths are used to control heavy outbreaks (Noga 2010). This organism is found in fresh and saltwater fish.

Tetrahymena is another opportunistic ciliate that can be found as a normal denizen of aquaria but will become parasitic on debilitated fish. These organisms encyst in the skin and tissues of the fish and are the causative agent of Guppy Disease in live bearers. The protozoa are tear-drop shaped, measuring 60–100 μm, free moving, and can be very difficult to treat. Formalin is often used to control outbreaks (Noga 2010). The analogous organism found in saltwater fish is called *Uronema*.

Epistylus is a small (micron) ciliate that is usually non-parasitic but is worth mentioning due to its unusual appearance and the fact that it can sometimes be found attached to fish that are debilitated (Figure 15.21). This organism has both a free-swimming and a stalked, sessile form. The cup-shaped body attaches to the fish or other object by means of a long, thin stalk, and when live specimens are viewed microscopically, their feeding cilia can easily be seen, beating the water for food items. They will jerk back, periodically, if threatened, but once danger has passed, they will elongate and feed once again. *Epistylus* species are often colonial. This organism can affect fresh and saltwater fish.

Chilodonella and its saltwater counterpart, *Brooklynella* (Figure 15.22) are large oval-shaped ciliates with the cilia found on the long axis. The organism has dorsoventral flattening and a notched anterior end. This organism moves slowly in a forward, rolling motion. It is found on the gills and skin.

Capriniana is a freshwater sessile ciliate that attaches to gills with a sucker.

Trematodes

There are parasitic trematodes that are of great concern in aquaculture. They can be divided into two main groups:

Monogenean trematodes have suckers, or a "hold-fast" structure for attaching to the host known as a haptor. The shape of the haptor helps speciate the organism. Haptors do not break down quickly after the death of the organism and can often be found on gill clips or skin scrapes of even heavily autolyzed fish. As a group, monogeneans can reproduce rapidly. Some are oviparous and some are viviparous. Affected fish may gulp air at the top of the tank, as their ability to absorb oxygen decreases. The key to treatment is determining if the parasite is oviparous or viviparous. Monogeneans are large, compared to the protozoa, and can measure anywhere from 300 to 2000 μm. Monogeneans have a simple, direct life cycle. *Gyrodactylus* is viviparous and fully formed young can sometimes be seen inside a gravid adult. It is primarily found on skin and fins. This organism is found on both fresh and saltwater fish, has no eye spots, and has two pairs of anchoring hooks. *Dactylogyrus* is oviparous. Its eggs hatch into ciliated larvae, which are in the infectious stage (Figure 15.23). This organism,

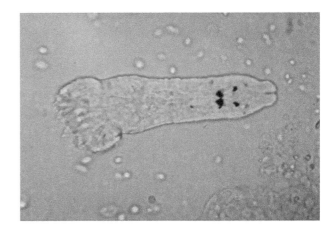

Figure 15.23 *Dactylogyrus.*

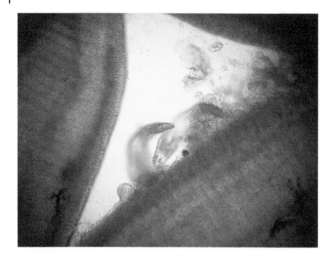

Figure 15.24 *Dactylogyrus.*

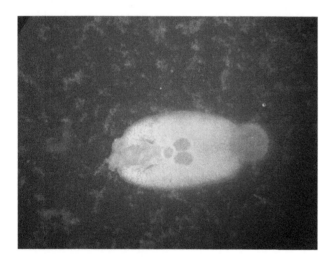

Figure 15.25 *Neobenedenia.*

found in fresh and saltwater fish, is found primarily on the gills (Figure 15.24). It has two to four eye spots and a pair of large anchoring hooks. The head is scalloped shaped.

Neobenedenia, a capsalid monogenean that affects saltwater fish, has three pairs of anchoring hooks and affects the gills and skin (Figure 15.25). Affected fish can be treated with praziquantel.

Treatment is usually performed with praziquantel or formalin as a bath or dip. Secondary bacterial infections may also occur (Noga 2010).

Digenean trematodes are the true flatworms and are endoparasites of fish and other animals. Also known as flukes, the adults have suckers for holding onto tissues. They have a complex life cycle, and fish can be either the primary, secondary, or final host, depending on the species. Adult digenean parasites are usually found in the intestinal tract but can also be found in organs such as the liver. Intermediate stages can encyst throughout the body, and cause "black spot disease" in aquarium fish. The preferred treatment is praziquantel (Noga 2010).

Nematodes

Nematodes, such as roundworms, can also be found as fish endoparasites. They have complex indirect life cycles, and fish can serve as both intermediate and final hosts. Nematodes can be found in the digestive system, swim bladder, and body cavity. In severe infestations, they may even be seen protruding from the vent. Treatment consists of oral fenbendazole, mixed with feed, but care must also be taken to eradicate any intermediate hosts, such as invertebrates, to break the life cycle and prevent reinfestation (Figure 15.26).

Cestodes

Cestodes, or tapeworms, also are endoparasites of fish, which can serve as intermediate or final hosts. Due to their complex life cycle, they are more common in wild or imported fish. One species, *Diphyllobothrium*, is of particular concern to humans, who are a definitive host and can become infected by eating raw or undercooked fish. Affected fish can be treated with praziquantel, but both a bath and oral route should be used to eliminate the parasites from all tissues.

Crustaceans

Crustaceans can also parasitize both fresh and saltwater fish. One of the most commonly seen is *Lernaea*, also known as anchorworm, which affects freshwater fish, most commonly in koi and goldfish production ponds. This

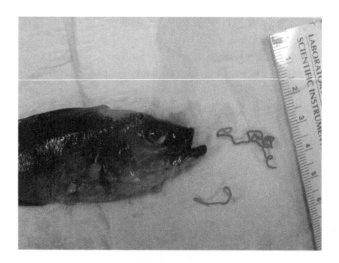

Figure 15.26 Nematode infestation.

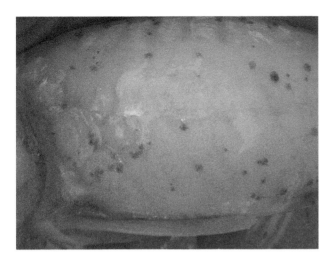

Figure 15.27 *Argulus.*

ectoparasitic copepod can be seen with the naked eye. The free-swimming copepodid is the reproductive stage. After mating, the female transforms into a worm-like shape and embeds into a fish's body, leaving a portion hanging outside of the fish's skin. The area of attachment becomes inflamed and can lead to secondary bacterial infections (Stoskopf 1993). Heavy infestations can kill young or small fish. Organophosphates can be used to treat large aquaria or ponds, but for small numbers of fish, the easiest (and most rewarding) treatment is to manually remove the parasite with tweezers, taking care to not to leave any portion still imbedded within the fish. *Ergasilus* is a parasitic copepod occasionally found in pond fish but rarely in home aquaria. It resembles an anchor worm. Ponds are treated with organophosphates. The fish louse *Argulus*, found on both fresh and saltwater fish, can be seen with the naked eye (Figure 15.27). Its size is roughly 5 mm to 8 mm in length. It has prominent eyes, sucking discs, and a stiletto. Because it is transparent, it tends to take on the color of the fish. It typically looks like dark spots or freckles on the skin. This organism is also treated with organophosphates.

Physical Examination

It is harder to examine a fish out of water than it is to examine a pet that will sit still and allow an exam to be done. A lot of the time one needs to rely on the patient's owner or primary care giver to explain what is going on, but with all exams one should try to be thorough and ask the right questions. The physical exam should be performed the same way as with other patients, beginning with an external overall view of the animal. A plan can then be put in place as to what will be needed for the rest of the exam. Will sedation be required? What equipment will

be needed? All supplies should be gathered and ready to go to minimize the amount of time the animal is being handled and, if sedated, under anesthesia.

Restraint

When restraining fish it is important to consider the stress to that patient and consequences to handling. Use latex or nitrile gloves that are powder free, otherwise one can cause the loss of their slime/mucus coat which could lead to the introduction of a disease. Chemical restraint may be needed to help gather information for a diagnosis (see Anesthesia section). Veterinary staff should be prepared to collect all samples to keep handling to a minimum.

The best way to handle a fish, depending upon its size, is to hold in one hand by placing a thumb over the front of their nose and forehead region and keeping the dorsal fin down with the palm of the hand and fingers on their underside (Figure 15.28). For larger specimens having help to restrain is beneficial. If they are venomous protective equipment should be worn, such as leather gloves or gauntlets covered with latex.

Chemical Restraint/Anesthesia

As fish medicine has increased in scope and knowledge, so has the need to immobilize fish for procedures. Advanced procedures such as laparotomy and tumor removal can now be performed relatively safely in the veterinary clinic. Even simpler procedures, such as skin scrapes and gill clips, are facilitated when a large or aggressive fish is sedated.

One of the most popular drugs used for chemical restraint is tricaine methanesulfonate. Formally known as MS-222,

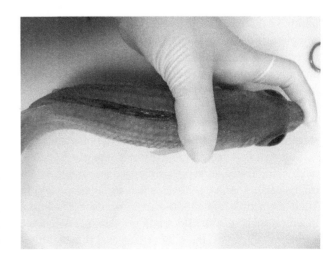

Figure 15.28 Restraint.

it is available from a variety of manufacturers as Tricaine or Syncane (from Syndel). While many other anesthetic drugs have been used in fish, tricaine methanesulfonate is the most commonly used drug and the only one approved in the United States for use in food fish (Boylan 2020). Although it is a very safe agent, it is also acidic, so it should be buffered with sodium bicarbonate to a pH level approximating that of the fish's original tank water. A concentration of 100–200 mg/L is used for induction, and 50 mg/L for maintenance (Noga 2010). A simple method for fish anesthesia is using multiple buckets, appropriate to the size of the patient. One bucket (the induction chamber) contains the fish in tank water, and another contains clean, non-medicated tank water. A measured amount of buffered stock solution of 10,000 mg/L is slowly added to the fish. Initial signs of anesthesia include an excitement phase, then slowing of opercular movement (gilling), and then loss of the righting reflex (the fish begins listing to the side). The ideal stage of surgical anesthesia is achieved when all loss of the righting reflex is obtained, and opercular movement has slowed or ceased. When the fish rolls onto its back the gills should be examined. They should have a bright red color. Pale gills are an indication of anemia or hypoxia. If this is observed, the anesthetic procedure should be discontinued or expedited depending on the reason for the procedure (Boylan 2019).

The heart rate and operulum/gill rate should be monitored when a longer procedure is performed. The trends of these are an indicator of the depth of anesthesia. The slower these are, the deeper the anesthesia. When the rate of these two increases, one should expect the patient to respond to noxious stimuli. A doppler or ultrasound can be used to monitor heart rate. The heart is typically located ventral to the gill cavity. If the depth of anesthesia needs to be reduced, this can be achieved by adding clean water to the anesthetic bath. This reduces the anesthetic concentration in the water (Boylan 2019). Once the procedure is complete, the fish can be placed in a bucket of clean water to recover. Gentle handling can be used to keep the fish in an upright position, and using a moderate, back-and-forth motion to increase water flow over the gills can speed recovery. Tricaine methanesulfonate leaches into plastic, so it is best to designate one bucket (or set of buckets) as an anesthesia chamber and keep the other equipment clean.

If the fish is to have a more invasive procedure such as more complicated surgery, a prolonged anesthetic device can be used. This is essentially a fish anesthesia machine. There are many types but most are homemade. The basics include a shallow tank sufficient for the size of the patient, a small water pump, and tubing connected to the outflow of the water pump. The patient is placed in the tank filled with medicated water and may be supported by porous

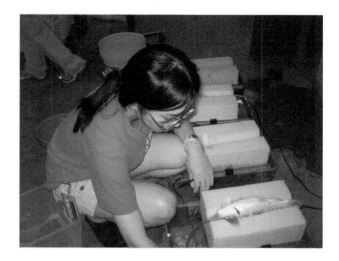

Figure 15.29 A fish being anesthetized. (Courtesy of Dr. Greg Lewbart.)

foam or a plastic "V" which cradles the fish in the water (Figure 15.29). The pump is placed into the water as well, and the tube from the pump is placed into the fish's mouth so that water flows over both sides of the gills and through the opercula. If any part of the fish needs to be exposed, for a surgical procedure, the tube in the mouth can be periodically removed and used to wet down the exposed area. Care must be taken to replace the tube immediately, to keep both anesthetic and oxygen flowing to the patient.

Pure clove oil or eugenol has been used for fish anesthesia. Its margin of safety is narrow compared to tricaine methanesulfonate, therefore it is not recommended as a commonly used anesthetic for fish (Boylan 2019). Due to the lower margin of safety, eugenol is often used for euthanasia, when the recovery of the fish is not necessary.

Both of these anesthesia agents may affect parasites upon the fish, causing them to drop off. Therefore, procedures such as skin scrapes and gill clips for parasite exams should be performed without anesthesia if possible (Stoskopf 1993).

Analgesia

Analgesia is a topic of interest in fish medicine; however, minimal research has been done on this subject. This means that the use of analgesics in fish is limited. Not only are fish kept as pets, but they have also become increasingly popular animal models in research. According to the Canada Council for Animal Care, fish are the most common animal research model, surpassing mice (Chatigny et al. 2018). This necessitates the use of analgesics for fish in research settings.

One reason for the limited use of analgesics in fish is that the capacity of lower vertebrates such as fish to experience pain remains a topic of debate. Despite the controversy professionals accept the fact that fish respond to noxious stimuli with a nocifensive response. Results of studies of neuroanatomy, neurophysiology, and neuroendocrine pathways reveal that fish are very similar to other vertebrates in their response to stress. Likewise, nociception travels via the peripheral nerves and is relayed through the spinal cord and then the thalamus just as it does in other vertebrates. Because veterinary expertise is sought more and more by owners of pet fish, for surgery in fish, catch and release sport fishing activities, and fish research, being cognizant of the fact that pain exists is important (Weber 2011).

While there may now be a general consensus that fish feel pain, one of the challenges is identifying the pain response in individual fish species (Chatigny et al. 2018). In other animals and in human infants, observing behavior is commonly used to identify pain in a patient. A challenge to using behavior as a pain indicator is that there is a lack of critical and comprehensive clinical data for the majority of fish species (Weber 2011). In order to know abnormal behavior, one needs to know what normal looks like. There is a lack of information regarding what normal behavior looks like in most species. The fact that fish lack facial expressions complicates the issue further.

Opioids are the most studied analgesics in fish followed by NSAIDs. Drugs such as amitriptyline, gabapentin, lidocaine, and medetomidine have been studied but less frequently. Opioid routes of administration include IM, IP injections, and bath immersion (adding the drug to water to achieve a specific concentration). Opioid administration results in few side effects with those reported being associated with cardiovascular and respiratory systems (Chatigny et al. 2018)

Morphine is the most studied analgesic and has shown the most beneficial effects on the fish it has been administered to compared to butorphanol, buprenorphine, and tramadol. It is one of the few analgesics for which pharmacological fish data is available. It can be given IM, IP, or by bath immersion. It also decreases the MAC of MS 222. This drug is considered to be a good choice for analgesia for a surgical procedure.

Few studies have been done using NSAIDs and only seven agents have been tested. Of those tested, NSAIDs have not proven to be very beneficial to fish. However, they do appear to be safe (Chatigny et al. 2018). A study in 2018 of meloxicam use in goldfish (*Carassius auratus auratus*) showed that a single IM injection caused no acute toxicity (Laronche et al. 2018).

Few studies have covered the use of local anesthetics in fish. Lidocaine has been used in the studies that have been conducted. Interestingly, lidocaine can be administered in the water in the same way MS 222 is, providing general anesthesia. The exact mechanism of action of lidocaine administered this way has not been completely explained. MS 222's safety, long-standing history of use in fish, ease of administration, availability, and relatively low cost have continued to make it the universally popular general anesthetic in fish (Chatigny et al. 2018).

Surgery/Wound Healing

Surgery is not uncommon in fish, but it can be tricky. Examples of surgeries that may be performed on fish include mass removal, enucleation, GI obstruction, and swim bladder repair (Shelley 2018). Trying to keep a surgical field sterile or out of the water can prove to be very challenging. Sometimes one has to become very creative. Sedation/anesthesia is required (see Anesthesia section) and depending upon how invasive the surgery is will help determine the anesthetic level required.

If an incision is required, scales will need to be removed to allow access to the skin. This can be accomplished by using forceps or hemostats to remove with a quick pull. To clean the area, it can be flushed with sterile water or saline and dried with sterile gauze. When performing surgery on fish, a true sterile field is not possible but a swipe of the incision site with dilute povidone–iodine or sterile saline can help to remove gross contamination. Plastic drapes can be placed over the fish to keep it moist and provide a working surface to decrease contamination of the surgical site (Shelley 2018).

Aquatic species are very prone to their suture lines dehiscing. It is up to the veterinarian to determine the best closing method for that animal. Keeping a close eye on that individual while healing is facilitated by keeping them in an isolation tank until healing is deemed sufficient.

Radiology

Typically, sedation of the patient will be required in order to obtain radiographs. Just like in other animals, creativity may be necessary to get the shot desired. It is best to practice with a dead specimen beforehand, if possible, to get the desired techniques and settings in place to minimize handling time. The plate should be covered with a plastic bag to prevent any damage from water (Figures 15.30 and 15.31).

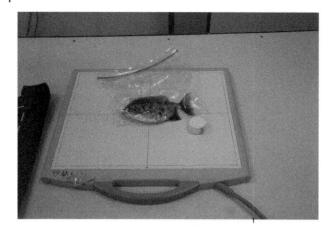

Figure 15.30 Radiographing a fish.

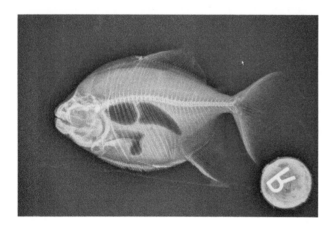

Figure 15.31 Lateral radiograph of a fish.

Basic Diagnostics

Some basic diagnostics that can be done on a patient without any sedation (unless too large or dangerous) are skin scrapes, fin clips, and gill clips. Sedation could make the parasites fall off or die, making the diagnostics unreliable. These techniques are called wet mounts, so one will want to use a dropper or pipet or fingertip to place small drops of water (tank water preferred) on a slide. The necessary sample is obtained, placed on a slide and then coverslipped to look under the microscope. One should start at low power and work up to higher magnification with any concerning areas. Most parasites can be seen at 100 total magnification.

External parasites can be seen on the animal itself and/or when a skin scrape is performed. Some external parasites do not work well with the cover slip method (Figure 15.32). To do the skin scrape, use the cover slip and slide it at a 45-degree angle with the lay of the scales to collect mucous from areas on the body, being sure to scrape any abnormal areas (Figure 15.33). One should either lay the coverslip

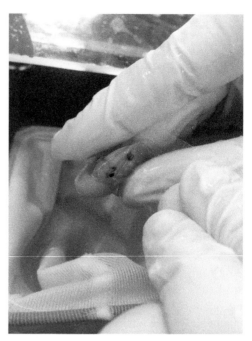

Figure 15.32 Skin scraping of a fish using a coverslip.

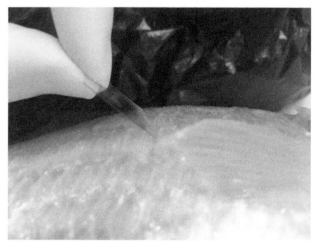

Figure 15.33 Close-up of a skin scraping.

down on a drop of water or place the mucous in a drop of water and look at it under the microscope. The preparation should be made to ensure that it is not too thick.

For fin clips, abnormal areas should be identified. A sample should be collected in a thin area of tissue (Figure 15.34). A pair of sharp scissors of an appropriate size for the patient should be used to snip a small sample of the fin. This sample should be placed in a drop of water and coverslipped.

Gills can be tricky, especially if the patient is small. Suture scissors works wonderfully for this, especially since

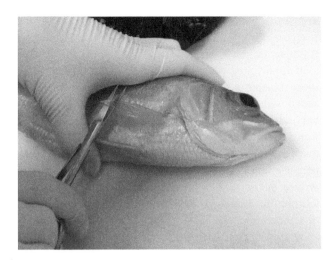

Figure 15.34 Fin clip.

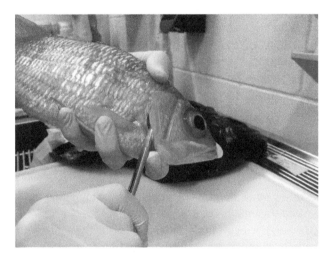

Figure 15.35 Gill clip.

they come in a wide range of sizes. The operculum will need to be lifted up first to allow access to the gill chamber (Figure 15.35). The operculum should be held there and then the hooked curved end of the scissors should be slipped under the tips of several primary lamellae taking care not to take too much to avoid hemorrhage. A small amount of blood is normal during this sampling; however, the sample should be placed in a drop of water and coverslipped. When using sharp pointy scissors, one should ensure that the fish is calm, otherwise a struggle could cause an unintended laceration.

If gills are not accessible, (closed operculum such as sygnathids) one can try flushing and aspirating with a small syringe and red rubber tube cut down to size and placing that fluid on a slide for examination.

Venipuncture

Blood samples can be a valuable diagnostic tool, for complete blood counts, chemistries, and possible cultures. When taking the sample, it is advised to use a syringe with heparin to prevent clotting, then placing the sample in a lithium heparin tube. Making slides for the complete blood count should be done as soon as possible as the heparin can cause morphological changes to the sample. If blood is taken for a culture, be sure to write the temperature in which the patient is housed for proper incubation of the sample to occur. One should be aware that the sample may take a long time to grow.

A preferred site for collecting the blood sample is the tail, using either a lateral or ventral approach. If the lateral approach is used, the needle is inserted under the scales just below the lateral line on the middle portion of the tail (Figure 15.36). The needle should be directed cranially and parallel with the lateral line, holding it at a 45-degree angle, inserting to the level of the vertebral bodies.

If the ventral approach is used, the needle should be inserted under the scale's midline of the ventral surface and posterior to the anus. Similar to the procedure in reptiles, if one should hits the vertebrae, the needle went a little too far and it needs to be backed out just a small amount.

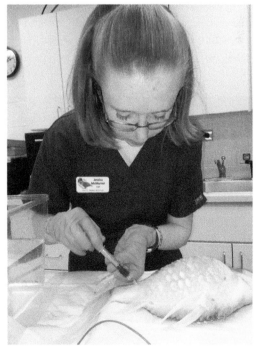

Figure 15.36 Venipuncture. (Courtesy of Dr. Greg Lewbart.)

Injections

There are times when an injection of medication would be advantageous to treat a problem in a fish. Just as in any other animal, the patient must be weighed first. This can be accomplished by using a container to place the fish in and a scale. One must first place aquarium water in the container. The container is placed on the scale and then the fish is added. The change in the weight is determined. This works best for small fish unless a large scale is available. One can weigh a large fish by placing them directly on the scale. Sedation should be used first. If appropriately sized netting is available, large tractable fish can be scooped up and weighed directly with a hooked hanging scale, such as those used in recreational fishing.

There are two ways to medicate a fish by injection, the intramuscular route or the intracoelomic route (ICe). Just as in other patients, the size of the needle corresponds to the size of the patient.

For the intramuscular route, the dorsal muscles just lateral to the dorsal fin provide an adequate site. Only small amounts of medication should be injected. This site is only used in fish larger than five inches in length.

The ICe requires that the fish be fasted for twenty-four hours prior to the injection so as to avoid inadvertently puncturing the stomach or bowel thereby causing peritonitis. The injection should be made on the ventral midline with the fish in dorsal recumbency (Figure 15.37A and B). The ideal area to inject is between the pectoral fins and the pelvic fins, avoiding the areas of the pectoral and pelvic girdles (Noga 2010).

Transportation

If transportation is needed for a fish, the primary goal is to maintain good water quality and keep the fish alive. For short transports, a suitable plastic bag with air or oxygen added with a good seal is adequate. For longer transports maintaining temperature, lighting (natural cycle) and water quality is important. This is accomplished by using twice as much air space with oxygen as water in the transport bag and tying it with a tight seal. Once the fish has arrived at the new destination, if this is the permanent location, acclimation time will be needed for the difference in temperature, pH, and salinity. To acclimate the fish, allow the unopened bag to float in the new tank for at least 15 minutes but no more than 30 minutes. If introducing the fish to a pond, do not allow the bag to remain in direct sunlight. Then open the bag and let a small amount of new water into the bag with the fish. Repeat this several times until there is at least 50% bag water to 50% new water in with the fish. This process should take no more than an hour. When the fish is deemed acclimated, slowly tilt the bag into the water so the fish can swim away unassisted. Some people prefer to net the fish out to lessen the chance of introducing pathogens into the system via the transport of water.

Euthanasia

Like any other animal, fish may need to be humanely euthanized. Past methods of euthanasia, such as cold stunning (freezing) or hypoxia (leaving it out of the water) are not certain or quick for the animal and are not considered

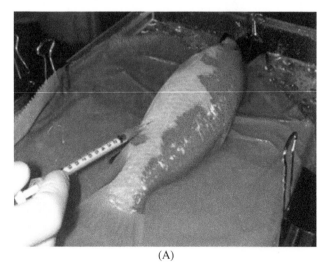

(A)

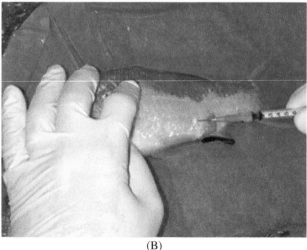

(B)

Figure 15.37 (A, B) Coelomic injection. (Courtesy of Dr. Greg Lewbart.)

humane. So it follows that "flushing" is not acceptable, either! Below the steps to euthanize a single fish are discussed. Different protocols apply to fish intended for human consumption.

To euthanize a fish, preparations for euthanasia should be similar to the preparations made for anesthesia. The environment should be quiet and nonstimulatory. Light intensity should be reduced. This can also be accomplished by placing the fish in a dark or opaque container. Alternatively, red light illumination can be used. The water the fish was housed in should be used with supplemental aeration and temperature provided if needed.

As stated in anesthesia, eugenol in high doses may be used for euthanasia. Overdosing of the anesthetic agent, tricaine methanesulfonate, is also effective. The immersion euthanasia solution can be prepared using water from the fish housing system and the fish placed in it. Alternatively, a concentrated form of the anesthetic agent as a solution can be introduced directly into the container the fish is in which can minimize stress. One should ensure that the fish stays in the euthanasia solution as long as necessary to guarantee death.

Because of the thousands of types of fish reliable methods of determining death may not be available for all. However, loss of movement, loss of reactivity to stimulus, and cessation of opercular activity for 30 minutes are good indicators. Also, the loss of the vestibuloocular reflex (movement of the eye when the fish is moved from side to side) can be checked as it is no longer present in fish that are deeply anesthetized or euthanized. Absence of a heartbeat is not a reliable indicator as the heart can continue to beat after brain death or removal from the body (AVMA 2020).

Secondary methods of euthanasia are recommended when appropriate after the fish is anesthetized (AVMA 2020). An example would be using an overdose of an intravenous or intracardiac barbiturate. This is especially effective in large fish such as koi, whose heart is easily accessible when the fish is dorsally recumbent, located just between the pectoral fins. As with any euthanasia, it is important to be humane. One should be mindful of the stress levels on the animal and perform euthanasia as quickly and comfortably as possible.

Necropsy

If a necropsy is to be performed, it is best to start as soon as death is ensured. Fish autolyze more quickly than mammals (Stoskopf 1993). Also, ectoparasites may begin to die or fall off the fish immediately after death. It is best to perform diagnostics such as skin scrapes or gill clips in a timely manner. The drawback to this is, a fish with absolutely no

signs of life or doppler readings may still have a beating heart upon internal exam. The heart can either be removed or injected with barbiturate euthanasia solution. If unable to perform the necropsy immediately, the fish should be refrigerated.

As with any necropsy, begin with a thorough external exam. The condition of the scales and fins should be noted, as also an increase or decrease in slime production. Unless preformed pre-mortem, this external exam should also include a skin scrape and gill clip, although external parasites may be absent in the presence of euthanasia solutions. Reddening of the skin can indicate sepsis. Wounds may indicate tankmate trauma. Look in the fish's mouth for signs of trauma, debris, or red discoloration. Carefully examine the gills, which should be bright, deep red. Pale or pink gills may indicate hemorrhage; excessive mucus, clumped, or brown gills may indicate gill irritation due to poor water quality (such as high levels of ammonia or nitrites) or parasites. White patches are a sign of gill necrosis.

Most aquarium fish are laterally flattened; therefore, a lateral approach to the necropsy is best (Figures 15.38 and 15.39).

With the fish lying on its side, a scissor is inserted into the vent (rectum), with the tip of the blades pointed cranially. A ventral midline incision is made, going between the paired pelvic and pectoral fins, and up to the ventral junction of the gill plates (opercula) if possible. Some fish have bony protective pectoral plates and may be difficult to incise; utility scissors may be required. The next cut returns to begin again at the vent. Direct the scissors dorsally while cutting. Resistance will be felt when the blades attempt to cut solid muscle, but much less when cutting only through the thinly muscled wall of the coelomic cavity. This naturally directs the scissors in a curve following the outline of the cavity and opens a "window" into the side of the fish. To ensure not incising the GI tract or the swim bladder, the

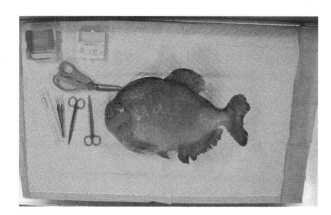

Figure 15.38 Instruments and supplies for a fish necropsy.

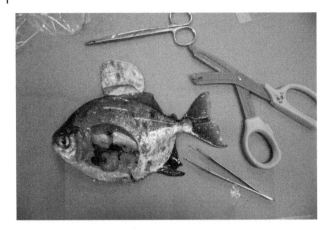

Figure 15.39 Initial step in performing a necropsy.

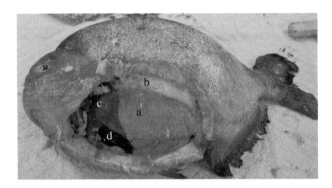

Figure 15.40 (A) Ova (B) fat occluding the swim bladder (C) liver showing fatty changes (D) spleen.

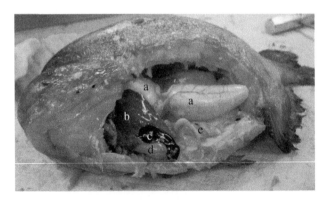

Figure 15.41 (A) Swim bladder, two-chambered, (B) liver (C) spleen (D) stomach (E) mesenteric fat.

blades of the scissors should be directed upward against the coelomic muscle.

A healthy fish will usually have some coelomic fat present. Fish are capable of obesity; however, due to the scaly exterior, obesity may not be apparent until internal examination reveals copious adipose. Fatty tissue will

need to be removed carefully to ensure visualization of the organs.

If the fish is female, the coelomic cavity may be filled with eggs or fry. These will need to be removed for the necropsy to proceed. Even a nonreproductive female will have tiny, undeveloped ova. In a male, the testes may be reproductive or nonreproductive. A male fish in breeding condition will have enlarged, firm testes. Outside of the breeding season, the testes may shrink dramatically, making them difficult to visualize. In most fish, they will be a long, thin, paired organ running dorsally just beneath the swim bladder.

The swim bladder varies in shape between different species, but it is often two-chambered (Figure 15.40).

It is situated on the dorsal wall of the coelomic cavity (Figure 15.41). The walls of the swim bladder can be clear or opaque and may also contain speckles or stripes of white. Note whether the swim bladder is intact or not. The kidney lies retro-coelomically, cranial to the swim bladder and is closely associated with the spine. The normal kidney is difficult to visualize, as it appears to be pressed up into the vertebral column. The fish kidney is paired but often joins to appear singular and is comprised of anterior and posterior segments (Helfman et al. 2009), distinguishable only by histological exam. They should be deep red in color.

The first, largest organ often noted is the liver (Figure 15.42). Analogous to other vertebrates, the liver should be deep, and brick red in color. However, the high-fat diets of most aquarium fish usually result in a yellowed or nutmeg liver color. Be sure to also note the texture of the liver, such as firm, rubbery, or friable. If sepsis is suspected, the liver is the preferred site of culture, if the necropsy has been performed in as clean a manner as possible up until this point. Most species of fish have a gallbladder; however, sharks and rays do not. An enlarged, firm gallbladder may be a sign of prolonged fasting.

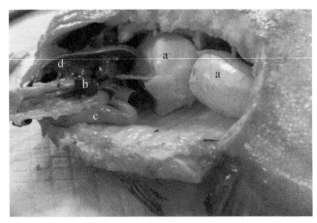

Figure 15.42 (A) Swim bladder (B) gall bladder (C) stomach (D) liver.

Figure 15.43 Kidneys along the spinal column.

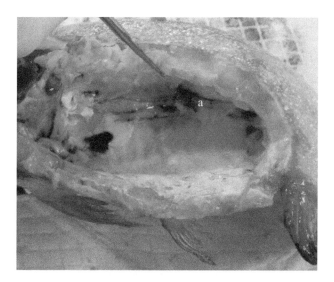

Figure 15.44 Fish gastrointestinal tract.

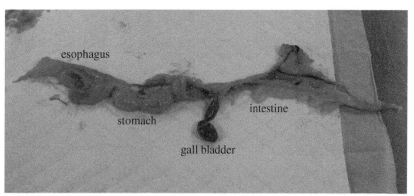

The spleen shape varies among species, from spherical to elongate. The spleen should also be deep red in color.

The GI tract will differ from species to species (Figures 15.43 and 15.44). Herbivorous fish, as in other vertebrates, tend to have more complex intestines than carnivorous fish. Especially of note are the pyloric caeca, found in many fish, most notably trout and bass. These numerous, fingerlike projections give the intestines more surface area for nutrient absorption. They can be quite bizarre-looking and may not appear to contain ingested food. During exam of the GI tract, intestinal samples can be taken at different points to examine later for the presence of endoparasites. If the fish has been inappetence for some time, the GI tract may contain only bile or mucus.

The heart in most fish is located directly behind the gills, between the pectoral fins, and may be difficult to access (Figure 15.45). Bone cutting scissors may be necessary.

Muscle tissue can be evaluated by incising the skin in different areas. Some parasites embed into the muscle and can only be found by thorough examination.

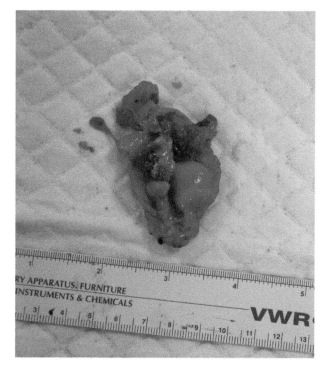

Figure 15.45 Fish heart.

References

Andrews AE. 2003. *Manual of Fish Health*. Firefly Books.

AVMA. 2020. *AVMA Guidelines for the euthanasia of Animals 2020*. Schaumburg, IL, American Veterinary Medical Association. https://www.avma.org/sites/default/files/2020-02/Guidelines-on-Euthanasia-2020.pdf

Boylan S. 2019. Fish anesthesia. In: *Proceedings of the VMX Conference, Orlando, Florida*, pp. 959–960.

Brunner B. 2003. *The Ocean at Home*. New York: Princeton Architectural Press.

Chatigny F, Creighton C, Stevens E. 2018. Updated review of fish analgesia. *J Am Assoc Lab Anim Sci* 57(3): 5–12.

Helfman GS, Collette BB, Facey DE, Bowen BW. 2009. *The Diversity of Fishes*, 2nd edn. Wiley-Blackwell.

Laronche C, Limoges M, Lair S. 2018. *J Zoo Wildlife Med* 49(3): 617–622.

Mortimer CH. 1956. The oxygen content of air-saturated fresh waters, and aids in calculating percentage saturation. *Intern Assoc Theoret Appl Commun* 6.

Nelson JS. 2006. *Fishes of the World*. Hoboken, New Jersey: John Wiley & Sons, Inc.

Noga EJ. 2010. *Fish Disease and Treatment*. Blackwell-Wiley Publishing.

Shelley J. 2018. Tropical fish medicine. In: *Proceedings of the VMX Conference, Orlando, Florida (1102)*.

Stoskopf M. 1993. *Fish Medicine*. Philadelphia: Saunders.

Romer AS, Parsons TS. 1985. *The Vertebrate Body*, 5th edn. Philadelphia: Saunders.

Weber E. 2011. Fish analgesia: pain, stress, fear aversion, or nociception? *Vet Clin North Am Exot Anim Prac* 14(1): 21–32.

Williams R 4th,, Neubarth N, Hale ME. 2013. The function of fin rays as proprioceptive sensors in fish. *Nat Commun*.

Section VI

Exotic Companion Mammals

16

Ferrets
Colleen Roman

Introduction

The art of veterinary medicine has extended itself into many families of creatures. Among small mammals, also known as "pocket pets," and more recently, exotic companion mammals, the ferret has become one of the more popular pets in today's society. Although the practice of medicine in ferrets is still viewed as being different from the traditional feline and canine practice, the same techniques that are used in small animal practice may be easily applied to small mammal practice. It is important for the veterinary team to recognize that there will be similarities and differences in the application of these techniques compared to small animal practice. Other novel medical approaches may also be utilized to provide solutions to problems.

The domesticated ferret found in the United States is commercially raised for the pet industry and medical research. It is conjectured that they arrived in North America as pets from early English settlers over 300 years ago. They are most likely a domesticated variety of the European ferret (*Mustela putorius furo*). The black-footed ferret (*Mustela nigripes*) is an indigenous species of the southwestern United States. There are strict fish and wildlife regulations that vary from state to state regarding the possession of these animals. Veterinary facilities, which often serve as the first point of contact for the pet-owning public, need to be acutely aware of these requirements.

Anatomy

Conformation

The ferret has an elongated body that allows the animal to enter small areas and holes for the pursuit of prey. This feature provides challenges for both owner and veterinary staff in caging and handling. Remember: wherever the head goes so follows the rest of the body. The males are larger than the females and their weight fluctuates according to season similarly to dogs and cats (Hillyer & Quesenberry 1997, 4).

Skin and Hair Coat

There are three naturally occurring coat color patterns. Sable is the most commonly observed but albino and cinnamon are also seen. The sable ferret, known also as "fitch," has been reported as a cross between the European polecat and ferret. They typically have black-tipped guard hair, a cream undercoat, black feet and tail, and a black mask. In the United States, enthusiasts have developed over 30 color combinations. Some of these include silver, chocolate, panda (Figure 16.1), and Siamese (Figure 16.2).

One of the first observations that handlers of ferrets make about this animal is that there is a distinct odor. This odor is primarily from oil glands and not from the anal glands, as many people tend to think. This odor may become more obvious when they are excited or during breeding season. There are numerous commercial bathing products that help to make these creatures more "house friendly." Descenting at a young age is a popular procedure performed at breeding farms but unfortunately, it has limited effects in preventing the odor. Ferrets have no sweat glands in their skin. As a result, the veterinary staff must be aware of the possibility that hyperthermia may occur.

Skeletal System

The vertebral formula for the ferret is C7, T15 (14), L6 (5-7), S3, Cd18 (Quesenberry et al. 2021). The anatomical considerations of interest include a small sternum and thoracic inlet, non-retractable claws and a J-shaped os penis. Skeletal anatomy is depicted in Figure 16.3.

Digestive Tract

The ferret has 30 deciduous teeth and 34 permanent teeth. The permanent teeth erupt between 50 and 74 days. The

Exotic Animal Medicine for the Veterinary Technician, Fourth Edition. Edited by Bonnie Ballard and Ryan Cheek.
© 2024 John Wiley & Sons, Inc. Published 2024 by John Wiley & Sons, Inc.
Companion Website: www.wiley.com/go/ballard/4e

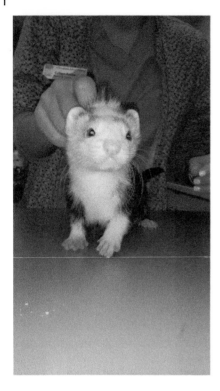

Figure 16.1 Panda colored. (Courtesy of Colleen Roman, DVM.)

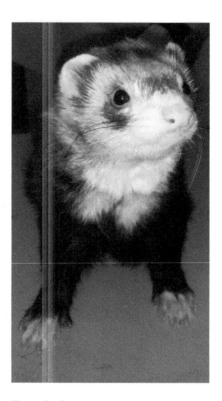

Figure 16.2 Siamese colored. (Courtesy of Colleen Roman, DVM.)

upper teeth are as follows: 6 incisors, 2 canine, 6 premolars, and 2 molars. The bottom arcade has 6 incisors, 2 canine, 6 premolars, and 4 molars (Fox & Marini 2014). (See Figures 16.4 and 16.5.)

Ferrets have five pairs of salivary glands. Care must be taken not to confuse the mandibular salivary gland with the lymph nodes in that area. The stomach of the ferret is simple and can expand to accommodate large amounts of food (Figure 16.6). The small intestine is short in length and has an average transit time of 3–4 h (Fox & Marini 2014).

Heart and Lungs

The heart lies approximately between the sixth and eighth ribs. In comparison to other mammals such as cats and dogs, the location of the heart in ferrets is relatively more caudal than expected for auscultation. The lungs consist of six lobes. The left lung has two lobes and the right has four (Fox & Marini 2014).

Spleen

The ferret spleen varies greatly in size, depending on the animal's age and state of health. When enlarged, the spleen extends in a diagonal fashion from the upper left to the lower right quadrant of the abdominal cavity. An enlarged spleen tends to be a very distinct finding during physical examination (Hillyer & Quesenberry 1997, 9).

Urogenital Tract

The right kidney is cranial to the left kidney and is covered by the caudate lobe of the liver. The bladder holds approximately 10 mL of urine. In the male, the prostate is found at the base of the bladder.

Gender is easily determined in males, who have a ventral abdominal preputial opening (Figure 16.7A) similar to dogs. In females, the urogenital opening has the appearance of a small slit (Figure 16.7B). During estrus, the vulva becomes enlarged. The natural breeding season is from March to August.

Fertility in both genders is dependent on the photoperiod. Females are seasonally polyestrous and induced ovulators. Ovulation occurs 30–40 h after copulation. Gestation typically lasts 41–42 days. If fertilization does not occur, pseudopregnancy often occurs and that will last 41–43 days. If such females are not bred, a large percentage of these individuals will remain in estrus with the potential for developing bone marrow suppression secondary to elevated estrogen levels (Hillyer & Quesenberry 1997, 10).

Adrenal Glands

Both adrenal glands lie in the fatty tissue anterior to the cranial pole of the kidneys. The left gland is located medial to the kidney and is approximately 6–8 mm in length. The right adrenal gland is more dorsal than the left. It is covered

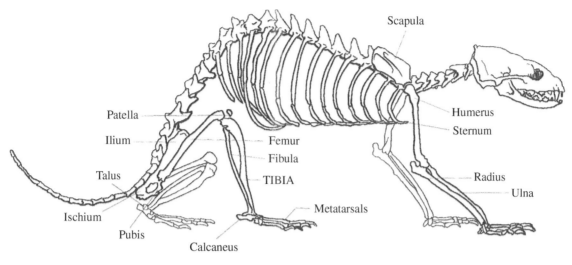

Figure 16.3 Ferret skeletal anatomy. (Drawing by Scott Stark.)

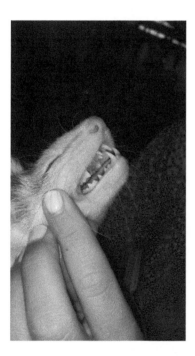

Figure 16.4 Ferret dentition. (Courtesy of Colleen Roman, DVM.)

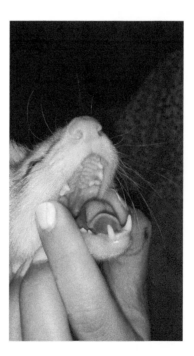

Figure 16.5 Ferret oral anatomy. (Courtesy of Colleen Roman, DVM.)

by the caudate lobe of the liver and is attached to the caudal vena cava. It is larger than the left with an overall length of 8–11 mm. This knowledge is important when assessment of adrenal gland disease is attempted either surgically or ultrasonographically.

Biologic and Reproductive Data

Table 16.1 provides basic biologic and reproductive data necessary for proper examination of a ferret or for answering common client questions.

Behavior

Ferrets are active little animals and the trouble that they can get into is limited only by the size of their head. The adult males are called hobs, intact females are called jills, spayed females are sprites, and juveniles are called kits. The ferret has been and still is used for hunting, biomedical research, and most recently as a pet. The domesticated ferret does not fear humans or unfamiliar environments, unlike its counterpart, the European polecat (Fox & Marini 2014). In pairs, they constantly play fight, expelling sounds

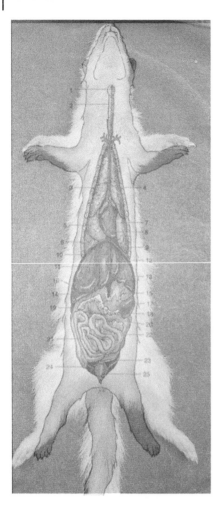

Figure 16.6 Ferret visceral anatomy. (Quesenberry Ferrets, Rabbits and Rodents 3rd edition.)

Table 16.1 Selected biologic values for the domestic ferret.

Adult weight	Male 1–2 kg
	Female 600–950 g
Life expectancy	5–11 years
Rectal temperature	Mean 101.8°F (38.8°C)
	Range 100–104°F (37.8–40°C)
Heart rate	200–400 beats/min
Blood volume	Male 60 mL
	Female 40 mL
Noninvasive blood pressure	Systolic: 95–155 mmHg
	Diastolic: 51–87 mmHg
	Mean: 69–109 mmHg
Respiratory rate	33–36 breaths/min
Urinary output	1 mL/h
Urine pH	6.5–7.5
Maintenance fluid needs	Unknown, estimated 60 mL/kg/day
Maintenance caloric needs	200–300 kcal/kg/day

Source: Quesenberry et al. 2021, 7

Husbandry

The word "ferret" means to search out something, to ferret it out, or to find something. This is a pet ferret's whole existence and an extremely important factor in providing a safe and an environmentally rich habitat for these animals. Assume that ferrets can go anywhere. The limiting hole diameter for escape is usually less than 1 inch; anything over that they can easily explore. Cages in the home setting and the veterinary hospital must reflect this attitude. All potential openings to the outside such as heating and air conditioning vents and tubing, dryer vents, doors, and windows are all possible routes of escape.

A ferret will not fare well outdoors because of its domestication. Inside the house, reclining and other furniture, bedding, appliances, and electrical cords offer potential injury and even death as a possibility. Owners must be acutely aware of the dangers of ingestion of household items such as insulation for wiring and pipes, packing material, rubber bands, and soft rubber material for shoes or other pet toys. These latter items are particularly dangerous as ferrets seem to have an affinity for materials made out of rubber. Gastrointestinal obstruction is a common problem seen in young ferrets.

Ideal caging should provide multiple levels and a hiding or den area (Figure 16.9), sufficient area for a litter box, and space for food and water. However, some owners may also set aside an entire room as living quarters for their ferrets. Food bowls should be made of a nontoxic product and safe

from a low growl to a high-pitched scream when challenged or in pain. They will continuously roll and bite their opponent on the face and feet, their favorite spot being the nape of the neck. Domestic ferrets are highly social and enjoy playing, exploring, and sleeping with other ferrets (Figure 16.8) (Quesenberry et al. 2021).

Many times in the heat of play with humans or companions, they will back up across the room chattering and hissing at the same time. They are attracted to quick movements, an instinct developed primarily for hunting prey. Their eyesight is only good up to short distances, and they depend upon their excellent sense of smell and acute hearing to help them maneuver in their environment. Due to their sense of smell, they constantly keep their nose close to the ground. This predisposes them to loud sneezing, which often alerts their owners to their location. Ferrets are active about 25–30% of the day and asleep the remaining 70–75% (Hillyer & Quesenberry 1997, 12).

Figure 16.7 (A) Male reproductive anatomy. (B) Female reproductive anatomy. (Drawings by Scott Stark.)

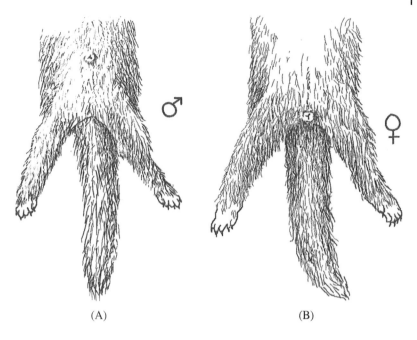

(A)   (B)

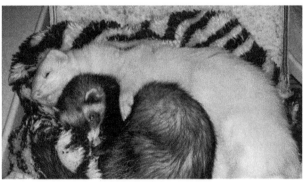

Figure 16.8 Bonded ferrets sleeping together. (Courtesy of Colleen Roman, DVM.)

water bottles are available commercially. Litter pans in a household setting may consist of a small plastic litter box similar to cat pans but may require lowering one side of the pan for entry. Also ferrets commonly back into corners to eliminate so boxes with rear sides higher than the front may prove to be beneficial. In a veterinary hospital, small, low cardboard boxes are useful for debilitated or post-surgery animals. They are also conveniently disposable.

Toys should be "ferret" approved; hard, nonchipping rubber balls, metal toys that make noise, and "ferret" jungle gyms made of PVC pipes provide good entertainment.

Nutrition

The domestic ferret, European polecat, and black-footed ferret are predatory animals that feed primarily on small mammals and birds. Early ferreters fed their animals bread or corn meal soaked with milk. They survived on this diet as long as it was supplemented with fresh meat.

Most ranch ferrets are fed commercial pelleted foods. Initially, mink diets were fed but they lacked important nutritional components due to their protein base of fish (Bell 1999, 169).

The ferret is an obligate carnivore with a very short intestinal tract. Compared to a cat, the ferret has relatively about one-half the intestinal length. They are spontaneous secretors of hydrochloric acid like humans and unlike dogs, cats, and many other predators. These animals will often hide food in various locations in their environment for future consumption. Because of the inefficiency of the ferret's digestive tract, ferret diets need to be high in protein and fat and low in fiber. Traditional ferret diets include 30–40% protein and 15–30% fat. The type of diet used depends on the ferret's health status and life stage, such as if they are growing kits or lactating jills (Bell 1999, 172).

It is important to feed a high-quality domestic ferret food in dry form. Dry food is preferred over moist due to the health benefits for the mouth, teeth, and gums. Young kits will require some moistening of the kibble foods until they get their adult teeth. At about 10 weeks of age, they should begin to handle dry kibble. There are numerous commercial foods available from pet stores, veterinary clinics, or the Internet. If food availability is difficult, a high-quality dry kitten food may be substituted. Some ferret food manufacturers also have senior diets available.

In some situations, such as medical problems, surgery recovery, or cold environmental conditions, supplements may be warranted. Products such as Nutrical

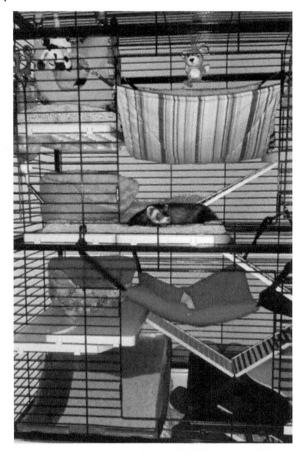

Figure 16.9 Ferret multi-level habitat with enrichment items. (Courtesy of Colleen Roman, DVM.)

(Vetoquinol) are available through veterinary offices. A common over-the-counter product, Ferrevite (8 in 1 vitamin supplement), is also a good choice. Snacks and treats should be held to a minimum since this animal will over-indulge in its favorite foods and run the long-term risk of malnutrition. Commercial meat or liver snacks for cats or ferrets are acceptable, and an occasional raisin may add a little variety to a ferret's diet. In some medical conditions, such as insulinoma, treats or supplements that are high in sugar may need to be avoided except at the direction of a veterinarian.

Water should be fresh and available at all times and may be preferred in a bowl and/or bottle.

Common Diseases

There are many disease syndromes found in ferrets. Canine distemper is occasionally found manifesting itself in various forms. Early signs include mucopurulent ocular nasal discharge, crusty facial and eyelid lesions, and hyperkeratosis of the footpads. In some individuals, there

is an orange color change to the skin. These animals are often anorexic, and in advanced cases may show central nervous signs such as ataxia, torticollis, and nystagmus.

Intestinal obstructions are very common in young inquisitive ferrets. These individuals present with or without vomiting, they may have diarrhea, they are lethargic, and in most situations, there is a palpable abdominal mass. Bruxism, which is when a ferret gnashes its teeth from side to side and may froth at the mouth, is a common sign of pain.

Epizootic catarrhal enteritis (ECE) or green slime disease is a debilitating disease of young and old ferrets. ECE is usually brought into the house via introduction of a new young ferret. It is a highly contagious disease of ferrets characterized by profuse green diarrhea, dehydration, anorexia, and progressive wasting.

Tumors present themselves in many ways with ferrets. The most common tumors involve the adrenal gland. These tumors may be benign or malignant. Adrenal gland disease most often presents as a dermatologic concern (Figure 16.10). Hair loss on the tail, bilateral hair loss along

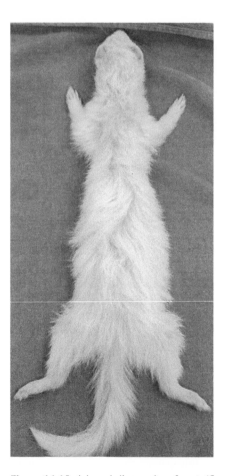

Figure 16.10 Adrenal disease in a ferret. (Courtesy of Colleen Roman, DVM.)

the abdomen, and vulvar enlargement in spayed females are consistent findings with adrenal gland involvement. Adrenal tumors can also cause behavior change and generalized muscle wasting. Secondary complications of the disease found in male ferrets involve the prostate in the form of prostatic hyperplasia or cysts, and they commonly present with dysuria. Bacterial or fungal bladder infections can be a sequela to prostatic disease in males with adrenal disease. This problem may be extremely challenging to treat.

Lymphoma is found in the ferret in numerous forms. It may involve the lymph nodes, spleen, liver, intestines, kidneys, lungs, and bone marrow. Squamous cell, mast cell, basal cell, and sebaceous gland tumors are the most common tumors of the skin.

Insulinoma, a type of pancreatic cancer, is very challenging to manage. Ferrets present very weak and sometimes seizing. Due to the excessive insulin produced by this pancreatic tumor, blood glucose levels in affected ferrets are very low. These animals often present with significant weight loss, dehydration, moderate to severe depression, anorexia, or in a comatose state.

Renal cysts are found in many ferrets and often are only coincidental findings.

Ectoparasites such as fleas, ear mites, sarcoptic mites, and ticks are common in ferrets and are easily treated. Endoparasites are uncommon but coccidia and giardiasis are occasionally found. There is some geographic prevalence to ringworm (mycotic) in some individuals.

Posterior weakness is a frequent observation in sick or debilitated ferrets. This is also a common sign seen in hypoglycemic animals.

Disseminated idiopathic myofasciitis also known as myofasciitis is a disease of unknown etiology first documented in 2003. This disease is characterized by severe inflammation of muscles and surrounding fascia. Ferrets with this condition tend to be young (6–24 months of age). Clinical signs are often nonspecific and may include inappetence, pyrexia, lethargy, pain, reluctance to move, and diarrhea. Individuals also develop anemia and neutrophilia with a left shift. Supportive care is necessary and should include analgesics, fluids, and nutritional management. Successful treatment using chloramphenicol, cyclophosphamide, and prednisolone was used in three confirmed cases (Quesenberry et al. 2021).

Zoonotic Diseases

Influenza (orthomyxovirus) is the only documented zoonotic disease of ferrets. In most cases, the transmissibility from humans to ferrets is much higher than from ferrets to humans. Owners should be aware of that risk to their pets when they have upper respiratory problems. Other potential zoonotic diseases include leptospirosis, listeriosis, salmonellosis, campylobacteriosis, tuberculosis, and rabies. There are no known cases of transmission of rabies to humans from ferrets.

Cryptosporidiosis has been found in ferrets; however, it may not cause clinical disease. While the zoonotic potential of *C. parvum* is unknown, ferret owners should be advised of transmission potential if oocysts are found during a fecal examination (Quesenberry et al. 2021).

History and Physical Examination

The procedure for taking a history and performing a physical examination on ferrets should follow routine small animal veterinary protocol. Questions should include: Has your ferret been coughing, sneezing, vomiting, or having diarrhea? Has there been any discharge from the eyes, nose, or any other body orifice? What is your pet's diet and how is its appetite? Does your ferret drink water excessively, have increased urination, or is it straining to urinate? Is your ferret active and alert?

Physical examination should also be consistent. The initial examination should be evaluated "hands-off" with observation of the patient prior to handling. This includes the patient's overall mentation status, posture, gait, and evaluation of signs of pain. The latest approach in the assessment of pain in animals is the species-specific grimace scales that appear to utilize our tendency to focus on the face of an animal. Also, grimace scales can easily and rapidly be taught to animal caretakers and appear to be less time-consuming than other pain assessment methods. Grimace scales are based on the Facial Action Coding System (FACS) for humans, which describes changes to the surface appearance of the face using action units (AUs) such as brow lowering, tightening and closing of the eyelids, nose wrinkling, and upper lip raising (Reijgwart et al. 2017). These changes in facial conformation prior to handling, during handling, and after handling should be noted for the evaluation of pain (Figure 16.11).

A hands-on physical examination should begin at the facial region and work caudally. Make sure that all areas are searched. Look for discharge from the eyes, nose, or ears. Examine the ears for masses or signs of mites. Remember, dirty ears do not necessarily need to be cleaned. A certain amount of discharge is normal and is present for protection. Are the eyes uniform in appearance and are there any signs of cataracts? Are all adult teeth present or are there remaining deciduous teeth? Does the rest of the oral cavity appear normal? Gingivitis and tartar are common

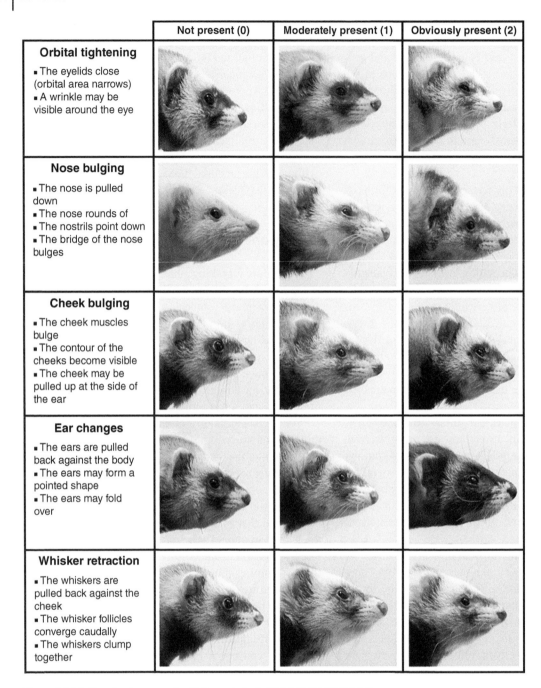

	Not present (0)	Moderately present (1)	Obviously present (2)
Orbital tightening ▪ The eyelids close (orbital area narrows) ▪ A wrinkle may be visible around the eye			
Nose bulging ▪ The nose is pulled down ▪ The nose rounds of ▪ The nostrils point down ▪ The bridge of the nose bulges			
Cheek bulging ▪ The cheek muscles bulge ▪ The contour of the cheeks become visible ▪ The cheek may be pulled up at the side of the ear			
Ear changes ▪ The ears are pulled back against the body ▪ The ears may form a pointed shape ▪ The ears may fold over			
Whisker retraction ▪ The whiskers are pulled back against the cheek ▪ The whisker follicles converge caudally ▪ The whiskers clump together			

Figure 16.11 Ferret grimace scale. (Reijgwart et al. (2017)/PLOS/CC BY 4.0)

findings in the oral cavity that should be noted if present. Often the best way to evaluate the oral cavity is by gently scruffing the nape of the neck and waiting for the ferret's characteristic yawn reflex.

Do you see any signs of lymph node enlargement? Heart and lung fields are evaluated in the same respect as with other small animals, with one slight change. Due to the more caudal location of the heart, auscultation of the heart in ferrets typically occurs at the caudal chest area as opposed to the mid-chest area. Are the lung sounds normal and is there any indication of a heart murmur? Does the animal appear normal and of good conformation? Muscle and skeletal systems should be symmetric and show no sign of dysfunction. Do the limbs move in a normal manner? How is the appearance of the skin and hair coat? Thinning of the hair and/or alopecia along the body as well as the tail is a sign of adrenal disease. Ferrets do go through a photoperiod, where they molt their summer coat in order to prepare for their winter coat. This can be commonly misdiagnosed as a clinical disease. Canine distemper may cause crusty lesions on the skin or an orange color change. Hydration is also measured by skin turgor. Always be aware of masses of the skin and subcutaneous tissue.

Abdominal palpation is best accomplished by elevating the ferret above the examination table by the nape of the neck or by gently holding it around the neck. Most of these individuals will accommodate the examination without too much struggle. Keep in mind that the spleen in many ferrets may be enlarged with no other indication of disease or illness. Examination of the prepuce and penile region in the male and vulvar area of the female is important to look for infection or any indication of endocrine problems.

For neurologic problems consider the overall behavior of the ferret. Is the ferret aware, alert, and curious or does it appear to be star gazing and unconcerned with its surroundings? Is the ferret having trouble standing? Ferrets with evidence of neurologic disorders, depending on the clinical signs, may have a life-threatening illness that requires immediate medical intervention.

Anxiety and Stress-free Techniques

There is a movement in veterinary medicine focused on making the veterinary visit as stress and anxiety-free as possible for the patient. While techniques were created with dogs and cats in mind, they can be used in other pets. There is no "one way" to make a visit an anxiety and stress-free experience. Individual animals and clients will have individual preferences. While performing procedures we often have to touch our patients in sensitive areas. Creating a plan of action for each patient can be a quick process that saves time and creates a more pleasant experience for the veterinary healthcare team, the patient, and the client.

Considerate Approach, Gentle Control, and Touch Gradient

The following are definitions from the Fear Free^SM Certification Program for dogs and cats. The principles can be applied to ferrets. Considerate approach encompasses the interaction between the veterinary team and the patients and inputs from the environment while veterinary care is being administered. Gentle control is how the veterinary team comfortably and safely positions the patient to allow the administration of veterinary care. The goal of considerate approach and gentle control is to alleviate fear, anxiety, and stress (FAS) in patients.

Key concepts with gentle control include: restraint is frightening and creates FAS; use the least amount of restraint as needed. In general, it is beneficial to use treats before, during, and after procedures. Constant communication between team members is critical.

Touch gradient is a term used to describe how to touch canine and feline patients to minimize FAS during veterinary procedures. This can easily be applied to ferrets. Touch gradient encompasses both gentle control and considerate approach has two components:

- It begins by maintaining continual physical hands-on contact throughout the entire procedure or examination whenever possible.
- It includes acclimating a patient to an increasing level of touch intensity, while continuously measuring the patient's acceptance and comfort.

Plan of Action

There are multiple components to creating a plan of action for a procedure.

1. Assess the patient.
   a. Observe and notate body language and behavioral indicators of FAS.
   b. Notate the current level of FAS based on the FAS scale.
   c. Continuously reassess throughout the procedure.
2. Assess yourself.
   a. Are you utilizing a considerate approach?
   b. Ask for help if you are feeling uncomfortable.
3. Assess the environment.
   a. Remove stressors in the environment.
   b. Set up a calming environment.
4. Create a veterinary plan for care.

When creating the veterinary plan for care, first determine a reinforcement hierarchy/reward ladder for the patient. Next, procedures should be ranked as most to least important procedure. The veterinarian will be responsible for determining the importance of procedures. Then the most important procedures in order of least to most aversive should be ranked. Determine if there are stopping points for breaks in the procedure and what behavioral indicators for this patient will be considered a stopping point.

Once a high-level re-enforcer is discovered for the patient, a plan for which order the procedures will be performed should be decided upon including stop points. Now the 3Ws can be considered:

- **Where** will the procedure be performed? The exam room, treatment area, and housing area?

- **Who** will be present? If possible, it is usually best for the owner to be present.
- **What** do you need to make the environment as pleasant as possible? What items do you need for the procedure? Everything should be ready before the patient is brought to the area.

Stress-free visits start at home and utilizing a safe hard-sided carrier that eliminates the need for forced loading and unloading can start any appointment off for better success (Figure 16.12A and B) (Martin 2017).

Preventive Medicine

The primary focus for preventive care in ferrets should be centered on annual or bi-annual physical examination. An early vaccination program is imperative in young ferrets. These individuals should be vaccinated at 6 to 8 weeks, 10 to 12 weeks, and 13 to 14 weeks for distemper (Purevax Ferret Distemper, Boehringer Ingelheim). Purevax is a canarypox-vectored recombinant vaccine that does not contain complete CDV or adjuvants; thus, post-vaccination risks are reduced. (Quesenberry et al. 2021, 15) Rabies vaccination is strongly recommended in environments with risk of infection and may also be required by law in individual states or municipalities. A rabies vaccine (Imrab®-3/TF, Boehringer Ingelheim or Defensor 1/3, Zoetis) may be given as early as 3 months of age. Both canine distemper and rabies boosters are given yearly along with a physical examination.

Vaccine reactions still can occur in some ferrets. Vaccine reactions seen include lethargy, depression, vomiting, seizures, and cardiac arrhythmias. Veterinary hospitals have adopted various protocols for dealing with newly vaccinated ferrets. Some hospitals will monitor these ferrets at least 30 min after vaccination. Other hospitals may provide premedication with an antihistamine prior to vaccination. Whatever the protocol, be aware that vaccine reactions have been known to occur at least 24 h post-vaccination. Owners should be alerted to the clinical signs and take appropriate measures to seek veterinary care should these signs appear after discharge from the hospital.

Heartworm disease is found in ferrets. Currently, there is only one FDA-approved form of heartworm prevention for ferrets on the market. The drug, Advantage Multi® for Cats (imidacloprid and moxidectin), is manufactured by Elanco Animal Health Inc. and approved to prevent heartworm disease in ferrets. Applied monthly, it also treats flea infestations by killing adult fleas (FDA.gov website 2018).

Prevention of heartworm disease may be accomplished by off-label use of Heartgard® Plus 68 µg (Heartgard® Plus, Boehringer Ingelheim). One-fourth tablet should be given once monthly. The remainder of the tablet should be discarded since the remaining preparation will deteriorate. A liquid ivermectin preparation may also be used by mixing 0.3 mL of injectable ivermectin (Ivomec® 1% Injection for Cattle, Boehringer Ingelheim) in 28 mL (1 oz) of propylene glycol. This should be administered at 0.2 mL/kg PO (20 µg/kg) once per month. This preparation is light-sensitive and should be stored in a light-blocking container. The expiration date is 2 years as long as the time period falls within the expiration date of the stock bottle (Hillyer & Quesenberry 1997, 70).

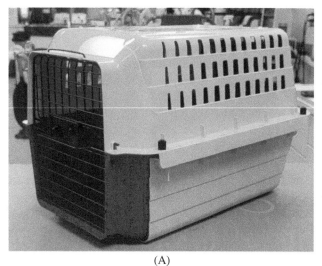

(A)

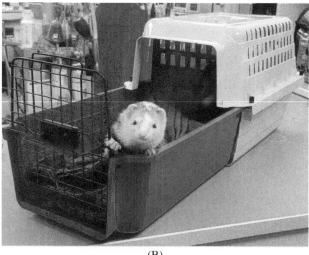

(B)

Figure 16.12 (A) Closed carrier (B) Carrier opened to show easy-loading hard-sided design for stress-free travel. (Courtesy of Colleen Roman, DVM.)

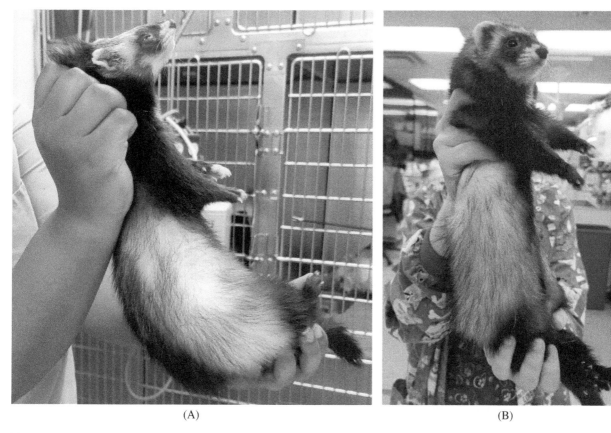

(A)   (B)

Figure 16.13 (A) Ferret restraint using the scruffing method. (Courtesy of Colleen Roman, DVM.) (B) Ferret restraint without scruffing. (Courtesy of Colleen Roman, DVM.)

Internal parasites are not commonly seen in ferrets and when found are usually protozoal such as coccidias and flagellates. An annual fecal examination is strongly recommended as part of a wellness checkup (Marini 2013).

Restraint

As with any animal, proper restraint involves the humane handling of the patient with consideration for the safety of the assistant. Although ferrets are usually active creatures, they are easily managed in the clinical setting. Young ferrets and occasionally adults that are less frequently handled may have a tendency to nip. Some of these individuals may latch onto a finger and require a gentle extraction.

The preferred methods for injections and examination are scruffing the neck (Figure 16.13A) or forming a ring around the neck using the index finger and thumb and supporting the thoracic cavity with the dominant hand while supporting the hind limbs with the non-dominant hand (Figure 16.13B). The rear legs and rear quarters are firmly pulled caudally but not at full extension. Another method involves wrapping the ferret in a towel "burrito" style (Figure 16.14). This is very effective for jugular

venipuncture. Many ferrets may be vaccinated or treated without any physical restraint other than using a treat as a distraction.

More appropriate stress-free handling methods are preferred. These can be more efficiently accomplished by using a distraction such as a liquid diet like Royal Canin Recovery

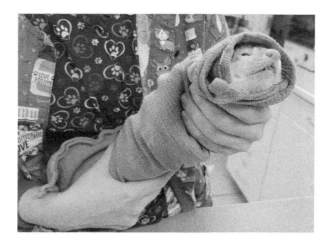

Figure 16.14 Ferret restraint using the "burrito" method with a hand towel. (Courtesy of Colleen Roman, DVM.)

diet, Emeraid or Oxbow Carnivore care, or nutritional supplements such as Nutri-Cal or Furo-Tone Skin and Coat supplements. These can be bottled-fed, syringe-fed, or even applied to an inanimate surface such as the examination table or a feeder toy.

A few individuals may require restraint with light sedation prior to the performance of any procedure. Chamber or mask induction with gas anesthesia is usually all that is needed. Besides the risks of anesthesia, minor changes may occur in the results from blood drawn in the anesthetized patient. The advantages are that procedures may be performed quickly and with less stress and struggling on the part of the patient and handler.

Radiology and Ultrasound

As with many small animals, it is difficult to radiograph a part without radiographing the whole individual. Obviously, one should measure the body part of interest and set the machine according to the thickness and the machine's technique chart. Small mammal technique charts need to be tailored to each clinic's equipment. Contrast radiography is employed as a diagnostic tool in ferrets. The most common use is in gastrointestinal studies. The protocol, though similar to the cat, should keep in mind the fast gastrointestinal transit time of the ferret. (See Figures 16.15 and 16.16.)

Ultrasound studies are easily performed and readily tolerated by ferrets with only light restraint. Whole-body scans are performed often with special attention to the stomach, pancreas, lymph nodes, liver, kidneys, adrenal glands, bladder, and the prostate in males.

Anesthesia and Surgery

Inhalation anesthesia has historically been the recommended method for induction of ferrets. Isoflurane is the most common product in use. Sevoflurane has more recently been used and lacks the irritating taste of isoflurane. The main disadvantage is the cost of sevoflurane. Intubation may be a challenge with ferrets but is similar to that in cats. The technique may require the use of a stylet. Gas anesthesia is then continued for the duration of the procedure. Use of a forced-air patient warming system (Bair Hugger, Arizant, Eden Prairie, MN) will help to prevent hypothermia. Pulse oximeters, respiratory monitors, and cardiac monitors work well with ferrets.

Sedation with a combination of pre-anesthetics such as benzodiazepines, alpha-2 agonists, and analgesics can provide adequate sedation for intravenous catheter placement. Induction can, therefore, be performed with injectable anesthetics such as propofol or Alfaxalone and maintained either after intubation of gas anesthetics or with constant rate infusions (CRIs) of injectable anesthetics.

Analgesia is an important element in the recovery of postsurgical ferret patients. Opioids such as hydromorphone (0.05–0.3 mg/kg SQ, IM q6-8 h), butorphanol (0.05–0.5 mg/kg SQ, IM, IV q 2–4 h) or buprenorphine (0.01–0.03 mg/kg SQ, IM, IV q6–12 h) are effective in ferrets (Quesenberry et al. 2021, 551–553).

Common procedures in ferrets include gastrotomies, enterotomies, adrenalectomies, cystotomies, partial pancreatectomies, lymph node biopsies, and mass excisions of the dermis. Most orchiectomies and ovariohysterectomies are performed at the breeding farms prior to entry of the ferret into the pet population. Every state has its own regulations regarding breeding, spaying, and neutering. Hepatic and splenic biopsies are employed as diagnostic tools and may be performed surgically or through the use of ultrasound-guided biopsy forceps. Ferrets often have enlarged spleens that may or may not be the origin of disease. Many orthopedic problems common in dogs and cats are not found in the ferret. However, fractures and dislocations do occur in pet ferrets.

Parasitology

Fecal examination is routinely performed in young ferrets and in ferrets presenting with clinical signs of illness. Intestinal parasites are uncommon compared to dogs and cats. Coccidiosis (*Isospora* spp.) when found occurs in young animals. The oocysts are shed between 6 and 16 weeks of age and can be demonstrated in fecal examination. The *Isospora* spp. that affects cats and dogs may cross-infect ferrets. *Eimeria* can also be found in ferrets (Marini 2013).

Giardiasis may be seen in ferrets housed in pet store settings. Cryptosporidiosis is a common finding in young ferrets and may persist in immunosuppressed individuals for months. No treatment exists in ferrets and one must keep in mind the zoonotic potential in the immunocompromised human population.

Ear mites often produce a persistent brown-red aural discharge without clinical significance. These parasites also cross-infect dogs and cats. Ear swabs are the key to diagnosis.

Heartworm disease (*Dirofilaria immitis*) occurs in ferrets, especially in endemic areas.

Flea infestation (*Ctenocephalides* spp.) is a common finding in ferrets housed with dogs and cats. Flea control methods for cats, particularly Advantage Multi® (Elanco

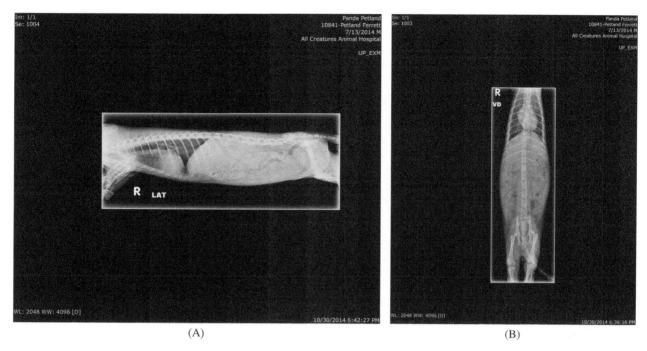

Figure 16.15 (A) Full body lateral radiograph. (Courtesy of Colleen Roman, DVM.) (B) Fully body V/D radiograph. (Courtesy of Colleen Roman, DVM.)

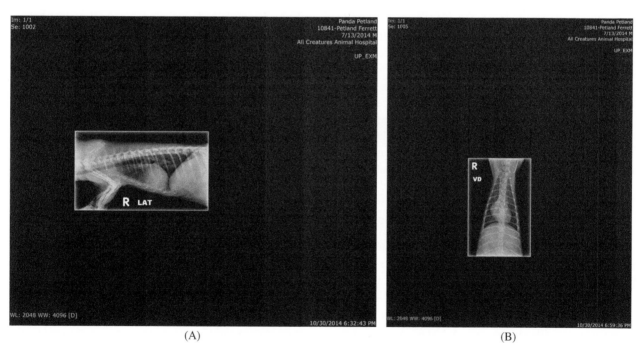

Figure 16.16 (A) Thoracic radiograph lateral view. (Courtesy of Colleen Roman, DVM.) (B) Thoracic radiograph V/D view. (Courtesy of Colleen Roman, DVM.)

Animal Health Inc), Revolution® (Zoetis), and Frontline products (Boehringer Ingelheim) have been used but are not approved. These topical medications are usually applied in smaller doses (Hillyer & Quesenberry 1997, 17–18).

Urinalysis

Collection is achieved by one of three methods. Gentle expression, catheterization, and cystocentesis have all been successfully used. Catheterization is difficult in both males

Table 16.2 Urinalysis normals for ferrets.

Color	Clear to yellow
Specific gravity	1.015–1.055
Ph	6.0–7.5
Protein	0–1
Glucose	0–Trace
Ketones	Negative
Bilirubin	Negative
Occult blood	Negative
WBC	0–5
RBC	0–3
Casts	Occasional
Crystals	Occasional
Epithelial cells	0–Few
Bacteria	Negative
Urine volume (mL/24 h)	8–140 mL (Mean 26–28 mL)

Source: Antech Diagnostics.

and females due to the small size of the urethra and the anatomically challenging os penis. Some manufacturers produce specialized equipment for this purpose (Cook Veterinary Products, Queensland, Australia). However, size 3.5 French red rubber catheters have been successfully used to catheterize male ferrets.

Due to the activity of the animal, cystocentesis may be best performed under anesthesia using a 25-gauge needle attached to a 1 mL or 3 mL syringe. Care should be taken to avoid using a large needle as it may lacerate the bladder.

Urine dipstick, specific gravity, and sedimentation are utilized for standard analyses. Urinalysis normal values are presented in Table 16.2. Urine culture should be performed in cases of suspected kidney or bladder infection preferably using a sample obtained via cystocentesis or sterile catheterization.

Emergency and Critical Care

The normal lifespan of a ferret is 5–8 years. In an emergency, as with any animal, a history and physical examination are crucial in determining the magnitude of the situation. Insulinoma, adrenal gland disease, and cardiomyopathy occur most often in older ferrets. Mediastinal lymphosarcoma, diarrhea, or foreign body ingestion are found commonly in emergencies of young animals. Infectious diseases affect ferrets of any age and are a consideration in an environmental setting where people have respiratory illnesses or where new ferrets have been introduced.

Ill ferrets require minimal handling. Young and old ferrets are susceptible to green slime disease (ECE). Vaccine reactions were more common with previous vaccine protocols but had improved with the introduction of the new ferret distemper vaccine (Purevax Ferret Distemper, Boehringer Ingelheim).

Standard methods of restraint for ferrets include wrapping the ferret in a towel or grasping the nape of the neck. Temperature, pulse, respiration, physical examination, and history are important to establish a good baseline.

Hospitalization of critical ferrets requires a quiet, temperature-controlled cage with oxygen capabilities.

Anorexic ferrets are at risk due to hypoglycemia or hepatic lipidosis. The gums of the lethargic ferret may be rubbed with supplements containing high levels of sugar in order to provide an immediate energy boost to the ferret until other life-saving measures may be performed. Later on, assist feeding A/D Diet (Hill's Pet Nutrition, Inc., Topeka, KS), Royal Canin Recovery Diet (Mars, Inc.), or Critical Care Diet for Carnivores (Oxbow, Murdock, NE) via syringe or tongue depressor will provide good nutritional support. Other preparations are available or can be formulated in the hospital.

Basic diagnostic tests include a blood chemistry, hematology, and fecal examination. A blood glucose can be performed on a human glucometer, blood chemistry analyzer, or with less accuracy using a blood glucose stick. The blood chemistry analyzer offers the best accuracy providing the blood sample has been properly processed. The primary venipuncture site in ferrets is the jugular vein with the saphenous and cephalic veins serving as secondary sites.

Catheter placement is intravenously either in the lateral saphenous or cephalic veins. Jugular catheterization can be utilized but is not tolerated well by the ferret. They often become depressed due to the required bandaging around the neck. Cutdowns of the jugular and cephalic veins in severely dehydrated ferrets may be a consideration. Sometimes, the vascular system of the dehydrated patient may require rehydration with fluids delivered via the subcutaneous route hours prior to attempted placement of intravenous or intraosseous catheters.

Intraosseous catheter placement can be performed in the humerus, femur, or tibia with the femoral placement being the best. This procedure is best performed under anesthesia. In animals that are severely debilitated anesthesia may not be a safe option. This procedure is painful and may require local block of the periosteum and surrounding soft tissue.

Fluid administration requirement for ferrets is 60 mL/kg/day. Dehydration and losses are the same as other small animals. With critical animals, it is important to use the IV or

IO route. It is recommended that an IV pump designed for small mammals is used.

Medications are administered via IV or IO catheters, IM injection in the quadriceps, and oral routes. Oral preparations are accepted best in liquid form since pill medication is difficult to administer in ferrets. Oral medications may be made more palatable with special flavorings that encourage better compliance from the patient by compounding pharmacies.

Cystocentesis may require sedation due to the thin wall of the bladder and the potential for laceration. Ultrasound-guided centesis is also a consideration.

Urethral catheterization requires anesthesia in all patients regardless of condition. Locating the urethral opening is a challenge in both males and females. Male ferrets present more often in an emergency situation due to urethral obstruction from prostatic disease secondary to adrenal gland problems or cystic calculi (Orcutt 1998, 99–107).

Sex Determination

Sex determination is not as difficult as in many small mammals. Adults are similar to the dog. Neonate males have a urogenital opening on the ventral abdomen. Female ferrets have a narrow anogenital distance (Fox & Marini 2014) (see Figure 16.7).

Clinical Techniques

Nail Trimming

Ferrets have non-retractable claws, five on each paw. When they grow long, they are prone to catch on household items such as carpeting, bedding, and clothing. Nails should be trimmed monthly to prevent such hazards. Human nail clippers or scissor-like trimmers for ferrets work well (Figure 16.17). Ferret nails are always transparent and caution should be taken to avoid clipping the nail blood supply.

Urine Collection

Cystocentesis

Use a small syringe attached to a 25-gauge needle. Palpate the bladder in the caudal abdomen or use an ultrasound-guided technique.

Urinary Catheterization

Use a 3.5 French red rubber or other specialty catheters, nasolacrimal cannula or small gauge needle, a water-based

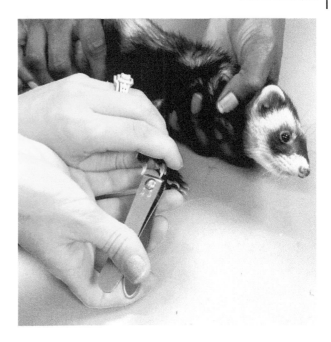

Figure 16.17 Nail trim. (Courtesy of Colleen Roman, DVM.)

lubricant, sterile gloves, hemostats, forced-air warming blanket, and gas anesthesia.

Males The male anatomy is complicated by the J-shaped os penis and the small diameter penile urethra.

a. Prepare supplies and anesthetize patient.
b. Estimate length of catheter from center of urinary bladder to the urethral entrance.
c. Position ferret into ventral recumbency and retract the prepuce.
d. Use a nasolacrimal cannula or a blunt-tipped needle as a stylet, insert the lubricated tip of the cannula or catheter into the urethra orifice. Keep in mind that the orifice is not directly at the tip of the penis but ventral to the end of the penis. There is often a small flap of penile tissue that must be elevated in order to access the urethral opening.
e. Advance the catheter until urine begins to flow.

Females
a. Prepare supplies and anesthetize patient.
b. Place animal in ventral recumbency with elevated hind quarters.
c. Aseptically prepare vulva and perivulvar area.
d. Locate urethral opening using vaginal speculum or otoscopic cone.
e. View the urethral opening on the ventral floor of the vaginal vestibule, approximately 1–1.5 cm cranial to the clitoral fossa.
f. Insert catheter and advance until urine flow is achieved.

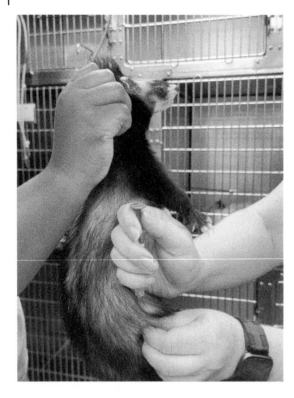

Figure 16.18 Subcutaneous injection. (Courtesy of Colleen Roman, DVM.)

Collect Voided Sample from Examination Table or Empty Litter Box

Many ferrets will urinate and defecate after their temperature is taken.

Temperature, Pulse, and Respiration

The same procedure employed with the dog and cat is used in the ferret.

Medication Administration

Injectable medications and fluid administration require proper restraint.

IV Sites Normally given via IV catheter.

a. Jugular vein
b. Cephalic vein
c. Lateral saphenous vein

IM Sites
a. Quadriceps
b. Lumbar epaxials
c. Triceps
d. Semitendinosus and semimembranosus. Caution needed to avoid the sciatic nerve.

Subcutaneous Sites Can be given in a fold of skin anywhere along the dorsum (Figure 16.18).

Per os Administered by tilting head back and placing syringe through the side of the mouth or placing syringe inside of mouth while ferret is standing.

Venipuncture

Jugular Vein

a. Sternal recumbency with one hand pulling front legs off the table and the other pulling the head back.
b. Using a towel, wrap the ferret tightly with only the animal's head exposed. With the animal in dorsal recumbency, the ferret's head is flexed dorsally toward the person responsible for drawing the blood sample (Figure 16.19). The assistant should apply light pressure to the vein on either side of the manubrium and the sample is drawn from the jugular vein.
c. Ferret may be positioned similar to a cat for a jugular venipuncture. The head is elevated dorsally, the front legs are extended downward, and blood is drawn with the needle approaching the same direction as the head.

Cephalic Vein

a. Normal restraint using the scruff of the neck.
b. Extend the foreleg.
c. Hold off the vein.
d. Draw sample using a 25- or 22-gauge needle (Figure 16.20).

Saphenous Vein

a. Used as last resort.
b. Technique is the same as for the cephalic vein.

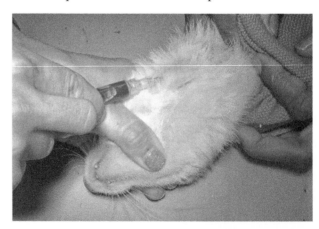

Figure 16.19 Jugular venipuncture. (Courtesy of Colleen Roman, DVM.)

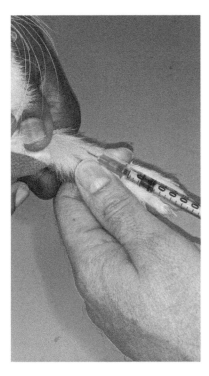

Figure 16.20 Cephalic venipuncture. (Courtesy of Colleen Roman, DVM.)

Cranial Vena Cava

This site has become more and more popular as veterinary personnel become comfortable with its utilization. The risk of cardiac puncture is low due to the length of the vena cava and caudal thoracic placement of the heart along with the proper use of short needles and proper placement. Sedation or anesthesia may be required unless the patient is calm and adequately restrained. Practice with an anesthetized ferret can aid in mastery of this venipuncture (Lennox 2009).

a. The ferret is restrained in dorsal recumbency with its neck extended or held upright as shown in Figure 16.21. Alternatively, it can be wrapped in a towel.

b. Choose a one-half-inch needle of 25 or 27 gauge.

c. Insert the needle in the area to the right or left of the manubrium of the sternum at a slight angle aiming it toward the opposite hip.

d. While applying negative pressure, advance the needle. Deep penetration is not necessary as the vessel is fairly close to the surface at the cranial aspect of the sternum.

e. Look for a flash. Once one is obtained blood should be obtained with ease. If no blood is seen, redirecting the needle may be necessary or the needle may go through the vessel.

f. Use of this technique is strongly recommended only by experienced veterinary team members.

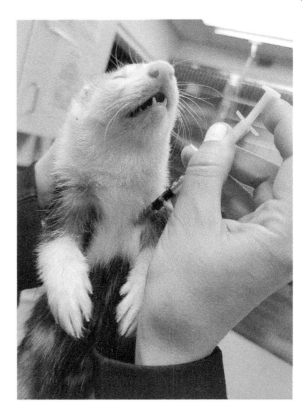

Figure 16.21 Cranial vena cava venipuncture. (Courtesy of Colleen Roman, DVM.)

Intravenous Catheter Placement

Sites Include Jugular, Saphenous, and Cephalic Veins

See Figure 16.22.

Technique

a. Materials required: 24- or 26-gauge IV catheter, clippers and surgical preparation supplies, tape, flush, tourniquet, if needed.

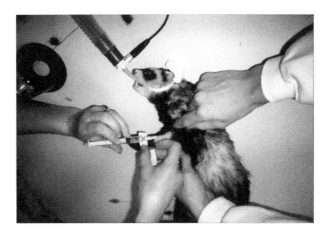

Figure 16.22 Cephalic catheter placement. (Courtesy of Dr. Sam Rivera.)

b. Prepare site using aseptic technique.

c. Apply tourniquet as needed.

d. Use a 22-gauge needle to penetrate the skin lateral to the vein in the area where the catheter will enter just prior to entering the vein. In general, ferret skin is difficult to penetrate.

e. Visualize the vein, insert the needle, and advance the catheter until blood enters the hub of the needle.

f. When the catheter is properly seated in the vein and blood is flowing freely from the catheter, flush the catheter thoroughly with about 0.2 to 0.3 mL heparinized saline and replace the cap. Remember that a smaller amount of flush will be used to accommodate the smaller patient.

g. A small drop of surgical glue may be placed at the catheter–skin junction. Tape the catheter in place, taking care not to apply too much pressure to the skin leading to constriction of the vein.

h. Connect IV line to patient using a mini drip set and/or an IV pump with the potential to calibrate fluid rates for smaller patients.

Intraosseous Catheter Placement

Sites Include Humerus, Tibia, and Femur
See Figure 16.23.

Technique

a. The femur is the best site that causes the least restriction in movement.

b. Use 20- or 22-gauge catheters. A stylet or larger needle may be used to create a pilot hole, or entry point, for the catheter.

c. General anesthesia is recommended except in debilitated individuals. Local anesthetic blocks may be used for the surrounding soft tissue and periosteum.

Enema

1. Materials needed: Small rubber urinary catheter, water-based lubricant, enema solution (warm soapy water), and syringe

2. Insert lubricated tip of the rubber urinary catheter into the rectum of the restrained animal.

3. Attach syringe full of enema solution to the end of the catheter and gently flush the colon using constant steady pressure.

4. Remove the catheter and cleanse the surrounding skin.

Bandage and Wound Care

The same procedures used on other small animals may be used with ferrets. A separate small mammal bandage

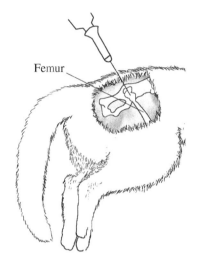

Figure 16.23 Intraosseous catheter location. (Drawing by Scott Stark.)

box with ready-to-go materials may be used. The materials should include small-scale items, such as small scissors and 1/2 inch tape or materials cut to scale from larger-diameter supplies.

Blood Transfusion

Blood transfusions may be used if a local donor system is in place. Many facilities that see large numbers of ferrets may keep healthy donor ferrets on site in case a transfusion is needed. Other ferrets may be privately owned and available as needed on an emergency basis.

Donor ferrets, similar to their canine and feline counterparts, require regular screening for disease through physical examination, baseline blood work evaluation, fecal examination, assessment of adrenal hormone levels, and possibly radiographic and ultrasonographic examination. These ferrets will also need preventive medical care, including heartworm prevention, regular deworming, and vaccination for rabies and canine distemper viruses.

The amount of blood available for transfusion is based upon body weight. The compatibility of donor and recipient ferrets should be determined according to previously described methods in canine and feline practice. The donor ferret should be sedated with gas anesthesia to avoid any struggling and to provide a complication-free needle stick, which will prevent contamination of the sample with disruptive clotting factors. The transfusion recipient may receive the blood sample via fluid pump. Prior to transfusion, necessary premedication with antihistamines may be performed to minimize transfusion reactions.

The donor ferret should be kept warm, should receive replacement fluids and, depending upon the amount of

The figure label reads: Femur

blood removed, will then be designated as unavailable for transfusions for a period of time as determined by the veterinary facility.

Dental Prophylaxis

Periodontal disease is quite common in ferrets, in which preventative care is the best measure. The gold standard is daily tooth brushing with "pet-safe" toothpaste and a soft-bristled brush Figure 16.24A and B). Topical cleansing gels that can be placed on the gum lines, such as TDC and Maxi/Guard (Addison Biological Laboratory, addisonlabs .com), are also available. However, given ferrets' mischievous behavior, water additives such as healthy mouth (Healthy Mouth, healthymouth.com) or cat dental treats may be suitable off-label options. Sealants such as OraVet (Merial, merial.com) or Sanos (Allaccem, allaccem.com) can be applied but may be difficult to start later in life because application requires the ferret to be anesthetized. An oral examination, including a pain score that may be associated with periodontal disease or trauma, should be part of every annual examination (Cooper, 2017).

The steps for dental prophylaxis in ferrets are similar to those in cats. Awake examination of the face and extraoral anatomy is performed to assess for erythema, excoriations, masses, and swellings. This includes full examination of the eyes and orbital sockets, cheeks, nose, lips, and mandibular lymph nodes. Anesthetized examination includes a more thorough evaluation of the oral cavity including the tongue, soft and hard palate, lingual frenulum (as with cats this is a common location for linear foreign bodies), arytenoids, and epiglottis. The dental arcade is assessed for malocclusions and the same dental grading system for dogs and cats is used to evaluate and record the varying levels of gingivitis, plaque, calculus, and mobility. Assessment and measurement of each tooth's sulcus depth and notations of fractures/trauma/missing teeth are recorded (Cooper, 2017). See Figure 16.25).

The standard protocol for dental cleaning is performed; flushing the oral cavity with dilute chlorhexidine solution to reduce aerosolized bacteria, hand scaling, ultrasonic scaling, polishing, and fluoride treatment. The use of dental radiography has become a crucial component in oral health care of all species pre-dental cleaning and post-dental cleaning if it is available.

Euthanasia

Euthanasia can be performed by sedating the patient using chamber or mask induction with gas anesthesia (isoflurane or sevoflurane) or a combination of injectable medications for sedation (such as midazolam 1–2 mg/kg + butorphanol 0.2–0.3 mg/kg IM). After the ferret has been sedated, an intravenous catheter can be placed in either the cephalic veins or lateral saphenous veins and the euthanasia

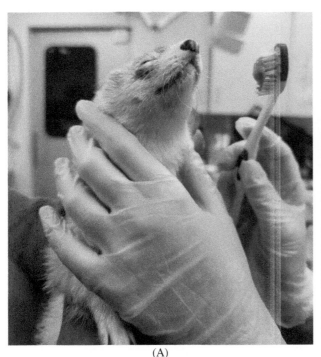

(A)

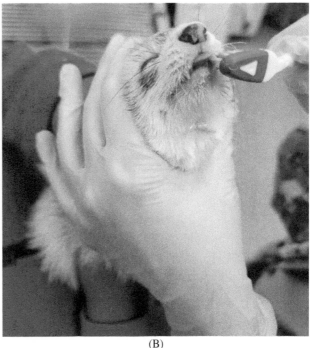

(B)

Figure 16.24 (A, B) Teeth brushing in ferrets. (Courtesy of Colleen Roman, DVM.)

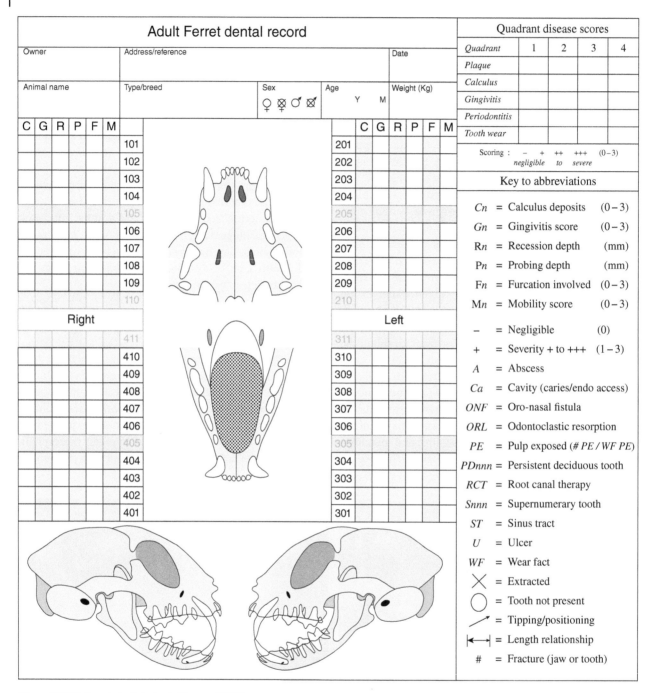

Figure 16.25 Ferret dental chart. (Cooper (2017).

solution can be administrated for attended euthanasia. Alternative methods, if venous access is not available, is to anesthetize the ferret first, then euthanasia solution can be administered directly into the heart with an intra-cardiac injection (not recommended to be performed during an attended euthanasia).

References

Bell JA. 1999. Ferret nutrition. *Vet Clin North Am Exotic Anim Pract Crit Care* 169–192.

Cooper J. 2017. Ferret dentistry: No weaseling about it! *Today's Vet Nurse* 2(1): 8–15.

Fox JG, Marini RP. 2014. *Biology and Diseases of the Ferret*, 3rd edn. Chichester: Wiley-Blackwell.

Hillyer EV, Quesenberry KE. 1997. *Ferrets, Rabbits, and Rodents: Clinical Medicine and Surgery*. Philadelphia: W.B. Saunders.

Lennox AM. 2009. Blood from turnips: the art of diagnostic testing. In: Proceedings of the North American Veterinary Conference, Orlando, FL, pp. 1867–1870.

Marini R. 2013. Ferret ectoparasites. In: *Clinical Veterinary Advisor: Birds and Exotic Pets*. St. Louis, MO: Elsevier.

Martin, D. 2017. Fear Free[SM] techniques for common veterinary procedures. In: Proceed World Small Animal Veterinary Association Congress. Copenhagen, Denmark; September 25–28.

Orcutt CJ. 1998. Emergency and critical care of ferrets. *Vet Clin North Am Exotic Anim Pract* 99–126.

Quesenberry KE, et al. 2021. *Ferrets, Rabbits, and Rodents: Clinical Medicine and Surgery*, 4th edn. Missouri: Elsevier.

Reijgwart ML, Schoemaker NJ, Pascuzzo R, Leach MC, Stodel M, de Nies L, et al. 2017. The composition and initial evaluation of a grimace scale in ferrets after surgical implantation of a telemetry probe. *PLoS One* 12(11): e0187986.

17

Rabbits

Vanessa K. Lee, Douglas K. Taylor, and Deborah Mook

Introduction

The domestic rabbit (*Oryctolagus cuniculus*) is a lagomorph in the Leporidae family. The early domestication of the rabbit began in Western Europe and northwestern Africa in the first century B.C. By the mid-1600s, rabbits were raised in Europe for meat and fur and disseminated around the world via sailing vessels that stocked them as a source of meat. Female rabbits are called "does," males "bucks" and neonates are "kits." Those raised for food are termed "fryers."

Rabbits are attractive as pets because they are quiet, gentle, rarely bite, are relatively odor-free, and can be trained to use a litter box. They generally enjoy good health with appropriate husbandry and protection from predators, environmental extremes, drafts, and trauma. Today in the United States, in addition to being kept as pets, rabbits are exhibited for show, and show jumping competitions (Figure 17.1), used in scientific research, and utilized for food and fur production.

Behavior and Reproduction

Rabbits are a generally timid and submissive prey species with a propensity for chewing and gnawing. If given space and social opportunities, they will chase, jump, gambol, rear, bat at objects, gnaw, and explore (Bayne 2003). Episodes of cavorting and exploration tend to be intermittent and interspersed with longer periods of huddling or resting against a wall or surface. Overall, rabbits are quiet, not particularly playful with humans, and tend to urinate and defecate in a chosen area, which facilitates litter box training. If caged and not accustomed to people, rabbits might retreat to the back of the enclosure when approached and thump a hind foot—the latter being a general warning or alarm call. Aggressive rabbits may growl or grunt, charge, flail with the front feet, and attempt to bite and scratch, especially with the powerful rear limbs. They

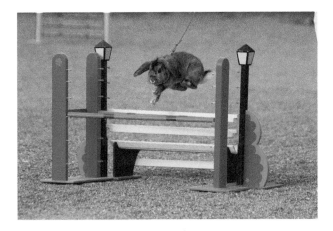

Figure 17.1 Rabbit show jumping. (Fruitpunchli/Wikimedia Commans/CC-BY-SA 4.0.)

scent mark by rubbing the chin on objects and frequently chew on caging wire, wood, cardboard, paper, hay, or other materials they encounter.

Although rabbits are considered a social species, housing in groups must be done cautiously. Sexually mature, intact rabbits tend to be more aggressive than neutered animals. Intact rabbits of either sex may also spray urine and demonstrate destructive behaviors, although these behaviors are more common in intact males (Stein & Walshaw 1996; Crowell-Davis 2007). Intact does can demonstrate aggression toward other females, but compatible groups, particularly if formed in small clusters while young, can often be maintained successfully (Bayne 2003). Intact, adult males can rarely be housed together safely, but neutered males may live peacefully in groups (Raje & Stewart 1997). Rabbits of either sex may be behaviorally incompatible with other animals even if neutered.

Abnormal and stereotypic behaviors that might be revealed during acquisition of a history include cage bar chewing, excessive fur plucking, psychogenic water consumption, head swaying or weaving, head pressing, obsession with pawing or digging at the cage floor or food hopper, rapid circling, or sitting with the head lowered (Bayne 2003; Crowell-Davis 2007). Although backed by no scientific evidence, stereotypies, and abnormal behaviors may be disproportionately high in rabbits kept singly and confined to hutches. The rabbit hutch should therefore be designed and outfitted to encourage species-typical behavior and enhance well-being. In confined conditions, enrichment devices decrease the incidence of undesirable behaviors and increase overall activity (Bayne 2003; Johnson et al. 2003). Devices that have been used most successfully to encourage the species-typical nudging, playing, digging and investigative behaviors of rabbits are boxes filled with hay, chew-resistant plastic toys and balls, Nylabone® products, sections of PVC tubing, metallic washers suspended from chains, stainless-steel rabbit rattles on spring clips and hay and other food items specially formulated for rabbits (Bayne 2003; Johnson et al. 2003; Crowell-Davis 2007). One study suggests classical music might even decrease stress in rabbits (Pevelar & Hickman 2018). Rabbits will make frequent use of hiding places such as crates or boxes, and the boxes can provide additional chewing enrichment.

If rabbits are to be mated, pairing should be done under supervision as does may be aggressive toward bucks. The female should be taken to the buck's cage to reduce the chance of aggression. A buck will circle a receptive doe and then quickly mount and copulate. A buck may also demonstrate mildly aggressive behaviors, such as ear biting, but is unlikely to cause significant trauma. Does can rebreed within 24 h of parturition—termed "kindling"–and produce up to 11 liters per year. However, rebreeding prior to removing the kits is not recommended. Kits are born in a nest constructed from hair plucked by the doe from the dewlap and other materials that she may scavenge from the environment. Kits are altricial, born hairless and blind—an attribute differentiating them from hares, which are precocial and born fully furred with open eyes. A doe typically nurses the kits only once per day. Kits may show growth rates of up to 35–40 g per day. Lactation peaks at 3 weeks postpartum. The kits start eating solid food at 2 weeks of age and cecotrophy, the consumption of feces directly from the anus, commences about a week later. Weaning should be done at 5–6 weeks.

Anatomy and Physiology

Rabbits possess a number of distinguishing morphophysiological attributes that make them interesting and differentiate them from more traditional pets. The ears are highly vascularized which helps dissipate heat. The ears are fragile and should never be used for restraint or carrying an animal. Rabbits have a high muscle-to-bone ratio. While 13% of the body weight is comprised of bone in the cat, only 8% is bone in the rabbit (Harkness & Wagner 2010). Because they possess large muscle masses, the long bones and lumbar spine are particularly susceptible to fracture or luxation, respectively. The skeletal anatomy of the rabbit is shown in Figure 17.2.

Does have a duplex uterus with dual cervix and 8–10 mammary glands. The inguinal canals remain open for the life of the buck and the testicles may be found either in the scrotum or retracted into the abdomen. Herniation of other intrabdominal organs is prevented by large fat depots immediately covering the inguinal canals (Swindle & Shealy 1996). Figure 17.3 shows rabbit visceral anatomy.

The rabbit digestive tract anatomy and physiology is interesting and unique. It is a nonruminant herbivore preferring to consume the tender, succulent parts of plants. The teeth are open-rooted and grow continuously. The normal dental formula is I2/1, C0/0, PM 3/0, M3/3 and is unique because the upper dental arcade includes two sets of incisors with a small, secondary pair, the peg teeth, situated immediately to the lingual side of the larger labial pair. The single pair of lower incisors occludes with the upper secondary incisors. The void between the incisors and premolars is called the diastema (Figure 17.4). The incisors may grow at a rate of up to 1 cm per month.

Rabbits have a glandular stomach that functions essentially as a storage organ. The cardiac sphincter has significant tone such that true vomiting does not occur. The stomach is never empty, remaining more than half full even after a 24-h fast (Griffiths & Davies 1963). The stomach pH of an adult rabbit is significantly lower than that of other species (Cheeke & Cunha 1987). This acidic environment renders the upper gastrointestinal tract sterile and functions partly to protect against pathogens. The gastric pH is higher in sucklings, permitting bacterial colonization of the hindgut by cecotrophs from adults in the population. Unfortunately, it also provides a window of opportunity for entry of bacterial pathogens particularly around the time of weaning.

The small intestine is similar to most species in form and function serving as the major site of acid neutralization, protein and carbohydrate digestion, fat emulsification, and absorption of many nutrients. Rabbits are hindgut fermenters, similar to the horse, with digestion characterized by selective excretion of fiber, cecal fermentation, and reingestion of cecal contents. The cecum, comprising about 40% of the total gastrointestinal capacity, is a site of constant peristalsis with mixing and remixing of its contents. Within the cecum exists an intricate and delicate balance between nutrients, the microflora, and motility. It is the primary site of bacterial fermentative digestion

Figure 17.2 Rabbit skeletal anatomy. (Drawing by Scott Stark.)

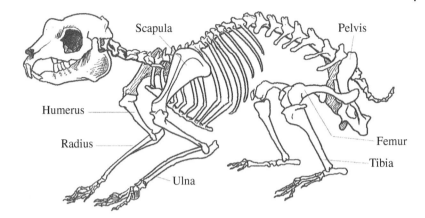

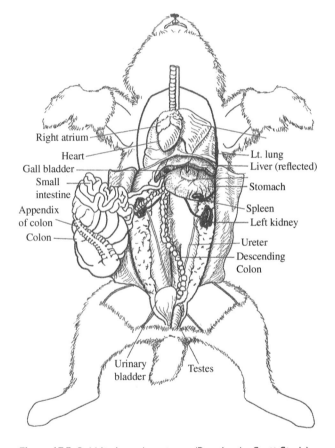

Figure 17.3 Rabbit visceral anatomy. (Drawing by Scott Stark.)

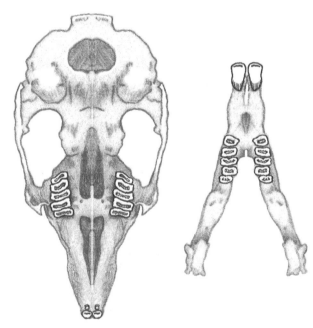

Figure 17.4 Rabbit dentition. (Drawing by Scott Stark.)

and water absorption. The anaerobic flora important in cecal fermentation are comprised of *Bacteroides* and other species (Cheeke & Cunha 1987; Davies & Davies 2003).

Cecal fermentation of carbohydrates results in the production of volatile fatty acids (VFA) in a process similar to that which occurs in ruminants. VFAs are absorbed through the cecal wall and used as an energy source (Cheeke & Cunha 1987). The colon is characterized by serial sacculations (termed haustrae), and the fusus coli, a muscular thickening at the termination of the transverse

colon unique to lagomorphs that regulate contractions (Davies & Davies 2003). Contractions move fluid and small digestible particles back into the cecum and propel large pieces of fiber distally where they are formed into the excreted hard pellets that are typically observed. At intervals, the cecum contracts and the fluid, protein, and vitamin-rich cecal contents are expelled into the colon to form the cecotrophs, also called night feces, which are small, soft, mucin-coated balls consumed directly from the anus and swallowed whole (Davies & Davies 2003). The mucus-like membrane serves to protect the cecotrophs, and fermentative commensals contained therein, from the gastric pH. This cecotrophy serves to recycle vitamins, amino acids, volatile fatty acids, and digested bacteria to the upper GI tract for absorption or further digestion (Davies & Davies 2003). As a rule, cecotrophy occurs about

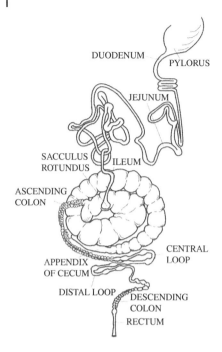

DUODENUM

PYLORUS

JEJUNUM

SACCULUS
ROTUNDUS

ILEUM

ASCENDING
COLON

CENTRAL
LOOP

APPENDIX
OF CECUM

DISTAL LOOP

DESCENDING
COLON

RECTUM

Figure 17.5 Rabbit GI tract. (Drawing by Scott Stark.)

4 h subsequent to meal consumption (Davies & Davies 2003). Wire bottom caging has no effect upon cecotrophy given the consumption of the cecotrophs directly from the anus, but the application of an Elizabethan collar can be disruptive to the process. The presence of a lymphoid mass, the sacculus rotundus, at the termination of the ileum, is another unique anatomic feature of the GI tract. Lymphoid tissue is also found in the appendix at the cecal tip (Figure 17.5).

Laboratory and Biological Data

Normal reference ranges for the species provided by the diagnostic laboratory that has processed the samples should be used when interpreting data. When such values are not available from the laboratory, the ranges in the tables that follow can be used as an approximation of normal in a healthy rabbit (Tables 17.1–17.3). However, "normal values" may be influenced by laboratory variation, sample collection technique e.g., extent of restraint, type of anesthesia, hemolysis, post-collection sample handling e.g., refrigeration, breed and age of the subject, and other factors. The numeric data provided herein are obtained from research populations of rabbits that were uniform in genotype and age and maintained under standardized conditions. The interpretation of laboratory data, as in any other circumstance with any other species, should be done with consideration of the history, findings from a physical examination, and results of other diagnostic tests. The predominant circulating white blood cells are lymphocytes

Table 17.1 Hematology and blood coagulation values.

Parameter	Normal distribution	Reference
Total WBC (10^3/µL)	4.6–13.2	Wolford et al. 1986
Heterophils (%)	<50	
Lymphocytes (%)	>50	
Monocytes (%)	0–3	
Eosinophils (%)	0–2	
Basophils (%)	0–7	
Platelets (10^3/µL)	300–700	
PCV (%)	33–45	
RBC (10^6/µL)	5.5–7.5	
Hemoglobin (g/dL)	11–15	
MCV (fL)	56–66	
MCHC (%)	32–36	
MCH (pg)	19–22	
Reticulocytes (%)	<4	
Bleeding time (min)	0.8–2	Livio et al. 1988
Clotting time (min)	1.1–5.5	
OSPT (s)	7.9–17.9	Gentry 1982
APTT (s)	19.5–22.5	
Prothrombin time (s)	6.9–8.1	Lee and Clement 1990
Thrombin time (s)	5.7–14.1	

APTT, activated partial thromboplastin time; MCH, mean corpuscular hemoglobin; MCHC, mean corpuscular hemoglobin concentration; MCV, mean corpuscular volume; min, minutes; OSPT, one-stage prothrombin time; PCV, packed cell volume; RBC, red blood cells; sec, seconds; WBC, white blood cells.

and heterophils, the latter being the neutrophil equivalent which may be mistaken for an eosinophil because of its numerous small intracytoplasmic eosinophilic granules (Figure 17.6). Unlike cats and dogs, lymphocytes are generally more common than heterophils, especially in young animals. Basophils (2–10%) are also more common in rabbits than other species (Harkness & Wagner 2010). Reticulated red blood cells may also be observed more frequently in rabbits than in dogs or cats.

Clinical chemistry values are comparable to those of other species with the exception of serum amylase and calcium levels. Calcium is efficiently absorbed from the gut. Consequently, blood levels directly reflect dietary levels often resulting in nonpathogenic hypercalcemia with values exceeding 15 mg/dL in animals consuming a high calcium diet. Rabbits are susceptible to arteriosclerosis resulting from dietary calcium imbalances or vitamin D excess. Serum amylase is considerably lower in rabbits than in dogs and cats (Nowland et al. 2015).

The urine pH ranges from 6 to 8.2 with alkaline urine (pH > 8) generally associated with good health and acidic pH with anorexia or fasting. The normal range of urine

Table 17.2 Clinical chemistry values.

Parameter	Normal distribution	Reference
AST (U/L)	0–30	Yu et al. 1979
ALT (U/L)	0–60	
GGT (U/L)	0–8	Hewitt et al. 1989
SAP (U/L)	0–139	
CPK (U/L)	<700	
BUN (mg/dL)	9–22	
Creatinine (mg/dL)	0.6–1.5	
Glucose (mg/dL)	86–137	
Amylase (U/L)	270–700	Yu et al. 1979
Total bilirubin (mg/dL)	0.4–9.2	
Sodium (mEq/L)	138–150	Gillett 1994
Chloride (mEq/L)	92–120	
Calcium (mg/dL)	6–15	Yu et al. 1979
Phosphorus (mg/dL)	3–5	
Potassium (mEq/L)	3.5–7	Gillett 1994
Total protein (g/dL)	5.3–7.6	Yu et al. 1979
Albumin (g/dL)	3.1–4.7	

ALT, alanine aminotransferase; AST, aspartate aminotransferase; BUN, blood urea nitrogen; CPK, creatine phosphokinase; GGT, gammaglutamyltransferase; SAP, serum alkaline phosphatase.

Table 17.3 Normative and reproductive values.

Parameter	Normal distribution	Reference
Lifespan (years)	5–7 (15 max)	–
Gestation (days)	31–32	
Litter size (kits born)	4–10	
Weaning age (weeks)	5–6	
Rectal temperature (°F)	101–104	
Heart rate (bpm)	200–300	
Respiratory rate (bpm)	30–60	
Blood pressure, systolic (torr)[a]	90–130	
Blood pressure, diastolic (torr)[a]	80–90	
Food intake (g/kg/day)	50	Harkness and Wagner (2010)
Water intake (mL/kg/day)	100	

[a] Blood pressure values are given for instrumental conscious rabbits with central arterial catheters. Values average 0 torr less if the central auricular artery is used (Edwards et al. 1959).

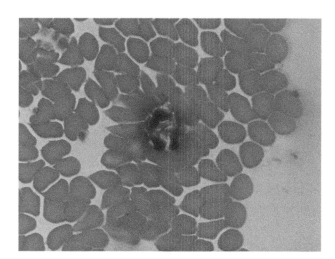

Figure 17.6 Rabbit blood smear showing heterophil (Courtesy of Dondrae Coble.)

specific gravity is 1.003–1.036 with 1.015 representing the normal mean in a healthy population of rabbits (Nowland et al. 2015). Calcium is cleared from the blood by the kidney and excreted in the urine (Cheeke & Cunha 1987) and the urine is therefore often turbid due to calcium carbonate excretion. Urine is also commonly pigmented, ranging from light yellow to orange to various combinations of red with brown. Certain porphyrin pigments in the urine may cause a reddish appearance and elicit unfounded concerns for hematuria (Garibaldi et al. 1987). Consequently, any suspected cases of hematuria in the rabbit should be confirmed by a complete urinalysis. The most likely causes of hematuria are uterine adenocarcinoma, uterine polyps, uterine hyperplasia, abortion, urolithiasis, cystitis, septicemia, disseminated intravascular coagulation, and certain renal diseases.

The urine should be free of protein, casts, blood, glucose, ketones, and bilirubin. An occasional white blood cell per high-powered field in an examination of the sediment is normal. The urine output ranges from 20 to 350 mL/kg/day and is influenced by many factors related to the diet, animal, and environment, with the typical production from 50 to 75 mL/kg (McLaughlin & Fish 1994, Nowland et al. 2015). Ammonium magnesium phosphate (struvite) and calcium carbonate are the two most common uroliths of rabbits (Brock et al. 2012). Struvite uroliths are usually the consequence of a urinary tract infection. Calcium carbonate may precipitate and form uroliths when the urinary pH exceeds 8.5 (Leck 1988). Infection, inadequate water intake, genetic predisposition, metabolic disturbances, and nutritional imbalances enhance the development of urolithiasis.

Husbandry

While rabbits are frequently housed indoors nowadays, they can be kept outdoors, with the appropriate shelter from the elements. Rabbits can be litter box trained and make suitable indoor pets; however, their proclivity for gnawing can become destructive if directed toward household items. Regardless of the arrangement, it is critical to protect rabbits from drafts, temperature extremes, predators, flying insects, and environmental intoxicants. Rabbits are cold weather tolerant and are best kept at temperatures of 60–72°F or slightly below and 30–70% relative humidity (Harkness & Wagner 2010, Quinn 2012). If housed outdoors, protection from cold below 40°F in the winter and excessive heat in the summer is vital. The provision of a covered nesting box containing straw, shavings, or other insulative bedding provides protection in cold weather. Shade and plenty of cool water are paramount when temperatures exceed 85°F. Heat stress is a significant risk at this temperature and above. In extreme heat, the hutch should be moved to an area such as a breezy garage or patio with a fan. Air-conditioned areas should be avoided, as the drastic temperature changes could be too stressful.

Plans for constructing rabbit hutches and nesting boxes and sources for commercial units are readily found online. At a minimum, rabbits should be provided with floor space sufficient to allow an animal to stretch out to full length and vertical space that allows sitting on the haunches. Hardware cloth of 1.25×2.5 cm grid is suitable for flooring, but the animal should have access to solid surfaces as well to reduce the risk of pododermatitis. Wire flooring should be cleaned regularly to remove suspended hair and feces. Attempts at environmental enrichment should focus on providing hiding places, material for chewing (cardboard, paper), nutritional supplements such as hay, and other devices that promote species typical behaviors (refer to the "Behavior" section for additional information).

Nutrition

Rabbits should be fed a pelleted ration supplemented with free choice hay and small amounts of fresh foods. Pelleted feed, made primarily from timothy or alfalfa hay, is readily available in pet and farm supply stores. Pelleted diets are nutritionally complete and typically contain 14–18% crude protein, 40–50% carbohydrate, 2–4% fat, 10–22% crude fiber, and appropriate vitamins and minerals

in the proper balance. Alfalfa hay is higher in protein, calories, and calcium than timothy. Timothy hay-based pellets are generally preferred because the higher calcium of alfalfa will increase urinary calcium that can predispose the animal to urolithiasis and excessive urinary sludge. Indigestible fiber, although discriminately excreted and not an important source of nutrients, is important in digestion, normal health, and the prevention of fur pulling, gastric trichobezoars, enteritis, mucoid enteropathy, and other gastrointestinal maladies (Cheeke & Cunha 1987). For growth, 10–15% dietary fiber is optimal and adults should be fed rations containing 15–22% fiber. Fiber promotes peristaltic activity critical to the hindgut fermentative process. Without sufficient long particle length (>0.5 mm) fiber, resultant hypomotility and micro floral alterations can lead to disease.

A variety of good quality hays can be the majority of the diet, particularly for overweight animals (Clauss 2012). Fruit should only be used as an occasional treat, and preferably those with a higher fiber content such as apples. A wide variety of greens including cabbage, cauliflower leaves, broccoli leaves, kale, turnip greens, mustard greens, sunflower leaves, carrot tops, or green bean vines, can be offered. High-calcium greens, such as kale, should be limited. Fresh herbs such as parsley, cilantro, and basil are also safe. Overfeeding of fresh greens and fruits predisposes to starch overload, cecal pH extremes, and enteric diseases. Rabbits seemingly enjoy grazing on lawns, which is best done under supervision in a yard free of fertilizers, herbicides, and pesticides. It is important to prevent access to any toxic plants (Cheeke & Cunha 1987). Human breakfast cereals, such as shredded wheat biscuits can be offered occasionally as a treat, but grains and products high in fat or sugar should be avoided (Davies et al. 2003). It is not necessary, and may actually be harmful in some cases, to supplement a proper diet with minerals.

A rabbit will typically consume 5% of its body weight in dry feed and 10% in water. Rabbits kept as pets or used in research are usually fed limited rations, while those grown for food production or breeding are fed *ad libitum*. Peak food consumption in *ad libitum*-fed rabbits is biphasic occurring in the interval from late afternoon to approximately midnight and again shortly after dawn (Davies & Davies 2003). Controlled feeding is done by offering 50–75% of the *ad libitum* consumption once per day and is important in preventing obesity and urolithiasis. For a medium-sized adult rabbit weighing 4–6 kg, 120–180 g (approximately 2/3 of a cup) per day of pelleted diet is appropriate. Limit feeding is especially important at weaning during the dietary transition from milk-based diet to plant-based food when there may not be sufficient enzymes in the gut to digest plant carbohydrates and protective maternal antibodies are waning. Limit feeding of weanlings also protects them from osmotic overload, pH extremes, and enteric disease. 60 g per kilogram per day up to a maximum of 120–180 g per day is usually sufficient.

Rabbit kits are entirely dependent upon milk until 10 days of age and then progressively begin to consume solid foods and maternal-origin cecotrophs up until weaning at around 4 weeks of age (Davies & Davies 2003). Kits typically nurse once daily with ingested milk forming a semi-solid curd protected in the stomach by an antimicrobial fatty acid product called "stomach oil" or "milk oil" (Davies & Davies 2003). This curd gradually passes into the intestine between feedings (Davies & Davies 2003). Rabbits fed on milk substitutes or milk from another species fail to develop protective fatty acid products and are devoid of colostral antibodies making them susceptible to bacterial enteric infections (Davies & Davies 2003).

Water should be provided *ad libitum* and is generally consumed at twice the feed intake quantity or about 100–120 mL/kg/day. Water consumption varies with factors such as environmental temperature, diet composition, and physiological demands (e.g., lactation). Lactating will consume water up to 90% equivalent of their body weight daily (Harkness & Wagner 2010).

Common and Zoonotic Diseases

The medical management of rabbits can generally be accomplished by meeting a few basic goals. The tenets of preventive care are good nutrition and sanitation combined with protection from predators, drafts, environmental extremes, environmental intoxicants, and trauma.

The health status of commercially reared rabbits can vary. *Pasteurella*-free flocks exist, but most sources have some problems with coccidiosis, encephalitozoonosis, and, on occasion, internal and/or external parasites. New Zealand White and Dutch Belted rabbits are often available as specific pathogen-free animals from rabbitries. Other outbred stocks or domestic breeds may not be pathogen-free and typically are colonized by *Pasteurella multocida*. Rabbits obtained from pet stores, unless the vendor can make a specific claim otherwise, should be assumed to be *Pasteurella*-infected. In private practice, one is most likely to encounter a domestic or wild rabbit in the clinic for interventional purposes rather than preventive medicine. The most common presentations to a veterinary clinic will be for anorexia, abscesses, malocclusion, elective surgical procedures such as ovariohysterectomy (OHE) and orchiectomy, and nail trimming. Rabbits also may experience respiratory, gastrointestinal, or integumentary illnesses, as well as neoplasia. The diseases of greatest clinical importance are grouped into those affecting the respiratory, digestive, and integumentary systems and by infectious, inherited, or traumatic/environmental etiology.

Respiratory Infectious Diseases

Bacterial upper respiratory tract disease in rabbits is commonly referred to as "snuffles," and is characterized by sneezing, mucopurulent nasal discharge, and conjunctivitis. Dacryocystitis can also cause these clinical signs, and although often caused by the same bacteria, the veterinarian may need to determine if the nasolacrimal duct is affected in order to determine the best clinical management or if malocclusion or other dental diseases may be the inciting cause of nasal discharge/conjunctivitis instead of a primary bacterial infection. These syndromes are the most common infectious illness in pet rabbits, and if a bacterial etiologic agent is involved, it is likely to be *Pasteurella multocida*. *P. multocida* can also be associated with ear infections, causing a head tilt and other associated clinical signs. It can also be found as a secondary, or commensal, pathogen, and one not causing the primary disease. The organism is part of the normal nasal flora of cats, as well, but the serotypes that cause disease in rabbits differ from those in cats. Other bacteria have been identified in cases of rabbit snuffles, including *Bordetella bronchiseptica*, the second most common cause, Staphylococcal species, and *Pseudomonas* (Hedley 2014). Pasteurella can be enzootic in large groups of rabbits, such as in rabbitries or pet stores, and up to 90–100% of adults will be infected. Inapparent carriers of *Pasteurella* occur frequently, and subclinical infections localized to the nasal passages or tympanic bullae are common. On the other side of the clinical spectrum, the bacterium may cause a chronic, progressive, incurable, potentially fatal multi-systemic disease, starting with the upper respiratory tract. Most commonly, the syndrome presents with frequent sneezing or mucopurulent nasal discharge (Langan et al. 2000, Hedley 2014). *Pasteurella* may be transmitted by direct contact, close contact aerosol, vertical transmission, or, less frequently, venereal routes. The role of fomites in transmission is unclear. *Pasteurella multocida* is harbored in the nasal cavity and/or tympanic bullae where it may remain localized. Harborage in these areas protects the bacterium from antibodies and administered antibiotics. The organism is capable of dissemination from the nasal passages to other parts of the body leading to a constellation of clinical manifestations including conjunctivitis, skin abscesses, inner ear infection, pyometra, orchitis, pneumonia, or septicemia.

In a rabbit with suppurative clinical signs, a presumptive diagnosis of pasteurellosis can easily be confirmed by bacterial culture or PCR. Deep nasal swabs should be done under sedation/anesthesia to submit for either or both of these tests. In cases where septicemic Pasteurellosis is suspected, the organism should be recoverable from the blood. Culture and PCR of deep nasal swabs can also be useful in detecting carriers, although it will be negative if the bacteria are localized to the tympanic bulla. Alternatively, the serum can be assessed for antibodies against *Pasteurella multocida* that may be suggestive of exposure and infection (Sanchez et al. 2004). There are no effective vaccines, commercially available or otherwise, to prevent pasteurellosis or control its clinical signs, although there have been many attempts at generating them. Veterinary care is primarily supportive and may be dissatisfying for all parties. Antibiotics, such as marbofloxacin (Rougier et al. 2006), sulfas, chloramphenicol, tetracyclines, or enrofloxacin, may be given for a month or more and result in improvement of clinical signs, but it is difficult to eliminate the organism, and upon completion of a course of therapy, symptoms may recrudesce and worsen over time. Less severe cases may improve and stabilize, but animals may remain carriers. Supportive care may include regular cleaning of obstructed nares, flushing of the nasolacrimal duct in cases of dacryocystitis, nebulization or vaporizer treatments, and excision or incision/drainage of abscesses.

Experimental infection with SARS-CoV-2 has been documented (Mykkytyn et al. 2021), but preliminary studies indicate natural infection to be rare (Fritz et al. 2022).

Diseases of the Digestive System

Rabbits, particularly weanlings and young kits, commonly experience diarrheal disease. Infectious agents that play an important part in the gastrointestinal illnesses of rabbits include coccidia, rotaviruses, and coronaviruses, and the bacterial agents *E. coli*, *Lawsonia*, and *Clostridium*. Husbandry practices, including diet and sanitation, play a vital role in maintaining gastrointestinal health, and the provision of a high-fiber diet will in many cases be preventative or ameliorative.

Coccidiosis, caused by enteric or hepatotrophic species of the genus *Eimeria*, is a major disease problem in young rabbits. Infection can be subclinical or mild, but clinical disease is characterized by fulminant diarrhea, and occurs in juveniles, especially recent weanlings, kept under poor conditions or stressed by transportation. Unlike enteric coccidial species, *Eimeria stiedae* parasitizes the liver and bile duct. Infection is often subclinical, but in young rabbits, the agent may cause fatal hepatic failure characterized by icterus, hepatomegaly, elevated hepatic enzymes, wasting, and anorexia. The transmission of coccidia in rabbits is by the fecal-oral route and the diagnosis is made by fecal examination for oocysts or at necropsy. Administration of sulfa drugs, ivermectin and/or toltrazuril, are treatment options (Cam et al. 2008); however, treatment may only reduce coccidian burden and not eliminate it (Harkness & Wagner 2010). Because oocysts require a day or more to sporulate at room temperature, the ingestion of night feces is not considered to play a role in the dissemination of disease, and aggressive sanitation is important in controlling the spread of infection. If housing and fomites are not cleaned effectively, oocysts remaining in the environment may be a source of reinfection for months. Most rabbits that are housed in well-sanitized and stress-free environments will not show clinical signs and may develop life-long immunity. Vitamin E deficiency may potentiate coccidiosis.

Rotavirus is enzootic in many rabbitries where it is mildly pathogenic. It destroys enterocytes that synthesize disaccharidases consequently causing diarrhea due to maldigestion. Infection may be fatal in young kits that are not protected by maternal antibodies under epizootic conditions. As with enteric viral diseases of other species, treatment is directed at supportive care.

Coronaviruses have been found in association with diarrhea in young rabbits. One survey of commercial rabbitries in North America showed a prevalence of antibodies detected by serology to be as much as 40% (Deeb et al. 1993). In an outbreak situation, morbidity and mortality can be high (Oglesbee & Lord 2020). Definitive diagnosis requires demonstration of coronaviral particles in gut contents by electron microscopy. Thus, diagnosis of pet rabbits is unlikely, and treatment will remain directed at supportive care.

Bacterial enterotoxemia is caused primarily by *Clostridium* spp. (*e.g., C. spiroforme, C. perfringens*), although other enteropathogenic bacteria are less commonly involved (Rosentthal 2004). Clostridial species are Gram-positive, anaerobic bacteria that are either not normally a part of the gastrointestinal flora or are suppressed to a very low and nonpathogenic level in healthy adults. The normal gut microflora is protective, and its disruption appears to be required for colonization by *C. spiroforme*. Changes caused by weaning, environmental stress, or by disruption of the normal flora through concurrent infection or the use of antibiotics with anaerobic and Gram-positive spectra can be predisposing factors. Beta-lactam antibiotics and lincosamides carry the highest risk, with ampicillin, clindamycin, and lincomycin being the classically associated antibiotics, although erythromycin has also been associated with the disease. Oral administration of antibiotics is more likely to be causative than parenteral administration. For example, penicillin and cephalosporins can be safely administered parentally while oral administration is not advised. All antibiotics, but particularly those with a known link to bacterial enterotoxemia, should be used with caution in rabbits, with the informed consent of the client, and not on a herd-wide basis. Clinical signs include anorexia, wasting, and diarrhea and are usually the result of enterotoxins which damage normal gut function. The disease is suspected based on a combination of a history of recent change in environment or antibiotic use and clinical signs. Gram stains of gut contents may show typical coiled bacteria. Anaerobic culture can positively identify the organism, and several methods exist to assay for the enterotoxin. Treatment consists of a combination of nursing and supportive care aimed at normalizing the gut microflora. Fluid therapy and increasing the fiber content of the diet are critical. Antimicrobials may carefully be brought to bear, particularly metronidazole (Oglesbee & Lord 2020). The importance of sanitation, for removal of spores from the environment, should be stressed to the client.

Tyzzer's disease is caused by *Clostridium piliforme*, a Gram-negative obligate intracellular bacterium having vegetative and spore forms. Like coccidiosis, it causes disease most commonly in recent weanlings, especially in the face of crowding, poor sanitation, or deprivation of food or water. Immunocompetent rabbits maintained in sanitary settings may show no clinical signs but may also shed spores for a few weeks until they clear the infection (Barthold et al. 2016). Natural infection is thought to be caused by ingestion of spore-contaminated food or bedding. The spores are hardy and can persist in the environment for years. In susceptible animals, mortality can be acute and high, and the diagnosis can be difficult to establish and is often made using special stains (silver) of specimens obtained at necropsy. Serologic assays exist for the agent but suffer from non-specific cross-reactivity leading to false positives.

Enteropathogenic strains of *E. coli* are also important pathogens of young rabbits, particularly in colony settings. The bacterium is normally found as part of the commensal flora but proliferates in the cecum in disease-causing yellow diarrhea and high mortality within 48 h (Wales et al. 2005). Factors increasing susceptibility to disease include stress or concomitant infection with another disease (Swennes et al. 2012). Sucklings within 2–8 days of birth and weaned kits less than 3 months of age are most at risk. The organism can be identified by culture, and characterization of the isolate will assist in predicting its virulence. Good sanitation, fluid therapy, body temperature maintenance, and antibiotics are important in treatment. Vaccines have been attempted but are complicated by the variability in bio/serosubgroups of the agent (Zhu et al. 2006).

Lawsonia intracellularis is the cause of proliferative enteropathy and typically afflicts young rabbits. Although infection is characterized by a 1–2-week course of diarrhea, depression, and dehydration, it is rarely fatal. The organism, relatively prevalent in diarrheic rabbits (Lim et al. 2012), is difficult to culture; histopathology or molecular diagnostic assays are usually necessary (Horiuchi et al. 2008). Severely diarrheic rabbits require fluid therapy and body temperature management.

There are few helminth parasites of clinical importance in domestic rabbits. The common rabbit pinworm, *Passalurus ambiguus*, is not zoonotic and is largely nonpathogenic. It is found in the cecum and large intestine of wild rabbits and occasionally domestic or laboratory rabbits and can be found at a prevalence of as high as 75% in healthy rabbits (Abdel-Gaber et al. 2019). The life cycle is direct and infection is acquired by ingestion. The diagnosis may be made by demonstration of oocysts by fecal floatation examination techniques or observation of expelled adult nematodes on the feces. The eggs (43 μm × 103 μm, flattened on one side) are laid in embryonated, infective form. Common anthelmintic agents used in dogs and cats, such as ivermectin, fenbendazole, and pyrantel pamoate have high efficacy in rabbits (Carpenter et al. 2001, Curtis & Brooks 1990; Düwel & Brech 1981).

Mucoid enteropathy syndrome is a mucoid diarrheal disease with a grave prognosis, particularly in weanling rabbits. The pathogenesis remains largely conjectural, but dietary factors have been implicated. Commercial rabbit feed is high-energy and low in fiber, and rabbits fed this type of diet have a higher incidence of this syndrome than rabbits fed high-fiber diets (Barthold et al. 2016). Some studies have suggested an infectious etiology of as-yet unknown origin: the syndrome can emerge as an epizootic, and inoculation of healthy rabbits with cecal matter from rabbits with the syndrome recapitulates the disease (Hu et al. 2018). Affected rabbits are thin with a hunched posture, anorectic, dehydrated, hypothermic, mildly bloated, and have abundant gelatinous mucus excretions. Dietary change and other stressors, such as painful injections, overheating, or inadvertent water deprivation (including excessively warm, yet plentiful, water in the summer months) may also predispose to disease. Treatment is generally unsuccessful with the case fatality rate approaching 100% making prevention a key strategy. Mucoid enteropathy can largely be prevented by feeding high fiber rations and maintaining quality husbandry practices of clean environment and minimization of stress.

Ileus may occur in rabbits of all ages, is common, and generally presents as an anorectic rabbit with decreased or no fecal production but otherwise appears normal. This syndrome is usually associated with gastric stasis and/or cecal impaction and can be a primary or secondary condition. It may be possible to palpate a doughy mass in the cranial abdomen (the stomach) or more caudal in the ventral abdomen (cecum), but abdominal palpation may also be normal. Gut stasis can be caused by environmental changes, stress (including postoperative stress or concurrent disease), malocclusion or excessive amounts of a high-energy, and low-fiber diet. The stomach contents may or may not be predominantly composed of hair, and the presumptive diagnosis of trichobezoar may occasionally be made. Due to gastric hypomotility, the stomach contents, whether hair or ingesta, become dehydrated and difficult to pass. The bacteria inside the gut may produce excessive gas, further exacerbating the discomfort.

Treatment consists of rehydrating the contents of the stomach, maintaining hydration of the animal, and stimulating motility. The rabbit may need assisted feeding, and several commercially available critical care diets for herbivores are available. Syringe feeding is preferable if possible because the large fibers needed to stimulate motility can clog feeding tubes, but nasogastric or esophagostomy tubes can be placed if needed (Makidon 2005; Fisher 2010; Rosen 2011). Subcutaneous fluids are often helpful, and intravenous fluids may be necessary in severe cases. Provided there are no signs of impaction, motility modifiers, and appetite stimulants can be administered to assist in restoring normal gastrointestinal motility. Classically, metoclopramide and cisapride were used. Although cisapride is no longer available on the commercial market, it can be obtained through compounding pharmacies. Mirtazapine, a tricyclic antidepressant with appetite-stimulating properties, has been shown to increase appetite in other species (Quimby & Lunn 2013) and may be of use (Ozawa et al. 2022). Mirtazapine has the advantage of availability in a transdermal formulation and may be applied to the ear pinna of the rabbit. If this formulation is used, gloves should be worn during application and the pinna should be monitored for erythema. Pain medications should be considered as well, although some veterinarians are leery of them because of potential gastrointestinal side effects. Buprenorphine can cause ileus and associated inappetence in rabbits, but this effect is not universal, and many rabbits can receive an appropriate dose without or with minimal gastrointestinal side effects (Cooper et al. 2009; Goldschlager et al. 2013, Deflers et al. 2018). Nonsteroidal anti-inflammatories such as meloxicam, could theoretically predispose the animal to gastric ulcers, however, generally, they are well-tolerated. Meloxicam has the additional advantage of being available in an oral formulation that is easy to administer. Cerenia has been considered by some to provide analgesia in veterinary patients, with some promising results in rabbits (Ozawa et al. 2019). Additional treatments that may be useful include simethicone to decrease the amount of gas, exercise to stimulate motility,

and abdominal massage (Fisher 2010). It is critical to differentiate ileus from intestinal obstruction, as the latter can occur as a result of hair obstructing the small intestine and may require surgical intervention (Harcourt-Brown 2007).

Additionally, it is important to appreciate that healthy rabbits commonly harbor gastric trichobezoars without pathologic effect. Slaughter checks of 208 healthy rabbits in one study showed that 23% had trichobezoars (Leary et al. 1984). In the same study, infusion of rabbit stomachs with latex causing a large space-occupying mass had no effect on the immediate or long-term health of the rabbits. Consequently, trichobezoars can be incidental findings in rabbits and should not be considered to be pathologic until proven otherwise.

Integumentary Infectious Diseases

Additional dermatologic infectious diseases are described under "Zoonotic infectious diseases." The most important integumentary disease of rabbits is ear mite infestation by the ectoparasite *Psoroptes cuniculi* (Figure 17.7). Pet owners may refer to the condition, formally called otoacariasis, as ear mange or ear canker. The classic presentation in advanced cases is thick crusts encasing the ear. Exudate and inflammation in the ear canal can be extensive with lesions also appearing on the face, neck, and occasionally around the perineum (Bulliot et al. 2013). Infestation causes pruritus, head shaking, stress, and competition for nutrients. Transmission of the parasite is direct and the life cycle requires 21 days for completion. Mites can survive off the host for weeks at a time (Varga & Patterson 2021). Subclinical infections can be present for an extended period, which explains the sudden onset of clinical signs in the absence of recent contact between animals (White et al. 2002). Tens of thousands of mites may infest a single

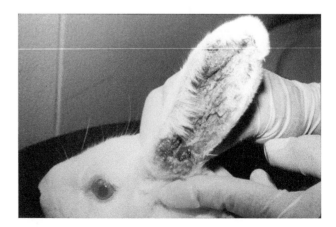

Figure 17.7 Ear mite infestation.

animal (Bowman et al. 1992) making them readily obtained from samples of the lesions. The mites are large enough to be seen with the unaided eye, but the diagnosis usually is made by identifying the large adults in the aural canal using an otoscope or observation of mites from exudate swabbed from the ear observed under a microscope. Treatment with ivermectin, selamectin, and moxidectin is effective when combined with aggressive environmental sanitation (Curtis & Brooks 1990; Wright & Riner 1984; Kurtdede et al. 2007; McTier et al. 2003; Wagner & Wendlberger 2000; White et al. 2002). Oral fluralaner has also been used successfully for treatment (Sheinberg et al. 2017). The ear crusts are best left alone as they will resolve with treatment and manipulating them can cause excessive bleeding and pain. Alternative treatments, including topically applied ivermectin and oils, have been advocated (Fichi et al. 2007). *Leporacarus gibbus* is a mite that less commonly infests rabbits, causing pruritus, alopecia, and dermatitis typically on the dorsal lumbar and ventral tail areas. Selamectin or imidacloprid and permethrin are effective treatments (Birke et al. 2009).

Rabbits are susceptible to infestation with the cat and dog flea species, *Ctenocephalides felis and C. canis*, as well as others when housed outdoors. The most common clinical signs include pruritus and dermatitis. Diagnosis is made by observing either the fleas or 'flea dirt.' Several products including imidacloprid, selamectin, and lufenuron have been safely used to manage flea infestations in rabbits, although selamectin may need to be applied weekly to be consistently effective (Hawkins, 2014; White et al. 2002). Fipronil has been associated with toxicities and should be avoided (White et al. 2002).

Venereal spirochetosis is caused by the bacterium, *Treponema paraluis cuniculi*. The disease is known by a number of synonyms including treponemiasis, cuniculosis, vent disease, and rabbit syphilis. Transmission may be venereal through coitus or extragenital through facial-genital contact. Fomites may also play a role. In contrast to many other infectious diseases of rabbits, young rabbits are relatively resistant to infection, and incidence increases with time spent in a breeding program. Following contact, organisms localize and proliferate at mucocutaneous junctions causing erythema and edema of the prepuce, vulva, scrotum, perineum, or anus. The nose, eyelids, lips, and extremities can also be affected. The lesions become vesicular, exude serum, and then become dry, scaly, and crusty. In the natural course of the disease, lesions persist for 1 to 5 months (Delong 2012). The bacterium colonizes regional lymph nodes where it remains even after lesions dissipate, and subsequent stress in the absence of treatment may again precipitate clinical disease.

Treponemiasis must be differentiated from traumatic or chemical dermatitis, localized nontreponemal bacterial pyoderma (e.g., "hutchburn"), dermatophytosis, and ectoparasites. The diagnosis is made through history, physical examination, and *in vitro* tests such as darkfield microscopy and various serologic assays. Penicillins given for periods ranging from 5 to 28 days is the treatment regimen of choice. A less intensive penicillin regimen involving weekly injections for a total of three treatments has also been advocated (Delong 2012). Lesions generally resolve and the organism is eliminated within 3 weeks of treatment initiation.

Moist dermatitis, sometimes called "hutch burn," may be seen in the perineal area subsequent to urine or diarrhea scald. Lesions around the face, neck, or dewlap are the consequence of malocclusion or continual moistening of the fur by drinking from a water bowl and may be referred to as "slobbers." The initial physical insult may lead to secondary bacterial dermatitis caused by *Pseudomonas aeruginosa*, which originates from feces or fecal-contaminated drinking water. *Pseudomonas* species elaborate a blue-green pigment that discolors the affected fur and hence the condition is occasionally called "blue fur disease." The treatment is aimed at correcting the initiating cause, drying the environment, clipping fur in the area of any lesions, and treating the lesions with astringents and topical or systemic gentamicin. Good sanitation practices, controlling obesity, and abstaining from offering water in bowls or crocks will aid in prevention.

Necrobacillosis (Schmorl's disease) is a syndrome presenting as dermatitis of the face and neck caused by excessive salivation, usually due to malocclusion or other dental disease. Secondary infection with the Gram-negative anaerobic bacterium, *Fusobacterium necrophorum*, may then become established. This bacterium is a normal inhabitant of the gastrointestinal tract and infection is often associated with unsanitary housing conditions. Fecal contamination from cecotrophy may be a source of oral inoculation. A combination of clinical signs and anaerobic bacterial culture are sufficient for diagnosis. Treatment consists of debriding wounds and applying topical antibiotics. Systemic penicillins, cephalosporins, or chloramphenicol may be used in severe cases. Prevention is achieved by maintaining a high level of sanitation, providing dental care where indicated, and eliminating sources of trauma such as course feed or sharp edges in cages.

Fly strike can occur in rabbits exposed to the outdoors, especially when housed in outdoor enclosures. About 1–3 cm swellings in the subcutis with a small hole may be caused by a single larva of *Cuterebra* species. The larvae should be surgically removed to avoid damage as crushed larvae can cause an anaphylactic reaction. Maggots of non-cuterebral species may be found anywhere on the body but have a predilection for the perineal skin folds of aged or obese rabbits. For all fly species, the treatment is to remove the larvae, clean the wound site under sedation, administer antibiotics, and continue wound care and fluid therapy as needed. Preventive strategies consist of fly control measures including screening outdoor pens.

Mastitis can occur in lactating does, and occasionally independent of lactation. The offending bacteria are typically *Staphylococcus aureus*, *Streptococcuss* spp., or *Pasteurella* (Girolamo & Selleri 2021). Antibiotics, warm compresses, and fluid therapy, with incision and drainage are curative.

Zoonotic Infectious Diseases

Domestic rabbits harbor few zoonotic agents of any significance, with dermatophytosis (ringworm) debatably the most important. *Trichophyton mentagrophytes* is most common, but *Microsporum canis* and other species may cause infection (Brock et al. 2012; Vogtsberger et al. 1986). Red, raised lesions are usually found around the head and ears, and a skin scraping placed in dermatophyte test medium or cleared with 10% KOH will confirm a diagnosis. Marginal husbandry practices, poor nutrition, environmental or internal stress factors, overcrowding, excessive heat and/or humidity, genetics, ectoparasites, age, and pregnancy can all predispose animals to infection. Direct contact or fomite transmissions are possible and rabbits may be asymptomatic carriers (Lopez-Martinez et al. 1984). The disease is readily transmissible to humans. Individual animals should be isolated and treated locally with miconazole or clotrimazole, and more generalized infections may require topical lime sulfur, or systemic griseofulvin or lufenuron (Brock et al. 2012; White et al. 2002; Hoppman & Barron 2007).

Certain ectoparasites, such as the fur mites *Cheyletiella parasitovorax*, *Leporacarus gibbus,* and burrowing sarcoptid mites may be transmissible to humans. *C. parasitovorax* is often called "walking dandruff," as it resembles white flakes that are visible to the naked eye. It typically causes mild lesions in both rabbits and humans. Selamectin, moxidectin, and imidacloprid have been used as treatments (Hawkins 2014; d'Ovidio & Santoro 2014).

Salmonellosis caused by *Salmonella typhimurium* presenting as a peracute fatal disease subsequent to a stressor (e.g., anesthesia, environmental extremes), has been reported most commonly within meat-producing facilities (Schadler et al. 2021). The diagnosis is made via culture and identification of the organism from blood, bile, feces, lymph nodes, or affected organs. Treatment is ineffective in eliminating the carrier state and, due to the public health risks, euthanasia of affected animals should be considered. *Yersinia pseudotuberculosis* is acquired by ingestion and causes emaciation and swollen lymph nodes with variable incidence of septicemia or diarrhea. *Listeria monocytogenes* causes acute, sporadic disease in many species. In rabbits, it most commonly causes septicemia, abortion, and fatality of pregnant does.

Rabies virus has been reported in pet rabbits, serving as a reminder that any pet animal with access to the outdoors requires adequate protection (Eidson et al. 2005; Karp et al. 1999). Unfortunately, there is currently no available rabies vaccine.

The protozoan *Encephalitozoon cuniculi* has a tropism for the brain, kidneys, and eyes. Ingestion, usually of food contaminated with infected urine, or nasal inoculation are the typical routes are infection. Although most infections are subclinical, the manifestation will depend on the primary organ affected. A head tilt and other neurologic signs are most commonly observed, but kidney failure and intraocular lesions such as cataracts and uveitis can also occur (Harcourt-Brown 2004). It may also infect immunocompromised humans, manifesting as diarrhea, renal disease, and keratoconjunctivitis. *E. cuniculi* is found in up to 30% of asymptomatic rabbits, and 69% of pets with neurologic symptoms were seropositive (Harcourt-Brown & Holloway 2003). Definitive diagnosis has historically been reliant on identification of lesions in brain tissue or PCR, and antemortem diagnosis is based on clinical signs and serology. PCR has been used to detect organismal DNA from liquefied lens material in cases of uveitis and lens rupture, but PCR tests of urine and CSF have been unreliable (Kunzel et al. 2008; Rich 2010). Data regarding treatment of rabbits for encephalitozoonosis is scant, although benzimidazole derivatives such as albendazole, oxibendazole, and fenbendazole have resulted in improvement in some cases (Harcourt-Brown & Holloway 2003; Suter et al. 2001; Fisher 2010). Benzimidazoles should be used with caution as they have been associated with toxicosis in rabbits (Graham et al. 2014). Corticosteroids might be a useful adjunct but should be used judiciously as rabbits are particularly susceptible to their immunosuppressive and toxic effects (Harcourt-Brown & Holloway 2003; Rosentthal 2004).

Of lesser importance are diseases such as leptospirosis, tularemia, and endoparasitism. *Francisella tularensis*, the etiologic agent of tularemia, rarely infects domestic lagomorphs, but may cause acute, febrile disease. A history of exposure to wild rabbits is associated with the vast majority of human cases. Zoonoses generally can be prevented by wearing gloves and long-sleeved clinical garments when handling rabbits and handwashing upon the removal of gloves.

Other Infectious Diseases

Rabbit hemorrhagic disease (RHD), caused by a lagovirus (calicivirus family), has emerged as an agent of increasing concern. The disease is acute and highly fatal. Clinical signs can vary and may include hemorrhage from nose, mouth, or rectum, difficulty breathing, neurologic signs, or sudden collapse. A small number of animals may be asymptomatic carriers. The virus historically presented as an explosive outbreak with high mortality in rabbitries, with rabbits succumbing to a severe and widespread intravascular coagulopathy (Xu & Chen 1989, Percy & Barthold 2007). Slaughter and disinfection were standard procedures in rabbitries where outbreaks occurred. However, a new serotype, RHDV serotype 2 (RHDV2), emerged in Europe in 2010 and was first seen in the United States in 2018. This serotype has been associated with outbreaks in both wild and domestic rabbits. Infected rabbits shed the virus in urine, feces, blood, and secretions, and the virus is very hardy in the environment, surviving heat and freezing for weeks to months. Transmission can be by close contact, but also by contact with almost any contaminated surface, including feed, bedding, clothing or shoes, or equipment. Mechanical vectors such as insects or predators may also play a role (Calvete et al. 2022). Because the disease is found in both domestic and wild rabbits, the potential impact on wildlife populations is a source of concern. A vaccine is available in Europe and, as of this writing, is under emergency use authorization in the US while pending FDA approval. Domestic rabbitries are encouraged to vaccinate their rabbits. RHDV2 is a foreign animal reportable disease and, if suspected or diagnosed, must be reported to state agricultural authorities.

There is no treatment for RHD. Prevention involves attention to biosecurity practices, both in the field and in domestic settings.

Field necropsies for research purposes are discouraged, and any carcass that needs to be removed should be double-bagged with appropriate biosecurity precautions. In the home, do not allow wild rabbits to come into contact with domestic ones, and do not allow newly acquired rabbits to come into contact with established rabbits for at least 2 weeks.

Cerebral larval migrans and fatal central nervous system disease may be seen in rabbits that acquire aberrant infections with *Baylisascaris* species. Disease may occur where raccoons or skunks contaminate stored feed or hay, gain access to barns or cages housing rabbits and defecate from the cage top into the interior of the cage, or where pet rabbits have grazed contaminated forage (Deeb & Digiacomo 1994; Jensen et al. 1983; Kazacos & Kazacos 1983). Raccoons tend to harbor heavy burdens

as female Baylisascaris nematodes produce substantial numbers of eggs that remain infective for years (Bauer 2013). Thus, wherever there are raccoons, the possibility of Baylisascaris infection is present. Signs of infection include progressive torticollis, ataxia, tremors, and falling (Deeb & Digiacomo 1994). The diagnosis is based on clinical signs and histopathology, but fresh minced brain can be placed in a Baermann apparatus to separate the larvae for specific identification. The condition is untreatable. Rabbits are a dead-end host for this disease and cannot pass it on to humans.

There are a number of other infectious diseases of rabbits that are not likely to be encountered in pet rabbits but are worth mentioning. *Obeliscoides cuniculi*, the rabbit stomach worm, is common in wild rabbits and may be found in laboratory rabbits that are fed contaminated feed or grazed on contaminated forages. It is a trichostrongyle imbedding in the gastric mucosa with a direct life cycle with shedding for 61–118 days (Jenkins 2004). Common in the United States, this parasite has recently been found in Europe as well (Fanelli et al. 2020). Staphylococci may cause septicemia, suppurative disease (including cutaneous abscesses or mastitis), and conjunctivitis. It is most severe and common in young or distressed animals. Owners should be aware of the potential for any mammal, including rabbits, to harbor methicillin-resistant *Staphylococcus aureus*. Rabbits are susceptible to toxoplasmosis (Leland et al. 1992), with public health ramifications should undercooked rabbit meat be consumed (Almeria et al. 2021). They may be an accidental host for the canine heartworm (Narama et al. 1982) and other dirofilarial species if housed outdoors.

Inherited Diseases

Buphthalmia due to inadequate drainage of aqueous humor from the anterior chamber is not uncommon in New Zealand White rabbits (Tesluk et al. 1982). It occurs unilaterally or bilaterally and is usually detectable by 3–5 months of age. Buphthalmia is characterized by megaloglobus, increased intraocular pressure (IOP), and increased corneal diameter. It is generally not painful, at least in the initial stages, but may cause blindness. Medical treatment with antiglaucomatous agents generally is not successful. Consequently, patients should be regularly monitored for pain or distress, and clients should be advised against breeding affected rabbits.

Splay leg is a developmental musculoskeletal disorder seen in young rabbits; the rear limbs splay laterally and animals will not bear weight (Fisher et al. 2021). The condition varies in severity from mild with animals showing only clumsiness when ambulating to severe where animals are completely paralyzed. In the latter cases, euthanasia is warranted. As is the case with most inherited disorders, clients should be advised not to breed affected rabbits.

Any number of other genetic and metabolic diseases including epilepsy, hydrocephalus, arteriosclerosis, cataracts, Pelger-Huet anomaly, cleft palate, lymphosarcoma, and hypertension (Brock et al. 2012) occur dependent upon the breed and genotype. Arteriosclerosis is a polygenic or familial trait that can be seen in all breeds, with calcified vessels visible on radiographs. Clinical signs are vague and may include general malaise, lethargy and weight loss. Hydrocephalus is often associated with dwarfism and brachygnathia although vitamin A deficiency in pregnant does will produce identical clinical signs in offspring (Brock et al. 2012, Quinn 2012).

Skeletal, Traumatic, Idiopathic, and Environmental Diseases

Malocclusion is one of the most common clinical conditions for which an owner will bring a rabbit to the veterinarian. Incisor malocclusion (mandibular prognathism, walrus teeth, and buck teeth) in young rabbits is most likely inherited but may also be caused from tooth loss due to trauma. The inherited condition is secondary to the shortening of the maxillary skull relative to the mandible of normal length with the lower incisors extending cranial to the upper incisors and growing into the mouth. Incisor malocclusion in adult animals is more likely to be secondary to malocclusion of the cheek teeth. Cheek teeth malocclusion is common in older animals, and animals are more likely to develop the condition if they are on high-grain, low-fiber diets (Lenox et al. 2021). Malocclusion will lead to functional anorexia and wasting with variable drooling. Maloccluded upper cheek teeth grow toward the cheek while the lower grow toward the tongue, potentially causing wounds in the respective surfaces, and abscesses and dacryocystitis can also result from the abnormal elongation of the roots. Diagnostic approaches include oral examination, endoscopic oral examination, radiographs, and computed tomography (CT). Some success has been achieved in quantifying dental disease with anatomical reference lines and grading systems (Korn et al. 2016, Artiles et al. 2020). The treatment for malocclusion is periodic tooth trimming with an appropriate power dental bur or extraction. In cases where the cause is suspected to be genetic, the owner should be counseled against breeding the animal.

Traumatic vertebral subluxation or fracture may result from struggling against restraint, improper handling, or sudden jumping. Rabbits are quite adept jumpers, and some can clear obstacles over 4 feet high, but they seem more prone to injury if they jump in response out of fear or from being startled, even from low heights. Rabbits are predisposed to injury by the high muscle-to-bone ratio in rabbits. The lumbosacroal joint acts as a fulcrum for the hind limbs with subluxation or fracture generally occurring at L7 or the caudal vertebrae, although anywhere in the lower thoracic or lumbar vertebra can be affected. Diagnosis is made by clinical signs of posterior paresis or paralysis, loss of pain sensation, urinary retention, and fecal incontinence, palpation during physical examination, and/or radiography or computed tomography (CT). Possible sequellae include decubital sores and perineal dermatitis from urine scald, along with uremia from urine retention. In acute injury, high-dose methylprednisolone has historically been used to prevent further damage. However, the use of steroids is controversial as their value has not been proven and they have significant side effects, especially in steroid-sensitive species such as rabbits (Paul-Murphy 2007). Long-term prognosis depends on the degree of injury, with mildly injured rabbits more likely to respond to medical management, such as cage rest, anti-inflammatory drugs, bladder expression, and other supportive care as needed. Severely injured rabbits are likely incurable and may require euthanasia, but recovery has been documented for even paralyzed animals with months of medical management (McCullough et al. 2012). The use of carts has been described for paraplegic rabbits, but some suggest the stress associated with carts might be significant (Keeble 2014).

Older rabbits can develop osteoarthritis like cats and dogs. Osteoarthritis can cause spondylosis of the vertebra and cause hindlimb weakness or affect the leg joints. The subsequent reluctance to move predisposes animals to urinary sludge and dermatitis of the perineal region because of decreased activity and grooming. The diagnosis can be made based on signalment, physical exam, and radiographs. It is often managed using analgesics such as meloxicam, although exercise and chondroitin sulfate are also beneficial (Ma et al. 2018).

Ulcerative pododermatitis is a common condition in rabbits and presents as erythema and/or decubital ulcers typically on the plantar surfaces of the hind feet (Figure 17.8). Superficial ulcers and scabs may progress, without intervention, to abscesses or granulomas, and further progression leads to the involvement of deeper tissues like ligaments and bone. In rabbits, the skin of the foot is thin and protected by thick fur. The lesions arise due to ischemia caused by the soft tissues of the foot being compressed between the substrate and bony structures of the foot (Blair 2013). Contributing factors are excess body weight, lack of activity, poor sanitation, excessive environmental moisture, and improper substrate. Treatment

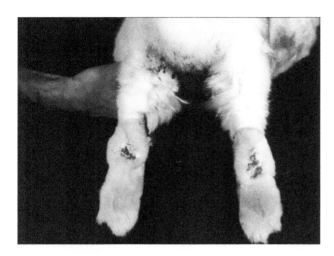

Figure 17.8 Pododermatitis.

consists first of correcting the underlying cause of the condition, if possible. Since the flooring of the enclosure is a common root cause, this should be changed, if indicated, to a soft substrate to reduce pressure on the foot. The substrate may be hay, straw, recycled paper, fleece, or a soft towel. All must be changed frequently. If obesity is a contributing factor, a weight loss program should be initiated. Toys and enrichment may be provided to encourage movement and an assessment of diet should be conducted.

Treatment consists of keeping the site dry and clean and commonly requires bandaging, with frequent bandage changes, often for weeks at a time. Systemic antibiotics may be effective, particularly those such as trimethoprim-sulfamethoxazole (TMS) or enrofoxacin that penetrate well to deep tissues (Blair 2013). The condition is painful and analgesics are likely to be necessary. Meloxicam is an effective NSAID in rabbits, and butorphanol can also be used. Successful treatment is lengthy and rechecks should assess effectiveness of treatment via observation and measurement of the wound. If underlying causes are addressed, treatment is often successful.

Because rabbits absorb and excrete large amounts of calcium, urolithiasis, and excessive urinary sludge, usually associated with calcium carbonate crystals, can occur. This predilection is exacerbated by inactivity and feeding high calcium diets and can be acutely precipitated by dehydration associated with any number of conditions. Clinical signs often include perineal dermatitis and an increased cloudiness in the appearance of the urine. The precipitate in the urine may become a "sludge" that is difficult to impossible to void, leading to acute urinary obstruction. Bladder sludge may be seen on the perineum and may be possible to express it in a sedated animal. Sterile conditions must be differentiated from bacterial cystitis, and this distinction informs treatment strategies.

Management includes flushing the bladder, pain medications, dietary modifications to decrease calcium, increased water intake (Fisher 2010), and appropriate antibiotics if bacterial overgrowth is associated.

Pregnancy toxemia is uncommon, but Dutch or Polish breeds may be predisposed. It is most common in pregnant does during the last week of pregnancy, but a similar metabolic toxemia may also be seen in pseudopregnant, postparturient, or obese does. Obesity and fasting are predisposing factors, and there is some evidence that hereditary factors play a role. There is often hepatic fatty infiltration and necrosis. Clinically affected animals are depressed, have acetone breath, dyspnea, and decreased urine production. Abortion, incoordination, convulsions, and coma may precede death. Death without premonitory signs can occur. Treatment with lactated Ringers or 5% dextrose, steroids, and empiric use of calcium gluconate may be attempted but is rarely successful. Prevention focuses on providing an adequate nutritional plane, including a high-energy diet late in gestation balanced with obesity prevention.

Idiopathic sebaceous adenitis is another cause of dermatitis and alopecia that must be differentiated from infectious conditions. Diagnosis is based upon consistent histologic findings and excluding bacterial, fungal, and other potential causes of these signs. Although it can be difficult to manage, successful treatment with cyclosporine and topical phytosphingosine has been described (Kovalik et al. 2012).

Neoplasia

Retrospective assessments of tumor incidence in rabbits are confounded by the fact that case reports and historical surveys have been largely derived from colonies of research animals where rabbits rarely live longer than 1–2 years of age. While tumor incidence increases with age, there exists no comprehensive tumor incidence information for aging rabbits.

Uterine adenocarcinoma is the most common spontaneous neoplasm of female rabbits with a high incidence in the Dutch, Californian, and New Zealand White breeds. The incidence is less than 5% in does under 2 years of age, but in certain populations, it may affect 80% of does over 5 years of age (Barthold et al. 2016). Clinical signs include vulvar bleeding, anemia, and a palpable abdominal mass. The prevention and attempted treatment of the disease is by OHE. Unless does are to be bred, OHE between 5 and 6 months is recommended universally. In young rabbits, the most common neoplasm is lymphosarcoma. Unlike other species, where lymphoid organs are the most common sites of involvement, in rabbits it is the kidney and gastric mucosa (Barthold et al. 2016). Interstitial cell tumors and seminomas have been reported in male rabbits (Tinkey et al. 2012). Other neoplasms that have been reported with some frequency in rabbits include thymoma, embryonal nephroma, leiomyoma/leiosarcoma, cutaneous papilloma, and mammary adenocarcinoma.

Taking a History

The fundamentals of collecting a history for rabbits are like those for other animals and are summarized in Table 17.4. The first information to gather should be the signalment. Certain rabbit breeds may be predisposed to particular diseases, so breed is an important component of the signalment as it would be for dogs. There are currently 50 breeds in the United States recognized by the American Rabbit Breeders Association (A.R.B.A.) ranging in size from 1 kg dwarf/small breeds to 5–8 kg or greater giant breeds. Many of these breeds can have multiple varieties. Rabbit breeds are made distinctive by a combination of body size and shape, ear carriage, and pelt coloration. If the ears "flop" down alongside the head, rather than stand erect, the breed is of the lop-eared variety. Some non-show grade lops may have one or both ears "helicopter" by projecting horizontally. Many rabbits presenting to a veterinary practice, particularly if acquired from a pet store, are not purebreds or do not meet the breed standards. However, there are breeds that may commonly be seen, such as the Dutch, Holland Lop, Mini-Lop, Lionhead, and Flemish Giant (see Table 17.5). The best method to become familiarized with rabbit breeds is to visit the ARBA website at: https://www.arba.net. (See Figures 17.9–17.15.)

The realities of rabbit medicine are that most animals present for a clinical problem and few are seen for wellness exams. This being the case, it is important to obtain a detailed history about both the presenting complaint and the routine care of the animal. In terms of diet, it is important to ask not only what is offered, but what the animal eats. Unfortunately, many commercial rabbit pellets are mixed with unhealthy items such as corn and seeds, and rabbits may selectively eat high carbohydrate and high fat items leading to obesity or gut stasis (Harcourt-Brown 2002). Pellets can also be composed of different types of hay that may have different nutrient values. It is also important to ask about the primary enclosure—determine flooring or substrate type and the ability of the animal to exercise, either within the primary enclosure or upon being given exercise opportunities outside of it. Beyond questions about husbandry, the general inquiries about the rabbit are like those made for other animals. Decreased appetite/anorexia is one of the most common presenting complaints for rabbits, but this can be symptomatic of

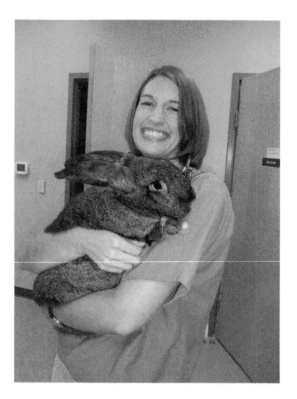

Figure 17.9 Flemish giant. (Courtesy of Dr. Stacey Wilkinson.)

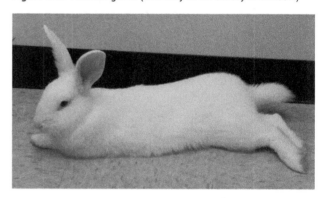

Figure 17.10 New Zealand White. (Courtesy of Dr. Stacey Wilkinson.)

a wide variety of issues or diseases. Respiratory, dental, dermatological, and gastrointestinal problems are common issues for rabbits presenting to the veterinarian. Sometimes rabbits, especially unspayed adult females, present because of increased aggression. The etiology for aggression can vary from hormonal, normal exploratory behavior, pain, deafness, and even infectious diseases, so questions specifically about behavior should be included when gathering a comprehensive history (Harcourt-Brown 2002).

Physical Examination and Preventive Medicine

Rabbits should be transported to the clinic in a secure carrier where they can remain in the exam room. A normal

Table 17.4 History questions for rabbit owners.

Topic	Questions	Comments
Signalment	Age Sex Neutered status Breed	Owners may not be correct about the sex of the rabbit and education might be necessary The age when the animal was neutered may also be relevant
Acquisition	Location (pet store, breeder, etc.) When the animal was acquired	How many owners the animal has had may be important for behavioral problems
Housing	Cage type Flooring substrate Exercise amount/frequency Frequency of cage cleaning	If the animals have wire-bottom cages, ask about access to areas away from the wire Amount of time peer day or week available out of the cage for exercise is important
Environment	Other animals in the house Indoors/outdoors Potential environmental hazards	Newly acquired rabbits or wild animals may be a source of infectious diseases Rabbits may like to chew objects when roaming the house
Diet	Types of food: hay, pellets, fresh foods Amount offered and eaten	Make sure to ask about treats and if the pellets are just pellets or have other items (corn, seed, etc.)
Animal	Changes in feces or urine Changes in appetite or diet preferences Changes in behavior Coughing, sneezing, or nasal discharge Any medications, including herbal and nutritional supplements	If there are changes in appetite/drinking, ask about any environmental changes such as a new diet, stressful situation, or new water or food dispensers

Table 17.5 Examples of common pet rabbit breeds seen in practice.

Breed	Size range (lb)	Color and markings	Other characteristics
Californian	8–10.5	White with colored nose, ears, tail, and feet	Compact body type and pink eyes
Flemish giant	15–22	Variable	Large back arch, gentle giant, glossy, dense fur
Dutch	3.5–5.5	White forequarters and thorax with ears, cheeks, and back half of body is colored	Short, blocky, compact body type
Lionhead	2.5–3.75	Variable	Petite, shaggy, wool mane
Holland lop	<4	Variable	Short, blocky, compact body type
English lop	9–12	Variable	Longest ears of all rabbit breeds, long slender body
Mini-lop	4.5–6.5	Variable	Short, blocky, compact body type
New Zealand White	9–12	Albino	Compact body type, ruby pink eyes

rabbit will rest compactly on all four limbs with mouth closed and regular twitching of the nostrils. Animals presenting with severe pain will show a hunched posture and immobility and may exhibit teeth grinding, known as bruxism. Those in acute pain or distress, especially upon handling, may emit a high-pitched cry. It is important to bear in mind that even an amiable rabbit will become aggressive if experiencing chronic pain.

Regardless of where the physical exam begins, a systematic, thorough, and consistent approach is important. Many prefer to start at the head, and this begins with an appreciation of the normal protrusion of the eyes, which varies among breeds, and is more prominent in males during breeding season and in fearful animals (Harcourt-Brown 2002). Rabbits may not exhibit a menace response because of their natural tendency to freeze, making this reflex an

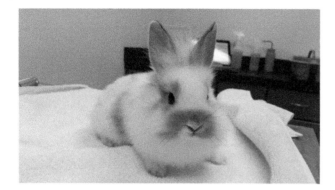

Figure 17.11 Juvenile lion head. (Courtesy of Dr. Stacey Wilkinson.)

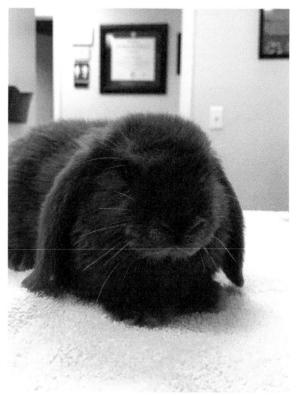

Figure 17.13 Mini lop. (Courtesy of Dr. Stacey Wilkinson.)

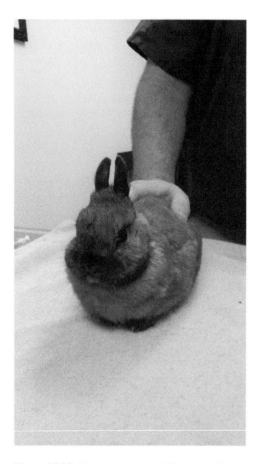

Figure 17.12 Netherland dwarf. (Courtesy of Dr. Stacey Wilkinson.)

inadequate test for vision (Vernau et al. 2007). Ocular examinations can be done for other species, keeping in mind that atropine may be unreliable or ineffective as a mydriatic due to the presence of serum atropinesterase in many rabbits. Ocular or nasal discharge should be absent. Periocular depilation or discharge may be suggestive of conjunctivitis or dacryocystitis/nasolacrimal duct obstruction

that can occur with bacterial infections or malocclusion. Dacryocystitis is usually secondary to dental disease, particularly of the incisors. Conjunctivitis can be associated with primary bacterial infections, environmental irritants, eyelid abnormalities, or secondary to dacryocystitis or an upper respiratory infection (Harcourt-Brown 2002). *Pasteurella multocida* is the most common cause of conjunctivitis with nasal discharge. One should take note of sneezing or evidence of obstructed breathing throughout the examination. Rabbits are fastidious groomers so while the eyes and nose may be clear, the inside of the front paws might show evidence of oculonasal discharge.

The ears should be examined for crusts or discharge indicating bacterial or mite infections. Lop-eared rabbits are prone to accumulations of exudate in the ear canals. The fur should be smooth and coat thick, but small areas of alopecia can occur normally with the molting process in some breeds. The scrotum of mature males and the internal pinnae of the ears are the only hairless areas on a normal rabbit. Mature females can possess a large fold of skin over the throat called a dewlap, an area prone to dermatitis in animals that drink from water bowls or have excessive saliva secondary to dental disease. Older castrated males can also develop skin folds like the dewlap. The hair should be examined, especially on the dorsum, for

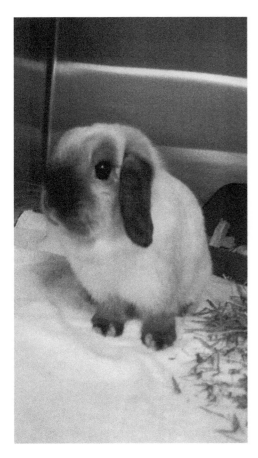

Figure 17.14 Holland lop. (Courtesy of Dr. Stacey Wilkinson.)

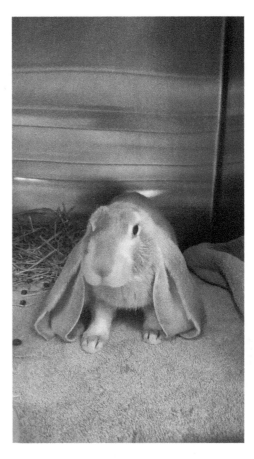

Figure 17.15 English lop. (Courtesy of Dr. Stacey Wilkinson.)

evidence of parasites. If the rabbit spends significant time outside, careful examination through the hair for signs of fly larvae. Skin turgor is a good indicator of hydration status. The hairless skin on the scrotum of the males or the inguinal skin in females/neutered males is the best place to assess skin tenting.

Vertebrae and ribs should be easily detectable, but not pronounced. The abdominal organs, such as the stomach, kidneys, and spleen, are easily palpated. Auscultation will reveal heart rates of 130–325 beats per minute and a normal respiratory rate is 30–60 breaths per minute. Rectal thermometers are poorly tolerated, and temperature is not usually taken during the exam unless the animal is critical, but the normal range is 101–104°F (Harkness & Wagner 2010). Animal and human tympanic thermometers can be used, but these produce more variable readings that are often lower than rectal temperatures. Ausculted airway sounds should be short, regular, and rapid in progression with dry bronchovesicular sounds. Auscultation of gut sounds may reveal problems if the rabbit has a decreased appetite, but reduced sounds can be present even in healthy animals.

As described in the restraint section, the patient should be cradled to lift the animal to look at the ventrum. The mammary glands of intact should be palpated for evidence of mastitis (Mullen 2000). The urinary and genital openings are located immediately below the anus (Figures 17.16 and 17.17). The testes descend at about 12 weeks of age in the buck but may be retracted partly into the abdomen due to the open inguinal canal. The testicles can be manipulated from the inguinal canals into the scrotum for palpation by applying light pressure in the cranial inguinal area. Look for any signs of crusts in the genital region. Rabbits have inguinal glands, which are folds of skin by the anal orifice that normally have a brown, foul-smelling deposit. At this time, the feet should be examined. Obese or mature, potentially arthritic animals may have urine scald or the presence of a fecal impaction in the fur and perineal skin folds because of their inability to groom themselves.

The oral exam is poorly tolerated, and so it is often saved for last. The incisors can be easily viewed for length and symmetry by retracting the lips. Saliva staining around the mouth can serve as an indicator of oral disease. Dwarf rabbits are prone to congenital incisor malocclusion

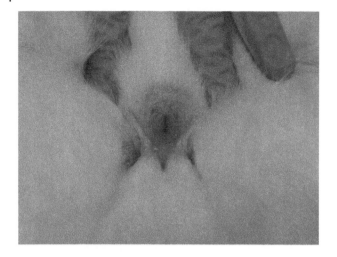

Figure 17.16 Sex determination of a female rabbit.

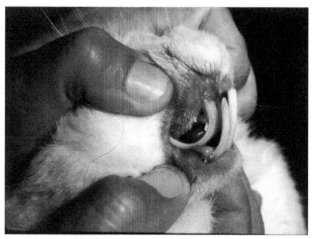

Figure 17.18 Malocclusion.

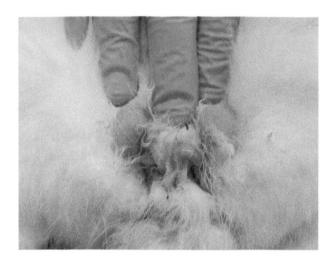

Figure 17.17 Sex determination of a male rabbit.

Handling and Restraint

Lifting and carrying rabbits is stressful for this prey species. In addition, rabbits are at significant risk of injury from improper handling. Something seemingly as innocuous as permitting a rabbit to leap from one's arms into a cage may result in vertebral luxation or fracture. If rabbits are improperly restrained, they may inflict painful scratches to a handler from the claws on their powerful rear limbs. Lifting rabbits should be minimized using appropriate enclosures and floor-based interaction. When carrying the animal is necessary, minimization of stress is key. Rabbits should never be handled by the ears or allowed to dangle their back feet. Use of an appropriately sized transport box can be a relatively stress-free method of transport. Using positive reinforcement, rabbits can be trained to enter a box, or the rabbit can be gently "scooped" into it. If the lid can be removed, physical exams can be accomplished with the rabbit in the base of the box. If a rabbit must be carried in a person's arms, use of a towel around the animal to help provide support and prevent struggling may be helpful (Figure 17.19). Always support the hindquarters with one arm, and the other hand may be placed around the shoulders (Bradbury & Dickens 2016). When returning a rabbit to its cage or setting it on a surface, do not allow it to leap or hop from the arms. If possible, place the rabbit down rear end first, especially when placing it back in the cage. This way, the rabbit is less likely to kick from the handler's arms, which predisposes it to back injury.

For the physical exam, if the rabbit is in a transport box, the exam can be conducted with the animal securely in the box. This is likely the ideal, and least stressful, method of examination. Otherwise, rabbits should be examined in such a way as to minimize stress. The rabbit can be placed on an examination table with a nonslip substrate

(see Figure 17.18). The molars are difficult to examine without sedation. An otoscopic cone or stainless steel nasal speculum with an attached light source will aid visualization in an awake and appropriately restrained patient.

At present, there are no standard vaccines or prophylactic dewormers for pet rabbits in the United States. A vaccination against *Pastuerella* has been studied but is not yet available (Suckow et al. 2008). Fecal exams should be considered in new or rabbits housed outdoors. The best preventative health measure is to spay female rabbits around 5 months of age, depending on the breed, to eliminate the potential for uterine adenocarcinoma. Neutering both males and females decreases the likelihood of aggressive behavior. Males can maintain fertile sperm for about 4 weeks after neutering.

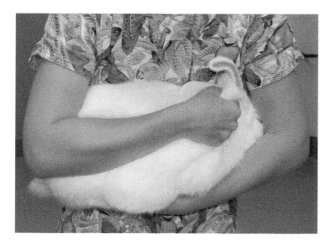

Figure 17.19 Restraint for transport.

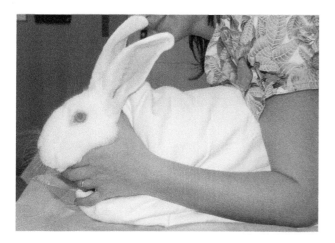

Figure 17.20 Restraint using a towel.

under them to help the animal have traction and be less likely to kick while trying to gain its footing. These exams are most easily conducted with two people, one to gently restrain the rabbit and the other to conduct the exam. The person restraining the rabbit should stand facing the flank of the patient placing one hand gently over the thorax and the other upon the hindquarters, with the purpose of maintaining the position of the rabbit should it attempt to make a sudden and dangerous jump forward. If a solo exam is necessary, the hindquarters can be braced against the restrainer's abdomen. With one hand on the thorax, the other can be used for the physical exam. At any point, the examiner or assistant can gently place their hand over the rabbits' eyes to reduce the likelihood the animal will try to jump.

Examining the ventrum and genital region is very important but can be difficult to do safely and is best done with an assistant. Some animals will become immobile

when placed in dorsal recumbency, which can be advantageous for the exam, but realize that the animal is likely "freezing" because of undue stress (Harcourt-Brown 2002; Brandao et al. 2021), and as such this technique is not recommended. An oral exam requires two people if the animal is not sedated. It is easiest to wrap the animal in a towel and tuck the back end into the restrainer's abdomen (Figure 17.20). Place each arm along the flanks to restrain the body, leaving the hands free to restrain the head and neck area. The restrainer should be careful not to occlude nasal passages because rabbits are obligate nasal breathers and will not breathe through their mouth even though is it open during the exam. Restraint for specific procedures is further described in "Clinical Techniques."

Imaging

The common indications for imaging include suspicion of dental disease, vertebral luxation, limb fracture, respiratory disease and gastrointestinal diseases, or other intrabdominal diseases such as uterine adenocarcinoma. Radiography and ultrasound are commonly available in clinical practice and may be early modalities of choice. Endoscopy, CT, and MRI are becoming more available and cost-effective, however, and may be available for rabbit patients. Positioning for most forms of imaging is facilitated using sedation or general anesthesia. Otherwise, it may be difficult to manipulate the animal in such a way as to avoid risking injury or movement, or to obtain the necessary view.

For respiratory or abdominal radiography, the DV view, rather than the VD, is preferred in rabbits because it minimizes the risk of torso rotation along its sagittal axis, enhances spino-sternal alignment and does not impair respiration. If the practice encounters a considerable number of lapine patients, it is worthwhile to develop a technique chart for the various anatomic structures. An alternative is to use a feline technique chart, but to shorten the exposure time, compensate with increased mA, and reduce the KVp to preserve resolution. Interpretation of abdominal radiographs in the rabbit is complicated by the low amount of abdominal fat available for contrast, and the constant presence of ingesta and gas in the GI tract.

Dental radiographs should include lateral, DV/VD, and two lateral oblique skull films; and rostral and intraoral views may also be helpful (Capello & Gracis 2005). Obliques are used to thoroughly evaluate the tooth roots and are obtained by placing the animal laterally and rotating the side of the mouth that is facing upwards dorsally at approximately 10–20 degrees. Care should be taken when positioning a sedated animal for radiographs, especially a rostral view, because flexing the neck can obstruct the airway. The neck should always be extended whenever possible (Figure 17.21 and 17.22). For a thorough discussion about radiographic technique in the rabbit, the readers are referred to *Clinical Radiology of Exotic Companion Mammals* (Capello & Lennox 2008). The addition of CT and potentially MRI can be helpful, particularly for dental, respiratory, and ear diseases. These modalities provide further differentiation of soft tissues, facilitating distinction between fat and associated tissue, for example, as well as allowing for assessment of individual teeth in the case of dental disease (Capello 2016).

Anesthesia

Rabbits can present an anesthetic challenge to veterinarians or veterinary technicians inexperienced with them. Rabbits are comparatively difficult to intubate, for example, but a veterinary technician who is knowledgeable and develops confidence will become proficient in all techniques necessary to safely anesthetize the rabbit patient. In all cases, it is most important to keep the patient calm and isolated from perceived threats such as noisy dogs. A distressed rabbit can be permeated with catecholamines to a degree that adversely affects anesthetic procedures (Jenkins 2000).

Pre-anesthesia

Obtaining a thorough history and a pre-anesthetic physical examination are important in detecting underlying medical conditions that may complicate anesthesia. Examination of the nares for rhinorrhea suggestive of bacterial respiratory disease, and careful auscultation of the thorax for evidence of cardiac or pulmonary disease, should be carried out. Once admitted to the clinic, rabbits should be kept in escape-proof cages in a quiet area. Rabbits have high metabolic energy requirements and are unable to vomit; therefore, preoperative fasting is a topic of debate. A short preoperative fasting period of 1–2 h is generally recommended to reduce the amount of food in the oral cavity that could be inhaled or complicate intubation, although cleaning of the mouth might still be necessary (Jenkins 2000; Hawkins & Pascoe 2021). Fasting rabbits for longer periods can predispose animals to a post-operative gastrointestinal disturbances, metabolic acidosis, and hypoglycemia, especially in young animals or adults of small breeds (Flecknell & Thomas 2015). Fasting of obese, pregnant, or post-parturient rabbits is contraindicated as it may predispose to ketosis and liver necrosis.

Anticholinergics can be administered prior to anesthesia if deemed necessary. One should bear in mind that serum and tissue atropinesterases found in many rabbits

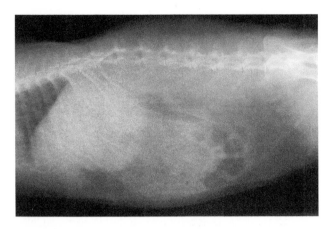

Figure 17.21 Lateral radiograph. (Courtesy of Ryan Cheek.)

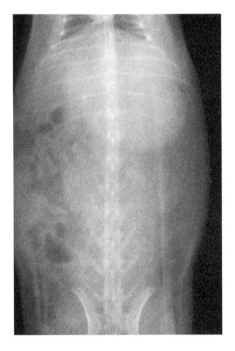

Figure 17.22 V/D radiograph. (Courtesy of Ryan Cheek.)

render the anticholinergic agent atropine sulfate relatively ineffective. In the presence of atropinesterase, atropine must be given in high doses (1–2 mg/kg) with redosing every 10–15 min (Lipman et al. 2008). Therefore, the administration of 0.01–0.02 mg/kg glycopyrrolate subcutaneously (SC) to reduce salivary and bronchial secretions and prevent vagal bradycardia is an advisable alternative.

Anesthetic Agents Used in Rabbits

Inhalant anesthetics are often the preferred primary mode of anesthesia for rabbits because it is precise, rapidly adjustable, safe, and effective. In addition, postoperative recovery is faster and less complicated than with injectable anesthetics. Sevoflurane and isoflurane are the two most used inhalant drugs used in rabbits. The minimum alveolar concentration (MAC) of sevoflurane is approximately 3.7–4% in rabbits, which is higher than the isoflurane MAC of approximately 2.5% (Scheller et al. 1988; Turner et al. 2006). The anesthetist should remember that these doses will not provide sufficient anesthesia for all rabbits and procedures, but also that the required doses are lower when given in conjunction with other drugs and in animals with some systemic diseases such as liver disease (Yin et al. 2012). The side effects of inhalants in rabbits are similar to those in other species, with one potential peculiarity being that isoflurane by itself can increase IOP in rabbits (Chae et al. 2021). However, this increased IOP can be mitigated by giving sedative drugs for premedication, which might explain why this effect is not seen in other species where isoflurane is rarely used by itself.

Injectable drugs should be used to pre-medicate and/or induce animals that will subsequently be maintained on inhalant anesthesia. Inhalant induction using a mask or induction chamber without premedication is possible but not widely recommended because struggling, distress vocalization, and breath-holding can occur (Flecknell 2015; Hedenqvist et al. 2001). Although sevoflurane is thought to have a less aversive odor than isoflurane, the aforementioned behaviors can occur with both inhalants (Flecknell et al. 1999). Mask induction with an inhalant after the administration of sedative drugs can be done without harm to the patient with proper restraint (Figure 17.23).

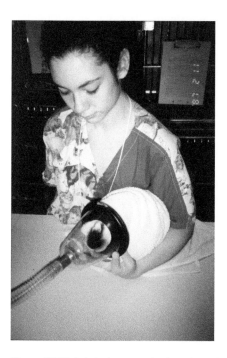

Figure 17.23 Inhalation anesthesia using a face mask.

Common premedications include an opioid with or without a benzodiazepine, such as butorphanol or buprenorphine with midazolam (Schroeder & Smith 2011). Alternatively, the anesthetist can administer an alpha2 agonist alone or in combination with ketamine hydrochloride or a benzodiazepine (Hedenqvist et al. 2015; Terada et al. 2014; Desprez et al. 2022). An alpha2 agonist with ketamine can be sufficient for full induction of anesthesia with an adequate dose. Intravenous propofol or ketamine are additional options for induction of anesthesia, assuming the patient has been sufficiently sedated with premedication for easy placement of a catheter. The published doses of propofol vary widely in rabbits, and it should be given slowly and to reduce the risk of causing apnea (Allweiler et al. 2010). Some example induction protocols for rabbits include: low-dose ketamine with xylazine or dexmedetomidine for sedation followed by mask induction with an inhalant, butorphanol, and midazolam followed by mask induction or dexmedetomidine with midazolam followed by ketamine induction. If injection is not feasible, the intranasal route is an option for administration of induction agents (Robertson & Eberhart 1994). The onset of effect is rapid (less than 3 min), and the duration of effect may be 30 min or more. Midazolam, opioids, and alpha2 agonists with and without ketamine can effectively induce low-grade sedation or anesthesia by this route (Robertson & Eberhart 1994; Santangelo et al. 2016). The technician should be aware that these injectable drugs have effects on rabbits like those seen in other species. These drug effects vary depending on the dose and drug combination used, but in general, the technician should expect effects on blood pressure, respiration and a lowered need for isoflurane (Chang et al. 2009; Turner et al. 2006; Schroeder & Smith 2011). If the animal will be undergoing a painful procedure, analgesics should be included as part of this process prior to starting surgery. Subcutaneous administration of anesthetic drugs is better tolerated by the patient than intramuscular, but any reversal drugs given at the end of the procedure might not work as quickly (Williams & Wyatt 2007).

Alfaxalone is a steroid anesthetic that has increased in popularity since it became available in the United States in a multidose formulation. Intramuscular alfaxalone is an effective sedative for minor procedures, and its sedative properties and duration are increased by combining it with other drugs such as opioids (butorphanol, buprenorphine, and hydromorphone), midazolam and dexmedetomidine (Huynh et al. 2015, Bradley et al. 2019, Costa et al. 2022, Knutson et al. 2022, Ishikawa et al. 2019, Marin et al. 2020; Reabel et al. 2021, 2022). An anesthetist can also use alfaxalone as an intravenous induction agent following premedication with drugs such as dexmedetomidine and midazolam (Bradley et al. 2022, Engbers et al. 2017). Hypoxemia is a risk, especially at high doses and in combination with other drugs (Rousseau-Blass & Pang 2020, Navarrete-Calvo et al. 2014, Tutunaru et al. 2013).

Once anesthesia has been induced, rabbits are often maintained on inhalant anesthesia either via a face mask or endotracheal intubation. A mask is easy to use and might be preferred, especially for short procedures. In contrast to a face mask, endotracheal intubation allows for assisted ventilation and easy access to the airway in event of an emergency but is sometimes avoided because the anatomy of the rabbit oropharynx makes endotracheal intubation challenging (Tran et al. 2001). The oral cavity is long and narrow, the mandible has a limited range of abduction, and entry into the oral cavity is partially occluded by the large incisors and cheek teeth. The tongue protrudes dorsally, the epiglottis is large, U-shaped, soft, and flexible, and the larynx slopes ventrally. Additionally, laryngeal tone and the propensity to laryngospasm are high. All these factors combine to obscure visualization, access to the glottis, and make endotracheal intubation of the rabbit challenging.

Despite the anatomical challenges, rabbits can be reliably and easily intubated by an experienced technician. Intubation should be carried out with an endotracheal tube of 3.0–4.0 mm internal diameter endotracheal tube for rabbits weighing 3–6 kg or 1.0–2.5 mm endotracheal tube for rabbits weighing less than 3 kg. Cuffed tubes can used but the cuff is often not inflated as rabbits are prone to postintubation tracheal strictures, which would be noted approximately 2–3 weeks later (Grint et al. 2006; Nordin et al. 1977; Phaneuf et al., 2006; Squire et al. 1990). Intubation can be accomplished by direct visualization aided by a laryngoscope or otoscope (Hawkins & Pascoe 2021). The key to intubation by direct visualization is to bring the mouth, larynx, and trachea into linear alignment (Figure 17.24). This can be accomplished with the animal in a sternal, dorsal, or lateral position with the head hyperflexed. The tongue should be retracted laterally through one of the diastema, the bilateral spaces between the incisors and premolars, to prevent laceration on the incisors.

A guide wire or rigid endoscope can be employed to assist with orotracheal intubation. If a 3.0 mm or larger internal diameter endotracheal tube is used, intubation can be achieved using the polypropylene guide technique (Gilroy 1981). A 56-cm, 8 Fr polypropylene catheter should be passed through the endotracheal tube lumen from the connector to the distal end until the blunt catheter tip extends 15–20 cm past the bevel. Under direct visualization using a laryngoscope, the tip of the catheter should be cautiously advanced through the diastema, past the vocal folds, and into the trachea. Once the guide is in the trachea,

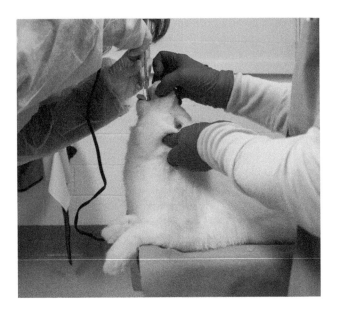

Figure 17.24 Body position for orotracheal intubation.

the laryngoscope can be removed and the endotracheal tube advanced as a sheath over the stationary catheter into the trachea. Following intubation, the stylet or guide should be immediately removed and the endotracheal tube secured. Alternatively, the endotracheal tube can be placed over a rigid endoscope, instead of using a laryngoscope, which aids in both visualization and guiding the tube for orotracheal intubation (Tran et al. 2001).

If preferred, intubation can be performed blindly. After induction, the rabbit should be placed in sternal recumbency with the head extended dorsally such that the alignment of mouth, larynx, and trachea is perpendicular to the table surface. An endotracheal tube should then be advanced to the proximal aspect of the larynx. This can be confirmed by visualizing the fogging of the tube interior with every exhalation and listening for respiratory sounds through the endotracheal tube. The position of the tube should be adjusted until the sounds are at maximal intensity. At this point, the endotracheal tube should be gently advanced into the trachea. If breaths are shallow, it is sometimes helpful to have an assistant administer gentle chest compressions and to advance the tube timed with the release of a compression (inhalation). A cough reflex often confirms correct insertion. A capnograph can also help to confirm proximity of the tube tip at the oropharynx. This blind technique carries a risk of trauma and should be abandoned in favor of direct observation if intubation is not successful. Regardless of the intubation technique, intubation should never be forced, because the trachea, tracheal bifurcation, and tissues of the oropharynx are easily damaged, and the vagus nerve may be stimulated. Correct placement in the trachea should be further confirmed by visualizing the respiration-associated condensation of water vapor on the internal surface of the endotracheal tube, by auscultation in conjunction with manual respiration using an Ambu bag, or capnography. Mechanical ventilation should not start until intubation is confirmed, because overzealous ventilation into the stomach can lead to acute dilatation and rupture.

There is no consensus on the use of topical anesthetics to enhance intubation. While spraying of the pharynx, larynx, and trachea will reduce the risk of laryngospasm and enhance passage of the tube, it also suppresses the convenient forward motion of the glottis during swallowing that may enhance intubation. If a topical anesthetic is desired, lidocaine 10% oral spray should be judiciously misted on the glottis to prevent laryngospasm and facilitate intubation. Topical benzocaine should not be used because it might cause methemoglobinemia.

Nasotracheal intubation and supraglottic airway devices are alternatives to traditional endotracheal intubation to maintain a patent airway during inhalation anesthesia. The principles of the nasotracheal approach are like those of the oral but might be less technically demanding for some people (DeValle 2009). Nasotracheal intubation is best accomplished with the animal in dorsal recumbency with the head over the edge of a table, and then gently passing the tube to avoid damage to the surrounding tissue (Figures 17.25 and 17.26). Supraglottic airway devices consist of a mask that covers the glottis, and this mask is connected to the anesthesia system via a tube in the same way that an endotracheal tube connects. These devices require less technical skill to place compared with an endotracheal tube, which is highly beneficial for those with little experience or in cases of emergency. The laryngeal mask airway (LMA) is a version of this device that has been used in human pediatric patients for many years and more recently successfully used in rabbits (Kazakos et al. 2007; Smith et al. 2004). The mask of an LMA inflates to provide a seal around the glottis that allows for assisted ventilation. This seal might not be complete, which does create small risks such as gastric tympany from anesthesia introduction into the esophagus, an unprotected airway in the event of regurgitation, and increased anesthetic waste gas accumulation. These reports indicate that LMA sizes 1–1.5 perform the best. A V-gel® is a branded supraglottic airway device that is a similar concept to an LMA, but it does not have an inflatable cuff and instead relies on its shape and material to form a seal over the glottis. V-gels® have been used successfully in rabbits, but respiratory function monitoring is essential as they have been associated with respiratory obstructions (Raillard et al. 2019; Engbers et al. 2017).

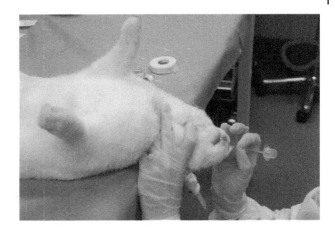

Figure 17.25 Body position for nasotracheal intubation.

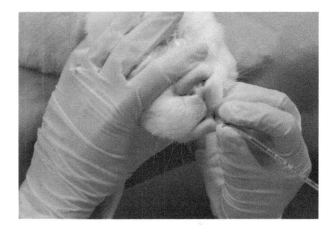

Figure 17.26 Nasotracheal intubation.

An Ayre's T-piece or other non-rebreathing circuit is most appropriate for rabbit inhalational anesthesia (Flecknell 2015). Once intubated, the rabbit should be connected to a gas anesthesia machine with a closed breathing circuit for ventilation with a mechanical respirator at a rate of 30 to 40 breaths per minute and a tidal volume of 11–15 mL/kg. The inspiration-to-expiration ratio should be 1:2 or 1:3 and airway pressures should not be permitted to exceed 20 cmH$_2$O as barotrauma will occur at higher pressure (Reuter et al. 2005). If mechanical ventilation is not available, spontaneous ventilation should be accommodated with a semi-closed pediatric breathing circuit. Spontaneous respirations should be regular and deep and occur at a rate of 15 or more breaths per minute. The anesthetist should be cognizant of the risk of apnea in this circumstance and be prepared to evaluate the depth of anesthesia and assist ventilations.

As an alternative to inhalation anesthesia, anesthesia can be maintained with injectable drugs alone. The disadvantages of anesthesia by injection include the lack of precision in anesthetic depth control, prolonged recovery time, and physiologic changes such as hypotension, hypoxemia, and acid–base disorders associated with some agents. Injectable drugs as sole anesthetic agents are best for uncomplicated procedures involving healthy animals. The anesthetist should consider administering supplemental oxygen to reduce the impacts of respiratory depression if relying on injectable anesthesia.

Combinations of ketamine hydrochloride with alpha2 agonists are the most common protocols for maintaining anesthesia with injectable drugs. These drugs are combined because ketamine as a sole agent does not provide sufficient analgesia or muscle relaxation, and alpha2 agonists alone drugs do not provide sufficient sedation or analgesia for surgical procedures. Effective doses include ketamine (35–45 mg/kg) with xylazine (5 mg/kg) and ketamine (15–25 mg/kg) with dexmedetomidine (0.25 mg/kg) (Flecknell 2015; Flecknell & Thomas 2015; Orr et al. 2005; Difilippo et al. 2004) given SQ. These protocols will typically induce anesthesia within 10–15 min and last 25–45 min, but total time of unconsciousness might be up to 2 h (Flecknell 2015). Even as a combination, ketamine and alpha2 drugs might not be sufficient for major surgical procedures such as a laparotomy or thoracotomy. Ketamine and xylazine combinations can be sufficient for ocular procedures and do not increase IOP (Holve et al. 2013). Premedication with an opioid or acepromazine can provide deeper anesthesia, and these triple combination regimens will provide anesthesia lasting 60–90 min. Acepromazine should be used with caution in ill animals because it may further contribute to hypotension, bradycardia, and respiratory depression. If it is necessary to extend anesthesia, incremental doses of one-half the original ketamine dose can be given as the xylazine will last longer than the ketamine. As an alternative to single or repeated injections, continuous infusion protocols have been described for ketamine and xylazine or dexmedetomidine (Wyatt et al. 1989; Sayce et al. 2020). General anesthesia can also be maintained with a constant rate infusion of alfaxalone if the rabbit is intubated to allow for respiratory support (Bradley et al. 2022). This method of anesthesia should be carried out with an infusion pump or precisely controlled mini-drip (60 drops/mL) and vital signs should be monitored closely. Infusion using propofol and ketamine has also been described (Cruz et al. 2010). Some studies have suggested that repeated use of alpha2 agonists could increase the risk of myocardial degeneration and fibrosis in rabbits, and this potential side effect should be considered, especially if repeated anesthesia is necessary (Hurley et al. 1994, Marini et al. 1999, Williams et al. 2017).

Telazol^R (Aveco Co. Inc., Fort Dodge, IA), tiletamine combined with zolazepam, has been shown to be nephrotoxic for rabbits at doses of 7.5 mg/kg and its use is contraindicated (Brammer et al. 1991; Doerning et al. 1992). It is possible that the reported toxic effects of Telazol are breed-specific and there are those who advocate its use. This being the case, the authors recommend judicious use of this anesthetic agent should it be chosen. While propofol is useful as an induction agent in combination with other drugs, it is not effective as a sole agent in maintaining anesthesia in rabbits.

Perioperative Considerations

While anesthetized, rabbits should have ophthalmic ointment placed in the eyes to prevent exposure to keratitis. The maintenance of normothermia from induction through recovery is especially important and can be accomplished using circulating water blankets such as the Gaymar-T (Gaymar, Orchard Park, NY) or hot air blankets such as the Bair Hugger (Arizant Healthcare, Eden Prairie, MN) (Sikoski et al. 2007). The temperature of the operating room also affects an animal's body temperature, but consideration must be given to the people who work in the room as well (Edis et al. 2021). An intravenous catheter should be placed for administration of parenteral fluids. Fluids should be given at a rate of 10–20 mL/kg/h via a 60 drop/mL intravenous fluid administration set. If it is desirable to gain arterial access for blood gas analysis or blood pressure monitoring, a 22-gauge catheter can be placed in the central auricular artery and secured with a heparin lock for blood gases or connected to a transducer for continuous arterial pressure monitoring.

Anesthesia Monitoring

Fundamental anesthesia monitoring includes an assessment of reflexes, heart rate, respiratory rate, mucous membrane color, and capillary refill time. Blood pressure can be a useful addition as it combined with heart rate are the most reliable measures of anesthetic depth, with changes of 20% or more from baseline usually requiring action to ensure an adequate plane of anesthesia. Traditional reflexes used in the monitoring of rabbit anesthesia include righting, palpebral, corneal, pedal withdrawal, jaw tone, and pinna reflex. The pinna reflex is the most accurate measure of depth of anesthesia followed by pedal withdrawal (especially of the hind leg) and jaw tone. Corneal and palpebral reflexes are not reliable indicators of adequate anesthesia. Rabbits can retain corneal and even palpebral reflexes sometimes when in a surgical plane of anesthesia. When reflex assessment is used as the sole determinant of anesthetic depth, more than one reflex should be monitored to ensure adequate anesthesia.

Blood pressure can also be a useful indicator of overall cardiovascular status. The systolic/diastolic arterial pressure of an anesthetized rabbit is approximately 95/75 (Huerkamp 1995). As a general guideline, arterial pressures should not be permitted to decrease below 80/60. The monitoring of heart rate and rhythm can be performed with an esophageal stethoscope or by electrocardiography. Indirect blood pressure monitoring can be attempted with cuffs placed on a forelimb, but accurate readings can be difficult to obtain given rabbit anatomy. Direct blood pressure is more accurate but requires catheterization of the central auricular artery and specialized equipment so can be more time-consuming and complicated to perform. Capnography, blood gas analysis, and pulse oximetry are useful in evaluating the adequacy of ventilation. Pulse oximetry probes can be placed on the cheek, base of tail, tongue, or rectal probes used. Ventilation-perfusion efficiency can also be assessed through observation of mucous membrane color and capillary refill time.

Post-anesthetic Care

Rabbits should be recovered with their head in an extended position and frequently monitored to ensure that their head remains in that position, as a hyperflexed head can impede respiration. The rabbit should also be turned during recovery, approximately every 15–30 min, to avoid pulmonary congestion. Following completion of surgery under inhalation anesthesia, recovery is rapid, and rabbits typically are conscious and regain the righting reflex within 20–30 min. The most likely causes of delayed or complicated recovery from general anesthesia are hypothermia and anesthetic overdosage followed by sequela related to lengthy procedures such as hypoglycemia, or dehydration. Yohimbine or atipamezole can be given to reverse the effects of alpha2 agonists and speed recovery. Anesthetic agents impair central and peripheral thermoregulatory mechanisms and rabbits are prone to radiative and conductive heat losses because of their high body surface area to body weight ratio. Because the pharmacokinetics of anesthetic metabolism are partially temperature dependent, maintaining body temperature is critical to recovery from anesthesia. Ideally, recovering animals should be kept in an escape-proof incubator on a clean, dry towel or blanket. The use of an incubator permits careful control of the ambient temperature. Recovery should not take place on metal flooring or in suspended wire cages because heat loss will be accelerated. Where an incubator is not available, supplemental heating can be provided with a water-circulated heating pad or a forced air warming device as used during surgery. It is important to remember that rabbits tend to gnaw and, if left unattended, they may mutilate heating pads or wiring. The ambient temperature in the recovery area should be 84–90°F (29–32°C). The temperature of the animal and the recovery area should be monitored regularly throughout recovery to ensure that thermal burns or hyperthermia do not occur. Supplemental oxygen should be provided if the anesthetist has any concern that oxygen levels were not adequate during surgery or at risk of declining during recovery. Extubation should take place only when chewing begins or coughing is elicited. If warranted, respiratory depression can be treated with 2–5 mg/kg doxapram subcutaneous or intravenous every 15 min.

After animals have regained consciousness from anesthesia, the technician should shift attention to providing palatable food sources, reducing stress, and monitoring for pain and wound healing in the post-surgical patient. As rabbits are prone to hypoglycemia because of high metabolic rates and, in juvenile animals, limited fat reserves, a nutritious diet should be provided as soon after surgery as feasible. Hay should be immediately available for the rabbit in addition to their normal pelleted diet and spraying the hay and cage walls with water can encourage food and water consumption. Inappetant animals can be offered additional supplements or treats as described in the "Nutrition" section, or herbivore liquid dietary products. Prolonged anorexia and ileus should be treated as described in other sections of this chapter. Rabbits may self-mutilate areas that are painful or irritating and if self-mutilation is a concern, a 12-inch Elizabethan collar can be used in conjunction with administration of analgesics. Be aware that rabbits typically tolerate these collars very poorly and long-term maintenance will prevent cecotrophy which could lead to B vitamin and other nutritional deficiencies. The animal should continue to be assessed and managed for pain as described below, along with wound healing, daily or more frequently as warranted.

Pain Assessment and Management

Rabbits experiencing pain will often exhibit changes in appetite, activity, and behavior (Kohn et al. 2007; Weaver et al. 2010). Following acute recovery from anesthesia, the technician should perform a frequent assessment of these parameters to effectively detect and manage pain. Appetite can be determined by measuring both food and water intake along with fecal and urine output. Fecal quantity and quality are an excellent indicator of the status of gut motility, which can be affected by food intake, stress, and pain. Painful rabbits might also show reduced activity, such as a reluctance to move, slow postural movements, and less rearing up on their back legs, although they might hide some signs of pain in the presence of human observers (Weaver et al. 2010; Pinho et al. 2020; Leach et al. 2009). Bruxism behavior, the slow, rhythmic tooth grinding, can be a sign of pain. Bruxism should not be confused with the quick, infrequent tooth purring that rabbits can normally do. An extensive list of other behaviors and how surgical pain might affect them is available, and some are more subtle and will require more experience to note (Pinho et al. 2020; Leach et al. 2009).

Painful rabbits often have changes to their facial expressions including wincing or partially closed eyelids, flattened cheeks and whiskers, a pointed nose, and flattened ears (Keating et al. 2012; Leach et al. 2009). Several objective pain scoring systems have been developed that consider these changes to a rabbit's appearance (Figure 17.27). One of the most popular, the grimace scale, has variations that have been used in many species to assess pain (Mota-Rojas et al. 2020). Specific to rabbits, the grimace scale accounts for ear position and facial expressions (Keating et al. 2012; Hampshire & Robertson 2015, Raillard et al. 2019). However, some have criticized the grimace scale as too limited in application and have developed pain scoring systems that consider additional factors to the grimace characteristics, such as heart rate, respiratory characteristics, pupil dilation, response to manipulation of a potentially painful area, alertness, vocalizations, behavior, activity, and appetite (Banchi et al. 2020; Benato et al. 2021). Although a formal scoring system can be useful, it is most important that a technician is familiar with normal rabbit characteristics so they can recognize when a rabbit has pain that needs to be addressed.

Managing pain requires a multi-pronged approach leading to a comprehensive analgesia plan that also reduces external sources of stress. Generally, analgesics should be first administered before the start of the surgical procedure. Analgesia is most effectively achieved by using multiple analgesic agents in combination, although single-agent analgesia could be appropriate for procedures not expected to cause significant pain. Either an opioid or NSAID alone might not be adequate to completely relieve the pain associated with major surgeries (Leach et al. 2009; Weaver et al. 2010). For major surgeries, a pre-operative combination of an NSAID, opioid, and local analgesia can be used to reduce the development of pain from multiple sources. Multi-modal anesthesia will also allow for using lower doses of each drug and therefore reduce the side effects of any individual drug (Goldschlager et al. 2013). Local analgesics (e.g., lidocaine, bupivacaine) can be administered using similar principles as in other species, and commonly used in rabbits via topical creams or local infusion into the surgical site. Epidural injections might be more challenging in rabbits than in larger species and

limited descriptions of effective nerve blocks in rabbits are available (Ong et al. 2020; Kluge et al. 2017; Keating et al. 2012; Goldschlager et al. 2013; Garcia et al. 2020, Raillard et al. 2019).

NSAIDs inhibit the activity of the enzymes cyclooxygenase (COX) 1 and 2 and are sufficiently potent to treat musculoskeletal, incisional, and acute, mild visceral pain. More specific inhibitors of COX-2 activity such as meloxicam are preferred to reduce the effects of blocking COX-1 activity such as gastric ulceration and impaired clotting. Meloxicam is frequently chosen because both injectable and oral formulations exist, with the oral formulation available in an easy-to-dose liquid form (Benato et al. 2020). Rabbits metabolize oral meloxicam quickly and therefore higher doses might be needed than in other species, but it is unknown how much these higher doses might accumulate or how much that might vary between individuals (Turner et al. 2006; Fredholm et al. 2013; Delk et al. 2014). The authors recommend an initial dose of 1 mg/kg followed by 0.5–1 mg/kg daily. This dosing appears to be safe at least for the duration needed for surgical pain (Eshar & Weese 2014; Delk et al. 2014). If preferred, other NSAIDs such as carprofen and ketoprofen can be used (Hedenqvist et al. 2015).

Opioid agents act by binding to specific receptors in distinct parts of the nervous system. Those most used in rabbits are buprenorphine, butorphanol, and fentanyl; but morphine, meperidine, and oxymorphone will also be effective. Respiratory depression is a common concern with opioids in rabbits, especially with mu agonists, making partial mu agonists such as buprenorphine and agonist-antagonists like butorphanol popular choices for pre-operative analgesics. Injectable opioids are typically used prior to the start of surgery. Buprenorphine can be used safely pre-operatively even when given with injectable anesthetics but will still exert a mild respiratory depressive effect that is greater than butorphanol (Shafford & Schadt 2008; Schroeder & Smith 2011, Murphy et al. 2010). Fentanyl is also available as a dermal patch, which is advantageous as it abrogates the need to handle the patient for drug administration and provides consistent drug delivery. A 25 µg/h fentanyl patch can be used on the outer ear surface or back of the rabbit. The location and skin preparation can affect absorption rates and the inner ear should be avoided (Foley et al. 2001; Mirschberger et al. 2020). A 12 µg/h patch might be more appropriate for small rabbits (less than 4–5 kg). An adhesive dressing placed over the patch can help keep it in place. Because 24 h is required for dermal fentanyl to reach therapeutic levels, an additional agent such as an NSAID and/or alternate opioid during that time should be provided if pain is expected. Buprenorphine is also a popular choice for post-operative

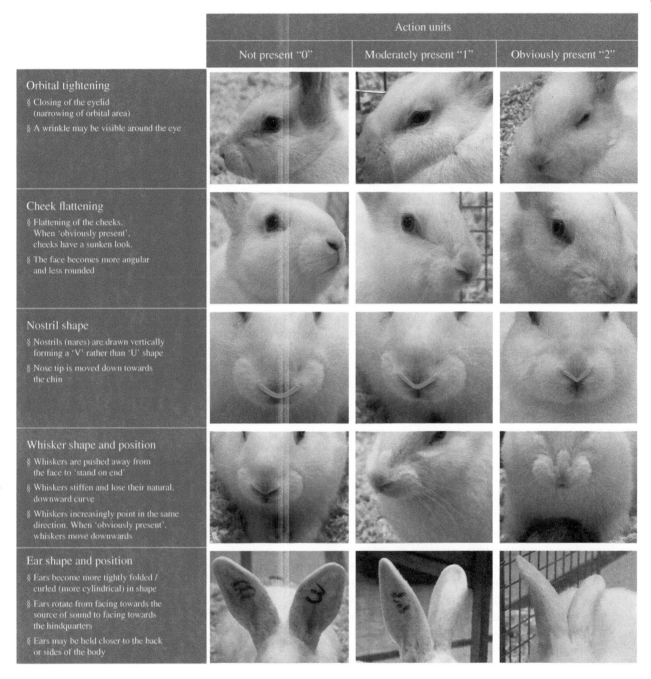

Figure 17.27 Rabbit Grimace Scale. Additional information is available from the NC3rs/National Centre for the 3Rs in the UK. (Courtesy of National Centre for the Replacement, Refinement, & Reduction of Animals in Research.)

pain relief and can be given by injection every 6–12 h to rabbits (0.01–0.05 mg/kg IM, SC) (Benato et al. 2020). A sustained-release formulation of buprenorphine is also available for rabbits and can provide approximately 3 days of analgesia with one dose but can take 15 h to reach adequate levels (Andrews et al. 2020; DiVincenti et al. 2016). Opioids decrease gastrointestinal motility and attempts to reduce this impact with motility-modifying drugs have been unsuccessful (Deflers et al. 2022; Feldman et al. 2021; Martin-Flores et al. 2017). Although studies of the clinical significance of buprenorphine in ileus show varying results, the lower end of the dose range (0.02 mg/kg) might be necessary to minimize gastrointestinal stasis and respiratory depression (Deflers et al. 2018; Schnelbacher et al. 2017; Cooper et al. 2009). Tramadol is a convenient oral opioid that has been used in other species, but to the author's knowledge, no effective dose of oral tramadol has been identified in rabbits (Souza et al. 2008).

Common Surgical Procedures

Preparation of a rabbit for surgery is not particularly novel to the species and will consist of steps identical to those used for other species. The fur at the surgical site will be clipped and the skin should be decontaminated with alcohol and disinfectant scrubs such as povidone iodine or chlorhexidine. Rabbits have thick hair coats, fine fur, and thin skin, which make hair removal laborious and put a premium on clipper maintenance. It is ideal to have spare blades available. Rabbit skin easily lacerates when clipping if performed carelessly or with dull clipper blades. Concentration should be kept on the skin being taut in front of the clipper blade and the head of the blade flat against the skin. The best skin preparation comes from using a combination of no. 10 and no. 40 blades to prepare the skin. Gentle handling of the skin perioperatively is helpful in reducing the incidence of postoperative auto-mutilation of incisions, for which rabbits are notorious.

The surgical procedures most performed in rabbits include OHE, castration, drainage of abscesses, cutaneous mass excision, and exploratory laparotomy. Enucleation, perineal dermatoplasty in cases of unresolving urine scald, cystotomy, large bowel, and renal surgical procedures have also been described in rabbits (Mullen 2000; Guzman et al. 2021). Castration and OHE are often performed for the same reasons that these procedures are carried out in dogs and cats. Castration should be recommended to clients as a measure for bucks housed indoors to prevent urine spraying and mounting, to reduce aggression toward other rabbits and owners, and to eliminate the risk of testicular cancer. OHE is recommended with group housing situations and to prevent uterine diseases such as uterine adenocarcinoma. Both procedures are performed with the patient in dorsal recumbency. The surgical approaches for these two procedures are like those used for dogs and cats, with castration commonly performed by the scrotal approach, prescrotal approach, or by abdominal midline incisions for crytorchidism (Guzman et al. 2021, Swindle & Shealy 1996). The OHE requires a standard, midline abdominal approach, and surgical site preparation should reflect this. It is important to express the urinary bladder during preparation for an OHE to avoid complications during surgery. Oophorectomy is an option if only sterilization is desired, and an endoscopic approach has been described (Divers 2010).

A variety of other surgical procedures can be safely performed in rabbits, and the preparation of the surgical site will vary by location and surgeon preference. Cystotomy is indicated for urolithiasis. Although the bladder wall is thin, which may be discouraging to some surgeons, it holds suture well (Mullen 2000) and can be closed in a single layer (Swindle & Shealy 1996). Most rabbits with urolithiasis are overweight and probably over-consuming calcium (Mullen 2000), therefore the postoperative instructions given to the owner should include instructions regarding nutrition. An exploratory laparotomy is required in cases of gastrointestinal obstruction from foreign bodies or space-occupying lesions. Enucleation may be necessary for ocular trauma, severe buphthalmia, or retrobulbar abscess. The retrobulbar venous sinus is extensive and the risk of severe and difficult-to-control hemorrhage exists (Mullen 2000). It is important to have considerable sterile methylcellulose on hand to pack the ocular defect. Likewise, bulla osteotomy for drainage of middle ear infections, such as for pasteurellosis, is fraught with risks of postoperative pain and drainage complications (Swindle & Shealy 1996) and is a procedure probably best referred to a specialty surgical practice.

Absorbable polymer suture materials, such as monofilament polyglyconate, are preferred by many for internal use, owing to their minimally reactive nature. Because they are not exposed and are less likely to be chewed, subcuticular sutures are preferred for skin closure. Generally, sutures in sizes appropriate for cats (3/0, 4/0, and 5/0) are suitable for rabbits. Cyanoacrylate tissue adhesives also provide satisfactory closure providing they are used in clean, dry incisions. Regardless of which material is used for skin closure, it is important to keep in mind the proclivity of rabbits for chewing at their wound closure materials which necessitates close monitoring during the wound healing period.

Clinical Techniques

Analgesia for Clinical Procedures

The technician should consider pain management for noxious procedures to make the procedure easier to perform and reduce stress for the animal. Analgesia options are discussed above in the "Pain Assessment and Management" section. Specifically, topical anesthetic creams, such as EMLA or lidocaine cream, might be useful for techniques such as catheter placement. These topical anesthetics might reduce the restraint that is required, but the technician must account for the substantial time for these to have an effect and ensure the animal does not ingest the cream (Flecknell et al. 1990). For example, if applying EMLA cream to the ear, a layer of the cream should be applied and covered with an occlusive dressing while waiting for the 20 min needed for the drug to take effect (Keating et al. 2012).

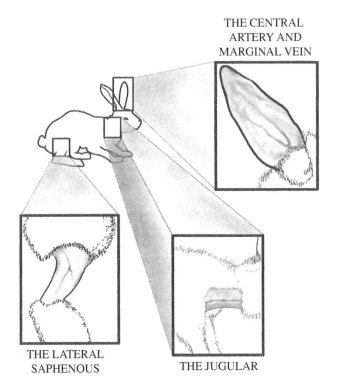

THE CENTRAL
ARTERY AND
MARGINAL VEIN

THE LATERAL
SAPHENOUS

THE JUGULAR

Figure 17.28 Venipuncture sites. (Drawing courtesy of Scott Stark.)

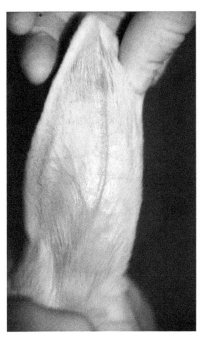

Figure 17.29 Marginal lateral ear vein on the left and the prominent central auricular artery. (Courtesy of Ryan Cheek.)

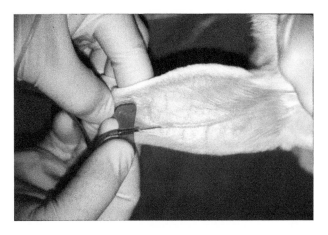

Figure 17.30 Blood sampling using the central auricular artery with a butterfly catheter. (Courtesy of Ryan Cheek.)

Blood Collection

Blood is most often obtained from the ear arteries or veins, jugular or saphenous vein, and may also be collected from the cephalic vein (Figure 17.28). Blood collection from the ear vessels carries a risk of hematoma or bruising that may be unacceptable to an owner. There is also a small risk of thrombosis and subsequent sloughing of the skin, which is more likely in breeds with small ears or if using the artery (Brandao et al. 2021; Harcourt-Brown 2002). The preferred location depends on the techniques developed by the phlebotomist. Rabbit blood can clot quickly, so heparinizing the syringe and needle may be helpful.

The auricular artery is central while the veins are found along the margins of the ear (Figures 17.29 and 17.30). The hair may be shaved and the application of a warm towel will help dilate the vessel. The size of the needle depends on the size of the vessel, and generally a 22- to 27-gauge needle is used. The needle is inserted into the vessel and if the vessel is large enough may be aspirated with a syringe. For small breeds, suction from a syringe may collapse the vessel and so blood can be collected as it drips from the needle hub. Upon removal of the needle, it is necessary to apply pressure for 3–5 min if using the artery and monitor thereafter for 10–15 min.

The lateral saphenous vein is easily accessible in an appropriately restrained rabbit. The restrainer should hold the animal wrapped in a towel in their lap and hold off the back leg just below the stifle. The vein is seen where it crosses from medial to lateral, usually around the middle third of the lateral tibia. Sometimes the vessel can be seen with just alcohol but shaving the hair will assist with visualization. A butterfly catheter attached to a syringe is often the easiest way to obtain blood (Figure 17.31).

The jugular vein can be used in some cooperative awake patients, but this technique may require sedation. If the animal is sedated, place the animal in dorsal recumbency and shave the neck area. A fully awake animal can be restrained in the same way as a cat for jugular venipuncture, wrapped

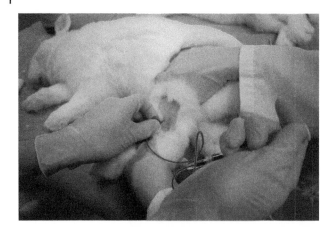

Figure 17.31 Approach for blood collection from saphenous vein.

in a towel and held at the edge of the table using one hand to hold the head up while the other restrains the front legs. Venipuncture of the cephalic vein is difficult, particularly in small breeds.

Placing a Catheter

The marginal ear veins and cephalic vein are the easiest and most frequently used to place an intravenous catheter. As with venipuncture, catheterization of the ear vessels carries a small risk of necrosis, so the cephalic vein is often used (Brandao et al. 2021; Harcourt-Brown 2002). The lateral saphenous vein can also be used for venous access, and the central ear artery can be used if arterial access is needed for direct blood pressure measurement or periodic blood gas analysis in surgery. For any catheter, an Elizabethan collar may be used to prevent the animal from removing it but should be avoided in cooperative animals. Elizabethan collars can be stressful and prevent the animal from engaging in cecotrophy, so they are not ideal for long-term use.

The principles of preparation are the same as for other species and the patient will be more cooperative with sedative drugs. A 24-gauge catheter is appropriate for most rabbits, but a 22-gauge may be used in large vessels of some large rabbits. Occlude the vessel by compressing proximal to the location of the catheter. After puncture of the vessel wall, the catheter should be advanced over the stylet and into the vessel lumen. The thin walls of the vessel make it easy to visualize the threading of the catheter into the lumen of the vein to the hub. Owing to the small volume of blood in the vein and the low venous blood pressure, it is unlikely to obtain a backflow of blood into the catheter flange or hub. If in doubt, a small quantity of saline can be injected via the catheter for observation of the vessel blanching with infused fluid. A roll of four or five gauzes 4×4 sponges should be placed in the concave pinna and

the catheter secured using tape in a butterfly application followed by a circumferential wrap of tape over the roll of gauze in the ear. The IV line should also be secured with a circumferential wrap of tape. (See Figure 17.32A–C.)

Urinalysis

Urine may be collected from a clean cage pan, by catheterization, cystocentesis, or from anesthetized rabbits by expression. As the bladder wall is thin and susceptible to trauma or puncture, cystocentesis, manual expression, or catheterization should be performed with care. For cystocentesis, use a small needle appropriate for the patient (23- to 25-gauge).

Parasitology

The tools used in the diagnosis of parasitism in rabbits are often available in the small animal practice. With the ability to perform fecal flotation examination, fur examination, skin scraping, and an examination of the ear canals, nearly any diagnosis can be made effectively. With skin scrapings, bear in mind that the skin of rabbits is comparatively thin and may lacerate easily. An otoscope should be used to assess for *Psoroptes cuniculi*. The diagnosis can be confirmed by gently swabbing exudate from the canal with a cotton-tipped applicator and mineral oil for examination under a microscope. For rabbits housed outdoors, one important consideration is that flies are attracted to rabbit droppings and owners may confuse the recently hatched fly larvae with parasites. PCR tests are available from multiple commercial laboratories for the most common internal and external parasites.

Administration of Medications

Intravenous Injection

The marginal ear veins are the easiest to access for intravenous injection, but the cephalic and saphenous veins can also be used. The technique is the same as described for venipuncture. Typically, volumes of up to 5 mL/kg can be given as a slow bolus by this route (Pekow 2012). One needs to be careful not to inject into the central auricular artery, which may be fatal (O'Malley 2005).

Subcutaneous Injection

The methodology for a subcutaneous injection is the same as that for other species, with the interscapular region preferred. A 21- to 25-gauge needle should be inserted under the lifted loose skin over the scapulae and parallel with the

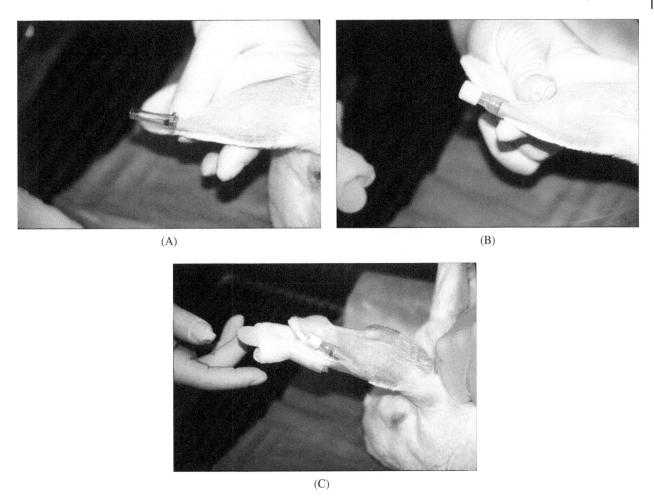

Figure 17.32 (A) Initial insertion of the catheter in the vein; note the "flash." (B) The catheter seated into the vein and cap has been applied. (C) A tongue depressor was added for additional support.

underlying muscle. Volumes of 10–20 mL/kg can be given by this route (Harcourt-Brown 2002).

Intraperitoneal Injection

This route is rarely used in rabbits but should be considered in neonates or moribund, hypothermic animals where vasoconstriction may be pronounced and there is a need to rapidly attempt fluid therapy or administer medications. For intraperitoneal injection, the rabbit ideally should be held on its back with the head slightly lower than the hindquarters to allow the stomach and intestines to fall cranially. However, if dorsal recumbency is at all resisted, the animal can be positioned on its side or in ventral recumbency. A second individual should insert a 21- to 25-gauge needle at a 45° angle through the skin and abdominal wall slightly to the right and just caudal to the umbilicus. Aspirate before injecting to reduce the chance of injecting into an organ. For fluid therapy or injection of a volume of material of more than a few milliliters and

to prevent accidental laceration of the internal organs, a catheter can be inserted and the stylet immediately removed after puncture of the abdominal wall. Volumes of up to 100 mL of warmed fluids can be given to a 5-kg rabbit by the intraperitoneal route (Pekow 2012).

Intramuscular Injection

Restraint technique for injection is comparable to that for examination. A solo restrainer should hold the animal with the flank against their side or abdomen and the head tucked into the elbow of the dominant arm, with the dominant arm wrapped around the exposed flank of the animal and the hand curled around and restraining the hindquarters. The free hand is then used for the injection. Fractious rabbits may need two people for injection or to be wrapped in a towel. Lumbar muscles (cranial to the pelvis) or the cranial aspects of the rear leg (quadriceps) are the sites of choice to avoid damage to the sciatic nerve (Brandao et al. 2021). Aspiration should be performed to confirm that blood is not obtained before injecting. Any volume >0.5 mL/kg should be divided and given in two sites.

Intraosseous Infusion

Intraosseous infusion is indicated in situations where intravenous access is not possible, or difficult, and a delay in therapy may affect survival. The common locations for catheterization are the humerus, tibial crest, and femur. A 20- to 22-gauge spinal needle that is about half the length of the bone is appropriate for most situations. If a spinal needle is not available, use an appropriately sized hypodermic needle. If the hypodermic needle plugs, a thinner, sterile Kirschner wire can be used as a plunger to push the bone cortex from the needle lumen (Anderson 1995). The procedure can be undertaken in kits as small as 200 g, although potential risk of injury to active growth plates must be considered in juvenile animals (Bielski et al. 1993; Harcourt-Brown 2002). Preparation of the area should follow strict aseptic technique because of the risk of osteomyelitis, and if it is necessary in an emergency in a conscious animal, a local anesthetic such as lidocaine can be used. The proximal humerus may be the easiest location for placement, where the needle is inserted through the greater tubercle (Harcourt-Brown 2002). For the tibial crest, the needle should be inserted at the medial aspect of the proximal tibia of the flexed stifle at an angle of about 30° (Anderson 1995; Bielski et al. 1993; Otto & Crowe 1992). Because of the curved cortex of the tibia, it may be difficult to keep the needle in the medullary cavity and instead go into the cortex. The femur can be difficult because of the well-developed trochanteric fossa, and the catheter often needs to pass through three layers of cortical bone. Although placement of the catheter may be more difficult in the rear leg, some rabbits may be less inclined to disturb a catheter that is not by the face (Jenkins 2004). For any location, the needle should be advanced in a distal direction away from the physis until there is a dramatic reduction of resistance indicating penetration of the marrow cavity, and one aspirates slightly to obtain marrow to confirm that the needle is in the desired location. Once in the marrow cavity at the desired depth, the needle should be sutured to the skin and protected, and further immobilized with a sterile wrap and bulky bandage. Any drug, agent, or fluid that can be safely given intravenously can be given by the intraosseous route. The maximal rate of infusion is about 10 mL/min by this route (Anderson 1995).

Medication per os

Rabbits may accept oral medications when mixed with small amounts of preferred food items, such as bananas.

Alternatively, a medication can be given in suspension using a syringe. The rabbit might ingest suspensions or liquid medications from the syringe if palatable, and rabbits usually like sweet formulations such as juice, applesauce, or fruit baby foods. For rabbits who will need to be on long-term medication, the technician should consider teaching a client to acclimate a rabbit to taking medications from a syringe by starting with only palatable solutions. Importantly, any high-carbohydrate fruits or treats used to administer medications must be limited to avoid dysbiosis.

Uncooperative patients can be restrained as previously described and manually given the drug. Solution volumes should be limited to less than about 5 mL of liquid. In some cases, it may be tempting to give drugs via the drinking water; however, dosing is imprecise. Depending on their level of consumption, the palatability of the liquid, and stability of the drug, animals may be over or underdosed. Rabbits can be difficult to pill but may accept palatable medications when placed through the diastema as far back in the mouth as possible. A pill "gun," as used in cats, may be useful for this procedure.

Teeth Trimming

Conventional dog nail trimmers should not be used for trimming the incisors because of the risk of complications, including longitudinal fissures, periodontal abscesses, and damage to the germinal tissue (Gorrel 1996; Malley 1996). Nail trimmers can also leave sharp edges that may lacerate the tongue, cheek, or lips. Ideally, the teeth should be reduced using high-speed dental equipment with a water-cooling system (Capello & Gracis 2005). Alternatively, a Dremel® tool (Dremel, Racine, WI) is frequently used, but these have a lower speed and increased torque that increases the chance of thermal damage to tissues without careful use. These procedures generally require sedation. There is specialized equipment available that significantly aids rodent and rabbit dentistry (Capello & Gracis 2005), but readily available items can also be useful, such as a tongue depressor or the barrel of a syringe through the diastema to serve as a gag to open the mouth slightly and as a backstop when trimming the incisors. Extraction is also an option for severely affected teeth but is much more difficult for cheek teeth than incisors. Rabbits can do very well with all their incisors extracted, by using their lips for prehension. In cases of malocclusion, teeth trimming may need to be repeated every 6–8 weeks for the lifetime of the animal (Swindle & Shealy 1996).

Nail Trimming

Nails can be trimmed with any conventional nail trimmer used for dogs or cats. The quick is typically easy to visualize and overly aggressive trimming causing bleeding should be managed as for dogs and cats. Owners can be taught to trim the nails of their pets as nails may grow long with rapidity in sedentary animals. Declawing should not be done in rabbits unless medically necessary for a particular digit. Unlike cats, rabbits use the last phalanx for weight bearing and traction, and removal can lead to abnormal weight distribution and foot injuries. Excessive scratching should be handled through behavior management and frequent nail trims.

Assist Feeding

Nutritional support is important for rabbits that are anorexic because they are predisposed to hepatic lipidosis. Critical care diets specifically for herbivores are available (Critical Care, Oxbow Animal Health, Murdock, NE), but ground-up pellets can be used as well if necessary. Many rabbits can be syringe fed by restraining the animal with a towel and gently placing a catheter tip syringe in the diastema as previously described. Syringe feeding is highly preferred over tube feeding to reduce stress and provide more fibrous foods, but tube feeding can be done if rabbits do not accept the syringe. Animals will typically need to be sedated for tube feeding to reduce the risk of the rabbit chewing tube and to allow easy passage of the tube through the well-developed esophageal sphincter. Select a tube that should be larger than the trachea and premeasure to the last rib on the left side and mark the tube. Once the tube is passed, proper placement can be confirmed by aspirating stomach contents or injecting 5–10 mL of air through the tube while auscultating the stomach for the tell-tale sounds of bubbling fluid or turbulent airflow. This procedure could be attempted in a conscious animal with appropriate restraint, using an oral speculum so that the tube is not bitten and being certain that the tube has passed into the stomach and not curled back into the esophagus because of resistance from the sphincter.

If a permanent tube is needed, nasogastric tubes can be placed using techniques like those used in cats (Rosen 2011). The disadvantage of nasogastric tubes is that solutions designed for nutritional support of rabbits will clog such a narrow tube. Although it is common to use human nutrition products such as Ensure for rabbits, these are not ideal for herbivores. There are solutions available for herbivorous reptiles that will pass through these tubes, although no solution will be able to provide appropriate insoluble fiber because it would clog the tube (Paul-Murphy 2007). Surgical placement of pharyngostomy and gastrostomy tubes has also been described (Smith et al. 1997; Rogers et al. 1988).

Although of arguable value given the bactericidal gastric pH, assisted feeding may be attempted for transfaunation in cases of cecal dysbiosis. This procedure is accomplished by outfitting a healthy donor rabbit with an Elizabethan collar overnight to prevent cecotrophy. The collected cecotrophs should be mixed and suspended in warmed (37°C), non-bacteriostatic saline, and strained through gauze prior to administration with a stomach tube. A volume of 40–60 mL of this suspension can be safely given to a 4- to 5-kg rabbit using a 12 Fr, 16-inch Sovereign Feeding Tube (Kendall Co., Mansfield, MA).

Sex Determination

Determining the sex in rabbits is like cats. The vulva in does is located directly below the anus (Figure 17.16). The ensheathed penis of the buck is located directly below the anus, adjacent to an obvious scrotum with palpable testes (Figure 17.17). However, due to open inguinal canals the testes may migrate back and forth from the scrotum to the abdomen. The penis has a more circular appearance than the pointed shape of the vulva and the anogenital distance is greater in males than females. Mature females have a pronounced dewlap, although obese males can have a skin fold in the same area that could cause confusion. Females have pronounced nipples while they are rudimentary in males.

Emergency and Critical Care

Emergency care is intended to stabilize the rabbit and afford the opportunity to pursue the diagnosis of the primary problem. Common presentations requiring critical care include gastrointestinal disorders, trauma, environmental exposure (hypothermia, hyperthermia), intoxications, respiratory distress, neurologic symptoms, and urinary obstruction. The tenets of care include fluid therapy, body temperature maintenance, oxygen administration, and control of hemorrhage. If in shock, rabbits rarely present in a compensatory stage as may be seen in dogs and birds, and instead usually have signs of decompensation such as hypothermia, bradycardia, hypotension, pale mucous membranes, and prolonged capillary refill time (Lichtenberger 2007). Rabbits are obligate nasal breathers, so a rabbit that is open-mouth breathing is in severe respiratory distress. Acute respiratory distress can occur with bacterial infections of nasal passages, bacterial pneumonia, trauma, or cardiac disease (Paul-Murphy 2007).

If cardiopulmonary resuscitation is required, immediate action is directed at the "ABCs" of emergency care: airway, breathing, and circulation. An airway should be established via intubation or a tracheostomy tube and the animal placed on oxygen. If an airway cannot be established, high-flow oxygen with tight-fitting mask can be used at a rate of 20–30 breaths per minute while monitoring the animal for signs of bloat (Lichtenberger 2007; Buckley et al. 2011). Chest compressions at a rate of at least 80 per minute and medications are used to address circulatory issues but bear in mind that atropine is not the preferred anticholinergic if one is indicated. More advanced care and monitoring include intravenous fluids, ECG, blood gas analysis, end-tidal CO_2 measurements, and temperature. The use of corticosteroids in shock therapy is not recommended for rabbits (Lichtenberger 2007). The treatment may also need to include addressing metabolic disturbances that may be the cause or consequence of the shock.

Hypothermia is possible in sucklings, those rabbits housed outdoors in winter, and those recovering from anesthesia, especially if fluids at room temperature were administered. Slowly restoring normothermia and circulation with warm, isotonic fluids in conjunction with an external heat source such as warm water bottles, water-circulated heating pads, or a Bair Hugger is the primary objective. A rapid rise in body temperature without control may increase brain metabolic demands above that which can be provided and expose the heart, liver, and lungs to cold, acidotic blood from the periphery. Overzealous body warming also could result in hyperthermia. Failure to restore fluids in any hypothermic animal can result in acute tubular necrosis. Hypoxemia should be considered as a possible complication in downer and hypothermic animals, and animals may require oxygen delivered via a face mask.

Hypoglycemia may be seen in neonatal or small breed animals either on an inadequate nutritional plane or recovering from surgery. High metabolic energy demands and small fat reserves coupled with postoperative anorexia make these animals particularly at risk. It could be a companion to hypothermia. In a pinch, however, response to glucose therapy can be used as a diagnostic tool. Acute hypoglycemia should be treated by intravenous or oral bolus of 50% dextrose (e.g., 2 mL/kg). Parenteral administration of glucose is preferred because excessive administration of oral carbohydrates may lead to cecal dysbiosis. For those animals that are both hypoglycemic and hypothermic, intravenous glucose will provide fuel to the brain during rewarming.

Hyperthermia is present when rectal temperatures exceed 104°F (40°C). Rabbits are prone to hyperthermia if housed outdoors because they cannot sweat or effectively pant. It may also be caused Iatrogenically by overzealous rewarming during anesthetic recovery or can be associated with certain toxicoses. The treatment is to cool the rabbit slowly. Hyperthermia can be treated with room temperature intravenous fluids and tepid water, especially on the ears. Animals need to be monitored for kidney failure and other metabolic abnormalities.

Rabbits may present with a variety of gastrointestinal emergencies, such as ileus, diarrhea, gastric dilation, and obstruction. Ileus and diarrhea can both lead to life-threatening enterotoxemia and dehydration. Ileus is more common than diarrhea, and is a frequent problem given the intricate, complex, and delicate interrelationship between diet, other environmental factors, the commensal, fermentative microflora, and gut motility in rabbits of all ages. Diarrhea can also occur due to these factors or be associated with other conditions, such as infection or antibiotic administration. Fluids and nutritional support are the most important aspects of treatment. Even if there is no appreciable fluid loss observed, colonic hypomotility leads to decreased water absorption and dehydration (O'Malley 2005). Cecotrophs contain high levels of vitamins B and K, so supplementation of especially B vitamins should be considered for animals that are unable or unwilling to eat their night feces. Additional treatment may include analgesics, pro-motility agents, antibiotics, anthelmintics, anti-ulcer medications or other agents as indicated. Specific treatment options are discussed in "Disease of the Digestive System" section. For diarrhea, transfaunation may be considered. It should be noted that yogurt and many commercial probiotics have not been shown to be effective in floral reconstitution for rabbits (Myers 2007). Gastric dilation is rare, but must be excluded in an anorexic rabbit, because the animal may need to be decompressed and prokinetic agents may be contraindicated. Gastric dilation can occur secondary to small intestinal obstruction because of the inability to vomit, leading to fluid and gas accumulation in the stomach. This must be differentiated from gut stasis based on radiographs. Initial treatment includes passage of a stomach tube to decompress and fluid therapy, with subsequent decisions regarding whether surgery is necessary (Harcourt-Brown 2007).

Trauma scenarios include fractured limbs, traumatic vertebral luxation or fractures, and fight-related lacerations. Limb fractures should be stabilized by splinting, if possible, but often this is difficult, and surgery may be indicated. Radiography should be performed to characterize the fracture. Rabbits presenting acutely for vertebral injury should be radiographed, kept in a clean, padded cage to retard the development of decubital ulcers, and provided fluid and dietary therapy as needed. While vertebral injuries typically have a poor prognosis for recovery, a positive outcome can result from surgery and intensive management (McCullough et al. 2012). Additional details are described in the section on skeletal diseases. Trauma to the scrotum or testes may require castration.

The principles of treatment for toxin exposure are like that for cats and dogs, with some notable exceptions. Emetics such as apomorphine are ineffective. It may be necessary to apply an Elizabethan collar for 72 h to keep the patient from eating cecotrophs that may still contain the toxic substance. Therapy should include fluid administration, gastric lavage, bathing, and activated charcoal as indicated depending on the substance and route of intoxication. Toxicoses have been associated with a variety of chemicals, pesticides/rodenticides, antibiotics, tiletamines, and various household plants (Johnston 2008). Although rabbits are resistant to many plant toxins, they are sensitive to aflatoxins that may be present in the feed (Harcourt-Brown 2002). Lead toxicosis can result from rabbits chewing baseboards in older homes with lead-based paint; anorexia or neurologic signs are presenting signs. Fipronil (Frontline®) or high doses of permethrins or pyrethrins can be toxic, especially in small rabbits.

The most likely causes of hemorrhage are trauma and internal hemorrhage or hematuria in intact does with uterine adenocarcinoma. Hemorrhage should be controlled with direct pressure or surgical intervention if needed. Fluids should be administered as previously described for significant blood loss. Transfusion can be considered for rabbits based on principles that apply to other small animals. Although blood groups have not been studied in rabbits, a crossmatch is recommended (Lichtenberger 2004). Rest, oxygen therapy, iron supplementation, and nutritional support may also be important in the treatment of anemia.

Euthanasia

Methods should conform to those listed as acceptable in the *AVMA Guidelines for the Euthanasia of Animals: 2020 Edition* (American Veterinary Medical Association 2020). In a practice setting, the preferred method is by injection of a barbiturate (50–100 mg/kg) into the lateral marginal ear vein. This can be facilitated by first sedating or anesthetizing the rabbit as described in the section "Anesthesia." If an ear vein is not accessible, the euthanasia solution can be administered via the intraperitoneal or cardiac route, with the latter performed only when the animal is in a surgical plane of anesthesia.

References

Abdel-Gaber, R., Ataya, F., Fouad, D. et al. (2019). Prevalence, morphological and molecular phylogenetic analyses of the rabbit pinworm *Passalurus ambiguous Rudolphi* 1819, in the domestic rabbits *Oryctolagus cuniculus*. *Acta Parasitol* 64 (2): 316–330.

Almeria, S., Murata, F.H., Cerqueira, C.K. et al. (2021). Epidemiological and public health significance of *Toxoplasma gondii* infection in wild rabbits and hares: 2010–2020. *Microorganisms* 9 (3): 597.

Allweiler, S., Leach, M.C., and Flecknell, P.A. (2010). The use of propofol and sevoflurane for surgical anaesthesia in New Zealand White rabbits. *Lab Anim* 44: 113–117.

American Veterinary Medical Association (2020). *AVMA Guidelines for the Euthanasia of Animals: 2020 Edition*.

Anderson, N.L. (1995). Intraosseous fluid delivery in small exotic animals. In: *Kirk's Current Veterinary Therapy XII: Small Animal Practice*, 1331–1335. Philadelphia: W. B. Saunders Co.

Andrews, D.D., Fajt, V.R., Baker, K.C. et al. (2020). A comparison of buprenorphine, sustained-release buprenorphine, and high-concentration buprenorphine in male New Zealand white rabbits. *JAALAS* 546–556.

Artiles, C.A., Sanchez-Migallon Guzman, D., Beaufrere, H., and Phillips, K. (2020). Computed tomographic findings of dental disease in domestic rabbits (*Oryctolagus conuculus*):

100 casees (2009–2017). *J Am Vet Med Assoc* 257 (3): 313–327.

Banchi, P., Quaranta, G., Ricci, A., and Mauthe von Degerfeld, M. (2020). Reliability and construct validity of a composite pain scale for rabbit (CANCRS) in a clinical environment. *PLoS One* 15 (4): e0221377.

Barthold, S.W., Griffey, S.M., and Percy, D.H. (2016). *Pathology of Laboratory Rodents and Rabbits*. Oxford: Blackwell Publishing.

Bauer, C. (2013). Baylisascariosis—infections of animals and humans with 'unusual' roundworms. *Vet Parasitol* 193 (4): 404–412.

Bayne, K. (2003). Environmental enrichment of nonhuman primates, dogs and rabbits used in toxicologic studies. *Toxicol Pathol* 31 (Suppl): 132–137.

Benato, L., Murrell, J.C., Blackwell, E.J. et al. (2020). Analgesia in pet rabbits: a survey study on how pain is assessed and ameliorated by veterinary surgeons. *Vet Rec* 186 (18): 603.

Benato, L., Murrell, J., Knowles, T.G., and Rooney, N.J. (2021). Development of the Bristol Rabbit Pain Scale (BRPS): a multidimensional composite pain scale specific to rabbits (*Oryctolagus cuniculus*). *PLoS One* 16 (6): e0252417.

Bielski, R.J., Bassett, G.S., Fideler, B. et al. (1993). Intraosseous infusions: effects on the immature physis – an experimental model in rabbits. *J Ped Orthop* 13 (4): 511–515.

Birke, L.L., Molina, P.E., Baker, D.G. et al. (2009). Comparison of Selamectin and Imidacloprid plus Permethrin in Eliminating *Leporacarus gibbus* Infestation in Laboratory Rabbits (*Oryctolagus cuniculus*). *JAALAS* 48 (6): 757–762.

Blair, J. (2013). Bumblefoot. *Vet Clin Exot Anim* 16: 715–735.

Bowman, D.D., Fogelson, M.L., and Carbone, L.G. (1992). Effect of ivermectin on the control of ear mites (*Psoroptes cuniculi*) in naturally infested rabbits. *Am J Vet Res* 53: 105–109.

Bradbury, A.G. and Dickens, J.E. (2016). Appropriate handling of pet rabbits: a literature review. *J Small Anim Pract* 57: 503–509.

Bradley, M.P., Doerning, C.M., Nowland, M.H., and Lester, P.A. (2019). Intramuscular administration of alfaxalone and in combination for sedation and anesthesia of rabbits. *JAALAS* 58 (2): 216–222.

Bradley, M.P., Doerning, C.M., Nowland, M.H. et al. (2022). Evaluation of alfazalone total intravenous anesthesia in rabbits premedicated with dexmedetomidine or dexmedetomidine and buprenorphine. *Vet Anesth Analg* 49 (3): 308–312.

Brammer, D.W., Doerning, B.J., Chrisp, C.E. et al. (1991). Anesthetic and nephrotoxic effects of Telazol in New Zealand white rabbits. *Lab Anim Sci* 41 (5): 432–435.

Brandao, J., Graham, J., and Quesenberry, K.E. (2021). Basic approach to veterinary care. In: *Ferrets, Rabbits and Rodents: Clinical Medicine and Surgery*, 4the (ed. K.E. Quesenberry, C.J. Orcutt, C. Mans, and J.W. Carpenter), 150–161. St. Louis: Elsevier.

Brock, K., Gallaugher, L., Bergdall, V.K., and Dysko, R.C. (2012). Mycoses and non-infectious diseases. In: *The Laboratory Rabbit, Guinea Pig, Hamster and Other Rodents* (ed. M.A. Suckow, K.A. Stevens, and R.P. Wilson), 504–529. Boston: Academic Press/Elsevier.

Buckley, G.J., DeCubellis, J., Sharp, C.R., and Rozanski, E.A. (2011). Cardiopulmonary resuscitation in hospitalized rabbits: 15 cases. *J Exot Pet Med* 20 (1): 46–50.

Bulliot, C., Mentre, V., Marignac, G. et al. (2013). A case of atypical psoroptic mange in a domestic rabbit. *J Exot Pet Med* 22: 400–404.

Calvete, C., Delacour, S., Oropeza-Velsquez, R.V. et al. (2022). Experimental study of the mechanical transmission of rabbit hemorrhagic disease virus (RHDV2/b) by *Aedes albopictus* (Diptera: Culicidae) and *Phlebotomus papatasi* (Diptera: Psychodidae). *J Med Entomol* 59 (1): 350–354.

Cam, Y., Atasever, A., Eraslan, G. et al. (2008). *Eimeria stiedae*: experimental infection in rabbits and the effect of treatment with toltrazuril and ivermectin. *Exp Parasitol* 119 (1): 164–172.

Capello, V. and Gracis, M. (2005). *Rabbit and Rodent Dentistry Handbook, edited by AM Lennox*. Lake Worth: Zoologic Education Network Inc.

Capello, V. and Lennox, A.M. (2008). *Clinical Radiology of Exotic Companion Mammals*. Ames: Wiley-Blackwell.

Capello, V. (2016). Diagnostic imaging of dental disease in pet rabbits and rodents. *Vet Clin North Am Exotic Anim Pract* 19 (3): 757–782.

Carpenter, J.W., Mashima, T.Y., and Rupiper, D.J. (2001). *Exotic Animal Formulary*, 2de, 301–326. Philadelphia: W.B. Saunders Company.

Chae, J.J., Prausnitz, M.R., and Ethier, C.R. (2021). Effects of general anesthesia on intraocular pressure in rabbits. *JAALAS* 60 (1): 91–95.

Chang, C., Uchiyama, A., Ma, L. et al. (2009). A comparison of the effects on respiratory carbon dioxide response, arterial blood pressure, and heart rate of dexmedetomidine, propofol, and midazolam in sevoflurane-anesthetized rabbits. *Anes Analg* 109 (1): 84–89.

Cheeke, P.R. and Cunha, T.J. (1987). *Rabbit Feeding and Nutrition*. Orlando: Academic Press.

Clauss, M. (2012). Clinical technique: feeding hay to rabbits and rodents. *J Exot Pet Med* 21: 80–86.

Cooper, C.S., Metcalf-Pate, K.A., Barat, C.L. et al. (2009). Comparison of side effects between buprenorphine and meloxicam used postoperatively in Dutch belted rabbits (*Oryctolagus cuniculus*). *J Am Assoc Lab Anim Sci* 48 (3): 279–285.

Costa, R.S., Ciotti-McClallen, M., Tilley, R. et al. (2022). Intramuscular alfaxalone with or without buprenorphine or hydromorphone provides sedation with minimal adverse effects in healthy rabbits in a randomized blinded controlled trial. *JAVMA* 15: 1–6.

Crowell-Davis, S.L. (2007). Behavior problems in pet rabbits. *J Exot Pet Med* 16 (1): 38–44.

Cruz, F.S.F., Carragaro, A.B., Raiser, A.G. et al. (2010). Total intravenous anesthesia with propofol and S(+)-ketamine in rabbits. *Vet Anaesth Analg* 37 (2): 116–122.

Curtis, S.K. and Brooks, D.L. (1990). Eradication of ear mites from naturally infested conventional research rabbits using ivermectin. *Lab Anim Sci* 40: 406–408.

d'Ovidio, D. and Santoro, D. (2014). *Leporacarus gibbus* infestation in client-owned rabbits and their owner. *Vet Dermatol* 25: 46–47.

Davies, R.R. and Davies, J.A. (2003). Rabbit gastrointestinal physiology. *Vet Clin North Am Exotic Anim Pract* 6 (1): 139–153.

Deeb, B.J., DiGiacomo, R.F., Evermann, J.F., and Thouless, M.E. (1993). Prevalence of coronavirus antibodies in rabbits. *Lab Anim Sci* 43: 431–433.

Deeb, B.J. and Digiacomo, R.F. (1994). Cerebral larval migrans caused by *Baylisascaris* species in pet rabbits. *JAVMA* 205: 1744–1747.

Deflers, H., Gandar, F., Bolen, G. et al. (2018). Influence of a single dose of buprenorphine on rabbit (*Oryctolagus cuniculus*) gastrointestinal motility. *Vet Anes Analg* 45 (4): 510–519.

Deflers, H., Gandar, F., Bolen, G. et al. (2022). Effects of a single opioid dose on gastrointestinal motility in rabbits (*Oryctolagus cuniculus*): comparisons among morphine, butorphanol, and tramadol. *Vet Sci* 9 (28): 1–11.

Delk, K.W., Carpenter, J.W., KuKanich, B. et al. (2014). Pharmacokinetics of meloxicam administered orally to rabbits (*Oryctolagus cuniculus*) for 29 days. *Am J Vet Res* 75 (2): 195–199.

Delong, D. (2012). Bacterial diseases. In: *The Laboratory Rabbit, Guinea Pig, Hamster and Other Rodents* (ed. M.A. Suckow, K.A. Stevens, and R.P. Wilson), 303–364. Boston: Academic Press/Elsevier.

Desprez, I., Pelchat, J., Beufrere, H. et al. (2022). Agreement of caudal aortic arterial blood pressure with oscillometry using two cuff widths placed on the thoracic or pelvic limbs of sevoflurane anesthetized rabbits. *Vet Anaes Analg* (Mar 17; online ahead of print).

DeValle, J.M.S. (2009). Successful management of rabbit anesthesia through the use of nasotracheal intubation. *JAALAS* 48 (2): 166–170.

Difilippo, S.M., Norberg, P.J., Suson, U.D. et al. (2004). A comparison of xylazine and medetomidine in an anesthetic combination in New Zealand white rabbits. *Contemp Top Lab Anim Sci* 43: 32–34.

DiVincenti, L., Meirelles, L.A.D., and Westcott, R.A. (2016). Safety and clinical effectiveness of a compounded sustained-release formulation of buprenorphine for postoperative analgesia in New Zealand white rabbits. *JAVMA* 248 (7): 795–801.

Divers, S. (2010). Clinical technique : endoscopic oophorectomy in the rabbit (*Oryctolagus cuniculus*): the future of preventative sterilizations. *J Exot Pet Med* 19 (3): 231–239.

Doerning, B.J., Brammer, B.W., Chrisp, C.E. et al. (1992). Nephrotoxicity of tiletamine in New Zealand white rabbits. *Lab Anim Sci* 42 (3): 267–269.

Düwel, D. and Brech, K. (1981). Control of oxyuriasis in rabbits by fenbendazole. *Lab Anim* 15: 101–105.

Edis, A., Pelligand, L., Baldrey, V., and Hedley, J. (2021). Effect of theatre temperature on body temperature during anaesthesia for routine neutering of domestic rabbits (*Oryctolagus cuniculus*). *Vet Anes Analg* Dec 2 (online ahead of print).

Edwards, A.W., Korner, P.I., and Thornburn, G.D. (1959). The cardiac output of the unanesthetized rabbit, and the effects of preliminary anesthesia, environmental temperature, and carotid occlusion. *Q J Exp Physiol* 44: 309–321.

Eidson, M., Matthews, S.D., Willsey, A.L. et al. (2005). Rabies virus infection in a pet guinea pig and seven pet rabbits. *JAVMA* 227 (6): 932–935.

Engbers, S., Larkin, A., Rousset, N. et al. (2017). Comparison of a supraglottic airway device (v-gel) with blind orotracheal intubation. *Fron Vet Sci* 4 (49).

Eshar, D. and Weese, J.S. (2014). Molecular analysis of the microbiota in hard feces from healthy rabbits (*Oryctolagus cuniculus*) medicated with long term oral meloxicam. *BMC Vet Res* 10 (62): 1–9.

Fanelli, A., Ghirardi, M., Meneguz, P.G., and Tizzani, P. (2020). First report of *Obeliscoides cuniculi* in the European rabbit (*Oryctolagus cuniculus*). *Acta Parasitol* 65 (3): 787–789.

Feldman, E.R., Singh, B., Mishkin, E.R. et al. (2021). Effects of cisapride, buprenorphine, and their combination on gastrointestinal transit in New Zealand white rabbits. *JAALAS* 60 (2): 221–228.

Fichi, G., Flamini, G., Giovanelli, F. et al. (2007). Efficacy of an essential oil of *Eugenia caryophyllata* against *Psoroptes cuniculi*. *Exp Parasitol* 115 (2): 168–172.

Fisher, P.G. (2010). Standards of care in the 21st century:the rabbit. *J Exot Pet Med* 19 (1): 22–35.

Fisher, P.G., Kunzel, F., and Rylander, H. (2021). Neurologic and musculoskeletal diseases. In: *Ferrets, Rabbits and Rodents: Clinical Medicine and Surgery*, 4the (ed. K.E. Quesenberry, C.J. Orcutt, C. Mans, and J.W. Carpenter), 233–249. St. Louis: Elsevier.

Flecknell, P.A., Liles, J.H., and Williamson, H.A. (1990). The use of lignocaine-prilocaine local anesthetic cream for pain-free venipuncture in laboratory animals. *Lab Anim* 24: 142–146.

Flecknell, P.A., Roughan, J.V., and Hedenqvist, P. (1999). Induction of anesthesia with sevoflurane and isoflurane in the rabbit. *Lab Anim* 33: 41–46.

Flecknell, P.A. (2015). *Laboratory Animal Anesthesia*, 4the. New York, NY: Elsevier.

Flecknell, P.A. and Thomas, A.A. (2015). Comparative anesthesia and analgesia of laboratory animals. In: *Veterinary Anesthesia and Analgesia, 5th Edition of Lumb and Jones* (ed. K.A. Grimm, L.A. Lamont, W.J. Tranquilli, et al.), 754–763. Ames, IA: Wiley Blackwell.

Foley, P.L., Henderson, A.L., Bissonette, E.A. et al. (2001). Evaluation of fentanyl transdermal patches in rabbits: blood concentrations and physiologic response. *Comp Med* 51: 239–244.

Fredholm, D.V., Carpenter, J.W., KuKanich, B., and Kohles, M. (2013). Pharmacokinetics of meloxicam in rabbits after oral administration of single and multiple doses. *Am J Vet Res* 74 (4): 636–641.

Fritz, M., de Riols de Fonclare, D., Garcia, D. et al. (2022). First evidence of natural SARS-CoV-2 infection in domestic rabbits. 9: 49–52.

Garcia, C.M., Doss, G., Travis, M.L. et al. (2020). Efficacy of greater auricular and auriculotemporal nerve blocks performed in rabbits. *Vet Anes Analg* 47 (4): 567–573.

Garibaldi, B.A., Fox, J.G., Otto, G. et al. (1987). Hematuria in rabbits. *Lab Anim Sci* 37: 769–772.

Gentry, P.A. (1982). The effect of administration of a single dose of T-2 toxin on blood coagulation in the rabbit. *Can J Comp Med* 46: 414–419.

Gilroy, B.A. (1981). Endotracheal intubation of rabbits and rodents. *JAVMA* 179: 1295.

Girolamo, N.D. and Selleri, P. (2021). Disorders of the urinary and reproductive systems. In: *Ferrets, Rabbits and Rodents: Clinical Medicine and Surgery*, 4the (ed. K.E. Quesenberry, C.J. Orcutt, C. Mans, and J.W. Carpenter), 201–219. St. Louis: Elsevier.

Goldschlager, G.B., Gillespie, V.L., Palme, R. et al. (2013). Effects of multimodal analgesia with low-dose buprenorphine and meloxicam on fecal glucocorticoid metabolites after surgery in New Zealand white rabbits (*Oryctolagus cuniculus*). *J Am Assoc Lab Anim Sci* 52 (5): 571–576.

Gorrel, C. (1996). Teeth trimming in rabbits and rodents. *Vet Rec* 139 (21): 528.

Graham, J.E., Garner, M.M., and Reavill, D.R. (2014). Benzimidazole toxicosis in rabbits 13 cases (2003–2011). *J Exot Pet Med* 23: 188–195.

Griffiths, M. and Davies, D. (1963). The role of soft pellets in the production of lactic acid in the rabbit stomach. *J Nutr* 80: 171–180.

Grint, N.J., Sayers, I.R., Cecchi, R. et al. (2006). Postanaesthetic tracheal strictures in three rabbits. *Lab Anim* 40 (3): 301–308.

Guzman, D.S.M., Szabo, Z., and Steffey, M.A. (2021). Soft tissue surgery: rabbits. In: *Ferrets, Rabbits and Rodents: clinical medicine and surgery*, 4the (ed. K.E. Quesenberry, C.J. Orcutt, C. Mans, and J.W. Carpenter), 432–445. St. Louis: Elsevier.

Hampshire, V.H. and Robertson, S. (2015). Using the facial grimace scale to evaluate rabbit wellness in post-procedural monitoring. *Lab Anim* 44 (7): 259–260.

Harcourt-Brown, F. (2002). *Textbook of Rabbit Medicine*. Oxford: Alden Press.

Harcourt-Brown, F.M. and Holloway, H.K. (2003). *Encephalitozoon cuniculi* in pet rabbits. *Vet Rec* 152 (14): 427–431.

Harcourt-Brown, F.M. (2004). *Encephalitozoon cuniculi* infection in rabbits. *J Exot Pet Med* 13 (2): 86–93.

Harcourt-Brown, T.R. (2007). Management of acute gastric dilation in rabbits. *J Exot Pet Med* 16: 168–174.

Harkness, J.E. and Wagner, J.E. (2010). *Biology and Medicine of Rabbits and Rodents*, 5the, 272. Ames: Wiley-Blackwell.

Hawkins, M.G. (2014). Advances in exotic mammal clinical therapeutics. *J Exot Pet Med* 23: 39–49.

Hawkins, M.G. and Pascoe, P.J. (2021). Anesthesia, analgesia, and sedation of small mammals. In: *Ferrets, Rabbits and Rodents: Clinical Medicine and Surgery*, 4the (ed. K.E. Quesenberry, C.J. Orcutt, C. Mans, and J.W. Carpenter), 536–558. St. Louis: Elsevier.

Hedenqvist, P., Roughan, J.V., Antunes, L. et al. (2001). Induction of anaesthesia with desflurane and isoflurane in the rabbit. *Lab Anim* 35: 172–179.

Hedenqvist, P., Jensen-Waern, M., Fahlman, A. et al. (2015). Intravenous sufentanil-midazolam versus sevoflurane anesthesia in medetomidine pre-medicated Himalayan rabbits undergoing ovariohysterectomy. *Vet Anaes Anal* 42: 377–385.

Hedley, J. (2014). Respiratory disease. In: *BSAVA Manual of Rabbit Medicine* (ed. A. Meredith and B. Lord), 160–167. Gloucester: British Small Animal Veterinary Association.

Hewitt, C.D. et al. (1989). Normal biochemical and hematological values in New Zealand White rabbits. *Clin Chem* 35: 1777–1779.

Holve, D.L., Gum, G.G., and Pritt, S.L. (2013). Effect of sedation with xylazine and ketamine on intraocular pressure in New Zealand white rabbits. *JAALAS* 52: 488–490.

Hoppman, E. and Barron, H.W. (2007). Ferret and rabbit dermatology. *J Exot Pet Med* 16 (4): 225–237.

Horiuchi, N., Watarai, M., Kobayashi, Y. et al. (2008). Proliferative enteropathy involving *Lawsonia intracellularis* infection in rabbits (*Oryctolagus cuniculus*). *J Vet Med Sci* 70 (4): 389–392.

Hu, B., Fan, Z., Wei, H. et al. (2018). Detection of mucoid enteropathy syndrome disease in rabbit farms in East China. *Res Vet Sci* 119: 259–261.

Huerkamp, M.J. (1995). Anesthesia and postoperative management of rabbits and pocket pets. In: *Kirk's Current Veterinary Therapy XII: Small Animal Practice*, 1322–1327. Philadelphia: W. B. Saunders Co.

Hurley, R.J., Marini, R.P., Avison, D.L. et al. (1994). Evaluation of detomidine anesthetic combinations in the rabbit. *Lab Anim Sci* 44 (5): 472–478.

Huynh, M., Poumeyrol, S., Pignon, C. et al. (2015). Intramuscular administration of alfaxalone for sedation in rabbits. 176 (10): 255.

Ishikawa, Y., Sakata, H., Tachibana, Y. et al. (2019). Sedative and physiological effects of low dose intramuscular alfazalone in rabbits. *J Vet Med Sci* 81 (6): 851–856.

Jenkins, J.R. (2004). Gastrointestinal diseases. In: *Ferrets, Rabbits and Rodents: Clinical Medicine and Surgery*, 2de (ed. K.E. Quesenberry and J.W. Carpenter), 161–171. St. Louis: W.B. Saunder Co.

Jenkins, J.R. (2000). Surgical sterilization in small mammals. Spay and neuter. *Vet Clin North Am Exot Anim Pract* 3 (3): 617–627.

Jensen, L.J. et al. (1983). Natural infection of *Obeliscoides cuniculi* in a domestic rabbit. *Lab Anim Sci* 30: 231–233.

Johnson, C.A., Pallozzi, W.A., Geiger, L. et al. (2003). The effect of an environmental enrichment device on individually caged rabbits in a safety assessment facility. *Contemp Top Lab Anim Sci* 42 (5): 27–30.

Johnston, M.S. (2008). Clinical toxicoses of the domestic rabbit. *Vet Clin Exot Anim* 11: 315–326.

Karp, B.E., Ball, N.E., Scott, C.R. et al. (1999). Rabies in two privately owned domestic rabbits. *JAVMA* 215 (12): 1824–1847.

Kazacos, K.R. and Kazacos, E.A. (1983). Fatal cerebrospinal disease caused by *Baylisascaris procynosis* in domestic rabbits. *JAVMA* 183: 967–971.

Kazakos, G.M., Anagnostou, T., Savvas, I. et al. (2007). Use of the laryngeal mask airway in rabbits: placement and efficacy. *Lab Anim (NY)* 36: 29–34.

Keating, S.C.J., Thomas, A.A., Flecknell, P.A., and Leach, M.C. (2012). Evaluation of EMLA cream for preventing pain during tattooing of rabbits: changes in physiological, behavioural and facial expression responses. *PLoS One* 7 (9): e44437.

Keeble, E. (2014). Nervous system and musculoskeletal disorders. In: *Manual of Rabbit Medicine* (ed. A. Meredith and B. Lord), 225. British Small Animal Veterinary Association.

Kluge, K., Menzies, M.P.L., Kloeppel, H. et al. (2017). Femoral and sciatic nerve blockades and incision site infiltration in rabbits undergoing stifle joint arthrotomy. *Lab Anim* 51 (1): 54–64.

Kohn, D.F., Martin, T.E., Foley, P.L. et al. (2007). Public statement: guidelines for the assessment and management of pain in rodents and rabbits. *J Am Assoc Lab Anim Sci* 46: 97–108.

Korn, A.K., Brandt, H.R., and Erhardt, G. (2016). Genetic and environmental factors influencing tooth and jaw malformation in rabbits. *Vet Rec* 1748 (14): 341.

Kovalik, M., Thoday, K.L., Eatwell, K. et al. (2012). Successful treatment of idiopathic sebaceous adenitis in a lionhead rabbit. *J Exot Pet Med* 21: 336–342.

Knutson, K.A., Petritz, O.A., Thomson, A.E., and Balko, J.A. (2022). Intramuscular alfaxalone butorphanol midazolam compared with ketamine butorphanol midazolam in New Zealand white rabbits. 61 (5): 475–481.

Kunzel, F., Gruber, A., Tichy, A. et al. (2008). Clinical symptoms and diagnosis of encephalitozoonosis in pet rabbits. *Vet Parasitol* 151 (2–4): 115–124.

Kurtdede, A., Karaer, Z., Acar, A. et al. (2007). Use of selamectin for the treatment of psoroptic and sarcoptic mite infestation in rabbits. *Vet Dermatol* 18 (1): 18–22.

Leach, M.C., Allweiler, S., Richardson, C. et al. (2009). Behavioural effects of ovariohysterectomy and oral administration of meloxicam in laboratory housed rabbit. *Res Vet Sci* 87 (2): 336–347.

Leary, S.L., Manning, P.J., and Anderson, L.C. (1984). Experimental and naturally-occurring gastric foreign bodies in laboratory rabbits. *Lab Anim Sci* 34: 58–61.

Leck, G. (1988). Removing a calculus from the urinary bladder of A rabbit. *Vet Rec* 83: 64–65.

Lenox, A.M., Capello, V., and Legendre, L.F. (2021). Small mammal dentistry. In: *Ferrets, Rabbits and Rodents: Clinical Medicine and Surgery*, 4the (ed. K.E. Quesenberry, C.J. Orcutt, C. Mans, and J.W. Carpenter), 514–535. St. Louis: Elsevier.

Langan, G.P., Lohmiller, J.J., Swing, S.P., and Wardrip, C.L. (2000). Respiratory diseases of rodents and rabbits. *Vet Clin North Am Small Anim Pract* 30 (6): 1309–1335. vii.

Lee, M.J. and Clement, J.G. (1990). Effects of soman poisoning on hematology and coagulation parameters and serum biochemistry in rabbits. *Mil Med* 155: 244–249.

Leland, M.M., Hubbard, G.B., and Dubey, J.P. (1992). Clinical toxoplasmosis in domestic rabbits. *Lab Anim Sci* 42: 318–319.

Lichtenberger, M. (2004). Transfusion medicine in exotic pets. *Clin Tech Small Anim Pract* 19: 88–95.

Lichtenberger, M. (2007). Shock and cardiopulmonary-cerebral resuscitation in small mammals and birds. *Vet Clin Exot Anim* 10: 275–291.

Lim, J.J., Kim, D.H., Lee, J.J. et al. (2012). Prevalence of *Lawsonia intracellularis*, *Salmonella* spp. and *Eimeria* in healthy and diahhheic rabbits. *J Vet Med Sci* 74 (2): 263–265.

Lipman, N.S., Marini, R.P., and Flecknell, P.A. (2008). Anesthesia and analgesia in rabbits. In: *Anesthesia and Analgesia in Laboratory Animals*, 2nde (ed. R.E. Fish, M.J. Brown, P.J. Danneman, and A.Z. Karas), 299–334. Boston: Academic Press (Elsevier).

Livio, M. et al. (1988). Role of platelet-activating factor in primary hemostasis. *Am J Physiol* 254: 218–223.

Lopez-Martinez, R., Mier, T., and Quirarte, M. (1984). Dermatophytes isolated from laboratory animals. *Mycopathologica* 88: 111–113.

Ma, N., Wang, T., Bie, L. et al. (2018). Comparison of the effects of exercise with chondroitin sulfate on knee osteoarthritis in rabbits. *J Orthop Surg Res* 13 (1): 16.

Makidon, P. (2005). Esophagostomy tube placement in the anorectic rabbit. *Lab Anim (NY)* 34 (8): 33–36.

Malley, D. (1996). Teeth trimming in rabbits and rodents. *Vet Rec* 139 (24): 603.

Marin, P., Belda, E., Laredo, F.G. et al. (2020). Pharmacokinetics and sedative effects of alfazalone with or without dexmedetomidine in rabbits. *Res Vet Sci* 129: 6–12.

Marini, R.P., Li, X., Harpster, N.K., and Dangler, C. (1999). Cardiovascular pathology possibly associated with ketamine/xylazine anesthesia in Dutch belted rabbits. *Lab Anim Sci* 49 (2): 153–160.

Martin-Flores, M., Singh, B., Walsh, C. et al. (2017). Effects of buprenorphine, methylnaltrexone, and their combination on gastrointestinal transit in healthy new zealand white rabbits. *JAALAS* 56 (2): 155–159.

McCullough, A.W., Guzman, D.S.M., Keller, D. et al. (2012). Medical management of multiple traumatic vertebral subluxactions and fractures in a rabbit (oryctolagus cuniculus). *J Exot Pet Med* 21: 172–180.

McLaughlin, R.M. and Fish, R.E. (1994). Clinical chemistry and hematology. In: *The Biology of the Laboratory Rabbit*, 2de (ed. P.J. Manning, D.H. Ringler, and C.E. Newcomer), 111–127. Orlando: Academic Press.

McTier, T.L., Hair, J.A., Walstrom, D.J., and Thompson, L. (2003). Efficacy and safety of topical administration of selamectin for treatment of ear mite infestation in rabbits. *JAVMA* 223 (3): 322–324.

Mirschberger, V., Diemling, C., Heider, A. et al. (2020). Fentanyl plasma concentrations after application of a transdermal patch in three different locations to refine postoperative pain management in rabbits. *Animals* 10 (1778): 1–12.

Mota-Rojas, D., Olmos-Hernandez, A., Verduzco-Mendoza, A. et al. (2020). The utility of grimace scales for practical pain assessment in laboratory animals. *Animals* 10 (1838).

Mullen, H.S. (2000). Nonreproductive surgery in small mammals. *Vet Clin North Am Exot Anim Pract* 3 (3): 629–645.

Murphy, K.L., Roughan, J.V., Baxter, M.G., and Flecknell, P.A. (2010). Anaesthesia with a combination of ketamine andmedetomidine in the rabbit: effect of premedication with buprenorphine. *Vet Anaesth Analg* 37 (3): 222–229.

Myers, D. (2007). Probiotics. *J Exot Pet Med* 16: 195–197.

Mykkytyn, A.Z., Lamers, M.M., Okba, N.M.A. et al. (2021). Susceptibility of rabbits to SARS-CoV-2. *Emerg Microbes Infect* 10 (1): 1–7.

Narama, I. et al. (1982). Pulmonary nodule causes by *Dirofilaria immitis* in a laboratory rabbit. *J Parasitol* 68: 351–352.

Navarrete-Calvo, R., Gomez-Villamandos, R.J., Morgaz, J. et al. (2014). Cariorespiratory, anaesthetic and recovery effects of morphine combined wit medetomidine and alfaxalone in rabbits. *Vet Rec* 174 (4): 95.

Nordin, U., Lindholm, C.E., and Wolgast, M. (1977). Blood flow in the rabbit tracheal mucosa under normal conditions and under the influence of tracheal intubation. *Acta Anaesthesiol Scand* 21 (2): 81–94.

Nowland, M.H., Brammer, D.W., Garcia, A., and Rush, H.G. (2015). Biology and diseases of rabbits. In: *Laboratory Animal Medicine*, 3rde (ed. J.G. Fox, G.M. Otto, M.T. Whary, et al.), 411–461. New York: Academic Press/Elsevier.

Oglesbee, B.L. and Lord, B. (2020). Gastrointestinal diseases of rabbits. In: *Ferrets, Rabbits and Rodents*, 174–187. Philadelphia: Elsevier Saunders.

Orr, H.E., Roughan, J.V., and Flecknell, P.A. (2005). Assessment of ketamine and medetomidine anaesthesia in the domestic rabbit. *Vet Anaesth Analg* 32: 271–279.

Otto, C.M. and Crowe, D.T. (1992). Intraosseous resuscitation techniques and applications. In: *Kirk's Current Veterinary Therapy XI: Small Animal Practice*. Philadelphia: W.B. Saunders Company Co.

O'Malley, B. (2005). Rabbits. In: *Clinical Anatomy and Physiology of Exotic Species: Structure and Function of Mammals, Birds, Reptiles, and Amphibians*, 173–196. Philadelphia: Elsevier Saunders.

Ong, B.H.E., Hidaka, Y., Kaneko, Y. et al. (2020). Effects of a single-bolus bupivacaine injection into the coccygeal spinal canal of rabbits. *J Vet Med Sci* 82 (2): 197–203.

Ozawa, S.M., Hawkins, M.G., Drazenovich, T.L. et al. (2019). Pharmacokinetics of maropitant citrate in New Zealand white rabbits (*Oryctolagus cuniculus*). *Am J Vet Res* 80 (10): 9630968.

Ozawa, S., Thompson, A., and Petritz, O. (2022). Safety and efficacy of oral mirtazapine in New Zealand White rabbots (*Oryctolagus cunniculus*). *J Exot Pet Med* 40: 16–20.

Paul-Murphy, J. (2007). Critical care of the rabbit. *Vet Clin Exot Anim* 10: 437–461.

Pekow, C.A. (2012). Basic experimental methods in the rabbit. In: *The Laboratory Rabbit, Guinea Pig, Hamster and Other Rodents* (ed. M.A. Suckow, K.A. Stevens, and R.P. Wilson), 243–258. Boston: Academic Press/Elsevier.

Percy, D.H. and Barthold, S.W. (2007). Rabbit. In: *Pathology of Laboratory Rodents and Rabbits*, 3de (ed. D.H. Percy and S.W. Barthold), 253–308. Ames: Blackwell Publishing.

Pevelar, J.L. and Hickman, D.L. (2018). Effects of music enrichment on individually housed male New Zealand white rabbits. *J Am Assoc Lab Anim Sci* 57: 695–697.

Phaneuf, L.R., Barker, S., Groleau, M.A., and Turner, P.V. (2006). Tracheal injury after endotracheal intubation and anesthesia in rabbits. *J Am Assoc Lab Anim Sci* 45: 67–72.

Pinho, R.H., Leach, M.C., Minto, B.W. et al. (2020). Postoperative pain behaviours in rabbits following orthopaedic surgery and effect of observer presence. *PLoS One* 15 (10): e0240605.

Quimby, J.M. and Lunn, K.F. (2013). Mirtazapine as an appetite stimulant and anti-emetic in cats with chronic kidney disease: a masked placebo-controlled crossover clinical trial. *Vet J* 197: 651–655.

Quinn, R.H. (2012). Rabbit colony management and related health concerns. In: *The Laboratory Rabbit, Guinea Pig, Hamster and Other Rodents* (ed. M.A. Suckow, K.A. Stevens, and R.P. Wilson), 218–242. Boston: Academic Press/Elsevier.

Raillard, M., Detotto, C., Grepper, S. et al. (2019). Anaesthetic and perioperative management of 14 male New Zealand white rabbits for calvarial bone. *Surgery* 9 (896): 1–13.

Raje, S. and Stewart, K.L. (1997). Group housing for male New Zealand white rabbits. *Lab Anim* 26 (4): 36–38.

Reabel, S.N., Queiroz-Williams, P., Cremer, J. et al. (2022). Comparison of blind and endoscopic-guided orotracheal intubation on laryngeal and tracheal damage in domestic rabbits (*Oryctolagus cunuculus*). *Vet Anaesth Analg* 49 (4): 398–406.

Reabel, S.N., Queiroz-Williams, P., Cremer, J. et al. (2021). Assessment of intramuscular administration of three doses of alfazalone combined with hydromorphone and dexmedetomidine for endoscopic-guided orotracheal intubation in domestic rabbits. *JAVMA* 259 (10): 1148–1153.

Reuter, J.D., Fowles, K.J., Terwilliger, G.A., and Booth, C.J. (2005). Iatrogenic tension pneumothorax in a rabbit. *Contemp Top Lab Anim Sci* 44 (4): 22–25.

Rich, G. (2010). Clinical update on testing modalities for *Encephalitozoon cuniculi* in clinically sick rabbits. *J Exot Pet Med* 19 (3): 226–230.

Robertson, S.A. and Eberhart, S. (1994). Efficacy of intranasal route for administration of anesthetic agents to adult rabbits. *Lab Anim Sci* 44 (2): 159–165.

Rougier, S., Galland, D., Boucher, S. et al. (2006). Epidemiology and susceptibility of pathogenic bacteria responsible for upper respiratory tract infections in pet rabbits. *Vet Microbiol* 115 (1–3): 192–198.

Rogers, G., Taylor, C., Austin, J.C. et al. (1988). A pharyngostomy technique for chronic oral dosing of rabbits. *Lab Anim Sci* 38: 619–620.

Rosen, L.B. (2011). Nasogastric tube placement in rabbits. *J Exot Pet Med* 20 (1): 27–31.

Rosentthal, K.L. (2004). Therapeutic contraindications in exotic pets. *Sem Avian Exot Pet Med* 13 (1): 44–48.

Rousseau-Blass, F. and Pang, D.S. (2020). Hypoventilation following oxygen administration associated with alfaxalone dexmedetomidine midazolam anesthesia in New Zealand White rabbit. *Vet Anaesth Analg* 47 (5): 637–646.

Sanchez, S., Mizan, S., Quist, C. et al. (2004). Serological response to *Pasteurella multocida* NanH sialidase in persistently colonized rabbits. *Clin Diagn Lab Immunol* 11 (5): 825–834.

Santangelo, B., Micieli, F., Marino, F. et al. (2016). Plasma concentrations and sedative effects of a dexmedetomidine, midazolam, and butorphanol combination after transnasal administration in healthy rabbits. *J Vet Pharmacol Ther* 39 (4): 408–411.

Sayce, L.J., Powell, M.E., Kimball, E.E. et al. (2020). Continuous rate infusion of ketamine hydrochloride and dexmedetomidine for maintenance of anesthesia during laryngotracheal surgery in New Zealand white rabbits (*Oryctolagus cuniculus*). *JAALAS* 59 (2): 176–185.

Schadler, J., Schwarz, J., Peter-Egli, J. et al. (2021). Survey of Salmonellae occurrence in meat-producing rabbitries in Switzerland. *Vet Rec Open* 9: e24.

Scheller, M.S., Saidman, L.J., and Partridge, B.L. (1988). MAC of sevoflurane in humans and the New Zealand white rabbit. *Can J Anaesth* 35 (2): 153–156.

Schnelbacher, R.W., Divers, S.J., Comolli, J.R. et al. (2017). Effects of intravenous administration of lidocaine and buprenorphine on gastrointestinal tract motility and signs of pain in New Zealand White rabbits after ovariohysterectomy. *AJVR* 78 (12): 1359–1371.

Schroeder, C.A. and Smith, L.J. (2011). Respiratory rates and arterial blood-gas tensions in healthy rabbits given buprenorphine, butorphanol, midazolam or their combinations. *JAALAS* 50 (2): 205–211.

Shafford, H.L. and Schadt, J.C. (2008). Respiratory and cardiovascular effects of buprenorphine in conscious rabbits. *Vet Anaesth Analg* 35 (4): 326–332.

Sheinberg, G., Romero, C., Heredia, R. et al. (2017). Use of oral fluralaner for the treatment of Psoroptes cuniculi in 15 naturally infested rabbits. *Vet Dermatol* 28: 393–394.

Sikoski, P., Young, R.W., and Lockard, M. (2007). Comparison of heating devices for maintaining body temperature in anesthetized laboratory rabbits (*Oryctolagus cuniculus*). *J Am Assoc Lab Anim Sci* 46: 61–63.

Smith, D.A., Olson, P.O., and Mathews, K.A. (1997). Nutritional support for rabbits using the percutaneously placed gastrostomy tube: a preliminary study. *J Am Anim Hosp Assoc* 33: 48–54.

Smith, J.C., Robertson, L.D., Auhll, A. et al. (2004). Endotracheal tubes versus laryngeal mask airways in rabbit inhalation anesthesia: ease of use and waste gas emissions. *Contemp Top Lab Anim Sci* 43: 22–25.

Souza, M.J., Greenacre, C.B., and Cox, S.K. (2008). Pharmacokinetics of orally administered tramadol in domestic rabbits (*Oryctolagus cuniculus*). *AJVR* 69 (8): 979–982.

Squire, R., Brodsky, L., and Rossman, J. (1990). The role of infection in the pathogenesis of acquired tracheal stenosis. *Laryngoscope* 100 (7): 765–770.

Stein, S. and Walshaw, S. (1996). Rabbits. In: *Handbook of Rodent and Rabbit Medicine* (ed. K. Laber-Laird, M.M.

Swindle, and P. Flecknell), 183–217. Tarrytown: Elsevier Science Inc.

Suckow, M.A., Haab, R.W., Miloscio, L.J. et al. (2008). Field trial of a *Pasteurella multocida* extract vaccine in rabbits. *J Am Assoc Lab Anim Sci* 4: 18–21.

Suter, C., Muller-Doblies, U.U., Hatt, J.M., and Deplazes, P. (2001). Prevention and treatment of *Encephalitozoon cuniculi* infection in rabbits with fenbendazole. *Vet Rec* 148 (15): 478–480.

Swennes, A.G., Buckley, E.M., Parry, N.M. et al. (2012). Enzootic enteropathogenus *Escherichia coli* infection in laboratory rabbits. *J Clin Microbiol* 50 (7): 2353–2358.

Swindle, M.M. and Shealy, P.M. (1996). *Handbook of Rodent and Rabbit Medicine* (ed. K. Laber-Laird, M.M. Swindle, and P. Flecknell), 239–254. Tarrytown: Elsevier Science Inc.

Terada, Y., Ishiyama, T., Asano, N. et al. (2014). Optimal doses of sevoflurane and propofol in rabbits. *BMC Res Notes* 7: 820.

Tesluk, G.C., Peiffer, R.L., and Brown, D. (1982). A clinical and pathological study of inherited glaucoma in New Zealand white rabbits. *Lab Anim* 16: 234–239. 1982.

Tinkey, P.T., Uthamanthil, R.K., and Weisbroth, S.H. (2012). Rabbit neoplasia. In: *The Laboratory Rabbit, Guinea Pig, Hamster and Other Rodents* (ed. M.A. Suckow, K.A. Stevens, and R.P. Wilson), 504–529. Boston: Academic Press/Elsevier.

Tran, H.S., Puc, M.M., Tran, J.L. et al. (2001). A method of endoscopic endotracheal intubation in rabbits. *Lab Anim* 35: 249–252.

Turner, P.V., Chen, H.C., and Taylor, W.M. (2006). Pharmacokinetics of meloxicam in rabbits after single and repeat oral dosing. *Comp Med* 56 (1): 63–67.

Tutunaru, A.C., Sonea, A., Drion, P. et al. (2013). Anaesthetic induction with alfaxalone may produce hypoxemia in rabbits premedicated with fentaly/droperidol. *Vet Anaesth Analg* 40 (6): 657–659.

Varga, M. and Patterson, S. (2021). Dermatologic diseases of rabbits. In: *Ferrets, Rabbits and Rodents: clinical medicine and surgery*, 4the (ed. K.E. Quesenberry, C.J. Orcutt, C. Mans, and J.W. Carpenter), 220–231. St. Louis: Elsevier.

Vernau, K.M., Osofsky, A., and LeCouteur, R.A. (2007). The neurological examination and lesion localization in the companion rabbit (*Orytolagus cuniculus*). *Vet Clin Exot Anim* 10: 731–758.

Vogtsberger, L.M. et al. (1986). Spontaneous dermatophytosis due to *Microsporum canis* in rabbits. *Lab Anim Sci* 36: 294–297.

Wagner, R. and Wendlberger, U. (2000). Field efficacy of moxidectin in dogs and rabbits naturally infested with *Sarcoptes* spp., *Demodex* spp. and *Psoroptes* spp. mites. *Vet Parasitol* 93: 149–158.

Wales, A.D., Woodward, M.J., and Pearson, G.R. (2005). Attaching-effacing bacteria in animals. *J Comp Pathol* 132 (1): 1–26.

Weaver, L.A., Blaze, C.A., Linder, D.E. et al. (2010). A model for clinical evaluation of perioperative analgesia in rabbits (*Oryctolagus cuniculus*). *JAALAS* 49 (6): 845–851.

White, S., Bourdeau, P.J., and Meredith, A. (2002). Dermatologic problems of rabbits. *Sem Avian Exot Pet Med* 11 (3): 141–150.

Williams, M.D., Long, C.T., Durrant, J.R. et al. (2017). Oral transmucosal detomidine gel in new zealand white rabbits (*Oryctolagus cuniculus*). 56 (4): 436–442.

Wolford, S.T. et al. (1986). Reference range data base for serum chemistry and hematology values in laboratory animals. *J Toxicol Environ Health* 18: 161–188.

Wright, F. and Riner, J. (1984). Comparative efficacy of injection routes and doses of ivermectin against *Psoroptes* in rabbits. *Am J Vet Res* 46: 752–754.

Wyatt, J.D., Scott, R.W., and Richardson, M.E. (1989). The effects of prolonged ketamine-xylazine intravenous infusion on arterial blood pH, blood gases, mean arterial blood pressure, heart and respiratory rates, rectal temperature, and reflexes in the rabbit. *Lab Anim Sci* 39: 411–416.

Williams, A.M. and Wyatt, J.D. (2007). Comparison of subcutaneous and intramuscular ketamine-medetomidine with and without reversal by atipamezole in dutch belted rabbits (*Oryctolagus cuniculus*). *J Am Assoc Lab Anim Sci* 46: 16–20.

Xu, Z.J. and Chen, W.X. (1989). Viral hemorrhagic disease in rabbits: a review. *Vet Res Commun* 13: 205–212.

Yin, Y., Ya, M., and Zhu, T. (2012). Minimum alveolar concentration of sevoflurane in rabbits with liver fibrosis. *Anesth Analg* 114 (3): 561–565.

Yu, L. et al. (1979). Biochemical parameters of normal rabbit serum. *Clin Biochem* 12: 83–87.

Zhu, C., Feng, S., Thatw, T.E. et al. (2006). Towards a vaccine for attaching/effacing *Escherichia coli*: a LEE encoded regulator (ler) mutant of rabbit enteropathogenic *Escherichia coli* is attenuated, immunogenic, and protects rabbits from a lethal challenge with the wild-type virulent strain. *Vaccine* 24 (18): 3845–3855.

18

Mice, Rats, Gerbils, and Hamsters

April Romagnano

Introduction

This chapter focuses on the mouse (*Mus musculus*), rat (*Rattus norvegicus*), gerbil (*Meriones unguiculatus*), and hamsters: golden or Syrian hamster (*Mesocricetus auratus*), European hamster (*Cricetus cricetus*), and Russian dwarf hamster (*Phodopus* spp.). They are described as follows:

Mice: Small, busy rodents; long, hairless tail; average adult 30 g (20–63 g)

Rats: Large, intelligent rodents; long, hairless tail; (225–500 g)

Gerbils: Desert-adapted rodents but need freshwater access; produce concentrated urine; long, hairy tail; (46–131 g)

Hamsters: Stocky, loose-skinned rodents; cheek pouches and short tail; (87–130 g) (Dwarfs 18–46 g)

Anatomy and Physiology

Basic anatomy and physiology of mice, rats, gerbils, and hamsters is like that of other mammals, so only the significant differences are addressed in this section (Figure 18.1). The reader should note the following. The spleen of the male mouse is 50% bigger than that of the female. Rats have no gallbladder and their Harderian glands are known to produce red porphyrin staining around the eyes; this is related to stress. Some gerbils have seizures, a thymus through adulthood, and a large adrenal weight-to-body ratio. Male hamsters have larger adrenals than females (Harkness & Wagner 2010). Rodents do not have sweat glands and should not be kept in heat (Quesenberry et al., 2021). They do not pant and so use other methods of heat dissipation like their tails, ears, and in mice salivation (Quesenberry et al., 2021).

The teeth of mice, rats, gerbils, and hamsters are divided into two separate functional units, the incisors and the

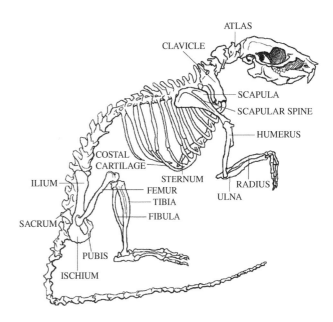

Figure 18.1 Rodent skeletal anatomy. (Drawing by Scott Stark).

cheek teeth, composed of molars only, no pre-molars. These two units are separated by a long gap called the diastema (Quesenberry & Carpenter 2021). The diastema is shorter in the mandible than in the maxilla, giving rodents their normal brachygnathic appearance (Quesenberry & Carpenter 2003).

Mice, rats, gerbils, and hamsters all share a dental formula of 2 (I1/1, C0/0, P0/0, M3/3), with hamsters having incisors at birth (Harkness & Wagner 1995). The incisors are open-rooted and grow continuously; the molars do not. Incisors develop a yellow–orange color as the animal ages. Classically the incisors are used for rostrocaudal gnawing during eating. A near-vertical biting motion also exists but is more common in defensive or offensive behaviors (Quesenberry & Carpenter 2003; Quesenberry et al., 2021). Gnawing naturally wears down the surface of the incisors, but a malocclusion of the incisors (Figure 18.8) precludes normal wear and makes trimming of the teeth necessary. Malocclusion is especially problematic in weanlings and if not caught early can lead to starvation and death. Malocclusion can be genetic, or it can occur secondary to a fractured tooth which grows back crooked, causing misalignment of teeth and preventing proper wear.

Rats, mice, and gerbils possess long tails; hamsters have very short tails. It is very important to exercise caution when handling the tail because improper restraint can cause trauma. In gerbils, the skin can actually slip ("tail-slip" or deglove) with improper handling (Harkness & Wagner 1995; Quesenberry et al., 2021). When held distal to the base, the animal can go into a spin and twist the distal part of the tail off in all three species, which is an escape mechanism. Further, rodents, mainly rats and gerbils, can regulate their temperature via thermoregulatory activities, such as tail extension. Hence, damage to the tail can indeed affect temperature regulation in these species.

Mammary tissue is extensive, reaching cranially between the front legs and up over the shoulders, and caudally toward the inguinal area. Therefore, mammary masses can be located well away from the teats. The mammary glands are paired, with rats having four to six pairs; mice, five pairs; gerbils, four pairs; and hamsters, six or seven pairs.

Harderian glands are specialized glands located behind each eye. They secrete a substance containing porphyrin, giving the secretion a red tinge. An animal experiencing stress or illness may have a buildup of the secretions around the eyes and may appear to the client to be bleeding from the eyes and nasolacrimal duct, and hence the nares. This collection of secreted material is also referred to as "red tears" and is most common in stressed rats.

Additional glandular structures include bilateral flank glands in the hamster and a ventral gland in the gerbil (Harkness & Wagner 1995). These sebaceous glands are brown in color and play a part in mating behavior, territorial marking, and marking of pups. The animals spend time grooming these areas and are often observed rubbing the glands over surfaces.

Small rodents are seasonally polyestrous and are spontaneous ovulators. Mating behavior results in the production of a whitish-tan collection of secretions, called a copulatory plug, that is often found lying in the bedding of the cage. Most male rodent species have an os penis and open inguinal canals, allowing them to retract the testicles into the abdominal cavity (Harkness & Wagner 1995). Gentle pressure on the caudal abdomen will force the testicles into the scrotal sac.

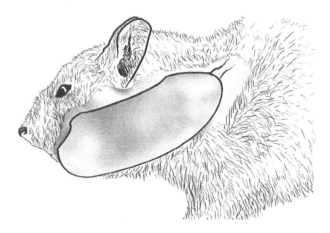

Figure 18.2 Cheek pouch. (Drawing by Scott Stark).

Hamsters have large cheek pouches that extend back to their scapulae (Figure 18.2). These pouches can distend to quite a large size, allowing the hamster to transfer food and bedding from one point to another. A startled mother may move her offspring from one area to another via her cheek pouches; however, the pups can suffocate inside a pouch. Hence, great care should be taken not to disturb females with litters.

The digestive systems of mice, rats, gerbils, and hamsters have some differences from other mammals, including an inability to regurgitate. Hamsters have an esophageal pouch that allows for pre-gastric fermentation of food prior to it reaching the stomach. Rodents are monogastric, with their stomachs divided into two areas: a glandular portion and a non-glandular portion. The practice of coprophagy is believed to assimilate certain nutrients, such as B vitamins that are produced by bacterial action in the colon (Quesenberry & Carpenter 2003; Hillyer & Quesenberry 1997). Rats do not have a gallbladder; therefore, bile continuously flows into the duodenum. The pancreas of rodents is arranged in diffuse lobes, making palpation difficult. Brown fat in rodents seems to provide a source of energy and is found deposited around the kidneys and thymus and between the shoulders. The rodent's visceral anatomy is shown in Figure 18.3.

Biologic and Reproductive Data

It is important for a technician to know physiologic data for small rodents (Table 18.1). This aids in determining an animal's state of health and also helps answer questions that owners commonly ask. It should be noted that gerbils form monogamous pairs, which should be set up before the animals reach maturity. Attempts to separate and repair a mated pair will result in fighting and may lead to death.

Table 18.1 Physiologic data for selected rodents

Data	Mouse	Rat	Gerbil	Hamster
Lifespan	1–3 years	2–4 years	3–4 years	18–24 months
Adult weight M/F	20–40 g/25–40 g	300–520 g/250–300 g	65–120 g/55–95 g	85–130 g/95–150 g
Body temperature (°F)	98–101	96.6–99.5	98.6–101.3	98.6–101.4
Heart rate (beats/min)	300–750	250–450	360	300–500
Respiratory rate (breaths/min)	60–220	70–120	90	35–135
Puberty	35 days	37–67 days	70–84 days	45–75 days
Estrous cycle	4–5 days	4–5 days	4–7 days	3–4 days
Gestation	19–21 days	21–23 days	24–26 days	15 days
Weaning age	21–28 days	21 days	21–30 days	20–25 days

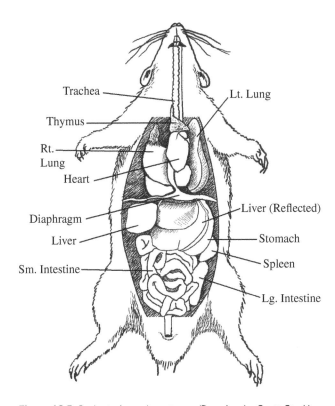

Figure 18.3 Rodent visceral anatomy. (Drawing by Scott Stark).

Husbandry

Rodent housing should be escape-proof, chew-proof, and easily cleaned. A variety of metal and plastic caging is available. Solid flooring is easy to clean and may help prevent trauma to the toes, feet, and legs. Breeding animals should be housed on solid flooring. Adequate ventilation is important because the buildup of ammonia from urea breakdown contributes to upper respiratory disease (Harkness & Wagner 1989). Wire caging promotes better ventilation than plastic shoebox-type or tunnel-type caging, but wire-bottom cages are dangerous for toes, feet, and limbs and are thus not recommended. Lameness is a common sequela to wire-bottom caging. Cleaning tunnel-type cages frequently solves some of their ventilation problems. Further, plastic caging with tunnels and toys provides more environmental enrichment and exercise for the animals than simple wire caging. If kept clean, these tunnel-type caging environments are best.

A variety of bedding materials have been available for some time, including ash and pine wood shavings and corncob. More recently, various absorbent paper products, developed for rodents and birds, have become available. The paper products are safer for rodents. They are not irritating to the feet and toes, and they are designed to break down if ingested and therefore usually do not cause impactions. Wood shavings can be too rough, or pointed, and cause lesions and abrasions, especially on the feet and toes, leading to pododermatitis. Due to the sensitive respiratory system of rats, wood shavings in general are not recommended because they produce so much dust. The use of cedar wood shavings is completely contraindicated; the aromatic oils are irritating and alone can cause pododermatitis. If cleaning is performed adequately (two or more times a week), scented bedding, such as dangerous cedar shavings, is unnecessary. Further, many wood shavings have chemical products in them that can adversely affect the liver and can also cause eye damage, among other problems. Corncob is the most absorbent but is prone to fungal growth and if fine can be ingested by some species, leading to fatal gastrointestinal impactions. In summary, the most important consideration is that the bedding be clean, dry, nonabrasive, non-nutritional, and supplied in ample quantities so that the animal can dig or burrow safely.

In addition to the bedding substrate, breeding animals should be provided with some form of nesting material. Lack of appropriate nesting material can result in the death of offspring (Harkness & Wagner 1995), either through abandonment or cannibalism, as can disturbing the nest in an effort to clean the cage. Commercial nesting products such as "nestlets" are available, or white tissue paper or paper towels can be used. Cotton towels should not be used because the animals can get entangled in the cotton fibers. This entanglement can cause constrictions leading to loss of toes, feet, or limbs. It is imperative that cages be cleaned just prior to parturition and stocked with all that the dam will need. One should also make sure that the soon-to-be lactating dam will have enough food to last about a week so that the nest will not be disturbed in any way during this time period. The young should not be handled during this time unless absolutely necessary, because cannibalism of offspring is most common within the first five days of parturition.

Exercise wheels and balls are popular with pet owners and provide the animals with a healthy activity. The wheels should be routinely checked for any rough or sharp areas, and owners using plastic balls should be cautioned to keep them away from stairs and from other pets. Most rodent species are more active at night, so placing the animal in an area other than the bedrooms might be a good idea. A small amount of vegetable-based oil applied on the axle of a metal wheel temporarily helps eliminate any squeaking.

Nutrition

Monogastric mice, rats, gerbils, and hamsters are omnivores and will eat anything—plant, animal, plastic, rubber, etc. if they get hungry enough or curious enough. Therefore, offer a fresh pelleted diet, such as those used for laboratory rodents, daily in ample amounts. One should be sure to buy the standard rodent chow pelleted diet from a reliable dealer who sells a lot and maintains fresh stock. In addition to the pelleted diets, all rodents are coprophagic and eat a fair amount of fecal pellets, providing them with B vitamins produced by their colonic bacteria.

Pelleted diets are preferred over seed mixtures, which contribute to nutritionally related diseases. Seeds can be given but are best saved for an occasional treat or a flushing food given during pre-breeding and breeding periods and as a supplement during lactation. A small amount of fresh food can be given daily as healthy snacks (carrots, sliced apple, and greens) but should be removed if not eaten within 4–6 hours. If fresh foods are not removed, spoilage can occur, fostering both fungal and bacterial growth, especially clostridium.

Crocks are recommended over plastic bowls that the animal may chew on and wire hoppers, which may cause facial abrasions (Harkness & Wagner 1989). Mothers with litters should have their food placed in a crock and directly in the cage on top of dry bedding for easier access.

Fresh water should be provided daily, and water bottle mechanisms need to be checked each day to ensure that they are functioning properly. Sipper tubes or drinking valves may become clogged with bedding or other foreign material, preventing the animal from having access to water. Intelligent, bored rodents, especially rats, are notorious for placing food or bedding directly into their water bottles through the valve. Alternatively, a malfunctioning water bottle may leak into the cage or not function at all, leading to dehydration. The bottle should be mounted on the outside of the cage with only the metal tube extending into the cage. This prevents the animal from chewing any plastic or rubber parts. The water bottle should never be filled completely. An air bubble is needed to ensure the water will come out of the sipper tube when licked.

Common Parasites, Diseases, and Zoonoses

Many of the medical problems seen in rodents, and especially pet mice, are associated with the skin.

Acariasis is the skin condition that results from mite infestation. Most species of mites are host-specific. Rodents can be affected by several species of skin mites; however, the most commonly encountered mites are the *Myobia* spp., *Myocoptes* spp., and *Radfordia* spp., which are spread through exposure to infected animals and bedding.

Signs include alopecia, dermatitis, rough hair coat, and skin lesions from excessive scratching. The rump area is typically involved and the lesions present as scaly, scabby dermatitis. These signs are most commonly seen in mice and hamsters. Further, geriatric male hamsters over 1.5 years of age typically develop dermatitis secondary to chronic kidney disease, lowered immune system, systemic disease, or malnutrition.

Some mite species can be visualized with a hand lens, or microscopically with a skin scraping. Ectoparasites can be treated with a variety of antiparasitic agents including ivermectin, selamectin, and milbemycin (Quesenberry & Carpenter 2021). Caging must be concurrently cleaned. Alopecia in mice housed in groups may be a result of barbering rather than an infestation with an ectoparasite.

Barbering behavior occurs when dominant mice chew on the whiskers and hair around the muzzle and eyes of subordinate mice. Usually, barbering occurs in a symmetrical pattern that is consistent with all animals in the cage. Barbering is not normally associated with dermatitis but can lead to it (Figure 18.4). Typically, a cage of mice will be suspected if one mouse in an affected group is not suffering

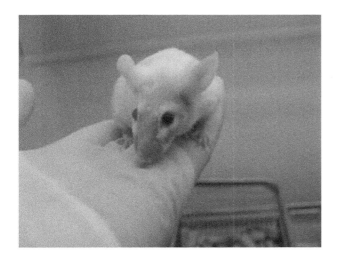

Figure 18.4 Barbering on a mouse.

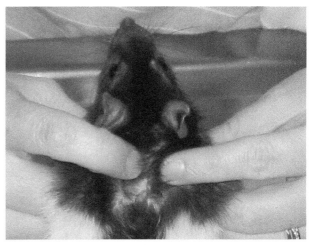

Figure 18.6 Bacterial infection on a rat. (Courtesy of Dr. David Martinez).

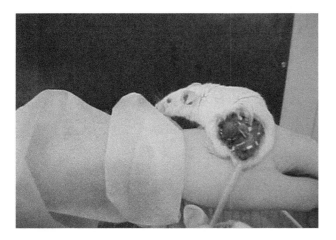

Figure 18.5 Male mouse with fight wounds on its back.

from hair loss. Usually, the unaffected mouse is the dominant mouse, and it should be removed from the group to stop the cycle. Barbering is most common in female mice and can also be seen in breeding pairs (including pups). Groups of male mice are usually fine, if litters are raised together from birth. However, unknown males put together in the same cage will fight ferociously. The most commonly affected areas during fighting are the rump, back, shoulders, tail, feet, and genitals (Figure 18.5). It is not uncommon for the entire penis (including the os penis) to be bitten off in severe cases of fighting. Any genital wounds should be monitored closely to ensure that the animal can urinate normally.

Mechanical abrasions result from self-trauma on cage bars, equipment, etc. This type of alopecia is husbandry related, and most commonly occurs around the lateral muzzle. Alopecia in this area is secondary to chafing on

drinking valves, metal feeders, or metal cage tops, and may be followed by dermatitis (Figure 18.6).

Mange is typically caused by *Demodex nanus* in rats but is a rare condition. This condition is also rare in gerbils. *Staphylococcus aureus* ulcerative dermatitis occurs in rats secondary to self-inflicted scratching of wounds or fur mite infestation, or over-inflamed salivary glands.

Avascular necrosis of the tail, or ringtail, occurs in both mice and rats. Ringtail can be caused by several factors but is most commonly associated with low humidity (less than 20%) and is more commonly seen during winter months when heating devices may be used. It is more common in laboratory rodents but can be seen in pet mice and rats. Treatment involves tail amputation below the necrotic annular constriction.

Common endoparasites include pinworms and tapeworms. Clinical signs may not be present but may include weight loss, diarrhea, and rectal prolapse in young animals. Detection of parasites is performed either through examination of fecal matter, through fecal flotation, or, for pinworms, by the cellophane tape test performed in the early afternoon around 2 p.m. The cellophane tape test is only about 30% accurate. A more accurate diagnosis is a cecal smear at necropsy.

To Perform the Cellophane Tape Test:

1. Assemble the following supplies: cellophane tape, microscope slide, microscope.
2. Press a small piece of the cellophane tape against the perianal area. For pinworms, testing is best done in the early afternoon, around 2 p.m., when the pinworm ova are exiting the animal's rectum.

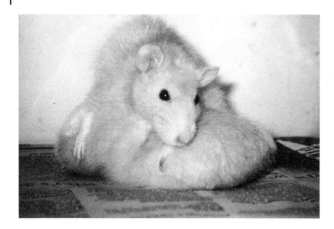

Figure 18.7 Neoplasia in a rat.

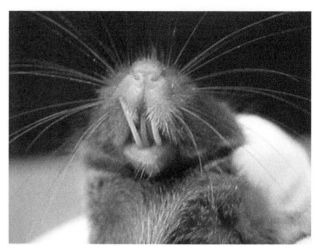

Figure 18.8 Malocclusion in a mouse.

3. Place the tape on a microscope slide, sticky side down, for examination (Quesenberry & Carpenter 2021; Hillyer & Quesenberry 1997).
4. Examine the slide for the slightly banana-shaped pinworm ova.

Note: Pinworm eggs are known to be sticky and very difficult to eradicate in the environment. Treatment is long and arduous. All bedding, food, and water must be replaced and everything else must be cleaned and disinfected, including the walls.

Neoplasia occurs in rodents, with mammary tumors a common finding in females (Figure 18.7). Rats develop predominately benign mammary fibroadenomas and mice develop predominately malignant mammary adenocarcinomas. Extensive mammary tissue may result in the tumor being located on the abdomen or shoulders. The tumors often interfere with the animal's ability to walk normally, and chronic mechanical irritation can cause them to become ulcerated (Harkness & Wagner 1989). Systemic and cutaneous lymphoma is common in hamsters both old and young. Young hamsters develop lymphoma secondary to hamster polyoma virus (HaPV). Male gerbils develop squamous cell carcinoma (SCC) of the ventral marking gland and female gerbils develop ovarian granulosa cell tumors.

Malocclusion results when the continuously erupting incisors are misaligned (Figure 18.8). This misalignment prevents the teeth from being worn down during normal daily activities. Common signs of malocclusion include weight loss, drooling, and oral trauma. Malocclusion is genetic. Breeding animals with malocclusion should be avoided at all costs. Other causes include malnutrition, disease, and injury (Harkness & Wagner 1989). Periodic trimming with a dental burr, clippers, or a sharp pair of scissors must be done carefully to avoid splitting the tooth;

rough edges should be filed smooth. Splitting teeth can result in the formation of abscesses.

Moist dermatitis commonly occurs in rodents that are chronically exposed to wet conditions, or in those with trauma to the skin from urine scalding, diarrhea, abrasions, cuts, or other breaks in the skin's integrity. The most common condition affecting gerbils, facial eczema or "sore nose," causes a moist dermatitis lesion on the face and nose caused by an accumulation of Harderian gland secretions (Quesenberry & Carpenter 2003; Hillyer & Quesenberry 1997). Other causes should be ruled out, such as malocclusion, damaged crockery or caging, and abrasive bedding. Treatment involves clipping the hair from the lesion, cleaning the area, and removing any known causative agents. The veterinarian may prescribe systemic and or topical antibiotics.

Hamsters with diarrhea are often referred to as having "wet-tail" (Figure 18.9). Young animals are particularly sensitive to proliferative ileitis, especially if recently weaned. Multiple bacteria are implicated in the cause, as well as improper diet and stress. Signs are hunched posture, matted hair, watery diarrhea, lethargy, rectal prolapse, and death. Careful husbandry may help prevent the disease, and the veterinarian may prescribe antibiotic therapy (Harkness & Wagner 1989).

Gerbils are susceptible to epileptiform seizures that can result from excitement related to handling. The seizures can be mild, resulting in a dazed or hypnotic appearance, or severe, and the activity may last only a few seconds to a minute or more. There is no treatment and anticonvulsant drugs are not indicated. Exposure to frequent handling at a young age may help prevent the seizures from occurring (Harkness and Wagner 1989).

From a zoonotic perspective, the following infectious diseases are of concern because they are common and

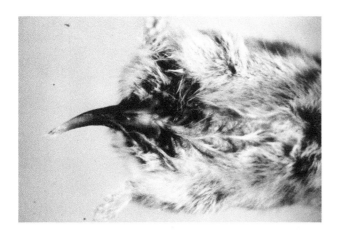

Figure 18.9 Wet tail.

transmissible to humans: lymphocytic choriomeningitis (LCM), a virus; and *Staphylococcus* spp., *Streptococcus* spp., *Pasteurella* spp., *Klebsiella* spp., and *Salmonella*, bacterial diseases.

Other relatively common diseases of rodents include mouse hepatitis virus (MHV), mouse parvovirus (MPV), mouse norovirus (MNV), mycoplasmosis, sialodacryoadenitis virus, and lymphocytic choriomeningitis.

LCM is found naturally in wild mouse populations and can be passed via arthropod vectors and through bodily secretions and bite wounds. Clinical signs, if present, include a hunched posture, unthrifty appearance, photophobia, and convulsions. LCM is zoonotic; humans can become infected through contact with infected tissue, urine, or a bite wound. Clinical signs are similar to those associated with influenza and include headache, fever, muscle aches, malaise, and meningitis.

MHV is a highly contagious disease that can cause severe diarrhea and death in very young (1–2-week-old) mice. MNV is a subclinical virus. MPV also results in enteritis but can be both subclinical and devastating.

Chronic respiratory disease (CRD) in rodents may be caused by *Mycoplasma pulmonis*. Animals can be carriers of *M. pulmonis* but never show any signs. CRD is very common in rats and clinical signs will be amplified if unsanitary living conditions, improper husbandry materials, and increased ammonia content are present. Respiratory disease, caused by infectious agents, is the most common health concern in rats. CRD is also referred to as murine respiratory mycoplasmosis in mice. Clinical signs include general upper respiratory signs; severe porphyrin staining around the eyes, nose, and mouth; as well as rhinitis and a possible head tilt associated with otitis. Antibiotics can be employed to help control the signs but will never completely eradicate the disease.

Sialodacryoadenitis virus is a coronavirus related to MHV and is spread through respiratory secretions. Infection causes the cervical lymph nodes to swell and the salivary glands to become inflamed. Affected animals may continue to eat despite swelling in the neck. A very noticeable sign is chromodacryorrhea or porphyrin staining, "red tears." The animal may be sensitive to light and develop ophthalmic lesions.

Tyzzer's disease is a fatal hepatoenteric infectious disease that hamsters and gerbils may also contract. Tyzzer's is caused by *Clostridium piliforme*. Mice and rats that contract this disease can overcome it. Clinical signs in hamsters and gerbils include listlessness, rough hair coat, weight loss, and sudden death. Stress is a major contributing factor in addition to exposure to infected bedding. In general, gerbils do not contract many diseases, when compared to other rodents,

There are diseases with zoonotic potential aside from LCM, *Staphylococcus* spp., *Streptococcus* spp., *Pasteurella* spp., *Klebsiella* spp., and *Salmonella*, many of which are more common in wild rodent populations than in domestic rodents. According to the Centers for Disease Control, the risk of a human contracting Korean hemorrhagic fever or the organism responsible for bubonic plague from a pet rodent is extremely remote in the United States (CDC, personal communication). People with immunosuppression are at higher risk and practicing good hygiene is essential. Rat bite fever is a bacterial infection causing chills, fever, myalgia, localized swelling at the wound site, and headache. It is also possible to contract hymenolepid tapeworm infection, which causes enteric disease in humans (Quesenberry & Carpenter 2003; Hillyer & Quesenberry 1997; Harkness & Wagner 1989). Other zoonotic concerns include rabies, which is extremely rare in rodents, and rodent allergies from urine and dander, which are very common and of great concern to the CDC.

Behavior

Most rodents are nocturnal but are easily awakened during the day. Gentle handling will prevent a startled animal from biting out of defense. Male mice, gerbils, and hamsters fight with each other and should be housed alone unless raised together from birth. Hamsters of either sex are better housed singly than in groups and should only be brought together for mating (Figure 18.10). Gerbils are known to establish monogamous pairs but fighting in older gerbils that previously seemed to peacefully coexist may develop and can result in serious wounds. Because many rodents are kept as pets for small children, separate

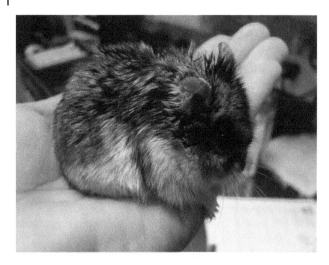

Figure 18.10 There are different species of hamsters that may be kept as pets. This is a Djungarian hamster. (Courtesy of Dr. Joerg Mayer, College of Veterinary Medicine, University of Georgia).

housing is recommended because witnessing such activity could be traumatic.

The exception to the housing recommendation is the rat. Rats are very social animals and tend to do better if housed with a cage mate (Figure 18.11). Rats of both sexes can be grouped together and females with litters can be left in communal housing with relative safety, provided conditions are not overcrowded. Females will share in caring for and nursing young animals.

Cannibalism of young may occur if nests are disturbed or the mother is overly nervous. This behavior is most often associated with hamsters and mice; gerbils seem less sensitive to disturbance and rats rarely cannibalize their offspring. It is imperative to ensure the cage is supplied with clean bedding and adequate food and water prior to parturition to prevent having to disturb the nest once the offspring have been born.

History and Physical Examination

Rodents should be brought to the hospital in the cage in which they are normally housed. The cage should be covered to protect the rodent from temperature changes, noise, and disease exposure. The person scheduling the appointment should advise the client not to clean the cage prior to coming into the hospital. This allows the staff to observe the condition of the cage, the presence of fecal material, type of bedding, and so on. Ideally, the client should sit away from cats and dogs, if not coming to an exotic clinic to prevent further stress. The examination room should be stocked with urine dipsticks for immediate

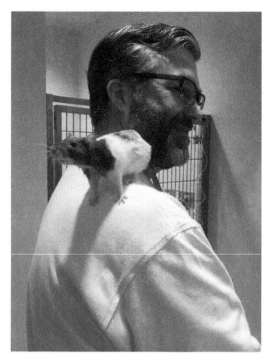

Figure 18.11 Rats are very social and make great pets. (Courtesy of Dr. Joerg Mayer, College of Veterinary Medicine, University of Georgia).

sampling because most rodents urinate as soon as they are handled or touched in the genital area (Quesenberry & Carpenter 2003; Hillyer & Quesenberry 1997).

As with any patient, clients should be asked where they obtained the pet, how long they have had it, what they feed it, and if this is the first time they have owned this particular species. Discuss with clients when they first noticed any signs of illness, how long the problem has existed, and what, if anything, they have done in response to the signs. Rodents must be weighed using a gram scale, and in a small container to prevent escape. Unless the practice has a thermometer specifically designed for use in rodents, forgo obtaining a rectal temperature. Standard thermometers are too large to use safely.

Restraint and Handling

Firm but gentle handling is important when working with rodents. They may bite out of fear, and also jump or run quickly in an effort to escape. Falls to the floor are survivable but could easily result in fracture of the liver, feet or limbs, ribs, or spine.

Most rodents are amenable to being gently scooped up into the hands to lift them from their cages. This is indeed the best way to pick them up. Rats and mice can be briefly lifted by the tail base and onto a table or other surface if scooping does not work with the animal in question. Gerbils should never be restrained or held by their tail. Prolonged handling of the tail can cause trauma, such as sloughing of the skin and exposing the vertebrae, especially in gerbils. Sloughing can also occur in rats and mice. Grasping the tail at its base prevents tail trauma. Use of a towel, screen, or barred lid of the animal's cage gives it something to hold onto when being restrained on a table. Rodents showing signs of aggression or agitation (chattering, vocalizing, rolling onto their backs, and in gerbils, thumping of the hind feet) can be picked up with an empty plastic container or lifted with a small towel folded for thickness. Gloves may be needed to handle some rats, but they are often unwieldy and can make it difficult to feel what the animal is doing. Therefore, care must be taken to observe the animal for any respiratory difficulty. Laboratory animal supply companies (e.g., Kent Scientific, Torrington, CT) have plastic restraint devices.

To Handle Gerbils, Mice, and Rats:

1. The animal should be scooped up. The base of the tail should be gently grasped only if need be, prior to scooping.
2. The animal should then be lifted out of its enclosure, and the animal's body allowed to rest on a hand, arm, or table. A hold should be maintained on the tail while supporting the animal's body to prevent escape (gerbils are excellent jumpers) (Figure 18.12A, B, C).
3. Rats can be lifted out of their enclosure by placing a hand over the dorsum and gently pressing their forelimbs together using the thumb and index finger.

To Handle a Hamster:

1. If the animal is awake, it can usually be scooped up gently using both hands; use caution if the hamster is sleeping because startled hamsters may bite.
2. If there is concern that the hamster may react aggressively, a piece of toweling or an empty plastic container may be used to lift the animal up.

For injections or other procedures that the rodent may object to, the animal may be scruffed, as follows.

1. It is helpful to place the rodent on a towel or the top of a wire cage while maintaining a gentle hold on the tail.
2. Slight traction should be applied to the base of the tail, which will encourage the animal to grip onto the surface with its front feet.
3. Grasp the loose skin over the neck, using the little finger of the restraining hand to hold the tail.

4. Scruffing a hamster can be more difficult; the abundance of loose skin can still permit the animal to turn and bite if the restrainer has not grasped a sufficient amount. An indication of a sufficient amount of skin grasped is when the hamster "smiles" (Figure 18.13A, B).

Radiology

Sedation is usually needed for most radiography in order to achieve proper positioning. Whole-body studies are often employed due to the size of the patient. Animals may be placed in radiolucent tubing or briefly positioned with painting tape. Exposure times of 1/60th of a second are best due to the rapid respiratory and heart rates of rodents.

Surgery, Anesthesia, and Pain Management

Common surgical procedures include ovariohysterectomy, castration, tumor excision, and abscess draining. Surgical preparation is similar to that of any small animal, except that prolonged fasting of the animal prior to anesthesia is not necessary and could result in hypoglycemia, because fasting reduces glycogen stores in the liver. Surgical scrub solutions should be warmed, as should the surgical tables (using a warm water circulating pad), the perioperative fluids, and the recovery incubator. This prevents unnecessary heat loss by the patient. Hypothermia is the number one killer of rodents, especially mice that undergo surgery. All rules of aseptic technique apply, and the surgical suite and equipment should be prepared accordingly. Sterile surgical tape can be used to restrain the animal on the table post-induction.

Rodents can be chambered or facemask-induced using isoflurane. Intubation is difficult in rodents, but induction can be maintained using a face mask or a plastic syringe case modified as a nose cone. A non-rebreathing system should always be used (Quesenberry & Carpenter 2003; Hillyer & Quesenberry 1997).

The technician should monitor the depth and quality of respiration. The deeper the animal's anesthetic plane becomes, the more the abdominal muscles will move with each breath. The animals normally breathe with their abdomen and/or diaphragm. When they start to use their chest and move their forelimbs, they are having problems. Lightly anesthetized rodents will still blink when the eyelashes are touched. The palpebral reflex will be diminished as the animal enters a surgical plane. The ears or toes can be pinched to evaluate the animal's ability to react; if the animal reacts, the plane of anesthesia is still light

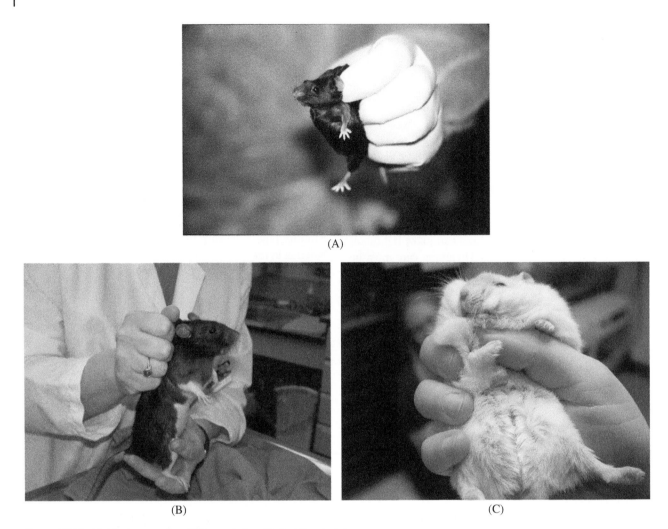

Figure 18.12 (A) Mouse restraint. (B) Rat restraint. (C) Gerbil restraint.

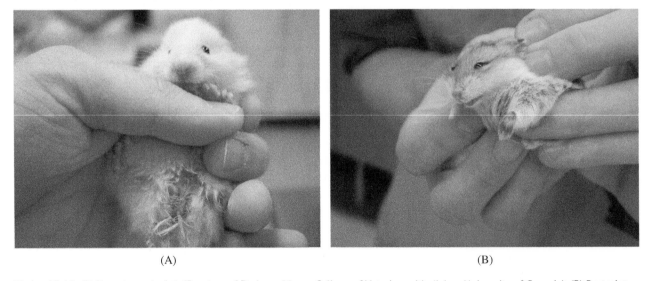

Figure 18.13 (A) Hamster restraint. (Courtesy of Dr. Joerg Mayer, College of Veterinary Medicine, University of Georgia). (B) Restraint using the scruffing method. (Courtesy of Jody Nugent-Dean).

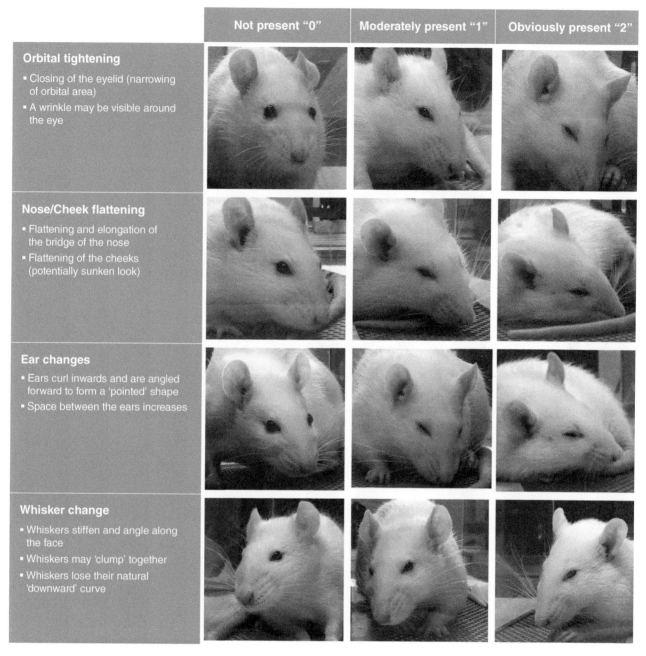

	Not present "0"	Moderately present "1"	Obviously present "2"
Orbital tightening • Closing of the eyelid (narrowing of orbital area) • A wrinkle may be visible around the eye			
Nose/Cheek flattening • Flattening and elongation of the bridge of the nose • Flattening of the cheeks (potentially sunken look)			
Ear changes • Ears curl inwards and are angled forward to form a 'pointed' shape • Space between the ears increases			
Whisker change • Whiskers stiffen and angle along the face • Whiskers may 'clump' together • Whiskers lose their natural 'downward' curve			

Figure 18.14 Rat Grimace Scale. (Courtesy of The National Centre for the Replacement, Refinement, and Reduction of Animals in Research).

(Quesenberry & Carpenter 2003; Hillyer & Quesenberry 1997). Pinching the ears is best on mice, and toes on rats.

Mucous membranes should be pink, and the color can be evaluated using the pads of the feet, ears, and eyes of albino, and gingiva. Pulse oximeters are commonly found in most small animal hospitals and can be placed on the tail, tongue, or foot pad.

Recovery from surgery should be in a pre-warmed incubator as described above; the incubator should be situated in a quiet area. The technician should gently turn the animal from side to side every few minutes to prevent pooling of blood on the dependent side. Rodents will attempt to chew sutures and bandages; surgical glue, staples, or subcuticular sutures are best. Elizabethan collars are available commercially. Those with Velcro closures are tolerated the best. The sedative effects of opioid analgesics, such as buprenorphine, often are enough to prevent self-trauma at the surgical site. Nonsteroidal anti-inflammatory drugs,

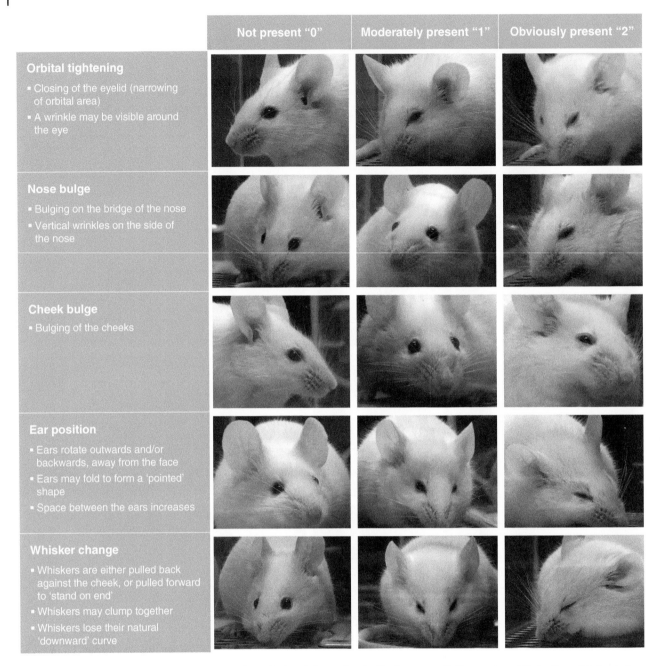

Figure 18.15 Mouse Grimace Scale. (Courtesy of The National Centre for the Replacement, Refinement, and Reduction of Animals in Research).

such as meloxicam, may also be used in rodents for minor surgery to manage post-operative pain.

Pain can be assessed by using the NC3Rs Grimace Scale. This scale attempts to define a visual Grimace Scale for Rats and Mice that help assess post-procedural/surgical pain. The scale units progress from 0 to 1 to 2 using 4 subcategories for rats and 5 subcategories for mice (Figures 18.14 and 18.15). More information is available from the NC3rs/National Centre for the 3Rs in the UK.

Bandaging and Wound Care

Rodents easily become stressed and daily wound care may do more harm than good. Wounds should be cleaned as thoroughly as possible during the initial treatment phase. The use of intact white paper towels for the first 48 hours post-surgery allows for easier observation, keeps the wound cleaner, and enables better drainage. After this initial time period, advise the owner to increase the frequency of bedding changes to keep the healing wounds as clean as possible.

Emergency and Critical Care

Unfortunately, many of the infectious diseases of rodents are challenging to treat, and, historically, harsher antibiotics were known to cause fatal reactions. Today, enrofloxicin is an example of a safe and effective rodent antibiotic. It can easily be delivered through the drinking water, thus decreasing the stress of handling. Supportive care in the form of subcutaneous fluids, dextrose, calcium, adequate dietary support such as diet gel (a fluid and food combination choice), and heat and oxygen must be administered immediately.

Wet tail or proliferative ileitis in hamsters may respond to improved diet, sanitation, and aggressive supportive care and antibiotics, such as enrofloxicin, after diagnostics are performed. Initially, enrofloxacin is given parentally and then in the drinking water, but the animal's prognosis is guarded (Plunkett 1993).

Animals suffering from bite wounds or lacerations may be extremely stressed and vocal. Be cautious when attempting to pick up an animal in this condition, because it may respond aggressively. Such patients should be kept warm and quiet until they can be anesthetized with isoflurane, if necessary, for wound care.

Sex Determination

Males and females can be distinguished by comparing anogenital distance. The distance from the anus to the genital papilla is greater in the male than in the female. This can be difficult to assess if there are no other animals present for comparison purposes. In hamsters, the male has a rounded posterior when viewed from above due to the scrotum, whereas the female's posterior appears squarer (Figure 18.16 A, B). Male gerbils have a larger mid-ventral scent gland (Figure 18.17).

Clinical Techniques

Administration of Medications

Parenteral administration sites include intravenous (difficult), intramuscular (may cause necrosis and usually not recommended due to the small muscle mass), intraperitoneal (common in lab animal medicine), and subcutaneous (preferred site, safest, and easiest).

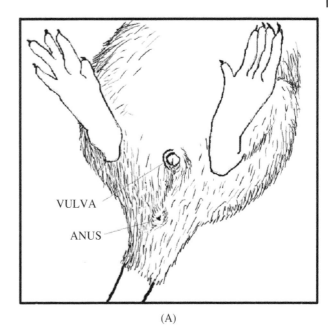

(A)

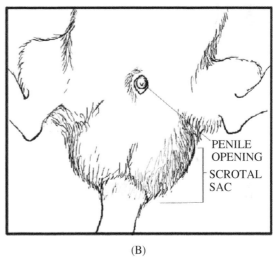

(B)

Figure 18.16 Sex determination. (A) Female. (B) Male. (Drawing by Scott Stark).

Intravenous Injection

Intravenous injection of drugs is difficult to accomplish in rodents. The most commonly used site is the lateral tail vein in mice, rats, and gerbils. Four vessels are present on the tail, two veins, and two arteries. Veins are located laterally on the tail and arteries are dorsal/ventral.

For Intravenous Injection:

1. Assemble supplies: 27–30-gauge (mice) or 22–25-gauge (rats and gerbils) needles, tuberculin syringes, chlorohexidine, and alcohol swabs.
2. Unless a restraint device is used, a second individual will need to restrain the animal.

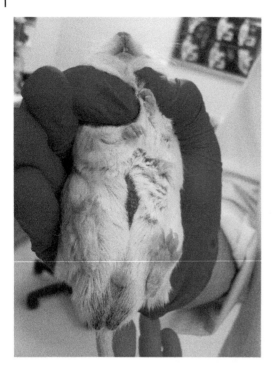

Figure 18.17 Gerbil scent glands. (Courtesy of Dr. Cheryl Greenacre).

3. Clean the venipuncture site with chlorohexidine and alcohol. Warming the tail with a focal heat light (penlight) may be useful to help visualize the vein and cause vasodilation.
4. Always slowly aspirate to ensure proper placement. Note that due to the low blood pressure of the mouse, there will not always be a flash of blood when in the vein.
5. Once the injection is completed, apply gentle pressure as the needle is removed to allow for clot formation.
6. Dispose of the needle into a puncture-proof biohazard container.

Intramuscular Injection

The quadriceps muscle can be used to administer injections in all four rodents discussed. Only very small amounts of drug can safely be injected into this site due to the small size of the patient (0.05 mL in mice, up to 0.3 mL in rats) or muscle necrosis will result. Care must be taken not to inject into the posterior thigh because irritation of the sciatic nerve may result. It may help to "pinch up" the muscle mass between the fingers of one hand while injecting with the other.

For Intramuscular Injection:

1. Assemble supplies: 25-gauge needles for mice, up to 22-gauge needles for larger rats, tuberculin syringes, chlorohexidine, and alcohol swabs.

2. Have an assistant restrain the animal if a commercial restraint device is not available.
3. Always aspirate prior to administering any medication to ensure correct placement.
4. Inject drug and withdraw the needle.
5. Dispose of needle into a puncture-proof biohazard container.

Intraperitoneal Injection

Intraperitoneal injections allow for larger volumes of drug to be injected than can be safely given by the intramuscular or intravenous routes. However, subcutaneous injections are safer than all of the above-mentioned injections and allow for larger volumes of drugs to be injected. Intraperitoneal injections are not without risk and should have limited applications in pet rodent medicine. Care must be taken not to puncture any abdominal organs. Intraperitoneal injections in rats require injecting into the left caudal quadrant, rather than the right, as in gerbils, mice, and hamsters. The rat's cecum is located in the right caudal quadrant. Slight resistance may be felt as the needle penetrates the abdominal muscles.

For Intraperitoneal Injection:

1. Assemble the following supplies: 21–27-gauge needles, syringes, chlorohexidine, and alcohol swabs.
2. Restraining the animal in one hand by scruffing the loose skin over the back of the neck and shoulders is required. The little finger of the same hand can be used to keep the tail pressed against the palm of the hand.
3. The animal's head should be tilted lower than the rest of the body to cause the abdominal organs to fall forward.
4. The needle should be inserted, bevel up, at an angle of about 20° into the right caudal quadrant unless it is a rat, in which case use of the left caudal quadrant is required.
5. The syringe should be aspirated to ensure that no organs have been punctured with the needle. If any yellow or greenish–brown fluid or any blood is aspirated, the needle and syringe should immediately be withdrawn and discarded. The procedure should be attempted again with a new needle and syringe, and the animal should immediately be started on parenteral antibiotics.
6. The needle should be disposed of in a puncture-proof biohazard container.

Subcutaneous Injection

Larger drug volumes can also be given subcutaneously (1–3 mL in mice, up to 5–10 mL in rats). The injection can be given under the skin along the flank, or in the loose skin of the neck, which is simultaneously being scruffed for restraint purposes.

For Subcutaneous Injection:

1. Assemble the following supplies: a 22–25-gauge needle for mice, 20-gauge needle for rats, syringes.
2. The animal's loose skin over the neck should be scruffed. This is the best area for subcutaneous injections.
3. The needle should be inserted into the tented skin between the fingers. It is often easier to position the syringe over the animal's head and point the needle toward its hindquarters if doing this alone.
4. Aspirate prior to injecting the medication to ensure proper placement.
5. The needle should be disposed of in a puncture-proof biohazard container.

Oral Administration

Unprofessionally compounded medications mixed into food or water can affect the taste, leading to the animal's refusing to eat or drink. Liquid medications can be more accurately administered to awake animals by gavage, or slowly and carefully by a 1 cc syringe. Gavage needles have ball-like tips to prevent trauma to the animal, and may be straight, curved, or bent (depending on the operator's preference). Compounded medications can be made up without flavor, color, or odor, or they can be made up in the flavor, color, and odor of the rodent's own pelleted diet. These options increase palatability and decrease stress because the animal can receive its medications in its own food or water without knowing it.

Gavaging

For Gavaging:

1. Gather the following supplies: a gavage needle of appropriate gauge and length attached to a syringe large enough to hold the entire dose of medication.
2. The top of the gavage needle should be lined up with the animal's nose, and the ball of the needle lined up with the animal's last rib to gauge depth of gavage needle insertion.
3. Wetting the ball of the needle with water may help it slide down more easily.
4. The animal should be restrained by scruffing the loose skin over the back of the neck, tucking the tail under the little finger. The animal should be held vertically with the head up (Figure 18.18).
5. The gavage needle should be inserted into the space behind the incisors, and the needle gently pushed into the animal's mouth, allowing it to follow the curve of the mouth down into the esophagus.
6. If any resistance is felt, or the animal becomes cyanotic (indicating that the needle is probably in the trachea),

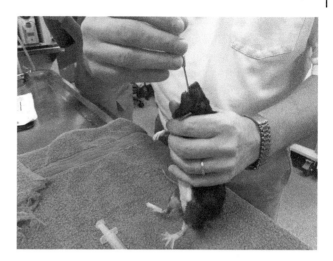

Figure 18.18 Gavaging a rat. (Courtesy of Dr. Joerg Mayer, College of Veterinary Medicine, University of Georgia).

immediately remove the needle, put the animal in oxygen, treat it with parenteral antibiotics, and repeat when the animal fully recovers.

7. When inserted to the level measured in step 2, inject the contents of the syringe and withdraw the gavage needle.

Blood Collection

In all rodents except the hamster, blood can be collected from the tail veins located laterally on the tail (Figure 18.19). It is recommended that no more than 0.14 mL of blood be collected from mice, 0.3 mL from a gerbil, 0.65 mL from a hamster, and 1.3 mL from a rat (Quesenberry & Carpenter 2003; Hillyer & Quesenberry 1997). The saphenous vein is another option and works quite well in rodents.

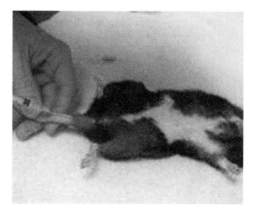

Figure 18.19 Venipuncture of the tail vein of a rat. (Courtesy of Dr. Joerg Mayer, College of Veterinary Medicine, University of Georgia).

To Collect Blood:

1. Assemble the following supplies: 23–27-gauge needles, tuberculin syringes or 3 mL syringe if a rat, chlorohexidine and alcohol swabs, and restraint device if available (rodent restrainers that leave the tail free are commercially available and work quite well).
2. Have an assistant restrain the animal if no restraint device is available.
3. Warming the tail with a warm water compress or low-wattage light may help to visualize the vein and will cause vasodilation.
4. Pressure must be applied proximally to the venipuncture site and can be accomplished using a rubber band and hemostats.
5. The needle should be inserted bevel-up into the vein and gently aspirated to prevent collapsing the vessel.
6. After blood collection, apply pressure to the venipuncture site as the needle is withdrawn to prevent hematoma formation.

Blood can also be collected retro-orbitally by puncturing the venous sinus or plexus with a microhematocrit tube (Figure 18.20A, B) or a beveled micropipette tip inserted into the medial canthus of the eye. This procedure requires the animal to be anesthetized briefly with isoflurane. There is a risk of causing damage to the eye, so this procedure should only be performed by highly skilled personnel and never with the owner present. Alternatively, submandibular bleeds can be performed on the mouse and the rat. This method is easier and safer. It also enables more blood to be collected and is best performed without anesthesia.

To collect blood at the medial canthus of the eye:

1. Assemble the following supplies: microhematocrit tubes or beveled micropipette tips, gauze sponges, ophthalmic ointment, and isoflurane machine.

2. Insert the microhematocrit tube into the eye at the medial can thus, rotating the tube gently to puncture the sinus.
3. Blood will fill the tube by capillary action.
4. Following the collection of blood, the tube should be removed, excess blood wiped from the site, and the eyelids gently held shut until hemostasis occurs.
5. Apply a sterile ophthalmic ointment into the eye (Quesenberry & Carpenter 2003; Hillyer & Quesenberry 1997).

The jugular vein is the preferred and recommended site for venipuncture and blood collection in rats. While not a common venipuncture route, blood can be drawn from the cranial vena cava in rats. Further, anesthesia is required for venipuncture of the cranial vena cava, the method has inherent risks, and is generally highly discouraged (Figure 18.21). Additional information about venipuncture using the cranial vena cava can be found in the "Techniques" section of Chapter 16.

Euthanasia

The owner may request to be present during the euthanasia procedure. An overdose of isoflurane is effective but can be followed by IC euthosol (pentobarbitol sodium and phenytoin sodium). If the induction chamber is relatively large, pre-fill it with the anesthetic to decrease the amount of time it will take before having the desired effect. Staff members not fond of rodents must keep in mind that pet rodent owners can be just as emotionally attached as the more familiar dog and cat owners. Remains should be treated with the same respect afforded to all deceased pets.

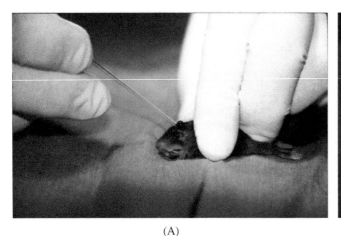

(A)

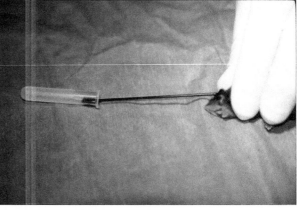

(B)

Figure 18.20 Blood collection from the venous sinus. (A) Restraint of a mouse during the initial insertion of a microhematocrit tube into the medial canthus. (B) Blood collection after successful puncture of the venous sinus with the microhematocrit tube.

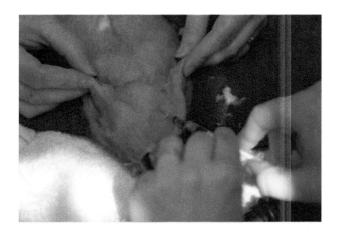

Figure 18.21 Blood being drawn from a rat using the cranial vena cava, an uncommon route. (Courtesy of Dr. David Martinez).

Acknowledgment

Dr. Romagnano would like to express gratitude to James B. Nichols, DVM, MS, for his critical review of the chapter and his expertise. She is also grateful to Shannon Sunday, CVT, SRA, LAT, for her critical review of the chapter and expertise, and would like to thank both Shannon and Raul Ortiz-Umpierre, DVM, for taking pictures for the chapter. She would also like to thank Dr. Tarah Hadley for her assistance.

Additional Reading

AALAS. 2016. *Laboratory Animal Technologist: LATG Training Manual.* American Association for Laboratory Animal Science.

AALAS. 2021. *Laboratory Animal Technician*: LAT Training Manual.

American Association for Laboratory Animal Science.

Harkness JE, Wagner JE. 1989. *The Biology and Medicine of Rabbits and Rodents*, 3rd edn, pp. 2–179. Philadelphia: Lea & Febiger.

Harkness JE, Wagner JE. 2010. *The Biology and Medicine of Rabbits and Rodents*, 5th edn, pp. 28–34. Philadelphia: Williams & Wilkins.

Hillyer EV, Quesenberry KE. 1997. *Ferrets, Rabbits and Rodents: Clinical Medicine and Surgery*, pp. 296–389. Philadelphia: 1st edn. St. Louis, MO: W.B. Saunders Co.

Langford DJ, Bailey AL, Chanda ML, Clarke SE, Drummond TE, Echols S, Glick S, Ingrao J, Klassen-Ross T, LaCroix-Fralish ML, Matsumiya L, Sorge RE, Sotocinal SG, Tabaka JM, Wong D, van den, Maagdenberg AMJM, Ferrari MD, Craig KD, Mogil JS. 2010. Coding of facial expressions of pain in the laboratory mouse. *Nat Methods* 7(6): 447-449.doi:10.1038/nmeth.1455

Oglesbee BL. 2011. *Blackwell's Five-Minute Veterinary Consult: Small Mammal*, 2nd edn. Ames, IA: Wiley-Blackwell.

Plunkett SJ. 1993. *Emergency Procedures for the Small Animal Veterinarian*, p. 177. Philadelphia: W.B. Saunders Co.

Quesenberry KE, Carpenter JW. 2003. *Ferrets, Rabbits, and Rodents: Clinical Medicine and Surgery*, 2nd ed. St. Louis, MO: W.B. Saunders Co.

Quesenberry KE, Carpenter JW. 2012. *Ferrets, Rabbits, and Rodents: Clinical Medicine and Surgery*, 3rd ed. St. Louis, MO: W.B. Saunders Co.

Quesenberry KE, Orcutt CJ, Mans C and Carpenter JW. 2021. *Ferrets, Rabbits, and Rodents: Clinical Medicine and Surgery*, 4th ed. St. Louis, MO: Elsevier.

Sotocinal SG, Sorge RE, Zaloum A, Tuttle AH, Martin LJ, Wieskopf JS, Mapplebeck JCS, Wei P, Zhan S, Zhang S, McDougall JJ, King OD, Mogil JS. 2011. The Rat Grimace Scale: a partially automated method for quantifying pain in the laboratory rat via facial expressions. *Mol Pain* 7: 55. doi:10.1186/1744-8069-7-55

19

Chinchillas
Ashley McGaha

Taxonomy/Common Species Seen in Practice

The chinchilla is classified as a rodent and is most closely related to the guinea pig. There are three subspecies of chinchilla; *Chinchilla langier* is the most commonly available in the pet trade. These animals inhabit the Andes Mountains of South America in Peru and Chile and are well adapted to living on cold and rocky slopes. Their average life span in captivity is 10 years, but they can live to the age of 20. Because they are closely related to the guinea pig, similarities in their physiology, care, and treatment will be apparent. See Table 19.1 for biological data.

Anatomy and Physiology

External Anatomy

There are two distinctive features in the external anatomy of the chinchilla. The first is the very dense fur that covers the entire body. It is so dense, in fact, that up to 90 individual hairs can come from each root (Hayes 2000). The second is the locomotory apparatus, which can be compared to the rabbit but is closer to that of the nutria. Chinchillas have very short front legs that are used for support and to hold food. These small legs have four digits (numbers 2, 3, 4, and 5; digit 1 is lost). The rear legs, however, are very large and powerful. Designed for jumping, they have three digits varying in size (numbers 2, 3, 4). The first and fifth digits are rudimentary only.

Digestive Tract

The mouth is largely filled by the tongue. The two lateral areas of the tongue are wider than the dorsal side, giving it an unusual shape.

The adult chinchilla has four incisors and sixteen molar-type teeth. The upper incisors usually have a right-angle indentation, while the lowers are ground down to a point. Only about one-third of the incisors protrude from the jaw. The grinding and cutting teeth have open roots, which means that they grow continuously. Therefore, the correct positioning of each tooth is crucial because it assures that each tooth is being constantly ground down. There may be slight differences in dentition among the different species. The most distinctive part of the mouth is the palatal ridges. Each chinchilla, no matter how closely related, has palatal ridges that distinguish it from any other chinchilla (Kraft 1987). Their dental formula is 2 (I1/1, C0/0, PM1/1, M3/3) = 20 (Quesenberry & Carpenter 2004).

The stomach is located in the abdominal cavity behind the diaphragm. It is similar in shape to that of a horse or pig. The duodenum has several afferent ducts from the pancreas as well as the bile duct. The longest portion of the small intestine is the jejunum and, in conjunction with sections of the large intestine, it takes up a large portion of the abdominal cavity. The ileum is the shortest section of small bowel that makes up the transition to the cecum. The cecum in chinchillas is similar to that in other rodents; it is located on the left side of the abdomen and under normal conditions, its contents are of liquid consistency. The cecum and the ascending colon help to fill the remainder of the abdomen, as it is the segment with the greatest volume. The ascending portion of the colon is also the longest section of the large bowel. The descending portion of the bowel and the rectum are usually filled with compact fecal matter and can be easily palpated if the animal is relaxed. It is difficult to determine the end of the colon and the beginning of the rectum. The end of the rectum widens slightly before reaching the anus. The posterior end of the rectum is surrounded by glandular packets; these packets in females appear to be thicker ventrally. In males, these packets are twice the

Exotic Animal Medicine for the Veterinary Technician, Fourth Edition. Edited by Bonnie Ballard and Ryan Cheek.
© 2024 John Wiley & Sons, Inc. Published 2024 by John Wiley & Sons, Inc.
Companion Website: www.wiley.com/go/ballard/4e

Table 19.1 Biological values for chinchillas.

Life span	10–15 years (up to 22 years reported)
Adult weight	450–900 g
Rectal temperature	94.8–100.2°F
Heartrate	200–300 bpm
Respiratory rate	40–80 breaths/min

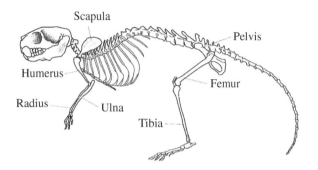

Figure 19.1 Skeletal anatomy. (Drawing by Scott Stark.)

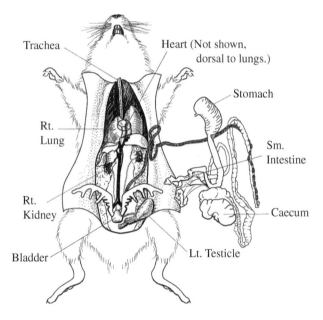

Figure 19.2 Visceral anatomy (Drawing by Scott Stark.)

circumference of the female packets. The skeletal anatomy is shown in Figure 19.1; the visceral anatomy is shown in Figure 19.2.

Liver

The liver is located between the diaphragm and stomach. There is very little lobulation visible and the gallbladder is located between the right and median sides. In the adult chinchilla, the liver weighs about 8–10 g (Kraft 1987).

Pancreas

In the chinchilla, the pancreas can be difficult to locate because it has many lobes. In addition, the surrounding fatty tissue and lymph nodes can make it difficult to distinguish with the naked eye.

Spleen

The spleen is of similar shape and location to other rodents. It is triangular in cross-section and the shape of an "L." The bottom of the "L" is located near the last rib on the left side.

Respiratory Tract

Starting with the head of the chinchilla, the first portion of the respiratory tract visualized is the nostrils. To the outside of each narrow, nostril is a "false" nostril. The nasal cavities arch upward and are interconnected along the upper portion. The chinchilla's nasal cavity is very large for an animal of this size. The trachea is dorsoventrally compressed as it moves down toward the lungs. The trachea splits at the level of the fourth and fifth vertebrae, descending toward the lungs. The right lung has four distinct lobes and the left only three.

Reproductive Organs

Female sex organs (ovaries) are located just below each kidney and are very small, about the size of a grain of rice. As the female reaches maturity, small lumps appear on the ovary, giving it an unusual shape. These lumps are caused by eggs migrating to the surface of the ovary. Several eggs mature at the same time, which means that several eggs can be fertilized at the same time. Unlike other mammals, as the eggs migrate down the oviduct they do not go into the ovarian pouch. They remain in the wall of the pouch where they are fertilized. After fertilization, the eggs move via peristaltic action to the uterus. The reproductive tract ends with the vagina, which becomes very visible when the animal is in heat. It is visualized as a horizontal slit between the anus and the urethra. Unlike many other mammals, the urethra of the female chinchilla terminates outside the vagina. There are no labial folds present.

The male sex organs are somewhat different from most other mammals. The testicles do not descend down into the scrotum and are considered incomplete. Only the epididymis is located outside the abdominal cavity and there is no scrotum. The sperm cells mature in the epididymis before they move to the sperm duct, and from there they move across the mesentery of the urinary bladder. The sperm ducts open right next to each other into the urethra, along with the openings of the other sex glands. The penis is S-shaped when in the normal resting position, with the glans penis terminating below the anus. Because the foreskin extends all the way to the anus, the actual opening is very narrow. A small bone about 1 cm long supports the penis during copulation. As blood fills the penis, pushing the tip forward, small backward-facing spines can be seen. These ensure better attachment during copulation.

Urinary Tract

The chinchilla's urinary system is similar to that of other mammals, in that it has two kidneys, two ureters, a bladder, and a urethra.

Anal Sacs

Located just inside the lower corner of the anal slit is a yellow nodular anal sac. Similar to dogs and cats, the chinchilla can expel the contents of this sac. It is a foul-smelling substance, which is probably used as a defense against natural enemies.

Reproduction

The following are average numbers for the different species of chinchillas:

First "heat": 3–4 months of age
Gestation period: 110–138 days
Number of young: one to three per pregnancy
Number of litters: one or two per year
Young: born precocial

The female returns to heat every 25–35 days if she does not conceive. The most reliable method of determining if the female is in heat is the behavior of the male (Johnson-Delaney 1996; Kraft 1987).

Husbandry

Because the chinchilla's normal habitat is the Andes Mountains in South America, it does not tolerate heat or humidity. Therefore, they should not be housed in a location where there is no protection from the heat. The enclosure should be large and made of material that they cannot chew through. The enclosure must have ample hiding places to mimic the caves that wild chinchillas live in. It is in their nature to jump, so it is recommended that the enclosure have multiple levels; small platforms on which they can perch are also helpful. All items should be made of materials that are easily cleaned.

Suitable bedding includes aspen shavings, newspaper, or recycled newspaper products. Because of their aromatic oils, pine and cedar shavings are not recommended and can lead to respiratory issues (Mitchell & Tully 2009).

Although chinchillas tend to keep their enclosure cleaner in comparison to most hindgut fermenters by defecating and urinating less frequently, the cage should still be cleaned at least once a week.

Chinchillas have hypsodont teeth, meaning they grow constantly. Objects for gnawing create great enrichment and allow for the teeth to maintain a more natural length. Branches, wood blocks, pumice stones, and salt blocks are all good choices.

The most specific requirement for chinchilla care is making a "dust bath" available on a daily basis. This helps to keep the coat and skin healthy. There are several commercial dust baths on the market. The bath mixture should be dry before allowing the chinchilla to use it. The mixture of choice should be placed about 1 to 2 inches deep in the bottom of a litter box, large bowl, or glass jar (one gallon or larger).

Nutrition

Chinchillas are herbivorous hindgut fermenters with a monogastric simple stomach. As in other rodents, chinchillas are coprophagic Because their digestive tract is similar to that of horses, the majority of their diet should consist of hay. In captivity, a diet of hay supplemented with a good quality pelleted diet should be offered. Pellets that have 16–20% protein, 2–5% fat, and 15–35% bulk fiber should be obtained for feeding (Quesenberry & Carpenter 2004). If the amount of hay is inadequate, the low amount of fiber may lead to enteritis. The quality of the hay must be monitored closely. Small amounts of fruits, vegetables, seeds, and grains may be offered as treats. Finally, as with all animals, fresh water must be made available at all times. Chinchillas, because they are so active, can be messy when it comes to water bowls. They will either knock them over or manage to get substrate in them. A water bottle is a preferable way to provide water because it keeps the water and cage cleaner (Quesenberry & Carpenter 2004).

Common and Zoonotic Diseases

Dental Diseases

A common problem in chinchillas is "slobbers," or malocclusion (Hayes 2000). This can occur in the incisors, premolars, or molars. As the teeth overgrow, they cause ulcers of the buccal mucosa and the tongue. Clinical signs

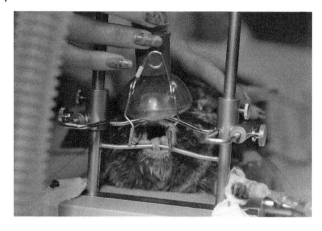

Figure 19.3 Chinchilla receiving a dental examination using an endoscope.

may be drooling, pawing at the mouth, weight loss, poor coat condition, anorexia, a decrease in stool volume, constipation, soiled or wet fur around mouth, chin, and forefeet, and lethargy (Mayer & Donnelly, 2013). Malocclusion can be caused by hereditary factors or a lack of objects in the environment to gnaw on. Since chinchilla teeth are open-rooted, meaning they continuously grow, routine teeth trimmings may be necessary in cases of hereditary problems. (See Figure 19.3.)

Skin Diseases

Poor husbandry is the leading cause of skin disorders in chinchillas. Bite wounds, traumatic injuries, fur chewing, fur slip, and unthrifty coat can all occur when the environmental conditions are poor. These disorders can appear rapidly if chinchillas are housed in a cage that is too small or if two incompatible animals are housed together. The animals may chew on themselves or their cage mates, which may lead to other injuries. Inadequate access to a dust bath may also cause a poor coat quality. Alopecia can also occur secondary to dental disease and hypersalivation (Mayer & Donnelly 2013).

Dermatophytosis is a disease usually caused by the introduction of contaminated hay or bedding to the chinchilla's housing. As in other species, scaly, circular areas of hair loss around the face, feet, and ears are the most common presentation. A skin scrape and fungal culture should be performed to confirm the diagnosis. This disease has zoonotic potential.

Gastrointestinal Diseases

Choke

Like rabbits and rats, chinchillas cannot vomit. Esophageal choke can result if the animal ingests an object too large to swallow. The most common objects are bedding and treats. The animal usually presents with excessive salivation, dyspnea, and anorexia. The object may be palpated on physical examination or diagnosed with diagnostic imaging.

Bloat

Bloat can occur for many reasons including inappropriate diet or sudden change in diet, dental disease, unkempt cage, stress, or pain (Mayer & Donnelly 2013). The chinchilla presents similarly to other animals with a distended and painful abdomen, dyspnea, and reluctance to move. Many treatments are recommended, from exercise in mild cases to decompression by transabdominal trocar.

Hairballs

Hairballs can occur in chinchillas just like they do in rabbits. They are usually caused by low dietary fiber in combination with excessive fur chewing. The animal usually presents with lethargy, reluctance to move, and anorexia. The hairball may be palpated on physical examination or diagnosed with contrast radiographs or fluoroscopy.

Enteritis

Proper diet for chinchillas is one of the most important factors when discussing their care. An improper diet can be one of the most likely causes of enteritis, although a sudden diet change may also be a factor (Hayes 2000; Kraft 1987; Ritchey et al. 2004). If the animal is not offered hay, if the hay is of poor quality, or if the animal is eating a large amount of pellets or fruit and green vegetables, this may cause a change in the normal flora and fauna of the gastrointestinal tract. The motility of the gut and the fermentation process may also be altered, leading to an overgrowth of pathogenic bacteria. Other less common causes of enteritis are parasitic infection and prolonged or inappropriate use of antibiotics (Hayes 2000; Lightfoot 1999). Animals may present with anorexia and bloating. Those who have had chronic enteritis may present with constipation, impactions, intussusceptions, and rectal prolapse.

Determining the cause may be difficult because of the multiple factors involved. Radiographs, fecal flotation for parasites, and fecal cultures may be needed to determine an etiology. Symptomatic treatment is usually best with fluid therapy, antibiotics, and anti-parasitics given as indicated.

Constipation

In most cases, owners feed a diet of pellets almost exclusively, which can lead to many of the problems stated before. The pelleted diets are high in protein as well as calories but are low in fiber. This low-fiber diet can also lead to constipation, which may be seen more often than diarrhea (Hayes 2000; Kraft 1987; Johnson-Delaney 1996). Clinical signs are straining to defecate and fecal pellets that may be small, hard, and in some cases bloodstained. Treatment involves slowly increasing the amount of fiber in the chinchilla's diet by feeding a small amount of fresh vegetables or high-quality grass hay.

Respiratory Diseases

Chinchillas are susceptible to pneumonia; however, these cases usually occur when there are large numbers of animals housed together and the husbandry is poor (Kraft 1987). Most pet owners should not have any problems in this area. Clinical signs include depression, dyspnea, and a nasal discharge. The treatment protocol includes antibiotics administered by nebulization if conditions allow.

Neurologic Diseases

Chinchillas are highly susceptible to *Listeria monocytogenes* infection; however, it is unlikely that pet chinchillas would be exposed (Hayes 2000). Ataxia and circling are usually followed by convulsions and death. Treatment protocols have been ineffective once clinical signs are noticed.

Penile Disorders

Male chinchillas are susceptible to developing penile disorders that can either be an incidental finding on a normal physical examination or the cause of clinical disease. During a full physical examination, the penis should be manually everted from the prepuce.

"Fur ring," or accumulation of fur wrapped around the base of the penis, can be a common finding and should be gently removed if possible. Most penile diseases including balanoposthitis, infection of the prepuce and glans penis, and paraphimosis, swelling and inflammation of the prepuce and/or glans penis, can both be a secondary complication of a fur ring (Mayer & Donnelly 2013).

Heat Stroke

Chinchillas are very prone to heat stroke and should not be housed in temperatures over 80°F (26.7°C) with high humidity. A chinchilla's cage should be away from windows that provide direct sunlight as well as heater vents. Just as with any other pet, they should never be left in a car during hot weather. The treatment for this condition is the same as would be given to a dog or cat (Quesenberry & Carpenter 2004, Mitchell & Tully 2009).

Zoonotic Diseases

Pet chinchillas may be exposed to *Baylisascaris procyonis* in contaminated hay (Ness 1999). This nematode infects the cerebrospinal fluid, causing ataxia, torticollis, and paralysis. There is no treatment for this condition and there is zoonotic potential for anyone handling the contaminated bedding and feed. Strict hygiene practices, including wearing gloves and washing hands, should be followed.

While not common, dermatophytosis has been diagnosed in chinchillas. It is treated with oral or topical medications just as in dogs and cats. And also just as in dogs and cats, this disease poses a zoonotic risk for the owner. Owners should be instructed to wear gloves when treating their pets and cleaning their cages. Children should not handle their pets during treatment.

Salmonellosis has occurred in fur-production herds of chinchillas, but healthy chinchillas have had *Salmonella* isolated from them as well. It is not recommended that clinically normal chinchillas be treated, but owners should practice strict hygiene when handling them (Mitchell & Tully 2009).

Behavior

Chinchillas are naturally nocturnal but may be active during daylight hours. They have become popular as pets because of their inquisitive personality, gentle nature, and the fact that they rarely bite. They are very entertaining to watch because of their athletic nature and, if given the materials to do so, will jump high in the air to reach a ledge or run around the walls of their enclosure. Their level of activity does not seem to diminish with age. Because by nature their means of defense is flight, they are very fast on their feet. If a chinchilla is allowed to get loose in a house, they will be a challenge to catch.

Taking the History and Performing the Physical Examination

An accurate history is vital when working with chinchillas because husbandry is often the most significant factor. These animals can be difficult to handle, because they are very quick and agile, and in most cases do not want to be touched. A good preliminary examination should be done prior to actually handling the animal. A visual examination may be performed if the owner has brought the pet in a wire cage. If not, then placing the chinchilla on the floor of the examination room and allowing it to move around normally is the best option. One should be sure that all doors are closed, because they are very curious about their surroundings. A healthy chinchilla should be alert with bright eyes and a twitching nose. It may breathe rapidly, but it should not breathe with an open mouth.

The tail should be erect and its hair coat should be thick, soft, and smooth.

Handling and Restraint

Chinchillas can be very difficult to restrain and should be handled with care. Because they are very excitable and nervous, handling a sick or debilitated patient can pose a challenge. The base of the tail and hind legs should be held gently with one hand while the other hand supports the chest and shoulders (Figures 19.4 and 19.5). Some patients may be easier to handle if allowed to hide their face in the bend of the handler's elbow. Making the patient feel secure is of the utmost importance; if not, they may attempt to jump from the handler's grasp. If this is the case, sitting on the floor while completing the examination may be necessary. This allows for better support and, if the chinchilla does get away, it will not fall and sustain a traumatic injury. If the patient is frightened while being restrained, it may

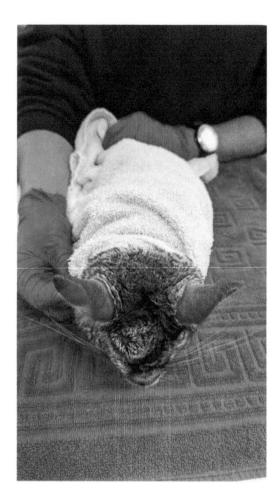

Figure 19.5 The technician is restraining the chinchilla for an oral and aural examination.

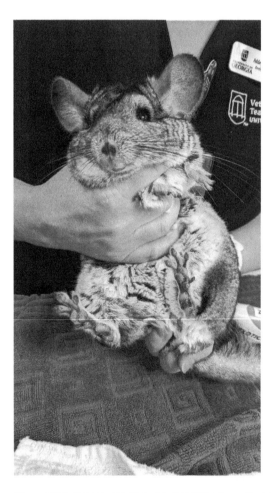

Figure 19.4 Proper restraint of a chinchilla for a physical examination.

release a large portion of fur in areas where it is being held. This is called a "fur-slip" (Lightfoot 1999). This can also occur due to rough handling and scruffing the patient. Great care should be taken while handling chinchillas as clients are very aware of "fur slip" and do not appreciate their pet losing fur during an exam.

Once the patient is comfortably restrained, the examination can begin. The average weight of a chinchilla is 400–600 g, with the male usually being smaller than the female (Johnson-Delaney 1996; Lightfoot 1999). The temperature can be taken rectally; however, an ear thermometer is less stressful and is usually accurate enough for a healthy physical examination (Figure 19.6). If the patient is very ill, then a rectal temperature will give the most accurate reading. The normal temperature is 97–102°F (36–39°C) (Johnson-Delaney 1996; Lightfoot 1999). The heart rate and respiratory rate can be obtained by normal means. The normal heart rate is 200–350 beats/min and the normal respiratory rate is 40–80 breaths/min (Johnson-Delaney 1996; Lightfoot 1999).

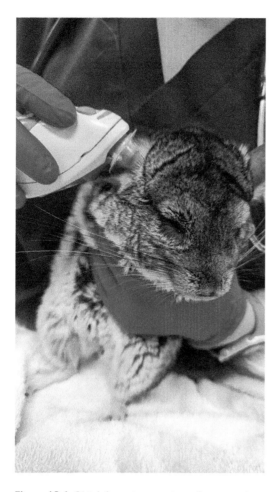

Figure 19.6 Obtaining a temperature via an ear thermometer.

Radiology

Diagnostic imaging is most easily obtained if the animal is sedated or anesthetized. Imaging that includes a contrast study such as magnetic resonance imaging (MRI) and computed tomography (CT), may require heavier sedation via intravenous or intraosseous catheter placement.

Anesthesia and Surgery

Chinchillas may need heavy sedation or anesthesia for a multitude of minor and surgical procedures. Chinchillas are extremely difficult to intubate due to a narrow palatial ostium formed by the soft pallet, palatoglossal arches, and tongue (Johnson 2010). Intubation without visualization via endoscope is not recommended due to potential trauma associated with blind intubation, which can lead to epiglottal edema and dyspnea. Therefore, gas anesthesia is often maintained via facemask (Figure 19.7). Injectable anesthetic protocols are preferred for venipuncture, diagnostic

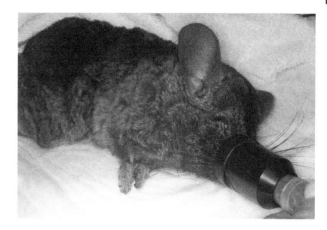

Figure 19.7 Isoflurane anesthesia by mask with a rodent circuit.

imaging, catheter placement, and minor procedures. While keeping the triad of anesthesia in mind, creating an anesthetic protocol with a combination of analgesia, amnesia, and muscle relaxation drugs is preferred.

Combinations of drugs that may be used include but are not limited to; alfaxalone/midazolam/buprenorphine, dexmetatomidine/ketamine, alfaxalone/butorphanol, midazolam/butorphanol/ketamine (Parkinson & Mans 2017). Meloxicam, butorphanol, buprenorphine, and oxymorphone have been used as analgesic agents in chinchillas (Hawkins and Pascoe, 2021).

Parasitology

Fecal flotations and direct smears should be performed, although intestinal parasites are uncommon in chinchillas. Depending on the organism, the patient may be asymptomatic or present with diarrhea. Protozoal infestations by *Trichomonas* spp., *Balantidium* spp., *Cryptosporidium*, and *Eimeria chinchillae* may occur. The latter is the chinchilla coccidian that has been shown to be transmissible to other rodents. Nematode infestations by *Physoloptera* and *Haemonchus contortus* have been reported. It is also possible for chinchillas to have flea infestations, so they may also have tapeworms, usually *Hymeolepsis nana* (Ness 1999). One unusual aspect of the life cycle is that the same animal can be the intermediate and permanent host.

Urinalysis

Normal urine values are as follows:

Color: yellow to slightly red
Turbidity: most often cloudy
pH: 8.5
Protein: negative to trace
Glucose: negative

Ketones: negative
Bilirubin: negative
Urobilinogen: 0.1–1 ng/dL
Nitrates: negative
Blood: negative
Specific gravity: usually >1.045

During a urine sediment examination of a normal chinchilla, some calcium carbonate crystals may be found along with amorphous debris. Casts, bacteria, erythrocytes, and leukocytes are rare in a normal patient, but occasional squamous epithelial cells are common (Ness 1999).

Emergency and Critical Care

Most of the diseases and ailments discussed previously are not considered emergencies. However, in the case of an emergency with a chinchilla, protocols similar to those of other small mammals should be followed. For example, an IV catheter can be very helpful in an emergency as well as in a critically ill patient. Once the patient has been stabilized, a calm and quiet environment is very important for the recovery process.

Sex Determination

Determining the sex of a chinchilla can be challenging, especially in young animals. The testicles can be visualized in adult males but the lack of a scrotum can make this more of a challenge. The fact that the clitoris, because of its size and shape, can often be mistaken for a penis provides another obstacle when sexing chinchillas. The location of the penis versus the clitoris can often be the determining factor because the distance from the rectum to the penis is greater than that of the clitoris.

Clinical Techniques

Venipuncture

For a procedure of this nature, it is preferable to have a chinchilla anesthetized or heavily sedated. There are several sites for venipuncture; the jugular vein being the most common site, and it allows larger blood volumes to be obtained. There are five other sites for venipuncture: the cephalic, saphenous, femoral, lateral abdominal, and tail veins (Figure 19.8).

The process for collecting blood from the jugular is as follows (Ness 1999).

1. Place the patient in sternal recumbency.
2. Extend the head and neck to make the lateral aspect of the lower cervical region accessible.

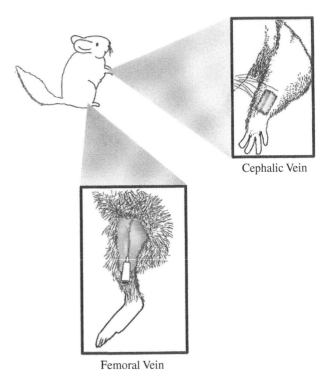

Figure 19.8 Venipuncture sites. (Drawing by Scott Stark.)

3. Apply gentle pressure to one side of the thoracic inlet to occlude the vessel.
4. Wet the area with an alcohol swab and visualize the distended vein.
5. Using a 23- to 25-gauge needle attached to a 1 to 3 mL syringe, insert the needle into the vein at approximately a 45° angle.
6. Draw back slowly if using a 3 mL syringe so as not to collapse the vein.

A 25- to 27-gauge needle on a 0.5 to 1 mL syringe should be used to collect samples from the other sites mentioned above. The femoral and cephalic veins are the most commonly used of those mentioned.

Intravenous Catheter Placement

The cephalic and lateral saphenous veins are the most common sites used for catheter placement (Figure 19.9). The procedures are the same as in any other small animal (see the "Techniques" section in Chapter 16). Note that a small cutdown may not be necessary, but some intact males may have tougher skin.

Intraosseous Catheter Placement

While in most cases, the chinchilla's peripheral veins are readily accessible; in an emergency, it may be necessary to

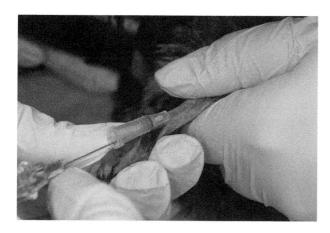

Figure 19.9 24 gauge catheter placement in the left cephalic vein.

place an intraosseous catheter. If the patient is moribund, sedation or anesthesia may not be an option. However, analgesia or local anesthesia is always recommended when placing a very painful intraosseous catheter. The steps for placement are as follows:

1. Locate the site for placement of the catheter. The two sites used in chinchillas are the femur or tibia. The femur is preferred due to its size and location, so this one will be discussed.
2. Locate a syringe needle or spinal needle with a metal stylet of the largest bore possible for the patient (usually 22 gauge is sufficient). A syringe of heparinized flush will also be needed.
3. Clip and surgically prepare the site.
4. Once the site has been prepared, the greater trochanter should be palpated and stabilized for insertion of the needle. The needle is then inserted and with a gentle twisting motion, advanced slowly. The needle should continue to be advanced through the bone and into the marrow cavity. Aspiration with the flush syringe, until blood is visualized in the hub, should be performed. It should be flushed quickly because the marrow can clog the needle.

5. The needle should be secured with tape, and in some cases, it may need to be sutured in place to provide more stability.
6. This catheter may be used for up to 72 h, after which a replacement in another location will be required.

Once the catheter is in place, great care must be taken to maintain it. Its location may inhibit normal movement and cause some discomfort. This in turn may cause the patient to attempt to remove the catheter by chewing or rubbing.

Administration of Medication

In the event that medications need to be given, there are several routes of administration. As with many other exotics, one must make sure to downsize the equipment and the volume of medications used.

Per os: Medication is usually liquid and can be given by needleless syringe on the side of the mouth just behind the incisors.
Subcutaneous: 23- to 25-gauge needle under the skin in the flank or neck area.
Intravenous: 25- to 28-gauge needle, preferably an insulin syringe in the lateral saphenous or cephalic vein.
Intramuscular: 23- to 25-gauge needle with no more than 0.3 mL/site. Recommended sites include the semimembranosus, quadriceps, and semitendinosus muscles (Ness 1999).

Euthanasia

As with most other small animals, the preferred method of euthanasia is lethal injection. If an IV catheter has been placed in the cephalic vein, it can be used for administration of the euthanasia solution. If a catheter is not available, either an IV or intracardiac injection (after the animal is anesthetized) with a syringe may be used. It is frequently easiest to first use isoflurane or sevoflurane to anesthetize the patient and then follow up with injectable euthanasia solution.

References

Hawkins MG, Pascoe PJ. 2021. Anesthesia, analgesia, and sedation of small mammals. In: *Ferrets, Rabbits and Rodents: Clinical Medicine and Surgery*, 4th edn. p. 552. St Louis, MO: Elsevier.

Hayes PM. 2000. *Diseases of Chinchillas*. Philadelphia: W.B. Saunders Co.

Johnson DH. 2010. Endoscopic intubation of exotic companion mammals. *Vet Clin North Am Exot Anim Pract* 13(2): 273–89.

Johnson-Delaney CA. 1996. *Exotic Companion Medicine Handbook for Veterinarians*. Lake Worth, FL: Wingers Publications.

Kraft H. 1987. *Diseases of Chinchillas*. Neptune City: T.F.H. Publications.

Lightfoot TL. 1999. Clinical examination of chinchillas, hedgehogs, prairie dogs, and sugar gliders. *Vet Clin North Am Exot Anim Pract* 2(2): 447–454.

Mayer J, Donnelly T. 2013. *Clinical Veterinary Advisor: Birds and Exotic Pets*. St. Louis, MO: W.B. Saunders Co.

Mitchell M, Tully T. 2009. *Manual of Exotic Pet Practice*. St. Louis, MO: W.B. Saunders Co.

Ness RD. 1999. Clinical pathology and sample collection of exotic small animals. *Vet Clin North Am Exot Anim Pract* 2(3): 591–619.

Parkinson L, Mans C. 2017. Anesthetic and postanesthetic effects of alfaxalone–butorphanol compared with dexmedetomidine–ketamine in chinchillas (*Chinchilla lanigera*). *J Am Assoc Lab Anim Sci* 56(3): 290–295.

Quesenberry K, Carpenter J. 2004. *Ferrets, Rabbits, and Rodents:Clinical Medicine and Surgery*. St. Louis, MO: W.B. Saunders Co.

Ritchey L, Cogswell EL, Cogswell M. 2004. *Joy of Chinchillas*. Self published.

20

Guinea Pigs

Liz Vetrano

Introduction

The domestic guinea pig, *Cavia porcellus*, is a hystricomorphic rodent indigenous to South America. Also called cavies, guinea pigs were first domesticated between 500 and 1000 AD. Historically, guinea pigs, or *cuy*, were raised by the Incas for food and use in religious ceremonies (Pignon and Mayer 2021). They were brought to Europe about 500 years ago. They remain a food source today in South America, specifically in the Andean mountains (Pignon and Mayer 2021).

Common Types

Today guinea pigs are a common laboratory and companion animal. Their popularity in research is declining, however, due to the use of genetically engineered rodent models and alternative live-animal models (Pritt 2012). In Europe and North America, pet guinea pigs are increasing in popularity due to their small size and docile nature. The American Cavy Breeders Association recognizes 13 breeds of guinea pigs with a variety of coat colors. Those guinea pig breeds most commonly seen in companion animal practice are the American or English, the Abyssinian, and the Peruvian. English cavies have a short, smooth hair coat (Figure 20.1), while Abyssinians (Figure 20.2) have a short, rough hair coat with rosettes along the shoulders, sides, and back, and Peruvians have a long, smooth hair coat that requires regular grooming. Some hairless breeds are also popular including the skinnies who only have hair on their head and lower legs (Capello & Lennox 2012).

Anatomy and Physiology

A member of the Caviidae family, the guinea pig has a short, stocky, tailless body, with hairless pinnae (Harkness et al.

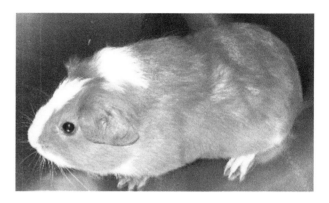

Figure 20.1 American guinea pig with a smooth hair coat. (Courtesy of Jill Murray.)

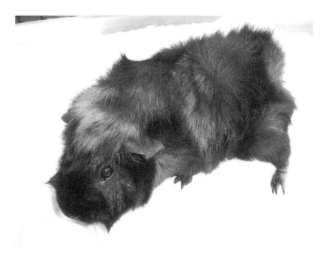

Figure 20.2 Abyssinian guinea pig, showing rosettes in hair coat. (Courtesy of Jill Murray.)

2010). Males are larger than females and typically average 900–1200 grams in body weight, compared to 700–900 grams for females. Obesity is very common in guinea pigs (Pignon and Mayer 2021). They have four digits on their forefeet and three on their hindfeet. Guinea pigs have large tongues, a small, narrow oral cavity, and fleshy cheek folds that invaginate the oral cavity, obscuring visualization. Like all rodents, they are monophyodont, with an elodont (continuously growing) dentition, and aradicular (rootless) cheek teeth (Yarto-Jaramillo 2011). The incisors are normally white in the healthy animal, unlike most rodents (Yarto-Jaramillo 2011). The dental formula is 2(*I* 1/1, *C* 0/0, *P* 1/1, *M* 3/3) = 20 (Harkness et al. 2010). The maxillary cheek teeth of guinea pigs have a palatal convexity, and the mandibular cheek teeth have a buccal convexity, which in severe cases may result in tongue entrapment. This results in a 30° oblique occlusal plane of the cheek teeth, with shorter crowns compared to the rabbit (Capello & Lennox 2012; O'Malley 2005). The soft palate is continuous with the base of the tongue forming a membranous covering of the posterior pharynx. Food, water, and air pass through an opening called the palatal ostium (Hawkins & Pascoe 2021; Yarto-Jaramillo 2011). The larynx lies dorsally within the oropharynx, in close association with the nasopharynx, making them obligate nasal breathers. This, combined with the small size of the oral cavity, challenges orotracheal intubation and predisposes guinea pigs to respiratory disease (Yarto-Jaramillo 2011).

Guinea pigs are monogastric hindgut fermenters. They have a large cecum occupying the center and left side of the abdomen, containing about 65% of the gastrointestinal contents (Harkness et al. 2010). Unlike rabbits, guinea pigs do not practice cecotrophy. They are still coprophagic; however, the nutritional benefit of this practice is still not well understood. Rabbits benefit by ingesting more Vitamin B and protein. Guinea pigs still require 7–10 Vitamin B dietary sources daily. When coprophagy is prevented, the guinea pig experiences difficulty digesting fiber, weight loss, and more minerals are excreted in the feces. The gastrointestinal transit time (excluding coprophagy) is approximately 20 hours (Harkness et al. 2010). When coprophagy is factored in, GI transit time can take as long as 66 hours (Pignon and Mayer 2021). The gastrointestinal flora is primarily Gram-positive and anaerobic.

Boars have an os penis and open inguinal canals allowing them to retract their testicles into the abdominal cavity. Sows possess two uterine horns and a single os cervix opening into the vagina (Trewin & Hutz 1998). Both species possess a single pair of inguinal mammae (Harkness et al. 2010; O'Malley 2005). A thin membrane covers the vagina except during estrus and parturition. The pubic symphysis is fibrocartilaginous and is capable of separating during parturition. Failing to breed the sow prior to 7 months of age increases the risks of dystocia as the pubic symphysis is less able to separate.

Other anatomic characteristics of note in the guinea pig include their large tympanic bullae; large, bilobed

Table 20.1 Physiologic data for the guinea pig.

Physiologic data	Range
Lifespan	5–7 years
Average adult weight (M/F)	900–1,200 g/700–900 g
Sexual maturity	Males: 3 months; Females: 2 months
Estrous cycle length	15–17 days
Ovulation	Spontaneous
Gestation period	63–68 days
Litter size	2–4 pups
Normal birth weight	45–115 g
Weaning age	21 days
Respiratory rate per minute	40–120 rpm
Heart rate	240–310 bpm
Rectal temperature (°F)	99.0–103.1 (37.2–39.5 °C)
Average blood volume	70 mL/kg

Source: Adapted from Quesenberry (2021), p. 271.

adrenal glands; and functional thymus (Harkness et al. 2010) (Table 20.1).

Sex Determination

Anogenital distance can be a reliable method for sexing many rodents; however, it is not reliable for sexing guinea pigs. To determine a guinea pig's gender, gently restrain the animal and examine the external genitalia. In the female, the genital area will have a "Y" shape. The male will have more of a straight slit. Intact adult males will possess testes, although retraction into the abdominal cavity is possible. Applying gentle pressure caudally and cranially to the genitals will cause extrusion of the penis in the male animal for confirmation of sex (Harkness et al. 2010).

Behavior

Guinea pigs are docile animals that with gentle handling and petting, can become quite affectionate and responsive pets (Bays et al. 2006). It is essential to become familiar with their common behaviors. Recognizing and educating clients on how to do this as well, will be beneficial when abnormal behaviors come to light. This may indicate the early stages of a medical condition or behavioral a concern. They are highly social and prefer group housing. In the wild, they live in small social groups, and bonding amongst guinea pigs has been shown to be very important for domestic pets (Bays et al. 2006). It is important to note, however, that over-crowding, aggressive breeding, and animals introduced later in life may have increased risk of intraspecies aggression. Most intraspecies aggression can occur when intact males are in the presence of females or when the pigs have not been raised together. It is essential to hold introductions in a neutral territory with adult supervision (Bays et al. 2006). Switching enclosures and allowing them to familiarize themselves with each other's scent is another tactic. Ovariohysterectomies and castrations can also limit hormonal influence of behaviors, thus making introductions easier, and eliminate the possibility of reproduction (Bays et al. 2006).

Guinea pigs produce a wide variety of vocalization patterns that have been categorized into 11 distinct call types (Harkness et al. 2010). Often, cavies will vocalize in response to hearing their food being prepared and in social interactions with other guinea pigs and their owners. Some common sounds include chutting, which indicates curiosity, grunting, which can indicate a mating sound of arousal or can be associated with anger, or squealing which can signal fear, pain, or hunger (Bays et al. 2006). When frightened or excited, guinea pigs may "stampede" around their enclosure, trampling anything in their way. Another typical fear response is to suddenly freeze and remain immobile for a brief period of time (Harkness et al. 2010).

Behavioral enrichment is extremely important for domestic guinea pigs. This provides them with physical exercise, mental stimulation, and catering to their natural instincts. This can be accomplished by providing them with plenty of time outside of their enclosures. Physical exercise and allowing them to roam can decrease the chances of obesity and allow for exploration. A shallow plastic pool or portable folding pen can be transformed into a safe play area. Newspaper, PVC piping, tubes, cardboard, and sheets can be used to create tunnels. Hiding treats and greens amongst the tunnels and under newspaper will encourage natural foraging behaviors (Bays et al. 2006).

Biologic and Reproductive Data

Guinea pigs are polyestrous, breeding year-round. They reach sexual maturity at approximately 2 months of age for the boar and 3 months for the sow and a body weight of 350–400 grams (Trewin & Hutz 1998). The sow experiences a postpartum estrus of 2–15 hours and will likely become pregnant if mated (Harkness et al. 2010). Finding a copulatory plug in the bedding of the cage suggests breeding has occurred. This plug is an accumulation of secretions that will fall from the vagina shortly after breeding takes place. This plug is used to prevent semen from falling out and to prevent other boars from mating with the sow.

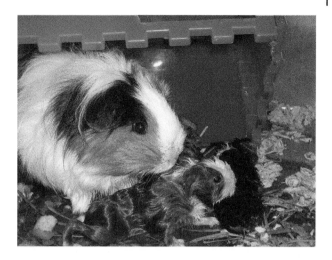

Figure 20.3 Guinea pig pups are precocious at birth. (Courtesy of Jill Murray.)

The gestation of the guinea pig averages 68 days, with a range of 59–72 days (Harkness et al. 2010; Trewin & Hutz 1998). Sows do not practice nest building like other rodents. Litters of two to four pups are typical, although larger litters are possible. Milk supply from the sow does not increase with demand, and therefore smaller litter sizes are desirable. Pups are precocious, born fully furred, with eyes open, and all teeth erupted (Figure 20.3).

Within a few hours of parturition, the pups are able to walk, and may begin eating solid food. Because they are eating solid foods, hand rearing is not as difficult as in altricial species, but they should be allowed to nurse from the sow for the first 3 weeks of life. Pups that do not receive sow's milk during the first 3–4 days of life often do not survive. Voluntary micturition does not occur until the second week of life and the sow must lick the pups' anogenital region to stimulate urination and defecation (Harkness et al. 2010).

Like the placenta of humans, guinea pig sows have a labyrinthine hemochorial placenta that has been well studied. The disk-shaped organ connects to the uterine wall and placental sac as the main fetal-maternal exchange organ. The pup receives all of its maternal antibody from the placenta and not from the colostrum. Concurrent blood flow through the placenta allows for more efficient transport of oxygen across the fetoplacental unit. The disk is composed of different zones to serve the fetal and maternal needs during gestation (Trewin & Hutz 1998) (Figure 20.4).

Husbandry

Guinea pigs require relatively simple caging with large floor space to allow for exercise and paired housing. Caging should be escape-proof, chew-proof, and be easily

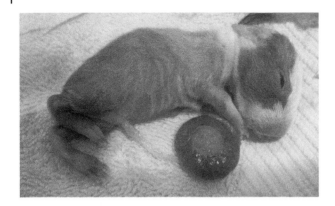

Figure 20.4 Hemochorial placenta of the guinea pig sow. (Courtesy of Jill Murray.)

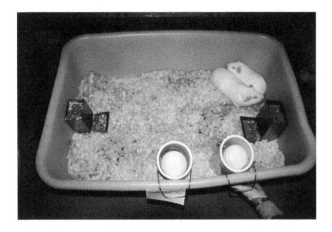

Figure 20.5 An appropriate housing setup for guinea pigs. (Courtesy of Ryan Cheek.)

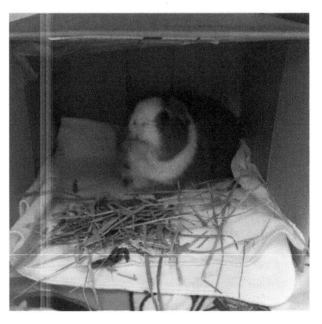

Figure 20.6 Guinea pig resting in a hide house during a hospital stay. (Courtesy of Liz Vetrano.)

cleaned. Being unable to jump, a cage with 25-cm (10-inch) walls is often sufficient to contain the bedding material and keep the guinea pig contained (Harkness et al. 2010). However, a cage with a secure lid is necessary if the owner has other pets that could be a potential threat to the guinea pig. Solid cage flooring is preferable to reduce the risks of injury and pododermatitis. A non-irritating, soft, non-aromatic substrate like recycled newspaper, yoga mats, or fleece should be provided to reduce the risk of pododermatitis and respiratory irritation. As with other rodents, guinea pigs are thigmotactic. They prefer to avoid open spaces, showing a preference for confined spaces, and should be provided with hide boxes (Hargaden & Singer 2012) (Figure 20.5 and Figure 20.6).

Guinea pigs are comfortable at a room temperature of about 65–79°F (18–26°C) (Harkness et al. 2010). Higher temperatures can increase risks of heat stress, while lower temperatures increase susceptibility to respiratory infection and other diseases as a result of immunosuppression. Owners should be cautioned to keep cages away from drafty areas, windows, and home heating sources. Good ventilation is essential to help reduce prevalence of respiratory diseases.

Water should be provided in a bottle with a sipper tube, as guinea pigs typically prefer this over bowls. The bottle and spout should be cleaned and evaluated regularly for patency and function. An improperly functioning water bottle should be replaced. Fresh water may need to be provided more frequently than for other rodents as guinea pigs tend to play with the sipper tube and spit food particles from their mouth back into the bottle (Harkness et al. 2010). Food should be provided in a weighted bowl to prevent spillage, waste, and contamination of foods with waste products. Fresh foods should be offered in a separate bowl.

Abyssinian and Peruvian guinea pigs will benefit from regular grooming as fecal pellets and bedding may become stuck in the long fur. Spot baths with a mild shampoo, followed by thorough rinsing can be given making sure to dry the animal thoroughly, and keep it warm.

Nutrition

Guinea pigs are strict herbivores who require a diet high in fiber to maintain appropriate hind-gut fermentation. The recommended daily diet for pet guinea pigs is a high-quality grass hay (ad lib), commercial guinea pig pellets (1/4 cup per healthy animal daily), and a small amount of fresh greens compromising no more than 10%

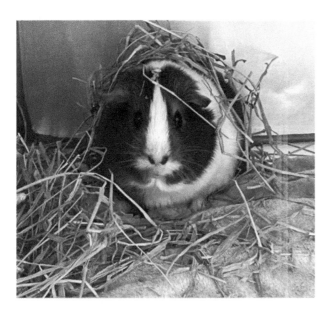

Figure 20.7 A variety of hay should be offered ad lib while in the hospital. (Courtesy of Liz Vetrano.)

of the daily diet (Figure 20.7). Fruits should be offered only as treats due to their high sugar content. Pellets should contain a minimum level of 10% crude protein. For growth and lactation, the pellets should contain 18–20% (Pignon and Mayer 2021). Guinea pigs digest fiber more efficiently than the rabbit. Food intake and satiety in the guinea pig are achieved through gastric distension as opposed to metabolic energy needs. Vegetables and fruits should be washed thoroughly prior to feeding to remove any pesticide residue. They should be removed from the cage after a few hours to prevent spoilage. Edible enrichment may also be provided, making sure to avoid those that are high in carbohydrates, fats, and sugars (Figure 20.7).

Lacking the enzyme, L-gulonolactone oxidase required for the synthesis of ascorbic acid (vitamin C) from glucose, guinea pigs require a daily exogenous source of vitamin C. Scurvy is a common condition in guinea pigs which is a result of not providing appropriate pellets or supplementation. Although commercial guinea pig pellets are fortified with vitamin C, most is oxidized or lost within 90 days of manufacturing (Gresham & Haines 2012). Pellets should be stored in a cool, dry, dark container to further reduce breakdown of vitamin C. Because of their instability, pellets should not be relied on as the sole source of vitamin C. Fresh vegetables, such as dark leafy greens, red and green peppers, broccoli, and small amounts of fresh fruits such as kiwi, oranges, and tomatoes, are good sources of ascorbic acid. Many Vitamin C-rich foods are also high in calcium or oxalates and should be offered in small amounts which can contribute to other conditions such as urinary calculi (Pignon and Mayer 2021). Commercial

vitamin C-enriched treats and tablets are also available for exogenous supplementation. Supplementation of vitamin C in the water is discouraged due to the instability of vitamin C in the environment, and the change in palatability of the water, potentially leading to dehydration in the animal. Non-breeding adults require 10–25 mg/kg of supplemental ascorbic acid daily, while growing and pregnant animals require higher levels of 30 mg/kg daily (Harkness et al. 2010; Pignon and Mayer 2021; Yarto-Jaramillo 2011).

Guinea pigs prefer to drink water from a nipple drinker than from a water bowl (Pignon and Mayer 2021).

History and Physical Examination

A complete physical exam and review of dietary practices and husbandry should be performed at least annually in the healthy guinea pig. A thorough patient history should be collected with any new patient, including the origin of the animal, detailed information pertaining to the patient's diet, husbandry practices, past medical history, and presenting complaints. History collection in existing patients may be tailored to the presenting complaint and any recommendations and changes made since previous visits.

Guinea pigs should be brought to the veterinary hospital in an enclosed transport carrier, protected from extreme temperatures and exposure to potential predators. In a busy and noisy clinic waiting room, clients and their pets should be placed in an exam room to reduce patient stress until the hospital staff can tend to the client and patient.

Unless medically urgent, the animal should be observed in the cage on presentation to better assess normal behaviors. Visual observation will provide information on appetite, fecal pellet production and quality, gait, stance, and overall attitude. Respiration rate should be the first vital observed prior to handling since this can increase the value. A healthy guinea pig will be engaging, inquisitive, vocal, active, and exhibiting a normal gait. A sick animal may mask signs of illness and disease initially, but may eventually hide, and/or appear tired and unwell.

Following the visual exam, the guinea pig may be systematically examined. The patient should be weighed on a gram scale to obtain an accurate body weight. While gently restraining the guinea pig, all vitals should be obtained. This includes a heart rate, respiratory rate, mentation, mucous membrane color (can be obtained by visualizing the gums or genitals), and rectal body temperature. The technician will need to restrain the guinea pig for a cursory examination of the oral cavity and the teeth; most animals resist oral examination, and the technician should be prepared for the patient to squirm and vocalize its objection.

Restraint

Guinea pigs are generally docile and respond better to gentle restraint (i.e., a "less is more" technique). Inappropriate handling can lead to stress and potential injury. Guinea pigs should never be scruffed, but should always be restrained with two hands, ensuring to support both the thorax and abdomen. Alternatively, the animal may be held along the arm of the restrainer against their body with the other hand placed on top of the animal to prevent falling or jumping. This method may be more comfortable for pregnant animals by avoiding any pressure on the abdomen. The guinea pig should be placed onto a towel for additional padding and to prevent slipping. The towel may also be used to gently wrap the guinea pig (like a burrito) to add more gentle restraint, especially during the oral exam (Figures 20.8 and 20.9).

Diagnostic sampling (imaging and blood work) may be collected with gentle manual restraint alone, but more commonly requires sedation or general anesthesia to expedite the procedure, reduce patient stress, and increase the success of sample collection. If the animal becomes stressed during restraint, the procedure should be aborted and alternative options for sample collection considered.

Radiology

Proper radiographic positioning typically includes whole body right lateral and ventral dorsal views (Capello et al. 2008; Silverman and Tell 2005). Whole-body views are usually achieved to reduce patient stress, although adding sedation is sometimes necessary to obtain proper

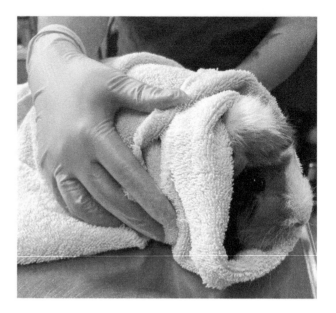

Figure 20.9 Guinea pig "burrito" towel restraint. (Courtesy of Liz Vetrano.)

positioning (Pignon and Mayer 2021). This can be achieved by either injectable sedation or light general anesthesia. This may be necessary if the patient is extremely stressed, compromised, or having another procedure performed (i.e., a molar trim). Abdominal ultrasounds are another diagnostically valuable tool. The patient will most likely have to be sedated to reduce movement and stress. Injectable sedation is typically adequate unless needle aspirates are required, in which case general anesthesia may be necessary (Pignon and Mayer 2021). Computed tomography (CT) scans have become increasingly more common to assess the entire body cavity and potential disease processes. Sedation is usually required to reduce movement artifact, especially when contrast is administered intravenously to enhance visualization of the internal organs.

Hematology

Guinea pigs have Kurloff cells which are large, mononuclear, granular lymphocytes that may be seen on evaluation of peripheral blood smears. They resemble a lymphocyte but contain oval or round inclusions known as Kurloff bodies (Campbell 2012). More commonly seen in reproductively active females, these cells are produced under estrogen stimulation by the thymus or spleen (Figure 20.10). Kurloff cells may also be seen in low numbers in boars and non-reproductive sows and are rarely seen in young animals (Campbell 2012). They are also found in the trophoblast region of the placenta (Hargaden & Singer 2012; Harkness et al. 2010).

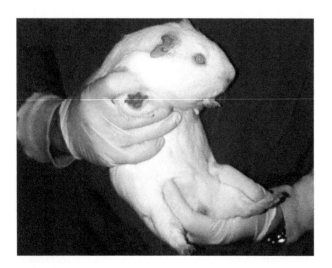

Figure 20.8 Proper guinea pig restraint. (Courtesy of Ryan Cheek.)

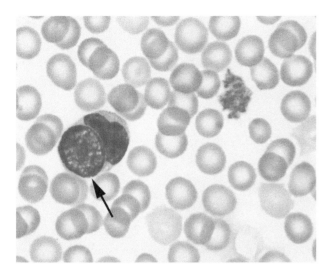

Figure 20.10 Kurloff cell seen in a peripheral blood smear of a sow. Inclusion is identified by the arrow. (Courtesy R. Cowell MRCVS, DABVP.)

Anesthesia, Surgery, and Analgesia

Anesthesia can be challenging in any small mammal, including rodents. Although difficult, it is important to provide appropriate care by performing pre-anesthetic examinations, determining an ASA status, and developing an appropriate anesthetic protocol in collaboration with a clinician. Unlike some other mammals, guinea pigs cannot vomit due to a lower esophageal sphincter, lack of emetic neurologic pathways, and limiting ridge of the stomach (Pignon and Mayer 2021). Prolonged fasting can lead to peri-anesthetic ileus, hypoglycemia, and a negative energy balance (Hawkins & Pascoe 2021). Many rodents, such as guinea pigs, are coprophagic and store feces and food in their oral cavities. Rinsing the mouth by gently syringing water and using cotton-tipped applicators is important to do while the patient is still awake and prior to sedation to reduce risk of aspiration (Pignon and Mayer 2021). "Boxing" or "gasing down" any patient is an outdated technique that can cause an increase in stress, pain, and inhibit the ability to reach and maintain an appropriate plane of anesthesia. There is a significant amount of literature supporting the use of injectable pre-anesthestics that allow for a smooth induction in addition to multimodal pain management. Examples of injectable pre-anesthetics used in guinea pigs include alfazalone, midazolam with an opioid or ketamine. There appears to be a less uniform response using ketamine with an alpha -2 agonist in guinea pigs. Because it may produce less than sufficient anesthesia, it should only be used for minor, less painful procedures (Hawkins and Pascoe, 2021).

Vascular access is essential for administration of fluid therapy, additional medications, and/or emergency medications (Pignon and Mayer 2021). Typical sites for catheterization include the cephalic and lateral saphenous. The author prefers the cephalic due to accessibility and better positioning. Depending on the patient's status, their already smaller vessels can be challenging to access. In these cases, intraosseous catheterization may be necessary. See Clinical Procedures for details on their placement.

Preoxygenation should be performed for 5 minutes via a facemask or oxygen cage prior to a gas inhalant, especially for patients with compromised respiratory function (Pignon and Mayer. 2021). After induction, the patient can be maintained on an inhalant gas anesthetic administered by a pediatric face mask and a non-rebreathing circuit (Hawkins & Pascoe 2021). Sevoflurane has a less pungent odor than the other inhalants and tends to take effect faster than isoflurane. All inhalants can cause respiratory and cardiovascular depression, which can be life-threatening (Pignon and Mayer 2021). It is important to keep the patient at the lightest plane possible to prevent death due to overdosing of an anesthetic. Premedications assist with the overall reduction of MAC of the inhalant. Due to the long soft palate, small size, and risks of laryngospasm, orotracheal intubation is not generally performed in private practice. When orotracheal intubation is needed, the use of visual aids (endoscope) greatly aids in intubation and reduces risks associated with blind intubation. Due to the small size of tracheal tubes, careful monitoring is needed to ensure the tube does not kink or obstruct with a mucus plug. This can be accomplished with a capnograph. Although anticholinergics will reduce the production of mucus, they also increase the viscosity of the mucoid secretions and subsequently increase the risk of mucoid plugs, making it harder to clear secretions. Due to guinea pigs being obligate nasal breathers, if intubation is not feasible, it is possible to administer possible pressure ventilation via a small facemask if there is a tight enough seal (Pignon and Mayer 2021).

Depth of anesthesia in most rodents can be evaluated partially by pinching of the toes or the ear for reaction to pain; however, there is concern that pedal reflexes may not be reliable depth indicators in guinea pigs and may actually indicate the animal is too deeply anesthetized. Slight corneal and palpebral reflexes are commonly maintained at a surgical plane of anesthesia in the guinea pig (Hawkins & Pascoe 2021). The patient's head and thorax should be slightly raised above the patient's abdomen to reduce the stress of the large abdomen resting on the patient's small thorax and restricting respiration (Yarto-Jaramillo 2011).

Any anesthetized patient should be closely monitored from induction through recovery. At a minimum, the patient's heart rate, respiratory rate and character, temperature, and anesthetic depth should be monitored. Additional anesthetic monitoring to include continuous electrocardiography (ECG) and pulse oximetry (SpO_2) can provide added information about the patient's circulatory and respiratory functions. Pediatric cuffs are available and can potentially be used for indirect blood pressure monitoring. Sometimes, these values can be challenging to obtain, but trends can still be monitored. Direct blood pressure would be more accurate; however, accomplishing arterial access is usually difficult. Hypothermia in a surgical patient can occur rapidly and be devastating. The use of forced-air warmers is preferred for thermal support in the anesthetized patient, while being cautious to carefully monitor the environmental and patient core temperature (Hawkins & Pascoe 2021). Due to their small size, their temperature can fluctuate rapidly. The author prefers Bair Huggers for appropriate heat support in small exotic species. The patient's eyes should be well lubricated to prevent corneal ulceration due to drying from the warm air. Direct heat sources (hot water bottle) should be used cautiously as they lead to vasodilation, resulting in increased heat loss, and can result in local burns.

The patient should be closely monitored on anesthetic recovery and in the perioperative period. Once adequately recovered, the patient may be placed in a small, single-level, solid wall enclosure for continued observation. Whenever possible, a temperature-controlled and oxygen-enriched incubator is ideal. Body temperature should still be monitored closely (especially since heat support is typically still necessary during recovery). Due to their small body size, their temperature should be recorded every 15–20 minutes until normothermic. Once the patient is stable, oriented to their environment, and able to ambulate unrestricted, a hide box, food, and water should be added to the enclosure. Care should be taken to ensure that food and water are easily accessible to the patient following surgery. The water bottle may need to be lowered and a shallow food bowl may be needed for easier access. The patient should be closely observed for pain, appetite, and fecal production. Syringe feedings with Oxbow Critical Care® should be administered once the patient is ambulatory and awake to decrease the chances of ileus by stimulating gut motility and increasing hydration. The cage and bedding should be kept clean and dry to prevent any surgical wound contamination.

Pre-emptive analgesia should be provided to the patient whenever pain is anticipated. Advantages of pre-emptive analgesia include anesthetic-sparing effects, improved anesthetic recovery, and reduced risk of complications

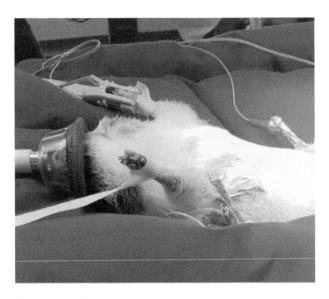

Figure 20.11 Guinea pig placed in ventrodorsal recumbency for an abdominal surgery. (Courtesy of Liz Vetrano.)

associated with pain (ileus, anorexia). Assessing pain in the rodent can be challenging as the animal may deliberately attempt to mask signs of pain to prevent unwanted attention from predators. Whenever possible, multimodal analgesia is preferred to enhance pain relief and allow the use of lower drug doses and subsequent decreased risk of administration (Miller & Richardson 2011). (Figure 20.11)

Analgesic agents that can be used in guinea pigs include buprenorphine, butorphanol, oxymorphone, and morphine. Meloxicam can also be used (Hawkins and Pascoe, 2021).

Urinalysis

A urine sample collected by cystocentesis may be needed if there are concerns of urinary calculi or cystitis. Whenever possible, the use of ultrasound to guide sample collection is preferred. The technique is the same as that described for small animals, although a smaller gauge needle (25-gauge) and sedation may be required (Harkness et al. 2010). Evaluation of a free-catch urine must be done with caution due to the high risk of environmental sample contamination.

Emergency and Critical Care

With the exception of acute trauma, most guinea pigs will present in an advanced state of illness following a prolonged state of disease that has gone mostly unnoticed by owner. This results from the animal's instinctive

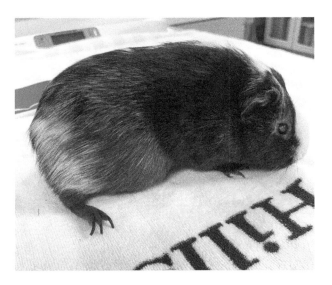

Figure 20.12 Guinea pig displaying abdominal pressing upon presentation through an emergency service. (Courtesy of Liz Vetrano.)

behavior, which is to mask signs of illness and disease in order to reduce risks of predation. Therefore, most ill animals presenting will likely be dehydrated, weak, and immunocompromised. The additional stress of transport and intervention may be further devastating. Whenever possible, the patient should be placed in an oxygen-enriched incubator, allowed to adapt to the environment and to recover from the stressors of travel prior to handling. In cases of life-threatening disease such as hemorrhage, seizure activity, penetrating wounds, and open fractures, immediate stabilization may be necessary, followed by further evaluation and treatment once the patient is stable (Figure 20.12).

Poor diet, husbandry deficiencies, and stress are all major factors in the development of illness and disease seen in pet guinea pigs. Some of the more common diseases and causes of veterinary presentation will be described. It is important to accurately triage a patient to evaluate their current status and proceed accordingly. Like other exotic species, guinea pigs are no exception when it comes to difficulty evaluating pain. Following a pain scale is helpful when determining an appropriate evaluation of their presentation. Signs such as orbital tightening, grinding teeth, abdominal pressing, and increased respiratory effort can all be signs of significant pain and should be observed and recorded. Obtaining a TPR is one of the most crucial steps during triage. This includes collecting a respiratory rate, heart rate, mucous membrane color, assessing hydration (skin tenting, sunken eyes, etc.), mentation, and rectal temperature. Becoming knowledgeable of the normal vital ranges is imperative in order to appropriately evaluate the patient's status and determine initial treatment.

Common and Zoonotic Diseases

Gastrointestinal

Gastrointestinal Hypomotility

Gastrointestinal stasis occurs as a primary or secondary condition to almost any other disease process (DeCubellis & Graham 2013). The GI tract is specialized for a high-fiber, herbivorous diet. Any minor changes can disrupt the normal functionality resulting in hypomotility which then results in dehydration, a decrease in fecal output, impaired cecal fermentation, disruption of bacterial microflora, and/or accumulation of gas within the GI tract (DeCubellis & Graham 2013). Signs of GI hypomotility include a decrease in appetite, small/misshapen droppings, lethargy, splinting, a decrease in GI sounds, dehydration, abdominal distention, and/or hypothermia (DeCubellis & Graham 2013). Depending on the progression, this can eventually result in hypovolemic shock, a decrease in body temperature, perforation, and death (DeCubellis & Graham 2013). Diagnosis is typically achieved by two-view (lateral and ventrodorsal), whole-body radiographs, and/or ultrasound to evaluate anatomy, GI motility, and gas patterns. Bloodwork including a full chemistry to evaluate organ function and complete blood cell count to evaluate inflammation and infection are usually necessary. Options for treatment include pain management, fluid therapy, and nutritional support. It is imperative to provide pain control in addition to stimulating GI motility with syringe feedings and fluid therapy. GI decompression may be indicated if an obstruction is suspected, and the case becomes emergent. This is accomplished by passing a red rubber tube through the oral cavity and into the stomach to remove any food material or debris (Pignon and Mayer 2021). This may require sedation with injectables (i.e., a benzodiazepine such as midazolam) and a light inhalant depending on the patient's condition and mentation.

Gastric Dilation and Volvulus

Gastric dilation and volvulus, otherwise known as GDV, is when the stomach fills with gas and fluid, followed by rotation on the mesenteric axis (Pignon and Mayer 2021). This can be acute and fatal in guinea pigs. Signs of GDV include depression, pain on abdominal palpation, hypovolemic shock, weak pulses, hypothermia, dyspnea, inappetence, pale mucous membranes, lethargy, etc. Typical diagnostics include whole-body radiographs which would demonstrate a large, gas-filled stomach silhouette sometimes caudally displaced. A gastric rotation between 180° and 540° has been reported in guinea pigs previously (Pignon and Mayer 2021). The prognosis for this condition is very poor. Surgical intervention is an option, but the survival rate is less than 25% (Pignon and Mayer 2021).

Gastrointestinal Dysbiosis

Guinea pigs possess a predominantly gram-positive gastrointestinal flora. Antibiotics effective against gram-positive organisms, such as penicillin, ampicillin, chlortetracycline, clindamycin, erythromycin, and lincomycin, destroy the gram-positive flora. This can lead to overgrowth of *Clostridium difficile*, a gram-positive bacterium. This overgrowth of *C. difficile* alters the guinea pig's normal gastrointestinal flora, resulting in enterotoxemia (Hawkins & Bishop 2012). Affected animals will exhibit a secretory diarrhea, and without prompt and aggressive intervention this may result in acute death. Non-antibiotic-induced dysbiosis can also occur due to abrupt dietary changes, stress, and ingestion of contaminated food. Signs of dysbiosis include anorexia, dehydration, hypothermia, and/or diarrhea. Dysbiosis is usually treated with supportive care including fluid therapy, nutritional support, and antibiotics.

Fecal Impaction

Fecal impaction can be common in older, intact boars. This can occur when an enlarged flacid anus becomes impacted with bedding and feces. If the condition goes unnoticed for a longer period of time, it can progress and result in inguinal sebaceous gland infections. Treatment for fecal impaction includes cleaning the area via manual evacuation and potentially diet change.

Dental Disease

Dental disease is a common problem in guinea pigs and other hystricomorph species due to their elodont dentition. Dental disease may be caused by diets deficient in fiber or Vitamin C, genetic predisposition, infection, or trauma (Pignon and Mayer 2021). A thorough oral exam is always warranted to not only check the incisors, but the cheek teeth (premolars and molars) as well. Sedation and or general anesthesia would be required to obtain an adequate examination of the oral cavity. Overgrowth of the cheek teeth can cause ulcerations (either buccal or lingual) or tongue entrapment. The cheek teeth have a sloped angle with an occlusion surface of 30° (Pignon and Mayer 2021). Animals experiencing dental disease are often presented with complaints of decreased appetite or anorexia, bruxism, epiphora, weight loss, drooling, and ptyalism. Treatment and prognosis will be dependent upon the underlying disease process and the severity of disease. Treatment may include reshaping teeth to normal length and occlusion, extraction of diseased teeth, pain management, dietary management, and supportive care as indicated. Some patients may require life-long dental care to manage the disease.

Reproductive Disease

Dystocia

Dystocia is one of the most common reproductive problems in guinea pigs. Sows that are bred after 7 months of age for the first time are at high risk for dystocia, due to fusion of the fibrocartilaginous joint of the pubic symphysis, and the large size of the pups (Gresham & Haines 2012; Hawkins & Bishop 2012). Straining, abnormal vaginal discharge, depression, and/or failure to produce a pup within 30 minutes after onset of contractions are all suggestive of dystocia (Hawkins & Bishop 2012). In cases of dystocia, cesarean sections are often necessary to deliver the pups.

Pregnancy Ketosis

Pregnancy ketosis is most commonly associated with obesity and stress and is seen in the 2 weeks prepartum or 2 weeks post-partum. It is most commonly the result of a negative energy balance due to the demands of the fetuses on the sow, and those animals with a large litter size, excessive stress, and obesity are at higher risk. There is rapid onset of signs including anorexia, lethargy, dyspnea, convulsions, and death. Some animals may decline over a few days while others will experience acute collapse and death. Treatment is often unrewarding, and most animals die despite aggressive medical intervention (Hawkins & Bishop 2012). Stress reduction and weight management during gestation are key elements for prevention of pregnancy ketosis.

Ovarian Cysts and Neoplasia

These reproductive conditions are very common in intact sows. There are two different types of ovarian cysts: serous or hormone-producing follicular cysts. Ovarian cysts can cause anorexia, weakness, depression, and pain upon abdominal palpation. Hyperkeratotic nipples are another common sign seen on physical examination in addition to swelling of the mammary glands (guinea pigs possess one pair). Serous cysts can be resolved by surgical intervention involving removal and an ovariohysterectomy. Follicular cysts can be managed with gonadotropic hormone agonist injections or longer-lasting hormonal implants.

Neoplasia typically presents with the same signs as symptoms as ovarian cysts. Additional signs may include vaginal bleeding, abdominal distention, and/or displacement of internal organs. Diagnostics such as radiographs, ultrasound, and/or CT scan can determine the difference between cysts and/or neoplasia. A fine needle aspirate under sedation can also determine the specific type of neoplasia if present. Uterine leiomyomas are the most common uterine tumors in guinea pigs (Pignon and Mayer 2021).

Treatment method includes surgical removal of the tumor along with an ovariohysterectomy. The best method of prevention is an early-age ovariectomy.

Respiratory Disease

Guinea pigs have a relatively small thoracic cavity compared to their body mass. They have a particularly sensitive respiratory tract, with a predisposition to disease of bacterial, viral, and fungal origin/pathogens. Common bacterial respiratory diseases seen in guinea pigs include those caused by *Bordetella bronchiseptica* and *Streptococcus pneumoniae*. Both organisms have zoonotic potential (Hawkins & Bishop 2012; Yarto-Jaramillo 2011). Transmission is via aerosolization, fomites, direct contact with another sick guinea pig, or in the case of *Bordetella*, any animal capable of carrying the bacteria: dogs, cats, rabbits, and non-human primates. *Streptococcus pneumoniae* can cause pleuropneumonia, pleuritis, and peritonitis (Hawkins & Bishop 2012; Yarto-Jaramillo 2011). Signs of respiratory disease include dyspnea, tachypnea, respiratory sounds, lethargy, coughing, weight loss, and/or an unthrifty coat. Upon presentation, it's also important to observe the medial aspect of the front legs where nasal discharge may be present. Treatment of bacterial respiratory disease may include antibiotics, anti-inflammatories, and supplemental vitamin C in anorexic animals. In advanced cases of disease, additional supportive care such as oxygen therapy and nebulization may also be needed. Crackles, minimal air movement, and wheezing observed via thoracic auscultation can indicate severity of disease.

Urinary Diseases

Urolithiasis

The alkaline urinary pH and high mineral content of the urine may be predisposing factors to crystal formation and urolithiasis in adult guinea pigs (Hawkins & Bishop 2012). Most recent data report a high incidence of calcium carbonate calculi (Hawkins et al. 2009). The direct causes have been unclear. Most calculi are found in the bladder, although calculi may be found in the kidneys, ureters, seminal vesicles (males), and the vagina. In males, the stone will typically get lodged at the bladder neck at the seminal colliculus (Pignon and Mayer 2021). Affected animals are more likely to have been fed a diet of concentrated pellets with high levels of calcium. Clinical signs are often related to the location and size of the calculi. Changes in micturition, hematuria, stranguria, and anuria may be present along with non-specific signs like pain, anorexia, and lethargy. Diagnosis is often made radiographically as most stones are radiopaque. Medical treatment is often unrewarding due to the high urinary pH, and surgical removal followed by dietary correction is needed. The prognosis is favorable if the underlying cause of urolithiasis is identified and corrected (Hawkins & Bishop 2012). Reoccurrence is very common. Prevention can be attempted by increasing water intake by offering water in nipple drinkers instead of water bowls.

Cystitis and Urinary Tract Infections

Cystitis and UTIs can frequently be identified with urolithiasis. The bacteria typically responsible is *Corynbacterium renale*, *E. coli*, or *Enterococcus*. The patient will usually present with stranguria, anorexia, hematuria, depression, and/or pollakiuria. Radiographs are usually performed first in order to rule out urolithiasis prior to urinalysis and urine culture and sensitivity. Identifying the specific species of bacteria causing the infection will determine the antibiotic appropriate for treatment. In addition to antibiotics, non-steroidal anti-inflammatories, and supportive care such as fluid therapy and syringe feedings may be warranted.

Integumentary

Alopecia

It is important to note that there is minimal to no hair between the nose and lips, outer pinnae, and behind both ears. This is normal for the breed. True alopecia can be caused by husbandry concerns, such as nutritional deficiencies and/or poor sanitation. Certain hormonal conditions such as adrenal disease or follicular ovarian cysts can also cause alopecia typically bilateral on the flank. Barbering is another condition that is observed upon close examination when the hair shaft is broken. Barbering can be self-inflicted which is usually caused by boredom or poor nutrition including lack of fiber. It can also be caused by a dominant cage mate. They may need to be separated to prevent further complications.

Dermatophytosis

This condition typically presents as scaly, patchy lesions on the face, feet, or dorsum. These lesions usually have crusty edges and can also be pruritic. A fungal culture is required for a definitive diagnosis and treatment with an antifungal. This condition is zoonotic, and it is important for the staff to wear appropriate PPE when suspected.

Pododermatitis

Pododermatitis is often associated with obesity and animals housed on wire flooring. The plantar surfaces of

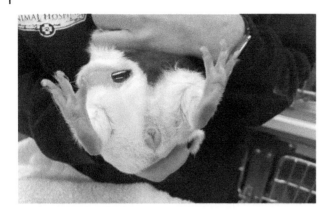

Figure 20.13 Example of bilateral pododermatitis on the plantar surface of the hind foot. (Courtesy of Liz Vetrano.)

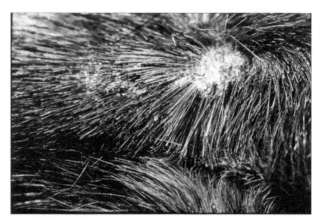

Figure 20.14 A guinea pig with mange. (Courtesy of Dr. Chris King.)

the feet become irritated, thickened, and ulcerated, and a secondary bacterial infection may ensue. Affected animals may vocalize and be unwilling to move due to pain. Treatment consists of appropriate antibiotic therapy, surgical debridement, topical cleaning, analgesic therapy, laser therapy, and correction of the underlying cause (Hawkins & Bishop 2012). (Figure 20.13).

Ectoparasites

Acariasis *Trixacarus caviae*, a common ectoparasite of guinea pigs, can result in severe dermatitis and pruritus. A hallmark sign of infection with *T. caviae* is profound pruritus resulting in seizure-like activity (Hawkins & Bishop 2012). In many cases these animals will also have alopecia, dull hair coats, excoriations on the skin, and possibly a secondary bacterial or fungal infection, increasing the suspicion of ectoparasitism. Severe pruritis can also lead to self-induced trauma. Diagnosis is made based on history, clinical signs, and microscopic examination of skin scrapings. Treatment should include administration of antiparasitic medication and treatment of any secondary bacterial or fungal infections.

Lice and Fur Mites The fur mite *Chirodiscoides caviae* is the most common ectoparasite of guinea pigs. There are also several species of lice such as *Gliricola porcelli* and *Gyropus ovalis* which may also cause infection (Figure 20.14). Unlike *T. caviae*, lice tend to be species-specific and typically require direct contact for transmission. Although lice tend to cause a less severe dermatitis, they can cause restlessness, alopecia, and crusty lesions. Antiparasitic medications such as ivermectin or selamectin are typically required for treatment. Severe cases may also require antibiotic therapy and non-steroidal anti-inflammatories.

Musculoskeletal

Osteoarthritis

Osteoarthritis can be a common occurrence in guinea pigs as a secondary condition to ulcerative pododermatitis. Severe cases of pododermatitis can lead to osteoarthritis due to obesity, inadequate exercise, and/or improper substrate (i.e., wire bottom caging). It should also be noted that recent studies have indicated that too much ascorbic acid supplementation may also result in osteoarthritis. Treatments may vary depending on the severity of the case. For mild cases, changes in substrate, antibiotics, non-steroidal anti-inflammatories, laser therapy, and/or proper exercise and weight loss can be sufficient. More severe cases may require amputation.

Vitamin C Deficiency

Scurvy, a musculoskeletal disease, develops as the result of a vitamin C deficiency. Guinea pigs are incapable of exogenous synthesis of vitamin C, possessing a mutated gene for L-gulono-γ-lactone oxidase. This prevents the conversion of L-gulonolactone to ascorbic acid, resulting in deficiency. Ascorbic acid is essential for collagen synthesis. Scurvy may develop in as little as 2 weeks following deficiency. Young, growing animals are more susceptible. Clinical signs of deficiency include anorexia, rough hair coat, diarrhea, weight loss, painful/swollen joints, petechia and hemorrhages of the mucous membranes, and pain, which may be manifested as vocalization, teeth grinding, biting, and reluctance to move (Gresham & Haines 2012; Hawkins & Bishop 2012; Yarto-Jaramillo 2011). Immunosuppression can lead to secondary complications that may require additional treatment in advanced disease.

A presumptive diagnosis of ascorbic acid deficiency can be made based on clinical signs and history of dietary deficiency. Radiographs of deficient animals may show enlargement of the costochondral junctions of the ribs and widening of long bone epiphyses (Hawkins & Bishop 2012). Serologic levels of ascorbic acid may be tested for confirmation. Treatment with parenteral ascorbic acid, coupled with good supportive care, usually results in a rapid recovery (Gresham & Haines 2012; Hawkins & Bishop 2012; Yarto-Jaramillo 2011). This needs to be followed with lifelong exogenous dietary supplementation and husbandry adjustments. This includes offering commercial guinea pig pellets with stabilized Vitamin C levels and fresh foods including red and/or yellow peppers (Pignon and Mayer 2021).

Other Common Diseases

Cervical Lymphadenitis

Swellings on the neck are usually due to inflamed or abscessed lymph nodes caused by *Streptobacillus* spp. or *Streptococcus* spp. Infection, which is a normal oropharyngeal and nasal flora of guinea pigs. Cervical lymphadenitis, or "lumps" as it is commonly called, may result from oral abrasions caused by malocclusion, abrasive feed, or bite wounds which lead to the bacteria gaining access to the cervical lymph nodes which results in abscessation (Pignon and Mayer 2021). The patients typically present with swellings in the ventral neck region. Diagnosis is based on clinical signs, bacterial culture of the purulent material, and/or aspirates of the lymph nodes (Pignon and Mayer 2021). Treatment of abscesses typically includes surgical excision, systemic antibiotics, and supportive care.

Clinical Techniques

Administration of Medication

Medications can be administered in a variety of ways which is typically dependent on routes, doses, volumes, and duration of therapies. Different routes are considered not only based on these factors but also on time, effectiveness, and practicality, as well. Oral medications are the easiest to administer; however, may not be as effective depending on the patient's condition and disease process (i.e., gastrointestinal stasis, dysbiosis, hypothermia, etc.). Other routes to consider would be intravenous, intramuscular, or subcutaneous. The intravenous route will deliver the medication at a much quicker rate. This is desirable for most critical patients; however, due to their small size and depending on how debilitated the patient is, this may not be a possible choice if venous access cannot be obtained. Intramuscular is another option for injectable medications in these cases. Subcutaneous routes are also viable options which may take longer to take effect but are always easy to administer. It is important to remember that each case may be different depending on patient condition and the desirable treatment chosen by the clinician. Be mindful that specific medications may also only be delivered via specific routes and may have adverse affects if not delivered correctly.

Subcutaneous (SC or SQ)

Subcutaneous injection of medications allows for slightly larger volumes to be administered than with intramuscular administration. Fluid therapy may also be administered via the subcutaneous route in between the scapulae. It is important to note what the body temperature is prior to administration of fluids. The patient may require warmed fluids if they are hypothermic. Most guinea pigs will rest on the exam table and can be restrained by cupping your hands around them. A towel placed on the table provides the animal with some traction.

The skin should be tented away from the underlying muscles, and the needle inserted at a slight angle (30°), being careful not to pass all the way through to the other side of the skin. The area between the scapulae tends to have the most subcutaneous space and is the desirable location for subcutaneous fluids and injections. The syringe plunger should be withdrawn slightly for negative pressure to ensure subcutaneous placement. The medication or fluids should be administered efficiently. A butterfly catheter may be easier to use if the animal is very active.

Intramuscular (IM)

Intramuscular injections are usually given in the epaxial muscles which are located along the spine. The large gluteal muscles of the hindlimbs are another option if the epaxial muscles are not as prominent. Volumes exceeding 0.3 mL should not be instilled into any one site.

Have an assistant gently restrain the patient, being aware that the patient might squirm or vocalize in response to the injection. The muscle belly should be isolated, and the needle inserted at a 30° angle. When administering into the epaxial muscle, it is important to palpate the spine and the muscle to determine correct placement (avoiding the spine). Aspirate the syringe prior to injection to ensure correct placement. Administer the medication promptly and withdraw the needle. It is also important to note that the restrainer plays a huge role when administering IM injections. Supporting the hind end and using a towel to wrap around the patient can reduce injury.

Intravenous (IV)

Intravenous injections can be challenging. The lateral saphenous and cephalic veins are most accessible, but sedation is often needed to decrease patient movement and objection. The area over the vessel should be shaved and aseptically prepped. The assistant restraining the animal will extend the limb and provide proximal pressure to the injection site to distend the vein. The needle is inserted into the vessel gently, taking into consideration the small size, superficial location, and fragility of the vessel. Blood may or may not be seen in the hub of the needle upon appropriate placement due to the small size. Care should be taken to stabilize the needle within the vessel and ensure the medication is not administered perivascularly. Apply direct pressure to the venipuncture site as the needle is withdrawn to prevent formation of a hematoma. A light pressure bandage may need to be applied to the site for 15–20 minutes to prevent hematoma formation.

Venipuncture

Collection of hematologic samples in guinea pigs is challenged by their short legs and thick necks. The lateral saphenous and cephalic veins may be used for

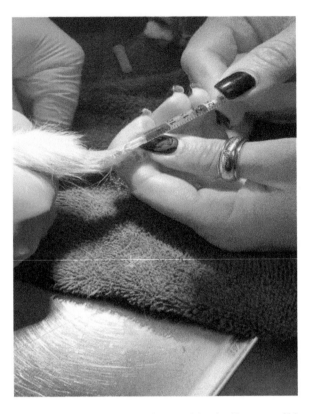

Figure 20.16 Venipuncture of the pedal vein. (Courtesy of Liz Vetrano.)

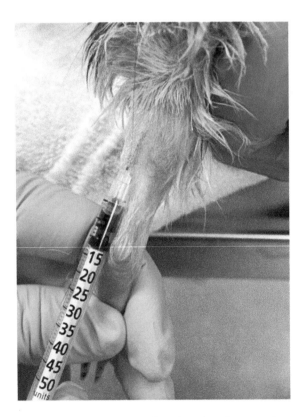

Figure 20.15 Venipuncture of the lateral saphenous vein. (Courtesy of Liz Vetrano.)

small-volume sample collection appropriate for blood smears or blood glucose evaluation. For a saphenous venipuncture, the caudal end of the patient can be placed on the edge of the exam table allowing the hind legs to hang over the edge. One of the legs is held off by the restrainer to better visualize the vessel which runs around the caudal aspect of the hind leg. See Figure 20.15. The pedal vein located on the dorsal aspect of the hindfoot is another option for venipuncture. See Figure 20.16.

Jugular or cranial vena cava venipuncture allows for collection of larger sample volumes. For jugular venipuncture the patient may be manually restrained using methods similar to those applied to other mammals; however, the author's preference is to use sedation as the animals generally resist restraint and there is a risk of lacerating the vessel. Alternatively, the experienced phlebotomist may utilize the cranial vena cava under sedation or general anesthesia. For this, the patient is in dorsal recumbency, and the needle is inserted into the thoracic cavity between the first rib and the manubrium at a 45° angle to the body, advancing caudally to the opposite rear limb (Figure 20.17). The plunger is withdrawn as the needle is slowly advanced until blood enters the syringe. Caution must be taken not to lacerate the vena cava or advance into the heart (Campbell 2012; Harkness et al. 2010; Huneke 2012).

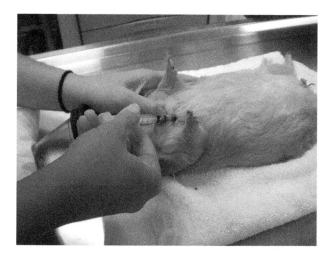

Figure 20.17 Blood collection form the cranial vena cava. (Courtesy of Jill Murray.)

No more than 1% of the healthy patient's blood volume should be collected or 10% of the patient's body weight in grams (Pignon and Mayer 2021). For example, if a patient weighs 800g, you may collect up to 8 ml of blood. Sometimes, due to small sample volumes, diagnostic testing may need to be prioritized. Various hematologic references are available for the guinea pig, and some are listed in the "References" section of this chapter.

Catheter Placement

Intravenous catheterization in guinea pigs can be difficult due to the small size and fragility of the vessels. Catheters may be placed in the cephalic, lateral saphenous, or even pedal veins as described above for intravenous injection, ensuring asepsis during placement and maintenance (Figures 20.18 and 20.19). The author prefers not to saline flush the catheter prior to placement as this reduces the flow of blood into the catheter hub. The skin tends to be very thick, especially in intact boars. The author prefers to penetrate the skin prior to placement next to the vessel with a small gauge needle (such as a 27g) after aseptically prepping the area. This decreases the chances of burring the catheter and allowing for a smoother placement. Sedation may be required prior to placement to decrease movement and patient stress. Midazolam is an injectable benzodiazepine used in small patients for mild sedation and is especially desirable due to its ability to be reversed. Tape (typically 1") should be placed underneath the catheter and around the extremity initially to secure the catheter in place. Care must be taken to make sure it is not too tight but is attached to the skin. Once the t-set or injection port is attached, confirming patency by flushing the catheter should be done in a timely fashion as these catheters tend to clot quickly. This can be accomplished with a small amount of saline flush. Since they are small patients, it's important to be mindful of how much flush is being used during this process. The author prefers to use

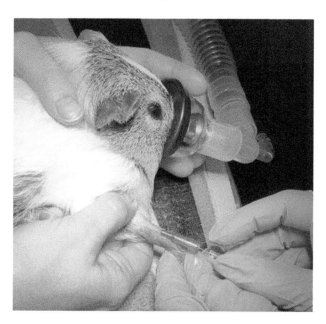

Figure 20.18 Cephalic IVC placement in the front leg. (Courtesy of Liz Vetrano.)

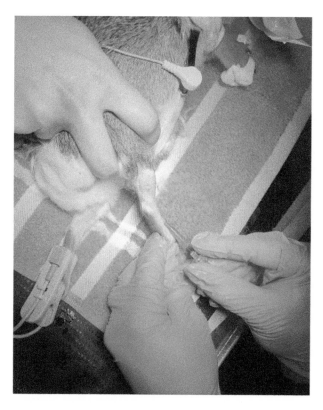

Figure 20.19 IVC placement in the pedal vein of the right hind foot. (Courtesy of Liz Vetrano.)

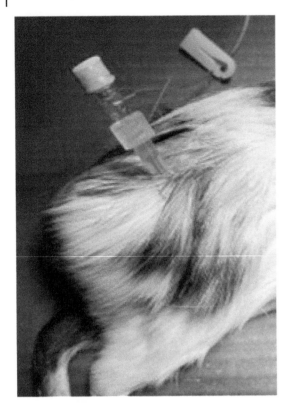

Figure 20.20 IO catheter placement via the greater trochanter of the right femur during CPR. (Courtesy of Liz Vetrano.)

1 ml syringes with saline for these cases. Once patency is confirmed, 2 small anchors (1/2" tape) should be placed to secure the t-set or injection port followed by another piece of 1" tape around the extremity. The author prefers to use Elasticon at the proximal portion of the tape to prevent the entire catheter from slipping (this can be removed safely with adhesive tape remover). It's important to ensure the bandaging remains clean and dry. Some patients require a soft e-collar or catheter guard to prevent chewing.

When rapid fluid delivery is necessary in times of circulatory collapse, intraosseous catheter placement into the proximal tibia or the femur (via the greater trochanter) (Figure 20.20). The location is shaved and prepped using chlorhex scrub followed by alcohol or saline. An 18–25-gauge spinal needle or hypodermic needle can be used. The length of the catheter should be the length of one-third to one-half of the medullary cavity and a wire stylet should be used to reduce the potential of a bone core (Pignon and Mayer 2021). A local anesthetic such as lidocaine can be used for additional pain management during placement. The point of insertion is palpated, and the needle is inserted with gentle, consistent pressure until the medullary cavity is penetrated. The catheter is flushed with a small amount of saline (usually IO catheters will

have more pressure than an IV catheter when flushing). A two-view radiograph should also be taken to confirm correct placement Once placement is confirmed, the catheter is secured with tape and stay sutures. Antibiotic ointment should be placed around the insertion site prior to bandage wrap placement. Placement of any catheter may need to be completed under sedation and/or general anesthesia.

Bandaging and Wound Care

Superficial wounds are best managed with topical cleansing and lavage to obtain a clean wound for second-intention healing. Application of topical medications and continued wound care will cause additional stress to the patient. The administration of systemic antimicrobial, anti-inflammatory agents, fluid therapy, and nutritional supplementation (i.e., syringe feedings) may also be necessary. Providing a clean environment with reduced cage furnishings to help reduce further contamination and trauma is advised.

In larger, contaminated wounds, surgical exploration, debridement, and/or closure may be necessary. External sutures and bandages are not well tolerated and difficult to place and maintain. Whenever possible, subcuticular sutures are a better alternative for wound closure. Penetrating wounds and fractures can be difficult to manage and require creativity, owner compliance, and diligence in monitoring. An Elizabethan collar may have to be placed to prevent chewing of the incision and/or suture removal.

Euthanasia

As guinea pigs are often a child's pet and companion, end-of-life decisions can be difficult. As a result of illness, disease, age related health problems, and poor quality of life, the owner and clinician may conclude that humane euthanasia is the best course of action to end the animal's suffering. As with other mammals, humane euthanasia may be accomplished with an overdose of a barbiturate anesthetic agent. Administration of a pre-anesthetic agent to calm the animal prior to euthanasia is required to ensure the patient is pain-free and without stress. The administration of an opioid and benzodiazepine may be given IM or SC, allowing for the owner to hold the animal while they become sedate. This is followed by IV or IC (intracardiac) administration of an overdose of a barbiturate anesthesia. In some cases, depending on the patient's condition, an IVC may be placed so the owner may be present. It is important to communicate with the owner that vascular access may not be possible, and it may be too stressful to attempt multiple times. Once the euthanasia agent is delivered, the animal will pass slowly as the medication is taken up in the body, ceasing circulatory function.

Alternatively, the patient may be anesthetized with a high dose of an inhalant anesthetic followed by an IP or IC injection of a euthanasia agent (Leary et al. 2020). This is typically not performed in the owner's presence.

References

Bays T, Lightfoot T, Mayer J. 2006. *Exotic Pet Behavior*. St. Louis, MO: Elsevier

Campbell TW. 2012. Mammalian hematology: laboratory animals and miscellaneous species. In: *Veterinary Hematology and Clinical Chemistry*, 2nd edn (eds MA Thrall, G Weiser, RW Allison, et al.), pp. 225–237. Ames, IA: Wiley-Blackwell.

Capello V, Lennox A. 2012. Small mammal dentistry. In: *Ferrets, Rabbits, and Rodents: Clinical Medicine and Surgery*, 3rd edn (eds KE Quesenberry, JW Carpenter), pp. 452–471. St Louis, MO: Elsevier.

Capello V, Lennox A, Widmer WR. 2008. *Clinical Radiology of Exotic Companion Mammals*. Ames, IA: Wiley-Blackwell.

DeCubellis J, Graham J. 2013. Gastrointestinal disease in Guinea disease in Guinea pigs and rabbits. *Vet Clin Exot Anim Pract* 16: 421–435.

Gresham VC, Haines VL. 2012. Management, husbandry and colony health. In: *The Laboratory Rabbit, Guinea Pig, Hamster, and Other Rodents* (eds M Suckow, K Stevens, R Wilson), pp. 603–619. Waltham, MA: Elsevier.

Hargaden M, Singer L. 2012. Anatomy, physiology and behavior. In: *The Laboratory Rabbit, Guinea Pig, and Other Rodents* (eds M Suckow, K Stevens, R Wilson), pp. 575–602. Waltham, MA: Elsevier.

Harkness JE, Turner PV, VandeWoude S, et al. 2010. *Harkness and Wagner's Biology and Medicine of Rabbits and Rodents*, 5th edn, Ames, IA: Wiley-Blackwell.

Hawkins M, Bishop C. 2012. Diseases of guinea pigs. In: *Ferrets, Rabbits, and Rodents: Clinical Medicine and Surgery*, 3rd edn (eds KE Quesenberry, JW Carpenter), pp. 295–321. St Louis, MO: Elsevier.

Hawkins MG, Pascoe PJ. 2021. Anesthesia, analgesia and sedation of small mammals. In: *Ferrets, Rabbits, and Rodents: Clinical Medicine and Surgery*, 4th edn, pp. 537–541. St Louis, MO: Elsevier.

Hawkins MG, Ruby, AL, Drazenovich TL, et al. 2009. Composition and characterisitics of urinary calculi from guinea pigs. *JAVMA* 234(2): 214–220.

Huneke RB. 2012. Basic experimental methods. In: *The Laboratory Rabbit, Guinea Pig, Hamster, and Other Rodents* (eds M Suckow, K Stevens, R Wilson), pp. 621–635. Waltham, MA: Elsevier.

Leary S, Underwood W, Anthony R, et al. 2020. *AVMA Guidelines for the Euthanasia of Animals*, p. 57. AVMA.

Miller AL, Richardson CA. 2011. Rodent analgesia. *Vet Clin North Am Exot Anim Pract* 14: 81–92.

O'Malley B. 2005. Guinea pigs. In: *Clinical Anatomy and Physiology of Exotic Species* (ed B O'Malley), pp. 197–208. Philadelphia, PA: Elsevier Saunders.

Pignon C, Mayer J. 2021. In: *Ferrets, Rabbits, and Rodents: Clinical Medicine and Surgery*, 4th edn (eds KE Quesenberry, JW Carpenter), pp. 271–294. St Louis, MO: Elsevier.

Pritt S. 2012. Taxonomy and history. In: *The Laboratory Rabbit, Guinea Pig, Hamster, and Other Rodents* (eds M Suckow, K Stevens, R Wilson), pp. 563–574. Waltham, MA: Elsevier.

Silverman S, Tell LA. 2005. *Radiology of Rodents, Rabbits and Ferrets*. St Louis, MO: Elsevier Saunders.

Trewin AL, Hutz RJ. 1998. Guinea pig, female. In: *Encyclopedia of Reproduction*, vol. 2 (eds E Knobil, JD Neill), pp. 583–588. San Diego, CA: Academic Press.

Yarto-Jaramillo E. 2011. Respiratory system anatomy, physiology, and disease: guinea pigs and chinchillas. *Vet Clin North Am Exot Anim Pract* 14: 339–355.

21

Degus
Stacey Leonatti Wilkinson

Introduction

The degu, *Octodon degus*, is a hystricomorph rodent from north-central Chile, with a diverse natural habitat ranging from the coastal regions to the Andes mountains. It belongs to the family Octodontidae, which also includes cavies, porcupines, and chinchillas (Najecki & Tate 1999; Nowak 1999; Woods & Boraker 1975). Degus may also be referred to as a brush-tailed rat or trumpet-tailed rat due to the black tuft of fur at the tail tip (Johnson 2002; Woods & Boraker 1975). They are highly social animals, naturally living in large community burrows. Unlike most rodents, degus are diurnal, long-lived (up to 15 years in the wild and 5–8 years in captivity), sprecocious, and have a low incidence of disease, making them desirable pets. Degus are a commonly used species in the research of diabetes, cataracts, and circadian behavior (Colby et al. 2012; Johnson 2002; Najecki & Tate 1999).

Anatomy and Physiology

Recognizing that degus share many anatomic and physiologic similarities with other rodents, this section will focus on the differences and key points specific to the degu.

An adult degu will reach a body weight ranging from 170 to 300 g and a body length of 250 to 310 mm (excluding the tail) (Jekl 2021). Their fur has a gray-brown coloration with a cream-colored ventrum. They have a long, thin, haired tail, with a black tuft of fur at the tip. The pinnae are darkly pigmented with sparse fur. The feet have four well-developed digits with a smaller fifth digit possessing nails instead of claws. The forefeet are highly dexterous and used to hold food and other objects (Colby et al. 2012; Woods & Boraker 1975).

As mentioned, degus belong to the family Octodontidae, where "octodon" refers to the figure-of-eight shape of their cheek teeth. Degus have a total of 20 elodont (continuously growing) teeth, which includes the premolars. The dental formula of the degu is: 2 (I 1/1, C 0/0, P 1/1, M 3/3). The long aradicular incisors of a healthy adult animal possess an orange pigment to the enamel on the superficial rostral edges. This is the result of iron deposition and results in increased enamel strength for chewing wear. The cheek teeth are aradicular (rootless) and hypsodont (high crowned) (Colby et al. 2012; Long 2012; Najecki & Tate 1999; Woods & Boraker 1975). They are hindgut fermenters, possessing a simple glandular stomach, and a functioning cecum. The gastrointestinal transit time of the degu is approximately 5.1 h. Degus practice coprophagy, reingesting most of their nighttime fecal pellets (Colby et al. 2012; Edwards 2009) (Figures 21.1 and 21.2).

Due to their natural habitat's arid climate and seasonal scarcity of water, degus have adapted to water conservation in times of decreased availability. Their urine is normally turbid and a dark yellow color (Colby et al. 2012; Johnson 2002).

Degus have dichromatic vision and can distinguish between some colors. Age-related changes in the eye (cataracts) are frequently observed in mature animals (Colby et al. 2012; Richardson 2008).

Sex determination of the degu is similar to that of other rodents in that the anogenital distance of the male is approximately twice that of the female. The testes are intra-abdominal and there is no scrotum (Capello & Sjoberg 2005; Richardson 2008). Gentle pressure may be applied to the prepuce to extrude the penis. Females have four pairs of mammary glands (Colby et al. 2012; Johnson 2002; Najecki & Tate 1999) (Figure 21.3).

Behavior

Wild degus live in large social groups (Colby et al. 2012; Richardson 2008). Pet degus should be housed in pairs or small social groups to reduce behavioral problems and

Exotic Animal Medicine for the Veterinary Technician, Fourth Edition. Edited by Bonnie Ballard and Ryan Cheek.
© 2024 John Wiley & Sons, Inc. Published 2024 by John Wiley & Sons, Inc.
Companion Website: www.wiley.com/go/ballard/4e

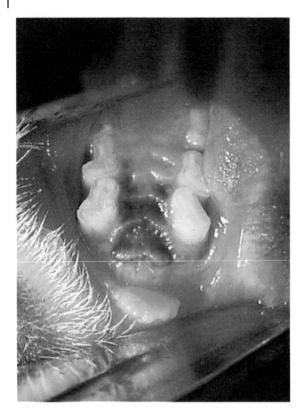

Figure 21.1 A healthy adult degu exhibiting the normal orange pigmented enamel on the rostral aspect of the incisors. (Courtesy Dr. Dan Johnson.)

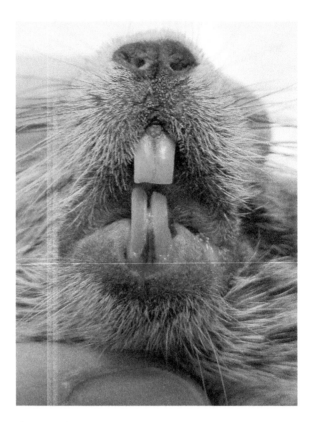

Figure 21.2 The characteristic figure-8 shape of the cheek teeth. (Courtesy Dr. Dan Johnson.)

stress from isolation. They utilize a variety of sensory modalities in communication. Tactile communication, mutual grooming, scent marking, and vocalization are frequently observed. Degus can produce a variety of individualized vocalizations and courtship calls that assist in identification of individual animals. They have a highly developed olfactory system, and unlike most rodents, the females engage in more scent marking than the males (Colby et al. 2012; Najecki & Tate 1999).

Reports of intraspecies aggression are rare, yet in the absence of social interaction, physical stimulation, and enrichment, aggressive behaviors, and self-mutilation may be observed (Johnson 2002; Najecki & Tate 1999).

Biologic and Reproductive Data

Degus are spontaneous ovulators with regular estrous cycles and functional corpora lutea. Both males and females are reproductively mature at approximately 4 months of age, but breeding should not begin until 6 months of age when the animals reach their adult body weight (Colby et al. 2012; Najecki & Tate 1999). Sexual maturity of the sire can be assessed by the presence and

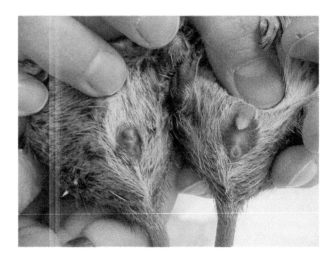

Figure 21.3 Sex determination in the male and female degu. The anogenital distance of the male (right) is approximately double that of the female (left). (Courtesy Dr. Dan Johnson.)

size of spikes on the glans of the penis (Colby et al. 2012). Breeding of a mature animal not previously bred is not recommended due to an increased risk of pregnancy toxemia and dystocia (Johnson 2002). Reproduction is noted to decline in animals after 4 years of age (Colby et al. 2012).

The sire remains with the dam during gestation and parturition. The gestation of the degu is long for a rodent of similar size, ranging from 87 to 93 days. Litter size can range from 1 to 12 pups, with an average of 6 to 7 pups (Colby et al. 2012; Richardson 2008). The dam experiences a post-partum estrus and is receptive to male copulation during this time. Both males and females participate in the care of the pups. Unlike most rodents, neither the male nor the female normally exhibits aggression or cannibalism towards the pups. Pups are precocial at birth, being fully furred and with their teeth erupted. Their eyes and ears will open within 1–3 days postnatally. Pups begin to nibble on solid food by 14 days of age but continue to nurse until 4 to 5 weeks of age (Colby et al. 2012; Edwards 2009).

Husbandry

Degus are diurnal, social, and very active animals. They adapt easily to new environments and are easy to keep as pets (Jekl 2021). Caging should be escape-proof, chew-proof, easily cleaned, and of appropriate size to allow for exercise and group housing. A minimum cage size of 24 × 48 inches (60 × 120 cm) is recommended for social housing of two degus. Whenever possible, larger cages are recommended, and the size of the cage should increase with an increase in the number of animals (Colby et al. 2012; Najecki & Tate 1999). Edible enrichment may also be provided, making sure to avoid foods and commercial products that are high in carbohydrates, fats, and sugars due to increased risks for diabetes and hepatic lipidosis (Colby et al. 2012; Johnson 2002; Najecki & Tate 1999; Richardson 2008).

The ideal enclosure will be of adequate size for social housing with multiple levels including hide boxes and a running wheel for exercise. Wire mesh cages with solid floors are preferred to glass aquaria in order to allow for ventilation (Richardson 2008). An absorbent, non-irritating, non-aromatic substrate like recycled newspaper should be provided to reduce the risk of pododermatitis and respiratory irritation. Wire flooring in cages increases the risks of pododermatitis and accidental trauma (Johnson 2002).

The enclosure should be kept away from drafts and extreme temperatures. Degus have difficulty with thermoregulation and may struggle with temperatures greater than 32°C (90°F). A relative environmental humidity of 30–60% is considered adequate (Colby et al. 2012). As is the case with chinchillas, a twice-weekly dust bath is recommended to assist with grooming of the coat to remove oils and debris (Najecki & Tate 1999; Colby et al. 2012).

Water should be provided in a bottle with a sipper tube. The bottle and spout should be cleaned and evaluated regularly for patency and function. An improperly functioning water bottle should be replaced. Food should be provided in a weighted bowl to prevent spillage, waste, and contamination of foods with waste products.

Nutrition

Degus are herbivorous animals, in the wild consuming a diet of foliage, flowers, fruit, and seeds (Colby et al. 2012; Edwards 2009; Jekl et al. 2011; Woods & Boraker 1975). Limited studies on the nutritional requirements of captive degus have been performed. Feeding the pet degu a high-quality commercial rodent or guinea pig pellet supplemented with unlimited high-quality grass hay and a small amount of fresh produce is recommended (Edwards 2009; Johnson 2002; Richardson 2008). Offering a variety of food items from an early age will help to prevent rigid food preferences from forming. The degu does produce the enzyme L-gulonolactone oxidase and therefore does not require daily supplementation with ascorbic acid (vitamin C) (Colby et al. 2012; Edwards 2009). Timothy and other grass hays are preferred to alfalfa hay. The hay should be fresh and free of moisture and mildew. Vegetables and fruits should be washed thoroughly prior to feeding to remove any pesticide residue and should be removed from the cage after a few hours to prevent spoilage and bacterial growth. Fruits and vegetables high in sugars and carbohydrates should be avoided; instead offer vitamin- and fiber-rich produce in moderation, such as bell peppers, leafy greens (dandelion, herbs, carrot tops, romaine lettuce), pumpkin, cucumber, squash, cauliflower, broccoli, green beans, and sweet potatoes.

Restraint and Handling

Whenever possible, rodents should be brought to the hospital in their normal cage. The client should be instructed not to clean the cage prior to their appointment so the veterinary staff can observe the animal's normal habitat and fecal output. When this is not possible, a small, escape-proof carrier should be used for transport, and the client should bring a list of the supplies, feed, and pictures of the enclosure. The cage should be protected from the elements during travel. Stress reduction during transport and hospitalization should be practiced whenever possible, limiting the animal's exposure to predators, extreme temperatures, and excessive handling.

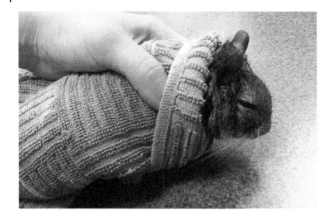

Figure 21.4 Gentle restraint of the pet degu in a hand towel. (Courtesy Erica Mead RVT.)

Degus respond well to gentle handling and restraint whereas inappropriate handling may lead to stress, trauma, and potential aggression. Degus should never be picked up by their tails. As part of their prey response, when grabbed by the tail, the degu will spin, resulting in a degloving injury of the tail, possibly requiring surgical amputation. With their highly social nature, degus should be picked up by scooping and restraining the body in the cup of the hand or lightly wrapped in a towel. Handling should be expedited to reduce the risk of hyperthermia and stress (Colby et al. 2012; Johnson 2002) (Figures 21.4 and 21.5).

Restraint for diagnostic sample collection and therapies may require the use of sedation or general anesthesia to limit stress and movement and to expedite the procedure.

Common Diseases

Stress, poor diet, and poor husbandry are major factors in the development of illness and disease. Often, the presenting complaint in the sick animal will be a combination of non-specific signs.

Common causes of presentation to the veterinary hospital include dental disease, skin disease (self-mutilation, barbering, trauma), cataracts, gastrointestinal disease, trauma, and bacterial infection (Johnson 2002; Long 2012).

Dental disease is one of the most commonly reported reasons for veterinary presentation of the pet degu. In a 2011 retrospective study, Jekl et al. reported that approximately 60% of pet degus presenting to the veterinary hospital are suffering from an acquired dental disease (Jekl et al. 2011). Due to the elodont dentition, malocclusion and subsequent overgrowth can lead to clinically appreciable dental disease requiring veterinary care. Patients with dental disease will often present with a history of anorexia or reduced feed intake, epiphora, hypersalivation,

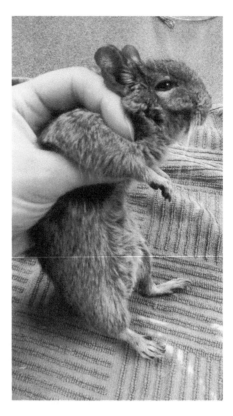

Figure 21.5 Gentle restraint of the pet degu in the hand, showing control of the head. (Courtesy Erica Mead RVT.)

and other manifestations of pain. Dietary deficiencies and general health can be directly linked to dental health and discoloration of the incisor enamel, most notably iron metabolism. Molar elodontoma as a result of coronal and apical elongation has also been reported in the maxillary and mandibular cheek teeth, causing irreversible damage to the nasal passages and sinuses (Jekl et al. 2011; Long 2012). Incisor malocclusion may be the result of trauma, congenital abnormalities, and abnormal chewing behaviors. Often, this progresses to malocclusion of the cheek teeth.

Skin problems, the second most common disease presentation of pet degus, are most often the result of barbering, self-mutilation, trauma, and aggression (Jekl et al. 2011). Cataracts, gastrointestinal diseases due to dietary deficiencies, and trauma are also commonly reported (Jekl et al. 2011; Richardson 2008).

A diagnostic workup and treatment of the sick degu will be determined in consultation with the owners in consideration of the patient's clinical presentation, disease process, age, prognosis, and monetary investment.

Pharmaceutical therapy in degus, like any rodent, should receive careful consideration. There are no pharmaceuticals labeled for use in rodents, although many references provide anecdotal doses and references.

History and Physical Examination

A complete physical exam and review of dietary practices and husbandry should be performed annually (Johnson 2002). A thorough patient history should be collected whenever a new patient presents to the hospital. During follow-up visits, questions may be tailored to the presenting complaint and any recommendations and changes made from previous visits. A thorough history will include the source of the animal, detailed information pertaining to the patient's diet, husbandry practices, past medical history, and presenting complaints.

Unless medically urgent, the animal should be observed in the cage on presentation to better assess normal behaviors. Careful observation will also provide information on appetite, fecal pellet production and quality, gait, stance, and overall attitude. A healthy degu will be engaging, inquisitive, active, and have a normal gait. A sick animal may mask signs of illness and disease initially, but may eventually hide, and/or appear tired and unwell.

Following the visual exam, the patient may be removed from the enclosure and carefully examined. The patient should be weighed on a gram scale to obtain an accurate body weight for patient monitoring and accurate dosing of medications. Careful restraint of the degu is necessary to prevent tail degloving, trauma, and unnecessary stress.

Hematology

Due to the clinical challenges of venipuncture, there are limited hematologic references for the pet degu. The University of Michigan has developed limited hematologic references from their small, captive, laboratory degu colony and may be referenced when applicable (Colby et al. 2012). The International Species Identification System (ISIS) has reported limited complete blood count values for captive degus (Teare 2013).

Sample collection in the degu, due to their small size, is challenging and may not be feasible for clinical practice. The lateral saphenous and cephalic veins may be used for small-volume sample collection appropriate for blood smear or blood glucose evaluation. The experienced phlebotomist may utilize the cranial vena cava as a site for collection of larger hematologic samples under general anesthesia (Jekl et al. 2011). Other methods of collection used in the research setting are not clinically appropriate in the pet degu due to high risks of complications. No more than 1% of the healthy patient's blood volume should be collected. This equates to approximately 1.7–3 mL in the adult degu with a body weight of 170–300 g. Due to small sample volumes, diagnostic testing may need to be prioritized.

Radiology

Whole-body imaging studies are common in most rodents. For accurate interpretation, two views taken at 90° angles from one another are needed. Lateral and ventrodorsal whole-body radiographs should be the minimum radiographic database. The need for additional radiographic views is based on clinical presentation and evaluation of survey radiographs, which may reveal an area(s) of interest.

The use of general anesthesia is often necessary to obtain diagnostic images. Light adhesive tape along with restraint aids (foam wedges, sandbags) will assist in proper patient positioning.

The use of dental radiographic equipment or a mammography unit can provide more detailed images in the small patient and may be of greater diagnostic value in these small animals.

Anesthesia and Surgery

Most information on anesthesia and surgery is extrapolated from other hystricomorph rodents. Although degus cannot vomit due to their highly developed cardiac sphincter, whenever possible, degus should be fasted 1–2 h prior to anesthetic administration. Many rodents store food in their oral cavities; cleaning out the oral cavity with a moistened cotton-tipped applicator following induction is recommended to prevent aspiration. Fasting patients for more than 1–2 h may increase the risks of hypoglycemia and peri-anesthetic ileus (Richardson 2008).

Anesthesia may be accomplished with injectable anesthetic agents and supplemental oxygen or through the delivery of inhalant anesthetic agents via a precision vaporizer (Colby et al. 2012). The small patient size restricts endotracheal intubation in the clinical setting. Anesthetic gases and oxygen may be delivered via an induction chamber, facemask with a non-rebreathing circuit, or commercial rodent anesthetic unit.

Any anesthetized patient should be closely monitored from induction through recovery. At a minimum, the patient's heart rate, respiratory rate, temperature, and anesthetic depth should be monitored. Additional anesthetic monitoring to include continuous ECG and pulse oximeter can provide supplemental information about the patient's circulatory and respiratory functions. Depth of anesthesia in most rodents can be evaluated partially by pinching the toes or gently pinching the ear for reaction to a painful stimulus.

Hypothermia in an anesthetized patient can occur rapidly and be devastating in such a small patient. The use of radiant heat is preferred for thermal support in the anesthetized patient, with careful monitoring of the environmental and patient temperatures to ensure the patient does not experience hyperthermia. Direct heat sources (hot water bottle) should be avoided as they lead to vasodilation, resulting in increased heat loss (Richardson 2008).

The patient should be monitored closely on anesthetic recovery and in the perioperative period. While minimal research exists, analgesic drugs used in chinchillas have been used in degus. When appropriate, the patient may be placed in a small, single-level, solid-wall enclosure for continued observation. Whenever possible, a temperature-controlled and oxygen-enriched incubator is ideal. Once the patient is stable, oriented to their environment, and able to ambulate unrestricted, a hide box, food, and water may be added to the enclosure. Make sure the food and water are easily accessible to the patient following surgery. The water bottle may need to be lowered and a shallow food bowl may be needed for easier access. The cage and bedding should be kept clean and dry to prevent any surgical wound contamination.

Parasitology

Fecal examination should be conducted on any new or ill animal that is exhibiting signs of gastrointestinal distress or unthriftiness. Infection with intestinal protozoal parasites is uncommon, but may result in diarrhea, weight loss, and in extreme cases, death. Immunocompromised animals, weanlings, or those experiencing overcrowding or inappropriate environmental disinfection may present a higher risk of parasitism. Treatment of intestinal parasitism is based on findings.

Emergency and Critical Care

Most sick degus presenting to the veterinary hospital are highly compromised and the stress of transport and intervention may be devastating. Whenever possible, the patient should be placed in an oxygen-enriched incubator, allowed to adapt to the environment, and, prior to handling, recover from the stressors of travel. In cases of life-threatening diseases such as hemorrhage, penetrating wounds, and open fractures, immediate stabilization may be necessary, followed by further evaluation and treatment once the patient is stable.

With the exception of acute trauma, most rodents will present in an advanced state of illness following a prolonged state of disease that has gone mostly unnoticed by the owner until recently. This is the result of wild behaviors used to reduce risks of predation, by masking signs of illness and disease. Therefore, most rodents presenting for illness and disease will likely be dehydrated, weak, and immunocompromised as a result of prolonged illness.

Clinical Techniques

Administration of Medication

The indications, drug, volume, risks, and skill of personnel are some of the factors that are considered in the selection of medications and route of administration. There are no pharmaceuticals labeled for use in rodents, although there are a number of references that provide anecdotal recommendations on dosages, routes, and duration of therapies. In general, dosages used for other rodents (such as guinea pigs) can be used for degus. Administration of oral medications, when compounded to an appropriate concentration, volume, and flavor, may ease administration and compliance by the owner and patient. When medications are to be sent home, consultation with the owner should be done to ensure they are able to administer the prescribed treatments.

Parenteral sites of medication administration include subcutaneous, intramuscular, intraperitoneal, and intravenous routes.

Oral (PO)

Oral administration of medications allows for at-home administration and avoids the risks of parenteral administration. Commercially prepared pediatric suspensions, when available and appropriate, should be used. Working with a veterinary compounding pharmacy can be beneficial when commercial products are not available. The pharmacist can create a palatable, oral suspension that is of appropriate concentration and volume for the small size and needs of the degu patient. Similar to guinea pigs, certain oral antibiotics can cause fatal dysbiosis of the intestinal flora and their use should be avoided. These include beta-lactams, lincomycin, clindamycin, and erythromycin.

In an anorexic degu, syringe feeding is needed in order to facilitate GI motility, promote a positive energy balance, and prevent hepatic lipidosis. Commercial herbivore hand-feeding formulas are available for this purpose, and the amount given daily may vary based on the animal's presentation and severity of illness. The total amount can then be divided into multiple smaller feedings throughout the day, and the amount gradually reduced as the animal's normal appetite returns.

Subcutaneous (SC)

Subcutaneous injection may be chosen for the administration of subcutaneous fluid therapies, pre-anesthetic agents, or therapeutics. The absorption of subcutaneous medications is slightly prolonged compared to intramuscular and intravenous routes.

Subcutaneous fluids should be warmed to body temperature prior to administration. A butterfly catheter may improve administration in an active patient. The dose of fluids administered will be dependent upon the patient's clinical presentation, dehydration (if present), and fluid calculations for maintenance, resuscitation, and ongoing losses. Subcutaneous dosing may be repeated once the body has absorbed the fluid bolus and there is medical indication for repeated therapy.

Intramuscular (IM)

Intramuscular injections are most easily administered in the quadriceps muscles of the hindlimbs. Care must be taken to avoid injection into the sciatic nerve. Only small volumes of medication can be administered at this site, and it is recommended not to inject volumes greater than 0.1 mL into any one site.

Intraperitoneal (IP)

Intraperitoneal injection allows for administration of larger volumes of medication compared to IV or IM. Risks of IP injection include accidental puncture of abdominal organs or the administration of tissue/mucosa-irritating substances into the abdominal cavity. For IP injections, the animal should be restrained in dorsal recumbency with the back legs pulled caudally. Due to the cecum, the needle is inserted at a 30° angle into the lower right quadrant (left in rats) of the abdomen.

Intravenous (IV)

Intravenous injection in rodents is difficult and often impractical in the clinical setting due to the extremely small size and friability of the vessels. The lateral saphenous and cephalic veins are recommended intravenous injection sites in the pet degu. Intravenous injection will require the patient to be sedated or anesthetized to reduce movement. A delicate approach and advancement into the vessel is necessary. A small flash of blood in the needle hub may or may not be seen due to the small size and vascular collapse. The medication should be administered slowly after releasing proximally applied pressure (high pressure can result in perivascular administration). The injection site should be closely monitored during administration to ensure the medication is not going perivascular; the animal may respond negatively to delivery of medication (pain) or a proximal swelling may be noticed.

Catheter Placement

Intravenous catheterization is most likely reserved for the research setting. When rapid fluid delivery is necessary in times of circulatory collapse, intraosseous catheter placement into the proximal humerus or trochanteric fossa of the femur is recommended using a hypodermic needle of appropriate size. Intraosseous catheters should be placed aseptically under general anesthesia as this procedure is painful (Jekl 2021). Radiographs should be performed following placement to confirm adequate placement within the marrow cavity.

Wound Management

Superficial wounds are best managed with topical cleansing and lavage to obtain a clean wound for second-intention healing. Application of topical medications and continued cleaning will cause stress to the animal and irritation that may lead to self-mutilation and delayed wound healing. The administration of systemic antimicrobial and anti-inflammatory agents may also be necessary. Providing a clean environment with reduced cage furnishing to help reduce further contamination and trauma is advised.

In larger, contaminated wounds, surgical exploration, debridement, and/or closure may be necessary. External sutures and bandages are not well tolerated and are usually chewed and removed by the patient (Richardson 2008). Whenever possible, subcuticular sutures are a better alternative for wound closure. Penetrating wounds and fractures can be difficult to manage and require creativity, owner compliance, and diligence in monitoring.

Euthanasia

Owners are often very attached to their pet degus due to their degus' long lifespan and highly social behaviors. As a result of illness, disease, or age-related health problems, the owner may request humane euthanasia to end the animal's suffering. As with other mammals, humane euthanasia may be accomplished with an overdose of a barbiturate anesthetic agent. Administration of a pre-anesthetic agent to calm the animal prior to euthanasia is preferred. The administration of an opioid or benzodiazepine may be given IM or SC, allowing for the owner to hold the animal while they become sedate. This is followed by an IP administration of an overdose of a barbiturate anesthesia. The animal will pass slowly as the medication is taken up in the body, ceasing circulatory function. Alternatively, the patient may be anesthetized with a high dose of inhalant anesthetic and an IP or IC injection of barbiturate anesthesia given to cease circulatory function.

References

Capello V, Sjoberg JG. 2005. Two techniques for neutering in a degu. *Exotic DVM* 6(6): 27–30.

Colby L, Rush H, Mahoney M, et al. 2012. *The Laboratory Rabbit, Guinea Pig, Hamster, and Other Rodents* (eds M Suckow, K Stevens, R Wilson). Waltham, MA: Elsevier.

Edwards MS. 2009. Nutrition and behavior of degus (*Octodon degus*). *Vet Clin North Am Exot Anim Pract* 12: 237–253.

Jekl V. 2021. Degus. In: *Ferrets, Rabbits, and Rodents Clinical Medicine and Surgery* (eds KE Quesenberry, et al.), 4th edn. St. Louis, MO: Elsevier, pp. 323–333.

Jekl V, Hauptman K, Knotek Z. 2011. Diseases in pet degus: a retrospective study in 300 animals. *J Small Anim Pract* 52: 107–112.

Johnson D. 2002. What veterinarians need to know about degus. *Exotic DVM* 4(4): 39–42.

Long CV. 2012. Common dental disorders of the degu (*Octodon degus*). *J Vet Dentistry* 29(3): 158–165.

Najecki DL, Tate BA. 1999. Husbandry and management of the degu (*Octodon degus*). *Lab Anim* 28(3): 54–57.

Nowak RM (ed). 1999. *Walker's Mammals of the World*, 6th edn. Baltimore, MD: Johns Hopkins University Press.

Richardson VCG. 2008. *Diseases of Small Domestic Rodents*, 2nd edn. Oxford, UK: Blackwell Publishing.

Teare JA (ed). 2013. *Octodon degus*. In: *ISIS Physiological Reference Intervals for Captive Wildlife: A CD Rom Resource*. Eagan, MN: International Species Information System.

Woods CA, Boraker DK. 1975. *Octodon degus. Mamm Species* 67: 1–5.

22

Hedgehogs
Ashley McGaha

Taxonomy, Anatomy, and Physiology

Hedgehogs belong to the order of Insectivora, which includes the most primitive of all living placental mammals today (Storer 1994). There are many different species of hedgehogs, including the European, African, Pruner's, Algerian, long-eared or Egyptian, and Ethiopian or desert hedgehog. There are slight differences between these species, including ear size and times of hibernation. For the most part, the various species can be treated medically in a similar way. The Egyptian hedgehog is noted for its surly disposition (Lightfoot 1997). The most commonly encountered species are the African pygmy hedgehog (*Atalerix albiventris*) and the European hedgehog (*Erinaceous europaeus*). African hedgehogs are slightly different from their European cousins in that they do not hibernate (Storer 1994). Unless otherwise noted, this chapter refers to pet African Pigmy hedgehogs (Figure 22.1).

Hedgehogs' brains are small and primitive and are smooth, not fissured. The sensory parts of the brain, including the olfactory and tactile areas, are very well developed. They have vibrissae, which are long, stiff hairs around the mouth, and nostrils that are used for their sense of touch (Storer 1994).

Their digestive tract consists of a simple stomach with no cecum. The transit time averages twelve to sixteen hours (Johnson 2004).

Most species of hedgehogs have five toes on each foot, except for the four-toed hedgehog, which only has four toes on the back feet (Storer 1994). They have very strong legs that are used for digging, and they have a nonexistent tail.

The reproductive anatomy of the hedgehog can be seen in Figure 22.2A and B. Note that the distance from the penis to the anus is much greater than the distance from the vulva to the anus. The penis of the male hedgehog can be seen in Figure 22.3.

Hedgehog skeletal anatomy is shown in Figure 22.4.

Dentition in these animals is unique because they are insectivores (Figure 22.5). The top row of teeth includes three incisors, one canine, three premolars, and three molars on each side, and the bottom consists of two incisors, one canine, two premolars, and three molars, for a total of thirty-six (Storer 1994, Johnson 2004). The incisors are sharp, the canines are small, and the molars and premolars are broad and flat for grinding. The first set of incisors has a large gap for appending and killing insects. Hedgehogs' teeth are very small and sharp. The baby teeth erupt at about 23 days and permanent teeth erupt at 7–9 weeks (Storer 1994).

Hedgehogs' senses, including smell and hearing, are very developed. Their eyesight is of moderate ability with limited color vision. They are highly resistant to many toxins (Storer 1994).

Their face, underbody, and legs are covered with cream- to brown-colored soft hairs. The rest of the body is covered with quills (also called spines) that emerge from the dorsal surface of the body called the mantle. Each quill is connected to a small muscle, which can help pull the quill erect. When the animal is frightened, the quills are erect and crossed, making a very formidable barrier (Storer 1994).

Hedgehogs are mostly terrestrial. They tend to walk slowly, looking for food, but can scurry at about six feet/second (4 miles/h). They can also use their spines as a cushion for rolling or dropping from high places (Storer 1994, Johnson 2004).

Biologic and Reproductive Data

Table 22.1 includes biological and reproductive information. Clinical pathology data is also included.

Exotic Animal Medicine for the Veterinary Technician, Fourth Edition. Edited by Bonnie Ballard and Ryan Cheek.
© 2024 John Wiley & Sons, Inc. Published 2024 by John Wiley & Sons, Inc.
Companion Website: www.wiley.com/go/ballard/4e

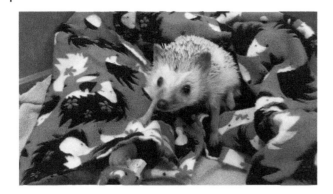

Figure 22.1 Hedgehog patient. (Courtesy of Dr. Stacey Wilkinson.)

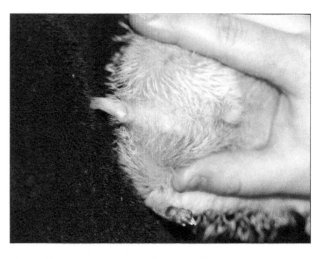

Figure 22.3 Male hedgehog. (Courtesy of Ryan Cheek.)

The urogenital opening of females is not connected to the anus but is directly anterior (toward the animal's head). The male's penis is more anterior than the female's genitalia (Storer 1994). The males have a prominent penis sheath. The testes are intraabdominal and not readily visible. Pressure can be placed on the abdomen to push the testes into the inguinal area. Internally, males also possess complex accessory reproductive glands, which may account for as much as 10% of body weight during the breeding season (Johnson 2004).

Pregnancy detection is often accomplished by monitoring body weight. Typically if a female gains more than 50 g within three weeks of being with a male, then she is considered pregnant. During pregnancy and lactation, nutritional demands may increase up to threefold. The female may cannibalize, kill, or abandon her newborn young if she is stressed or disturbed. Therefore, the male must be removed before parturition and the mother should not be disturbed for 5–10 days after parturition (Johnson 2004). Dystocia is rare and passive transfer of immunity occurs through colostrum in the first 24–72 h of life. Orphaned young can be raised on puppy or kitten milk replacer (Johnson 2004).

Behavior

Hedgehogs are usually solitary animals and they can be aggressive when housed together. However, captive animals can become quite tame over time (Storer 1994).

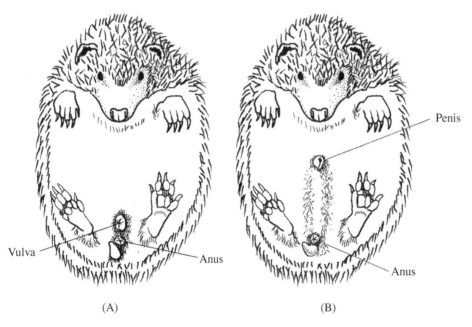

(A)   (B)

Figure 22.2 Sex determination in a hedgehog. (A) Female. (B) Male. (Drawing by Scott Stark.)

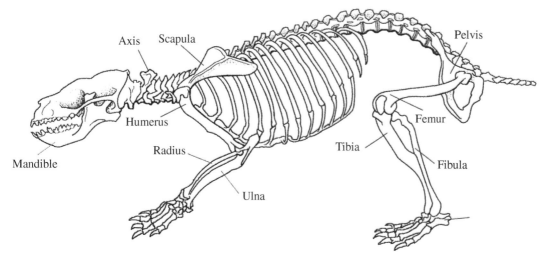

Figure 22.4 Skeletal anatomy. (Drawing by Scott Stark.)

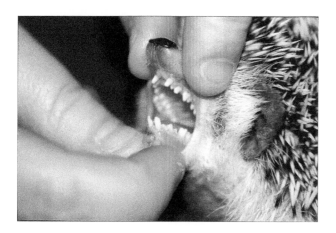

Figure 22.5 Dentition. (Courtesy of Ryan Cheek.)

Interestingly, a group of hedgehogs is called a prickle (Figure 22.6).

Typical defense postures include rolling into a ball with erect spines. Hedgehogs will hiss and spit to try to scare off potential predators. The spines will stay erect and will vibrate, in an effort to try and drive the spine into anything that touches it. This posture makes it very difficult for hedgehogs to be picked up either by a human or another animal (Storer 1994).

Hedgehogs are also good at wedging themselves into very small places. This can make it difficult to examine these pets. It is best to ask the owners to bring them in an easily accessible carrier, not in balls or other transport apparatuses that will make it difficult to remove them if they become frightened.

Hedgehogs can become excited when encountering smells or substances. They will engage in a behavior that is called self-anointing or anting (Ivey and Carpenter 2012). When they encounter an unusual odor or substance, they

Table 22.1 Biologic and reproductive data.

Sexual maturity	3–9 months (Storer 1994, 53)
Litter size	2–6 (Storer 1994, 53)
Gestation	32–48 days (Storer 1994, 53)
Weaning	5–6 weeks (Storer 1994, 53)
Breeding	1–2 times/year spontaneous ovulates, but depends on environmental conditions (Storer 1994, 54)
Lifespan	3–4 years in the wild (Gregory 1992, 63)
WBC	$5.8–21 \times 103/mL$ (Ness 1999, 596)
Neutrophils (%)	49–70
Lymphocytes (%)	22–38
Monocytes (%)	0
Eosinophil (%)	2–11
Basophils (%)	0–5
Hematocrit (%)	28–38
Hemoglobin (g/dL)	9.9–13.1
RBC ($\times 106$/mL)	4.4–6
MCV (fL)	60–67.4
MCHC (g/dL)	25.1–48.3
Platelets ($\times 103$/mL)	200–412
MCH (pg)	21.2–23.4
ALT (IU/L)	39.7–68.9 (Ness 1999 2:3, 600)
T. Bill (mg/dL)	0–0.1
T. Protein (g/dL)	5.3–6.3
Albumin (g/dL)	2.6–3.4
Glucose (mg/dL)	81.5–116.1
BUN (mg/dL)	21.3–32.9
Creatinine (mg/dL)	0.2–0.4
Calcium (mg/dL)	9.5–10.9

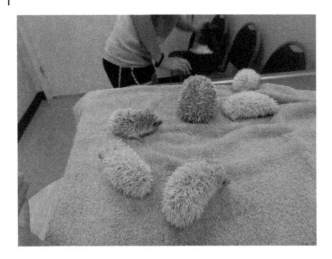

Figure 22.6 A prickle of hedgehogs. A female (the large one) with her litter. (Courtesy of Dr. Stacey Wilkinson.)

will become stiff and begin to make licking motions with their tongues, which are very long. They can start to bite or tug and produce large amounts of saliva. They can then get into extremely contorted positions by stiffening their front legs and pinning their heads back between their shoulder blades. The hedgehog then mixes the smell or substance with its saliva and applies it to its quills. This behavior can look much like a seizure and can continue for a long period of time (Figure 22.7A and B). Considerable controversy

exists about this behavior, but the most plausible theory is that the hedgehog is trying to transmit odor to other animals, or its current surroundings (Doss & Carpenter 2021).

Husbandry

The optimal temperature is between 65°F and 90°F, with the best temperature at 80°F. If the temperature is too low, these pets may start to hibernate, and if too high, they can have significant health problems related to heat stress. Hedgehogs can tolerate temperatures of up to 100°F for short periods of time (Storer 1994, Johnson 2004).

It is best to keep adults in individual cages because they can become aggressive if housed together. Plastic or fiberglass crates work well due to ease of cleaning. Aquariums make great housing, but care must be taken to monitor for overheating. Twenty-gallon aquariums are of adequate size and can be purchased with wire covers. Recycled/shredded paper or aspen shavings are a very good substrate and should be changed twice a week (Storer 1994). Litter box training is possible and hedgehogs tend to use the bathroom in one area of the cage. Once that area is found, a small litter pan can be placed in the cage. Dust-free litter seems to work best because these pets roll and scratch the litter (Storer 1994). Self-clumping litter can pose a problem for hedgehogs, because if they become wet

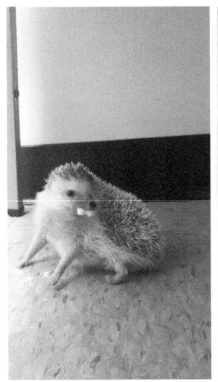

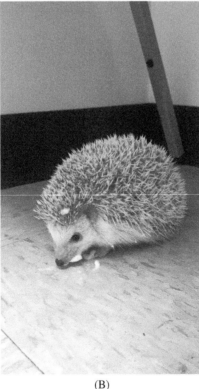

(A)   (B)

Figure 22.7 A hedgehog exhibiting self-anointing behavior. (A) Froth can be seen coming out of its mouth. (B) The substance can be seen on the mouth, on the head, and on the floor. (Courtesy of Dr. Stacey Wilkinson.)

for any reason, the litter can stick in the spines and be very difficult to remove. They should be kept on a 12-h light cycle (Johnson 2004).

Hedgehogs like security and they feel quite secure if they have a place to hide. A piece of PVC piping can be used for sleeping quarters. One side of the tube can be capped off, providing a small and secure place for them to sleep. However, should more than one hedgehog be housed together, the tube should not be capped, because they may pile on top of one another and become trapped inside (Storer 1994).

Regular rabbit or guinea pig water bottles work well. Bowls or saucers are potentially hazardous, because hedgehogs may climb inside and could drown.

Solid surface exercise wheels designed for hedgehogs can be used (Johnson 2004).

Nutrition

Hedgehogs are insectivores, which means that they require a high-protein diet (Storer 1994). For nonbreeding hedgehogs, feeding live food is acceptable. Crickets, mealworms, grasshoppers, snails, slugs, pinkie mice, and small nontoxic frogs are good sources. Small amounts of fruit may also be fed. Feeding live food can also add enrichment to their lives (Johnson 2004). The dietary calcium: phosphorus ratio should be 1.2–1.5:1 (Carpenter 2002).

Nonbreeding hedgehogs can become overweight or obese on regular diets, so care must be taken with the quantity that is fed. Kitten food (wet or dry) may be used, as well as high-quality dog food mixed with cottage cheese in a 5:1 ratio (Storer 1994). Chopped meat or hard-boiled eggs can be given as an occasional treat.

Commercial diets are also available. Mazuri manufactures an insectivore diet that can be fed to hedgehogs.

Common Diseases

Lameness

Often hedgehogs are presented for reluctance to move or weak gait. There are many causes of lameness, including overgrown toenails, constriction of toes with foreign material, fracture of long bones from trauma, and even neoplasia. Systemic disease causing weakness can be perceived as lameness (Lightfoot 1999).

Anorexia

Because hedgehogs do not have continuously erupting teeth, malocclusion is a problem that is seldom seen. However, gingival and periodontal disease do occur in older hedgehogs. Gingivitis may improve with ascorbic acid (50–200 mg/kg PO, SC every 24 h) (Johnson 2004). Husbandry problems, such as changing food, are often the cause of anorexia. If this does not seem to be the case, then blood work may be needed to determine whether there are any significant liver problems such as hepatic lipidosis or neoplasia (Lightfoot 1999).

Diarrhea

Diarrhea can be caused by many types of problems such as husbandry, parasites, bacterial infection, and even salmonellosis. After reviewing correct feeding techniques and food with the owner, other appropriate diagnostics, such as fecal floats, should be done. Other systemic illnesses can present with diarrhea as well.

Salmonella infections are well-documented in hedgehogs. Symptoms include anorexia, mucoid diarrhea, dehydration, and weight loss (Johnson 2004).

Dermatologic Problems

Many forms of diseases can cause problems with skin or quill loss. The problems can range from ectoparasites, hypersensitivity, dermatophytosis, and neoplasia. Fungal infections can be found with normal fungal culture techniques and are most likely to be *Trichophyton* or *Microsporum* (Lightfoot 2000, Johnson 2004). Zoonotic transmission has been documented (Johnson 2004).

Generalized infections are characterized by crusting around the base of the spines. They can be treated with either griseofulvin (25–50 mg/kg by PO every 24 h for 30 days) or ketoconazole (10 mg/kg PO every 24 h for 6–8 weeks) (Johnson 2004). If one hedgehog in a group is diagnosed, the entire group should receive treatment (Johnson 2004).

Ectoparasites are also common in the African Hedgehog (Figure 22.8). Mite infestations with *Caparinia* or *Chorioptes* species are routine (Johnson 2004).

Neurological Problems

Wobbling hedgehog syndrome is a fatal neurodegeneration disease that effects the brain and spinal cord of African pygmy hedgehogs (Mayer & Donnelly 2013). It is characterized by progressive ataxia and weight loss, eventually leading to paralysis and death. Animals that begin to show signs are usually under the age of two years old, although this disease can occur at any age (Mayer & Donnelly 2013). It starts in the hind legs and gradually ascends until only the head can move. The progression can occur over weeks to months. There is no definitive treatment and no etiological agent has been found (Johnson 2004).

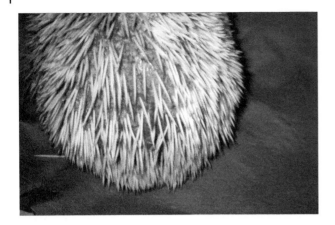

Figure 22.8 Mange. (Courtesy of Dr. Sam Rivera.)

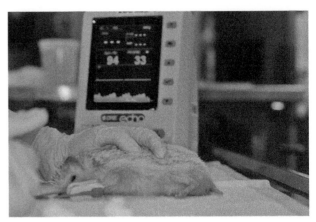

Figure 22.9 Obtaining a SpO$_2$ in a hedgehog with respiratory disease.

Progressive paralysis has been noted in hedgehogs. A viral encephalopathy has been noted in European hedgehogs (Ness 1999). Nutritional deficiencies can also cause many of the same signs. Rabies as well as *Baylisascaris* migration and polioencephalomyelitis are among the causes of neurologic disease.

Ophthalmologic Trauma

Due to the fact that these pets ball up, eye problems are usually associated with trauma and are not noticed until later in the course of the disease. These pets are also very difficult to treat. Enucleation is common and they do quite well with only one eye (Lightfoot 2000).

Liver Disease

Liver disease also occurs. Fatty liver disease and hepatic adenocarcinoma are two of the most common. Anorexia may be the only sign of liver disease (Johnson 2004).

Urinary Disease

Cystitis and urolithiasis are the most common types of urinary disease found in pet hedgehogs. As in other animals, a urinalysis with culture and radiographs should be obtained when urinary disease is suspected (Ivey and Carpenter 2012). Renal disease is also common and can be secondary to systemic disease. Lethargy, weight loss, polyuria, and polydipsia may occur (Johnson 2004).

Internal Parasites

Hedgehogs are susceptible to internal parasites such as nematodes, cestodes, and protozoa. *Isopora* and *Eimeria* species coccidia can cause diarrhea. Lungworm infections can also occur and result in bronchopneumonia or even death. Internal parasites are diagnosed by fecal floatation and direct smear (Johnson 2004).

Respiratory Disease

Hedgehogs are susceptible to respiratory pathogens such as *Pasteurella*, *Bordetella*, and *Corynebacterium*. Nasal discharge and sneezing may result. Diagnostic procedures include radiographs and a culture and sensitivity. SpO$_2$ should also be obtained to measure the oxygen saturation in the tissues (Figure 22.9). Treatment should be supportive and include antibiotics, fluid therapy, bronchodilators, oxygen therapy, and nebulization if needed (Johnson 2004).

Neoplasia

Neoplasia in hedgehogs is common. They can develop a wide range of tumors. Specific neoplasms reported in the hedgehog include squamous cell carcinomas, cutaneous mast cell tumors, mammary gland tumors, cutaneous hemangiosarcoma, alimentary lymphosarcomas, and plasmacytoma (Carpenter 2002).

Obtaining a History and Physical Examination

It is important to obtain as much information as possible about the pet before any actual handling takes place. Because hedgehogs are frightened very easily, it is better to observe the pet while taking a thorough history, including what the pet eats and drinks, its cage environment, or any other significant findings. Much of the physical examination must be performed under anesthesia to prevent the pet from balling up.

Hedgehogs can be difficult pets to pick up, but an object such as a spoon or litter box scooper can be used to pick them up. One should be very gentle and make sure that a finger does not get caught if the pet is trying to ball up.

There are many techniques to get hedgehogs to unroll. One method is to hold the hedgehog over a flat surface with the head pointing downward. With time, the hedgehog will unroll and reach for the table. Once the pet has unrolled, gently grab the back legs and hold the animal suspended by the back legs over the table (Gregory 1992). If this fails, anesthesia is necessary. Isoflurane is very well tolerated by these pets (Lightfoot 1999). A mask or tank is the most effective way to administer anesthesia. Salivation is often encountered with isoflurane.

Hedgehogs have a wide variety of squeals, snuffling, and sneezes that should not be confused with abnormal respiratory sounds (Johnson 2004).

Radiology

Diagnostic imagining is most easily obtained if the animal is sedated or anesthetized. Imaging that includes a contrast study such as magnetic resonance imaging (MRI) and computed tomography (CT), may require heavier sedation for an intravenous or intraosseous catheter placement. Positioning is similar to that of other small animals (Figure 22.10).

Anesthesia, Analgesia, and Surgery

Anesthesia and sedation are an important part of the physical exam. Most hedgehogs will curl up into a ball with their quills erect to create a defensive wall against predators, which, in this situation, is the veterinary staff. There are many drug combinations including alfaxalone, midazolam, hydromorphone, and ketamine that will create heavy sedative or anesthetic effects by administering an IM injection in-between the quills into the epaxial muscles. This will allow the animal to uncoil and for the veterinarian to perform their full physical exam. Isoflurane and sevoflurane have historically been well tolerated when injectable drugs are not an option. This is best accomplished by using a large dog mask and removing the diaphragm. Place the entire mask over the hedgehog and then wait for sedation to occur. Once the hedgehog uncurls, it is preferable to switch to a smaller mask (Figure 22.11) (Lightfoot 1999). Atropine (0.4 mg/kg SC, IM) can be given to help reduce hypersalivation. Supplemental heat is essential (Johnson 2004).

While limited data exists on the subject of the use of analgesics in hedgehogs, agents such as buprenorphine and meloxicam have been used (Doss & Carpenter 2021).

The most common surgical procedure is toe amputation, secondary to a string or hair that creates a foreign body and cuts off blood circulation. However, routine procedures are also performed including castration and ovariohysterectomy (Johnson 2004).

Urinalysis

Extensive analysis of the urine of the African hedgehog has not been done but extrapolations can be made from research on the European hedgehog. Research showed that the urine was negative for glucose, acetone, and acetoacetic acid. Albumin was present in about half of the animals (Ness 1999).

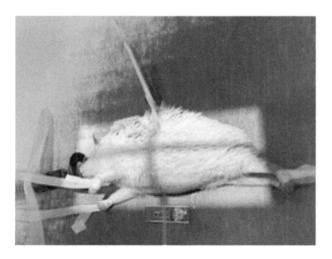

Figure 22.10 A hedgehog in right lateral recumbency for whole body radiographs with the mantle collimated out of view.

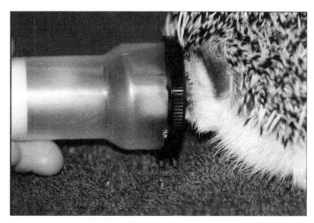

Figure 22.11 Anesthesia is maintained after initial induction by placing the patient in a face mask. (Courtesy of Ryan Cheek.)

Parasitology

Mites are a common problem with hedgehogs. The two major parasites commonly seen are *Caparinia* and *Chorioptes*. *Caparinia* is usually distributed over a significant portion of the body, and it may suddenly appear that entire hedgehog's skin is moving. Ivermectin is commonly used but must be used with proper shampoos as well. The Chorioptic species usually presents as a moderate to severe skin infection around the face and ears. Ivermectin is very effective (Lightfoot 2000).

Dermatophytes are also common causes of quill loss. *Trichophyton* is the most common dermatophyte found.

A variety of nematode, cestode, and protozoan parasites have been found in hedgehogs. Coccidia is present in as much as 10% of wild hedgehogs (Ness 1999). *Crenosoama striatum* is a common lungworm of the wild hedgehog.

Emergency and Critical Care

Many of the same techniques used in small mammals can be used in hedgehogs; however, with hedgehogs, anesthesia is still needed to perform a good physical examination. Intraosseous catheters are very useful in these small patients. Many must be monitored carefully because they will start to curl up and make further diagnostics quite difficult.

Clinical Techniques

Venipuncture

Venipuncture is next to impossible in the awake hedgehog. Supplies needed include a large face mask (diaphragm removed), small face mask; anesthesia machine; 1-mL, 25-gauge needle syringe; 3-mL, 22-gauge needle syringe; and blood collection tubes (preferably small tubes). See Figures 22.12–22.14. The technique for a jugular venipuncture is as follows:

1. A large anesthetic face mask with diaphragm removed is obtained.
2. The patient is placed under the face mask with the opening of the face mask tight against the table.
3. Oxygen and anesthetic gas are turned on.
4. Wait for the patient to become anesthetized.
5. Once the patient is asleep the face mask is changed to a smaller one.
6. The patient is placed in dorsal recumbence.
7. Gentle pressure is applied to the thoracic inlet.

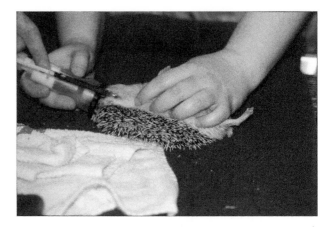

Figure 22.12 Jugular venipuncture. (Courtesy of Ryan Cheek.)

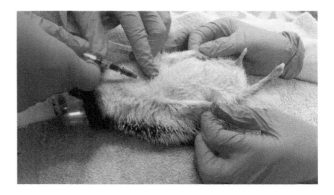

Figure 22.13 Anterior vena cava venipuncture on sedated animal. (Courtesy of Ian Kenda.)

8. A 3-cc, 22-gauge or 1-cc, 25-gauge needle is inserted into the jugular vein caudally and directed cranially to the point of the jaw. Alternately, the needle could be inserted into the proximal vein with the needle directed caudally (Figure 22.11). Gentle negative pressure is applied until blood is seen. **Note**: Many of these patients are obese so this technique is performed blindly.

TPR

Much of this information can be obtained while looking at the patient before it is handled; however, many times anesthesia is required. A large face mask with the diaphragm removed is placed over the patient and held tight to the table. Once the patient is anesthetized, a small face mask can be applied. The TPR can then be obtained along with a physical examination. A hedgehog's normal temperature is 95.7–98.6°F, heart rate is 180–280 bpm, and respiration is 25–50 breaths per minute.

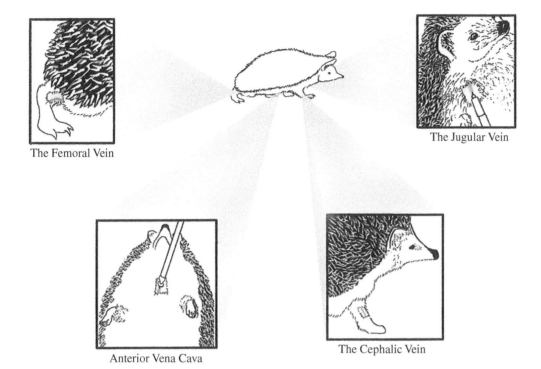

The Femoral Vein

The Jugular Vein

Anterior Vena Cava

The Cephalic Vein

Figure 22.14 Venipuncture sites. (Drawing by Scott Stark.)

Urine Collection

The patient is anesthetized as described in the previous techniques. The patient is then placed in dorsal recumbency. The bladder is palpated and stabilized while a 3-cc, 22-gauge needle is placed through the skin and body wall and then into the bladder. Once the sample collection is complete the needle and syringe are withdrawn.

Administration of Medications

Administration of fluids can be difficult. When hedgehogs are older, they do not take oral fluids easily, and they must be eating well if moistening the food is considered. Some oral medications can be injected into food but it must be certain that the patient is eating.

Injectable medications are tolerated well by these pets. Medications can be injected into the quill area subcutaneously (Lightfoot 2000). This is a high fat area for the hedgehog but absorption is sufficient.

Subcutaneous injections can be made in the rear legs or back. This is performed by carefully picking the patient up. A 25-gauge needle with a syringe is inserted between the quills and then under the skin. The medication is injected and then the needle and syringe are removed (Figure 22.15).

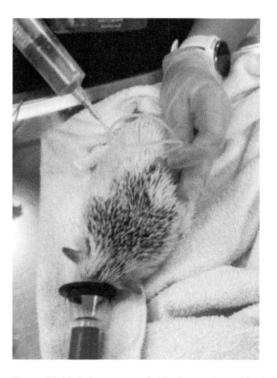

Figure 22.15 Subcutaneous fluids given using a 21 g butterfly catheter in between the spines.

Intravenous catheter placement can be done with the cephalic vein but can be very difficult due to the size of the patient. When the pet awakens from anesthesia, it may curl up and cause the catheter to function improperly.

Bandaging and Wound Care

Bandaging and wound care can be very difficult to manage in these pets. Being aware of what will happen to the bandage as the pet curls up is crucial. Anesthesia or heavy sedation is usually required and normal bandaging techniques are used.

In general, many of the techniques used in small animal medicine can be used in hedgehogs; however, one must always consider the possible complications if the animal should curl up.

Euthanasia

Euthanasia in hedgehogs is performed via an overdose of a barbiturate. First, the patient should be anesthetized via injection or gas anesthesia and then using standard IV injection protocols, the barbiturate should be administered.

References

Carpenter J. 2002. *Diseases and Medicine of the African Hedgehog*. Tufts Animal Expo.

Doss G, Carpenter J. 2021. In: *Ferrets, Rabbits, and Rodents: Clinical Medicine and Surgery*, 4th edn (eds KE Quesenberry, et al.), pp. 403–413. St. Louis, MO: Elsevier.

Gregory M. 1992. Hedgehogs. In: *Manual of Exotic Pets* (eds P Beynon, J Cooper), p. 63. Gloucestershire: British Small Animal Veterinary Association.

Ivey E, Carpenter J. 2012. In: *Ferrets, Rabbits, and Rodents: Clinical Medicine and Surgery*, 3rd edn (eds KE Quesenberry, et al.), pp. 413–414. St. Louis, MO: Elsevier.

Johnson D. 2004. Diagnosing and treating African pygmy hedgehogs. In: *Atlantic Coast Veterinary Conference*.

Lightfoot T. 1997. Clinical techniques of selected exotic species: chinchilla, prairie dogs, hedgehogs, and chelonians. *Semin Avian Exotic Pet Med* 6(2): 96–105.

Lightfoot T. 1999. Clinical examination of the chinchillas, hedgehogs, prairie dogs, and sugar gliders. *Vet Clin North Am Exotic Anim Pract* 2(2): 447–469.

Lightfoot T. 2000. Therapeutics of African pygmy hedgehogs and prairie dogs. *Vet Clin North Am Exotic Anim Pract* 3(1): 155–172.

Mayer J, Donnelly T. 2013. *Clinical Veterinary Advisor: Birds and Exotic Pets*. St. Louis: Saunders.

Ness R. 1999. Clinical pathology and sample collection of exotic small mammals. *Vet Clin North Am Exotic Anim Pract* 2(3):591–620.

Storer P. 1994. *Everything You Wanted to Know About Hedgehogs But You Didn't Know Who to Ask*. Columbus, TX: Country Store Enterprises, pp. 14–96.

23

Skunks

Serina Scott and Samuel Rivera

Introduction

Skunks are commonly kept as pets and are comparable to cats in regard to their temperament and size (Figures 23.1 and 23.2). They were originally classified within the family Mustelidae, which includes ferrets, weasels, badgers, mink, and otters. However, based on recent DNA work, it has been found that skunks are distinct from mustelids and are now in their own family, Mephitidae. The striped skunk (*Mephitis mephitis*) is the most common species found in the pet market. It is native to North America, ranging from southern Canada to the United States and northern Mexico. In the wild, skunks do not undergo true hibernation.

The most popular color pattern is black fur with white stripes along the dorsum. Different colorations including brown and white and albino may be seen in practice. They have extremely sharp teeth and their bite can cause severe injuries. The skunks in the pet market are usually descented at 2–4 weeks of age. In the United States, it is illegal to keep skunks as pets, in some states so it is essential for veterinary personnel to be familiar with state and local regulations.

Skunks are intelligent and adapt well to life in captivity. They commonly bond with their owners if obtained at a young age. When fearful or stressed, they can bite so it is important that they be socialized while young (Benato and d'Ovidio 2021).

They can be litter box trained and harness or leash trained. They are nocturnal animals but can adjust to a diurnal cycle.

Anatomy and Physiology

The anatomy and physiology of skunks are similar to those of other small carnivores. One key difference is their highly developed anal sacs, which can eject their contents for a distance of 6 m and with great accuracy.

Biologic Data

Average lifespan: 10–12 years
Body temperature: 102°F (38.9°C)
Heart rate: 140–190 beats per minute
Respiratory rate: 25–50 breaths per minute
Average body weight: 4.5 kg
Gestation: 63 days
Litter size: 4–10
Urine pH: 6.0

Husbandry and Nutrition

In the wild, adult males are solitary except during the winter months when they may share a den with several females (Wallach & Boever 1983). Spaying and neutering skunks between 3–6 months of age are recommended to prevent both behavioral and medical issues. Young skunks can be housed together, but as they get older, they often require separate enclosures. The cage should provide a nest box and a litter box. Skunks have a natural instinct to dig and their enclosure should be secured to prevent escape.

Wild skunks are omnivores with their natural diet consisting of invertebrates, small mammals and birds, fruits, vegetables, and grain. To date there is no formulated diet specifically for skunks; however, there are some commercially made diets marketed specifically for domestic skunks. Other commercial options would include a combination of omnivore and insectivore diets. A varied diet consisting of fruits, vegetables, eggs, dog food, mice, cereals, and insects is recommended. The diet should mimic their diet in the wild as closely as possible. Dairy products are a good source of calcium but should be fed in limited amounts as they can cause gastrointestinal upset. It is important to note that skunks have a tendency to become obese and their weight should be closely monitored. Skunks are less active and tend to gain weight in

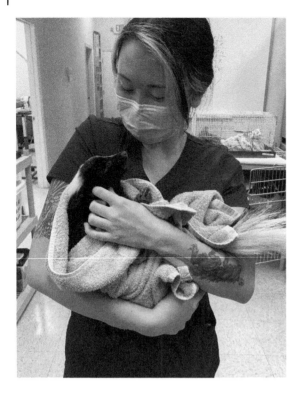

Figure 23.1 Skunk patient. (Courtesy of Serina Scott.)

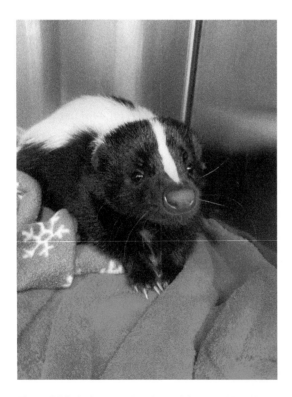

Figure 23.2 A skunk patient in a clinic cage. Note the long front nails. They can be clipped with a dog/cat nail clipper. (Courtesy of Serina Scott.)

the fall and winter months. Feeding an adequate diet will decrease the development of obesity and the associated health problems.

Common Health Problems

Obesity

This is the most common clinical presentation and the leading cause of morbidity in skunks. Most pet skunks are kept inside and fed an inadequate diet that leads to obesity. In most cases, correction of the diet and adequate husbandry practices can help to maintain an ideal body weight.

Hepatic Lipidosis

This disease is caused by an increased accumulation of triglycerides in the liver, which is due to an increased mobilization of fat from the body stores and the inability of the liver to process it expeditiously. The end result is the build-up of fat within the hepatocytes leading to compromised function. There is a close relationship between obesity and the development of hepatic lipidosis. Clinical signs include prolonged anorexia, lethargy, vomiting, weight loss, and jaundice. The presumptive diagnosis of hepatic lipidosis is based on the history, physical exam findings, and serum chemistry abnormalities. A definitive diagnosis is based on the cytologic evaluation of a liver fine-needle aspirate or biopsy. Treatment involves primarily supportive care.

Cardiomyopathy

Cardiac disease is not uncommon in skunks. The clinical signs are exercise intolerance, weight loss, dyspnea, lethargy, anorexia, coughing, ascites and/or edema, pale mucous membranes, and cold extremities. The diagnosis is based on radiographs, electrocardiogram, and echocardiogram. Cardiomyopathy is treated the same as in ferrets.

Dental Disease

The dental formula of skunks is 2 (I3/3, C1/1, PM3/3, M1/1). Common dental conditions seen in skunks are advanced periodontal disease and fractured teeth. Common clinical signs are changes in eating habits, halitosis, pawing at the mouth, hypersalivation, or facial swelling. Periodontal disease is usually a result of a poor diet. Treatment involves dental cleaning, antibiotics, and diet correction where appropriate.

Dermatitis

Skin problems are common in skunks, particularly in obese ones. Some of the most commonly seen lesions are dry and scaly skin, alopecia, papules, pustules, and excoriations. Dermatitis can be caused by nutritional deficiencies, ectoparasites, and fungal or bacterial infections.

Canine Distemper

Canine distemper has been reported in the ferret, skunk, mink, badger, weasel, sable, and grison (Wallach & Boever 1983). The clinical signs are fever, hyperemia of the face and ears, scleral inflammation, ocular discharge, depression, anorexia, diarrhea, dyspnea, hyperkeratosis of the foot pads, and neurologic signs. The incubation period is 5–7 days for the acute phase. The diagnosis is based on clinical signs and serologic testing. Treatment involves mostly supportive care. Fluid support and broad-spectrum antibiotics should be initiated. Unvaccinated skunks that contract canine distemper have a poor prognosis.

Feline Panleukopenia

Feline panleukopenia can affect skunks. This is an acute viral disease that can lead to high mortality in skunks. The clinical signs are hemorrhagic enteritis, anorexia, and depression. Death usually occurs within 3–5 days after the onset of the clinical signs. A presumptive diagnosis is based on the characteristic clinical signs accompanied by a low white blood cell count. The best treatment is supportive care.

Aleutian Disease

Aleutian mink disease parvovirus (ADV) is known to infect skunks (Pennick et al. 2007). Infection is characterized by hypergammaglobulinemia and immune-complex disease. Persistent infection is due to the inability of the animal's immune response to eliminate the virus. Clinical signs are non-specific and may include lethargy, erythema of the skin around the eyes, pyrexia, dehydration, and facial tremors. Lymphoplasmacytic infiltration and immune complex deposition in various organs may ultimately result in death. No effective treatment has been reported.

Zoonotic Diseases

Baylisascaris columnaris is a roundworm found in skunks. This parasite can cause visceral larva migrans in humans which is often fatal. Usual contamination is through the fecal-oral route. Strict hygiene and use of PPE when handling potentially contaminated material is the best prevention of transmission.

Rabies is a serious and fatal human health problem. The rabies virus can be transmitted to humans through saliva most commonly from wild infected skunks due to a bite. In North America, the wild striped skunk is the most prominent wildlife reservoir of rabies (Drenzek & Rupprecht 2000). The clinical signs of rabies in skunks are varied. Generally, any behavior considered abnormal for the particular animal should be considered suspicious. The incubation period for rabies varies from 2 weeks to 6 months. In the furious form of the disease, the virus can be shed in the saliva 1–6 days prior to death.

The diagnosis of rabies is based on the identification of viral antigen and/or characteristic lesions in the brain. Public health officials do not accept vaccination against rabies in pet skunks, and the animal may need to be euthanized and tested for rabies if it is involved in a biting incident. Although rabies is a great concern in the wild skunk population, the disease is relatively rare in captive-bred skunks. Pet skunks, as other common pets, can become infected with rabies if exposed to a reservoir in the wild.

Physical Examination

A healthy skunk should have a glossy, thick coat and bright clear eyes. Yellow coloring of the white fur is considered abnormal. The stools should be formed. Obesity or an underweight patient should raise a red flag as to the health status of the pet.

Signs of illness in a skunk include change in stool consistency, reduced appetite, dull hair coat, yellowing of the white fur, obesity, dry cracked feet, ocular or nasal discharge, coughing, sneezing, and bad breath.

Vaccinations

Pet skunks should be vaccinated against canine distemper, feline panleukopenia, and rabies (Miller 1995). For young skunks, a vaccination schedule and route of administration typically used for puppies can be employed. There are no vaccines licensed for use in skunks, however, vaccines licensed for use in ferrets can be used. It is important to note that if a skunk bites a person, public health officials will not accept rabies vaccination (as it is used off-label) and the animal may need to be euthanized and tested for rabies.

Restraint

Skunks can be restrained in a manner similar to that used for cats. One difference is that many skunks lack a significant scruff, making scruffing behind the neck difficult. Most tame skunks can be picked up by placing one hand on each side of the body caudal to the axillary region. The skunk's primary defense is the expression of its anal sacs. It is highly recommended that any skunk that has not been descented be examined outdoors as their spray is pungent and incredibly difficult to remove from most surfaces. Leather gloves can be used for handling fractious animals. Many fractious skunks will require chemical immobilization prior to handling. Use of a squeeze cage may be helpful.

Radiology

The radiographic techniques and positioning are similar to those used in domestic animals. Many skunks require sedation in order to obtain good-quality radiographs.

Anesthesia/Analgesia

Gas anesthesia is commonly used in skunks. Sevoflurane and isoflurane are among the safest anesthetic agents used being maintained on gas anesthesia via a face mask or endotracheal intubation. Skunks are commonly sedated first with parenteral drugs. A common sedation protocol consists of ketamine at a dose of 10–20 mg/kg in combination with midazolam at a dose of 0.5–1 mg/kg given IM. Buprenorphine may be added at a dose of 0.02–0.03 mg/kg if indicated for pain control. Dexmedetomidine and butorphanol as well as other drug combinations are also used, with doses typically extrapolated from dog doses and titrated as needed. IV induction is another option for anesthetizing skunk patients, using either propofol or alfaxalone at dog doses. This requires the use of a catheter, with the most common and feasible placement being the cephalic vein. Most skunks must be sedated before attempting to place a catheter.

As with all species, it is important to recognize and manage pain in skunk patients. Common signs of pain are similar to those of other exotics such as inappetence, lethargy, hunched posture, and squinting. Pain control is essential for the health and well-being of the animal. Preoperative and perioperative pain medications should be added to anesthetic protocols when indicated. Postoperative pain can be managed with medications such as meloxicam at a dose of 0.2 mg/kg by mouth every 24 h, gabapentin at a dose of 5–10 mg/kg by mouth every 8–12 h, or opioids such as buprenorphine or tramadol at dog doses.

Parasitology

Skunks are susceptible to a variety of internal parasites including roundworms, tapeworms, and coccidia. Roundworms and tapeworms are managed similarly to an infestation in domestic animals. Coccidiosis can cause severe disease in skunks. The clinical signs commonly seen are diarrhea, weight loss, anorexia, dehydration, and depression. The diagnosis is based on the identification of oocysts in the feces. Treatment involves the administration of antiprotozoal agents similar to those used in domestic species.

Toxoplasmosis has been reported in skunks, ferrets, and weasels. The clinical signs are fever, lymphadenopathy, splenomegaly, myocarditis, pneumonitis, hepatitis, hydrocephalus, encephalitis, dermatitis, and enlarged lymph nodes. The antemortem diagnosis is based on serologic testing. Antiprotozoal drugs are used to treat toxoplasmosis.

The lungworm *Crenosoma mephitidis* is a parasite that can affect the lungs of skunks. The clinical signs are coughing, dyspnea, depression, anorexia, and depression. The diagnosis is based on the identification of the infective larvae in the feces. Ectoparasites also commonly affect skunks. Fleas, ticks, and mites should be treated in the environment as well as topically with products approved for use in cats (Miller et al. 2015).

Clinical Techniques

Blood Collection

Blood sampling is an important diagnostic tool particularly when assessing a sick skunk. The sites most commonly used are the jugular, cephalic, lateral saphenous, and femoral veins. Manual restraint for blood collection is appropriate for tame skunks used to handle or with extremely debilitated animals. Fractious animals will need sedation for safe venipuncture. The size of the needle used will depend on the size of the animal and the vein used.

Jugular Vein

Skunks usually resist restraint for jugular venipuncture more than they do for cephalic or lateral saphenous collection. The restraint is similar to that used for cats. The animal should be restrained in sternal recumbency, with the front legs held over the edge of the table. The assistant can hold the head with one hand extended by holding the head from the dorsum, use the thumb and fingers, and wrap the head in the palm, placing the thumb and fingers on opposite sides of the head under the temporomandibular joint. Alternatively, if the skunk does not

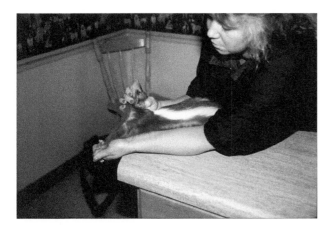

Figure 23.3 Restraint for jugular venipuncture of the skunk. (Courtesy of Ryan Cheek.)

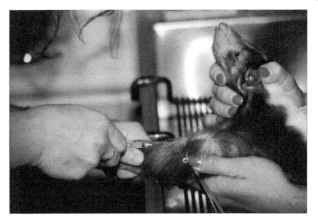

Figure 23.4 Cephalic venipuncture in a skunk. (Courtesy of Ryan Cheek.)

tolerate being stretched over the table, the skunk can be positioned at the edge of the table. The restrainer can then lift the head to allow the technician access to the jugular vein. This method is less stressful, and skunks tend to tolerate it much better. Gentle pressure is applied at the thoracic inlet lateral to the trachea. The needle is inserted bevel up at a 25° angle into the vein. After the sample is collected, pressure is released, the needle is withdrawn, and digital pressure is applied at the venipuncture site for 30 s (Figure 23.3).

Cephalic Vein

The animal is restrained in sternal recumbency. An assistant should restrain the patient's head by the scruff of its neck with one hand and the forelimb extended by the elbow. Alternatively, the head can be restrained as described for jugular venipuncture. Pressure is applied with the thumb around the elbow, rotating gently laterally. The limb is held with a free hand and the thumb is used to stabilize the vein. The needle is inserted at a 20–25° angle. Once the vessel is entered, gentle suction is applied until the desired amount is obtained. Too much suction can cause collapse of the vein. Once the needle is withdrawn, gentle pressure should be applied to the venipuncture site (Figure 23.4).

Lateral Saphenous Vein

This vein is located in the lateral aspect of the hindlimb. This is the third option if the other two vessels are not accessible. This vein is small and often yields a small volume of blood. The assistant can hold the skunk in lateral recumbency by holding the scruff of the patient's neck with one hand and the venipuncture leg with the other hand. The leg is held around the stifle with the leg extended. The leg

is grasped around the tarsus and the skin is gently pulled to stabilize the vein. The needle is inserted at a 20° angle and the blood sample is collected. Digital pressure is applied for 30 s afterward to prevent hematoma formation.

Femoral Vein

The femoral vein is located in the medial aspect of the thigh. Collection from this vein is performed similarly to the technique used in the cat. In obese skunks, the femoral vein can be very difficult to find.

IV Catheter Placement

The cephalic vein is the preferred vein for IV catheter placement. Cephalic catheterization in skunks is much like placing a catheter in a dog breed with short, stumpy legs (e.g., Corgis, Dachshunds, etc). Prior sedation will be necessary in most cases. They often have thick skin, so it may be helpful to nick the skin with a large gauge needle over the vein prior to catheter placement. With the patient properly restrained, the site should be shaved and prepped. Using an appropriately sized catheter, the catheter and stylet should be inserted into the cephalic vein at a shallow angle and slowly progressed until blood is flowing. After carefully inserting the catheter into place over the stylet, the catheter is then capped. Finally, the catheter should be secured with white tape and vet wrap and checked for patency before use.

Urine Collection

Urinalysis is an important part of the health assessment in skunks. The techniques for collecting urine are similar to those used in dogs and cats.

Voided urine: Urine can be collected from the bottom of the cage using a syringe. The disadvantage of this technique is that fecal and litter contamination affects the results.

Manual expression: With the animal sedated, transabdominal pressure is applied to the urinary bladder to overcome the sphincter pressure. The urine can be collected into a sterile container or from the tabletop.

Cystocentesis: With the animal sedated, the bladder is gently isolated. A 25- to 22-gauge needle on a 3- to 5-mL syringe is inserted into the bladder and the urine is collected. This is the preferred method when performing a culture and sensitivity test on the urine.

Fecal Analysis

The flotation and direct fecal smear techniques are performed as for domestic species.

Administration of Medications

There are several routes for administration of medications. Oral route: Liquids or powders mixed with food are the most common forms of oral medications. In many cases, the skunk's sharp teeth precludes the use of tablets. Liquid medications can be placed in the side of the mouth with a syringe. Powder medications can be mixed with a favorite treat or a small amount of soft food such as yogurt or cottage cheese.

Intramuscular route: Parenteral medications can be given in the thigh musculature or the biceps.

Subcutaneous route: This site is most commonly used for the administration of fluids to sick animals. The interscapular and lateral flank regions are the best sites for the administration of subcutaneous fluids.

Intravenous route: The cephalic, jugular, and lateral saphenous veins can be used for the administration of medications. In most cases, the skunk has to be sedated to facilitate the use of intravenous medications unless the animal is severely debilitated.

Euthanasia

Domestic skunks should be sedated or anesthetized using injectable or gas anesthetics prior to being euthanized. After they are sufficiently sedated, euthanasia should be performed via IV injection.

References

Benato D, d'Ovidio D. 2021. Skunks. In: *Ferrets, Rabbits, and Rodents Clinical Medicine and Surgery* (eds KE Quesenberry, et al.), pp. 419–423. St. Louis, MO: Elsevier.

Drenzek CL, Rupprecht CE. 2000. The rabies pandemic. In: *Kirk's Current Veterinary Therapy XIII* (ed JD Bonagura). Philadelphia: WB Saunders Co.

Fowler ME. 1986. Descenting carnivores. In: *Zoo and Wild Animal Medicine*, 2nd edn (ed ME Fowler). Philadelphia: W.B. Saunders Co.

Miller E. 1995. Immunization of wild animal species against common diseases. In: *Kirk's Current Veterinary Therapy XII* (ed JD Bonagura). Philadelphia: WB Saunders Co.

Miller RE, Fowler ME, Kollias GV, Fernandez-Moran J. 2015. Mustelidae. In: *Fowler's Zoo and Wild Animal Medicine*, vol. 8, pp. 476–490). WB Saunders Co.

Nowak RM. 1991. *Walker's Mammals of the World*, 5th edn, vol. 1. Baltimore: The Johns Hopkins University Press.

Pennick KE, Latimer KS, Brown CA, Hayes JR, Sarver CF. 2007. Aleutian disease in two domestic striped skunks (*Mephitis mephitis*). *Vet Pathol* 44: 687–690.

Wallach JD, Boever WJ. 1983. *Diseases of Exotic Animals: Medical and Surgical Management*. Philadelphia, PA: WB Saunders Co.

24

Sugar Gliders
Nia Chau and Samuel Rivera

Introduction and Natural History

Sugar gliders (*Petaurus breviceps*) are small marsupials native to Australia and New Zealand (Figure 24.1).

They are nocturnal arboreal animals that inhabit the trees of tropical and sclerophyll forests and create nests in tree hollows. In the wild, sugar gliders live in groups of up to 12 individuals (Booth 2000). They are very social animals that are best kept in pairs or small related groups in captivity to avoid clinical depression. They require a large enclosure with branches, nest boxes, and hiding areas. They are vocal and have a variety of yaps and screams. (Johnson-Delaney, 2021) Proper husbandry and diet are essential for a healthy pet. During extreme weather conditions or food shortages, sugar gliders conserve energy by going into torpor for up to 16 hours per day (Booth 2000).

Sugar gliders were first introduced to the United States companion pet industry in 1993 (Brust 2009). They have since gained popularity and are appealing to most due to their small size and "cute" appearance. People are also attracted to the species because of their innate desire for companionship. This can allow a pet owner and sugar glider to form a bond.

Anatomy

Sugar gliders have blue–gray fur with a dark line extending from the nose to the lower back. Various color morphs now exist due to selective breeding and demands from consumers in the pet industry. Each foot has five digits, but the second and third digits of the hind feet are partially fused (Figure 24.2). They are used as a comb for grooming and climbing.

Sugar gliders have a membrane (the patagium) that extends from the lateral aspect of the fifth digit of the forelimb to the tarsus (Figure 24.3).

This membrane allows the sugar glider to glide a fair distance. They then use their bushy tails like a rudder to lightly steer through the air while gliding. Sugar glider tails are also somewhat prehensile. Though they cannot support their entire body weight, gliders occasionally use them to carry things such as nesting material.

Males have frontal, sternal, and urogenital scent glands (Figure 24.4A, B, C, D).

The females have a pouch and urogenital glands. Scent glands are also found on the paws, corners of the mouth, and external ears. The scent glands are used for marking territory and members of the same group (Smith 1984). The males have a pendulous scrotum located cranial to the penis (Figure 24.5).

The female has a ventral abdominal pouch that is used for rearing joeys. It opens cranially and contains four teats. Unlike most marsupials, sugar gliders lack an epipubic bone which is believed to help support the pouch. This adaption may have evolved to reduce skeletal weight and make gliding easier. Sugar gliders have a cloaca where the gastrointestinal, urinary, and reproductive tracts empty. They have a large cecum that may assist in digestion of the sap eaten in the wild (Henry & Suckling 1984).

Sugar gliders have a short gestation period of 15–17 days in which the altrical joeys will migrate to the abdominal pouch where a longer development period of approximately 3 months occurs within the pouch. Once they outgrow the female's pouch, young sugar gliders remain in the nest and are cared for by parents until they are weaned at 110–120 days.

The incisors of sugar gliders are adapted for their diet. They often have to bite into tree bark to access food sources, so their mandibular incisors are designed to be slightly longer and protrude at a more forward angle. This alignment can sometimes be mistaken for a malocclusion but is a normal anatomical finding and should not be trimmed (Figure 24.6).

Exotic Animal Medicine for the Veterinary Technician, Fourth Edition. Edited by Bonnie Ballard and Ryan Cheek.
© 2024 John Wiley & Sons, Inc. Published 2024 by John Wiley & Sons, Inc.
Companion Website: www.wiley.com/go/ballard/4e

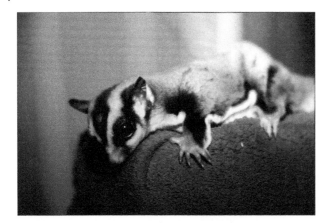

Figure 24.1 Sugar glider. (Courtesy of Ryan Cheek.)

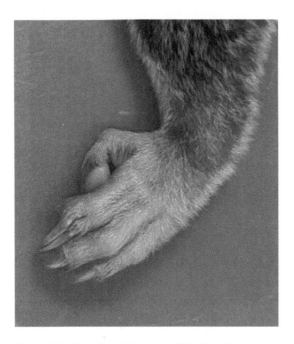

Figure 24.2 Hind foot. (Courtesy of Nia Chau.)

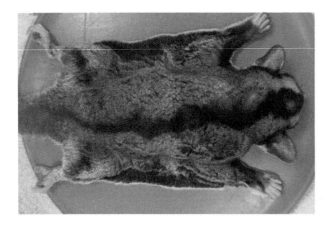

Figure 24.3 Patagium. (Courtesy of Nia Chau.)

Biologic Data

Weight range: 95–160 g
Body length: 16–21 cm
Heart rate: 200–300 beats per minute
Respiratory rate: 16–40 breaths per minute
Rectal temperature: 96.5–97.9 °F (35.8–36.6 °C)
Cloacal temperature: 89.6 °F (32 °C)
Gestation: 15–17 days, young leave the pouch at 70 days
Weaning age: 110–120 days
Lifespan: 9–12 years

Husbandry and Nutrition

Though small in size, sugar gliders need an enriching habitat with ample room. The larger the enclosure the better for the animal. An enclosure measuring a minimum of 2 × 2 × 2 meters is adequate for housing up to six animals (Dunn 1982). A nest box for sleeping and hiding must be provided. The nest box can be lined with a piece of cloth, shredded bark, or dried leaves, and this lining should be changed weekly and/or as needed when soiled. Newspaper and pine or cedar wood shavings are not recommended. Sugar gliders are arboreal animals; therefore, branches and furnishings suitable for climbing are essential. A pair is the minimum number to keep together, but small colonies are ideal since they are a social species.

The environmental temperature should be between 64 and 75 °F (18–24 °C). They can withstand temperatures in the mid to high 80s but higher temperatures can predispose them to hyperthermia.

In the wild, sugar gliders eat sap and gum from eucalyptus and acacia trees, nectar from eucalyptus blossom, and a variety of insects (Henry & Suckling 1984). Though they are mainly insectivores, consuming the sugar-containing sap from these plant sources make them an omnivorous species. The diet in captivity consists of a variety of fruits, commercial sugar glider pellets, commercial insectivore diets, insects supplemented with vitamins and minerals, nectar, and small invertebrates. Food and water should be provided in an elevated location. Nectar should be provided in covered feeders to keep the nectar from getting on the fur. The ideal amount of food to offer is 15–20% of their body weight (Booth 2000).

Common Diseases

Nutritional Osteodystrophy

This is one of the most common diseases seen in captive sugar gliders (Pye & Carpenter 1999). The clinical signs

Figure 24.4 (A) Gular scent gland in a standard gray sugar glider. (B) Frontal scent gland in a standard gray sugar glider. (C) Frontal scent gland in a leucistic sugar glider. (D) Abnormal gular scent gland in a leucistic sugar glider. (Courtesy of Nia Chau.)

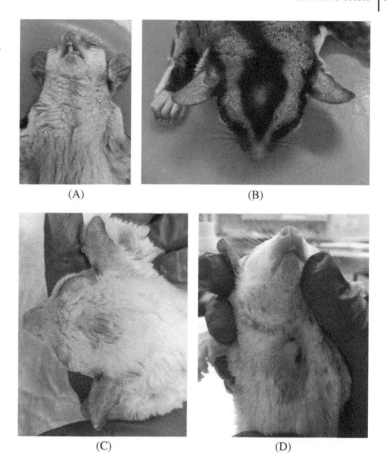

(A)　　　　　　　　(B)

(C)　　　　　　　　(D)

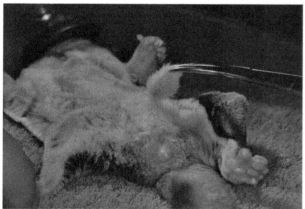

Figure 24.5 Pendulous scrotum in an intact male sugar glider. (Courtesy of Ashley McGaha.)

include acute onset of hindlimb paresis or paralysis. This disease is believed to be caused by feeding an inadequate diet low in calcium and vitamin D_3 and high in phosphorus. Too much fruit and muscle meat can predispose animals to this disease. The diagnosis is based on a thorough history and radiographs. The treatment includes cage rest, parenteral calcium, diet correction, and calcium and vitamin D_3 supplementation.

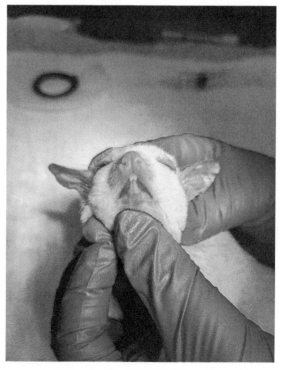

Figure 24.6 Incisors. (Courtesy of Nia Chau.)

Enteritis

Diarrhea is commonly seen in sugar gliders. The etiology is multifactorial. Common causes include bacterial infections, intestinal parasites, malnutrition, or stress. Fecal parasite checks and cultures are helpful diagnostic tests. Treatment is aimed at correcting fluid and electrolyte imbalances, and addressing the etiology if known.

Trauma

Trauma is most common in wild sugar gliders. In captivity, the most common cases of trauma involve cat and dog attacks. Some of the common injuries are lacerations, pneumothorax, hemothorax, spinal trauma, and ocular trauma. Other sources of trauma can include cage mate aggression or self-mutilation. The cause of the aggression or self-mutilation must also be addressed in these cases. Often cage mate aggression is a result of improper introduction among individuals. Self-mutilation may be a result of stress from being solitary or an indication of some other systemic disease process.

Dental Disease

Tartar buildup associated with periodontal disease is often seen. This has been associated with feeding carbohydrate-rich diets (Booth 2000). The teeth can be cleaned as needed. Feeding insects with a hard exoskeleton can help minimize tartar buildup (Figures 24.7A, B, and 24.8).

Obesity

Obesity is seen in sugar gliders fed an inadequate diet. Diets high in fat and proteins predispose animals to obesity. Lack of exercise can also contribute to obesity. Obese animals are predisposed to cardiac and hepatic disease.

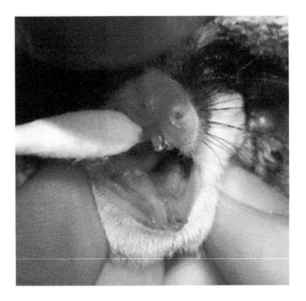

Figure 24.8 Dental disease seen during an oral examination. (Courtesy of Megan Partyka.)

Stress-related Disease

Animals under constant stress are prone to developing behavioral problems. Some of the clinical signs of stress-related disorders include alopecia, self-mutilation, coprophagia, hyperphagia, polyuria, pacing, and cannibalism. The source of the stress must be identified and eliminated to help correct the problem.

Rectal Prolapse

The rectum and/or cloaca can prolapse through the vent. Common causes include tenesmus secondary to enteritis, malnutrition, trauma, or stress. The prolapsed tissue should be kept moist and replaced as soon as possible. Prolonged exposure to prolapsed tissue can lead to necrosis, which carries a worse prognosis for successful replacement and

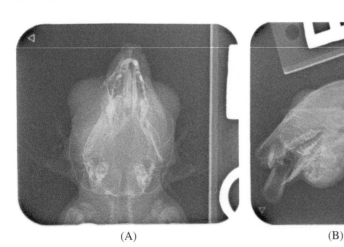

(A)   (B)

Figure 24.7 (A) Dental disease. (B) Evidence of osteomyelitis. (Courtesy of Megan Partyka.)

recovery. It is important to rule out and correct potential causes of the prolapse to prevent it from recurring.

Penile Prolapse and/or Self-mutilation

Prolapse of a male sugar glider's penis can be a result of stress-induced self-mutilation, sexual frustration, or an indication of a systemic disease. In severe cases, the penis may become necrotic and amputation is recommended. Sugar gliders have a forked penis and urinate from the base of the penis, so amputation of the distal necrotic portion will not impede urine elimination (Figure 24.9).

Neoplasia

Neoplastic disease is relatively common. Lymphoid neoplasia is the most common type of tumor reported (Booth 2000). Other tumors reported include mammary gland tumors, bronchogenic carcinoma, chondrosarcoma, masses in visceral organs, and oral tumors.

Malnutrition

Malnutrition is frequently seen in sugar gliders fed an inadequate diet. As a result, malnutrition leads to hypocalcemia, hypoproteinemia, and anemia. The clinical signs of malnutrition are non-specific and include lethargy, weakness, dehydration, pale mucous membranes, cachexia, and in some cases, seizures and pathologic fractures. The owner should be educated about the appropriate diet.

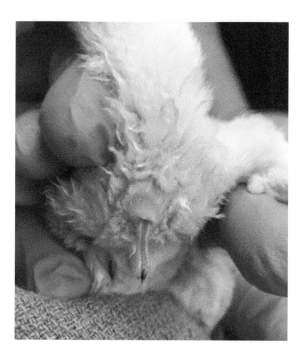

Figure 24.9 Penile prolapse. (Courtesy of Kelsey Trumpp.)

Treatment involves correction of the dietary inadequacies and supportive care. In these cases, it is imperative that the diet be corrected at home.

Physical Examination

Sugar gliders can be challenging to examine without sedation. A thorough history should be taken first that assesses the animal's enclosure environment, diet, and enrichment opportunities. One should ask about the number of animals kept and the enclosure size. The diet should be recorded. The owner should be asked whether there are other pets in the household, and where the animal was obtained. While taking the history, the animal's motor function and disposition can be visually observed. If a weight is needed, often the owner can place the animal on the scale, and then the weight can be recorded. If the animal is fractious, the weight can be obtained by placing it in a cloth bag. Body temperature can be obtained via aural, axial, or cloaca routes. Aural and axial routes may be preferred in a conscious patient (Figure 24.10A and B).

Measures should be taken to prevent over-stressing the animal while also protecting those handling the sugar glider from getting bitten. In particularly stressed or fractious animals, sedation should be strongly considered to safely obtain a full physical examination. This protects the safety of both the handlers and the patient.

Restraint

Prior to handling a sugar glider, care must be taken to secure all doors or other possible escape routes in the examination area. Sugar gliders can be fast and agile, so proper handling techniques and observation of the animal's body language and behavior are essential to prevent escape and injuries.

Depending on the animal's demeanor, when possible minimal restraint may be used to examine a sugar glider. Owners usually transport their sugar glider in a zippered pouch. If this method is used, it is advantageous to incorporate the pouch as part of effective restraint tools that can be used (Figure 24.11A and B). If the animal has a docile demeanor, visual examinations and other parts of a physical examination such as auscultation may be performed by minimally exposing the animal inside of the pouch prior to removal.

Treats can be used to reward the sugar glider for their participation in their veterinary care. Sedation should be considered whenever possible, particularly in fearful, nervous, and fractious patients. The sedation can be achieved via injectable agents.

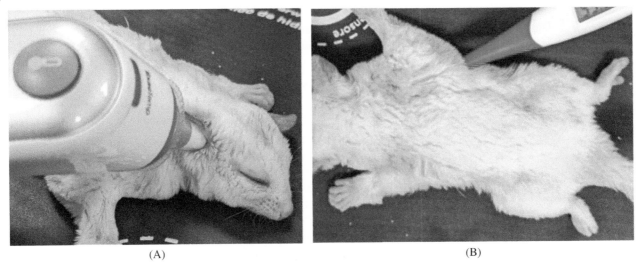

(A) (B)

Figure 24.10 (A) Obtaining an aural temperature. (B) Obtaining an axillary temperature. (Courtesy of Nia Chau.)

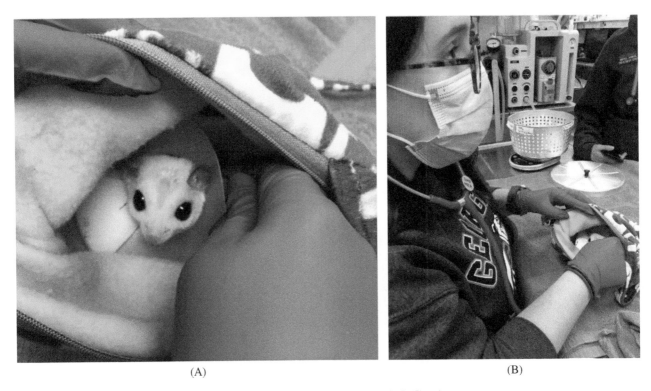

(A) (B)

Figure 24.11 (A) and (B) Use of a zippered pouch as a restraint tool. (Courtesy of Nia Chau.)

The best way to restrain sugar gliders is by holding the head between a thumb and middle finger and using the index finger to restrain the top of the head. The body is then placed in the palm of the restrainer's hand. Fractious animals can be restrained using a cloth bag or small hand towel. To accomplish this, the animal should be placed in a small enclosure (scale basket or box). Then a cloth bag or towel can be placed over the hand that will grasp the animal. The animal is then grasped and the bag slipped over the whole body. Once in the bag one can gently expose the head and restrain it. It is important to keep the seam of the bag toward the outside to keep the animal from injuring itself with the small threads.

Radiology

The radiographic techniques in sugar gliders are similar to those used in other domestic animals. A comparison of

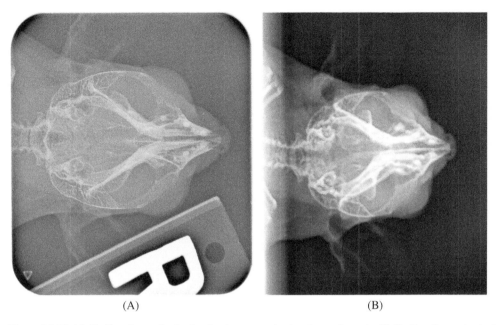

(A) (B)

Figure 24.12 (A) Skull radiograph obtained using a standard radiography unit. (B) Skull radiograph obtained using a dental radiography unit. (Courtesy of Nia Chau.)

radiologic techniques can be visualized in Figure 24.12A and B.

Anesthesia and Analgesia

Anesthetic preparation in sugar gliders involves a protocol with a combination of analgesic and anesthetic agents and a means of anesthetic monitoring. Sugar gliders should be fasted before undergoing anesthesia to minimize regurgitation and subsequent risks of aspiration. At least 4 hours is recommended but a longer duration may be required for surgeries of the gastrointestinal tract. Combinations of injectable analgesics and sedatives/anesthetics along with gaseous anesthetics such as sevoflurane and isoflurane are most commonly used. Injectable medications that are used include midazolam, hydromorphone, ketamine, and alfaxalone to name a few. When possible and indicated, venous access should be obtained via an intravenous catheter or an intraosseous catheter (Figure 24.13).

Induction can be accomplished by either face mask or chamber induction, but injectable induction agents are gaining popularity. A large face mask can be used as an induction chamber. The animal can be maintained via a face mask (Figure 24.14).

Intubation is strongly recommended when possible but may be difficult to achieve due to the size of the animal. Anesthetic monitoring is achieved through end-title CO_2, SpO_2, ECG, thermoregulation, and Doppler heart rate monitoring. SpO_2 can be attained via placing the probe on an

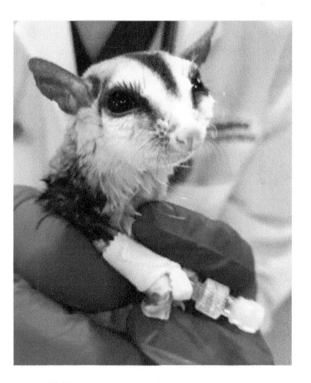

Figure 24.13 IV catheter. (Courtesy of Nia Chau.)

extremity, such as a foot, while a Doppler can be placed over the heart or on the femoral artery (Figure 24.15A, B, and C).

Thermoregulation should be provided via warming pads or a radiant heat source. Body temperature monitoring should be obtained via esophageal, rectal, or aural temperature monitoring.

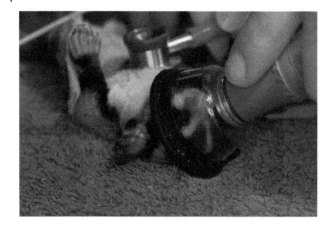

Figure 24.14 Isoflurane gas anesthesia by mask in a male sugar glider. (Courtesy of Ashley McGaha.)

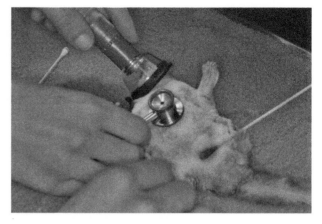

Figure 24.16 Preparation for castration of a male sugar glider. (Courtesy of Ashley McGaha.)

Surgery

The most common surgical procedures performed on sugar gliders are castration, ovariohysterectomy, and patagium repairs (Figures 24.16 and 24.17).

Other procedures include oral procedures such as dental extractions, phallectomy due to necrosis from a penile prolapse, abscess debridement, fracture repairs, and wound care from trauma due to aggression with cage mates or self-mutilation.

Parasitology

Coccidia and *Giardia* spp. have been identified in captive sugar gliders (Ness 1999). The diagnosis is based on the identification of the oocysts or trophozoites in the fecal sample. There is limited information on the incidence of gastrointestinal parasites in sugar gliders, but routine fecal examination should still be performed as part of an annual physical examination. This is particularly important when adding individuals into an existing population. Not only is it important to assess for internal parasite infections, but ectoparasites should also be monitored for and treated.

Clinical Techniques

Blood Collection

The blood volume that can be safely collected is up to 1% of the animal's body weight. Because of their active

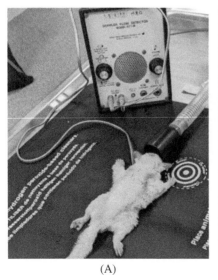

(A)

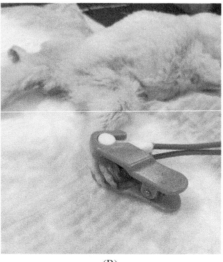

(B)

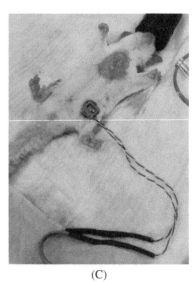

(C)

Figure 24.15 (A) Doppler placed on heart. (B) SpO$_2$ sensor on rear foot. (C) Doppler placed on the femoral artery. (Courtesy of Nia Chau.)

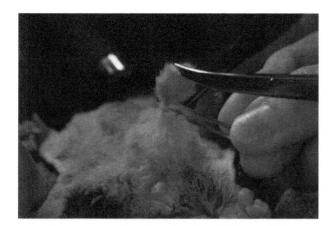

Figure 24.17 After using electrocautery to ligate the skin, vessels, and spermatic cord, the scrotum and testicles are removed with a scalpel blade. (Courtesy of Ashley McGaha.)

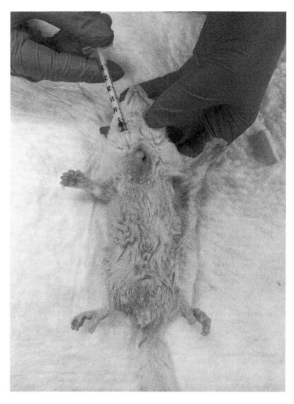

Figure 24.18 Venipuncture of the cranial vena cava. (Courtesy of Nia Chau.)

nature, sugar gliders often require sedation for blood collection, unless the animal is severely debilitated. They can be sedated using injectable sedative medications like midazolam or alfaxalone, or via gaseous anesthetics like isoflurane or sevoflurane via a mask or chamber induction.

Supplies needed include 27–30-gauge needles, 0.5- to 1-mL syringes, and 0.5-mL collection tubes.

Sites for venous blood collection include the jugular vein, cranial vena cava, medial tibial artery, cephalic vein, lateral saphenous vein, femoral vein, ventral coccygeal vein, and lateral tail veins.

Jugular vein: The animal is placed in dorsal recumbency. The forelimbs are aimed caudally. Gentle pressure is applied in the thoracic inlet. The fur is moistened along the jugular groove to allow better visualization. The needle is then inserted at a 30–45° angle in the jugular groove. Negative pressure is applied as the needle is advanced. The syringe will fill with blood as the jugular vein is entered.

Cranial vena cava: The animal is placed in dorsal recumbency. Both forelimbs are extended caudally. The needle is inserted at the angle formed by the manubrium and the first rib. The needle is aimed toward the contralateral hip joint at a very shallow angle. Suction is applied as the needle is advanced. It will fill with blood as soon as the vessel is entered. It is important not to reposition the needle in an attempt to find this vessel. If the vessel is missed, the needle should be withdrawn and another attempt made. Other vessels and nerves can be damaged inadvertently by excessive manipulation of the needle (Figure 24.18).

Medial tibial artery: The hindlimb is held in the extended position with the medial aspect exposed. The fur is slightly moistened with alcohol. The artery runs superficially from the stifle to the tarsus. The vessel should be visualized and the needle then inserted at a 30° angle. After the blood is

collected, gentle pressure should be applied to the site to avoid hematoma formation.

Other sites for blood collection include the cephalic, lateral saphenous, femoral, ventral coccygeal, and lateral tail veins (Figure 24.19).

The main disadvantage is that only very small amounts of blood can be collected from these sites due to their small

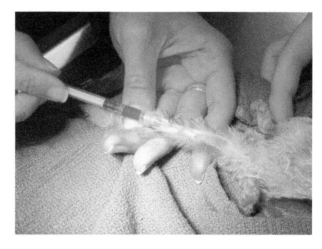

Figure 24.19 Ventral coccygeal vein venipuncture. (Courtesy of Nia Chau.)

size. In some cases, a small-gauge heparinized needle can be inserted into the vein and the blood collected directly from the hub using small collection containers or capillary tubes.

Urine Collection

Urinalysis is an important part of the health assessment in sugar gliders. The techniques to collect urine are similar to those used in dogs and cats.

Voided urine: Urine can be collected from the bottom of the cage using a small syringe. The disadvantage of this technique is that fecal and litter contamination affects the results.

Manual expression: With the animal sedated, gentle transabdominal pressure is applied to the urinary bladder to overcome the sphincter pressure. The urine can be collected into a sterile container or from the tabletop.

Cystocentesis: With the animal sedated, one should gently isolate the bladder. A 27- to 25-gauge needle on a 0.5- to 1-mL syringe is inserted into the bladder and the urine is collected. This is the preferred method when performing a culture and sensitivity analysis on the urine.

Fecal Analysis

The flotation and direct fecal smear techniques are performed as for domestic species.

Subcutaneous Fluid Administration

Subcutaneous fluid therapy can be administered to sugar gliders in the same manner as in other domestic species (Figure 24.20). The skin along the dorsum is tented and fluids are administered.

Intramuscular Injections

Intramuscular injections can be given into the epaxial or thigh muscles (Figures 24.21 and 24.22).

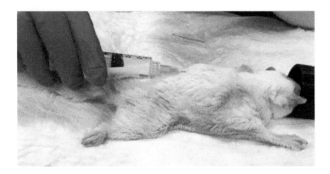

Figure 24.20 Subcutaneous fluid administration into the dorsum. (Courtesy of Nia Chau.)

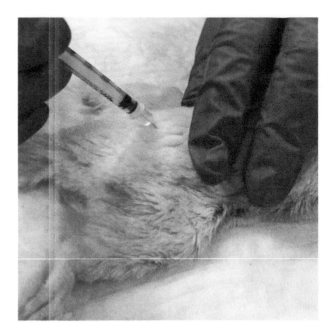

Figure 24.21 Epaxial injection. (Courtesy of Nia Chau.)

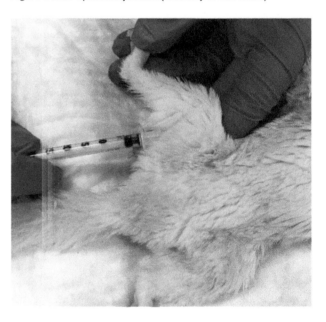

Figure 24.22 Hind limb intramuscular injection. (Courtesy of Nia Chau.)

Careful palpation and proper restraint are recommended when administering these injections. The muscles are small and care must be taken not to mistakenly hit important structures such as the vertebral column or sciatic nerves. Intramuscular injections are also important for administering sedative and analgesic agents. If a safe intramuscular injection is not able to be achieved, an alternative option can be a subcutaneous injection. In doing so, one must note that the onset of action of the drug will be slower and additional time must be allotted for the desired effect.

Euthanasia

Sugar gliders should be sedated or anesthetized prior to being euthanized. Injectable or inhalant anesthetics may be used for this procedure. Once sufficiently sedated, the euthanasia solution can be given by intravenous or intracardiac injection.

References

Booth RJ. 2000. General husbandry and medical care of sugar gliders. In: *Kirk's Current Veterinary Therapy XIII* (ed JD Bonagura). Philadelphia: WB Saunders Co.

Brust DM. 2009. *Sugar Gliders: A Complete Veterinary Care Guide*. Veterinary Interactive Publications.

Dunn RW. 1982. Gliders of the genus *Petaurus*: their management in zoos. In: *The Management of Australian Mammals in Captivity* (ed DD Evans). North Melbourne, Australia: Ramsay Ware Stockland.

Henry SR, Suckling GC. 1984. A review of the ecology of the sugar glider. In: *Possums and Gliders* (eds PA Smith, ID Hume). Sydney: Australian Mammal Society.

Ness RD. 1999. Clinical pathology and sample collection of exotic small mammals. *Vet Clin North Am Exot Anim Pract* 2(3): 591–620.

Pye GW, Carpenter JW. 1999. A guide to medicine and surgery in sugar gliders. *Vet Med* 94: 891–905.

Johnson-Delaney. 2021. In: *Ferrets, Rabbits, and Rodents: Clinical Medicine and Surgery*, 4th edn (ed KE Quesenberry, et al.), p. 388. St. Louis, MO: Elsevier.

Smith MJ. 1984. The reproductive system and paracloacal glands of *Petaurus breviceps* and *Gymnobelideus leadbeateri* (Marsupialia: Petauridae). In: *Possums and Gliders* (eds PA Smith, ID Hume), pp. 321–330. Sydney: Surrey Beatty & Sons with Australian Mammal Society.

25

Prairie Dogs

Stacey Leonatti Wilkinson and Samuel Rivera

Introduction

The black-tailed prairie dog (*Cynomys ludovicianus*) is a rodent native to North America, more specifically to the western plains of the United States (Figure 25.1). Over recent years, prairie dogs have become common in the pet trade. Prairie dogs are diurnal social animals that live in large groups in the wild. The ownership of wild-caught prairie dogs should be discouraged due to serious zoonotic potential. The source of a prairie dog should be investigated for this reason (Eshar and Gardhouse 2021). It is important to know that owning prairie dogs is illegal in certain regions in the United States.

Anatomy and Physiology

The anatomy and physiology of prairie dogs are similar to those of other rodents of comparable size. They are hindgut fermenters. The male has a prominent scrotum and the penis is relatively easy to exteriorize (Figure 25.2). The female has a short distance between the anus and the vaginal groove. Prairie dogs have a characteristic set of scent gland papillae that can be visualized on the anal margin when the animal is stressed.

Biologic Data

Average weight: 0.5–2.2 kg
Average lifespan: 6–10 years
Rectal temperature: 95.7–102.3 °F (35.4–39.1 °C)
Heart rate: 150–318 beats per minute
Respiratory rate: 40–60 breaths per minute
Breeding age: >2 years

Gestation: 30 days
Litter size: 1–10 (average 4)
Weaning age: approximately 6 weeks

Behavior

Prairie dogs are social by nature and can be affectionate pets (Figure 25.3). It is best if acquired at the age of 10 weeks, after they are fully weaned when they can then imprint on a new owner. This is not to say that an adult cannot make a good pet however more patience and time will be needed (Eshar and Gardhouse 2021).

Husbandry and Nutrition

Prairie dogs being very social animals are best kept in pairs or greater numbers. One male can be housed with multiple females. They require adequate room for digging. The cage should be well-ventilated and easy to clean. The enclosure should be made of heavy-gauge wire or stainless steel or plexiglass rather than wood so that it cannot be chewed. If made of metal mesh, it should be designed so that the snout or feet cannot fit through the bars. This can be accomplished by the mesh being very fine (0.5 in.) (Eshar and Gardhouse 2021).

It is important to provide a thick layer of substrate to allow the animals to burrow. Adequate bedding materials include recycled paper, non-aromatic wood shavings, and hay. The larger the enclosure the better.

The enclosure should be provided with a suitable hiding box. Multilevel cages are a consideration as it satisfies their desire to have a place to stand and look over their

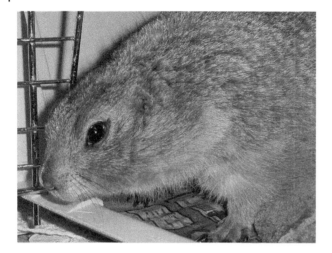

Figure 25.1 Prairie dog. (Courtesy of Dr. Dan Johnson.)

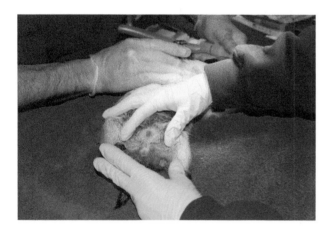

Figure 25.2 Male anatomy. (Courtesy of Dr. Sam Rivera.)

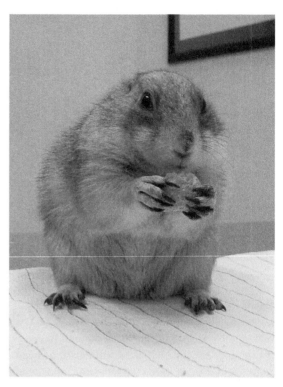

Figure 25.3 Prairie dog holding a treat. (Courtesy of Dr. Dan Johnson.)

Common and Zoonotic Diseases

Barbering

This condition often presents as areas of abnormal fur appearance with underlying healthy skin. It can be caused by the animal or a cage mate chewing the fur. It is often related to stress, and husbandry practices must be evaluated to help minimize fur barbering.

Obesity

Obesity is commonly seen in prairie dogs. As with other unusual pets, this condition is often due to inadequate diet and lack of proper exercise. Diets high in fat such as seeds and nuts lead to obesity and should be avoided. Obesity predisposes prairie dogs to other conditions such as heart, respiratory, and liver disease.

Nasal Dermatitis

This is a common condition in captive prairie dogs. It is most often due to rubbing the face on the cage wire. This results in abrasions and inflammation leading to secondary bacterial infections.

surroundings. They can also be provided with enrichment opportunities like tubing and pipes for tunneling, appropriate toys for chewing (cardboard, woven hay, etc.), and a solid-bottomed exercise wheel for running (Eshar and Gardhouse 2021).

Prairie dogs are not true hibernators. When exposed to low ambient temperatures, they may enter torpor, a state in which the body's physiologic activities are greatly reduced to conserve energy. The environmental temperature should be kept between 69 and 72 °F (20.5–22 °C) and the humidity at 30–70% (Johnson-Delaney 1996).

Prairie dogs are mostly herbivores. They should be fed high-quality grass hay ad lib, supplemented with a measured amount of a commercially formulated herbivore diet (such as rabbit pellets) as prairie dogs are prone to obesity. Fresh water must be provided on a daily basis.

Dermatomycosis (Ringworm)

Prairie dogs are susceptible to *Microsporum canis* and *Trichophyton mentagrophytes*. The most common clinical sign is alopecia. The diagnosis is based on a positive fungal culture. The treatment is similar to that of domestic animals and involves the administration of systemic antifungal drugs in addition to topical antifungal treatment.

Respiratory Disease

Respiratory disease is relatively common in prairie dogs. Obesity and poor ventilation are two common predisposing factors. Cedar bedding contains aromatic oils that can lead to irritation of the respiratory tract. Nasal foreign bodies (cage litter, hay, and carpet fibers) are common presentations. Overgrowth of the maxillary incisor teeth roots can lead to increased pressure and irritation in the nasal sinus passages. Pneumonia is often associated with bacterial and viral agents. The clinical signs of respiratory disease are similar to those seen in dogs and cats. They include dyspnea, nasal or ocular discharge, cyanosis, anorexia, and lethargy. The treatment includes appropriate antibiotic therapy and supportive care. Appropriate husbandry is important in the prevention of respiratory disease.

Elodontomas

Elodontomas (previously called odontoma or pseudo-odontoma) are a common cause of upper respiratory symptoms in captive prairie dogs (Phalen et al. 2000). Elodontomas are caused by inflammation of the periodontal bone as a result of dental disease or trauma. This repeated inflammation and trauma to the continuously growing tooth substance results in a mass-like growth at the apical root of the incisor tooth (Figure 25.4). This mass can invade the nasal passages leading to respiratory distress. The diagnosis is based on radiographic abnormalities of the incisor's root and surrounding soft tissue (Figure 25.5). Treatment involves removal of the affected tooth and debridement of the abnormal tissue. This is an extremely difficult surgery and requires intensive supportive care A stent may be placed during surgery to aid in breathing while the swelling and inflammation from the surgery subsides. Alternatively, the stent may be placed as a palliative treatment when surgery is not an option (Figure 25.6).

Heart Disease

Obesity is a predisposing factor for the development of heart disease. Clinical signs are lethargy, syncope,

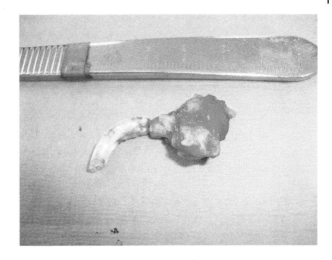

Figure 25.4 Excised elodontoma. (Courtesy of Dr. Dan Johnson.)

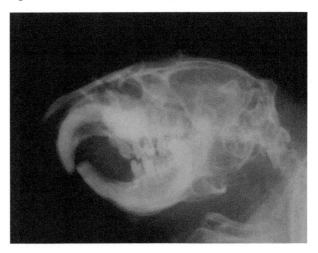

Figure 25.5 Radiograph of an elodontoma. (Courtesy of Dr. Dan Johnson.)

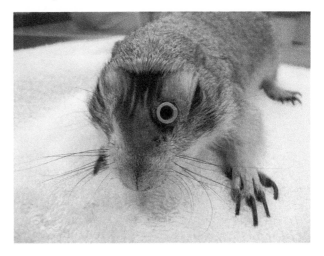

Figure 25.6 Prairie dog with a stent. (Courtesy of Dr. Dan Johnson.)

cyanosis, dyspnea, and cold extremities. The diagnosis is based on auscultation, radiography, echocardiography, and ultrasonography. Treatment is similar to other mammalian species.

Pododermatitis (Bumblefoot)

This condition is usually the result of poor husbandry. Animals kept in wire-bottom cages can develop small ulcers on the footpads that become infected. The infection results in severe swelling and abscess formation in the affected foot. In severe cases, tendonitis and osteomyelitis can develop. Bumblefoot is treated by debriding the affected lesions in conjunction with topical and systemic antibiotics. Correction of the underlying husbandry problem is essential for resolution and/or prevention of bumblefoot.

Zoonotic Diseases

Prairie dogs, particularly wild-caught animals, can be reservoirs of *Yersinia pseudotuberculosis*, *Yersinia pestis*, and *Baylisascaris* sp. *Yersinia pseudotuberculosis* can cause severe illness in humans. Affected humans can develop acute mesenteric lymphadenitis, fever, anorexia, vomiting, enteritis with diarrhea, and dehydration. This bacterium is transmitted to humans through the ingestion of contaminated material. *Yersinia pestis* causes sylvatic plague in humans, and the bacterium is transmitted to humans through the bite of fleas from carrier prairie dogs. Humans can also contract the infection from handling tissues from affected animals during necropsy. Flea control is essential to eliminate the human risk of exposure.

Baylisascaris sp. can cause serious disease in humans due to larval migration through the viscera, central nervous system, and eyes. This parasite is transmitted to humans through the ingestion of contaminated material or contact with open wounds on the skin.

Monkeypox is a zoonotic viral disease found primarily in wild mammals and in humans in the central and western African rainforests. The first report of this illness was in monkeys in 1958, hence the name, but many other mammals are susceptible to the virus. Monkeypox virus belongs to the Orthopoxvirus group. The majority of the viruses in this group can cause systemic disease characterized by fever and rashes and may be fatal in some species. In June 2003, an outbreak of monkeypox in people and pet prairie dogs occurred in the United States, primarily in the states of Illinois, Indiana, Kansas, Ohio, Missouri, and Wisconsin. These people began contracting monkeypox after handling sick pet prairie dogs. Transmission of the virus can occur through animal bites or direct contact with the animal's blood, body fluids, or lesions. It can also spread from person to person. Traceback investigations conducted by the Centers for Disease Control and Prevention revealed that those sick prairie dogs had been exposed to the virus through a pet distributor prior to sale. The prairie dogs had been kept in close proximity to imported African rodents. Laboratory testing revealed that some of those African rodents (Gambian giant rats, dormice, and rope squirrels) were also infected with the monkeypox virus.

Monkeypox is not a typical zoonotic disease associated with prairie dogs in the United States. However, this outbreak is a good example of how important it is for veterinary staff and pet owners to be aware of the risk of disease that can exist with pet ownership. The potential of acquiring a zoonotic disease depends on many factors, including:

- What is the origin of the animal (captive-born or wild, domestic or imported)?
- How much contact with other animals did it have during shipping or in the pet store or breeder?
- Is it housed outdoors and exposed to wild animals?

These are only a few of the factors to consider when evaluating the potential of a zoonotic disease in a sick pet. Veterinarians and veterinary technicians should strive to remain informed and proactive with their pet owners so that appropriate information and actions can be shared and taken in maintaining good health for the pet and its owners (CDC 2003, 2018).

Restraint

Prairie dogs are difficult to restrain. Animals that are used to frequent handling can be quite tame and examined awake. In many cases, sedation or full anesthesia is needed to perform a thorough physical exam. They do not have much loose skin around the neck making it difficult to scruff. Prairie dogs have sharp claws and teeth that can cause severe wounds to the handler (Lightfoot 1999). Tame animals used to being handled can be restrained by placing one hand around the chest and supporting the hind end with the other hand. Alternatively, the animal can be grabbed at the base of the tail and lifted gently with the forelimbs resting on a flat surface. The free hand is used to grab the animal on the back of the neck. This technique can be used to move the animal or to perform minor procedures such as nail clipping. Additionally, a thick towel can be used to wrap the animal. This allows for closer examination of the head and the administration of intramuscular injections in the hindlimbs. The towel also protects the handler from being scratched. Alternatively, thick leather gloves can be used (Eshar and Gardhouse 2021). Patients should be examined on the floor if possible as prairie dogs are not cautious about heights and will fall off an exam table, especially if they are frightened or upset during restraint.

Radiology

The radiographic techniques and positioning are similar to those used in domestic animals. Prairie dogs, unless severely debilitated, require sedation in order to obtain good-quality radiographs. The radiographic techniques are similar to those used in other small rodents.

Anesthesia and Analgesia

Sevoflurane and isoflurane gas are the most commonly used anesthetic agents. Induction can be accomplished by chamber induction. Tracheal intubation is difficult in prairie dogs. As a result, the animal can be maintained via a face mask (Figure 25.7). When the animal is anesthetized, its anterior end should be kept slightly elevated so the extensive viscera does not put excessive pressure on the diaphragm (Figures 25.8 and 25.9). Monitoring techniques used in other species (ECG, pulse ox, etc.) can be used similarly in prairie dogs (Figures 25.8 and 25.9). They should be maintained on supplemental heat similar to other rodents.

Analgesics that can be used on prairie dogs include buprenorphine and butorphanol. Ketoprofen and meloxicam are suitable for use as long as the patient is not azotemic (Eshar and Gardhouse 2021).

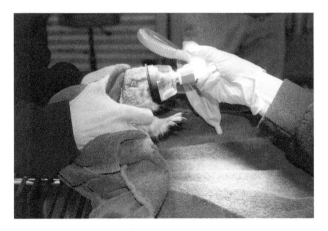

Figure 25.7 Mask induction of anesthesia. (Courtesy of Dr. Sam Rivera.)

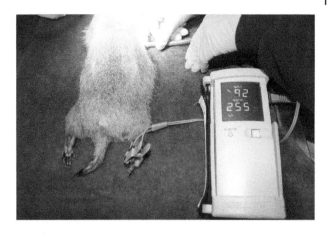

Figure 25.8 Pulse oximeter used on a prairie dog. (Courtesy of Dr. Sam Rivera.)

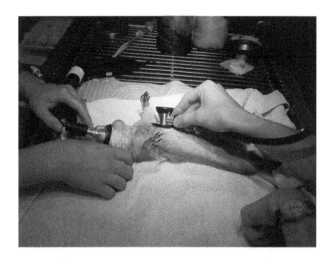

Figure 25.9 Anesthetic monitoring of a prairie dog with a submandibular abscess. (Courtesy of Dr. Sam Rivera.)

Clinical Techniques

Venipuncture

Many animals require sedation for blood collection. The jugular vein is the preferred site for blood collection. In obese prairie dogs, this vein can be difficult to visualize and is often approached blindly. The sedated animal is restrained in dorsal recumbency. The animal is kept with the anterior end elevated to facilitate breathing. In prairie dogs, the pressure from the abdominal organs on the diaphragm can compromise respiration. With the animal in dorsal recumbency, the forelimbs should be extended caudally. Gentle pressure should be applied at the thoracic inlet. The fur along the jugular groove should be moistened. A 23- to 25-gauge needle in a 1- to 3-mL syringe should be used. The needle should be inserted at a 45° angle and

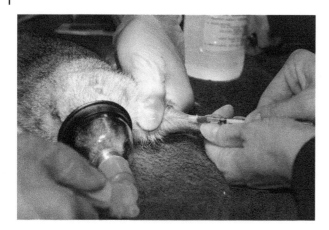

Figure 25.10 Cephalic venipuncture. (Courtesy of Dr. Sam Rivera.)

suction applied as the needle is advanced forward. In some cases, the needle may need to be redirected to either side in order to find the vein. Blood will immediately fill the syringe as the needle enters the vein. The cranial vena cava can also be used to obtain a blood sample in this position.

Venipuncture from the cephalic and lateral saphenous veins is done similarly to the way blood is drawn in other animals of comparable size. The cephalic vein is located on the dorsal aspect of the front leg and the lateral saphenous vein is located in the lateral aspect of the hindlimb, just proximal to the tarsus (Figure 25.10).

Urine Collection

Urinalysis is an important part of health assessment in sick prairie dogs. The techniques to collect urine are similar to those used in dogs and cats.

Voided urine: Urine can be collected from the bottom of the cage using a small syringe. The disadvantage of this technique is that fecal and litter contamination affects the results.

Manual expression: With the animal sedated, gentle transabdominal pressure is applied to the urinary bladder to overcome the sphincter pressure. The urine can be collected into a sterile container or from the tabletop. Excessive pressure should not be applied as this can lead to rupture of the urinary bladder.

Cystocentesis: With the animal sedated, one should gently isolate the bladder. A 27- to 25-gauge needle on a 0.5–1-mL syringe is inserted into the bladder and the urine is collected. This is the preferred method when performing a culture and sensitivity on the urine. One should take care to avoid the cecum; as such ultrasound may be beneficial to obtain a sample by cystocentesis.

Fecal Analysis

The flotation and direct fecal smear techniques are performed the same as for domestic species.

Administration of Medications

There are several routes for administration of medications.

Oral route: Liquids are the most common forms of oral medications. The prairie dog's small mouth and sharp teeth preclude the use of tablets. Liquid medications can be placed in the side of the mouth with a syringe.

Intramuscular route: Parenteral medications can be given in the thigh musculature or the biceps.

Subcutaneous route: This site is most commonly used for the administration of fluids to sick animals. The intrascapular and lateral flank regions are the best sites for the administration of subcutaneous fluids.

Intravenous route: The cephalic, jugular, and saphenous veins can be used for the administration of medications. In most cases, the prairie dog has to be sedated to facilitate intravenous medications, unless the animal is severely debilitated.

There are very few pharmacokinetic studies evaluating the use of medications in prairie dogs. In general, dosages used for other rodents can be used for prairie dogs. Similar to guinea pigs or other rodents, certain oral antibiotics can cause fatal dysbiosis of the intestinal flora and their use should be avoided. These include beta-lactams, lincomycin, clindamycin, and erythromycin.

In an anorexic prairie dog, syringe feeding is needed in order to facilitate GI motility, promote a positive energy balance, and prevent hepatic lipidosis. Commercial herbivore hand-feeding formulas are available for this purpose, and the amount given daily may vary based on the animal's presentation and severity of illness. The total amount can then be divided into multiple smaller feedings throughout the day, and the amount gradually reduced as the animal's normal appetite returns.

Euthanasia

As with other mammals, humane euthanasia may be accomplished with an overdose of a barbiturate anesthetic agent. Prairie dogs should be sedated or anesthetized prior to being euthanized. This can be done with an intramuscular injection of a benzodiazepine and/or opioid or with gas anesthesia as previously described. Once sufficiently sedated, the euthanasia can be performed using an intravenous, intracardiac, or intraperitoneal injection.

References and Further Reading

CDC (Centers for Disease Control and Prevention). 2003. Multistate outbreak of monkeypox – Illinois, Indiana, and Wisconsin, 2003. *MMWR* 52(23): 537–540.

CDC (Centers for Disease Control and Prevention). 2018. Monkeypox. Available at: http://www.cdc.gov/ncidod/monkeypox/.

Eshar D, Gardhouse SM. 2021. Prairie dogs. In: *Ferrets, Rabbits, and Rodents Clinical Medicine and Surgery*, 4th edn (ed KE Quesenberry, et al.), pp. 334–344. St. Louis, MO: Elsevier.

Johnson-Delaney CA. 1996. *Exotic Companion Medicine Handbook for Veterinarians*. Lake Worth: Wingers Publishing.

Lightfoot TL. 1999. Clinical examination of chinchillas, hedgehogs, prairie dogs, and sugar gliders. *Vet Clin North Am Exot Anim Pract* 2(2): 447–469.

Phalen DN, Atinoff N, Fricke ME. 2000. Obstructive respiratory disease in prairie dogs with odontomas. *Vet Clin North Am Exot Anim Pract* 3(2): 513–517.

26

Critical Care Feeding
Micah Kohles

Introduction

There will be times when a veterinary technician who works in an exotic practice is asked to care for a critically ill patient. As part of that care, a veterinarian may decide that a specific critical care diet needs to be fed. Not surprisingly exotic companion mammals (ECM) require unique diets specifically formulated for their nutritional needs. During times of anorexia or poor nutritional status assist feeding may be required. The individual pet's requirement for specifically formulated diets will need to be calculated and fed for a particular period of time. For many of these unique species, anorexic bouts of even 12–24 hours can have serious health implications and even lead to mortality. Providing vital nutrients when voluntary intake ceases is crucial. Powdered recovery diets mixed with water can provide essential hydration as well as provide routes to administer medication and nutritional support. Case-specific calculations of feeding amounts using animal body weight, appropriate metabolic factors, and activity/growth multipliers will help avoid over- or under-feeding. While duration of assist feeding can be variable, goals of recovery feeding should always be to return the animal to their standard diet consumed voluntarily.

What is Critical Care/Recovery Feeding?

Recovery or assist feeding products should be formulated and designed with the intent for hand feeding animals unwilling or unable to eat on their own. Calorically dense, nutritionally complete powdered products reduce volume intake while still providing key nutrients for recovery and health. Because these products are meant to be mixed with water, they are also supplying vital hydration to an animal in sub-optimal nutritional and dehydration status. When selecting a recovery/assist feeding formula, it is vital to use a formula that aligns with the species nutrient needs.

Since there are diets specifically formulated for ECMs, dog and cat products should be avoided. It is also important to select products formulated using ingredients that most appropriately mimic the species' normal diet to encourage voluntary food intake. Biologically relevant ingredients are easily digested by the animal and enhance palatability to stimulate appetite appropriately during recovery.

There are numerous products in the marketplace including the Critical Care Line from Oxbow Animal Health and Lafeber Company's Emeraid products (Figures 26.1–26.3). Ingredients are paramount to critical care. General ingredient recommendations specific to ECM nutritional needs are as follows: Artificial colors, preservatives, and flavors have no nutritional benefit and should be avoided.

- Herbivores: Grass hay-based formulas with added plant-based sources of protein, fat as well as omega fatty acids, stabilized vitamins, chelated minerals, prebiotics, and amino acids for recovery; natural flavors for appetite stimulation.
- Omnivores: Balance of plant, animal, and insect ingredients that are biologically relevant and appropriate for these species as well as omega fatty acids, stabilized vitamins, chelated minerals, prebiotics, and amino acids for recovery.

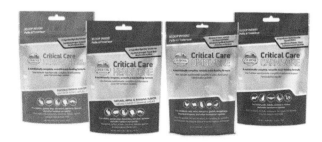

Figure 26.1 Examples of Oxbow critical care diets. (Courtesy of Dr. Micah Kohles/Oxbow Animal Health.)

Exotic Animal Medicine for the Veterinary Technician, Fourth Edition. Edited by Bonnie Ballard and Ryan Cheek.
© 2024 John Wiley & Sons, Inc. Published 2024 by John Wiley & Sons, Inc.
Companion Website: www.wiley.com/go/ballard/4e

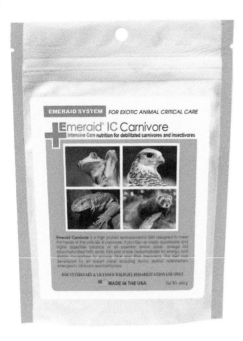

Figure 26.2 Lafeber's carnivore diet. (Courtesy of Christal Pollock.)

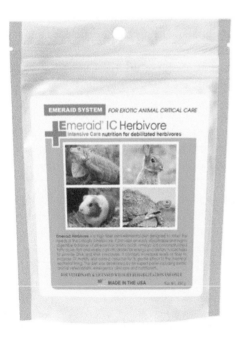

Figure 26.3 Lafeber's herbivore diet. (Courtesy of Christal Pollock.)

- Carnivores: Animal protein based with high caloric density and balanced amino and omega fatty acids profiles as well as stabilized vitamins, chelated minerals, prebiotics, and amino acids for recovery. Plant-based protein isolates should be avoided.

When to Assist Feed

Assist feeding in exotic companion animals is appropriate, or even vital, in a diversity of situations and should occur anytime an animal becomes anorexic. As anorexia is a non-specific symptom, investigation into root causes should begin immediately. For certain ECM species, especially hind gut fermenters such as rabbits, guinea pigs, and chinchillas, anorexia bouts lasting even 18–24 hours constitute a potential emergency (Figure 26.4) (Paul-Murphy 2007). Assist feeding can and should occur any time an animal is anorexic or has the potential to go off feed including, but not limited to use as/times of:

- Appetite stimulant
- Malnutrition
- Stress
- Support during specific disease states
- Gastrointestinal stasis
  - Dental disease
  - Anemia
  - Pancreatitis
  - Insulinoma

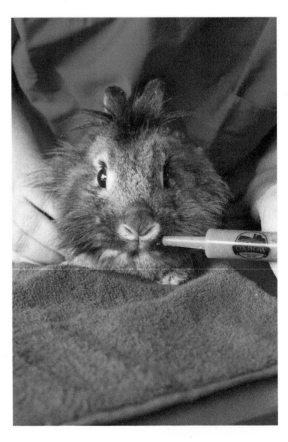

Figure 26.4 Syringe feeding a rabbit. (Courtesy of Dr. Micah Kohles.)

○ Metabolic disease
○ Cancer support
- Severe weight loss
- Geriatric patients
- Medication carrier
- Pre-surgery and post-surgery
- Receiving protocols

Approaches to Critical Care Feeding

While assist feeding in the clinical setting may be easiest, it is not always practical or optimal for long-term patients. Veterinary technicians can play an important role in teaching owners how to feed these diets at home. It is a good idea to educate owners on assist feed diets and feeding techniques for their pet before it is needed. This way both they and their pet are accustomed to the diet and its administration before it may be required. Also giving the owner handouts on how to perform the feedings and links to videos that they can view at home ensures the animal's best chance of recovery. This can also be made easier by having assist feeding products for sale in the clinic or on hand to send with patients. As stress alone can trigger anorexia in many ECM species, pets entering a new home, changing diets, and otherwise entering a period of stress may also benefit from 1 to 2 days of assist feeding.

The primary goal when determining the best approach to feeding critical pets is focused on pet and owner success. Key factors to keep in mind include level of underlying disease, patient and owner compliance and overall nutritional and hydration status. While not often successful in sick and diseased patients the goal should always be to give the animal an opportunity to self-feed. Owners and veterinary professionals should try various approaches to self-feeding before moving onto more invasive routes. This includes varying product consistency (dry, wet, etc.), feeding in combination with other known and palatable food items, utilizing the pet's normal feeding patterns and bowls, and minimizing environmental stress. It is surprising how many times a very sick and debilitated patient will begin taking in calories on their own when given the chance and the correct environment.

If not successful through less direct routes, there are numerous other options that can be considered including syringe feeding and more invasive options such as nasogastric and esophagostomy tube feeding. When tube placement is warranted, awareness of these routes and techniques as well as their applicability to specific species is good practical knowledge for veterinary professionals.

When preparing to syringe feed any animal the following important factors must be kept in mind. These

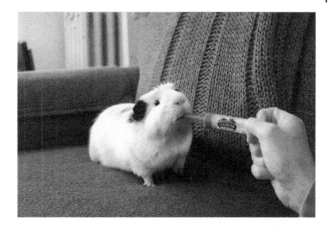

Figure 26.5 Syringe feeding a guinea pig. (Courtesy of Dr. Micah Kohles.)

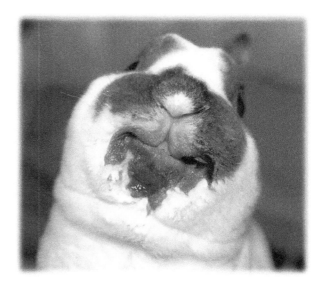

Figure 26.6 A rabbit after being assist fed. (Courtesy of Dr. Micah Kohles.)

include: ensuring the animal is stable enough to handle the associated stress, having the feeding products mixed up and ready to administer, having the correct equipment including multiple syringe options on hand and additional help if needed for animal handling (Figures 26.5 and 26.6).

Nasogastric tube placement has been reported in rabbits and other ECM species (Figure 26.7). Keys to success include utilizing the correct type and diameter feeding tube, understanding proper technique, usage of sedation and local anesthetic, proper tube maintenance, and using the correct products. It is important to use products with a small particle size to minimize the likelihood of tube occlusion. Oxbow's Fine Grind Critical Care and Lafeber's Emeraid Intensive Care are examples. Both diets are designed to go through as small as a 5 fr. tube keeping

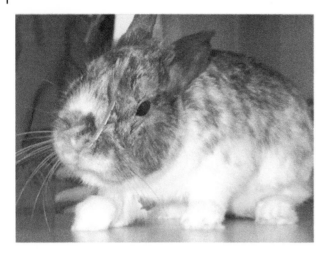

Figure 26.7 Nasogastric tube in a rabbit. (Courtesy of Dr. Micah Kohles.)

Table 26.1 RER multiplication factors for exotic patients.

Exotic Companion Mammals	Herbivore	Omnivore	Carnivore
Patient is eating other foods **and** being assist fed	70	70	70
Patient is **only** being assist fed	103–140	135–215	104–180
Reptiles and Amphibians			
Patient is eating other foods **and** being assist fed	25	20–40	20–30
Patient is **only** being assist fed	35	35–50	35–41
Birds			
Patient is eating other foods **and** being assist fed	100		175
Patient is **only** being assist fed	120		250
Chicken, Turkey, and Waterfowl			
Patient is eating other foods **and** being assist fed		100	
Patient is **only** being assist fed		120	
Psittacines and Other Birds			
Patient is eating other foods **and** being assist fed		175–180	
Patient is **only** being assist fed		200–250	

in mind that tube maintenance including appropriate flushing pre and post feeding is essential. Esophagostomy tube placement is fairly common practice in ferrets but not other ECM species. While parenteral nutrition has been reported in lab animal literature it is likely not relevant for most clinical practice applications (Graham et al. 2021).

How Much to Feed?

Most companies that make critical care feeding products will have charts and/or websites to calculate feeding amounts. Charts are often oversimplified for convenience's sake as they are typically used as a quick reference guide in clinical situations. The most accurate way to calculate feeding doses is via species and situation-specific calculations. Oxbow has reference information to calculate individual feeding recommendations on their website.

The first step to calculating an animal's energy requirement is determining metabolic body weight (MBW): $BW_{kg}^{0.75}$. Using Kleiber's law, this equation states, for the vast majority of animals, the metabolic rate scales to the 3/4 power of the animal's mass (body weight in kilograms). Using MBW, the resting energy requirement (RER) can be calculated by multiplying by a factor specific to species or groups of species: MBW × species-specific factor (Table 26.1). These factors are well-defined for dogs and cats in the literature, but for ECM and other exotic species, field metabolic rates have much more recently been investigated and validated (Nagy et al., 1999).

Final metabolic energy requirements (MER) are calculated by multiplying RER by an appropriate activity or growth multipliers: RER × multiplier. Research has been completed by Omaha's Henry Doorly Zoo, that determined

Table 26.2 MER activity and growth factors.

Maintenance adult	1.0
Young/growing	1.5
Weight gain[a]	1.2–1.8
Weight loss[a]	0.8–1.0
Seniors	Adjust as necessary

a) Use ideal MBW.

safe multipliers for exotic mammals and reptiles at 1-2 and 1-3 for exotic birds. Other multipliers may be used for various physiological states or metabolic goals (Table 26.2).

Once the MER (Kcal) is calculated, product feeding amounts can be calculated. Grams of product to feed are calculated by dividing MER by kilocalories per gram of product: MER/Kcal per gram. If one prefers to calculate feeding recommendations on a volumetric basis, dividing feeding grams by grams per tablespoon of product can be calculated: MER/Kcal per gram/grams per tbsp (Table 26.3).

Table 26.3 Kcal/gram and g/Tbsp of dry matter for common commercial diets.

	Oxbow Critical Care		Emeraid Intensive Care	
	Kcal/g	g/Tbsp	Kcal/g	g/Tbsp
Herbivore	2.67	9.0	2.95	6.9
Omnivore	3.6	8.0	4.086	8.1
Carnivore	6.0	4.0	4.979	8.5

Calculating dietary needs of a 0.5 kg, 3-month-old guinea pig using Oxbow's Herbivore Critical Care formula.

Step 1: Calculate MBW; BW$_{kg}$$^{0.75}$
  0.5 kg$^{0.75}$ = 0.59 kg
Step 2: Calculate RER; MBW × species-specific factor
  0.59 kg × 140 = 83.24 Kcal
Step 3: Calculate MER; RER × MER multiplier
  83.24 Kcal × 1.5 = 124.87 Kcal
Step 4: Calculate how much to feed per day
  Method 1: Calculate number of grams; MER/Kcal/g of product

$$\frac{124.87\ \text{Kcal}}{2.67\ \text{Kcal/g}} = 46.78\ \text{g/day}$$

  Method 2: Calculate number of tablespoons; (MER/Kcal/g of product)/g/Tbsp of product

$$\frac{(124.87\ \text{Kcal}/2.67\ \text{Kcal/g})}{9\ \text{g/Tbsp}} = 5.20\ \text{Tbsp/day}$$

Note that in the example above the total daily volume of dry product, in our Example 5.2 Tbsp/day, can and should be broken into as many feedings as appropriate for the patient and mixed with whatever amount of water to achieve desired consistency. It should also be noted that in some cases when an animal is completely anorectic it may not be advised or appropriate to feed 100% of their MER initially as their GI tract needs to slowly return to normal function.

How Long to Assist Feed

Duration of assist feeding is extremely case-specific. The most generic answer would be to continue assist feeding until the animal has returned to voluntary dietary intake. During this time, investigation into the root cause should be carried out to determine if further medical diagnostics or treatment is necessary. If after 3–5 days, the patient status has not improved, underlying issues are likely preventing full recovery. Primary clinical factors to monitor during feeding include body weight/BCS, fecal output (amount and frequency), hydration status, and other factors specific to feeding tube utilization when applicable. While most critical care and assist feeding formulas are designed to be short-term solutions, there are cases in which a recovery formula can be fed on a more long-term basis under close supervision. However, the goal of recovery feeding should always be to return the animal to their standard diet consumed voluntarily.

What About Hydration?

Chronic and acute dehydration are constant threats to ECM species. Understanding the role hydration plays in animal well-being and recovery is essential to properly support ill and diseased animals. Independent of the route of hydration support, constant diligence should be made towards monitoring patient hydration status and ensuring appropriate levels of hydration support.

Rabbits

- Typical water intake is about 50–150 mL/kg (22–46 mL/lb) daily.
- 2.5-kg rabbit on a dry diet will take approximately 160 mL of water, or 65 mL/kg, daily
  o It is interesting to note that this is approximately twice the intake of an average human adult derived from both food and drink.
- Summary: 50–100 mL water/kg body weight
  o Range: 50–150 (Fisher 2010).

Guinea Pigs

- 21.7 mL/100 g BW/day in 6-week-old male guinea pigs (312 ± 13 g) that were individually housed on sawdust.
- 7.5 mL/100 g BW/day in male guinea pigs (698 ± 19 g) fed a non-purified diet containing 20% crude protein.
- Summary: 75–125 mL water/kg body weight
  o Range: 75–215

Hamster/Gerbils

- Male and female golden hamsters consume, on average, 8.5 mL water/100 g BW/day
  o Males consume 5 mL water/100 g BW/day, while females consume 14 mL water/100 g BW/day.
- Chinese hamsters' water intake is 11.4 mL/100 g BW/day for males and 12.9 mL/100 g BW/day for females.
- Water intake for golden hamsters was found to be 4.5 mL/100 g BW/day in males and 13.6 mL/100 g BW/day for females.

- Summary: 75–125 mL water/kg body weight
  - Range: 45–140

Ferrets

- Typical water intake is about 25–50 mL/kg daily (Fox and Marini, 2014).

- This is highly dependent on life stage, activity level, and nutritional profile.
- Personal experience is that requirements are above and certainly the high end of this range in captive environments, on dry food (Author).

References

Fisher P. 2010. Standards of care in the 21st century: the rabbit. *J Exot Pet Med* 19(1): 22–35.

Fox J, Marini R. 2014. *Biology and Diseases of the Ferret*, 3rd edn. Chichester: Wiley-Blackwell.

Graham J, Doss G, Beaufrère H (eds). 2021. *Exotic Animal Emergency and Critical Care Medicine*. Ames, Iowa: John Wiley & Sons.

Paul-Murphy J. 2007. Critical care of the rabbit. *Vet Clin North Am Exot Anim Pract* 10(2): 437–461.

Additional Reading

de Matos R, Morrisey J. 2005. Emergency and critical care of small psittacines and passerines. *Semin Avian Exot Pet Med* 14(2): 90–105.

Hawkins M, Graham J. 2007. Emergency and critical care of rodents. *Vet Clin North Am Exot Anim Pract* 10(2): 501–531.

Lichtenberger M, Lennox A. 2009. Exotic companion mammal emergency medicine and critical care. In: Proceedings of the Association of Exotic Mammal Veterinarians Conference, 2009.

Nagy K, Girard I, Brown T. 1999. Energetics of free-ranging mammals, reptiles, and birds. *Annu Rev Nutr* 19(1): 247–277.

Section VII

Hematology

27

Avian and Reptile Hematology
Denise I. Bounous

Introduction

Birds and reptiles are not so different as one may suppose. Phylogenetically, these groups emerge closer to each other than to mammals (Gauthier et al. 1988). Hematology of both is similar, in that they have nucleated erythrocytes that develop and mature in the bone marrow sinusoids, unlike mammalian erythrocytes, which migrate into the sinusoids and into vessels after developing into mature anucleate erythrocytes (Campbell 1967). Automated hematology instruments do not accurately count nucleated erythrocytes. The morphology of blood cells may vary, not only between animal groups of birds and reptiles, but also between species within a group (e.g., iguanas and chameleons, or boas and rat snakes). Additionally, there are variations in the white blood cell differential among the different genera of birds and reptiles. In some snakes, such as the Boidae family (e.g., boa constrictors, pythons), the predominant leukocyte is the azurophil, whereas other snakes, such as rat snakes, have predominantly heterophils. Morphology of peripheral blood constituents can also vary. Thrombocytes of some birds and boid snakes are elongated and easily differentiated from small lymphocytes (Figure 27.1), but thrombocytes of the rat snake are small and round, very similar to lymphocytes (Bounous et al. 1996) (Figure 27.2). When performing a differential leukocyte count on birds or reptiles, it is advisable to scan the smear, examining each cell type, and identifying what characteristics can be used to classify the cell types before actually starting the count.

Blood Collection

Avian and reptilian blood volume is approximately 10% and 5–8% of body weight, respectively, and approximately 10% of blood volume can be taken from a healthy bird or reptile with no ill effects (Campbell 1995; Mader 2000). Therefore,

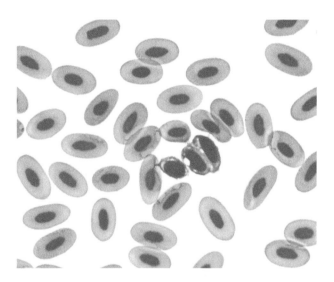

Figure 27.1 Blood smear from owl: cluster of elongated thrombocytes (Wright's stain, EDTA, original magnification ×100).

approximately 3.5 mL can be withdrawn from an Amazon parrot weighing 350 g, but only 0.35 mL from a budgerigar weighing 35 g. Thus, it is necessary to prioritize which assays are to be performed when only small volumes are available.

Blood for hematologic procedures must be collected in anticoagulant. Potential anticoagulants include ethylenediaminetetraacetic acid (EDTA), heparin, or sodium citrate. Heparin can interfere with staining of blood cells, and using sodium citrate causes dilution of the blood resulting in incorrect cell counts. Comparison studies with the three anticoagulants show that citrate causes significant changes in packed cell volume (PCV) as well as increased cell lysis. Samples for hematology that are collected into any of these anticoagulants should be evaluated within 12 h of collection for best results, as greater than 50% lysis can occur at 24 h. Heparin is frequently used as the anticoagulant for avian and reptile blood samples only because it allows both hematology and biochemistry analysis to be

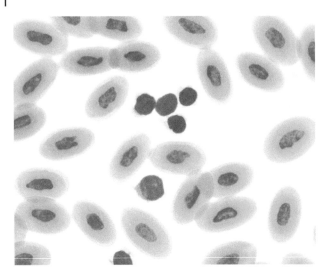

Figure 27.2 Blood smear from rat snake: cluster of small round thrombocytes, one lymphocyte (Wright's stain, EDTA, original magnification ×100).

performed on the same sample tube. Blood for biochemical analysis can be collected into lithium heparin or into "serum" tubes without anticoagulant. However, glucose, potassium, and chloride concentrations were shown to change significantly at 24 h in python samples collected in lithium heparin (Davidson et al. 2002). When possible, EDTA is the optimal anticoagulant for hematology analysis and serum for biochemistry; however, the volume of blood that can be removed from birds and reptiles frequently limits this optimization. Blood collected for biochemistry into heparin or into tubes without anticoagulant should be separated immediately to prevent artifactual changes.

Blood Smear and Assessment

Smears should be made as soon as possible after blood collection to avoid any deterioration of the cells. Methods for making smears include: (1) using a spreader slide across the slide containing the drop of blood, and (2) placing a cover slip on top of another coverslip containing a blood drop, then pulling the two coverslips apart. The cover slip method requires extra care in staining and must be fixed to a regular glass slide in order to evaluate microscopically. Blood smears are stained with classical Romanowsky-type stains, containing the dyes azure A, azure B, methylene violet, and methylene blue (e.g., Wright's stain, Giemsa stain, or rapid stains such as Diff-Quik or Accustain). A properly made smear can be used to assess the number of leukocytes and platelets, as well as evaluate erythrocyte morphology.

Leukocytes

Total Leukocyte Count

Leukocytes from birds are classified as heterophils, eosinophils, basophils, monocytes, and lymphocytes (Campbell 2000). Reptiles have an additional leukocyte, the azurophil (Frye 1991; Hawkey & Dennett 1989). In general, electronic counters cannot be used for avian and reptilian leukocyte counts. Avian and reptilian leukocytes are best enumerated using a hemocytometer. Various stains have been reported for use in differentiating and counting types of leukocytes from thrombocytes and erythrocytes. Using the Natt and Herrick's staining method, all leukocytes and thrombocytes stain varying degrees of a blue–violet color. One must be able to distinguish thrombocytes from leukocytes in the hemocytometer in order to calculate the leukocyte count. Use of the Leukopet eosinophil system containing phloxine B, which stains avian granulocytes (heterophils, eosinophils, and basophils) is an indirect method for leukocyte counting. This procedure requires an accurate differential to calculate the number of leukocytes. After counting the number of cells staining an orange–red color on both sides of the hemocytometer chamber, the count is corrected for all leukocytes (to include monocytes, lymphocytes, and azurophils) based on the differential as follows:

$$\text{Total WBC} = \frac{\text{Number of cells stained in the chamber} \times 1.1 \times 16}{\dfrac{\%\ \text{granulocytes}}{100}}$$

Example: $300 \times 1.1 \times 16/0.60 = 8{,}800$ cells/μL

Estimating the leukocyte count is highly variable and not very accurate. A "guestimate" of the number of leukocytes/μL blood can be made from a well-made smear by counting the number of leukocytes per high field (40× objective) in 10 fields, taking the average of the 10, and multiplying by 1,500.

Heterophils

Heterophils are functionally similar to the mammalian neutrophil. Heterophils are usually the most numerous leukocytes in pet bird blood (Figure 27.3). They are round cells with clear cytoplasm and prominent eosinophilic, rod-shaped to oval granules, which may partially obscure the nucleus. The nucleus of a mature heterophil usually has two to three lobes containing coarse, purple-staining chromatin. Immature heterophils are rarely present in peripheral blood of birds or reptiles, and usually are associated with inflammation (Bounous et al. 1989). The nuclei of these immature cells (toxic heterophils) have fewer

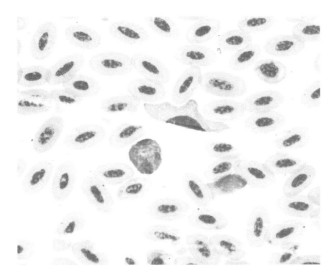

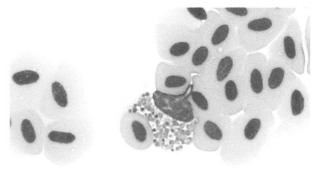

Figure 27.5 Blood smear from owl: toxic mononuclear heterophil with eccentric nucleus and both basophilic and eosinophilic granules (Wright's stain, EDTA, original magnification ×100).

Figure 27.3 Blood smear from hawk: heterophil, erythrocytes containing the hemoparasite *Leucocytozoon* (Wright's stain, EDTA, original magnification ×100).

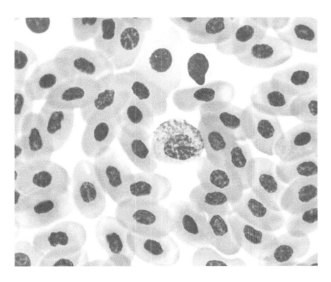

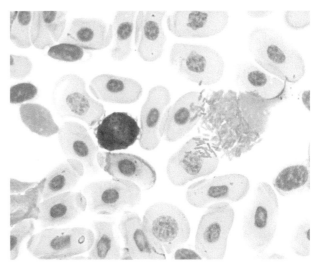

Figure 27.6 Blood smear from a tortoise: basophil with granules obscuring the nucleus, ruptured heterophil with loose granules (Wright's stain, EDTA, original magnification ×100).

Figure 27.4 Blood smear from tortoise: heterophil with band-shaped nucleus and area of basophilic cytoplasm (Wright's stain, EDTA, original magnification ×100).

reddish–orange granules can be pleomorphic across the species, ranging from needle-like to oval and from large to small (Figure 27.6). Heterophil cytoplasm of reptiles can frequently have a foamy appearance. As in birds, immature heterophils in the peripheral blood of reptiles indicate an increased demand for heterophils, such as in conditions of inflammation (Mateo et al. 1984).

Heterophilia—an increase in number of circulating heterophils—is usually a response to stress or inflammation. Heteropenia may also occur with severe inflammation that exceeds or affects bone marrow production.

lobes and may appear mononuclear with more basophilic cytoplasm and less mature granules (Figure 27.4). Very early granulocytes may be so poorly differentiated that granules are round and exhibit staining characteristics of both eosinophilia and basophilia (Figure 27.5).

Heterophils of reptiles are similar to birds, with some subtle differences. This cell can account for approximately 30–45% of leukocytes in reptiles. Mature heterophils of reptiles contain an oval-to-lenticular nucleus that can be eccentrically located in the cell with a chromatin pattern similar to that of birds. The nuclear color may range from more light blue in lizards to purple in other reptiles. The

Eosinophils

Eosinophils are uncommon to few in the peripheral blood of birds and reptiles. They are round, peroxidase-positive cells, with pale basophilic cytoplasm and many spherical

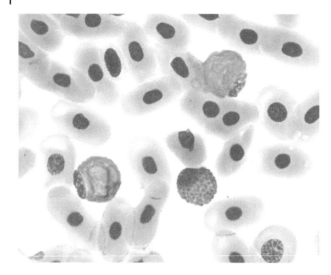

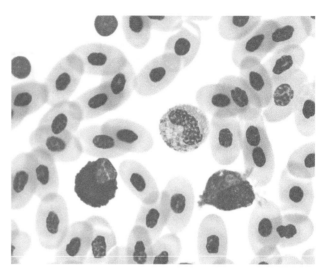

Figure 27.7 Blood smear from a tortoise: heterophil with ill-defined rod-shaped granules, eosinophil with round distinct granules, heterophil (Wright's stain, EDTA, original magnification ×100).

Figure 27.8 Blood smear from a lizard: basophil, band heterophil, monocyte (Wright's stain, EDTA, original magnification ×100).

reddish orange cytoplasmic granules (Figure 27.7). Eosinophil granules from birds may appear brighter than heterophil granules. The nucleus is eccentrically located, and nuclear lobulation is less than in heterophils. Reptilian eosinophil size varies with species, with snakes having the largest cells, turtles and crocodilians having intermediate-sized cells, and lizards having the smallest eosinophils. Eosinophils can make up from 7% to 20% of the leukocytes in healthy reptiles. Increased eosinophil numbers in pet birds have been associated with parasitism (Campbell 1994).

Basophils

Basophils are uncommonly seen in the peripheral blood of birds and most reptiles. Depending on the species, they may constitute from 0% to 40% of the leukocytes in reptiles, with turtles having the highest percentage. Basophils are easily identified because of their large, round, deeply basophilic granules. The round-to-oval nucleus is centrally or eccentrically located and frequently obscured by the granules (Figures 27.6 and 27.8). Reptilian basophils, as mammalian basophils, appear to be involved in processing immunoglobulin and histamine release (Sypek & Borysenko 1988).

Lymphocytes

Lymphocytes occur in different sizes and somewhat different morphologies. They are round or oval mononuclear cells with variation in the appearance of the nucleus and cytoplasm. Most are small to medium-sized (5–10 μm)

round cells with a centrally located nucleus containing densely aggregated chromatin. The nuclear shape is usually round to indented, and the cytoplasm is pale blue. The nuclear to cytoplasmic (N:C) ratio of small lymphocytes is high. Larger lymphocytes (15 μm) can have larger nuclei with more dispersed or reticulated chromatin and more cytoplasm so that the N:C ratio is less. Lymphocytes may have cytoplasmic blebs and sometimes deeper blue staining cytoplasm at the periphery of the cytoplasm. Occasionally a few azurophilic granules may be present. Lymphocytes may occasionally appear to be indented by surrounding cells on the smear. In some parrots (e.g., Amazons, *Eclectus*), lymphocytes are reported to be the most common leukocytes in peripheral blood. Reptilian lymphocytes are similar and can comprise up to 80% of the circulating leukocytes (see Figure 27.2). Reactive lymphocytes are larger cells with large nuclei containing dispersed chromatin and deeply basophilic cytoplasm. Reactive lymphocytes may result from antigenic stimulation of the immune system due to infection or inflammation. Lymphocytosis in reptiles can occur with viral diseases, inflammation, wound healing, and certain parasitic infections (Campbell 1996).

Monocytes

Monocytes are large mononuclear cells found less commonly than lymphocytes in the peripheral blood of birds and reptiles. These cells are more variable than most other types of leukocytes. They can be round to oval to rhomboid in shape. The nucleus may be small or large and round, indented, bilobed, or U-shaped. Monocytes may appear similar to large lymphocytes, but with finely granular

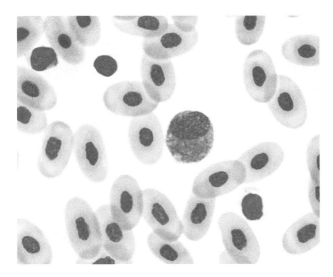

Figure 27.9 Blood smear from a lizard: monocyte with gray–blue cytoplasm and oval nucleus (Wright's stain, EDTA, original magnification ×100).

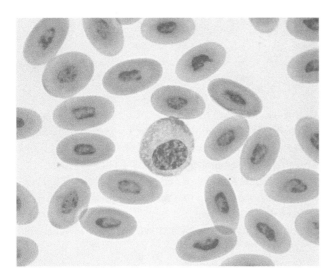

Figure 27.10 Blood smear from a rat snake: azurophil with granules at cytoplasmic periphery instilling a pinkish–purple hue (Wright's stain, EDTA, original magnification ×100).

cytoplasm that is blue–gray, and may also occasionally contain vacuoles. Monocyte nuclear chromatin is usually less clumped when compared to lymphocytes (Figure 27.9). Monocytosis in birds can occur with chronic illnesses, such as tuberculosis, chlamydia, and aspergillosis.

Azurophils

Azurophils are unique cells identified only in reptiles. (These cells eventually may be determined to be a type of monocyte.) They are similar in size to heterophils with abundant cytoplasm that is finely to coarsely granular and may sometimes contain vacuoles. Granules may impart

a purplish hue to the cytoplasm, particularly to the outer region (Figure 27.10). Occasionally azurophils are observed with vacuolated cytoplasm (Dotson et al. 1995).

Erythrocytes

Early erythrocytes are round with round nuclei. The cells and nuclei become more oval, and the nuclear chromatin becomes increasingly condensed as the cell matures. Mature avian and reptile erythrocytes appear oval to elliptical on the blood smear, with a centrally located nucleus that is also oval. It is not unusual for the erythrocyte nucleus to be irregularly shaped in some reptiles (Figure 27.11). The cytoplasm of the early erythrocyte is basophilic, becoming polychromatic, and then pale orange to pink when the hemoglobin and cell are mature. The change in color from basophilic to eosinophilic as the erythrocyte matures parallels the maturation of hemoglobin in the cell. The mature erythrocyte varies in size, and to some degree in shape, depending on the species of bird or reptile. A slight variation in the size of erythrocytes is normal. Polychromatophilic erythrocytes make up less than 5% of erythrocytes in the peripheral blood (see Figure 27.11). These cells can be identified and enumerated as reticulocytes by staining with a supravital stain, such as new methylene blue. Variation in the size of erythrocytes and number of reticulocytes can be used to classify anemia. A greater degree of anisocytosis in the presence of increased polychromasia is indicative of responsive anemia. A large number of hypochromatic erythrocytes

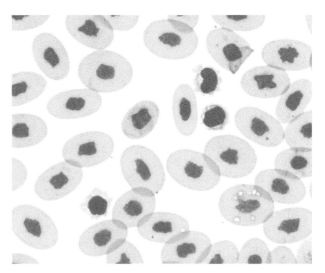

Figure 27.11 Blood smear from a lizard: basophilic erythrocyte in center, two thrombocytes. Note irregularly shaped erythrocyte nuclei, and tiny cytoplasmic vacuoles in erythrocytes (Wright's stain, EDTA, original magnification ×100).

is associated with an erythrocyte disorder such as iron deficiency anemia. Marked poikilocytosis may indicate a maturation dysfunction. Occasionally erythrocytes of reptiles may contain small, clear cytoplasmic vacuoles that are not associated with any pathology (see Figure 27.11).

Thrombocytes

Mature thrombocytes in birds and reptiles are round to oval with a round-to-oval nucleus containing clumped chromatin. Their shape can vary between species, but the cytoplasm is colorless to pale gray. Thrombocytes frequently contain a few small azurophilic granules. In some animals, thrombocytes are difficult to discern from small lymphocytes. Thrombocytes occasionally occur in closely associated groups in the smear, and this characteristic can be helpful in distinguishing thrombocytes from small lymphocytes (Figure 27.12). Thrombocytes have been reported to have potential phagocytic capabilities, but in general,

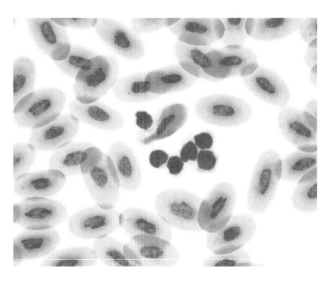

Figure 27.12 Blood smear from a rat snake: cluster of thrombocytes (Wright's stain, EDTA, original magnification ×100).

function as do mammalian platelets (Bounous et al. 1989).

References

Bounous DI, Dotson TK, Brooks RL Jr, Ramsay EC. 1996. Cytochemical staining and ultrastructural characteristics of peripheral blood leukocytes from the yellow rat snake (*Elaphe obsoleta quadrivitatta*). *Comp Haematol Int* 6: 86–91.

Bounous DI, Schaeffer DO, Roy A. 1989. Diagnosis of a coagulase negative *Staphylococcus* sp. septicemia in a lovebird. *J Am Vet Med Assoc* 195: 1120–1122.

Campbell F. 1967. Fine structure of the bone marrow of the chicken and pigeon. *J Morphol* 123: 405–440.

Campbell TW. 1994. Hematology. In: *Avian Medicine: Principles and Application* (eds BW Ritchie, GJ Harrison, LP Harrison), pp. 176–198. Lake Worth, FL: Wingers Publishing Inc.

Campbell TW. 1995. *Avian Hematology and Cytology*, 2nd edn. Ames, IA: Iowa State University Press.

Campbell TW. 1996. Clinical pathology. In: *Reptile Medicine and Surgery* (ed DR Mader), pp. 248–257. Philadelphia: W.B. Saunders Co.

Campbell TW. 2000. Hematology of psittacines. In: *Schalm's Veterinary Hematology* (eds BF Feldman, JG Zinkl, NC Jain), 5th edn, pp. 1155–1160. Baltimore: Lippincott Williams & Wilkins.

Davidson D, Harr K, Raskin R. 2002. Hematologic and biochemical changes caused by commonly used anticoagulants on Burmese python (*Python molurus bivittatus*) blood over time. *Vet Pathol* (in press).

Dotson TK, Ramsay EC, Bounous DI. 1995. A color atlas of blood cells of the yellow rat snake. *Compend Contin Educ Pract Vet* 17: 1013–1017.

Frye FL. 1991. Hematology as applied to clinical reptile medicine. In: *Biomedical and Surgical Aspects of Captive Reptile Husbandry* (ed FL Frye), 2nd edn, Malabar: Krieger Publishing Company.

Gauthier J, Kluge AG, Rowe T. 1988. The early evolution of amniota. In: *The Phylogeny and Classification of the Tetrapods* (ed MJ Benton), vol. 1: Amphibians, Reptiles, Birds. Oxford: Clarendon Press.

Hawkey CM, Dennett TB. 1989. *Color Atlas of Comparative Veterinary Hematology*. Ames, IA: Iowa State University Press.

Mader DR. 2000. Normal hematology of reptiles. In: *Schalm's Veterinary Hematology* (eds BF Feldman, JG Zinkl, NC Jain), 5th edn, pp. 1126–1132. Baltimore: Lippincott Williams & Wilkins.

Mateo MR, Roberts ED, Enright FM. 1984. Morphological, cytochemical, and functional studies of peripheral blood cells of young healthy American alligators (*Alligator mississippiensis*). *Am J Vet Res* 45: 1046–1053.

Sypek J, Borysenko M. 1988. Reptiles. In: *Vertebrate Blood Cells* (eds AF Rowley, NA Ratcliff). Cambridge: Cambridge University Press.

Section VIII

Zoo, Aquarium Medicine, and Wildlife

28

The Role of a Veterinary Technician in a Zoo
Sandy Skeba

Zoo medicine is like all the different types of veterinary medicine rolled into one. There is large animal and small animal care, with preventative medicine such as vaccinations, heartworm treatments, and routine bloodwork. Fieldwork is performed more often than not, as many zoo animals are either too wild or too large to come easily to the clinic. Research is a given at most zoos, and often the veterinary department plays a large role. Clinical laboratory work (see Figure 28.1) is also an important part of a zoo vet tech's day, as most of the animals in a zoo have nucleated red blood cells, and blood counts must be done by hand rather than with an analyzer. Emergency medicine cases are always lurking around the corner, as accidents can and do happen with zoo animals, and occasionally an injured human has to be patched up as well. Neonatology (see Figure 28.2) and geriatrics fall into the line of duty, from the joy of watching a giraffe calf take her first, tottering 6-foot-tall baby steps, to treating a geriatric cougar for renal failure. And most zoos perform necropsies on every animal that passes away, not just to diagnose what happened, but also as a measure of herd health, to find underlying problems that may be lurking in the rest of the collection. Any other specialty you can name (ophthalmology, oncology, surgery, and behavior) is performed at a zoo veterinary hospital. Because zoo veterinary staff need to know a lot of different disciplines, learning is encouraged, and is even included into the workday.

Typical Day

When people ask what a typical day is like for a zoo veterinary technician, the response is usually, "There is no typical day." And while this is true, there is some attempt to be structured. Much like private practice, appointments are made to see animals. Yearly exams, routine dewormings, and lumpectomies are all put on to the schedule. First thing in the morning, the technician usually

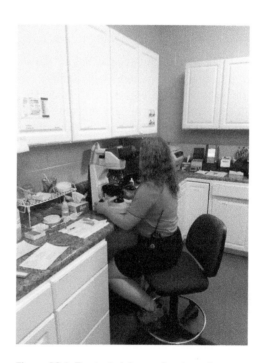

Figure 28.1 Zoo technician performing microscopy.

checks the schedule and prepares for procedures. Ongoing prescriptions are filled, and everyone meets briefly to go over what is expected will happen that day. But as the day progresses, the schedule is changed to meet the demands of emergencies, tours, and necropsies. An obstructed penguin may waddle in for a barium series, or a sudden outbreak of diarrhea in the meerkat exhibit may necessitate an hour at the microscope, looking for pathogens. A simple procedure may take only 15 minutes to perform, yet half an hour to setup and cleanup. One should never be too proud to pick up a broom or mop! And always, there is paperwork. Technicians fill out lab reports, write in animal's records, fill out daily reports, and file. Often, the veterinarian will have the technician fill prescriptions and write instructions to the keepers. Zoo veterinary technicians are increasingly

Exotic Animal Medicine for the Veterinary Technician, Fourth Edition. Edited by Bonnie Ballard and Ryan Cheek.
© 2024 John Wiley & Sons, Inc. Published 2024 by John Wiley & Sons, Inc.
Companion Website: www.wiley.com/go/ballard/4e

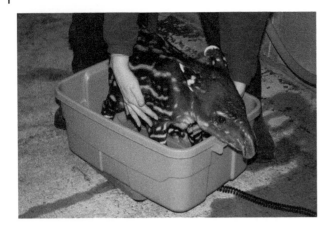

Figure 28.2 Weighing a baby Baird's tapir.

required to do some sort of public interaction, which can range from talking to an occasional tour through the veterinary clinic, to having the entire clinic on display, such as at Walt Disney World's Animal Kingdom, where all treatments and surgeries are performed in front of the visitors who can watch through large windows.

To make things even more challenging, technician duties vary from zoo to zoo. Some zoos have extensive in-house clinical laboratories, and technicians perform everything from hematology to cytology to reproductive research (such as sperm counts), while other zoos send everything to outside laboratories except for routine fecal exams. Necropsies are an important technician duty at some zoos, but if a zoo is close to a veterinary teaching hospital, they may send all their deceased animals there. At some zoos, keepers perform all animal restraint and hospitalized animal care, whereas at another, it is expected that the technicians will do all the capture and restraint, so the keepers are not associated with anything negative that happens to the animal. And although at most zoos, the veterinarians are the only personnel allowed to handle dangerous narcotics such as carfentinil, at a few zoos the veterinary technicians perform every aspect of chemical restraint, including using remote capture equipment (blowdarts) and firing of capture weapons. Some veterinary departments care for baby animals that are being hand-raised, including taking them home for overnight feedings. But in some zoos, this task is solely the purview of keepers and curators, unless the baby becomes ill. Some technicians even have the envious task of walking around their zoo at the end of the day just to look at the animals!

At most zoos, there is a 1:1 ratio of veterinarians to veterinary technicians. The usual number of vets and techs is two each. Often, the department hosts a veterinary resident (a recent veterinary school graduate who is learning zoo veterinary medicine from the permanent staff) for an allotted period of time, such as three years. Other individuals rotate through on a temporary basis, ranging from pre-veterinary students, technician students, and veterinary students in all stages of their schooling. Each individual has vastly different skill and experience levels, and teaching opportunities must be scaled to fit the student. For example, a fourth-year veterinary student may be allowed to give injections or take blood, while a pre-veterinary student needs to be taught how to hold a syringe correctly. At each level of training, there are people more adept than their peers. And always, there are volunteers, who spend their time filing or cleaning just to be part of the zoo team.

Veterinary staffing levels do differ, though. Some larger zoos host a "thundering herd" of veterinarians and technicians, with support staff ranging from hospital keepers, administrative staff, and nutritionists. But at the other end of the spectrum, a small zoo may have only one veterinary technician and a part-time, on-call veterinarian. In this case, the technician has constant responsibilities when it comes to coordinating animal care and triaging emergencies.

How Does a Zoo Differ From Private Practice?

A zoo veterinary clinic is much like private practice, but with more varied species, and some patients you cannot touch unless they are sedated. Of course, there are some of those in regular veterinary clinics! But it is *expected* that you can restrain a snarling, 120-pound rottweiler, or a maniacal 5-pound screaming cat. In zoo veterinary nursing, no one expects you to wrestle down a tiger or warthog (Figures 28.3 and 28.4). So in some ways, it is much safer for the technician! But in order to anesthetize some species, like zebras, powerful narcotics such as carfentinil or etorphine must be used. Accidental human exposure, such as a needle stick, from these drugs can be fatal. Also, most veterinary clinics do not have to see dangerous animals such as venomous snakes and non-human primates. Non-human primates are especially hazardous because of zoonotic diseases. Zoo veterinary technicians are exposed to far more potentially zoonotic diseases than domestic animal technicians. Herpes B, a virus that will kill a human from an exposure as innocuous as a splash of feces in the eye, causes nothing more than a cold sore in macaque monkeys. So protective equipment such as gloves, safety glasses, and masks should be used at all times around some animals. Conversely, zoo animals can catch human diseases, too, and may be far more affected than us. For instance, chicken pox is an irritating, itchy inconvenience most children experience. But a gorilla

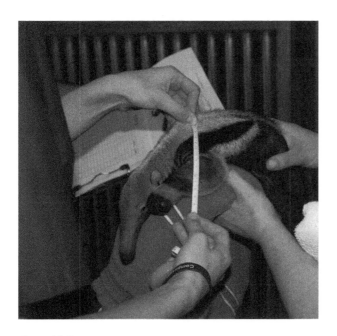

Figure 28.3 Taking body measurements on a baby anteater.

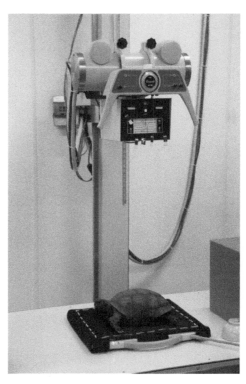

Figure 28.5 Tabletop technique for a tortoise radiograph.

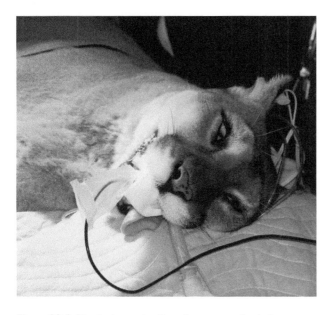

Figure 28.4 Physical examination of a cougar after being anesthetized.

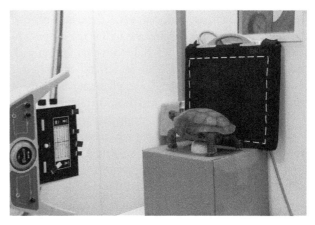

Figure 28.6 Horizontal beam technique used for a tortoise radiograph.

with chicken pox reacts with life-threatening tracheal and throat lesions. Even unusual animals, such as anteaters, can catch our flu virus. Imagine a giant anteater with a runny nose!

Radiology of zoo species can also be a challenge. Dogs and cats tend to lie down in fairly predictable positions on an X-ray plate, but there are animals that do not go into lateral recumbency easily, if at all. Once again the zoo technician is called upon to use his or her ingenuity to position

awkward patients such as a tortoise. Zoo animals that are considered dangerous are usually sedated for radiography, while mild-mannered patients can be expected to simply sit still for the procedure. It is uncommon for a zoo animal to be restrained during radiography as it is for dogs and cats, but appropriate protective and monitoring equipment must still be used (Figures 28.5–28.7).

One of the biggest differences between a domestic animal clinic and a zoo veterinary clinic can be seen in the pharmacy. Zoo clinics keep very little in stock of many of

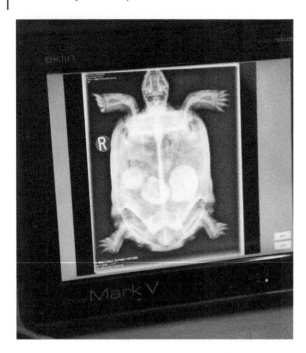

Figure 28.7 Digital radiograph of a tortoise with bladder stones.

the staples of dog and cat medicine, such as prednisone, Rimadyl, and Heartgard. For example, if a zoo has only one hypothyroid canid, it is only necessary for the hospital to carry the size of thyrosyn pill that treats that one animal, rather than have all sizes in stock for any hypothyroid dog that might walk in the door. A zoo pharmacy is a mix of small animal, large animal, and human medicines. For instance, human contraceptive drugs work well on apes, so a siamang's birth control prescription can be filled at the local pharmacy. Also, a zoo veterinary clinic relies heavily on compounding pharmacies. A medication such as metronidazole might be needed for a 120-gram lorikeet, and also a 100-pound anteater. Therefore it is useful to carry it, not only in different strengths, but different flavors as well. Liver flavoring might be perfect for a carnivore, but a fruit-loving psittacine would never take it willingly.

Even other equipment is affected by the diversity of the patients in a zoo veterinary setting. Typical dog and cat anesthesia masks may work well for some species, but a rhinoceros hornbill bird can be a challenge to fit. Because of this, zoo veterinary technicians must be resourceful. Old gallon jugs or empty fluid bags can be molded to a variety of faces, and even human infant masks can be used for small primates. One can imagine the size ranges of endotracheal tubes a zoo must have, to fit everything from shrews to elephants!

Zoo Veterinary Hospitals By Section

Treatment

Most medical procedures in a zoo occur in a main treatment room (Figures 28.8 and 28.9). For most zoo hospitals, this differs from private practice in that there is one central treatment area, not several rooms designed for accommodating multiple clients at once. Many zoo hospitals may have a large treatment area for most procedures and a smaller room for animals that are flighted or could escape easily (such as small primates) and may need to be recaptured. In a zoo hospital where the main treatment area is "on show," or visible to the public, the smaller, off-show room may also be used for planned euthanasia.

Within the main treatment area are all the typical instruments for complete physical exams, such as stethoscopes, ophthalmoscopes, and needles and syringes for sampling blood and lesions. In addition, most zoo treatment rooms have machines for performing anesthesia and monitoring vital signs, since many zoo patients must be fully anesthetized before a complete exam can occur (Figure 28.9). Zoos with an "on show" component to the veterinary hospital will perform most non-sterile surgical procedures before their public treatment window, in addition to routine treatments and exams. Most zoos have a "wet" or dental table with a tub component for performing teeth cleanings and extractions, and lancing abscesses.

Surgery

Many zoos have a dedicated surgical suite, where only sterile procedures such as laparotomies are performed. This room is usually sparsely furnished, with only the

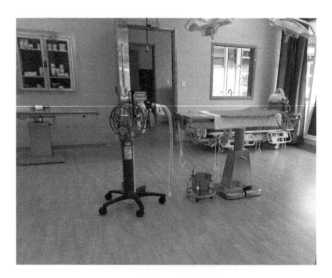

Figure 28.8 Zoo treatment room at an "on show" zoo with windows for the public to view procedures.

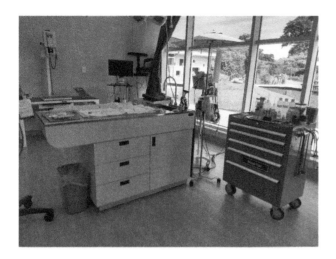

Figure 28.9 Zoo procedure set-up.

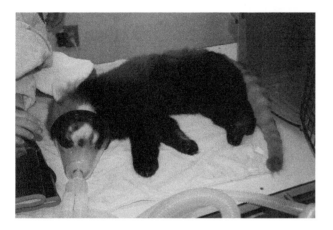

Figure 28.10 Red panda being anesthetized using a face mask.

surgical table and patient monitoring system residing within. Some hospitals keep specialized equipment, such as an endoscope system or an electrocautery unit, in the surgical suite for quick access. Newer zoo hospitals are often designed with pass-through cabinets for storing sterile instruments and equipment and drop-down hoses for oxygen and suction. Cabinets on the walls, suspended for ease of cleaning, may hold sterile items in smaller clinics. But all types of setups exist, and many fine veterinary teams work well with portable oxygen tanks fitted into the anesthesia machine and pump-style suction machines.

One of the biggest differences between private practice and zoo medicine is the variety of patients that are seen. So a surgical area may house a hydraulic large animal table and a small animal table. In many zoo surgical rooms, there is a drain so that the floor can be hosed down, particularly after a large animal procedure. Close at hand to the surgical area are a variety of face masks and different-sized endotracheal tubes required to keep exotic

animals safely under anesthesia (Figures 28.10–28.12). Zoos may have sterile surgical packs with differentiated sizes of instruments, as needed for "small," "medium," and "large" patient surgeries. Most zoos have ophthalmic and orthopedic packs, although they may call in specialists if those types of surgeries are indicated.

Radiology

Almost all zoos have digital radiology due to its ease of use and superior detail. Many zoos also utilize dental units for even finer detail of their smallest patients, such as poison dart frogs. It is becoming more common for zoos to have a computerized tomography (CT) scanner, which utilizes X-rays taken from several angles around the patient. Then, computer software creates three-dimensional images from these images. The amount of detail produced by a CT scanner aids greatly in the diagnosis of patients that are difficult to assess by regular radiographic images, such as bony-plated turtles and armadillos, and areas of the body that require fine detail to pinpoint medical issues, such as bone affected with osteomyelitis and the central nervous system. In lieu of having a CT machine on site, many zoos arrange access through a local specialty practice or veterinary university.

Regardless of the type of radiology used, detailed technique charts should be developed for the various views and species. Although some domestic animal settings can easily be translated to zoo animals, this is not the case with many, such as reptiles, amphibians, or even fish. Restraint during zoo radiography is almost always chemical, to keep both the veterinary staff and the patient as safe as possible. Only very docile patients, such as tortoises, may be safely radiographed awake. In most veterinary clinics, a human-standing chest plate is not installed as it would rarely be utilized and would add cost to the system. However, in a zoo, there are many species that can either be

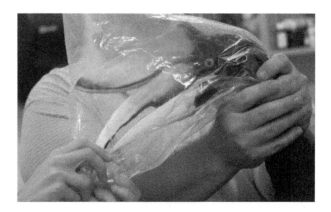

Figure 28.11 Induction of a rhinoceros hornbill using a plastic bag as a face mask.

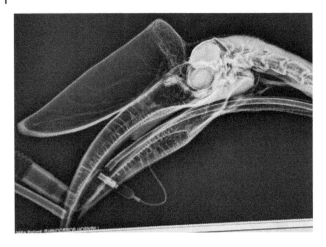

Figure 28.12 Radiograph of a rhinoceros hornbill showing anesthetic equipment used.

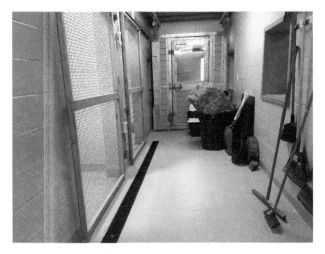

Figure 28.13 Zoo quarantine hallway.

set upon a table for an awake lateral radiograph, such as a rabbit in a plastic carrier, or even walked up to the chest plate, such as an alpaca. Almost all zoos have a portable radiology unit for fieldwork.

Another advantage of digital radiology is storage of images online in a cloud, or Picture Archiving and Communication System (PACS). This ensures images cannot be lost or damaged, and also enables veterinary staff to view radiographs on a computer monitor, eliminating the need for light boxes. Radiographs can be manipulated for clarity by the veterinarians and even shared via email with expert consultants.

Quarantine

Although many private practices have an isolation area for animals whose condition may be contagious, zoos tend to have quarantine areas, which can serve the same purpose (Figure 28.13). However, the primary reason for a quarantine area is to keep newly arrived animals separated from the rest of the collection. For a period that varies by type of animal, the patient is cared for and observed for any signs of illness which may have been precipitated by travel. Quarantine areas are usually sparsely furnished and purposely built as to be easy to clean, with impervious floors and shelves. To help the animal feel more comfortable, disposable items such as branches and cardboard boxes can be used as perching and enrichment. Easily disinfected plastic toys, appropriate to the species, may be utilized as well. For best quarantine practices, these animals are cared for by separate keeper staff. In smaller zoos, the regular keepers may either use coveralls and PPE to minimize cross-contamination with their other animals, or care for the quarantined species at the end of the day, on their way out. At the end of the quarantine period, an exam is

usually performed by veterinary staff to ensure the animal is healthy and thus safe to enter the zoo collection.

In a large enough zoo, separate areas may be set aside for avian, reptile, and mammalian species, or one area can be retrofitted for each type of species as needed. In most zoos, there is a dedicated "Class One" or dangerous animal holding, which is utilized for species that are extremely powerful and could damage and/or escape regular holding areas (such as lions or gorillas), or species that may be tractable but capable of demolishing unfortified housing, such as aardvarks. In most zoos, aquarium-dwelling animals are cared for in a separate area in the aquatics department by specialized keepers well-versed in water quality and signs of illness in those species (Figure 28.14). The veterinary team is still responsible for diagnosing infections such as parasites, approving and dispensing medications, and quarantine exit exams.

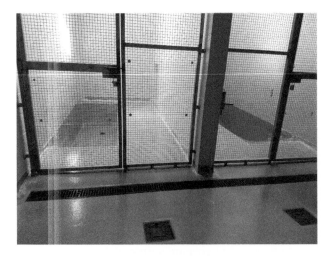

Figure 28.14 Zoo aquatic quarantine.

Intensive Care

Although many private practices have a specific "fluid ward" or other designated area for intensive care patients, a zoo must be able to either provide a wide variety of spaces in which to house very ill cases, or take the ICU to them! Although it is not usual that a zoo animal needs intensive care, it does happen, whether through illness or accident. A dedicated ICU area may have several small oxygen units to provide warmth and support to animals such as birds or reptiles. Larger oxygen units, such as those for housing dogs and cats, can be useful for many zoo species as well. It is helpful for ICU to be centrally located, so more people can easily watch the patients, yet closed off for decreased visual and auditory stimulus. In many zoo hospitals, a padded equine stall, such as those used for anesthesia and recovery, can double as a large animal ICU unit, complete with hookups on the wall or ceiling for coiled IV lines and equipment for monitoring vital signs. In some cases, the animal may not be capable of being transported to the hospital due to large size or danger to humans. Then the veterinary team must take fluid pumps, monitors, and medications to the animal's usual housing, and work within the confines of an often cramped and potentially dangerous space where healthy conspecifics still reside.

In newer zoo hospitals, in-stall cameras or mobile cams are utilized to help monitor patients, which reduces stress on a wild animal from being "watched" all the time and allows staff to perform other tasks while still keeping an eye on the patient. However, an intensive case means that zoo staff must rotate care if an animal requires around-the-clock nursing. In a small zoo, veterinary staff can be quickly fatigued by having to provide high levels of care, while also continuing with day-to-day preventative medicine for the collection. Fortunately, zookeepers are often willing and able to be taught basic veterinary care skills, such as changing fluid bags and checking IV catheter patency. Indeed, they often insist on helping with medical care of their charges, and a familiar presence can be calming to the patient, even with wild species. Once a critical case begins to stabilize, keepers can be rotated in as needed, depending on their individual comfort levels. Keep in mind that as a wild animal begins to recover from an illness, they can quickly become intractable and dangerous to handle without sedation! So, often therapeutics such as intravenous fluids or feeding tubes are pulled before medically ideal, and other means of treatment must be instituted, such as once daily restraint for administration of subcutaneous fluids and oral medications.

Nursery

Many zoos have some type of nursery, where baby animals are held if they are pulled for hand raising. The reasons for hand raising vary from zoo to zoo. Some institutions have a policy of only intervening if the infant or dam is in danger or ill. Maternal neglect or aggression or insufficient lactation are examples of situations requiring human interference. Other zoos routinely pull species that will go on to be "ambassador" animals, used in outreach programs to educate the public about the plight of their conspecifics in the wild. Some normally secretive species, such as clouded leopards, benefit from either hand raising or co-parenting with the natural dam, to increase their comfort levels around humans.

The staff performing the hand raising also differs between zoos; in some places, the veterinary team does all of the work with the baby, up until it is fully weaned. In others, members of the department from which the baby originated care for it, usually starting with higher level, experienced staff such as curators, and as the baby becomes more stable, keeper staff. Some institutions have both scenarios, with vet staff raising mammals and avian staff raising birds, or vet staff caring for the baby until it is stable, at which time it is passed to curatorial and keeper staff. In all cases, hand raising, though it can be rewarding, is also a delicate and exhaustive process (Figure 28.15). Many babies need to be fed every two hours around the clock for the first few weeks of life. Also, there are often issues with babies being reluctant to accept an artificial formula and nipple, especially if they spent some time with their natural dam. In these cases, tube feeding may be necessary initially. In all neonates, aspiration pneumonia due to fussy eating or inappropriate use of feeding methods is a fatal danger.

Equipping a nursery can be difficult, as one may not know which species are due to give birth. A zoo may know some of its gravid animals, but there are always surprise births. A well-stocked nursery has milk replacers for several species in general, and expected species in particular. For instance, if a domestic zoo animal such as a goat is expected to give birth, one can stock up on goat milk replacer as a precaution. But animals that are more difficult to assess for pregnancy, such as great apes, can give birth with no forewarning. A small amount of human formula can be kept at the zoo, and replaced as necessary from local grocery stores. Many carnivores can utilize puppy or kitten milk replacers as formula; these should always be on hand in zoos that breed these species. Some companies make exotic animal milk replacers, such as kangaroo formulas, that are expensive but necessary to stock when those species are in the collection in case of

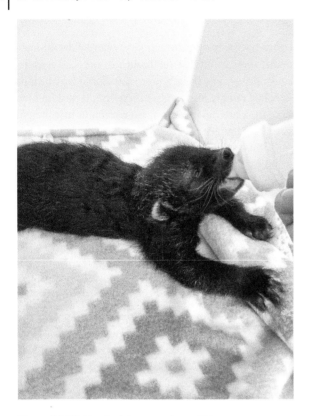

Figure 28.15 Hand raising a neglected binturong.

unexpected neonate rejection. A variety of different types of nipples and bottle sizes should always be kept on hand according to the zoo species present.

Laboratory

Almost all zoos have some semblance of an in-house laboratory, even if its only function is to perform fecals or to prepare shipments of specimens to outside labs (Figure 28.16). However, many zoo hospitals prefer to have as much labwork as possible performed in-house by their own experienced veterinary technicians. This is because of the diversity of animals within a zoo; a sample shipped to a laboratory that mainly performs diagnostics on domestic species may be misinterpreted as abnormal due to the unique features of the patient's physiology. For instance, rabbits do not have neutrophil white blood cells, but they do have heterophils, a neutrophil analogous cell that contains red granules. These granules mean the cells may be misconstrued as eosinophils, and be reported back as an eosinophilia and neutropenia. Primates, including humans, have low numbers of red granules in their neutrophils, which domestic species do not have. Birds and reptiles also have heterophils as their main bacterial-fighting white blood cell, and lack neutrophils.

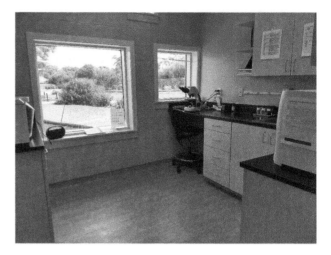

Figure 28.16 Zoo laboratory.

Even more interesting is the fact that mammals are the only vertebrates with non-nucleated red blood cells (with the exception of a few salamanders). Automated blood cell analyzers, developed from the technology of human blood analysis, are unable to correctly read avian, reptile, amphibian, and piscine blood cell counts. Thus, for accurate analysis, these species must have manual blood cell counts performed, usually on an etched glass hemocytometer. It takes some skill to perform this lab work, and having in-house trained technicians increases not only accuracy, but also decreases turn-around time of results. To do cell counts in house a diluent system is usually used, such as phloxine B dye that enhances the visibility of heterophils and eosinophils on the hemocytometer and utilizes an indirect formula to determine the total white blood cell count, or Natt-Herricks solution, which allows the technician to visualize all of the white blood cells for a direct count. However, this method runs the risk of confusing thrombocytes with lymphocytes and can have a larger margin of error depending on the skill of the technician.

Besides hematology, a zoo technician may also perform in-house urinalyses, cytologies (such as masses, abscesses, and post-mortem tissue impression smears), and blood chemistries on an automated analyzer. Gram's and acid-fast stains are often routinely performed on fecal and cytology samples to help the veterinarians to begin appropriate treatment before outside lab results, such as culture and sensitivity, arrive. A zoo technician may also be responsible for serum banking, often utilizing an ultra-low freezer and sample tracking systems/software. Often, there are outside researchers who place requests for samples from zoo animals, and the technicians are responsible for ensuring the sample is not only collected, but that it is stored and shipped correctly.

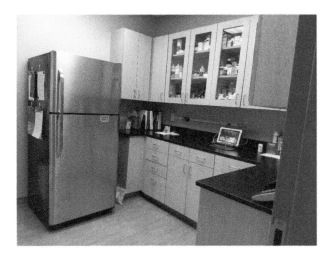

Figure 28.17 Zoo pharmacy.

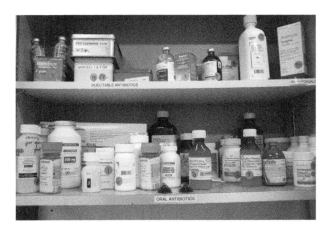

Figure 28.18 Zoo pharmacy showing common antibiotics. (Courtesy of Sandy Skeba.)

Examples of laboratory work that is usually shipped to reference specialty labs include DNA/RNA detection of pathogens, histopathology of tissues collected during necropsies or biopsies, serologic analysis of antibody levels, and clinical microbiology. But every zoo has a unique roster of lab duties; for example, some zoos have technicians that perform routine, weekly DNA sampling on their elephants to detect shedding viral loads of elephant endotheliotropic herpesvirus (EEHV). And often, if a veterinary technician has interest or skills in a particular laboratory procedure, the zoo may facilitate development of an in-house assay, which decreases both cost and turnaround time.

Pharmacy

Stocking a zoo hospital pharmacy is very different than that of a typical private practice! As mentioned in the main text, zoo medicine is focused on preventative care, and many medications typically found in large quantities in a

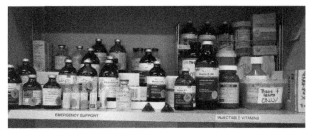

Figure 28.19 Zoo pharmacy showing emergency medications. (Courtesy of Sandy Skeba.)

small or large animal private practice are not even kept at a zoo (Figure 28.17). However, the veterinary technician or hospital manager must strive to keep the pharmacy stocked with any medications that may be needed in an emergency situation, as well as treatments and preventatives such as antiparasiticals, vaccines, antibiotics, nutritional supplements, and anesthetic agents, all for patients ranging in size and type from giraffes to songbirds to tigers (Figure 28.18). Many of the medicines in a zoo pharmacy are necessarily subjected to off-label use, since there are few formulations specifically approved for exotic species (Figure 28.19). Examples include using a combination feline vaccine for a clouded leopard, or a killed canine distemper vaccine in red pandas, which are exquisitely susceptible to that disease. The zoo veterinary technician may also perform in-house "compounding" of drugs when absolutely necessary, such as a five-gram poison dart frog needing a dewormer that is far too concentrated to measure out otherwise. Therefore, technicians in a zoo are expected to have above-average mathematical skills for drug dosages and dilutions.

Another facet of being a zoo veterinary technician is dealing with ultrapotent narcotics (Figure 28.20). These drugs are highly concentrated for use to quickly and safely anesthetizing large, dangerous animals such as zebras and rhinoceros. These drugs, such as etorphine and thiafentinil, are dangerous to handle, as even a small drop in the eyes, mucus membranes, or an open wound can paralyze a human, including respiratory muscles. Therefore, appropriate PPE must be worn at all times while handling, including safety goggles and nitrile gloves. An accidental needle stick with an ultrapotent drug is dangerous enough that human reversal agents should be present and ready to administer. Careful protocols and drills are necessary for mitigating possible emergency situations.

Many injectable drugs in a zoo pharmacy must be delivered by remote injection, via a darting system, due to the wild nature of zoo patients. This includes vaccinations, slow-release antibiotics, and anesthetic agents. So a zoo veterinary technician must learn how to load, pressurize, and even dart animals! Darts are flying syringes, with either pressurized air chambers that act as the delivery force, or a

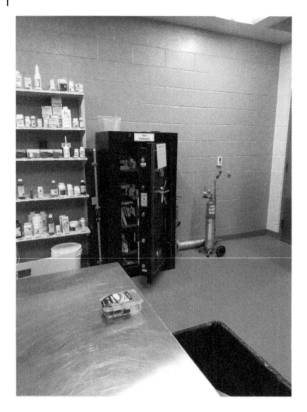

Figure 28.20 Controlled substance safe.

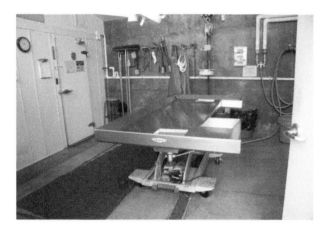

Figure 28.21 Zoo necropsy room.

carbon dioxide pellet that discharges when the dart strikes the animal. There are several types of guns used to deliver the dart to the animal, and there are different ranges for each type, since an animal that needs to be darted could be in a small enclosure (blowdart using breath to propel the dart), a large stall (compressed air pistol), or free ranging in a field (carbon dioxide rifle). The technician must be very comfortable with the zoo's chosen system before using it to administer drugs, especially ultrapotent narcotics. Practice

is very important, with both loading and preparing the darts and shooting practice with fake animal targets.

Necropsy

All zoos perform necropsies on just about every deceased collection animal unless precluded by severe autolysis. Thus, most zoo hospitals have a dedicated necropsy area ideally situated apart from any live animal holding, including the veterinary hospital, in case of infectious disease. A necropsy can shed light on not just what caused the individual animal's death, but disclose underlying issues not obvious while the animal was alive. Necropsy is also an important part of "herd health" in gregarious species; often, what is present in one member of the group is present in all of them. Different species of animals are susceptible to different illnesses, such as dilated cardiomyopathy in anteaters or amoebiasis in snakes and lizards. Knowing what is present in one member of the herd helps to better treat the remaining members.

A necropsy suite should be easy to clean and disinfect and be able to handle most zoo species. Stainless steel tables (small and large animal) and heavy-duty winches are utilized for handling carcasses (Figure 28.21). Tissues are often collected in formalin for histopathologic analysis and submitted to an outside pathologist with experience in exotic species. Small animals, such as lizards, frogs, or baby birds, may be incised, examined without removing organs, and submitted whole in formalin. Species with Endangered or Threatened status may have specific frozen and formalin tissue collection protocols that must be followed. As in the laboratory, it usually falls upon the technicians to ensure samples are properly collected, labeled, and sent to the correct facilities and researchers for processing.

Some larger zoos employ full or part-time pathologists, but otherwise the veterinary team, including technicians, performs all necropsies. A skilled technician with a special interest may even be relied upon to perform many smaller species' necropsies alone, calling for the vet as needed for consultation. Thus, the zoo technician should be comfortable with the anatomy of a wide variety of species.

Some zoos that are in close proximity to veterinary universities may have all of their necropsies performed there, with the exception of species too large for easy transport. Whether or not a zoo does necropsies in-house, the largest species, such as giraffes or elephants, are usually prosected on grounds, and often buried there. Disposal of carcasses otherwise can be through in-house or outside laboratory incineration, dedicated local landfill areas, or submission of carcasses for processing into teaching artifacts for zoo programs, including skulls and hides. In some cases, biomaterials may be requested by outside facilities,

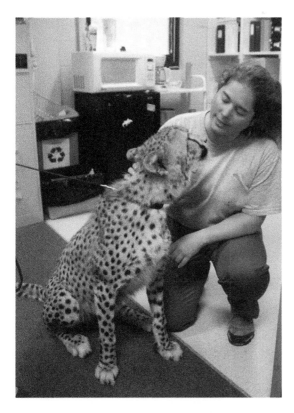

Figure 28.22 Physical examination of a habituated cheetah. Who is examining whom?

such as universities, for research or teaching projects. In these circumstances, approval must be obtained through an Institutional Animal Care and Use Committee, or IACUC, which determines the appropriateness of the request.

In a typical veterinary clinic, animals have owners. In a zoo, they have keepers. Zookeepers are much like the animals' owners in a zoo setting, in that they care for their charges every day, and are usually the first person to notice that something is wrong. After diagnosis, the keepers administer medications and care for the patient. They give the vet staff progress updates and make sure the patient is eating and drinking. An advantage to having zoo keepers instead of owners to deal with when it comes to patient care is that most keepers are better educated about animals than a typical pet owner. They understand drug dosing and why it is important to completely finish a medication. They are great at follow-up care and are trained to notice the first sign of health issues in wild animals, which are even better than their domestic counterparts at hiding their illnesses. Also, keepers are usually excellent at restraint and can be trusted to protect the veterinary staff as well as not injure the animal during an exam. Disadvantages to dealing with keepers are few, but they are there. A keeper who is very possessive of their animal ("my" elephant, "my" tiger)

can sometimes decide that they know what is best for the animal, even when it comes to veterinary care. This can also happen due to a keeper's higher education level, and the phenomenon known as "Dr. Google," where looking up diseases and their treatments is as easy as turning on your computer. Some keepers may sympathize with their animal so much that they are reluctant to call vet staff for a problem, because it will "scare" or "hurt" the animal. Keepers are only human, and working with their different personality types can be a challenge. A typical domestic animal nurse may only see a difficult client once in a while, and the clinic has the option of "firing" that client. But a zoo veterinary technician deals with the same ornery keepers, day in and day out. Still, a zookeeper is an important part of the healthcare team. Enabling zookeepers to express their opinion on veterinary issues such as whether or not an animal will take a particular medication better in pill or liquid form, or even as to when euthanasia is indicated by an animal's decreased quality of life, increases the trust between veterinary and keeper staff.

As for euthanasia, this is one area that is very different from private practice. Instead of an owner making the decision based on money or sentiment, medical decisions, for the most part, are made based on what is best for the animal. Many zoo employees get to have a say in this difficult decision. The veterinary staff gives as much information as possible to the keepers and curators, and discussion is not just encouraged but expected. Even when the decision is not unanimous, at least everyone feels they have had a chance to provide input.

Since zoo veterinary medicine is so specialized, there is no referral of off-hours emergency cases to another practice. When an animal needs care in an emergency situation, the entire veterinary team is expected to work. A giraffe C-section may take until 2 in the morning, and exhausted staff still needs to be at work the next day, even if the outcome was not positive. Not many zoos have enough veterinary personnel to rotate on-call duties, so a zoo veterinary technician is effectively on-call 24/7, no matter what the day or hour. Luckily, much of zoo medicine is preventative, and true emergencies are not a common event. But they do seem to come in waves!

Preventative medicine is a huge part of zoo work. Like dogs and cats, many exotic animals require vaccinations, although some may need these administered by remote injection (blowdarts). Zoo animals are checked for parasites twice yearly, and as would be expected, exotic animals have some very interesting parasites! Physical exams are performed, and in many species involve anesthesia in order to do a complete work-up (Figure 28.22).

Dental cleanings and extractions are common, in those species that have teeth. Examples of preventative care for different types of animals are as follows:

Primates – Physical exam every other year, including bloodwork (CBC, Chemscreen), full body radiographs, TB testing (intradermal, right upper eyelid), dental care, and ultrasonography of heart, kidneys, reproductive tract if female, and liver. Preventative care consists of yearly vaccines (rabies and tetanus), monthly oral ivermectin to prevent infection by *Baylisascaris* sp., and biannual fecal parasite exams.

Hoofstock – Physical exam every other year, including bloodwork (CBC, Chemscreen), fecal culture for Johne's Disease (*Mycobacterium paratuberculosis*), and TB test (intradermal, tailfold). Preventative care consists of yearly vaccines (rabies, clostridial combination) and biannual fecal parasite exams. Equids also receive vaccinations against equine encephalitis and West Nile virus, and their biannual parasite check includes a McMaster's quantitative exam.

Carnivores – Physical exam every other year, including bloodwork (CBC, Chemscreen), full body radiographs, dental care, and ultrasonography of heart, kidneys, reproductive tract if female, and liver. Preventative care includes monthly oral ivermectin for heartworm prevention, yearly vaccines including rabies, feline combination such as FVR-CP (cats), canine combination such as DHL-P2) (canids), and killed canine distemper (red pandas, bears, anteaters). Anteaters may also receive West Nile virus vaccines yearly.

Birds – Physical exam every other year, including bloodwork if large enough to sample safely (CBC, Chemscreen), and full body radiographs. Preventative care includes biannual fecal parasite exams, for raptors and corvids, and vaccination against West Nile virus.

Reptiles and amphibians – Physical exam every other year, including bloodwork if large enough to sample safely (CBC, Chemscreen), and full body radiographs. Preventative care includes biannual fecal parasite exams.

One of the biggest aspects of preventative medicine is quarantine. All animals coming into a zoo undergo a quarantine period of at least 30 days to prevent them from bringing disease into the animal collection. Some standard quarantine protocols include:

Mammals – 30 days. Exit exam includes bloodwork (CBC, Chemscreen), TB test if a primate or hoofstock, three negative fecal samples taken at least 1 week apart, updated vaccines, and full body radiographs.

Birds, not including psittacines – 30 days. Exit exam includes bloodwork if large enough for safe sampling (CBC, Chemscreen), three negative fecal samples, one negative fecal culture for *Salmonella*, and full body radiographs.

Psittacines – 90 days. Exit exam includes bloodwork (CBC, Chemscreen, parrot viral panel, and *Chlamydia* panel), three negative fecal samples with Gram's stain for normal flora, and full body radiographs. Parrot viral panel may include avian polyomavirus, psittacine beak and feather virus, and avian bornavirus.

Reptiles, not including snakes, and amphibians – 30 days. Exit exam includes bloodwork if large enough for safe sampling (CBC, Chemscreen), three negative fecal samples taken at least one week apart, and full body radiographs.

Snakes – 90 days. Exit exam same as other reptiles, but bloodwork includes testing for paramyxovirus.

One big disadvantage to keeping a closed collection is that there are usually no animal health care benefits for employee animals, such as is typical at a private veterinary practice. Many domestic animals carry diseases that can be especially injurious to exotic species, such as canine distemper. Because of this no outside pets are allowed to enter the zoo, even if they have a good vaccination record. A zoo veterinary technician can work with an excellent veterinary team, yet be unable to get help when his/her own pets need it.

Working for a zoo means working for a corporation, albeit usually a non-profit one. Many veterinary technicians will be used to this corporate life. However, this model differs from a privately owned practice, where the practice owner or practice manager makes all the final decisions as to hiring, firing, discipline, and patient care. A zoo veterinarian usually reports to a vice president or general curator. If there are personality conflicts, even within the veterinary team, they can be brought to the Human Resources department. Zoos usually have excellent employee benefits, such as health, dental/vision, and disability insurance. What zoos do not have, typically, is a good pay rate, although there are as many pay scales for zoo veterinary technicians as there are zoos, and salary usually increases with experience. Taking off for holidays is a problem, as most zoos are open on holidays; indeed, holidays are usually very busy days. So say goodbye to Memorial Day picnics with the family if you want to work at a zoo! Also, zoos usually try to maintain a sense of corporate ownership; that is, every employee is expected to put their best face forward to the public and promote the zoo's "brand" at all times. This includes when you are stopping at the grocery store on the way home; if you are wearing your uniform, you would be expected to smile and be polite when someone begins asking you about your job. All zoo employees are expected to pick up litter on the public path, assist with finding lost children, and answer questions from the public, no matter how inane. In some respects, this is similar to a private practice!

Most zoos rely heavily on "gate receipts" (visitors paying to see the zoo). Rainy days or hot weather can affect the operating budget. What this means for the veterinary technician is that diagnostic tests and animal health decisions may rely on the "value" of the patient, whether it is inherent (a rare Sumatran rhinoceros) or perceived (a beloved, geriatric pygmy goat with epilepsy). When times are tough, the veterinary team is expected to cut back on profligate expenses, yet still provide excellent veterinary care.

Most zoos adhere to strict guidelines of animal care. All zoos are also regulated by the USDA. Veterinarians from the USDA can show up unannounced to check such parameters as animal housing (parameters dictated by the Animal and Plant Health Inspection Service [APHIS]), controlled substance records, and the existence of expired drugs. These government agencies have a hand in controlling many aspects of animal care (Department of Agriculture 2013). In addition, many zoos aspire to become accredited by the Association of Zoos and Aquariums (AZA). The AZA sets even higher standards of animal care, and facilities wishing to obtain (or keep) AZA accreditation must meet those standards. Accredited zoos are inspected every five years by a committee consisting of members of other AZA-accredited institutions, including veterinarians, curators, and directors. They report their findings to the AZA accreditation committee, which decides if the facility in question remains (or becomes) accredited. If concerns are found, the AZA committee will attempt to correct them first via meeting with the zoo senior staff. Accreditation is not easy and requires true dedication and hard work.

AZA-accredited zoos usually adhere to guidelines set up by the Species Survival Plan (SSP), which keeps detailed genetic records of many endangered or threatened animal species. The SSP recommends breeding efforts for individual animals that are intended to produce genetically diverse and healthy offspring. Therefore, a female giraffe born at one institution is not just merely "up for sale" to the highest bidder, but may be put on "breeding loan" to a zoo that has a genetically compatible male. In a breeding loan, ownership of the animal remains with its original zoo; typically no money changes hands, but agreements are made as to which institution owns any resultant offspring. For example, "X" zoo that sends a male tapir to breed with another female at "Y" zoo will be guaranteed ownership of the second and fourth calves, while "Y" zoo will get the first and third. Breeding loans can be very complicated, and ensure not only genetic compatibility, but also that animals are not valued for strictly monetary purposes.

See Appendix 14 which contains a form used to transfer necessary data about an animal from one zoo to another.

Many zoos participate in conservation; indeed, conservation is mentioned in most zoos' mission statements as to why they exist! Participating in conservation may be as simple as adhering to SSP guidelines. But conservation efforts of endangered or threatened species can be taken much further, and often are. On a local scale, a zoo may support its neighborhood wildlife rehabilitation facility (money and/or supply donations, or volunteering). A zoo may also focus on an endangered species found in its home state, and perform fieldwork or sustain a captive population for breeding and reintroduction purposes. There are many opportunities for one organization to make a big difference in local conservation. International conservation efforts are also coveted, and some zoos boast field scientists in such remote locales as Madagascar or the Brazilian Pantanal. But if its resources preclude individual efforts, a zoo can contribute to an already established conservation organization, such as the Gorilla Rehabilitation and Conservation Education Center (GRACE) in the Democratic Republic of Congo; the International Rhino Foundation based out of Fort Worth, Texas; and the Tiger Conservation Campaign, initiated by the tiger SSP. Individual zoos can team up to pool resources for endangered species conservation. For example, in the 1990s several zoos founded the Clouded Leopard Consortium, which focuses on both conserving and breeding clouded leopards in Thailand, and importing captive-bred animals to the United States to diversify a population threatened by genetic bottlenecking.

With these conservation projects also comes a chance for a zoo veterinary technician to become involved with some exciting fieldwork! Local day trips to perform water quality testing or disease testing (such as chytrid swabbing for the deadly *Batrachochytrium dendrobatidis* fungus on amphibians) can be a fun change of pace from the regular workday. Some zoo technicians get to take their hematology and parasitology skills internationally to work on endangered species. A zoo veterinary technician can be a valued member of a research team. All it takes is the knowledge we already have, the wisdom to seize the opportunity when it comes along, and a sense of adventure!

Do You Have What It Takes to Be a Zoo Veterinary Technician?

As you have probably guessed by now, zoo veterinary medicine is a challenging yet rewarding career. The most important qualities of a zoo veterinary technician are flexibility and a thirst for knowledge. Unlike a private practice, a zoo vet technician is encouraged to investigate and learn during work hours. A private practitioner may forbid a technician from performing cytology on a mass or necropsying a deceased animal unless the owner has paid for the procedure. But as a zoo technician's knowledge increases, they become even more of an asset to their veterinary team. For example, most zoo technicians spend a lot of time performing parasitology exams. Zoo animals not only have interesting parasites, but also carry what can be thought of as a "micro zoo," commensal organisms that live within the intestinal tract yet cause no harm to the animal. Understanding the difference between these helps the veterinarian decide what should be treated and what can safely be left alone. A zoo technician familiar with gram staining can inform the veterinarian if there are gram-negative rods or gram-positive cocci in an abscess, enabling the correct antibiotic treatment to begin long before the culture results come back from the lab.

Often, the zoo technician is the first line of contact between the keepers and the veterinarian, and it is necessary to be able to decide which situations are emergencies and what can be scheduled for a later date. Keepers are only human and have a wide range of personality types. Professionalism with a sense of humor is key to a harmonious relationship. In fact, it behooves the technician to get along well with keeper staff, since a keeper that trusts the technician will also allow more freedom for animal contact. For instance, a keeper who likes the veterinary technician is more willing to allow them to feed the giraffes, or visit the tigers "behind the scenes" if they have guests or family visiting. A zoo veterinary technician can also be part of animal training for voluntary procedures, such as blood draws. A keeper who knows you have an interest in their animal and are easy to work with is much more amenable to having the technician participate in these exciting opportunities. See Appendices 15 and 16.

Being a zoo veterinary technician can be very difficult, emotionally. Many animals have short life spans; you may be enraptured by the birth of an animal, watch it grow, perform its annual exams, and visit it for training, then see its health decline until euthanasia is inevitable. Also, many zoos have problems with urban wildlife, and not only can raccoons and opossums physically damage collection animals, but they carry diseases that are deadly to animals naive to common North American infections, such as *Sarcocystis* or *Baylisascaris*. So trapping and euthanasia of otherwise healthy native wild animals is a fact of zoo life. Even domestic cats can be a problem if they wander onto zoo grounds; *Toxoplasma*, the ubiquitous protozoa many felines carry, is deadly to animals such as kangaroos. So diligent trapping is a must, although pet species are usually taken to a local shelter, rather than euthanized outright.

Job Description for a Zoo Veterinary Technician

Although most zoo job descriptions are similar, they will often emphasize the most usual, or important, duties by listing them first.

- Assist the veterinary staff with clinical procedures, including surgery, examinations, and necropsies (Figure 28.23).
- Monitoring of anesthetized patients (including intubation, catheter placement, and use of anesthesia machine).
- Dispense medications as prescribed by veterinarian.
- Obtain, handle, and process biological specimens from a variety of species, including birds, mammals, and reptiles.
- Perform radiography using both mobile and portable machines to accurately take diagnostic quality radiographs.
- Proficiency in clinical laboratory procedures, including maintenance and use of blood chemistry analyzers, and performing manual complete blood counts (CBC) with differential analysis on mammals, birds, reptiles, and fish.
- Prepare biological specimens for safe shipment to outside laboratories.

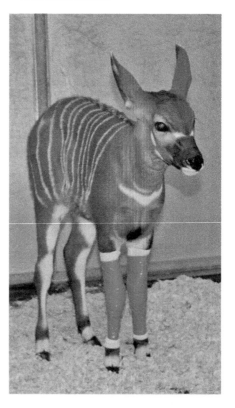

Figure 28.23 Bandages on a young Bongo antelope.

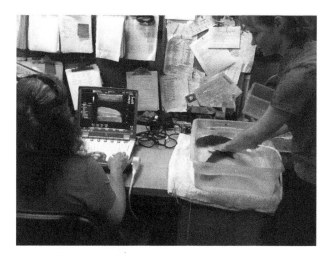

Figure 28.24 Ultrasound of a Hellbender.

- Familiar with the set-up, use, and maintenance of medical equipment, including endoscopy, ECG, ultrasound, dental unit, pulse oximetry, and doppler (Figure 28.24).
- Provide intensive and critical care to exotic animal patients, including restraint, handling, and medicating.
- Work with computer programs such as Outlook, Excel, and Word, and specialized medical record-keeping systems. The two main programs in use are ZIMS and TRACKS.
- Participate in guest interactions, such as hospital tours, and perform educational presentations.
- Ensure that the hospital facility is clean and well-maintained.

And, of course, the last duty is almost always the ubiquitous, "Perform other duties as assigned."

How Do You Become a Zoo Veterinary Technician?

An early interest in unusual animals is important, but one must have a solid knowledge of domestic animal medicine. This gives a technician a base of skills to extrapolate from. Having the opportunity to work with exotic animals in a veterinary practice gives exposure to animals beyond the dog/cat, horse/cow. Seek out any opportunity to work with wild or exotic species!

Volunteer work in an exotic practice or local zoo is helpful. By volunteering for a nearby zoo, one gets to know the veterinary team there. When there is a veterinary technician job opening, having had wild/exotic animal volunteer positions proves one has an interest. Strong laboratory skills are also an asset for a zoo veterinary technician. A little bit of networking helps, too! The key is to obtain experience, as that is what a zoo is looking for.

There are many options for following a zoo career path. Many zoos now have internships for veterinary technicians, both paid and unpaid. Working for a clinic that sees exotic animals is a great way to get experience, especially if you have none. Even watching exotic animal procedures helps, and most veterinarians, when they see you have an interest, are more than willing to train you to help them, as this only increases your usefulness to the clinic. Volunteering with wildlife is another great way to get exposure to non-domestic species. Wildlife rehabilitation is very hands-on, and veterinary technicians with even basic animal handling and medicating skills are coveted by a wildlife clinic. You will learn how to catch and restrain an owl, tube feed a rabbit, and care for exotic patients in emergency situations, such as hit-by-cars. It is also very rewarding to treat a wild animal and then get to release it to live its life free once again. Even increasing your knowledge by reading books about exotic and wild animal veterinary care helps. There is also an organization specifically for zoo veterinary technicians. The Association of Zoo Veterinary Technicians is run by, and for, technicians in the zoo (and aquarium) field. You do not have to work at a zoo to join! It is a great resource for technicians who want to learn more about the zoo field. Their website (azvt .org) has information about becoming a zoo veterinary technician, job listings, and suggested reference materials for aspiring zoo vet techs. There is a forum for technicians to post questions to each other about every aspect of zoo medicine, from how to raise a baby warthog, to what kind of hematology analyzers people like best. They have an annual conference, hosted by a different zoo each year, with lots of learning and networking opportunities. And there is even a scholarship program to assist veterinary technician students financially to attend the conference.

Many veterinary technicians enjoy a predictable day of spays and neuters, and explaining flea and tick prevention. There is comfort to routine, and the occasional incoming emergency is enough excitement for most. But a zoo veterinary technician enjoys the anticipation, every single day, of wondering just what will walk through the clinic door next!

Reference

Department of Agriculture. 2013. Animal Welfare Act, Volume: 1 Date: 1 January 2013 Original Date: 1 January 2013 Title: Subchapter A – Animal Welfare Title 9 – Animals and Animal Products. Chapter I Animal and plant health inspection service.

29

The Role of a Veterinary Technician at a Public Aquarium
Rachel Parchem

Introduction

Aquarium medicine is a multifaceted topic. There are many concepts that will be familiar for veterinary technicians as well as many unfamiliar concepts. No day is the same, and an aquarium veterinary technician will need to be flexible, creative, adept at triage, and proficient with time management skills. Preventive medicine such as quarantine, medical isolation, and routine physicals are key, and there is a heavy focus on these areas. These can include but are not limited to vaccinations, radiology, bloodwork, ultrasound, and parasite screening (Figure 29.1). A veterinary technician is responsible for knowing the varied types of anesthesia that will be performed on different species, restraint, and handling of different species, and relevant anatomical considerations for those species. Frequently, the technician must go to the patient due to factors such as patient size, and stress level, i.e., can this patient be transported to the hospital space? Will it harm itself during transportation? Having a mobile clinic set up is necessary. Most aquaria are involved in conservation efforts in the form of research or rehabilitation, and occasionally technicians are involved in these areas. Doing laboratory work, such as reading slide samples, fecal examinations, blood analysis, and microbiology is prevalent. Even though some samples can be sent to a reference laboratory, many may be done in-house since non-mammals have nucleated red blood cells. Working with neonates can be part of a technician's duties as well since animals will be born at the facility. Additionally, some species live longer in captivity due to access to good nutrition, medical care, and the absence of predators so geriatric care is also a consideration. With being responsible for a collection of animals, emergencies will happen. Triage skills and emergency/critical care skills are necessary and sought after. Necropsies are performed on deceased animals and technicians are responsible for performing them.

Typical Day

The day begins with treatments, preparation for exams, and communications with the veterinary team and husbandry staff to discuss the plan for the day and any case updates that need to be shared. When managing a large collection of animals, communication between staff is critical, and it is necessary for technicians to coordinate with animal care staff and veterinary staff frequently. Not unlike private practice, it is common for unscheduled procedures to happen—a lethargic otter, a bird favoring a leg, a case of severe conspecific aggression, or a shark lying at the bottom of a habitat.

A typical day might begin with scheduled anesthetic procedures or preventative physical exams. Preventative exams are crucial for the welfare of the animal collection. In an aquarium setting, these exams are done most frequently on avians, reptiles, and elasmobranchs. It is sometimes done on fishes and amphibians, but this is less frequent due to patient stress, limited diagnostic ability, and large number of these types of animals in the collection. In addition to keeping on track with an animal's welfare, it is especially important to do preventative exams to establish normals. When evaluating blood on a sandbar shark, if there is a routine history of bloodwork when healthy, one can better evaluate bloodwork performed on an urgent exam. Additionally, the knowledge obtained can be shared with other institutions bettering the welfare of the captive collection as a whole. It is the technician's role to set up, prepare, and facilitate these exams and procedures (Figures 29.2 and 29.3). Throughout the day technicians recheck patients from prior procedures, medicate patients who are under treatment, fill prescriptions, triage urgent and emergent calls, collect and run laboratory samples, and complete necropsies. Common laboratory samples include cytology, clinical microbiology (i.e., cultures and sensitivities), fecals, skin scrapes, gill clips, and hematology samples.

Exotic Animal Medicine for the Veterinary Technician, Fourth Edition. Edited by Bonnie Ballard and Ryan Cheek.
© 2024 John Wiley & Sons, Inc. Published 2024 by John Wiley & Sons, Inc.
Companion Website: www.wiley.com/go/ballard/4e

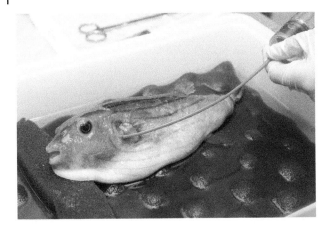

Figure 29.1 Pufferfish being ventilated using a syringe and a red rubber catheter to provide oxygenated water over the gills during a sedated exam. (Courtesy of Shedd Aquarium/Brenna Hernandez.)

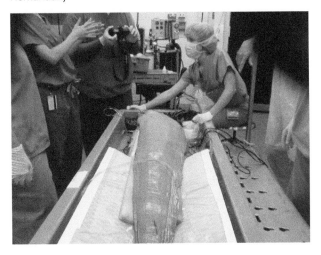

Figure 29.2 A large green moray eel (*Gymnothorax olyuranodon*) under general anesthesia for surgery. (Courtesy of Dr. Greg Lewbart.)

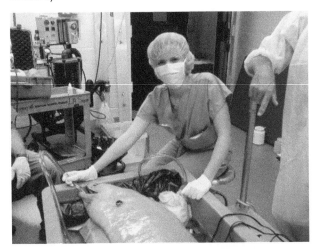

Figure 29.3 A close-up of the anesthetic equipment. (Courtesy of Dr. Greg Lewbart.)

Technicians are also responsible for hospital inventory, equipment maintenance, scheduling, and routine hospital stocking and cleaning. It is common for institutions that are education-focused for technicians to lead hospital tours, speak at conservation events, and host shadows, as well as students.

Every facility operates in a unique way. Facilities might have more than one technician and they will share the responsibilities. A common example of this is one technician being responsible for in-house laboratory samples and the other technician being responsible for clinical procedures. If there is only one technician, then that technician is responsible for both clinical procedures as well as laboratory procedures. There may be days when the technician is the sole member of the veterinary team present. It is expected that the technician is capable of functioning independently by demonstrating proficiency in triaging, performing diagnostics and procedures, and communicating with the off-site veterinarian if needed.

It is imperative that an aquarium technician facilitates trust with the animal care staff and the veterinary staff by communicating effectively and demonstrating competency.

How Does an Aquarium Differ from Private Practice?

Working at a public aquarium can be quite different from private practice. The technicians are expected to be familiar with a variety of species. Aquaria consists of teleosts (ray-finned fishes), elasmobranchs (sharks, rays, and skates), avians (waterfowl, penguins, psittacines, etc.), reptilians (chelonia, snakes, lizards, etc.), amphibians (frogs and salamanders, etc.), invertebrates and mammals both terrestrial and marine (Figure 29.4). Technicians need to be versatile in working with various species and understand the differences between them. There are skills and knowledge that are transferrable. These include but are not limited to basic veterinary medical principles like sterile fields, anticoagulants in blood collection tubes, sample handling, syringe handling technique, phlebotomy skills, and intubation. Much of this transferrable knowledge can be applied and built upon. For example, a veterinary technician is skilled at and understands intubation. At an aquarium, one would build on that knowledge by learning the differences in anatomy of the collection that will affect intubation as well as other considerations like when to use an uncuffed endotracheal tube. As a technician, it is expected that knowledge of the patients on multiple levels, especially when safety comes into play for the patient, technician, and staff is there.

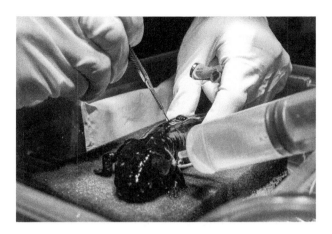

Figure 29.4 An anesthetized salamander undergoes surgery for a removal of a dermal mass. (Courtesy of Shedd Aquarium/Brenna Hernandez.)

Depending upon what species is being worked with—a fish with *Mycobacterium*, or a bird with aspergillosis, or a non-human primate—animal care staff need to be cognizant and cautious about zoonotic diseases and wear appropriate protective equipment. It is crucial to know the hazards of the species you are working with. Considering birds for example, for a raptor (red-tailed hawk, eagle, owls, etc.), animal handlers would be more concerned about the talons than the beak. For a psittacine (macaws, parrots, etc.) the beak poses much more of a risk than the talons. Not only do technicians need to be cognizant of the hazards to staff, but they also need to be aware of safety for the patient as well. Patient stress level is a constant consideration while working with these animals. Stress can lead to the patient injuring himself (flying into a habitat wall or attempting to jump out of a transport device) and can also lead to more severe risks such as capture myopathy and mortality.

The pharmacy is an area where many of the same medications used in small and large animal clinics are seen. It consists of analgesics, antibiotics, anesthetics, vitamins, supplements, antiparasitic medications, and contraceptives. An aquarium staple is MS-222 or tricaine methanesulfate. This is the powder used to sedate fish by adding it to the water. Due to the variety of species at an aquarium, as well as the variety in size of the patients, managing an aquarium pharmacy poses its challenges. Dilutions are key as many of the patients can be small. Think of a 1.5 gram dart frog that needs antibiotics! The pharmacy also needs to be equipped to accommodate a one-ton whale. There may be a need to order compounded medications, powdered medications, specific concentrations of medications, and specially flavored medications. US Food and Drug Administration (FDA)-approved medications for aquaculture can be used for treatments, but many medications

are used off-label (http://www.fda.gov/AnimalVeterinary/DevelopmentApprovalProcess/Aquaculture/ucm132954.htm). Medications can be purchased or made into a powder and added to the water in the habitat for medicated baths and this is routinely done. Medications can be placed in food items for patients who are reliably eating, and medications are also administered in routes such as topically, orally, intravenously, intramuscularly, and intracoelomically.

The equipment used in an aquarium setting can also be different. Equipment such as water pumps for ventilation are used, as well as air stones for oxygenating patients under anesthesia (Figure 29.5). Aquariums will have a small animal anesthesia machine and can have a large animal anesthesia machine as well (collection depending). This would be used on animals like dolphins or sea lions, whose lung capacities far exceed the small animal machine. Some equipment must be fabricated for a specific animal because it is not commercially made. Anesthesia masks for sea lions can include items such as traffic cones, or handmade face masks made for the specific patient's size. Intravenous catheters can be used to intubate small turtles and lizards. Clear tubes can be used to examine snakes, eels, and caecilians. Creative solutions must be made to meet the needs of the patient.

Finances are a large difference between an aquarium and private practice. Technicians will not be creating estimates and acquiring owner approval for specific costs of diagnostics and procedures, as these procedures are performed as needed. That is not to say that institutions are unlimited financially. Veterinary staff work with the financial department to decide the budget for the year, and budgets are dictated by the financial well-being of the institution. For large-budget items or procedures, these

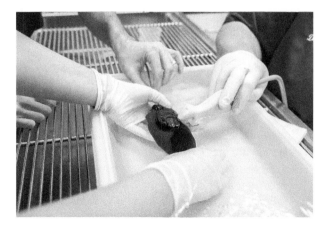

Figure 29.5 A sedated pufferfish is examined via ultrasound and ventilated using a red rubber catheter with oxygenated water. (Courtesy of Shedd Aquarium/Brenna Hernandez.)

will be discussed and may require approval. Veterinary teams are expected to provide an excellent standard of veterinary care with the budget they are provided.

Regulatory bodies of aquariums include The Association of Zoos and Aquariums (AZA), United States Department of Agriculture (USDA), Animal and Plant Health Inspection Service (APHIS), and Occupational Safety and Health Administration (OSHA). Aquariums are required to adhere to a strict standard of animal care as well as facility upkeep. Aquariums that are accredited by AZA are inspected every 5 years by a committee of animal care staff from other AZA institutions to retain their accreditation. USDA inspections can happen anytime, checking for animal welfare as well as medication usage like controlled drug logging and expired medication. Institutions also may have internal monitoring such as whistleblower systems, enrichment committees, welfare committees, and research approval committees.

An aquarium's clients are those who care for the animals daily. These clients are called husbandry staff. Biologists, aquarists, keepers, and trainers fall under this term's umbrella. Husbandry staff is responsible for providing proper husbandry such as an appropriate sized habitat, correct lighting, monitoring and testing water quality, temperature, and any other exhibit parameters. They are responsible for feeding and recording diets and monitoring their animal's behavior. The husbandry staff are the experts on their specific animals. They will typically be the first to notify staff of a medical concern with an animal, abnormal behavior, or water quality concerns. They can answer questions about the patient's history and provide useful information. They also will be able to restrain or handle their animal. Providing medical care for aquarium animals hinges on the teamwork of the veterinary staff and husbandry staff. It is imperative that trust is built and maintained between these groups.

Making the decision to euthanize an animal, unless it is an emergency-based decision, is usually done as a team. A group discussion would involve the husbandry staff, the director of that department, and the veterinarian to make the most informed and appropriate decision based on all the information provided.

The aquarium staff typically have first shift hours in the range of 7 a.m.–5 p.m. This includes veterinary staff. Veterinary staff are on-site seven days a week, meaning that weekend and holiday coverage is needed. Coverage methods vary by institution, an example is rotating weekends or a Tuesday–Saturday or Sunday–Thursday schedule. Veterinary technicians will be on call if anything were to happen while not on-site, additionally, if a critical care patient requires round-the-clock care, or a transport of animals is due to arrive after hours. If staffing allows, on-call will be rotated between technicians and veterinarians.

Quarantine can fall under the veterinary team or specific quarantine husbandry staff. Whether being cared for by the veterinary staff or husbandry staff, quarantine typically requires more medical attention than other areas. This is due to several factors. Stress can facilitate secondary issues by compromising their immune system. Transportation can be a stressful event. Water quality in the transport may not have been ideal. There is an adjustment period where the animals will need to get acclimated to a new habitat, diet, and routine. They may arrive with parasites, viral diseases, or bacterial infections. They may not want to eat initially after arriving. They may have been compromised prior to arrival. All these factors increase their rate of mortality and increase their medical care needs. Quarantined patients are cared for in specific areas that do not interact with non-quarantine areas. What is employed depends upon the animal's size and requirements. Quarantine is typically a range of 30–90 days, but this will vary on patient history and treatments that it may require. Any animal that arrives (aquatic and non-aquatic) goes through quarantine, and to minimize cross-contamination between habitats, foot baths, dips, or baths (bleach, fresh water, Virkon, and Roccal) for equipment (all equipment used—nets, pumps, buckets, hoses, air stones, and filters) and good hygiene are employed. Sick or diseased patients or systems are kept on a separate system from the rest of the population. This is necessary because aquarium medicine is akin to herd medicine. If a new trout arrives at the aquarium with an underlying parasitic, bacterial, or viral infection, placing this fish in the habitat with hundreds of trout could cause all trout to be affected. Quarantine plans can be a standard plan created by the veterinary staff per species, such as: reptiles have a 30-day minimum quarantine, with three fecals at least a week apart, then an exit exam to conclude quarantine which includes an exam, bloodwork, radiographs, ultrasound and sample collection for disease testing. Quarantine exams can also be created on a case-by-case basis. If the sending institution completed some of the requirements, then they may not need to be repeated. If an animal has no medical history, additional medications may be given prophylactically. For multispecies fish quarantines, or single-species fish quarantines that have a large number of fish, exit exams will be performed on a representative percentage of the population. This percentage is around 10% of the population depending on the institution's policy, and the specifics of that quarantine. For example, if a quarantine system consists of 12 parrotfish, 20 wrasse, and 10 hogfish, not every fish will receive an exam. You might sample 1 parrotfish, 2 wrasse, and 1 hogfish. Commonly the protocol for fish exit diagnostics is a sedated exam, a skin scrape (a sample of their mucous coating, not a sample of skin taken with a scalpel), a gill clip, and potentially a fin clip. All mortalities in that system will be reviewed, as well as their medical records and quarantine protocol. Then the decision will be made to release them from quarantine or keep them in quarantine for additional treatment or testing.

Working for an aquarium could mean working for a corporation or a non-profit facility, but in general, there is a hierarchy system in place: the technician reports to the veterinarian or technician manager, the veterinarian or technician manager reports to either a head veterinarian or the vice-president of a department, or the veterinarian reports to the owner of the facility. Most aquaria have an employee benefits system. However, a consideration of working in aquaria is that the financial compensation trends are lower than private practice.

Challenges of Large, Multispecies Habitats

Aquaria have multispecies habitats that can pose challenges. What if there is a parasitic infection in the fish, but adding the treatment to the water will cause mortality in sharks? Is it possible to empty hundreds of thousands of gallons to treat the habitat for parasites? How does one catch the one compromised fish in the school of hundreds? Certain species are more aggressive than others. How is the monitoring of every animal in an exhibit eating appropriately accomplished? Different species even in similar habitats can require different water quality parameters. Animal care staff need to know the species' demeanor (aggressive, docile), how they interact with others (will there be aggression?), if treatment is required for one animal, can all species handle it, what types of diet need to be fed (broadcast or target feed), and how can one be captured or handled if it needs an exam? Veterinary clinics have an owner bring in their pet either on a leash or in a kennel, but at an aquarium veterinary staff are more than likely going to have to go to the patient. There could be logistical complications involved depending upon the species and planning will be required.

Medication considerations regarding large habitats must be made. For instance, if several species of fish are affected by a parasite, should the whole habitat be treated, or should the fish most affected be separated and treated individually? Will the treatment be effective since these habitats are extremely difficult and logistically challenging to empty and disinfect? These types of considerations are discussed by the veterinary staff, husbandry staff, and building operations staff to create a feasible treatment plan. Treating a large exhibit may be very cost-prohibitive due to the amount of medication that would need to be added

to reach and maintain treatment levels. Some medications used in aquarium medicine such as chloroquine phosphate, have adverse effects on sharks and invertebrates and these animals would need to be removed and placed in appropriate reserve housing.

Husbandry staff are sometimes required to dive to separate animals that require medical intervention. That increases staff requirements and makes scheduling harder, as multiple people are usually needed to catch a specific animal, and a dive tender is required to monitor the safety of the divers in the exhibit. An additional consideration is that diving or netting an animal to catch it will cause stress not only in the targeted animal but in the entire habitat. If the animal is unable to be caught in a timely fashion, discontinuing the attempt to catch it may be elected for the welfare of the rest of the animals in that habitat. If managing a specific animal in a multispecies habitat, monitoring of this animal needs to be considered. Can the patient be reliably monitored, or will husbandry or veterinary staff be unable to locate and acquire the patient on a routine basis? If there are multiple rechecks or treatments required is there an appropriate reserve space to house the animal while it undergoes treatment? Sometimes, animals will not eat when they are not on exhibit, and that is a consideration that needs to be made as well.

Nutrition and oral medications can be difficult in these types of habitats. Most large, multispecies habitats are broadcast-fed. This means that an amount of food is determined by the population of the enclosure as a whole and fed out by being added to the habitat in a variety of locations. Difficulties in broadcast feeding include obtaining appropriate nutrition. There is no way to stop a food-motivated fish from eating as much as it wants and becoming overconditioned. There is also no way to aid a fish that is shyer in temperament from not getting an adequate amount or appropriate food items from becoming under conditioned. Monitoring appetite is difficult as staff will not always be able to see what animal is eating what food items and how often. If oral medications are required, there would not be a way to make sure that the current animal obtains the medications, and that other animals do not get accidentally medicated. On the other hand, target feeding is when animals are trained to feed at a target. A target can be a specific shape or colored object. When that object is placed in the water, the animal or animals will know that it is time to feed. With this method, individual diets can be monitored. Adjustments can be made to increase or decrease body condition appropriately and medication can be given orally. Target feeding requires a larger amount of time and is not always feasible. Animals can also be fed individually by divers. For some animals it is not in their natural behaviors to eat at the surface, so divers will take food to them. This method is time-consuming and more staff-intensive but it makes it easy to monitor food intake and medicate orally.

Sometimes these habitats will have a medical pool attached to the main habitat, or adjacent to the main habitat. This acts as a reserve space if any animal needs medical intervention, but it would not be ideal to have to dive to catch this animal for procedures and treatments. The medical pools will either be shallow, so procedures can be done in the pool itself, or some of them have a floor that can be raised and lowered to control the height of the water.

Marine Mammal Medicine

Marine mammal medicine is an important aspect of aquarium medicine. Marine mammals consist of cetaceans (whales and dolphins), pinnipeds (seals, sea lions, and walruses), sirenians (manatees and dukongs), and marine fissipeds (polar bears and sea otters). Marine mammals have the characteristics of mammals but live the majority if not all their lives in the water. Not all aquariums have marine mammals in their collection.

The husbandry staff that care for marine mammals are commonly titled trainers. Like the husbandry staff that work with non-mammals, they monitor the health and well-being of their animals every day. They are typically the first to alert veterinary staff of a medical concern. Working with marine mammals can be a high-stress environment. Everything around them must be gold standard. Technicians will also work with many different trainers and encounter a plethora of different personalities. The trainers and veterinary staff work together to train the animals in husbandry behaviors. Husbandry behaviors are trained behaviors that facilitate parts of a medical exam. For example, marine mammals can be trained to go into lateral recumbency and maintain that position to allow veterinary staff to perform an ultrasound. This allows a non-stressful and positive way for the animal to interact during its own medical care, as well as allows for frequent routine assessments of these animals. Other husbandry behaviors that are commonly trained are phlebotomy, radiographs, oral exams, ophthalmic exams, intramuscular or subcutaneous injections, and tactile exams (Figure 29.6) These trained behaviors are critical to their welfare. Not only does this allow for frequent monitoring with low handling and low stress, but it is also safer for the animal and the staff. If an animal does not willingly participate and diagnostics or treatment are required, manpower is used to obtain these animals from their habitat and restrain them. This poses an increased risk of injury for the animal

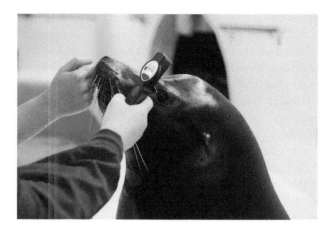

Figure 29.6 A California sea lion displaying voluntary husbandry behavior to allow veterinary staff to obtain intraocular pressures during an ophthalmic examination. (Courtesy of Shedd Aquarium/Brenna Hernandez.)

as well as the staff. This also requires many staff members and increases stress on the animal.

Preventative medicine is critical in all aquarium animals, but due to the high-profile nature of marine mammals, it is even more critical. Routine exams can include ultrasound, venipuncture, radiographs, and gastroscopy. Laboratory samples can be obtained and monitored including fecal monitoring and urine monitoring. Reproductive cycles and pregnancies are monitored regularly. Fissipeds are routinely sedated or anesthetized annually to complete their exams. Anesthesia, while not typically used for pinnipeds, cetaceans, and sirenians, can be administered if required.

Marine mammals have unique anatomy that veterinary technicians are required to be educated on while working with them. For example, during anesthesia on diving animals such as sea otters, end tidal carbon dioxide is routinely above 40 mmHg. This is normal for them while sedated and does not pose a concern. Beluga whales have very thick blubber that may require a spinal needle to give an intramuscular injection. Cetaceans have a unique structure called a goosebeak separating their trachea from esophagus that must be manually moved prior to intubation.

Marine mammals' births are also something the aquarium veterinary technician may be heavily involved in. Technicians are responsible for hospital preparedness and are involved in preparing, assisting, and monitoring any procedure that may take place. This could entail making sure everything is stocked, including formula supplies and all medications needed. Additionally, making sure that all equipment needed is staged in the marine mammal space, is functional, serviced, and all veterinary staff are comfortable operating it. Technicians can be on call for marine mammal births and stay extended hours if they require medical intervention or feedings.

Marine mammals are very high profile. Their welfare and health are paramount. Marine mammals in captivity are regulated by the USDA and institutions can be inspected to see if they are meeting the required standards. There are usually a large number of staff dedicated solely to working with marine mammals and monitoring their welfare daily.

Marine mammals and their welfare in captivity is a debated subject. Many people are against having marine mammals in captive environments because they are cognitively, emotionally, and socially complex animals. Protests of marine mammal captivity in aquariums do happen. Additionally, legislation can be passed altering what is allowed. Canada has passed legislation ending the public display of captive cetaceans. Conversely, marine mammals in captivity can inspire the public. This can motivate future generations into conservation efforts, and encourage people to make conservation changes in their daily lives, and when more guests enter the building, more financial capital is created for research and conservation efforts that can make a difference to these species in the wild. Additionally, research on wild marine mammals has its difficulties. By studying their captive counterparts, aquariums can use and share that knowledge to positively impact wild populations. It is imperative that a veterinary technician considers their own feelings on this subject matter before planning to work at an institution that houses marine mammals.

Do You Have What it Takes to Become an Aquarium Veterinary Technician?

Becoming an aquarium veterinary technician is a rewarding path. There are several approaches that can be taken. Volunteering is a very common way to get your foot in the door as well as networking. Zoos and aquariums typically take volunteers, and you can also investigate volunteering for wildlife clinics or exotic animal practices. Volunteering shows your interest in the field, helps you gain knowledge, and can put you in touch with mentors or people who can help you get started in this career. It can also help keep you in mind and in contact with the right people when job opportunities come along. You can also intern at zoos, aquariums, wildlife, or exotic animal practices. Most internships are unpaid, but they offer a wealth of knowledge and the ability to gain some of the necessary skills in addition to networking. Think of interning as an extended job interview!

Continuing to educate yourself can also be a good way to enter the field. The Association of Zoo Veterinary Technicians (AZVT) also includes aquariums, and you are not required to be working at an institution to join. Attending their conference will provide excellent networking within the zoo and aquarium community, help educate you on zoo and aquarium medicine, and fulfill your continued education licensing requirements.

Becoming a well-rounded, skilled veterinary technician is also a great way to enter an aquarium setting. Aquariums can have sea lions, whales, dolphins, and many other large animals, and knowing large animal medicine can help in these areas. Triage, urgent care, and emergencies happen, and having a background in emergency animal medicine is something that is looked for on applications. In-house sample evaluation, hematology evaluation, and necropsies are prevalent so having a laboratory background could be very beneficial. Sometimes institutions are willing to train technicians who do not have zoo or aquatic experience. You never know what an institution could be looking for, so it never hurts to apply.

Job Description for an Aquarium Veterinary Technician

A sample job description for a veterinary technician is as follows:

- Routinely assist with all aspects of preventative and emergency exams, anesthesia monitoring, radiology, ultrasonography, endoscopy, surgery, and dental work.
- Basic ability to perform a full range of veterinary technician skills including, but not limited to, phlebotomy, gavage feeding, fluid therapy, restraint, and other supportive care treatments (Figure 29.7).
- Basic ability to operate typical veterinary equipment such as X-ray, autoclave, diagnostic equipment, microscopes, blood chemistry analyzers, gas anesthesia, and laser therapy equipment.
- Ability to perform pharmacy-related skills including medical calculations involving, but not limited to, dilutions and dosages.
- Ability to dispense and administer medications as prescribed by a veterinarian.
- Basic ability to maintain medical packs, perform routine equipment maintenance tasks, and assist in the upkeep of the hospital supply inventories to ensure proper function of the hospital.
- Maintain respirator training to measure laboratory chemicals.
- Demonstrate knowledge of Microsoft Office or equivalent, including spreadsheet and database management.
- Maintain medical records in a medical database in a correct, timely, and orderly fashion.

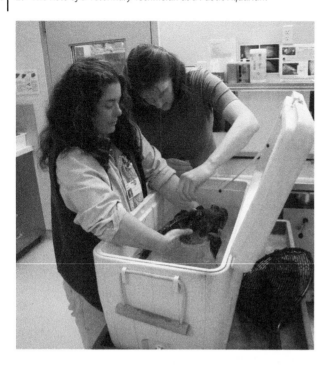

Figure 29.7 A physical exam being performed in the container it was placed in for the examination. (Courtesy of Sandy Skeeba, LVT.)

- Basic knowledge to assist with necropsies including collecting and preparing tissues for histopathologic evaluation.

- Obtain various samples from aquarium animals and prepare them for diagnostic laboratory testing such as skin scrapes/gill clips, fecal analysis, hematology, cytology, parasitology, urinalysis, and microbiology.
- Collaborate with team members in organizing, prioritizing, and delegating various hospital tasks.
- Communicate courteously and effectively with all husbandry staff regarding animal medical-related information and treatments.
- Serve as aquarium-wide support via educational, media, and conservation programs as requested.
- Support aquarium-wide rescue and rehab program and field research as requested.

There are many facets in the field of aquarium medicine and a technician can expect to be challenged on a regular basis. This challenge can be rewarding by having the opportunity to be creative, to problem solve, and to continually grow and learn. Aquarium medicine also offers the ability to work with many unique species. It allows for being part of innovative medicine, conservation, education, and research. Aquarium medicine can be competitive to enter as there are not as many openings as there are in-private practice. Due to this, it commonly requires relocation. Volunteering and interning are common methods to start your career in aquarium medicine or help figure out if aquarium medicine is the right fit.

30

The Role of the Veterinary Technician in Wildlife Rehabilitation
Melanie Haire

Introduction

Wildlife rehabilitation is the process of rescuing, raising, and treating orphaned, diseased, displaced, or injured wild animals with a goal of releasing them back to their natural habitats. For rehabilitation to be deemed successful, these released animals must be able to truly function as wild animals. This includes being able to recognize and obtain the appropriate foods, select mates of their own species and reproduce, and show the appropriate fear of potential dangers (people, cars, dogs, etc.) (Pokras 1995).

The veterinary technician is on the front line for receiving injured and/or orphaned wildlife. A background in veterinary medicine and animal husbandry makes veterinary technicians perfect candidates for this rewarding endeavor. In fact, the general public often assumes that the veterinary technician is knowledgeable about all species. This assumption could be detrimental to the wild animal's welfare if the technician does not have access to the proper instruction, facilities, and materials needed to care for these unique individuals.

This chapter is a compilation of pertinent information that will provide the veterinary technician with the resources and guidelines needed to provide temporary care for many of the wildlife species that are encountered in veterinary hospitals today. The chapter includes charts, instructional articles, networking contacts, product sources, suggested readings, and references taken from numerous literary sources on the topic of rehabilitation of North American wildlife. Interested technicians should note there are many books, seminars, web groups, and related organizational memberships available for anyone interested in quality wildlife care and a list of a suggested few is provided in Appendix 11.

The information in this chapter is primarily to be used as a starting reference point for the wild animal care technician working in a small animal clinic. It provides immediate information that can be used until more detailed information is obtained or the animal is transferred from the veterinary clinic to a licensed rehabilitator for long-term care and release.

Getting Started

For a veterinary technician, the level of involvement in wildlife rehabilitation can range from the care of an occasional orphan discovered by a hospital client to a career on staff at a wildlife center. The technician can rehabilitate wild animals as a full-time occupation, as a volunteer at a wildlife center, on the job at a veterinary clinic, or at home in addition to a separate career. Many zoological parks and aquariums also provide care to injured and orphaned wildlife and have separate facilities and staff designated for such activity.

Although the numbers and types of animals received by different wildlife technicians will vary, legal obligations are relatively consistent. To keep or possess in captivity any sick, orphaned, or injured wildlife, one must first obtain a wildlife rehabilitation permit from the state and/or federal government. Everyone, including the veterinarian, must have his or her own permit or be listed on someone else's permit to rehabilitate wildlife. Each state has its own laws and requirements but most require a permit to work with any indigenous species. A federal permit is required in addition to a state permit to work with migratory birds. A list of governmental departments that issue applications and permits is provided in Appendix 1 at the back of this book. The permitee is responsible for knowing what

Exotic Animal Medicine for the Veterinary Technician, Fourth Edition. Edited by Bonnie Ballard and Ryan Cheek.
© 2024 John Wiley & Sons, Inc. Published 2024 by John Wiley & Sons, Inc.
Companion Website: www.wiley.com/go/ballard/4e

species are covered on the permit and their individual regulations. The rehabilitator is responsible for keeping records on each animal and knowing its current listed status (nonthreatened versus endangered).

It is very important for anyone doing rehabilitation to build a reference library. The collection should contain literature on three basic topics: natural history, wildlife rehabilitation, and veterinary medicine as rehabilitation, which is a combination of all three. The veterinary technician should always keep in mind, when reading articles and talking to other rehabilitators, that there is more than one way to do things. New information is always coming out and it is the veterinary technician's responsibility to keep current as well as to learn to recognize what techniques might work better in different situations. Common sense and experience are the best ways to sort out contradictory suggestions and inaccurate information.

Networking with other rehabilitators is one of the most important sources of information. A list can be obtained from your state's special permits department with the names and contact numbers of all the rehabilitators in your state. These contacts can prove helpful for answering questions as they arise, helping to place animals that are not covered by your permit, placing animals when the clinic has reached full capacity, and building a network team to help with long-term animal care and releases.

Rehabilitating Wildlife in a Small Animal Veterinary Hospital

If the staff at a veterinary practice is interested in wildlife rehabilitation, it needs to establish a set of protocols. To accomplish this, the staff needs to first understand all that is involved. Rehabilitation can be both expensive and time-consuming. Profit-making is not a valid or realistic reason to do rehabilitation. Currently, there is no monetary assistance provided by any governmental departments to cover or reimburse rehabilitators for the costs of wildlife care.

Another crucial and difficult point that needs to be understood and accepted is that half of the animals that come in for rehabilitation will die or need to be euthanized. This is often extremely taxing emotionally on veterinary personnel, people who chose their profession in order to save lives. Deciding to euthanize an animal that could otherwise be saved but not returned to the wild with a good quality of life (such as releasing a one-legged hawk) may just be too hard for some individuals. Euthanasia is never an easy choice but keeping a wild animal alive because one "cannot handle" putting it to sleep is selfish and inhumane. Occasionally, nonreleasable wildlife can be

placed in appropriate educational facilities but quality of life should always be the highest priority.

Another issue concerns zoonotic diseases and learning to recognize them. Injured wildlife may expose hospital staff and animals to new risks. Proper personal hygiene as well as facility disinfecting techniques and protocols are critically important. Separate housing areas and separate clothing available for these areas provide safeguards against infectious or zoonotic cases. One method is to always treat the sick animals last so as not to transmit diseases to any other patient.

Hospital staff that have any contact with the wildlife should consider having the appropriate prophylactic vaccinations, such as tetanus and rabies, to protect them. Consultation with a personal physician is recommended.

Despite these cautions, there are many reasons to consider this volunteer work. It generates good clinic PR, provides a valuable service to the community and the clinic's clientele, is a kind act of giving something back to nature, and offers a personal reward for giving a living creature a second chance that it otherwise may not have had. Veterinarians benefit by gaining skill at performing new procedures (i.e., IM pin in an owl) by first learning on wildlife patients. Veterinary technicians can gain valuable experience in exotic animal handling from wildlife work such as restraint, anesthesia, blood collecting, bandaging, radiology, and necropsy.

Clinic Protocols

Selecting Types of Wildlife to Care For

If the decision to do rehabilitation is made, clinic procedures and protocols must be clear and written down. Among the decisions to make are what types and how many animals the practice can reasonably take in. Taking in more animals or more species than personnel are prepared to properly and safely handle can easily overwhelm a clinic. One way to set limits is to specialize in a particular species or area (i.e., take in only birds of prey or injured wildlife, no orphans, etc.) and refer the other calls to another qualified recipient.

Above all, the motto "Do No Harm" should always be remembered when working with animal patients and wildlife is no exception. Wildlife rehabilitation should not be attempted at a clinic without sufficient staff to do the feedings, treatments, cage cleanings, and so forth, as the animals will be the ones that suffer. The ability to realize one's limits shows professionalism. Hospital managers and owners need to make a clear decision about animal limits based on costs and expenses. Staffing and other business costs are very real factors that should be discussed ahead of time to help avoid staff "burnout" or resentment.

Stabilization or Long-term Rehabilitation—An Important Decision

Temporary stabilization verses long-term care should be determined by examining the layout of the buildings and grounds, available facilities, and the number and experience of participating staff. Barking dogs, staring cats, ringing phones, and exposure to people are unacceptable conditions for long-term rehabilitation. A treatment room might be a marginally acceptable area to keep an orphaned 2-week-old squirrel (both eyes and ears are closed at 2 weeks) but not a high-stress, imprintable, or easily habituated animal such as a deer fawn or raptor. Very few veterinary hospitals have flight cages of appropriate sizes and materials to adequately recondition a red-tailed hawk for release. Wildlife must be respected as wild and provided with suitable housing to reduce additional stress and fear and to promote natural behaviors that are necessary for successful release.

If there is no dedicated space for them, the clinic should provide temporary care only until the animal is stable and can be safely transferred to another rehabilitator. Veterinary hospitals without adequate facilities for rehabilitation can still perform a vital function for wildlife by becoming a drop-off and/or referral site for the public. This arrangement can benefit both the animal, by providing it proper temporary care away from the well-intentioned, but often detrimental, handling of the rescuer, and the rehabilitator by providing a valuable time-saver of a one-stop "pick-up" location.

Oftentimes the single most crucial role for the technician in a veterinary practice is simply to give the public accurate names and phone numbers of the appropriate rehabilitator. Putting the public in direct communication with the rehabilitation facility that will provide long-term care can eliminate the sometimes-fatal animal stress and delay of using the hospital as a drop-off site. This system allows the rehabilitator to be the clearing point and to have the opportunity to advise the finder how to return the animal if care is not truly needed or to have the caller transport the needy animal directly to the appropriate care provider. If the caller is willing to bring the animal to the clinic, chances are the caller will be willing to transport the animal directly to the rehabilitator. This method promotes the best use of time for both the veterinary staff and rehabilitators, thus allowing the medical personnel to best utilize their valuable expertise by caring mainly for the injured wild patients who must receive immediate medical attention.

Whether a hospital chooses to be a drop-off site, a referral center, or both, a current list of participating rehabilitators' names, locations, phone numbers, and species covered under each permit is a prerequisite. A prearranged plan for informing rehabilitators when a pickup or transport needs to be scheduled is a must to prevent unnecessary and often detrimental time delays before an animal can receive adequate care.

On the other hand, if the practice can provide adequate staff time and housing for the wildlife patients, then the hospital can consider becoming more involved in longer-term care such as surgery, wound care, emaciation, and hand rearing.

Choose your hospital's role wisely putting the animal's best interest foremost in the decision-making process.

Euthanasia

Before receiving animals, the hospital must have a clear euthanasia policy. Who will make the decision and do the actual procedure, what techniques will be used, and what criteria are used should be included in these protocols? There is a section on non-releasable criteria and euthanasia later in this chapter to help with this difficult topic.

Phone Protocols

So often overlooked, one of the most important areas in which the wildlife veterinary clinic personnel must be trained is the telephone procedure. Posting a clear protocol for handling wildlife calls near every phone will help ensure that the information received is accurate and consistent. The development of a wildlife phone call protocol should be a combined effort between the veterinary staff and the participating wildlife rehabilitators. Many animals come into rehabilitation that never should have been removed from the spot in which they were found. Educating the public is part of the responsibility of anyone participating in wildlife rehabilitation. Taking proper animal history information before the animal is even touched will drastically reduce the number of "orphans" that are kidnapped and end up needing to be hand-raised, thus reducing wasted time, money, and energy.

The caller should be asked if the animal appears to be orphaned or injured. What brought the finder to this conclusion? Many times it turns out that a little education in animal natural behavior can turn a "needy" or "nuisance" animal call into a lesson in living with wildlife. If the animal does appear to need assistance and the caller cannot handle it, advise the person to bring it in. One should never instruct or allow the caller to take care of the foundling himself or herself. If the caller cannot bring the animal into the clinic, the caller should be provided with phone numbers from the contact list for a rehabilitator, rescue volunteer, or a wildlife center in the caller's area.

Handling Phone Calls

In most instances, if an adult wild animal can be caught and picked up by a person, it has sustained some type of injury, shock, or is sick and is in need of some type of rehabilitation.

Conditions that require immediate medical attention include:

- Unconsciousness
- Bleeding
- Cold body temperature
- Open fracture
- Weakness, inability to stand (emaciated)
- Head swelling
- Head/eye twitching
- Eyes closed or matted shut
- Shock
- Puncture wounds from cat/dog bite
- Broken bones
- Flies, fly larva, or eggs present

If the animal found is an infant, have the caller describe the baby and its condition. It should be determined if the animal is truly an orphan. If warm, strong, and apparently healthy, the baby is probably not an orphan and every attempt should be made to return it to its mother or nest. If the baby is cold, weak, and emaciated, or if there are dead siblings nearby, the animal is probably orphaned. Mother animals do not abandon their young because humans have touched them.

Baby Songbirds

If the bird is naked or has a few body feathers but no tail feathers, the baby should be put back in the nest if at all possible. If the nest cannot be reached, instruct the caller to hang a homemade nest made from a basket or container near the old nest. The "surrogate" nest should be placed up off of the ground and protected from direct sunlight and rain. If the mother does not return by dark, advise the caller to bring the baby into the clinic. If the bird has body feathers with one inch or longer tail feathers, is hopping around and chirping, it is probably a fledgling. These youngsters have left the nest but the parents are still providing them with food. Instruct the caller to look around for a parent bird. If the baby is picked up and it vocalizes and attracts an adult bird's attention, leave it alone. If there are no parent birds in sight, the bird should be left and checked on several hours later. It may take 3–4 days for a "grounded" fledgling to learn to fly but a healthy one should be active, very mobile, and left where it was found.

Baby Raptors

If the nestling has eyes closed or has no feathers, return it to the nest if at all possible or make a surrogate nest. If the juvenile is hopping around or perching, has wing feathers and a short tail, it should be left alone. "Branchers" are young raptors that have left the nest but cannot yet fly. Both parents are still providing care to these birds on the ground or in low trees and shrubs. The only time to bring in a nestling raptor is if the caller cannot return it to its nest or secure a surrogate nest to the nesting tree. Refer the caller to a raptor rehabilitator for further instructions on how to replace a baby in its nest or make a surrogate one.

Baby Squirrels

Young squirrels are independent when they are about half the size of the adult and have bushy tails. If the baby does not yet have a fluffy tail, is crying or is cold, it might be orphaned. Mother squirrels often move their babies from nest to nest so a baby found at the base of a tree is not automatically an orphan. Even if there is no adult squirrel visible but the caller can stay nearby and watch for the mother, leave the baby unmoved. If the caller cannot watch, advise the caller to tie a small basket or box up off of the ground, with the baby inside, onto the possible nest tree out of reach of ground predators. The caller or someone must check the nest before dark and make sure that the infant has been reclaimed. If it is still in the box by dark, have the caller bring it in. Infant squirrels make a very high-pitched squeal or "chirp" when they are frightened, hungry, or cold and the mother can hear it from quite a distance.

Baby Rabbits

Baby cottontail rabbits should be left alone if uninjured and found in the nest. Even if the nest has been disturbed, the mother will usually come back. The deciding factor seems to be the extent of the nest disturbance. If the nest has sustained minimal disturbance of the nesting material, the babies should be covered back up and left alone. If the nest site has been destroyed or dug up by a predator, the mother may not come back. An attempt can be made to put the nest back together and a string placed on top of the nest. If, by morning, the string has been disturbed and the babies are warm and plump, the mother has come back to feed them. However, if the string is undisturbed over night or the babies are cold or look thin, the babies should be brought in. If the location of the nest is unknown and the baby's eyes are closed, it should be brought in. But if the young rabbit's eyes are open and its ears are upright and capable of rotating, they should be left undisturbed. Mother rabbits will not pick up and carry a baby back to the nest. Infants only feed at dusk and dawn and the mother will leave the nest in between feedings but stay nearby. Due to rabbits' secretive nature and infrequent visits to their nests, one should not automatically assume the babies are orphaned.

Baby Opossums

If an infant opossum is found that is less than 6 inches long and alone advise the caller to bring it in. Baby opossums that are old enough to leave the mother's pouch should cling to the mother's coat or follow along behind her. If they fall off or cannot keep up, they are sometimes left behind.

Baby Deer

Fawns should be left alone unless injured. The doe often leaves the fawn alone for hours at a time while she feeds.

Baby Raccoons

Baby raccoons are usually on their own by the time they are 4–5 months old and weigh 8–12 pounds. If a younger raccoon is discovered alone, the caller should leave the youngster where it was found and check on it periodically. Although nocturnal, the mother raccoon will look for her missing infant during the daytime as well as during the nighttime. If 24 hours passes with no sign of the mother, the licensed rabies vector rehabilitator should be called for instructions. One should be careful in advising the public to handle any rabies vector species.

Reuniting diurnal species' (active during the day) babies during the day light hours and nocturnal species' (active at night) babies during the night should be practiced. If the infant gets cold while waiting for the parent, a warm water bottle should be provided and placed with the baby. It may take several hours for a mother to reclaim her baby. If a diurnal species is found at night, it may be worth a try in the morning to reunite it with its parent.

Orphans that are brought in to the hospital will probably need to be taken home at night by a caretaker and brought back in the morning in order to provide the young animals with enough nourishment.

If the caller wants to try to take care of the animal themselves, explain to them why that is not in the animal's best interest. Some points to be made to argue this point include:

1. The problems of imprinting—the rehabilitators probably have more infants of the same species that they can put with the caller's animal and raise together as siblings.
2. The possibility of zoonotic or infectious diseases.
3. It is illegal for them to care for the animal without a permit.

4. Using the wrong formula or feeding technique can cause harm to or even the death of the animal.
5. Hand raising is very time-consuming—they should be given an idea of how often the animal needs to eat and how long the care time may be.
6. Acquiring and preparing the proper foods may be difficult, expensive, and not always pleasant (mealworms, grubs, killing mice, etc.).

If the caller has a raccoon, fox, bear, bobcat, owl, hawk, or any rabies vector species, or potentially dangerous animal, the name and phone number should be taken immediately in case he or she decides to keep it and not bring it in. This information should then be turned over to the appropriate authorities (county game protector, federal wildlife agent, etc.).

Intake Procedures

Under no circumstances should animals be handled or looked at in between the necessary feedings and treatments intervals. This rule needs to begin in the reception room with the arrival of the animal. Without lifting the lid or opening the transport cage, the receptionist should immediately transport the animal to the examination area while the rescuer fills out an intake form. This form should include the rescuer's name, address, phone number, animal type, and numbers, and finally the animal's circumstances for needing care. A detailed account of how, when, and where the animal was found can help determine the nature of the animal's problem. Also, information should be recorded as to how long the rescuer had the animal and if he or she attempted to medicate or feed the patient. This information helps the caretaker to investigate what happened to the animal and what the correct form of treatment should be. This form should be used as one would a pet's chart and record the physical exam findings, treatments, observations, and final disposition. The state and/or federal permit-issuing departments also require this information. A copy should be made and turned in to the rehabilitator who receives the animal to provide the new caretaker with all the available information. The original copy should be filed at the facility and used to help make the end-of-year report required by most states (see Appendix 2).

Meanwhile, back in the treatment room, the animal should have a quick visual exam to check for emergency conditions such as shock, hypothermia, or bleeding. If the animal appears stable and is not in a critical position, the animal should be allowed a little time to calm down from the previous handling and car ride before pulling it out of the box.

Ethical Considerations and Reducing Stress in Captive Wildlife

> "It is incumbent upon a person who takes the responsibility of manipulating an animal's life to be concerned for its feelings, the infliction of pain, and the psychological upsets that may occur from such manipulation."
>
> (Fowler 1986).

The wild nature of these animals should always be respected and one should be sensitive to the unique needs of these unusual patients. The number-one reason wild animals under human care die is from stress. All sick or injured animals need their strength to recover and cannot afford to use it up in attempts to escape from captive stress. Learning to recognize signs of early stress, with each species as well as between individuals, may possibly prevent or at least reduce such fatalities. Many birds have a natural escape pattern of moving up and away from danger and they feel threatened if they are housed down low and looked at from above. Typically, they are calmer if their cage is placed level with or above human eye level.

All prey animals fear direct eye contact or being stared or even looked at. One should consider the animal's viewpoint as typically the first thing a predator does while hunting is to keep its eye on the prey and then move directly toward it. When humans do this, it mimics the predator's behavior and frightens the animal. When walking past wildlife cages, it is a good idea to look in another direction.

Housing for different species is discussed further in each of their sections but a note on stress-reducing environmental factors should be mentioned here. Within each animal's enclosure, using something natural and familiar to the patient will help decrease stress. Housing away from sight or sound of predators (humans, domestic animals, wild predators—i.e., avoid housing hawks and cottontails in the same room) is of foremost importance. Second, providing something of a natural setting is calming to many species of captive wildlife. Many bird species need to feel hidden or protected from view by vegetated plant cover. By cutting a few small leafed branches off of a nearby tree or shrub and placing them inside the animal's enclosure (preferably before placing the animal inside), one can provide naturalistic hiding places for the recovering patient. Animals such as rabbits, squirrels, opossums, and chipmunks seek refuge by hiding under or inside something that cannot be seen through. Providing these types of patients with a nest box, hollow log, plastic tube, or even layers of cloth that they can burrow in will increase their sense of security and well-being as well as the chance of keeping them alive. Animals also equate having choices with comfort. Offering a bird several perches provides them with the opportunity to feel as if they have some control in their strange new captive world.

Initial Exam

The visual exam is the first part and perhaps one of the most important parts of the examination. Before even touching the patient, observe their posture, color, behavior, and stool quality. Look for discharges, level of alertness, body conditioning, head tilts, nystagmus, limping, or wing droops. Record all observations either on the intake sheet or on the examination form, whichever one the hospital's wildlife protocol calls for. There is an example of each form provided in Appendix 2. Many of these signs are not as obvious once the animal has been picked up and is held in an unnatural position. Also, an animal will try its best to conceal these "signs of weakness" to a predator if it knows it is being watched, so try to be sly about the visual exam. Sometimes using binoculars and watching from across the room gets the best results.

When performing the hands-on part of the examination, the examiner should be swift and thorough, reducing the handling time and the animal's psychological stress. Restraint should be performed on the animal quickly and with confidence, without a lot of repositioning. Prey animals view a predator's grip as fatal and frequent shifting of the animal's position only draws out the suffering.

Use of a systematic approach when doing exams insures that no area gets overlooked. Even though it may be obvious that the patient has a wing injury the exam should be performed in a systematic manner and all the animal's systems evaluated in order. The animal's eyes, ears, mouth, nose, skin turgor, limbs, body condition, and reflexes should be checked. Respiratory sounds should be observed and noted as well as any signs of bleeding. All anticipated supplies and medications must be ready before handling the animal so the patient does not have to wait unnecessarily. It is not uncommon to find secondary problems days later because they were initially overlooked due to the examiner's mistake of starting right at the big problem and then forgetting to follow through with the rest of the exam.

Restraining and examination techniques should be practiced as often as possible as this is the only way to become fast and efficient. Examine healthy live animals whenever possible to become familiar with "normals" in order to recognize the "abnormals." Information obtained from examining dead animals should not be underestimated. One can practice restraint positions, palpation, injection training, IO or IV catheter placement, bandaging, tube feeding, necropsy, and even surgical techniques on deceased patients.

Choosing Treatment Routes

When choosing appropriate treatment regimens, one should take into consideration the differences between the wild animal patient versus the domestic animals that are more routinely worked with. Domesticated animals can withstand more extensive procedures done with manual restraint alone. On the other hand, the use of anesthesia (i.e., isoflurane) should be considered when obtaining quality radiographs or performing even minor but painful procedures on wildlife.

Routes and frequencies of medication need to be carefully compared as well. Oral medications should be chosen, when appropriate, that can be injected into food items and fed to the patient. For example, enrofloxacin can be injected into a cricket and fed to a blue jay, or into a minnow and be fed to a heron. Every effort should be made to weigh the stress of handling and administering treatments against the benefits they provide. Although the first treatment of choice may recommend BID-TID treatments, realize that with wildlife this may not always be practical or possible. Wildlife medicine is a balance between what is effective and what the patient can tolerate. This sometimes calls for some creative medicine delivery ideas. Raptors can receive treatments of dexamethasone, LRS, vitamins, or antibiotics injected into a small or pinkie mouse that the bird can swallow whole at its normal eating time. Some pediatric suspensions have a more palatable taste and may be more readily eaten either right out of the medicine dropper or when mixed in with a favorite food item (i.e., Clavamox drops mixed in with fruit yogurt offered to an opossum). Another option is to have, frequently used, oral medications specially flavored or concentrated at a compounding pharmacy. Banana-flavored dewormers, meat-flavored antibiotics, alfalfa flavored anti-inflammatories just to name a few, have been very useful in both zoological and wildlife medicine.

Animals that do not swallow their food whole or eat food items in which medications are not easily hidden (i.e., adult squirrels, rabbits) may need to be hand injected. In these cases, effective medications with the longest action time to reduce multiple daily "catch-ups" should be chosen. Ideally, medications that need to be given only once daily should be sought.

In conclusion, it is not the role of veterinarians to know the best way to rehabilitate every wild animal. Their expertise is in anatomy, surgery, diagnostics, and treatment, not necessarily the natural history and behavior patterns of a southern flying squirrel. To assist the veterinarian in making more informed decisions, the technician should collect as much information as possible pertaining to the types of wildlife that the clinic decides to work with. Teamwork is crucial and the combined efforts of many individuals make up the best rehabilitation team. Each wildlife technician needs to form good working relationships with several veterinarians. One veterinarian cannot be expected to look at every baby squirrel but can advise on general treatment regimes and drug dosages.

A technician should always realize his or her limitations and should never feel as if networking makes one look incapable. Utilizing the experience of others is the best way to learn and can also prevent animals from suffering unnecessarily. No one should ever reinvent the wheel at the animal's expense. Always remember that the ultimate goal is to release the animal back into the wild with the best possible chance of survival. A technician can offer this to each and every animal that he/she works with if he/she learns to recognize when someone else may be more qualified. This may even mean transferring the animal to another person who may have a better rehabilitation setup, more experience or time, animal conspecifics, or better release sites.

While wildlife rehabilitation can be difficult, time-consuming, expensive, and many times downright frustrating, the benefits and personal rewards gained from this unselfish kind deed can be life-changing.

Release Criteria Versus Euthanasia

Some animals arrive at the clinic with injuries that warrant euthanasia. Other injuries and illnesses may not present themselves as life threatening but in fact are just as profound in terms of release and survivability in the wild. The veterinary technician should learn to recognize these less-obvious conditions that will ultimately lead to death of the animal if released back into the wild.

Merely saving a life for survival in captivity is not the goal. The animal must be capable of recognizing, obtaining, and processing food; recognizing and evading or defending against predators; acquiring shelter; acquiring and defending territories; performing normal seasonal movements and dispersal; and be capable of normal socialization with conspecifics (Diehl & Stokhaug 1991). Each type of animal, depending on its natural history and what it needs to do to survive, has different criteria, so a handicap considered relatively minor for one species may be life-threatening to another. For instance, a bird of prey must be capable of hunting and catching prey animals that may be as quick and fast as they themselves are. If a Cooper's hawk was released with any degree of flight defect, it would not be able to obtain prey that is often caught in midair. On the other hand, a mallard duck with a slight wing defect but flight capability, may be considered for release because it acquires its food while swimming and dabbling in the water, breeds in the water, and can also escape predators by diving as well as flying. Also, in some areas, mallards do not have to migrate so the need to fly great distances would also be reduced. Another example would be of an animal with impaired vision. An animal that does not depend on excellent sight to obtain food and avoid predation could also be considered releasable. For instance, a one-eyed, adult opossum might be considered releasable because in the wild it has few predators and relies on its sense of smell to find food items (carrion, insects, and vegetation) that do not require a great deal of visual acuity to acquire. However, a fox needs perfect vision to obtain its mainstay diet of live and very quick prey animals such as mice, chipmunks, birds, and rabbits.

The species of the animal involved should also be considered. An opossum with a fractured limb has a good chance for recovery. Opossums tend to tolerate bandages and splints well plus they are relatively inactive, which provides for optimal recovery. A deer with a fractured limb, on the other hand is a challenge. Many hospitals or centers do not have the facilities to deal with an injured deer. At best, these animals, even with adequate facilities, are difficult to maintain in captivity and they tend to further injure themselves trying to escape.

The potential for current handicaps to create new problems for an animal must be considered. For example, is a one-footed bird likely to develop bumblefoot or frostbite on the remaining foot? The bottom line is that the animal must have enough of the equipment and capabilities necessary to survive by means natural to its species if it is to be released (Diehl & Stokhaug 1991).

Being a careful observer, understanding the animal's natural history, performing a thorough physical exam, and being knowledgeable of the release requirements could spare an animal hours or days of suffering. Each animal deserves a careful and unbiased evaluation. If the releasability is in question, contact a rehabilitator immediately so a speedy decision can be made and the animal can begin to receive the treatment it deserves whether it turns out to be freedom by release or euthanasia.

Situations that may require euthanasia include:

- Compound or open fracture more than 48 hours old. These old injuries rarely can be properly repaired and the animal would lose full function of the limb making the animal nonreleasable.
- Complete loss of sight or hearing in any animal.

- Impaired vision in both eyes. Depending on the species, some animals can be considered for release if only one eye is affected.
- Nocturnal owls with hearing impairment.
- Amputated wings or legs: "Any birds that have sustained injuries requiring amputation of a wing at the elbow (humero-ulnar) or above, a leg or a foot…should be euthanized" (U.S. Fish & Wildlife—Rehabilitation regulation 50 CFR 21.27 #8). No animal should be put through the stress and pain of surgery only to be euthanized later because it can never be released.
- Raptors need unimpaired function of their feet to grasp, kill, and carry prey; therefore, any injury involving the unilateral loss of both the hallux (digit 1) and digit 2 on the same foot or the bilateral loss of both hallux.
- Fractures involving the wing or leg joints (or very near the joint) will never heal sufficiently enough for the animal to have normal use of the limb. The joint will heal by fusing in place and not allow for normal movement thus preventing the animal from flying or walking.
- Fractures with a significant piece of bone missing.
- Some wing fractures can heal out of alignment and result in a wing droop. Although flight may be possible, the wing cannot be allowed to drag on the perch/ground. The feather tips will become damaged and soiled and over time the bird may become non-flighted or develop an infection in the damaged follicles.
- Head trauma that results in abnormal posture in any animal.
- Back injuries that have resulted in loss of limb function in any animal.
- Animals imprinted on humans should never be released. These animals are not able to behaviorally fit into their own natural population and they could be dangerous to the public.
- Animals that have a highly incurable infectious disease.
- A rabies vector species from a rabies-endemic area (follow current state guidelines) should never be released.
- Mammals with two or more nonfunctional legs.
- Rodents or rabbits with a fractured jaw or any facial injury leaving permanently unaligned incisors. (Opposing incisor teeth must be able to be normally worn down or they will overgrow and eventually kill the animal.)

Nonreleasable animals can sometimes be placed in an approved educational, research program, or breeding facility. There are now several nonreleasable animal placement programs designed to help place these animals. Do not euthanize an endangered species without first contacting your local and federal authorities for authorization.

"We look to wildlife for the rules that we follow. Wildlife leads a life of quality, or it is not alive—it is one or the other for wildlife" (Moore & Joosten 1995).

Imprinting and Taming

Imprinting

The veterinary technician's code of ethics to "do no harm" could not be more pertinent to this subject. Understanding the definitions and what these two things mean to a wild animal under a technician's care can make the difference between life and death.

Imprinting is a socialization process by which an individual animal learns to identify itself with a species. This is a natural psychological process, which occurs early in life, during a restricted period of time called a critical period. Once this has occurred, the animal now identifies with the adult of its own species and learns by imitation and observation the methods for acquiring shelter, food, mates, and proper behaviors.

The route in which a mammal, bird, or reptile imprints is different and still not completely understood. In the area of wildlife rehabilitation, imprinting is probably only relevant to birds. The critical periods for most species of birds have not yet been determined. With ducks and geese, it occurs within the day of hatching and with smaller raptor species between day 8 and 21 after hatching. Larger raptor species usually imprint between day 12 and 28. The variations of days between species are largely due to their different rates of development. The most important period seems to be when the bird's visual focus develops. Before their eyes open, neonates also imprint on their parents' calls and vocalizations.

What this all means for the wildlife caregiver is that the animal could be improperly imprinted on humans if a great deal of care is not taken. Imprinting is not believed to be reversible so if the process is transferred to a person the animal will have a poor chance to survive. Birds that do not imprint on their own species will lack the survival skills they need, will not reproduce in the wild, and are often killed outright by their own species. A bird that has imprinted on a human is not releasable and will probably need to be euthanized.

To reduce the chances of improper imprinting, the baby should be returned to its nest and/or parents if at all possible. Sometimes orphans can be placed in foster nests and raised with like species of similar age. Many rehabilitation centers have nonreleasable surrogate parents (most commonly birds of prey) that raise same species' orphans that are not their own. If that is not possible, care should be taken to be sure all animals are raised with at least one other member of the same-aged species. Rehabilitators and nature centers that have permanent nonreleasable raptors can also house the young beside the adults to allow the juveniles a chance to observe, listen, interact, and possibly imitate the same species of adult. With some birds, a mirror may be helpful if the baby has no nest mates.

Birds (especially raptors) should be fed during their critical period, from behind a curtain-type blind or while wearing a hooded poncho with a mask to hide the human shape. By also using a hand puppet shaped like the head of the adult to feed raptor chicks, the young do not associate food with humans. Wildlife should be handled as little as possible, with limited talking, and housed out of sight or sound of humans, dogs, cats, and pet birds.

Taming

Taming is the process of an animal becoming socialized to humans by association with foods or other comforts over a prolonged period of time (Beaver 1984). Baby animals in a wide range of species are especially easy to tame. These tame animals have properly imprinted and identify with their own species but socialize with humans. Taming differs from imprinting in that the bond to humans is not as strong, takes longer to establish, and is more readily lost once human contact no longer occurs (Klinghammer 1991). The lack of fear tame animals show toward humans often leads to their deaths. These animals often get shot or trapped as few people trust a "friendly raccoon" and often misinterpret it to be diseased or rabid. Tame game species are often easy targets for hunters and trappers. Tame animals are also unsuitable for release due to possible dangerous encounters with humans. This process is usually reversible but should be done by a person other than the one who caused it before the animal is released. Taming can be avoided by minimizing human contact, especially human-associated positive stimuli such as food (Diehl & Stokhaug 1991). Wild animals no longer requiring hand-feeding should never be fed by hand. Food should be scattered around the enclosure when animals are sleeping and not likely to see the provider (i.e., feed opossums and flying squirrels 1–2 hours before dark when they are still asleep and out of view).

It is critical that the distinction be made between a true human imprint and a tamed animal with regard to the release potential. The animal's history must be traceable from the day it came in. Again, good record-keeping is essential as it will help determine if improper imprinting is even a possibility. If the animal can be proven to be tame but not imprinted on humans, it may still have a chance to be released.

Transporting Wildlife

A variety of containers can be used to transport wildlife. The two main considerations for choosing the appropriate transport container are the animal's safety and comfort. If someone is on the phone asking for advice on how to bring an animal into the clinic, someone should always ask for information about the animal such as, what type of animal is it, is it conscious, and is it a baby or adult? Each call should be taken on a case-by-case basis to determine what is the safest way to capture and transport each animal. After determining that the animal needs assistance, it should also be determined if the caller has the tools on hand to safely get the animal into the transport container, such as gloves, a blanket, or a broom. The caller's confidence and experience level should be ascertained before even suggesting that he or she attempt to handle a potentially dangerous animal. Human safety comes first. If in doubt, referring the caller directly to the rehabilitator may be the safest thing to do.

After capture an animal should be placed in a suitable lidded container with holes and kept in a quiet area before and during the transport. Unnecessary talking or playing the radio in the vehicle during transport should be avoided. Extreme temperatures should also be avoided by providing ventilation, shade from the sun, or extra heat if needed. Cardboard boxes make good temporary cages and can be quickly altered to suit many different types of animals. Ideally, the size of the container should be just large enough for the animal to comfortably fit into but not large enough for a great deal of activity. Cardboard boxes and pet carriers make the best types of transport containers because they offer solid sides and tops, which reduce visual stress for the patient, and are also disposable after use. Placing wildlife in a clear aquarium or plastic tote should only be done if there is a towel or blanket available to cover the enclosure to block out light and remove visual stimuli.

Proper nonslip material should be placed on the enclosure bottom to ensure proper footing and reduce stress as a result of slipping and sliding during the transport. Also, the cage should be secured down so it does not slide or flip over. No food or water should be provided during the time of the transport because the animals are usually too stressed to eat and the bowls often end up tipping over and spilling their contents getting the animal wet or dirty.

Adult Birds

Open-wire bird/rodent cages are not advisable for transporting because they need to be covered with a towel and the wire can be very damaging to the flight feathers. Songbirds can be placed in a wide-open paper bag with the top rolled tightly shut and clipped with a paper clip or clothespin. Several pencil-sized air holes should be provided in the bag for fresh air and ventilation. Plastic pet carriers work well for waterfowl, raptors, and the larger songbird species

(i.e., blue jays, robins), but care should be taken with the smaller species (i.e., wrens, warblers) that can fit through the holes on the cage door. Appropriate-sized cardboard boxes work equally well for small sparrows on up to large herons.

Carpet pieces, paper towels, or cloth towels serve as good cage flooring. Newspaper is too slippery as is the plain plastic bottom of a pet carrier. Alert and standing adult birds might use a perch to stand on if it is securely fastened and of proportional size to the bird's foot size. Tightly wedging a tree branch down low inside of a box before placing the bird inside can give the animal an option to perch. Raptors need a branch about 2–3 inches in diameter to properly perch on.

Provide soft material (i.e., rolled towel) to prop the animal up on if it is not capable of standing on its own.

If the rescuer describes a heron-type bird, warn the person of the dangers of the spear like beaks and advise them not to go near the bird without eye protection such as safety glasses.

If the caller describes a bird of prey, first warn them about the dangerous talons. It may be best to refer the caller directly to a raptor rehabilitator for an on-site rescue.

Baby Birds

Young featherless birds need supplemental heat and can be transported using a warm water bottle or a zip-lock bag (double bagged to prevent leaks) filled with warm water placed under or next to the baby's enclosure. The nestling bird can be placed in a small box, berry basket, or any plastic margarine-sized container lined with nonscented toilet or facial tissues as nesting material. The artificial nest, not the infant itself, should be placed on the heat source to prevent the chance of skin burns. It should be kept in mind that these types of portable warming devices stay warm for only 30–60 minutes. Covering the nest/carrier with a light cloth reduces drafts and helps hold the warmth inside. These young animals need to be transferred as quickly as possible to prevent chilling or further dehydration.

If the baby's nest falls also, advise the rescuer against bringing it with the baby due to the strong possibility of unwanted parasites living in the nest.

Adult Mammals

A wire cage or live trap is suitable to transport an adult squirrel, raccoon, opossum, fox, or groundhog, to name a few. Most of these animals can chew out of cardboard or plastic kennels in a surprisingly short period of time. The transporter's safety is of foremost importance so do not advise them to put themselves at risk over the animal. Also, be informed as to the status of rabies in the caller's area and of the vector species that carry the disease so the caller can be warned of any potential danger.

Injured medium to large mammals such as deer, coyotes, and bobcats may need chemical immobilization and special capture equipment, such as punch poles, dart guns, and snare poles, to prevent injury to the animal or the handler.

Flying squirrels and chipmunks are escape artists and need to be contained in a box or solid-sided container with the lid taped or snapped shut. Instruct the caller to make the air holes on the lid only and no larger around than a pencil or they could chew and enlarge the air holes to escape through them.

The cage bottom should be lined with ravel-free cloth and the entire cage draped for privacy. The cloth inside the cage provides better footing and a layer to hide under, which greatly reduces their stress. The transporter can be advised to protect the vehicle's floor or seats by placing an old blanket, if available, down first before setting the cage inside. The rescuer should be warned to use caution when handling these potentially dangerous animals and their cages.

Mammals

Cardboard boxes and pet carriers work well to transport these animals. Soft ravel-free cloth should be placed inside the cage and a heat source (warm water bottle) provided for hairless babies or those whose eyes are closed. The heat source should never go directly against the baby's skin but rather under the cage to warm up the cage bottom.

Turtles

Cardboard boxes or plastic buckets work for transporting these animals. Do not transport water turtles in a container filled with water because the turtle will bump against the sides of the container as it is moved about.

Snakes

Snakes are best transported in a pillowcase with the opening tied in a knot. The bag can then be placed into a box, cooler, or bucket. The handler should carry the bag by the tip of the knot because the snake could bite through the cloth bag. Snakes can also be gently swept with a broom into a lidded box or small trash can. Unless the caller has experience in identifying venomous snake species from nonvenomous ones, care should be taken in advising anyone to handle any snake. This may be a job for animal control or a reptile rehabilitator.

See Appendix 3 for additional information on handling and restraint of wildlife species.

Raptor Care

Birds of prey include eagles, falcons, condors, vultures, harrier, hawks, kites, osprey, owls, and the caracara. Raptors are legally protected by a number of federal acts such as the migratory bird treaty act of 1918, bald eagle protection act of 1940, and endangered species act of 1973. Many federal bird rehab permits do not automatically include birds of prey due to the special training and housing needed to work with these animals.

Raptor Handling

When handling any of these species of birds always keep in mind that their first line of defense is their talons. Be careful to safely secure the raptor's feet and legs before attempting to pick up or move the bird. Heavy gauntlet-type welding gloves, such as the type used for restraining aggressive cats, should be worn to catch a medium- to large-sized raptor. Small raptors such as screech owls and kestrels can be caught up using leather work gloves.

If a raptor feels trapped, it may either roll onto its back with feet up and talons ready or make a bold dash at its restrainer. A gloved hand should be kept ready at all times to deflect or grab such a bird in midair. If the bird flips onto its back, a rolled towel or a spare glove can be handed to it to grab with its feet and distract it long enough to allow a gloved hand to slip under the barrier and grab the animal by its legs.

To remove a raptor from a cage, one gloved hand should be used to block the bird from darting out around the other gloved hand as one reaches in. It is often helpful to drape a towel over the door to prevent the bird's from seeing a "get away" space around the restrainer's body. With medium and large birds of prey, it is best to grab both legs, up high against the bird's body, with one hand keeping a finger between the birds' legs. Once the legs are both contained, the wings can be folded up against the body with the other hand as the bird is pulled out. Every attempt should be made to avoid allowing the bird to beat its wings against the cage as it is extracted through the door.

When only one leg is grabbed, the natural reaction of the raptor is to grab back at the handler with its free foot. If the raptor manages to talon and hold onto a glove either the restrainer or someone else must first fully extend the leg in order for the toes to be opened back up. Then one by one each nail is removed with care taken to locate each of the other needle-sharp talons. It is very difficult to open up a foot on a raptor with a flexed leg.

Some birds will also attempt to bite, so securing the head or covering it with a towel may be necessary. The head must be secured when the eyes, mouth, nares, and ears are being examined. The handler needs to distract the bird with one hand and quickly grasp the head from behind with the other. Head restraint is accomplished by firmly holding the head between the thumb and index finger at the articulation of the mandible. Covering their eyes also tends to relax many raptor species and allows minor procedures to be more easily accomplished (giving injections, weighing, taking radiographs, or collecting blood). The use of an orthopedic stockinet to cover the head and body is another useful technique for raptor restraint when weighing. A Velcro strip can be used as leg restraints by first attaching around one leg, just above the feet, then wrapping around both legs.

If the bird is on the ground or in a large open-top box, a towel, blanket, or net can be draped over the bird and then the bird picked up after first feeling for and securing the legs through the draped material with a gloved hand. See Figure 30.1.

Raptor Initial Exam

Birds of prey are most commonly brought into veterinary hospitals with wing and/or leg fractures due to their frequency of colliding with motor vehicles. These birds tend to survive many of these collisions and due to their large size

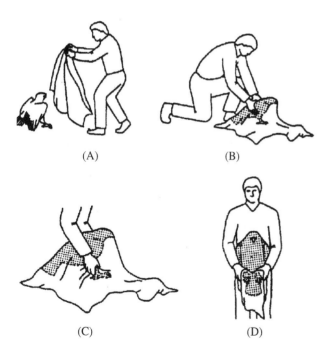

(A)   (B)

(C)   (D)

Figure 30.1 Picking a raptor up from the ground. (A) Blanket technique used to cover and catch a raptor. (B) Covered raptor is initially grasped with both hands over back shoulders. (C) Both hands secure legs just above the feet. (D) Restrain and carrying method with raptor held between arms against handler's body. (Permission for drawing use granted by the National Wildlife Rehabilitators Association.)

are more easily noticed alongside the road and thus rescued by other passing motorists. Two other common presentations are head or eye injuries.

Some of these animals, when presented to the hospital, may be in shock and will need to be treated accordingly. Usually, dexamethasone and lactated Ringer's solution (LRS) is the treatment of choice but only after first checking with the veterinarian. During the initial examination on any wild animal, one should be quick but thorough. A systematic method of examination that covers the patient from head to toe in the shortest time possible should be developed. Decreasing the handling time will dramatically reduce the bird's stress and increase its survival chances. Any cold bird should be placed on or under heat to allow the body temperature to reach normal range (98–102°F) before continuing with the exam.

Since raptors receive most of their water intake from the prey they eat, they easily become dehydrated when they are undernourished. Signs of dehydration include sunken eyes and thick, cloudy strands of mucous in the mouth. These birds should be immediately treated with warmed LRS by the oral, subcutaneous, intravenous, or intraosseous routes. One method is to tube feed small amounts of LRS with 5% dextrose into the bird's crop every 15 minutes for the first hour or two (Figure 30.2).

Next, the bird should be examined for fractures by palpation and radiology. Many raptors will tolerate a quick radiograph without sedation if properly held to the table with a combination of manual and paper tape restraint. Any potentially repairable broken limbs should immediately be stabilized with the proper splints or bandages. A bandage should be chosen that immobilizes the joint above and below the fracture site. The figure-eight bandage is good for immobilizing the wing and then can be wrapped to the body to eliminate joint movement (Figure 30.12).

If there is a fracture found in or very near any limb joint or if any two or more limbs contain a break, euthanasia should be strongly considered. These types of injuries often result in a nonreleasable animal and immediate euthanasia would be the most humane treatment. If the veterinarian is unsure of the releasability of any injured raptor, a raptor rehabilitator should be called first to help make the decision.

The bird's feather and muscle condition are two clues that are useful in determining the reason why the bird may have come in. If the feathers are ragged and soiled, that is evidence that the bird has probably been "grounded" for a long period of time so any injury is not likely to be fresh and wounds should be examined for fly eggs or larva. Any raptor that has been on the ground for several days or more will be dehydrated and potentially emaciated since these birds are unable to acquire live prey without flight.

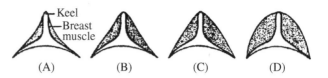

Figure 30.3 Subjective evaluation of a bird's condition based on pectoral muscle mass. (A) Severe muscle atrophy indicating a substantial amount of weight loss. (B) Moderate weight loss. (C) Severe weight loss, mild muscle atrophy. (D) Excellent condition with no detectable muscle atrophy. (Permission for drawing use granted by the Georgia Department of Natural Resources and Branson Ritchie, DVM, MS.)

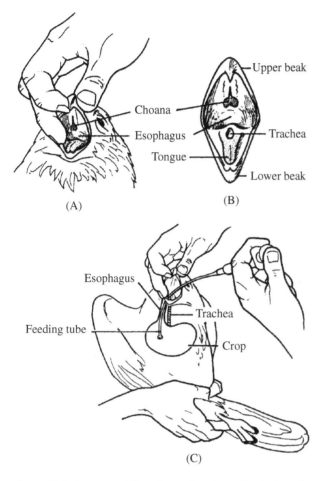

Figure 30.2 Anatomy of the avian oral cavity and technique for assisted feeding in birds. (A) Beak is held open by placing a finger in the corner of the mouth. (B) Close-up view of oral anatomy showing the esophagus at the back of the throat and trachea at the base of the tongue. (C) Proper placement of feeding tube in crop. (Permission for drawing use granted by the Georgia Department of Natural Resources and Branson Ritchie, DVM, MS.)

Dark green mutes (feces) are another sign of starvation. The bird's keel (sternum) can be palpated with fingertips to help assess the bird's level of health. A thin or emaciated bird's keel will feel "sharp" to the touch meaning that the keel bone is prominent and the breast muscles are atrophied (Figure 30.3).

Use a combination of physical condition, body weight, and degree of muscling on the keel to evaluate the bird.

Another all-too-common reason birds of prey end up in rehabilitation is gunshot injuries. Poisoning, whether intentional or unintentional, is also worth mentioning here because the veterinarian can sometimes determine toxicities with specific blood tests. Due to the nature of a raptor's eating habits, these birds may end up consuming a rodent or bird that ate poisoned bait and thus become secondarily poisoned. Emaciated juvenile birds often end

up in hospitals and wildlife care centers during their first winter due to their inexperienced hunting skills and the difficulties of surviving without an established hunting territory in the months when prey is most scarce.

Once the bird has been examined, it should be weighed (ideally in grams) so the medication, fluids, and food dosing will be accurate. The animal's weight is often the best indicator of how it is doing overall after being admitted for medical care. Good medical records that include all procedures, treatments, food intake, and weights should be maintained daily. A copy of these records can be made to give to the rehabilitator when the bird is transferred.

All treatments should be done as quickly as possible and with minimal talking. If any food, fluids, or medications need to be given orally, this should be done last after everything else has been done (injections, radiographs, venipuncture, etc.) to lessen the chances of regurgitation.

IM injections can be given in the leg or breast muscle. SQ fluids can be administered in either the axilla (wing web), lateral flank, or inguinal areas, doses divided into several sites, to provide maintenance or mild dehydration fluids. Intraosseous (IO) fluids are most often delivered via sterile catheter placed into the hollow cavity of the distal ulna or tibia for severe dehydration. This technique is described in Chapter 5 in this text. IV injections are given in the medial metatarsal or the right jugular vein. Once the patient is self-feeding, many medications can be injected or pilled into a food item that the bird can swallow whole, such as a pinkie or small mouse, and offered as part of the daily meal.

Raptor Caging

Most veterinary clinics can do short-term convalescent care with birds of prey but do not have the proper facilities for any long-term care or housing. All housing for raptors, as well as all wildlife, should be separate from the domestic patients and in a quiet area away from people and animal traffic.

Feathered healthy birds can be comfortably maintained at 60–85°F. Cages should have solid sides such as stainless sterile hospital rack cages or a large plastic pet kennel. A towel should be draped over the inside of the door opening to provide a complete visual barrier for the patients and to prevent them from catching their wings on the vertical door bars. The cage size should be large enough to allow the bird of prey to stand, turn around, and step up on a perch without touching its head or tail feathers yet not big enough for the bird to fly within and potentially further injure itself. Newspapers are adequate for lining the bottom of the cage.

Proper perching should always be provided for rehabilitating birds. Perches need to be of an appropriate size and well secured to the floor or cage sides. Large wooden tree branches or small logs can be used if the bird is only staying for several days. Cage perches can be made by combining PVC pipes into a "T" shape and then mounting it to a block of wood. These plastic perches should be wrapped with outdoor carpet or Astroturf and can be cleaned and reused. Raptors that require longer-term hospital stays should have padded perches to stand on to reduce foot injuries caused by the pressure of standing for long periods of time. The technician can wrap the perches with Vetrap to add cushioning and to provide an easy gripping surface. The perches should be secured at a height to prevent the bird's tail from dragging on the cage bottom but low enough to be easily stepped up.

The nature of the bird's injury should determine perch placement. No high perches should be available to a bird with a limb injury. To avoid any additional trauma, the perch should be 6–12 inches off the ground to begin with and gradually raised as the bird learns to step up and hop down from the perch. Ramped perches can cause problems if the injured bird climbs up to the top but "forgets" its handicap and jumps off. Most raptors never learn to descend from these learning perches the same gentle way they climbed up them.

A towel should be provided for padding to protect the bird's sternum if it is unable to stand. A rolled-up towel can be used to prop a weak bird up on its stomach at a 45° angle. The head should be level to prevent any fluids from the bird's nose or mouth from draining down into the lungs. Another caging method used for birds too weak to stand or with fractured legs is to place them in a box half full of shredded newspapers. This material not only supports the bird's body but also allows the feces to fall away from the bird.

The importance of keeping the feathers in good condition cannot be stressed enough. Wing and tail feathers, especially, are easily damaged if the birds are improperly housed. Even if the clinic is only holding the bird for a day or two, housing the bird in any cage where the feathers or feather tips can stick out will do some degree of damage. It only takes two or three broken flight feathers to deem an otherwise fit bird temporarily nonreleasable. If the damage in any way interferes with normal mobility, the bird must remain in captivity until it undergoes a molt and replaces the broken feathers with new ones. This is a normal process but may take up to a year to naturally occur.

In addition to proper housing, a tail guard can be easily applied. Some rehabilitation centers and veterinary clinics wrap tails as a common intake procedure. A tail-wrapping method is reprinted with permission from the North Carolina Raptor Center in Charlotte, North Carolina. (See Appendix 4.)

Raptor Feeding

As with any animal, the bird should be warm and hydrated before you offer solid food. If the bird appears in good condition and is not emaciated, it can be offered a natural prey item for its diet. Healthy diurnal birds of prey (hawks, falcons) need to be fed once a day during the daylight hours. Nocturnal birds (owls) should be fed once a day but only in the evening.

These birds eat a variety of rodents, birds, rabbits, fish, insects, and snakes in the wild but in short-term hospitalization, fresh-killed, or thawed adult mice will do. In some cases, it may take the new patient several days to accept the new surroundings and food. As long as the bird came in at a good weight this should not be a problem and the bird will start to eat when it gets really hungry. The food presentation may also confuse the bird and it may not recognize a dead white lab mouse as a food item. Offering brown or black mice sometimes helps, as well as cutting open the mouse cavity to reveal the organ tissue, which often stimulates the bird's appetite.

Occasionally a raptor needs a little help with one or two hand-feedings to get started. A mouse may need to be cut into small bite-size pieces depending on the size of the bird. The pieces can be offered from a hemostat while leaving the bird inside the cage. One should be quiet and not stare at the bird or make sudden movements. The food should be slowly held up to and allowed to touch the bird's beak. Sometimes the bird will bite at the food defensively and accidentally take the offering. One should stay still until the bird swallows it, which could take a minute or two for the first bite. This can be repeated several times, and then the remaining part of the meal can be left inside the cage with the bird. If the bird will not swallow the food or is too aggressive and tries to foot and bite the feeder, then it may need to be force-fed.

With the bird wrapped securely in a towel and properly restrained, the beak should be opened and pieces carefully placed one by one into the back of its mouth (past the glottis) with fingers or blunted hemostats. The bird needs to be allowed to swallow each bite one at a time. Care should be taken to open the beak at the base and not the biting curved tip. Once the beak is open, it can be kept open long enough to place the food by wedging a finger inside at the extreme base of the mouth. It should always be remembered that these birds can be dangerous and will foot or bite at any given chance. Once a stubborn raptor swallows several pieces of delicious rodent, even if it is a white one, it usually gives the bird incentive to start self-feeding.

If the bird is emaciated, dehydrated, or too weak to eat solid whole items, then tube feeding may be needed. Start first with SQ LRS fluids and then switch to the oral route once the bird has stabilized. Continue with liquid formula feeding (such as Lafeber's Emeraid Carnivore Care or Oxbow's Critical Care for Carnivores) until the bird has gained strength. Next, bites of skinless and boneless pieces of muscle or organ meat such as raw beef liver or muscle meat from a cut-up mouse or rat can be offered. Only after the bird has recovered its strength, which can take up to 3–4 days, should it be offered solid whole foods. Table 30.1 provides a feeding guideline for birds of prey.

Raptor Orphan Initial Care

The intake of many raptor "orphans" into the veterinary hospital can often be prevented by good phone protocols and animal history taking. Raptors have a stage of development between the nestling and fledgling stage referred to as "branching." At this age, young birds are feathered, still being fed by their parents, have left the nest, but are not flighted. Well-meaning people often discover these birds and believe them to be orphaned or injured because they will not fly away and there is no nest in sight. Because these birds are so easily captured, they are usually first picked up before the rehabilitator is notified. By asking the right questions, many of these "kidnapped" birds can be returned to the founding sight before any harm is done. If the clinic receives these calls, the best thing to do is to instruct the caller to leave the bird where it is and have the person call one of the raptor rehabilitators (on the referral phone list) to determine if the bird is truly orphaned or not.

Raptors are hatched with down but unable to leave the nest (semi-altricial). While hawks are born with their eyes open, owls are born eyes closed. Hatchling- and nestling-stage babies found on the ground should be replaced into the nest if at all possible. Some rehabilitators, nature centers, or wildlife agencies may have individuals to help with this process. If returning to the original site is not possible, the orphan should be temporarily cared for until a foster nest or captive foster parent can be found. Many of the larger wildlife rehabilitation centers have permanent foster parent birds that willingly feed many orphans each year.

Initial temporary care of orphaned raptors is similar to the care of all animal species (make sure they are warm and hydrated). The chick should first be provided with heat if it is not old enough to regulate its own body temperature.

One accepted rule for raptor brooding temperature is:

- Unfeathered birds should be kept at an ambient temperature of 85–90°F.

Table 30.1 Recommended feeding guideline for birds of prey.

Species	Avg. male/female wt (g)	Food type	Amount
American kestrel	M-111 g/F-120 g	1 mouse	25 g
Bald eagle	M-4,123 g/F-5,244 g	2 rats	200–300 g
Barn owl	M-442 g/F-490 g	2–3 mice	50–75 g
Barred owl	M-632 g/F-801 g	2–3 mice	50–75 g
Broad winged hawk	M-420 g/F-490 g	2 mice	50 g
Cooper's hawk	M-349 g/F-529 g	2–3 mice	50–75 g
Great horned owl	M-1318 g /F-1769 g	3–5 mice or 1/2 rat	75–125 g
Peregrine falcon	M-611 g/F-952 g	4 mice	100 g
Red-tailed hawk	M-1,028 g/F-1,224 g	3–5 mice or 1/2 rat	75–125 g
Rough-legged hawk	M-1,027 g/F-1,278 g	4 mice	100 g
Saw-whet owl	M-74.9 g/F-90.8 g	1 mouse	25 g
Screech owl	M-167 g/F-194 g	1 mouse	25 g
Sharp-shinned hawk	M-103 g/F-174 g	1–2 mice	25–50 g
Red-shouldered hawk	M-475 g/F-643 g	2–3 mice	50–75 g
Turkey vulture	1,467 g	6–8 mice or 1 rat	150–200 g

- Downey chicks with quills present can be kept at 80–85°F.
- Birds with feather quills and small feathers should be kept at 75–80°F.

Estimating actual raptor-chick age is beyond the scope of this chapter due to the sheer number of species and classifications of birds of prey. The raptor rehabilitator can be called with the bird's description and weight for age estimate and feeding instructions. After the chick is warm and active, provide hydration fluids orally by carefully placing two to four drops of solution into the throat beyond the glottis every 15–20 minutes until the bird becomes active.

Raptor Orphan Feeding

If the chick's transportation cannot be arranged before it needs to eat, the technician can offer it small pieces of rodent from tweezers or hemostats. Caution should be taken to avoid improper imprinting from the chick watching hand-feeding (refer to imprinting section). Imprinting within raptors occurs anywhere between 5 and 15 days of age. Raptor chicks do not gape for food like songbird babies do but they readily take food with the tips of their beaks and sometimes will even nibble on the feeding tool as they would their parent's beak.

If the chicks' eyes are closed, it is safe to hand-feed by touching the bird's beak with the feeding instrument containing small bites of food and trying to imitate the parents' feeding calls by whistling or chirping quietly. Because the chicks cannot see the person feeding it, one need only be concerned about the chicks' not hearing the person feeding talking.

If the bird's eyes are open and it demonstrates no fear or aggression, this is within the dangerous critical imprinting period and much care should be taken to prevent the youngster from seeing or hearing a human or any animal in the hospital. Some centers feed these birds with gloves and ski masks to partially hide the human shape or better yet feed with a hand puppet of a raptor-type bird (rubber bird hand puppets can sometimes be found at gift shops of nature stores and zoos). See Figure 30.4. Another option is to hang a towel, sheet, or curtain, to serve as a kind of blind, in front of the infant and feed by reaching around and peeking through a hole in the blind. These animals must never be available for "show and tell" and should be disturbed only for care taking until they can be transferred to the rehabilitator.

A juvenile raptor that shows fear or aggression is beyond the critical imprinting stage and, one hopes, has properly imprinted on its own species by now. These birds may also be capable of self-feeding, so try placing small pieces of food in with the bird. If it refuses to pick up the food on its own

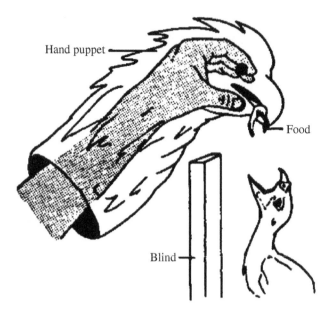

Figure 30.4 Hand-feeding puppet used for feeding neonates. During critical imprinting periods, hand-feeding puppets should be used in conjunction with blinds to prevent a young animal from associating food with humans. (Permission for drawing use granted by the Georgia Department of Natural Resources and Branson Ritchie, DVM, MS.)

after several feedings, refer to the above section on feeding adult raptors for hand-feeding ideas.

Raptor Orphan Food

Young raptors eat enormous amounts of food and often three to four times the amount of an adult. Weigh the chick in the morning before feeding and then feed 8–10% of body weight. The first few meals should be less to allow the digestive tract time to adjust to the changes. The crop should be allowed to fully empty before offering the next meal. Unlike hawks, owls do not have crops but tend to turn away from food when full (Crawford 1988).

Very young chicks, 0 to 7 days old, should eat just the soft muscle organ meat of prey foods dipped into vitamin water. The parents would remove all skin, fur, and bones initially from the meals. These young raptor chicks should eat, until they are satisfied, every 3–4 hours. Feed them until the crop is half to three-quarters full but not so full that it feels hard or extended. Meals should not be skipped, and birds should be fed for a 12-hour day.

Once they are 7 to 10 days old, one can begin to introduce small amounts of moistened hair, skin, and small bones into the diet, which will serve as roughage and later be cast up.

Around days 10–20, the chicks can be fed larger moistened pieces of meat with bones, skin, and fur for three feedings a day. Starting at 3 weeks of age, the young should be able to eat the entire mouse cut into three to four pieces and will start to pick these up on their own.

One should feed the 3-week-olds to fledge twice a day and offer whole-prey items for them to tear on their own. One should then continue to hand-feed them until it is certain that they are picking up enough food on their own to sustain themselves.

Once fledged, one can feed these birds once daily (owls in the evening, hawks in the morning).

Whether the baby is staying at the veterinary hospital for one meal or many, it is the clinic's responsibility to NOT allow this animal (or any wild animal) the opportunity to improperly imprint on human beings. If this is allowed to occur, the raptor will be deemed unreleasable and usually will need to be euthanized.

Raptor Orphan Housing

A small cardboard box lined with cloth works well for a very young raptor. A twisted towel made into a circle with the baby placed inside the "doughnut" serves well for support. Walls may need to be covered or cleaned daily because hawks and eagles tend to shoot when they excrete feces. Use of an incubator, heat lamp, or heating pad to provide external heat for the very young (2 weeks old or younger) will be necessary. Healthy raptors do not need as much heat as other birds, but if it seems lethargic or shivers, it may be cold. A panting chick is too warm. Housing temperatures are outlined below in the initial care section (Figure 30.5).

As the young become more active, pieces of branches can be placed on the nest bottom to provide the birds with foot-gripping exercise, which is necessary to develop coordination and strength.

When raptors fledge, they need a larger enclosure with stable perches that are larger around than the bird's grip. The enclosure should have solid sides to prevent the flight

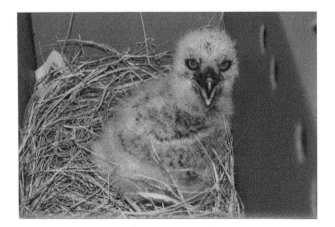

Figure 30.5 Baby hawk. (Courtesy of Melanie Haire.)

feathers from sticking out and becoming damaged. The growing chick will now need room to hop and flap its wings.

Misting these newly feathered birds daily with water will help stimulate them to preen and activate their uropygial gland for waterproofing. Once they are eating on their own, acclimated to the outside, and waterproofed, juvenile raptors are ready for outdoor flight caging. By now the bird should be transferred to a raptor rehabilitator to train on catching live food and prepare for release.

Altricial Orphan Songbirds Basic Care

This section is to be used as general information only. It should be kept in mind that every bird is slightly different in development and behavior. These guidelines are to be used by the veterinary technician until the bird can be transferred to a licensed rehabilitator.

Altricial birds are those that are hatched blind, naked, unable to control body temperature, and completely helpless (blue jays, robins, and mockingbirds).

Development

The development of the altricial bird is generally five stages. All species follow these stages but at different rates depending on their natural history.

1. Hatchling—0–4 days old, newly hatched, no voice, eyes closed, naked, or sparsely downy
2. Nestling—5–10 days old, eyes open, partially feathered, feeding call
3. Fledgling—11–14 days, almost fully feathered, can perch, hop, first attempts to fly, ready to leave the nest, able to thermoregulate, frequently preening, wing stretching, short tail feathers
4. Juvenile—fully grown, defensive, independence begins, lasts until sexual maturity
5. Adult—sexually mature

Initial Care

An animal should never be fed until it is warm. Use an incubator, a brooder, heat light, or heating pad to warm up a chilled infant and keep the baby on heat until it is feathered. Altricial baby birds' temperature guidelines are:

- Hatchlings—should be kept at 80–90°F
- Nestlings— should be kept at 80–85°F
- Fledglings—should be kept at 70–80°F

Once the bird is warm, it should be hydrated by offering drops of Pedialyte or LRS orally every 5–10 minutes until the baby passes a normal fecal sac. For most birds, this should consist of a dark solid part (stool) and a milky white softer part (urates) contained within a clear sac.

The baby bird should be examined for injuries, bruises, puncture wounds, bites, mites, and so on.

Identification of what species it is needs to be made to determine proper diet and feeding schedule.

Begin offering the infant hand-rearing formula.

Identification

To determine the type of bird, the bird rehabilitator should be called for help, and one can also refer to Appendix 5.

Information should be obtained about where and how the bird was found from the person who found it. These details not only help identify what type of bird it is, but also may help determine if the bird needs further help or if it can be returned to its parents.

The following items help to identify altricial nestling species:

1. Mouth color—The inside membranes of the mouth are usually brightly colored to attract attention from the feeding parent bird.
2. Gape flanges color—The fleshy "lips" that edge the mouth may be a different color than the inside of the mouth.
3. Beak description—The length and shape of the beak helps identify a species by what it eats. Insect eaters tend to have long, slender beaks, and seed eaters tend to have thick, short, and conical-shaped beaks.
4. Skin color or color of down—Presence or absence of down, natal down, and skin color are also species-specific.
5. Vocalizations—Many songbird species have unique feeding calls.
6. Location baby was found—Was the baby found in a tree cavity (woodpeckers, nuthatches), a fireplace (chimney swifts), and hanging planters (wrens, finches)?
7. Body size—When the tail feathers emerge from their sheaths, a baby bird has reached its full body size.

Housing Nestlings

The baby bird should be placed in a homemade nest constructed out of a berry basket, small plastic bowl, or margarine tub lined with unscented toilet or facial tissues.

A cuplike cavity with the nesting material can be constructed so the baby can nestle down but still receive support from all sides. The baby could develop leg problems if not properly supported during the nesting stage. For extra support, a paper towel can be rolled (snakelike) and coiled around the inside of the nest, and then the tissue placed over the top.

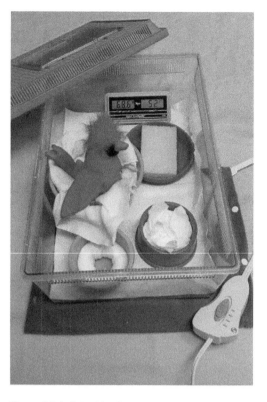

Figure 30.6 Baby bird incubator with hygrometer, wet sponge, nest with facial tissues and a heating pad.

If the tissue is piled high enough (within one-half inch of the nest container top), the baby can defecate over the side of the nest and help keep the inside clean.

Replace the tissue as it gets soiled.

Do not use the old natural nest because it may contain parasites and is too difficult to clean. Do not line the artificial nest with fresh grass because it is too cold and damp.

If the baby bird is very young, using an incubator with a wet sponge or other source of moisture for humidity may be necessary (Figure 30.6). A homemade incubator can be made out of a small plastic tote with air holes put in the lid. Care should be taken to provide enough ventilation so that the humidity does not build up and allow moisture to collect on the inside of the container, which in turn allows rapid growth of pathogens.

Instructions for how to make a homemade incubator are available on the International Wildlife Rehabilitation Council (IWRC) web page: www.iwrc-online.org.

If an incubator is not being used, the nest should be placed inside a safe container such as a lidded box or basket to prevent any unfortunate mishaps from babies falling out or pets getting into the nest. This especially applies to the technician who has the babies at work in a busy veterinary practice.

The nest should be kept on the heating pad or under the heat lamp at all times to keep the baby from chilling.

A thermometer should always be used to monitor the ambient air. The warmth should circulate around the infant.

A tissue or soft washcloth should be draped over the top of the baby to hold in the warmth and to simulate the security of a brooding parent.

Baby birds can usually come off the heat when they feather out as long as they are active and healthy.

Housing Fledglings

Once the babies are ready to leave the nest, they will require a larger cage. The nest can be placed inside a small flight cage so the youngsters can hop in and out of their nests until they no longer return to it. The cage should be large enough to allow the birds to take short flights and hop from perch to perch but small enough to be easily carried inside and out.

The sides should be constructed out of or lined with soft netting or nylon mesh to prevent injury to the bird or its feathers. Affordable commercially available soft-sided mesh cages can be purchased and successfully used to house fledgling and injured adult songbirds. Examples of such, are the Reptilariums® and pop-up laundry hampers or butterfly cages. These cages are available in different sizes and are easy to clean because in some (Reptilarium®) the mesh zips off the plastic frame and can be machine washed.

Wire bird or mammal cages should never be used. If the feathers stick out from between the cage bars they will fray, break off, and possibly become too damaged to support flight. At best these birds with damaged plumage will have to be held over until they molt out a new set of flight feathers. With many songbird species, this may take up to a year. Occasionally these birds develop permanent feather follicle damage and need to be euthanized.

The cage bottom can be lined with paper towels and should be changed out daily.

Several secured low branches should be included to allow for landing and perching practice.

If the weather is mild, the cage should be moved outside during the day but brought inside at night to start acclimating the birds to outdoor temperatures, sights, and sounds.

In addition to introducing the young bird to natural temperatures, the sunlight will provide vital and accurate doses of vitamin D_3. Birds require a proper balance of calcium and phosphorus in their diet for the development of normal, healthy bones. Vitamin D_3 is necessary to ensure that the body can absorb the dietary calcium. Without this proper absorption, the body cannot form normal bones, and the bones and the bill can become rubbery and soft. This deficiency, called metabolic bone disease, results in bone deformities or even stress fractures that are difficult at best to treat. Prevention is the best medicine, and a combination of 30 minutes a day of direct daylight or 30–60 minutes a day with artificial full-spectrum light plus a balanced diet will meet the requirements.

Plastic and glass filter out the necessary ultraviolet light so sunlight coming through a window or aquarium will not provide adequate light.

The entire cage should never be placed in direct sunlight. The babies can quickly overheat if a shaded area is not easily accessible. Ultraviolet rays from the sun are still available on cloudy days and in the shade.

The enclosure should never be left unprotected from possible predators. A screened porch or a fenced yard is no protection from a stray cat or hungry raccoon. Predator-proof caging can be affordably built but will not be discussed in this chapter. All hand-raised wild bird releases should be done by a licensed bird rehabilitator. Many of the rehabilitation manuals listed on the source pages have instructions for building prerelease and release caging.

Feeding Methods

There are many feeding methods in practice for feeding wild baby birds (Figure 30.7).

Blunt forceps, tweezers, pipettes, syringes, eyedroppers, small artists paint brushes, Popsicle sticks, blunted toothpicks, and fingers are just some of the tools that can be used for administering food.

A discussion of feeding techniques with a local avian rehabilitator will aid in choosing the one that works best.

Many of the above feeding implements only work with certain types of formulas, and sometimes a combination works well (Figure 30.7). Often the thickness of the formula depends on the age of the bird, so feeding several birds of different ages may require the use of more than one tool.

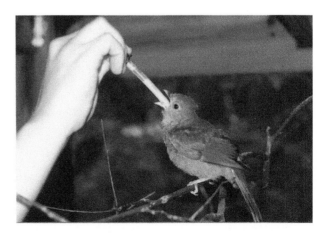

Figure 30.7 Hand-feeding a baby cardinal. (Courtesy of Melanie Haire.)

Many healthy nestlings and fledglings will gape readily and hungrily making feeding time for the caregiver much easier. These willing participants will continue to gape, for the most part, until their crops are full. Care should be taken to avoid overfilling the crop. If the bird is slow to swallow or flings food, it might be full or too dehydrated.

If the baby is hesitant to gape, it may be dehydrated or otherwise ill, not hungry, too frightened, or nervous, or it may not recognize the gesture as a feeding attempt.

One can tap on the side of the nest and whistle softly in an attempt to imitate the parent bird's arrival at the nest. This may require patience and several tries with different chirping sounds. Gaping nestmates often help stimulate gaping in all individuals including newcomers.

If the baby is hydrated and healthy but still will not gape, gently prying the beak open with fingers and placing a small amount of food toward the back of its mouth may be necessary. Some birds will get the picture quickly and only need one or two force-feedings to understand that they are being offered food and will not be harmed.

Once birds imprint on their parents and are old enough to have developed fear of humans in the wild, they become more difficult to hand-feed and may need to be force-fed until they become self-feeding. Introducing a bowl of food into their cage for this older fledgling group may be the answer.

Several altricial species of baby birds (i.e., some swifts, swallows, nighthawks, pigeons, and all doves) never gape, and knowing the identification of these species will save a lot of time and frustration. These individuals will need to be fed in a different manner.

The fledgling or juvenile swifts, swallows, and nighthawks are examples of birds that will probably need to be force- or tube-fed until release. Hatchlings and nestlings may adjust to hand-feedings but need to be fed by holding the food up to the bird's beak.

Pigeon and dove babies do not gape but they do beg. They naturally feed by sticking their beaks inside their parent's mouth, which is the opposite position of many songbirds. So the concept of willingly opening their mouths to the sight of an eyedropper full of food has no meaning to them. These birds will need to be tube-fed until they are self-feeding. Once the birds are 7 days old or older, a feeder can be made that resembles the feeding technique naturally used by this group.

Pigeon and Dove Feeder

A 12 or 20 cc syringe casing can be filled with a balanced parakeet seed mix (small seeds without a lot of hulls or shelled sunflower seeds) and tightly wrapped with Vetrap over the opened bottom of the case to keep the seeds in.

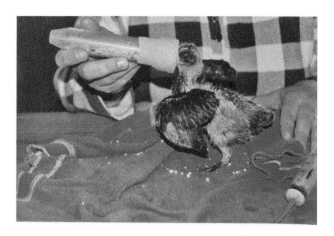

Figure 30.8 Pigeon feeder. (Courtesy of Melanie Haire.)

A quarter- to half-inch slit is then cut in the center of the Vetrap (long enough for the bird's beak to fit through but not too big to allow seeds to spill out around beak). Next, the bird's beak can be inserted into the slit in the Vetrap, and while holding the back of the bird's head to keep it from pulling out of the dispenser, the syringe can be tapped to simulate the movement of the parent bird. (Figure 30.8). It will take several attempts to get the bird to quit struggling and pulling away from the feeder. Once the baby swallows some seeds (probably by accident the first time), it will quickly start self-feeding right out of the dispenser. Then in addition to tube feeding into their crop with a hand-rearing formula, one can offer the baby the feeder several times a day to facilitate the self-feeding and weaning process.

A size 10 or 12 red rubber catheter cut to about 3 inches in length can be used to crop tube feed pigeons and doves. Exact, Pretty Bird, and Emeraid are examples of quality hand-rearing powdered diets commercially available at pet stores or veterinary clinics.

Food Prep

The bird formulas ideally should be made up fresh daily and refrigerated until use. Each feeding should be allowed to warm to room temperature before feeding it to the bird.

The consistency will vary depending on the diet and the age of the bird. Most diets are thick like oatmeal when hand mixed but can be blended down to a slurry that can be pushed through a syringe or dropper. Some formulas tend to thicken over the day during refrigeration, and a little water may need to be added to keep it at the proper consistency. Remember that baby birds need as many calories as possible so do not thin formulas down more than absolutely necessary. Runny or drippy formulas should never be fed because the food could drip down into the trachea and cause aspiration pneumonia.

Many diets can be made in batches and stored in the freezer for short periods of time. Making a week's worth of food at once and freezing it in ice cube trays can save a lot of time. One can thaw out as many cubes as needed for the day, and a backup supply is available if more babies are received.

One should be knowledgeable about nutrition because some ingredients lose dietary value when frozen or stored for long periods of time. One should always start with fresh, good-quality ingredients.

Feeding Frequency

Feeding frequency should follow this guideline:

Hatchling—Feed every 10–20 min (6 a.m.–10 p.m.)
Nestling—Feed every 20–30 min (6 a.m.–10 p.m.)
Fledgling—Feed every 45–60 min (7 a.m.–10 p.m.)
Juveniles—Feed every 2 hours (7 a.m.–9 p.m.)

In the wild, baby birds are fed from sunup to sundown. A technician should not make the mistake of thinking that they can be fed enough calories in a 9:00–5:00 workday. Hand-raising a baby bird is not a part-time responsibility. If the bird cannot be transferred over to a rehabilitator the same day, feeding arrangements must be made for the baby for a full 12–14-hour day. The biggest single mistake made, by well-meaning people, with hand-rearing baby wild birds is to underfeed them. The caretaker cannot make up for several missed feedings by feeding larger volumes at the next couple of feedings.

The only flexibility a caretaker has is to pick when the 12–14 hours begins and ends. By covering the cage and making it dark or leaving the lights on in the nursery past sundown, one can slightly alter the "daytime" if need be. This is not recommended for the long term or with older juvenile birds because they need to develop a sense of natural time.

Diets

It is ideal to feed the same diet that the rehabilitator will be using to prevent the stress of change to the baby's gastrointestinal tract. The recipes and ingredients should be kept on hand prior to the start of baby season in order to be always prepared. All too often the babies seem to come in at 10:00 p.m. on a Sunday night just as the pet stores close.

Proper bird species identification is necessary to choose the best diet recipe. By reading as much natural history information as is available, one can learn about food preferences, feeding methods, food presentation, and normal behavior.

The following are some examples of passerine hand-rearing formulas used at rehabilitation centers:

part soaked Hill's Science Diet Feline growth
1 part Gerber's High Protein Cereal
 1 tsp. bone meal
 Water to proper consistency (Evans 1986)
2. 1 cup soaked puppy chow
 1 T baby food beef
 1 T hard-boiled egg yolk
 3–4 drops balanced avian vitamins
 1/2 t ground egg shell
 (Johnson 1991)
3. 1 cup soaked Hill's Science Diet Feline growth (original recipe only)
 1/2 cup chick starter added to 1/2 cup boiling water
 3–4 drops balanced avian vitamins
 1/2 t Rep-cal (calcium w/vitamin D_3, phosphorus-free)
 1 t powdered Benebac

Mix cat food and hot chick starter together in blender. Add other ingredients after mix cools (Ivie 1999). Note: Science Diet Feline growth original recipe only is advised due to avian digestive problems associated with the other flavors.

These sample diets can be fed to a wide variety of species with the exception of doves and pigeons. These diets are a balanced base. Depending on the bird species, food items can be added to more closely match their natural diet.

- Insectivorous birds such as woodpeckers, swifts, and wrens should have insects added to the base. Mealworms, wax worms, crickets, and freeze-dried insects are examples of such supplements that should make up to 50% of the diet.
- Frugivores such as waxwings and orioles should have chopped fruit added.
- Birds with a tendency to develop a calcium deficiency such as mockingbirds, thrashers, and kingbirds should have food items rich in calcium or a calcium supplement added to the diet.
- Doves and pigeons being strictly seed and grain feeders can be tube fed with a commercial brand of baby bird food formulated for psittacines such as Kaytee's Exact Hand Feeding Formula. These powdered diets are available, ready to use after adding water, in most pet stores.
- Hummingbirds need a commercial nectar such as Nekton or Roudybush. Pet store or homemade sugar-water diets (although good for providing energy) only provide calories and will not keep a hummingbird alive long-term.

Additional Information

Avoid allowing formula to dry on the baby's beak, nares, or feathers. Remove any spilled food while it is still moist and easier to remove. If food is allowed to dry on feathers, it may cause feather loss or a skin infection. One should use a damp cotton swab to clean food off of the baby; wiping should be in the direction of the feather growth.

One should always try to house single baby birds with conspecifics. The rehabilitator should be contacted to help place the baby with other same-species orphans or, even better, into a foster parent situation. Arrangements should be made to get them together as soon as possible. The benefits of orphaned animals being raised with natural or foster siblings are immeasurable. They learn critical behavioral and social skills from interacting with the correct species.

Never forget that the goal of wildlife rehabilitation is to provide temporary care with the goal of releasing the animal with its best chances to survive. Technicians must above all do no harm and never release an animal that cannot properly care for itself.

- Limit talking around wildlife.
- Avoid improper imprinting.
- Adequate notes should be kept that can be used as reference material later. Good record-keeping may also prevent mishaps due to shift changes in caregivers.
- One should limit handling and activity to feeding and cleaning time only.
- Wild birds should never be housed near domestic pets, especially pet birds.
- All food containers and tools should be cleaned with hot soapy water after each use and allowed to air dry or towel dry before next use. Dip feeding instruments in 5% diluted bleach or soak in 10% diluted Nolvasan for 30 minutes once daily.

Caring for Adult Passerine (Song) Birds

Initial Care

The bird's history should be obtained on the intake form to help formulate the diagnosis of why the bird came into the clinic. The rescuer might know for certain that it was hit by a car, flew into a window, or was caught by a cat. If no cause is known, good "investigative" questions should help find the answer. If the bird was found in the driveway, it should be asked if there is a nearby garage with windows it might have collided with. If the bird was found under a bird feeder and has had its tail feathers pulled out, the founder should be questioned about the possibilities of outdoor cats in the area.

After the history taking, a visual exam should be performed first before touching the bird. The bird should be observed for signs of disease or illness such as ruffled feathers, squinted or closed eyes, sneezing, clicking, mouth breathing, dull feathers, lethargy, diarrhea, squatting instead of standing, and wing droops.

Next, a physical examination should be performed looking for obvious wounds and fractures along with more subtle signs of shock and dehydration. (See the section on performing the physical exam under "Initial Exam" above). Body and feather condition should be checked and noted. The keel should be palpated to determine if the bird is thin or emaciated. When checking for lacerations or bruising, feathers can be blown out of the way to better visualize the skin underneath.

Restraint for adult songbirds is relatively easy. Pressure should not be placed on a bird's sternum since they breathe by expanding their chest and abdominal cavities. Use of the "bander's" hold, enables the examiner to check the bird thoroughly while keeping a secure yet gentle hold on the patient (Figure 30.9). This hold should be used for any handling, medicating, or force-feeding procedures.

An accurate weight in grams should be obtained and monitored every 24–48 hours.

The bird should be kept warm and hydrated before attempting to feed it. If the bird feels thin, has bright green stools, sunken eyes, wrinkled skin, or is weak and lethargic, it should be offered two to four drops of rehydrating solution orally by placing the drops behind the glottis into the throat every 15 minutes for the first 1–2 hours.

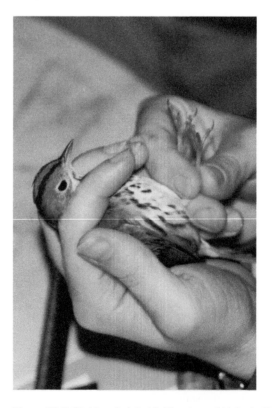

Figure 30.9 Bird bander's hold. (Courtesy of Melanie Haire.)

Dehydrated birds can receive SQ fluids injected into their wing web or into the loose medial skin folds where the legs join to the body. Injecting fluids, although more painful than delivering oral fluids due to the needle prick, may be less stressful in the end due to the larger volume that can be given at one time, which decreases the number of times needed to restrain the bird.

Immobilizing Fractures

Immobilization of any fractures should be performed as soon as possible so the bird does not further injure itself.

The wildlife veterinary technician should know how to apply all of the following bandages. The veterinarians may not be able to look at every bird that comes in with a fracture but if the proper stabilizing wrap is applied, the fracture may have all it needs to heal properly. Do not allow a bird with a fractured bone to sit in the hospital without a proper bandage. Waiting one or two days to apply the wrap could be too late.

If the bone needs more than a bandage to properly mend (long bones on larger birds such as ducks, owls, and hawks), the wrap should still be applied until the veterinarian can schedule the bone surgery procedure.

If the lower leg (tibiotarsus or tarsometatarsus) is fractured, on a small bird, a tape splint usually works well (Figure 30.10). The leg is held in a natural "perch" position and tape is placed on each side of the leg. One should seal the tape firmly up to the leg by pinching it with a pair of hemostats. The more tape applied, the more stable the splint but it should be kept in mind the weight of the apparatus versus the small size of your patient. The bird should be able to stand and perch with this type of bandage if it is properly trimmed.

The femur needs more than tape if it has been fractured. Cast padding and a splint (made of toothpicks, tongue depressors, halved syringe case, etc.) covered in Vetrap

depending on the size of the bird will be needed. The joint above and below the fracture site needs to be covered. If this is not possible, it is best not to bandage at all and arrange to have the bird transported to an experienced avian veterinarian or rehabilitator immediately.

Any leg bandage applied too tightly will prevent blood flow from leaving the foot, and the foot and toes may swell. The toes must be evaluated daily for swelling, loss of function, or discoloration.

Foot injuries can be bandaged in several different ways. In small songbirds, their toes can be taped down individually onto a cardboard "snowshoe." In larger birds, a padded ball bandage can be made to keep the toes aligned and the talons from puncturing the footpads (Figure 30.11). A circular piece of cardboard is cut that fits in the bottom of the bird's foot and is padded with cotton. The pad is taped in place by wrapping the cotton padding with Vetrap between the bird's toes. The toe tips should be slightly visible to be checked for bandage tightness. The bandages should be kept as clean and dry as possible because replacing the wrap before the bone is healed will delay or prevent healing.

For wing fractures, as with all fractures, the joint above and below the fracture site should be immobilized.

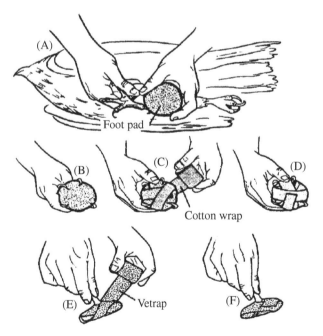

Figure 30.11 Padded bandage used in avian foot and leg injuries. (A) Cardboard plate is cut to fit the foot and is padded with cotton wrap and covered with tape. (B) Foot pad is placed against the bottom of the foot with the toes properly positioned and in extension. (C and D) Foot pad is wrapped in place with cotton padding. (E) Cotton padding is covered with Vetrap. (F) Completed bandage. (Permission for drawing use granted by the Georgia Department of Natural Resources and Branson Ritchie, DVM, MS.)

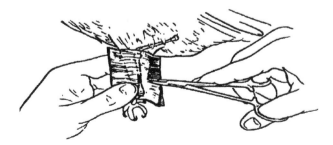

Figure 30.10 Tape splint used for fracture immobilization in the lower leg bones of small birds. Tape is placed on each side of the leg with the sticky sides facing each other. The tape is pressed together with hemostats. (Permission for drawing use granted by the Georgia Department of Natural Resources and Branson Ritchie, DVM, MS.)

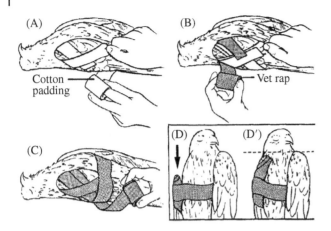

(A) Cotton padding

(B) Vet rap

(C)

(D) (D')

Figure 30.12 Figure-eight bandage used for the immobilization of the avian wing. (A) Cotton padding is wrapped from the carpus to the humerus and back to the carpus. (B) The same pattern is repeated with Vetrap. (C) Vetrap is passed around the midbody and taped in place. (D) A properly bandaged wing should be held at the same level as the normal wing. (D') If the wing drops below the level of the normal wing, the bandage should be removed and reapplied. (Permission for drawing use granted by the Georgia Department of Natural Resources and Branson Ritchie, DVM, MS.)

The figure-eight bandage holds the wing closed in a natural position and is adequate to immobilize a fracture on any portion of the wing as well as to reduce the weight of the wing on the shoulder. If the fracture involves the humerus, continue the wing bandage around the body to immobilize the shoulder joint (joint above the fracture).

If using the body wrap, one must be sure to pass the tape under the good wing on the opposite side and across the body on the upper keel (Figure 30.12). The fit should be snug but not tight enough to interfere with respiration or circulation.

When this bandage is properly applied, the bird should be able to stand and perch while holding the wing in a normal anatomic position. All wing feathers should be in alignment as well. If the bandage pulls the wing in an abnormal position, the bandage should be removed and reapplied.

Bird bones heal much more quickly than mammal bones do so bandages usually only have to remain on for 2–3 weeks as long as the bird is confined to strict cage rest for several days after the bandage is removed. After this cage-rest period, the bird should have manual limb massage and gradual limb extensions. After a good callus is formed, the bird can be placed in a flight cage.

Housing Adult Birds

Make sure the housing is as stress-free as possible. Cover the fronts of all bird caging and if possible give the bird natural materials to hide in. Reptilariums® (under mesh cages in Appendix 10) and the collapsible framed, mesh laundry hampers (available at discount stores) make excellent injured adult bird caging due to their soft-sided, feather-protecting material and lightweight. Reptilariums® have the additional benefit of being machine washable.

Perching of various heights should be provided if the bird is capable of standing.

As soon as its hospital stay is over, the patient should be transferred over to the rehabilitator in order to be housed in an appropriate aviary.

Feeding Adult Birds

Adult birds should be encouraged to eat on their own by providing natural food items that they may recognize. One can use whole berries, millet sprays, seed mixes, and live insects along with grains, cracked corn, bran, and chopped fruits. A stressed bird usually will not eat, so noise, bright lights, visual disturbances, and extreme temperatures should be reduced to allow the avian patient to settle down and eat.

If after one day the bird has not eaten, it must be force-fed at least four times a day. This can be performed by gently placing a thumb and forefinger at the corners of the mouth and either pressing it to open or by using the other hand to open the mouth and placing food carefully down the throat behind the glottis. Most birds will swallow when food is placed back far enough. Use one of the homemade diets in the nestling care section for hand-feeding or Lafeber's Emeraid Psittacine (powdered diet for debilitated birds) for tube feeding. For prey-eating birds powdered diets such as Emeraid Carnivore or Oxbow Critical Care for Carnivores are good products for tube feeding.

Sometimes force-feeding a bird several times is all it takes to get it to start self-feeding. One should make sure it is eating enough and maintaining a healthy weight.

Live insects (wax worms, mealworms, and crickets) should be "gut-loaded" with healthy, nutritionally rich ingredients and not fed off the shelf from a bait store. When insects are purchased, they usually have eaten much of the food that was in the container they have been living in so they will need to be provided with at least 24 hours of nutrition before feeding them to wildlife patients. Mealworms can be put into a plastic tub, with a ventilated lid, at room temperature with coarsely ground whole grains such as corn meal, rolled oats, wheat bran, or game bird starter. For moisture, a cut-up potato can be added to the top of the mixture. Crickets and wax worms can also eat this mixture.

Fresh-dug earthworms are also good to offer insectivorous or omnivorous birds, especially robins, thrashers, ducks, thrushes, jays, and mockingbirds.

See Appendix 6 for average weight of selected North American songbirds.

Precocial Bird Basic Care

At hatching, precocial birds are covered in feather down, are self-feeding, are ready to leave the nest, and can see, hear, run, and swim. These baby birds have no flanges on the sides of the mouth and have small, developed wings. The eggs of the precocial bird contain more nutrients and require more time to hatch, but the chick hatches out fully developed.

These birds (ducks, geese, killdeer, pheasant, quail, woodcock, and other shorebirds) have different dietary and housing needs from that of altricial birds.

Initial Orphan Care

One should never feed any animal until it is warm. An incubator, brooder, or heat light should be used to warm up a chilled infant. Despite their downy covering, precocial chicks need to be kept at slightly warmer ambient air temperature than altricial ones.

Newborn chick (0–7 days): 90–95°F
Chicks developing quills: 85–90°F
Birds with quills and developing feathers: 60–85°F

These chicks, if healthy, will usually readily eat and drink on their own. They are social and eat better in groups of similar species and ages.

If the chick is not eating, its dehydration and temperature should be checked. Some chicks can be quite nervous, and covering the box or cage with a towel may help them to eat.

If the bird is dehydrated, it can be offered drops of Pedialyte every 15 minutes for the first several hours or until it passes a normal stool. The fluid may have to be placed into the throat beyond the glottis if the baby is weak and dehydrated.

The bird should be examined for injuries, cuts, mites, or wounds.

Species identification should be determined in order to determine its proper diet and feeding schedule. One should begin offering the infant hand-rearing formula.

Identification

A bird rehabilitator should be contacted to help identify the species. Field guides may also be helpful. Ducks and some dabbling water birds have webbed feet or toes. Hatchling wood ducks have a visible egg tooth on the tip of the bill. Most shorebirds have very long legs and can run quite fast.

One should be sure to look at the beak shape. Ducks and geese have wide, flat bills while the killdeer have thinner, tapered beaks (Figure 30.13). Quails and pheasant have short, sturdy, and conical beaks.

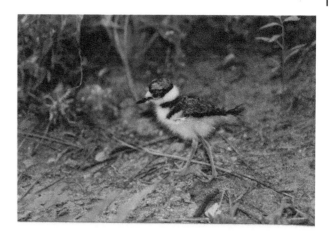

Figure 30.13 One-week-old killdeer. (Courtesy of Melanie Haire.)

Housing

A box or plastic tote lined with newspaper covered with either paper towels or ravel-free cloth towels will do. The container should be covered with a screen top because some ducks (wood ducks) can jump very high. These birds are messy and cardboard will become soiled and need to be replaced often.

A wild bird should never be housed in a wire pet bird or mammal cage. A ceramic brooder-heating element or a brooder heat light can be hung in one half of the cage, making sure the enclosure is large to allow the birds to move in and out of the heated area.

It is very important to provide these birds with hiding places, such as a small box on its side. One can hang a feather duster down inside the cage so babies can snuggle up under it for security, shelter, and comfort. All these cage items will get soiled and need to be cleaned and kept dry as possible.

Waterfowl will splash in the water bowl and then seek the heat lamp to dry off underneath. As the birds grow feathers and spend less time under the lamp, it can be gradually raised up until you wean the birds off of the supplemental heat.

Do not provide waterfowl with a pool unless directed to do so by an avian rehabilitator. Baby ducks and geese should never be left unattended during swimming time. If instructed to provide "swim time," a painter's roller tray can be used that will provide a ramp and shallow swimming area.

These young chicks need appropriate shelter and a quiet room to prevent stress that can oftentimes be fatal.

As they grow, so should their housing. Older juveniles and adults need to have a large outside predator-proof pen with a pool. This type of setup cannot usually be provided at a veterinary clinic or at most people's homes so transferring the birds to the rehabilitator or wildlife center is recommended.

Feeding

Food and water bowls should be placed on the side away from the heat.

Caution must be used with the selection of water bowl used to prevent babies getting soaked and chilled. Using a Mason jar filled with water and inverted over a shallow lid or a commercial chicken waterer (available at most feed and farm stores) works well. A small water bowl filled three-fourths full with rocks or marbles also provides a readily available drinking source and keeps the babies from jumping into the water.

Food varies slightly between species but most do well on crumbled unmedicated chicken starter. One can sprinkle some on the cage floor as well as provide some in a food bowl.

A very young, single chick may be unsure how and what to eat. It learns these skills by watching and imitating its mother. Other bird rehabilitators should be contacted immediately to locate another chick to place it with. Sometimes these birds will need to be force-fed until placement can be found. In the meantime, one can try to teach the youngster by "pecking" at the food with a finger. Food in motion also seems to help stimulate feeding behavior so the grain can be gently rolled around and tiny live mealworms, earthworms, or crickets offered to inspire the infant to begin to peck. Also, floating chopped greens and small amounts of chick starter on water tends to stimulate unsure waterfowl.

The food should be changed twice a day, and one can begin offering small live mealworms, chopped greens and berries, cracked corn, and crickets as the babies grow. Fresh food should always be available, as the birds will eat free choice.

Adult Precocial Birds (Including Waterfowl and Wading Birds)

Identification of the species and familiarity with its natural history, food preferences, and habitat is required.

An examination for injuries should be performed. Care must be taken of the water birds with long pointed beaks. Herons, cranes, kingfishers, loons, and egrets will stab at faces and eyes when feeling threatened. Smaller birds such as grebes, coots, gulls, and rails can strike very quickly with short sturdy beaks and give quite a pinch as well. Coots will kick and use the spurs on their legs to defend themselves.

Ducks, geese, and swans can be difficult to restrain as well due to their strength and size. These birds will bite and twist with their powerful bills as well as beat at their restrainer with their very powerful wings.

One should take precautions, wear goggles, secure their heads, and work in pairs when restraining these animals. Even the small species are surprisingly strong and difficult to restrain.

Examination, body temperatures, hydration, and treatments are similar to other adult birds. See Chapter 4, "Psittacines and Passerines."

These species are particularly susceptible to lead poisoning (from ingesting fishing sinkers and lead birdshot used for duck hunting), fish hook ingestion, monofilament entanglement, and botulism due to their aquatic nature.

Diving birds (grebes, some sea ducks, loons, etc.) are built for floating, swimming, and diving but not walking, so many times these birds are presented with "broken legs" because they will not or cannot stand. The legs of these birds are positioned far back on the body for propelling through the water instead of underneath the body for walking. Many times these birds get tired during migrational movements and come down for a rest. If a loon lands on a wet pavement or parking lot thinking it looked like water, it has no way to take off again. Many times these birds just need a few meals and to be placed on a large body of water to allow for takeoff. This is a good example of why learning about a patient's natural history is so important.

Housing

If a water bird needs to be housed, a plastic pet kennel works well. Due to the large volume of liquid stool they produce, keeping the pen clean can be challenging. If the bird is too weak to hold itself upright or has a fractured leg, placing it in a box half filled with shredded newspapers makes a good body support setup and also allows the feces to drop away from the bird, which keeps the feathers and vent clean.

Water birds must keep their feathers in perfect condition and naturally do so by constant preening and bathing. If the birds are strong enough and do not have a bandage on, they can be provided with a bath-water source either in the enclosure or in a sink or tub to allow them to bathe and keep their feathers waterproof. Caution should be used with pools because even ducks can drown, especially if they are weak or not waterproof. It may be best to transfer these birds out as soon as possible and allow the rehabilitator to do this process.

Many water-type birds do not have feet designed for long-term perching. A kennel, box, or mesh cage can have a flat "shelf-type" perch or a split log available to those who feel comfortable standing up off the ground.

These adult birds, especially the herons, rails, and egrets, are quite nervous and will pace and wear themselves out trying to escape if they do not feel secure and hidden. These birds should be provided with the quietest place possible with covering on all sides of the caging.

Feeding

Although the commercial game bird grain mixes are sufficient in nutrition for short-term care of many of these species, getting them to eat it is the biggest challenge. These birds, with the possible exception of some ducks and geese, tend to be very difficult captive feeders. One problem is that many are normally used to feeding in or while on the water. Sitting on a towel in a box is too unnatural for them, and they do not understand the concept of eating with a bowl of food in front of them. Also, due to their nervous nature, they might not ever feel secure enough to eat.

Oftentimes these species will need to be tube-fed or force-fed while they remain in captivity. Kingfishers, herons, and gulls must be fed fish, insects, and/or mice. To force-feed a fish, one must be sure to insert the fish head-first into the bird's mouth and gently push the fish down the throat until the bird swallows. Holding the head in an upright position for several moments after feeding each fish may help prevent the bird from regurgitating the meal.

Several tube-feeding formulas that can be used depending on the diet requirements of the species include Emeraid ground game bird pellets mixed with water, or blended fish.

All the medical procedures, cleaning, moving, and so on should be done before feeding is attempted. Feeding should always be the last procedure done on any animal and should be immediately followed by low-stress, quiet, and privacy to aid the animal in the digestion process. Sudden loud noises or big movements may cause the animal to regurgitate the food and possibly even aspirate it.

Some fish eaters will learn to fish live minnows or goldfish out of a pan or bucket. Ducks, geese, coots, shorebirds, and similar species may eat live insects and chopped greens if provided in addition to the grain diet. Another hint is to float grain, insects, and greens on top of a dish of water. Sometimes this more natural presentation stimulates the birds to stab or dabble at the groceries.

General Orphan Mammal Care

What to Do First

One should never feed any animal until it is warm and hydrated. A heat lamp, heating pad on low and always under cage not inside, or warm water bath to warm up a cold baby should be used. Once the baby is at normal body temperature, then one can start to rehydrate it.

Use of oral fluids such as LRS or Pedialyte is the preferred method of rehydration with infants. Subcutaneous fluids (LRS) can be used if the animal is moderately dehydrated. One should consider all animals that come into rehabilitation to be dehydrated to some extent. Fluids should always be warmed first before administering regardless of route.

The infant should be weighed and fluids provided at the rate of 40–50 mL/kg over a 12–24 period or until hydration is complete. See fluid chart in the glossary in Appendix 9 under "Dehydration."

Introducing Formula

Once the baby animal is warm and properly hydrated, feeding formula can gradually begin. It should be introduced slowly to prevent digestive problems.

One should never start an animal on full-strength formula. It should take 24–72 hours to introduce a milk formula depending on the degree of initial dehydration. A severely dehydrated animal's digestive tract cannot handle full-strength or solid foods. Feeding these food items prematurely could prove to be fatal.

The following dilution procedure should be followed:

Day 1: 25% full-strength formula/75% water or Pedialyte
Day 2: 50% full-strength formula/50% water or Pedialyte
Day 3: 75% full-strength formula/25% water or Pedialyte; or, 100% full-strength formula, if no diarrhea develops and infant remains hydrated

If diarrhea or bloating develops, at any stage, the concentration of formula should be reduced or replaced entirely with Pedialyte until the situation clears up. If problems persist for more than 24 hours, veterinary advice should be sought.

If bloating occurs, one can gently massage the infant's abdomen while submerging the bottom half of the infant's body in a warm water bath. One can also consider giving oral simethicone drops for gas relief if the massaging is not completely effective.

Using a probiotic (Lactobacillus) product, such as Benebac, can be helpful to reduce stress on the babies' intestinal tract and help prevent or treat diarrhea.

If the neonate regurgitates formula, feeding should be discontinued and that feeding skipped altogether. At the next feeding, the formula can be thinned with water by half and the volume reduced. If the vomiting continues, veterinary advice should be sought.

Preparing Formulas

Milk formulas should be mixed by the label's instructions using warm water to help dissolve the powdered

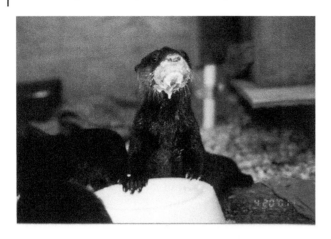

Figure 30.14 Three-month-old river otter enjoying a bowl of Esbilac milk formula. (Courtesy of Melanie Haire.)

milk. Ready-to-use liquid formulas are also available, but they tend to be more expensive. Once the can is opened, unused milk must be discarded after 72 hours making this sometimes wasteful (Figure 30.14).

Enough milk formula should be made up to last for 24 hours and kept refrigerated. When ready to feed, only enough should be heated for one feeding to 100–102°F (warm but not hot on a wrist). One way to warm formula is to drop formula-filled syringes into a mug of warm water. Using an electric coffee mug warmer may be helpful to keep multiple syringes warm. Also, one should remember to cap syringes or milk will leak out and mug water will refill syringe resulting in diluted formula.

Do not use the microwave to heat formula. This method tends to cook the milk and leaves contents unevenly heated.

The infant should be weighed and the species care pages in the appendix used to determine quantity of food intake.

Some infants prefer to be stimulated to urinate and defecate prior to feeding. Use of a cotton ball or soft facial tissue dipped in warm water to lightly wipe babies' abdomen and genitals will suffice. This process also seems to stimulate the nursing reflex in some species.

Selecting Milk Formulas

There are many brands of milk replacers available as well as many variations of how to use them. Again, this is where contacting a local rehabilitator becomes critical. The importance of using the correct diet cannot be stressed enough. One should try not to switch formulas unless the baby is having trouble digesting the milk replacer chosen. By using the same formula that the rehabilitator will be using, the animal transfer process will be made much easier on the infant.

Of the many commercial formulas available, no one milk substitute will meet the needs of all species. Substitute

domestic animal milk formulas for puppies, kittens, lambs, and foals have been successfully used. Recently a commercial line of milk replacers, formulated for wildlife, has become available. Due to space limitations, this chapter will not cover detailed wildlife nutritional requirements and comparisons. One should refer to the species care sheets in Appendix 7 for general diet guidelines. There are good reference articles and books available through the NWRA and IWRC on wildlife nutritional requirements.

The company Pet-Ag has been manufacturing milk replacer products since 1930 and most of the wildlife nutritional studies have been done on their products (e.g., Esbilac, KMR, Multi-Milk, Zoological Milk Matrix).

Homemade formulas are sometimes used but these rarely meet the complete nutritional requirements for wildlife. Cow's milk is not compatible with the natural milk of most wild animals and tends to cause gastrointestinal problems.

Syringe Feeding

Use the smallest size syringe that will hold the needed volume of formula. This provides the most accurate measurement of the animal's formula intake and the best flow control.

Many animals resist the first few feeding attempts due to the newness of the plastic feeder and the taste of the formula. However, after several feedings, they begin to accept their foster care (Figure 30.15).

Use of a soft rubber nipple (Catac) or silicone nipple (Mothering Kit) on the end of the syringe often helps facilitate the feedings. To help keep the nipple from slipping off the syringe tip, one needs to remember to wipe the syringe's slip tip dry and roughen the surface up slightly

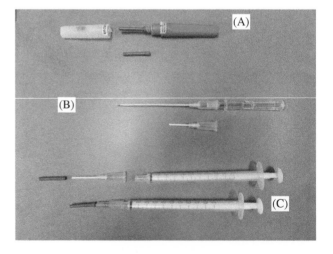

Figure 30.15 "Preemie" feeding nipple. (A) A multiple sample collection needle. (B) 16 gauge IV indwelling catheter. (C) Assembled. (Courtesy of Melanie Haire.)

with a hemostat before slipping the nipple on. One needs to make sure that an overeager youngster does not pull the nipple all the way off and choke on it. Also, once rodents' incisors appear, discontinued use of the nipple may be necessary due to their ability to chew the tip off and possibly ingest it.

In the case of the tiny neonate (i.e., newborn chipmunk, flying squirrels, mice), a handmade "preemie nipple" can be made from two common veterinary supplies. A size 16 gauge intravenous indwelling catheter cut off about one-half inch from the end can be used as the base for the nipple apparatus as it fits onto any slip-tipped syringe. The nipple is made from the rubber sleeve that covers the needle of a multiple-sample blood collection needle used to draw blood. First, the rubber sleeve should be pulled down and punctured with the collection needle to make the nipple hole. Then the sleeve is pulled off of the blood collection device and slipped over the cut catheter. A size 16-gauge catheter provides a snug fit for the nipple, and the apparatus is ready to attach to the feeding syringe (Figure 30.16).

Other feeding syringe attachment examples are tomcat catheters, feeding tubes, or teat infusion cannulas.

Any slip-tip syringe will work but the O-ring type syringe is much smoother, and the rubber plunger does not stick and wear out as fast as the regular plungers do. (See suppliers list in Appendix 10.)

Slow and steady pressure on the base of the syringe should be used to allow infants to drink small amounts at a time. Some species will nurse (i.e., squirrels, chipmunks, raccoons, and beavers) while others may lap (i.e., cottontails, opossums, and mink) at the tip of the nipple or syringe.

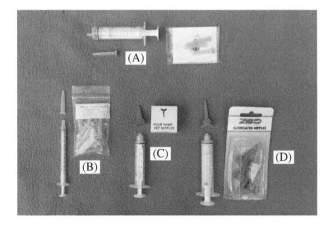

Figure 30.16 (A) Rubber Catac® nipples with slip tip syringe. (B) Silicone nipples with slip tip syringe. (C) Four Paws Vet nipples with Luer lock syringe. (D) Zoologic elongated nipple with Luer lock syringe.

Use the following methods to help control the formula flow rate:

To increase flow rate

- Apply more pressure on syringe.
- Allow air into the syringe.
- Enlarge the opening of the syringe tip or nipple.
- Thin down the formula.
- Use a larger size syringe.

To decrease flow rate

- Hold back on the syringe plunger.
- Remove air from syringe.
- Use another nipple with a smaller hole.
- Add rice baby cereal to thicken formula.
- Use a smaller-size syringe.

Each animal is different, and one may need several different syringes and nipple combinations even when feeding littermates. Individual infants may drink too quickly regardless of what is done and the syringe will have to be moved away every few seconds to reduce the chance of the baby choking or aspirating formula.

Other Feeding Implements

Bottle feeding can be used for some species of animals. Pet nursers and puppy and kitten bottles are sometimes used with small wildlife such as squirrels and rabbits. Human baby bottles and nipples will work for such species as large felids, canids, older raccoons, and otters. Neonatal carnivores should be started out on a human premature-infant-sized nipple. Hoofstock prefer a goat/foal-type nipple and bottle due to the size and shape of their mouths. This method offers a faster formula delivery system but less control over milk flow speed and quantity.

One needs to remember to make the size of the nipple hole appropriate for the animal at hand. Holes can be made in the nipple by several methods. By cutting the tip off with scissors or cutting an "x" into the tip, different flow patterns are created. To create a very small round hole, an appropriate-sized gauge needle is heated with the beveled tip in the flame. When the needle tip is hot, allow it to melt through the center of the end of the nipple. With the needle still in place, the entire apparatus should be placed in cold water until cool. Once the needle is removed, the hole remains approximately the same size as the needle gauge.

Eyedroppers can be used for hand-feeding but tend to produce air bubbles and make the milk flow difficult to control.

Gavage feeding, or stomach tubing, is another option for difficult feeders, such as armadillos, opossums, and nervous cottontails, who do not suck or drink consistently from other implements.

Stomach tubing can also be a lifesaving technique used with older juveniles and adult mammals but can also be the most difficult to do correctly and safely. When using the stomach tube method, one should never feed more than the calculated stomach capacity volume. It should be kept in mind that an emaciated animal's stomach capacity may be reduced by as much as 50%. Due to space limitation of this chapter, the gavage technique will not be covered here. This method is covered in chapter 9 under "Techniques."

Feeding Procedure

Infant mammals should be fed in an upright position on a soft, warm surface. Some babies like to feel secure and be wrapped in a cloth. They should never be fed on their backs as this could result in aspiration of the formula (Figure 30.17).

Mammals should be fed their calculated amounts until their stomachs are rounded but not tight. One should never overfeed a baby as it can lead to diarrhea, bloating, and perhaps death.

Even with every effect made, occasionally babies will aspirate formula and get milk in their nose or lungs. If this happens, feeding should immediately be discontinued, and the baby should be turned nose down and lightly tapped on its back. Any bubbles or drops should immediately be wiped off as they come out of the infant's nose or mouth to prevent reinhalation.

Once fed, all formula needs to be wiped off of the mammal. Allowing the milk to dry on the skin or hair of an infant can result in hair loss or skin infections. If the baby was not stimulated to eliminate before the feeding, it should be done afterward. One can gently stroke the belly

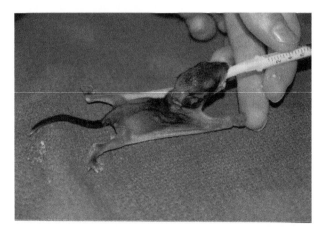

Figure 30.17 Three-week-old flying squirrel being fed with a silicone nipple and syringe. (Courtesy of Melanie Haire.)

and anal area with a warm, moist cloth until the flow stops. After about a minute, stimulation should be discontinued whether the baby has defecated or not. When the infant's eyes are open and there is evidence that it is eliminating on its own, stimulation can be discontinued. Any uneaten formula should be thrown away, as reheated milk should never be saved.

All feeding implements should be cleaned with hot soapy water after each feeding and a bottlebrush used to remove milk residue from hard-to-reach places inside the syringes/bottles. Syringes, bottles, and nipples should be disinfected once daily by soaking in an appropriate cleaning solution such as diluted 10% Nolvasan or 5% bleach for 10–15 minutes followed by a thorough rinse.

All items should be allowed to completely dry before each use to reduce the chance of bacterial overgrowth. Once they are cleaned and rinsed, feeding materials should be stored on an absorbent material such as a clean hand or paper towel or in a drying rack until the next feeding.

Orphan Mammal Housing

Most eyes-closed mammal infants can be housed in an incubator generally kept at 85–95°F. A set of plans to make an incubator is available online at the IWRC website: www.iwrc-online.org. A homemade incubator can be made from a lidded plastic tote with ventilation holes. Some rehabilitators use glass or plastic aquariums, cardboard boxes, plastic pet carriers, or laundry baskets, of appropriate height and size, for this stage. A heating pad set on low, placed a quarter of the way to halfway under the tote, can provide the heat, and a water-soaked sponge placed in a plastic container with holes for evaporation can provide the humidity. One should make sure that moisture does not collect on the inside of the incubator by providing enough ventilation. A heat lamp can be used in place of a heating pad but both should never be used at the same time (Figure 30.18).

A soft, ravel-free cloth such as cotton T-shirt, sweatshirt, or flannel or fleece material can be considered for bedding. Terry cloth should never be used because their fingers, toes, and nails are too easily caught and twisted in the loops.

When the mammals become more active, they can be placed in a larger enclosure to allow for more room to exercise, dig, or climb. Once their eyes are open, baby mammals tend to become more active and they begin to explore their surroundings. One needs to be careful that the adventurous youngster cannot escape out of too-large kennel door holes or unsecured cage lids. The supplemental heat and humidity can be removed when the baby is

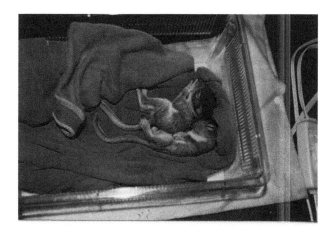

Figure 30.18 Two four-week-old gray squirrels on supplemental heat. (Courtesy of Melanie Haire.)

furred, able to thermoregulate, and spends most of its time away from the heat. This time varies from species to species and even from individual to individual.

Once the heat is no longer needed, one should begin to acclimate the babies by placing their cage outside for short periods of time at first and then gradually lengthening the time. Caution and common sense should be used with the placement of the cage, and one should be watchful for predators and sudden inclement weather and be sure to provide shade. The acclimation process usually can wait until the animal has been transferred to the rehabilitator's facility. Features such as nest boxes, hammocks, shelves, and natural items can be added to the cage at this stage.

The next phase usually begins once the mammals are weaned, eating natural foods, acclimated to the outside temperatures, and grown out of their cage. Preparing them for release by placing them in the large prerelease cages should be done at the rehabilitator's facility.

Recommended housing materials, sizes, and standards are also available online at the IWRC website, www.iwrc-online.org.

Species Care Sheets

The species summary sheets provided in Appendix 7 are meant for quick reference only. Entire books have been written on the care of each of these species and, whenever possible, one should refer to more than one source for more complete and detailed care. The charts are included to serve as a summary of age determinators and growth characteristics to provide the technician with enough general information to accurately confirm age and thus temporarily care for the most common species. Due to regional variations, standardized weights and infant developmental patterns are difficult to predict. Factors such as geographical location, subspecies, weather, season, and quantity and quality of food are just a few things that determine how fast or large an animal can grow. The species care sheets in Appendix 7 should only be referred to after reading the general orphan mammal care section. See Appendix 10 for a list of products mentioned in this chapter.

Acknowledgments

Avian illustrations (Figures 30.2, 30.3, and 30.4): Illustrated by Linda A. Orebaugh, MS, AMI, from the *Care and Rehabilitation of Injured Native Wildlife training manual*. Permission for use granted by the Georgia Department of Natural Resources & Branson W. Richie, DVM, MS.

Raptor Tail Wrap Procedure (Appendix 4): from *Raptor Rehabilitation, A Manual of Guidelines Offered by the Carolina Raptor Center*. Permission to use granted by Mathias Engelmann and Pat Marcum.

State and Federal Wildlife Permit Offices Lists (appendix 1): International Wildlife Rehabilitation Council Membership Directory 2001. Names and numbers are likely to change.

Raptor Restraint Illustration (Figure 30.1): Illustrated by George Carpenter. *Raptor Restraint, Handling, and Transport Methods* by Terry A. Schulz from the NWRA Volume 8 Symposium Proceedings. Permission for use granted by the National Wildlife Rehabilitators Association.

Photos: by Melanie Haire

Admission, Examination, and Animal Care Record Forms (Appendix 2): by Janet Howard

Handling and Restraint of Wildlife Species Paper: by Florina S. Tseng, DVM, from IWRC 1991 Conference Proceedings. Permission granted for use by International Wildlife Rehabilitation Council.

Guide to Identification of Hatchling and Nestling Songbirds (Appendix 5): by Marty Johnson from *NWRA Principles of Wildlife Rehabilitation, The Essential Guide for Novice and Experienced Rehabilitators*. Permission granted for use by the National Wildlife Rehabilitators Association.

Special Thanks: To Michael Haire, Veola Herron, Michael Ellis, Mike Fost, and Sue Barnard for all their help.

References

Beaver P. 1984. *Imprinting and Wildlife Rehabilitation*. Suisun, CA: International Wildlife Rehabilitation Council.

Crawford WC. 1988. Hand rearing birds of prey. In: *IWRC Proceedings*, pp. 1–6. Suisan, CA: International Wildlife Rehabilitation Council.

Diehl S, Stokhaug C. 1991. Release criteria for rehabilitated wild animals. In: *Symposium Proceedings*, pp. 159–81. St. Cloud: National Rehabilitators Association.

Dunning JB. 1984. *Body Weights of 686 Species of North American Birds*. Suisun, CA: IWRC.

Evans RH. 1986. Care and feeding of orphan mammals and birds. In: *Current Veterinary Therapy IX* (ed RB Kirk). Philadelphia: W.B. Saunders Co.

Fowler ME. 1986. *Zoo and Wild Animal Medicine*, 2nd edn. Philadelphia: W.B. Saunders Co.

Ivie D. 1999. Individual bird rehabilitator personal communication.

Johnson V. 1991. *Wild Animal and Rehabilitation Manual*. Kalamazo: Beech Leaf Press, Kalamazoo Nature Center.

Klinghammer E. 1991. Imprint and early experience: how to avoid problems with tame animals. *Symposium Proceedings*. St. Cloud: National Wildlife Rehabilitators Association.

Moore AT, Joosten, S. 1995. Euthanasia—the three stages of euthanasia. In: *NWRA—Principles of Wildlife Rehabilitation, The Essential Guide for Novice and Experienced Rehabilitators*. St. Cloud: National Wildlife Rehabilitators Association.

Pokras M. 1995. *NWRA—Principles of Wildlife Rehabilitation, Introduction*. St. Cloud: National Wildlife Rehabilitators Association.

Additional Reading

Adams P, Johnson V, Goodrich P, Haas R. 1991. *Wild Animal Care and Rehabilitation Manual*. Kalamazoo: Beech Leaf Press, Kalamazoo Nature Center.

Campbell TW. 1995. Raptor rehabilitation in the private veterinary hospital. In: *Exotic Animals: A Veterinary Handbook*, pp. 121–25. Trenton: Veterinary Learning Systems Co., Inc.

Chapman JA, Feldhamer, GA (eds). 1982. *Wild Mammals of North America*. Baltimore: Johns Hopkins University Press.

Ehrlich PR, Dobkin DS, Wheye D. 1988. *The Birder's Handbook, A Field Guide to the Natural History of North American Birds*. Fireside: Simon & Schuster.

Engelmann M, Marcum P. 1993. *Raptor Rehabilitation, A Manual of Guidelines Offered by the Carolina Raptor Center*. Charlotte: Carolina Raptor Center.

Evans AT, Evans RH. 1995. Rearing raccoons for release: Part II: Rehabilitation and diet. *Vet Tech* 6(6): 296–306.

Evans RH. 1987. Rearing orphaned wild mammals. *Vet Clin N Am Small Anim Pract* 17(3): 755–783.

Fowler ME. 1979. Care of orphaned wild animals. *Vet Clin N Am Small Anim Pract* 9(3): 447–70.

Fowler ME. 1983. *Restraint and Handling of Wild and Domestic Animals*. Ames: Iowa State University Press.

Hanes PC. 1988. Hand-rearing infant tree squirrels. In: *IWRC 1988 Proceedings*, pp. 77–93. Suisun, CA: International Rehabilitation Council.

Merritt JF. 1987. *Guide to the Mammals of Pennsylvania*. Pittsburgh: University of Pittsburgh Press.

Morzenti A. 1998. *Captive Raptor Management*. Madison: Omnipress.

Raley P. 1991. *Primer of Wildlife Care and Rehabilitation*. Troy: Brukner Nature Center.

Rue LL. 1981. *Furbearing Animals of North America*. New York: Crown Publishers, Inc.

Schwartz CW, Schwartz ER. 1974. *Mammals of Missouri*. Columbia: University of Missouri Press.

Stokes D, Stokes L. 1979. *Stokes Nature Guides, A Guide to Bird Behavior*, Vols 1–3. Boston: Little Brown & Co.

Stokes D, Stokes L. 1986. *Stokes Nature Guides, A Guide to Animal Tracking and Behavior*. Boston: Little Brown & Co.

Wasserman J. 1988. Raising orphaned flying squirrels. In: *IWRC 1988 Proceedings*. Suisun, CA: International Wildlife Rehabilitation Council.

White J. 2000. *IWRC—Basic Wildlife Rehabilitation 1AB Skills Manual*. Suisun, CA: International Wildlife Rehabilitation Council.

Section IX

Appendices

Appendix 1

State/Federal Wildlife Permit Offices

State and U.S. Territory Wildlife Permit Offices

Listings are alphabetical by state or territory.

Alabama Dept. of Conservation, Division of Wildlife/Freshwater Fisheries, 64 N Union St., Ste 584, Montgomery, AL 36134; 334-242-3467; Marianne.Hudson@dcnr.alabama.gov.

Director of Wildlife Conservation, Department of Fish and Game, PO Box 115526, Juneau, AK 99811-5526; 907-465-4148.

Mike Delmong, Wildlife Center Coordinator, Arizona Game and Fish Department, 50000 W Carefree Hwy, Phoenix, AZ 85086-5000; 623-582-9806; mdelmong@azgfd.gov.

Karen Rowe, Wildlife Permit Officer, AR Game and Fish Commission, PO Box 529, Casscoe, AR 72026; 870-873-4302; krowe@agfc.state.ar.us.

Nicole Carion, CA Department of Fish and Game, 601 Locust St., Redding CA 96001; 530-357-3986; Nicole.carion@wildlife.ca.gov.

Libby Henits, CPW/Special Licensing, 6060 Broadway, Denver, CO 80216; 303-291-7143; libby.henits@state.co.us.

Wildlife Permit Officer-Laurie Fortin, Department of Env. Protection, Wildlife Division, 79 Elm St., Hartford, CT 06106-5127; 860-424-3011; laurie.fortin@ct.gov.

Program Manager, Division of Fish and Wildlife, 6180 Hay Pt Landing Rd, Smyrna, DE 19977; 302-735-3600; Dawn.Webb@state.de.us.

Wildlife Permit Officer, Florida Fish and Wildlife Conservation Commission, 620 S. Meridian St., Tallahassee, FL 32399-1600; 850-488-6253; Loren.lowe@myfwc.com.

Special Permit Unit, Georgia DNR, Wildlife Resources Division, 2065 US Hwy 278 SE, Social Circle, GA 30025; 770-761-3044; Jamie.hawkins@dnr.state.ga.us.

HI Div of Forestry and Wildlife, 1151 Punchbowl St., Rm 325, Honolulu, HI 96813; 808-587-0163; james.m.cogswell@hawaii.gov.

Jon Rachael, Idaho Department of Fish and Game, PO Box 25, Boise, ID 83707; 208-287-2795; jon.rachael@idfg.idaho.gov.

Brian Clark, Department of Natural Resources, 1 Natural Resources Way, Springfield, IL 62702-1271; 217-785-5740; brian.clark@illinois.gov.

Linnea Petercheff, Wildlife Permit Officer, IN DNR, 402 W. Washington St., #W273, Indianapolis, IN 46204-2781; 317-233-6527; lpetercheff@dnr.in.gov.

IA DNR, Wallace State Office Bldg., 502 E 9th St., Des Moines, IA 50319-0034; 515-281-8524; Kelly.poole@dnr.iowa.gov.

Wildlife Permit Officer, FW Division, KS Department of Wildlife and Parks, 512 S.E. 25th Ave., Pratt, KS 67124-8174; 620-672-5911; becky.doyle@ksoutdoors.com.

Wildlife Permit Coordinator, KY Department of Fish and Wildlife Resources, #1 Sportsman's Ln, Frankfort, KY 40601; 502-564-3400; steven.dobey@ky.gov.

LDWF Non Game Program, PO Box 98000, Baton Rouge, LA 70898-9000; 225-763-3557, mcollins@wlf.lousiana.gov.

Susan Zayac, Department of Inland Fish and Wildlife, 284 State St., Station #41, Augusta, ME 04333-0041; 207-287-5240; susan.zayac@maine.gov.

Connie Roberts, DNR Wildlife & Heritage Services, 11701 Mountain Rd, Flintstone, MD 21530; 410-260-8540; croberts@dnr.state.md.us.

Tom French, Asst. Dir., Division of Fisheries and Wildlife, 1 Rabbit Hill Rd, Westbourough, MA 01583; 508-389-6355; tom.french@state.ma.us.

Casey Reitz, DNR Wildlife Division, PO Box 30444, Lansing, MI 48909-7531; 517-284-6210, reitzc@michigan.gov; www.michigan.gov/dnr.

Lori Naumann, DNR Nongame Wildlife Program, 500 Lafayette Rd., Box 25, St., Paul, MN 55155-4025; 651-259-5148; lori.naumann@dnr.state.mn.us.

Scott Peyton, Department of Wildlife, Fish and Parks, MS Museum of Nat. Science, 2148 Riverside Dr., Jackson, MS 39202-1353; 601-354-7303; scott.peyton@mmns.state.ms.us.

Exotic Animal Medicine for the Veterinary Technician, Fourth Edition. Edited by Bonnie Ballard and Ryan Cheek.
© 2024 John Wiley & Sons, Inc. Published 2024 by John Wiley & Sons, Inc.
Companion Website: www.wiley.com/go/ballard/4e

Tara Jennings, Missouri Department of Conservation, 2901 W Truman Blvd, PO Box 180, Jefferson City, MO 65102-0180; 573-751-4115, Tara.jennings@mdc.mo.gov.

Wildlife Permit Officer, MT Fish, Wildlife and Parks, 1420 E. Sixth Ave., PO Box 20071, Helena, MT 59601; 406-444-4595; fwpgen@mt.gov.

Nebraska Games & Parks, 2200 N 33rd St., Lincoln, NE 68503-1417; 402-471-0641; stephanie.patton@nebraska.gov.

License Office-Special Licenses, Nevada Dept of Wildlife, 6980 Sierra Center Pkwy St. 120, Reno, NV 95118; 775-688-1512; jmeadows@ndow.org.

Lt. Heidi Murphy, Wildlife Permit Officer, NH Fish & Game Dept., 11 Hazen Dr., Concord, NH 03301; 603-271-3127; Heidi.murphy@wildlife.nh.gov.

NJ Dept of Environmental Protection, Division of Fish & Wildlife, Mail code 501-03, PO Box 420, Trenton, NJ 08625; 609-984-0530; Krista.moser@dep.state.nj.us.

NM Department of Game and Fish, Special Use Permits Program, PO Box 25112, Santa Fe, NM 87504; 505-476-8066; dgf.permits@state.nm.us.

Paul R. Stringer, NYS Department Env. Con., 625 Broadway, Albany, NY 12233-4752; 518-402-8985; prstringer@gw.dec.state.ny.us.

North Carolina Wildlife Resources Commission, 1722 Mail Services Ctr, Raleigh, NC 27699-1722; 919-707-0050; tammy.rundle@ncwildlife.org.

Steve Dyke, ND Game and Fish Department, 100 N. Bismarck Expressway, Bismarck, ND 58501; 701-328-6347; ndgf@nd.gov.

Melissa Moser, Law Enforcement Division of Wildlife, 2045 Morse Rd., Bldg G, Columbus, OH 43229-6693; 614-254-6439; Melissa.moser@dnr.state.oh.us.

Law Enforcement Division, OK Department of Wildlife Conservation, PO Box 53465, Oklahoma City, OK 73152-3465; 405-521-3719; Sharon.lookabaugh@odwc.ok.gov.

Randi Lisle, Oregon Department of Fish and Wildlife, 4034 Fairview Industrial Dr. SE, Salem, OR 97302; 503-947-6303; Randi.j.listle@state.or.us.

Chad Eyler, Chief Special Permits, Enforcement Div. PA Game Commission, 2001 Elmerton Ave., Harrisburg, PA 17110-9797; 717-783-8164; pgccomments@pa.gov.

Wildlife Permit Officer, Division of Fish and Wildlife, 277 Great Neck Rd, West Kingston, RI 02892; 401-789-0281; Charles.brown@dem.ri.gov.

Wildlife Permit Coordinator, Sandhills Research and Education Center, PO Box 23205, Columbia, SC 29224-3205; 803-419-9645; licensing@dnr.sc.gov.

Wildlife Permit Officer, Game, Fish and Parks Department, Division of Wildlife, 20641 SD Hwy 1806, Fort Pierre, SD 57532; 605-773-4191.

Captive Wildlife Coordinator, Walter Cook, TWRA/Boating & Law Enforcement Division, 7294 Florence Rd, Smyma, TN 37167; 615-781-6652; walter.cook@tn.gov.

Megan Nelson, Wildlife Permits Specialist, Texas Parks and Wildlife Department, 4200 Smith School Rd., Austin, TX 78744-3291; 512-389-4481; wpoffice@tpwd.state.tx.us.

DNR Division of Wildlife Resources, 1594 W. North Temple, Suite 2110, PO Box 146301, Salt Lake City, UT 84114-6301; 801-538-4701; karencaldwell@utah.gov.

Hope Kanarvogel, Agency of Natural Resources, Fish and Wildlife Department, 1 National Life Dr., Davis 2, Montpelier, VT 05620-3702; 802-828-1254; Hope.kanarvogel@vermont.gov.

Dianne Waller, Virginia Dept of Game & Inland Fisheries, Permit Section, PO Box 90778, Henrico, VA 23228-0778; 804-367-9588; dgifweb@dgif.virginia.gov.

Judy Pierce, Division of Fish and Wildlife, 6291 Estate Nazareth 101, St. Thomas, VI 00802-1104; 340-775-6762.

Patricia Thompson, WA Department of Fish and Wildlife, 16018 Mill Creek Blvd., Mill Creek, WA 98012; 425-379-2302; patricia.thompson@dfw.wa.gov.

Wildlife Permit Officer, Division of Natural Resources Wildlife Resources, 1900 Kanawha Blvd., Bldg. 3, Rm. 816, Charleston, WV 25305; 304-558-2771; dnr.wildlife@wv.gov.

Wisconsin Dept of Natural Resources, Amanda Kamps, Wildlife Health Conservation, Specialist-Bureau of Wildlife, Management Division of Fish, Wildlife and Parks; 608-712-5280, amanda.kamps@wisconsin.gov.

Permitting Officer, Game and Fish Department, 5400 Bishop Blvd., Cheyenne, WY 82006; 307-777-4579; mark.nelson1@wyo.gov.

United States Migratory Bird Permit Offices

The following list includes only the US Fish and Wildlife Service Migratory Bird Permit Offices.

Region 1: HI, ID, OR, WA
Pacific Region Migratory Bird Permit Office, 911 N.E. 11th Ave., Portland, OR 97232-4181; 503-872-2715; permitsR1MB@fws.gov.

Region 2: AZ, NM, OK, TX
Migratory Bird Permit Office Southwest Region, PO Box 709, Albuquerque, NM 87103-0709; 505-248-7882; jmeadows@ndow.org.

Region 3: IL, IN, IA, MI, MN, MO, OH, WI
US Fish and Wildlife Service Migratory Bird Permit Office, 5600 American Blvd W, Bloomington, MN 55437; 612-713-5436; permitsjmeadows@ndow.org.

Region 4: AL, AR, FL, GA, KY, LA, MS, NC, SC, TN, VI, PR

Carmen Simonton, US Fish and Wildlife Service, Migratory Bird Permit Office, 1875 Century Blvd NE, Atlanta, GA 30345; 404-679-7049 permitsR4MB@fws.gov.

Region 5: CT, DE, ME, MD, MA, NH, NJ, NY, PA, RI, VT, VA, WV

Linda McKenna, Migratory Bird Permit Office Northeast Region 5, 300 Westgate Center Dr., Hadley, MA 01035-0779; 413-253-8643; linda_mckenna@fws.gov.

Region 6: CO, KS, MT, NE, ND, SD, UT, WY

US Fish and Wildlife Service, Migratory Bird Permit Office, PO Box 25486 DFC 60154, Denver, CO 80225-0486; 303-236-8171; permitsR6MB@fws.gov.

Region 7: AK

Beth Pattinson, US Fish and Wildlife Service, Migratory Bird Permit Office, 1011 E. Tudor Rd., Anchorage, AK 99503; 907-786-3459; beth_pattinson@fws.gov.

Region 8: CA, NV

Jennifer Brown, Migratory Bird Permit Specialist, Migratory Bird, Permit Office, 2800 Cottage Way, Room W-2606, Sacramento, CA 95825; 916-978-6183; Jennifer_c_brown@fws.gov.

National Permit Coordinator

Susan Lawrence, Division of Migratory Bird Management, 4401 N Fairfax Drive MBSP 4107, Arlington, VA 22203; 703-358-2016; susan_m_lawrence@fws.gov.

Appendix 2

Wildlife Admissions/Exam/Care Forms

Reproduced with acknowledgment to Janet Howard.

Admission Form

Clinic Name · Address · Phone Number

Date Admitted: _____ / _____ / _____   Case No. _____

Time Admitted: _____ AM / PM

Rescuer Information

Name: _____

Address: _____

City: _____ State: _____ Zip _____

Phone: _____

Do you wish to be contacted via email about the animal's status? ☐Yes ☐No

Email Address: _____

Animal Information

Species: _____   ☐ Young ☐ Adult

Date and time found: _____ / _____ / _____   Time: _____ AM / PM

Have you fed or medicated the animal? ☐No   ☐Yes, I gave it _____

Location Found: _____

Describe circumstances found: _____

Was anyone bitten or scratched by the animal ? ☐ Yes ☐No

Did you come in contact with blood/urine/feces/saliva? ☐ Yes ☐No

Other treatment/ comments: _____

Condition (Mark all that apply):

Cause of Admission:
(circle one)
- ☐ Cat / Dog Attack
- ☐ Hit by car
- ☐ Found on ground
- ☐ In road
- ☐ Abused
- ☐ Exposed to Chemicals
- ☐ Disease suspected
- ☐ Nest disturbed
- ☐ Hit window
- ☐ Shot
- ☐ Other: _____

Observations:
- ☐ Easy to catch
- ☐ Limping
- ☐ Can't stand
- ☐ Can't walk
- ☐ Panting
- ☐ Bleeding
- ☐ Wet
- ☐ Oiled
- ☐ Cold
- ☐ No apparent injury
- ☐ Other: _____

Describe condition: _____

_____

Disposition:

Date: _____ / _____ / _____

Circle One: R   TR   TD   TE   P   DOA   DIC   EOA   E

Location: _____

☐ US F&WS Notification (Illegal activity, E/TH species, B/G eagle) Date: _____

Examination Form
Clinic Name • Address • Phone Number

Case No.: _____
Date: _____ / _____ / _____   Time: _____ AM / PM

Basic Information:

Species: _____   Age: _____
Sex: ☐ Male ☐ Female   Weight: _____

Visual Observation:

Weight Distribution: ☐ Even ☐ Abnormal   Notes: _____
Movement/Attitude: ☐ Walks in circles ☐ Head tilt Notes: _____
Alertness: ☐ Comatose ☐ Lethargic ☐ Normal ☐ Excitable   Notes: _____
Body Condition: ☐ Emaciated   ☐ Underweight   ☐ Normal   ☐ Overweight

---

Temp: ☐ Hypothermic ☐ Cool   ☐ Normal ☐ Warm   ☐ Hyperthermic
Hydration: ☐ Severely dehydrated   ☐ Moderate dehydration ☐ Normal

---

Mouth: ☐ Normal ☐Plaque/lesions   ☐ Cap refill _____ seconds
    Notes:_____
Eyes: ☐ Follows movement ☐ Proper dilation ☐ Abrasions/Cuts ☐ Consensual
                                                                                      response
    Notes: _____
Ears: ☐ Normal ☐ Parasites ☐ Discharge/bleeding   Notes: _____
Nose: ☐ Normal ☐ Discharge/bleeding ☐ Cuts/abrasions Notes: _____
Fur/Skin: ☐ Cuts/wounds ☐ Abrasions ☐ Bald spots   ☐ Parasites Notes: _____

Gastrointestinal: ☐ Normal   ☐ Mouth odor ☐ Vomiting ☐ Blood
Urogenital: ☐ Normal   ☐ Discharge ☐ No urine/stool
Notes_____
Anal Area: ☐Normal ☐ Clogged ☐ Loose ☐ Parasites Notes: _____
Abdomen: ☐ Normal ☐ Bloated ☐ Painful ☐ Cuts/abrasions Notes: _____

Cardio/Pulmonary: ☐ HR _____/min.   ☐ RR _____/min.
    ☐ Cough ☐ Chest sounds Notes: _____
Muscular/Skeletal: ☐ Swelling ☐ Lameness ☐ Fractures/dislocation ☐ Pain
                                                                                      response

Animal Care Record

Clinic Name • Address • Phone Number

Case No.: _____

Species: _____   Description: _____

Weight Record

Date	Weight	Date	Weight	Date	Weight	Date	Weight

Feeding Chart

Date	Food Description	Amount per feeding	# Feedings Daily	Feeding Frequency	Comments

Treatment

Date	Medication/ Treatment	Comments/ Observations

Veterinary Care

Date	Description

Appendix 3

Handling and Restraint of Wildlife Species
Florina S. Tseng DVM

Introduction

Wildlife rehabilitation involves the care of sick, injured, and orphaned wildlife. These animals, while in captivity, require special husbandry practices—they must be transported, housed, and fed. When they are ill, they must be examined and treated. In addition, it will sometimes be necessary to relocate "nuisance" wildlife to more appropriate locations. All of these situations will necessitate the handling and restraint of wildlife species.

Considerations

Restraint can be as direct as holding the animal in your hands or as indirect as restriction of an animal's movement by fencing. The responsibility for the animal's welfare is in the hands of the rehabilitator. The amount of restraint on the animal should be as minimal as possible, yet enough to accomplish the purpose of the restraint and afford the handler maximum safety.

There are four basic considerations in the selection of a restraint technique:

A. Human safety always comes first in the execution of any capture or restraint plan. If a person is injured during an attempt to handle the animal, all attention will be focused on the care of that person and the capture will be unsuccessful.
B. Animal safety if the animal is hurt or dies during the capture/handling, you will not have achieved your goal!
C. Choose the proper technique to accomplish the desired result. Have you chosen a technique that is likely to work given the environment and the expected behavior of the species?
D. Can the animal be observed during and after the procedure? Observation of the animal during and after capture/handling and transport will allow you to act in a timely manner if problems arise, e.g., breathing difficulties, hyperthermia, etc.

In addition to the above basic considerations, there are also environmental, behavioral, and humane factors in handling and restraint. A major environmental consideration should be the possibility of hyperthermia generated during the capture procedure. In order to restrain an animal, you usually have to chase and catch it, which means increased muscle activity for the animal. This, in turn, translates into heat generation, especially if the air temperature and humidity are high. Smaller species tend to overheat faster than larger species because they have a higher metabolic rate. So, keep these factors in mind when planning restraint, e.g., try to plan activities for cooler times of the day, if possible, and try to work quickly and efficiently if it is necessary to work during the hotter times of the day. Animals dissipate heat by a variety of methods, including excretion of moisture via urine, feces, and evaporation. Moisture can be evaporated from the skin (as long as the relative humidity is not too high) and the skin can become wet from sweat glands, from the animals' licking themselves, etc. Evaporation also takes place from the lungs of all breathing animals, so panting serves to increase cooling from the respiratory tract. Be aware of restraint techniques that inhibit heat dissipation—e.g., stockinette placed around a bird's body will prevent them from spreading their wings to allow convection cooling; wrapping a mammal in a heavy towel will decrease evaporative cooling, or taping a beak shut will inhibit the ability of the bird to pant.

Clinical signs of hyperthermia include increased heart and respiratory rates, open-mouth breathing, and increased salivation/sweating in those species that are capable of sweating. These signs may, in turn, lead to dehydration and subsequent loss of cooling ability, weakness, depression, incoordination and, if the temperature rises above 108°F, eventually convulsions, collapse, and death will occur.

Exotic Animal Medicine for the Veterinary Technician, Fourth Edition. Edited by Bonnie Ballard and Ryan Cheek.
© 2024 John Wiley & Sons, Inc. Published 2024 by John Wiley & Sons, Inc.
Companion Website: www.wiley.com/go/ballard/4e

The converse side is hypothermia or low body temperature. This occurs when you are working outdoors in cold temperature, or when you have animals housed in outside areas on cold concrete or other surfaces. It may also occur when you have a weak or sedated animal that has lost the ability to shiver and generate heat. Be wary of placing these animals on a cold exam table because their body temperature will quickly drop.

Be aware of the immediate surroundings you are working in. You may be able to use the physical environment to your advantage in capturing an animal—for instance, herding an animal using portable barriers (plywood) into a large pen or shed or against a fence or cliff, will make the final capture much easier. You must also be aware of physical hazards in the environment that the animal may encounter during a capture episode.

You can also use the physical environment to decrease the animal's sense perceptions. If, for instance, the animal is nocturnal, try to capture it during daylight hours. Conversely, if they are diurnal, try to work at night or dim the lights during the capture attempt.

What are some behavioral considerations in deciding on your capture technique? You must know the natural history of the species—is it nocturnal or diurnal, when is the breeding season, when are young raised, what are the food habits, what is the habitat occupied, etc. These factors will aid in your decisions—e.g., if you capture an adult of the species, will you potentially be leaving young behind?

Animals have a natural fear of predators—this fear is what drives the flight or fight response. As you approach an animal, the first response will be to flee, if this is possible. If this is not possible and/or you come within a critical distance of the animal, the fight response will then be initiated. You may be able to use long-handled nets, poles, or projectiles to extend the effective range of capture by staying outside of this critical distance until the animal is effectively restrained.

Know what the animal's fight response will be! Wild felid kits respond to being grabbed by the nape of the neck much as a domestic kitten does. However, this is not true of adults! Raccoons will turn and bite if you hold them in this manner. Knowing the behavior of the species helps you to determine what an animal will do next—e.g., buteo hawks will use their feet more than their beaks whereas falcons will use both feet and beaks; eagles are perfectly willing to bite, too, whereas vultures will regurgitate. Pigeons and waterfowl will beat their wings when alarmed etc. If you understand behavior, you will be able to give more complete and better care to your patients.

Never underestimate the power of confidence on your part! Your voice, eye contact, and body language can all be used to psychologically restrain an animal or, conversely, let the animal know that you are afraid. Be sure of yourself, but never let yourself become overly confident.

"Every restraint procedure should be preceded by an evaluation as to whether or not the procedure will result in the greatest good for that animal" (Fowler, Handling and Restraint of Wild and Domestic Animals, p. 5). Lastly, you must consider the most humane method of capture. You should try to reduce stress on the animal as much as possible during the capture. These stressors include visual, auditory, olfactory, tactile, or psychological factors. Be sensitive but do your job. This means being prepared ahead of time so you can work as quickly as possible. In addition, try to minimize exacerbating any preexisting injury or condition during the capture and handling episode.

Preparation

Try to work in pairs whenever possible. Having a backup person ensures the safety and efficacy of the plan. Next, decide on the technique you will use beforehand—talk it through to make sure that everyone understands their role. Be prepared for all eventualities—especially the worst-case scenario! Then, make sure all necessary equipment is ready and in working order before you attempt the capture. Protective clothing is helpful in most situations—long pants, long-sleeved shirt, boots, gloves, and goggles.

Tools of Restraint

The first tool of restraint is psychological restraint—have confidence in your abilities. Everyone is aware that animals can sense when a person is afraid of them and react accordingly. Next, consider diminishing sensory perceptions. The more you can decrease or eliminate visual, auditory, or other sensory stimuli during the restraint episode, the easier it will be on both humans and animals.

Physical barriers include using items such as shields made of plywood, Plexiglas, blankets, etc. to herd animals from one area to another and provide a protective device between the handler and the animal. Confinement techniques include the use of squeeze cages, restraint bags, plastic tubes for holding snakes, etc.

It is also possible to use equipment to act as extensions of your arms—e.g., nets, snares, and tongs.

Nets: come in all sizes and shapes. By placing a net on the animal, many manipulative procedures, such as injections, examinations, or obtaining samples for blood work can be carried out. Hoop nets with long handles are commonly used. Be aware that the hoop edge can injure the animal. Better to allow the animal to enter the net than to swing the net at the animal. The net should be of sufficient depth to allow the hoop to be twisted, trapping the animal in the bottom of the net. If it is too shallow, the animal will be able to climb out. If you place the net on the ground or against the wall, it will help to restrict escape. Birds with talons or animals with claws are difficult to handle in large mesh nets. They may poke their limbs through the netting, possibly causing feather damage and fractured bones.

They may also cling to the netting with their talons, making it difficult to extract them. Try to use smooth netting for birds. If the mesh is too large, the animal may also force a head through the mesh and strangle. Know the characteristics of the materials with which the net is constructed. Nylon, cotton, and manila all withstand different degrees of stretch and wear. Inspect for flaws before use!

Rectangular nets can be placed in the path of various types of animals. As the animal runs towards it, the net is extended, and then dropped over the animal. Mist nets are used to capture small birds and bats. Cannon nets are shot over the top of the animal or herd. Nets can also be suspended over feeding areas and dropped over the animal to entangle it.

Snares: used carelessly can cause unnecessary pain or strangle an animal. Commercial snares are designed with swivels for humane and effective manipulation. Quick-release snares (Ketch-all TM) permit the animal to twist without being suffocated. Always try to include one front leg through the snare as well as encircling the neck to decrease any problems with twisting. Do not catch the animal around the chest or abdomen because you may cause crushing injuries to this part of the body and because this also allows too much mobility of the head. Animals with good forelimb dexterity, like raccoons, are sometimes difficult to catch with snares. Once you have the animal snared, grasp the tail and bring the animal taut to the pole, control the head, and remove the snare as quickly as possible.

Tongs: vise tongs grasp an animal at the neck. They act like snares but do not completely encircle the neck—they clamp behind the back of the head. These are used for initial control.

The use of physical force involves using your hands to grasp the animal. You must know where and how to grasp, how much pressure to use, and how this varies from species to species. The greatest protection you have is detailed knowledge of the animal. Gloves vary from thin cotton gloves to heavy, double-layered coarse leather gloves. Leather welder's gloves are good for general use. The thicker and heavier the glove, the less ability you have to determine how tightly you are grasping the animal or to feel the animal's response. Try to keep the glove loose on your hand so you can slip your fingers up or out of the way if teeth penetrate the leather. Gloves do not protect from crushing injuries! Chain mail gloves alone or within leather gloves offer more protection against the tearing effects of large canine teeth. Lastly, chemical restraint can be administered via injection, pole syringe, blow-dart, or pistol. These techniques and the restraint drugs used are further detailed in Restraint and Handling of Wild and Domestic Animals by Murray E. Fowler.

Specific Techniques by Species

Opossums

Danger potential: harp claws and 50 small sharp teeth! Technique—Fortunately, they usually move slowly during the daytime and will oftentimes "play possum" when stressed. Be careful if there are fetuses in the pouch, you may cause the fetuses to pull away from the nipples and they will need to be replaced right away. Opossums can be netted, snared, tonged, or manually handled by covering the head with a towel, grasping at the base of the tail and supporting under the chest, or grasping at the scruff of the neck.

Rabbits

Danger potential: will scratch with sharp claws and have powerful back legs. Technique—be aware that rabbits can kick so strongly with their rear legs that they can fracture their spines! Grasp the loose skin over the back of the neck, lift the hindquarters with the other hand for added support, and cradle the animal against your body. Rabbits can be induced into a torpid state by placing and holding them on their backs for a few seconds or blindfolding them.

Rodents

Danger potential: those sharp incisor teeth especially adapted for chewing and gnawing and sharp claws for burrowing. Technique—be aware that rodents possess no specialized thermoregulatory mechanisms—they achieve homeostasis by a high level of behavioral activity. Therefore, they are predisposed to hyperthermia when handled and hypothermia when sedated or anesthetized.

Squirrels, chipmunks: can use fine mesh net, though claws sometimes become entangled. Can use a towel and gloves (they can bite through gloves!), and try to grasp behind the neck and one foreleg.

Beaver: do not lift them up by their tail, since they are so heavy, you can cause spinal injuries. Restrain with a snare or tongs around the neck, then lift up and hold at base of tail. Or some people feel that they do not have much in the way of a neck and prefer to wrap them up in a blanket and just pick them up manually; they do not tend to be very aggressive

Porcupine: separate porcupines that are in a group before attempting to capture one or they may bump into one another, cause quill discharge and injury to one another. Approach from the rear when the porcupine is facing into a corner, reach under the tail and grab the underhairs, pull backward, and do not let the tail flip up or it will discharge quills into you. Then, slide your other hand beneath the tail and up under the body. You can also use a snare around the base of the tail and other snares on each foot to stretch the animal if you need to get a blood sample for any reason.

Carnivores

Danger potential: teeth designed for grasping and tearing prey with well-developed jaw muscles. Claws can rip and tear. Technique—in general, control the head first then the body. Wear gloves to guard against scratches, most can bite through gloves.

Fox, coyote, wolf: smaller canids can be netted or grasped by the base of the tail, and then manipulated until the scruff of the neck can be grasped. Can also use tongs around the neck for initial control, and can muzzle for further control of the mouth (though you are decreasing their ability to pant).

Bear: these animals have extremely powerful paws and limbs. Immature bears less than five months old may be hand-held or controlled with nets or snares. Mature bears can be handled only with squeeze cages and chemical restraint.

Raccoons: nets, squeeze cages, tongs, snares. Great forelimb dexterity.

Skunks: use a shield of plate glass or plastic, wear goggles, or protective clothing. Use a net to capture, then sedate or anesthetize to handle further.

Mink, weasel: snares or manually grasping at base of tail, pulling up and out of cage, then grasping behind the neck you must move quickly! Sometimes it is best to simply try to pin them behind the neck and then sort out where the rest of the body is.

Otters: river otters can be netted or snared. Sea otters require specialized techniques. They are trapped in the wild using basket nets from beneath while the otters float on the surface of the sea. The net is closed with a drawstring, then lifted out of the water. They are extremely susceptible to stress and have no insulating blubber layer. They are protected from hypothermia by their dense fur coats. You must prevent soiling of the coat.

Cats: infants are easily handled manually or wrapped in towels or canvas restraint bags. If the cat is under 30 lbs., they can be netted with a fine mesh net, snare, or tongs, then the tail is grasped with a gloved hand. Squeeze cages can be used for the larger species. One of our secret techniques for luring them into cages is to use catnip!

Hoofed Stock

Danger potential: antlers, sharp hooves. Technique— small cervids without antlers can be handled manually. With one arm, hold under the abdomen in front of the rear legs, and with the other arm, hold under the neck, lift the animal up and away from the ground and point the legs away from the handler's body. Larger cervids usually need to be chemically immobilized in order to work on individual animals. For herding or transporting, be aware that deer do not recognize chain link or wire net fences as barriers, therefore you should drape these with opaque plastic sheeting. You can also use plastic sheeting to herd them toward a certain area. Most injuries occur during herding and transport—try to arrange it so that you can funnel them via chutes into their new enclosure or a transportation crate. You must select the correct sized crate—if it is too large, they may try to turn around and injure themselves. Capture myopathy is a big problem in cervids.

Birds

Waterfowl: can be captured with nets or hooks or manually. Drape a towel over the wings to hold them against the body, then grasp behind the head. To carry, support the body, restrain the head, and let the legs dangle.

Shorebirds: will try to bite and stab with long, sharp bills. Protect your face with goggles if necessary. Can net birds like gulls or place a towel over them. Control the wings first, then the head.

Herons, cranes, etc.: their long, thin legs are easily broken by rough handling. They will aim for your eyes with their beaks and are fully capable of spearing an extremity—exercise extreme caution and always control the head first.

Raptors: beaks and talons are adapted for grasping and tearing flesh. Vultures will employ their beaks but have very weak feet. Wear heavy leather gloves and use a hood or towel on their heads to decrease visual stimuli. If a bird is on the floor of an enclosure, throw a towel or heavy cloth over the bird, wrap the bird in the fabric, and then grasp the feet, then the head. Try to remove the gloves after the initial capture to facilitate handling. The feet should be grasped with one hand above the talons (but not too far above the foot or you will lose control of the talons) and with your finger between the two feet, the head should be grasped from behind without obstructing the trachea. If the bird is perched, it can be approached from in front or in back. If coming from the front, grasp the legs first, one in each hand, then transfer the legs to one hand and grasp behind the head. If coming from the back, grasp the wings, body, and legs together, then separate the legs in one hand and the head with the other hand.

Galliform birds: usually docile but have claws and some males have well-developed tarsal spurs. Do NOT grab them by the feathers, especially the tail feathers, as the bird will release them into your hand. Hold the wings close to the body and try to control the legs.

Pigeons/doves: do not scratch, do not peck, and have mild dispositions. Will attempt to beat their wings when alarmed. Grasp them from above and behind and press the wings close to the bird's body.

Small passeriformes: capture with a net in the aviary, hold cupped in one hand with fingers around the base of the head. Do not completely surround the sternum and interfere with respiration. Sometimes it helps to darken the room and approach from behind.

Reptiles and Amphibians

Chelonians: small species can be handled manually. Hold them on either side of the carapace, you may need to insert a finger between carapace and plastron to prevent the shell from completely closing. Do not rapidly turn the animal upside down then right-side up again as it is possible to cause a torsion of the bowel by this sudden movement. Snapping turtles are capable of inflicting serious bite wounds—grasp them at the base of the tail, lift them off the ground then grab the carapace just behind the head.

Reference

Fowler, M.E. (1985). *Restraint and Handling of Wild and Domestic Animals.* Ames: Iowa State University Press.

You can turn them over onto the carapace; they usually relax in this position.

Snakes

Danger potential: can bite, produce venom, or constrict. Technique—grasp behind the head (if nonpoisonous), then support the body. If unsupported, the snake can thrash so much that it dislocates or fractures its vertebrae. Snake hooks can be used to pin the head to the ground. Snakes can be cooled for procedures that require only mild restraint but respiratory ailments are a possibility after prolonged chilling. Handling poisonous snakes is beyond the scope of this talk—suffice it to say that you must be extremely careful, always have antivenin on hand, and know what you are doing!

Amphibians

Danger potential: toothless but can bite with hard-keratinized plates in mouth. None are venomous. Technique—they can be netted, then surround the body with your hand—two fingers surround the neck and the rest of the hand encircles the body and back legs.

Conclusion

Just as there are a myriad of different animal species that the wildlife rehabilitator may be called upon to handle, there are similarly a wide variety of handling and restraint techniques that are available for use. Our job as knowledgeable rehabilitators should include familiarity with the proper techniques to use for each individual animal in each individual situation. In this way, we will best serve the interests of our unique patients.

Appendix 4

Tail Wrapping

A. Standard wrap (to be used with tail feathers, not in molt)
1. Materials
   a. 1–2 tongue depressors
   b. Spray bottle with water (set on mist)
   c. Gummed paper packaging tape (sticky when wet)
   d. Used X-ray film or other plastic
   e. Scissors
   f. Stapler
   g. Adhesive tape
2. Procedure
   a. Tear or cut off several strips of paper tape (2–3 inches long for American kestrel, 6–8 inches red-tailed hawk).
   b. Cut a strip of X-ray film about $1/3$ the length of the tail and about the same width as the folded tail. Fold it in half and staple it at the fold.
   c. Gather all tail feathers fairly close together without bending them—the narrower the tail wrap, the stronger and less cumbersome it will be.
   d. Place the tongue depressor along the center of the tail so that one end is flush with the feather tips and the other end almost reaches the bird's body. You may have to trim the tongue depressor.
   e. Fit X-ray "sleeve" over the tips of the tail and tongue depressor.
   f. Wet the first strip of paper and fold it around the end section of the tail making sure no feathers are bent (Figure A4.1).
   g. Repeat with as many strips as necessary to cover the tail to the bare shafts making sure that each strip overlaps the previous one; do not include tail coverts (downy feathers on underside of tail). Try to conform shape of wrap to natural curvature of tail feathers.
   h. Finally, fold one long strip lengthwise around the tip of the tail wrap and press all strips firmly together, making sure they all stick well (Figure A4.2).

3. Notes
   a. For long-tailed birds (cooper's hawk, etc.), you may have to tape two tongue depressors together.
   b. For American kestrels, you may have to cut one off a little.
   c. Make wraps as lightweight as possible.
   d. Press edges together firmly and dry the tail wrap. A wet or loose wrap will slide off as soon as the bird is returned to its cage.
   e. Tail wraps will have to be repaired or replaced periodically.
4. To remove this tail wrap
   a. Soak the whole tail in a pitcher or bucket filled with warm water. Gently begin separating the tape from feathers with your fingers. After 30–45 seconds, the whole wrap will often slide off in one piece. Do not try to cut or tear the wrap off dry—it will permanently damage feathers.

B. Modified wrap (To be used with tail feathers in molt)
1. Materials
   a. Piece of used X-ray film or similar light-weight plastic
   b. Masking tape
   c. Stapler
2. Procedure
   a. Cut a piece of plastic as long as the tail and twice as wide as the folded tail (not fanned out).
   b. Fold this piece in half lengthwise so it now matches the shape of the folded-up tail fairly well.
   c. Place a few staples along the long edge (where two edges meet) and along one short edge. You should now have an "envelope" with one short side still open.
   d. Carefully slide this sleeve over the folded-up tail.
   e. Attach the sleeve to some of the downy coverts on the underside and backside with some strips of masking tape. Be sure not to cover up the oil gland or the feathers covering the vent area.

Exotic Animal Medicine for the Veterinary Technician, Fourth Edition. Edited by Bonnie Ballard and Ryan Cheek.
© 2024 John Wiley & Sons, Inc. Published 2024 by John Wiley & Sons, Inc.
Companion Website: www.wiley.com/go/ballard/4e

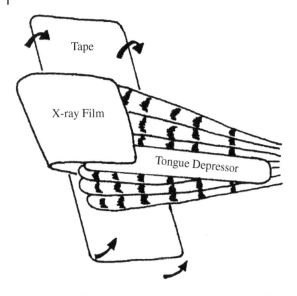

Figure A4.1 Wrapping the paper tape around the tail feathers.

3. Notes
   a. Depending on the material used this wrap may be stiff enough without the addition of tongue depressors.

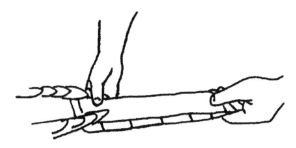

Figure A4.2 The completed tail wrap.

   b. If the bird is active or when the masking tape wears out, this wrap will have to be repaired/replaced.
   c. Standard-size sleeves can be prepared and kept on hand for quick applications.

Tail wrapping article reprinted with permission from the Carolina Raptor Center, www.birdsofprey.org, Raptor Rehabilitation, A Manual of Guidelines, pp. 30–31.

Appendix 5

Guide to Identification of Hatchling and Nestling Songbirds

Exotic Animal Medicine for the Veterinary Technician, Fourth Edition. Edited by Bonnie Ballard and Ryan Cheek.
© 2024 John Wiley & Sons, Inc. Published 2024 by John Wiley & Sons, Inc.
Companion Website: www.wiley.com/go/ballard/4e

Table A5.1 Yellow to orange mouth birds.[a]

Species	Mouth color	Gape flanges	Beak contour	Down	Legs/feet	Approximate weight in grams			Feeding call	Feathers	Special features
						Hatchling	Nestling	Adult (F)			
Starling	bright yellow	bright yellow, very prominent, lower larger than upper	very wide	grayish-white, long and plentiful on head, back, and wings	long legs	5.5–30	40–60	80	hatchling—single squeaky note	gray-black	
Mockingbird	yellow	yellow	wide	dark gray, plentiful	long legs	5–18	20–32	43	hatchling—single, clear, piping note; then throaty bark	gray and white striped wings and tail	gray, irides., crescent marking on roof of mouth
Robin	yellow to yellow-orange	pale yellow	wide	sparse, cream on head, back, legs	long legs	5–35	40–60	77	hatchling—staccato trill	rust-tipped speckly chest	skin often yellowish
Black phoebe	bright yellow-orange	bright yellow	wide, flat, tapering to a point	gray and sparse	long, thin legs	2–5	7–15	18	peep-peep	brown-tipped black feathers	insect eater
Pacific-slope flycatcher	bright yellow-orange	yellow	flat, wide, pointy tip, "arrowhead" look	white on head, back, and wings in a "star" cluster	long, thin, delicate, dark blue-gray, white toenails	2–6	7–8	11	insistent—crowlike squawk, frog-like when older	buff abdomen, buf, and white striped wings	insect eater
Cliff swallow	orange-yellow	flesh	very wide, flat, pointy beak	light gray head and back	short legs, small chubby feet	2–13	13–15	22	barking type chirp	nestlings—light tan on back by tail; otherwise adult	insect eater, cavity nest
Violet-green swallow	orange-yellow	cream	very wide, pointy beak	cream on head, shoulders, and back	short legs	1.5–8	8–10	14		white eyebrows	insect eater, cavity nest
California thrasher	orange-yellow	cream	curves down as nestling grows	dark gray on head, back, wings, thighs, plentiful	long legs	6–35	40–60	84		medium gray	
Chestnut-backed chickadee	orange-yellow	very yellow, prominent	flat, wide	gray on head and back	long, pale bluish-purple	1–4	6–8	10	squeaky cheep	buff abdomen, black head, buff—white circles on side of head	insect eater
Bewick's wren	orange	yellow	flat, wide, pointy	long, gray on head only	long, delicate	1–4	6–8	10		circles	
Bushtit	deep orange-yellow	yellow	short	none	long, delicate	1–3	3.5–4	5	3 syllable "locator" call, "mohawk" look	gray, first feathers on crown of head	females have blue eyes, cavity nesters
Wrentit	deep orange	yellow	pointy	none		1.5–6	7–11	14		gray-brown	yellow irides.

a) Bushtits, chickadees, creepers, dinners, flycatchers, mockingbirds, robins, shrikes, starlings, swallows, thrashers, thrushes, titmice, wrens, and wings

Table A5.2 Pink to red mouth birds.

Species	Mouth color	Gape flanges	Beak contour	Down[a]	Legs/feet	Approximate weight in grams			Feeding call	Feathers	Special features
						Hatchling	Nestling	Adult (F)			
House sparrow	pink	med. yellow, prominent	short-cone-shaped	none	short, chunky	2–13	14–20	27	melodic, single chirp	smooth, gray–white chest	
Rufous-sided towhee	pink	pale yellow	conical and pointed	dark gray	long legs, big feet	3–18	20–29	39		dark back, white spots on wings, and tail	
California towhee	pink to red	pale yellow not prominent	conical and pointed	long, brown–gray on head, back, and wings	long legs, big feet	4–20	25–39	52	high-pitched repeated, like crickets, changes to single peep	brown	
Brown-headed cowbird	deep pink	white to cream not prominent	heavy, to a point narrower than a towee's	long, snow-white	long legs, big feet, black tipped nails	2–20	25–30	39	continuous, high-pitched vibrating sound	breast yellowish when coming in	bald face, parasitic, often found in nests of towhees
Northern oriole	deep pink	pale yellow	long, pointed, narrow	long, white-lt. gray on back, wings, 2 rows on head	long, slate-gray legs	2.5–18	20–25	33	high, staccato, repeated notes, similar to blackbird	yellow breast, gray back, white wing bars	insect eater
Lesser goldfinch	red	pale yellow	similar to finch	grayish	short, pink, stubby	1–6	7–8	10		green to rust back, yellow abdomen	red dot at corner of gape flanges
Red-winged blackbird	red	yellow, not prominent	long, pointed	scant, white on back, lower wings, and thighs	long legs	3–15	20–30	42		bald face, similar to cowbirds	
Brewer's blackbird	red	white, not prominent	long, pointed	blackish-gray fairly plentiful	long legs, white toenails	3–15	20–30	42	raucous, repeated call, sounds like a rusty hinge	black	
Scrub jay	red	white, not prominent	long and wide	none	long legs, grabby feet, white toenails	6–30	35–70	87	hatchling- short repeated peeping, later a single squawk	ruddy skin furry gray head, blue wings, and tail	
House finch	red	white to yellowish	short, conical	white, long, and plentiful. 4 rows on head	short, stocky	1.5–8	10–15	21	none when newly hatched, then high-pitched peeping	stripey, gray/	white chest
Crow	red	white	very long, large, heavy	sparse, gray–brown on head, underparts	long, heavy	18–70	70–328	438		black	ruddy skin

a) Blackbirds, cowbirds, crows, finches, goldfinches, grosbeaks, jays, orioles, sparrows, tanagers, towhees, and waxwings.

Source: Marty Johnson, Wildlife Rescue, Inc., Palo Alto, CA 94303, 1995.

Appendix 6

Average Body Weights of Selected North American Songbirds

Bird species	Weight range (g)	Avg. weight (g)
American robin		77
Bluebird, eastern		31
Cardinal	33.6–64.0	45
Carolina wren		21
Chickadee, black-capped	8.2–13.6	10.8
Crow, American		448
Dove, mourning		126
Duck, mallard	720–1580	1,082
Finch, house	19–25.5	21
Flicker, yellow-shafted	130	106–164
Goldfinch, American	8.6–20.7	12.6
Grackle, common		115
Hummingbird, ruby-throated	2.4–4.1	3.0
Jay, blue	64.1–109	85
Mockingbird	36.2–55.7	49
Oriole, orchard	16.0–25.1	19.6
Pigeon		270
Purple martin		49.4
Sparrow, house	20.1–34.5	27.4
Swallow, barn	13.4–23.4	19
Thrasher, brown	57.6–89.0	69
Titmouse, tufted	17.5–26.1	21.6
Warbler, pine	9.4–15.1	11.9
Woodpecker, pileated		290
Woodpecker, red-headed	56.1–90.5	72

Exotic Animal Medicine for the Veterinary Technician, Fourth Edition. Edited by Bonnie Ballard and Ryan Cheek.
© 2024 John Wiley & Sons, Inc. Published 2024 by John Wiley & Sons, Inc.
Companion Website: www.wiley.com/go/ballard/4e

Appendix 7

Species Care Sheets

Raccoons

Raccoon Diet and Feeding

Formula: 1 part powdered KMR: 2 parts water.

- Stomach capacity is 50–66 mL/kg (5–7%) Use 50 mL/kg to reduce chances of diarrhea. (.05 × B.W. in g =_____ mL.) There are 30 mL/fluid ounce.
- Do not allow free choice formula feeding because some raccoons will overeat and develop diarrhea or bloat.
- Very young raccoons can be fed with a dropper, pet nurser bottle, or nipple attached to a syringe. The pet nurser has the least amount of flow control so use them with caution.
- Older juveniles are often fed with preemie baby bottles and nipples. After bottle feeding always remember to burp the baby by patting firmly between the shoulder blades and down the infant's back.
- New incoming infants may take several days to become accustomed to the new diet and feeding instrument.
- Scratching the back of a raccoon's neck, while holding the nurser in its mouth, usually stimulates a suckling reflex.
- Once baby raccoons get the idea of bottle nursing, the rest of the feeding times are spent trying to slow them down. They tend to drink very fast and you must pull the bottle away after they have received the measured formula amount or they will swallow air.
- Stimulate before feeding until eyes open and self-elimination is evident (4–5 weeks).
- Add baby rice cereal to formula as a thickener to slow down overzealous nursers.
- Gradually begin introducing solid foods (applesauce, yogurt, baby foods, softened puppy food), either in with the formula or separately, once raccoons have their eyes open and are beginning to get teeth (4 weeks).
- Once they have a taste for the puppy food in the formula, start offering it dry.
- Gradually decrease the bottle feeding until weaned (7–12 weeks).

- Begin to offer drinking water when raccoons begin to eat solid foods but plan to refill water bowl several times a day because they love to climb in and also dunk their food items in bowl.
- Some rehabilitators prefer to teach the babies how to lap formula out of a bowl. This method takes patience and a lot of washcloths to clean up afterward.
- Raccoons may resist weaning and lose weight at first.
- Dry puppy food (Science Diet Canine Growth) should constitute 90% of the post-weaning diet.
- Remaining 10% of diet should be apples, grapes, berries, eggs, vegetables, sweet potatoes, fish, worms, clams, small rodents, chicks, and crayfish.
- By 12 weeks old raccoons should be able to kill crayfish.
- By 14 weeks old raccoons should be able to kill young rats.
- Some individuals need to be fasted for 24 hours before they will try new foods.
- Use caution and protective clothing when handling raccoons since they are a rabies vector species.

Raccoon Housing

- From 0–5 weeks old, a cardboard box or pet carrier works best because it can be thrown out after it becomes soiled. Due to the zoonotic concern with the internal parasite *Baylisascaris procyonis*, any fecal-contaminated materials should be burned or thrown out. Never reuse any cages or caging materials used with raccoons with any other species since disinfectants are ineffective in killing the raccoon roundworm. Fresh feces are not infective, but becomes so in 3 to 4 weeks. Intake procedure for raccoons should include weekly dewormings of pyrantel pamoate suspension 4.5 mg/mL at 0.5–1 cc/lb.
- Use soft, ravel-free cloth as bedding. No terry cloth because their fingernails get caught in the loops too easily.
- Provide supplemental heat until they are 4 weeks old.

Exotic Animal Medicine for the Veterinary Technician, Fourth Edition. Edited by Bonnie Ballard and Ryan Cheek.
© 2024 John Wiley & Sons, Inc. Published 2024 by John Wiley & Sons, Inc.
Companion Website: www.wiley.com/go/ballard/4e

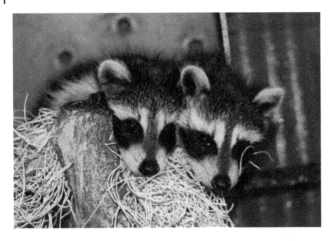

Figure A7.1 Raccoon babies.

- At 6 weeks provide animal with a wire cage with logs, natural substrate, tree limbs for climbing, and a hammock made from canvas or tight-weave netting should be hung near the top of the enclosure. The hammocks are a good substitute for wooden nest boxes because they can be changed and washed.
- By 8 weeks, raccoons are very active and need a large cage with lots of natural items to help keep them from getting bored (i.e., hollow logs, rocks, live plants, dirt for digging, water bowls for dunking food, pine cones, small pool).
- Outdoor acclimation usually starts at 6 weeks and finishes by 12 weeks (Figure A7.1).

Raccoon Release

- Release age is 4–5 months when they are self-feeding and acclimated to the outdoors.
- This page will not cover raccoon release due to the regulations on possessing rabies vector species in many states and the numerous difficulties one can face with this procedure. Turning all raccoons over to a licensed rehabilitator, vaccinated against rabies, is recommended.

Flying Squirrels

Flying Squirrel Diet and Feeding

Formula: 1 part powdered Esbilac: 2 parts water.

- Feed with a 1 or 3 cc O-ring syringe with silicone nipple.
- Flying squirrels have a good suckling reflex and the formula may need to be thickened to prevent aspiration.
- Gradually thicken formula with rice baby cereal starting at 3 weeks.
- Stimulate after each meal until the eyes are open and there is evidence of self-elimination in cage.
- Once eyes are open begin to introduce solid food items.

- Start decreasing number of formula feedings as solid food is being consumed (4–5 weeks).
- Wait at least 4 days between feeding reductions.
- A useful weaning tool is to add powdered rodent or primate chow to the formula starting at 5 weeks.
- Examples of weaning foods include dog chow, raw nuts, fresh corn on the cob, apple, grapes, rodent blocks, primate chow, seed mix, vegetables, sweet potatoes, carrots, broccoli, wheat germ, etc.
- Natural food items to offer include mushrooms, lichens, bark, buds, insects, acorns, hickory nuts, pine cones, beech nuts, berries, green buds, etc.
- Diet ratio of food groups should be: 80% rodent mix (dog, primate, and rodent chow); 20% fruit and vegetable matter; 1 nut/squirrel/day; 2–3 insects/squirrel/day.
- Offering squirrel "nutri-bites" (recipe under grey squirrel diet) until release will help assure proper nutrition.
- Provide drinking water in a bowl or water bottle when babies are weaned down to twice a day formula.
- Once weaned, feed the squirrels at night (since they are nocturnal) and scatter food around the cage.

Flying Squirrel Housing

- Supplemental heat is needed until they are 5–6 weeks old. Using a heating pad under half of the enclosure is recommended.
- Masters of escape, flying squirrels need to be housed in a secure enclosure with a tight lid.
- 1–4 weeks in aquarium or small box.
- 4–6 weeks in a larger wire portable cage (begin to acclimate to the outdoors).
- Provide a nesting box since these squirrels live in tree cavities in the wild.
- 6–14 weeks in outdoor prerelease pen (once acclimated). This pen needs to be large enough for the young flying squirrels to practice jumping and gliding. Minimum size of 6′ H × 6′ W × 8′ L.

- The pen needs both horizontal and vertical branches to assimilate the trees.
- Flying squirrels move from tree to tree and rarely go to the ground.

Flying Squirrel Release

- Release age is 14–16 weeks.
- Release criteria: Fully acclimated to outdoors, nocturnal behaviors, running from humans, opening shelled nuts, and eating natural food items.
- Whenever possible, raise and release flyers with a group since these animals live in colonies. Also, release in a well-wooded area where other flyers have been seen or heard.
- Release by closing animals up inside their nest box 1 hour before dark outside (tape hole shut). Tie box to tree trunk (6 ft or higher up) and remove tape from nest box entrance at dusk. Flyers will exit box and explore the treetops then sometimes return to the nest box until they find another cavity to sleep in.
- Supply backup food by having a nearby feeding station or putting bowl on top of nest box.

Flying Squirrel Miscellaneous Information

- When startled, flying squirrels flip on their backs and box at the invader with all four feet. Wake the sleeping baby up slowly and gently to prevent this aggressive display.
- Do not worry if the infant does not eliminate each time it is stimulated. Discontinue stimulation after about a minute. As long as the squirrel has at least one bowel movement a day bloating should not occur.

Opossums

Opossum Diet and Feeding

Formula: 1 part powdered Esbilac : 2 parts water

- Stomach capacity is 50–66 mL/kg or 5–7% of BW. (.05 × BW in g =____mL)
- Opossums have a poorly developed suckling reflex, which makes gavage feeding the most effective method to feed young animals under 45 g.
- Gavage tube size ranges from size $3^1/_2$–5 French feeding tube.
- Pinkies should be started on very dilute formula (1:5 w/water) and gradually built up to full strength formula over 3–5 days. Until infant is on full strength, feed more often.

- 0–75 days: tube feed q 2 hours at 5% BW. Belly should be rounded but not tight after a feeding and a milk line in the stomach should be visible through the skin.
- By the time they weigh 50 g, they do not tolerate tube feedings. Even before their eyes open a jar lid of warm formula can be placed in with baby opossums. By dipping their noses in the milk and allowing them to walk through the formula they will clean the milk off of themselves (and their littermates) and learn to self-feed faster.
- When able to lap up formula out of bowl, start thickening with rice baby cereal.
- Foods to help facilitate the weaning process: fruit yogurt, meat baby foods, bananas, grapes, cooked sweet potatoes, and apple sauce. These items can be mixed with milk formula in the bowl to encourage self-feeding.
- By 10–12 weeks gradually start adding puppy or cat chow to formula.
- By 16 weeks opossums should be weaned and eating solid food items such as fresh carrion, live crickets, mealworms and earthworms, fruit and vegetables native to area, raw eggs, dead minnows, and crayfish. Lightly sprinkle diet with a calcium supplement. Offer food in the evenings.
- Make sure there is always fresh drinking water available during and after weaning. Opossums have a habit of defecating in their food and water bowls so offer a water bottle to guarantee a clean water source.

Opossum Housing

- Housing: Small box or pet carrier with soft, ravel-free cloth, heating pad set on low, and a source of humidity until 8 weeks old. Careful to use cage lids and small (less than $1/_2$ in.) ventilation holes due to opossum's ability to easily escape.
- Maintain nest humidity at 70%.
- Move to $1/_4''$–$1/_2''$ mesh hardware cloth 2′ × 2′ × 4′ cage at 8–10 weeks.
- Use heating pad until 10 weeks or 80–90 g at external temperatures of 95°F.
- At 12 weeks begin outdoor acclimation. Opossums need exercise and a daily dose of vitamin D_3, naturally provided by sunlight, to help prevent metabolic bone disease (MBD). Opossums are very prone to MBD and must receive daily dietary calcium in addition to 30–60 minutes of unfiltered U/V light.
- Use caution when putting animals in sunlight. Opossums are prone to overheating and can die quickly if not provided with some shade and proper ventilation. They do not need to be in direct sunlight to benefit from natural U/V, just placed outside during daylight hours. Beneficial U/V rays are blocked out by glass windows.

- Move to release cage at 4 months.
- Becoming nocturnal and sleeping during the day by 4 mos.
- Small groups of same-age preweanlings can be housed together. Cannibalism can result when housing together older juveniles.

Opossum Release

- Consider release when the opossums are 5 mos. old and 8–10 in. in body length, 1.5 lb., self-feeding, acclimated to weather and outside temperatures, and baring teeth at caretaker.
- If the cage is on a suitable release site, open cage door 1 hour before dark and allow opossum to come and go. Provide backup food until the animals move on.
- Some opossums will leave the cage and explore at night but come back to the nest box by morning and sleep until the next dusk.
- If the cage is not on a suitable site, be certain the animals are ready and release them near cover and trees right before dark.

Opossum Miscellaneous Information

- Opossums are sensitive to corticosteroids and Levamisole is dewormer of choice.
- Opossums tolerate sutures, bandages, and splints well.
- Orphans have immature immune systems so wash hands before/after feeding.

Grey Squirrels

Grey Squirrel Diet and Feeding

Formula: 1-part powdered Esbilac: 2 parts water

- Stomach capacity is 50 mL/kg (.05 ml × BW in g =____mL)
- Use O-ring syringe with a silicone or Catac nipple to feed orphan squirrels.
- Stimulate after each feeding until 5 weeks.
- A healthy squirrel should gain 4–7 g/day once established on Esbilac formula.
- Squirrels should be fed lying on their stomachs with heads slightly raised.
- Add rice baby cereal to thicken formula at about 3 weeks.
- Add powdered rodent blocks to further thicken formula at about 5 weeks.
- When eyes open and the squirrel is eating rodent blocks or monkey chow, start offering self-feeding diet items such as: cracked nuts, small pieces of fresh corn on the cob, apple, grapes, broccoli stems, cauliflower, and rodent seed mixes.
- Start to wean at 8 weeks and finish by 10–11 weeks.
- Diet offered ratio should be: 80% rodent/primate chow: 20% other items. Do not allow the animal "to choose" a balanced diet for itself; stick with ratio.
- Limit nuts to 1 nut/squirrel/day or they will not eat enough more nutritious foods.
- Make sure squirrel is off milk and eating solid and natural food items for at least 2 weeks prior to release.
- Post-weaning foods: rodent blocks, high-quality dog chow (i.e., Purina One, Proplan, Eukanuba), uncracked acorns, hickory nuts, pecans, buds, bark, pine cones, fungi, sunflower seeds, insects, fresh vegetables; and rodent seed mixes.
- Healthy weaning tool: "squirrel nutri-bites" recipe:
  $1^1/_2$ cups powdered rodent or primate chow
  $^1/_3$ cup powdered Esbilac
  $^2/_3$ cup warm water
  $^1/_3$ cup chopped pecans
  $^1/_3$ cup crushed cuttlebone, if needed.
  Mix together and roll into small meatball-size balls.
  Keep refrigerated for up to 3 days or freeze for up to 6 months.
- These "squirrel nutri-bites" can be offered in place of a milk feeding and once the squirrels start eating them they can be offered free choice. Due to the milk content, do not leave them in cages long enough to spoil.

Grey Squirrel Housing

- From 0–4 weeks: lidded box, cardboard pet carrier, plastic or glass aquarium with heating pad on low under $^1/_2$ of cage.
- Use soft, ravel-free cloth for bedding such as cotton T-shirt, flannel, sweatshirts, fleece.
- At 5–6 weeks discontinue heating pad use.
- Around 6–8 weeks move to a small wire flush bottom cage ($^1/_2$″ × 1″ mesh or smaller) with tree limbs for climbing and provide a nest box inside cage.
- Start acclimating to outdoor temperatures by placing cage outside during warm days and bringing back in at night. Gradually leave out for longer periods of time until squirrels can comfortably be left out overnight. Baby squirrels do not have to be brought inside if a heat lamp can be provided near one of the nest boxes.
- At 8–12 weeks move squirrel to large outdoor wire release cage (minimum size 4′ × 4′ × 6′), the larger the better. Covered waterproof roof, back, and 1 side. Hang water bottle on cage. Attach nest box to the top of cage. Natural substrate on cage bottom and inside nest box.
- House animals with similarly aged conspecifics.

Grey Squirrel Release

Release Criteria:

- At least 12–14 weeks of age and acclimated to the outdoors for at least 2 weeks.
- Squirrels should hide at the sight or sound of approaching people and not allow any handling even from the hand raiser.
- Squirrels should be weaned for a minimum of 2 weeks, nest building, eating natural food items, and able to crack open whole-shelled raw nuts.
- If so, open cage door and allow animal to come and go. Continue to supply food until squirrels move on or at least for 3–4 weeks.

Cottontail Rabbits

Cottontail Rabbit Diet and Feeding

Formula: 1-part powdered KMR: 2 parts water

- Feed with O-ring syringe and nipple or tube feed rabbits.
- Stomach capacity = 100–125 mL/kg (10–12.5%) of BW. Safer to use 100 mL/kg or .1xBW in gm = _____ mL
- Cottontails benefit by receiving daily Benebac to aid with digestion and diarrhea prevention.
- Rabbits can be fed with a syringe but they seldom suckle. Some will lick formula from the tip of syringe drop by drop or swallow milk as it is dripped onto their lips.
- If your new cottontail refuses to eat, try a drop of Karo syrup on the end of the nipple or adding a bit of baby food (no sugar added) applesauce to the formula. Another trick used is to add orange-flavored Pedialyte to the formula to enhance the flavor.
- Allow cottontails to drink as much formula as they want per feeding. Better to feed these babies in as few feedings as possible. Twice a day is the goal as long as they get enough calories and are gaining weight.
- Gavage feeding is a faster method and ideal if there are many babies to feed or if the babies are frightened of handling and refuse to nurse. Be sure to watch a veterinarian or an experienced rehabilitator do this method before first trying it yourself. Although faster, tube feeding can be potentially lethal if done incorrectly. The rabbit's pallet skin is very fragile and can be punctured by the soft end of the feeding tube resulting in SQ delivery of formula followed by death.
- Stimulate baby rabbits before feeding until their eyes open.
- Keep a secure hold on baby rabbits when handling. Rabbits have a habit of suddenly jumping out of your hands or off the table.

- When eyes are open, start offering diced (easily done with scissors), fresh natural greens (clover greens and flowers, grass, dandelion leaves, alfalfa, privet) twice daily. No stems of plants should be given until rabbits are approximately 3 weeks old. Offer only a small amount at first and be sure greens are clean and chemical-free.
- Once they have adjusted to the new food items (3–4 days after they begin to sample it), offer larger amounts. There should always be some left over. After a week of eating solid foods, discontinue dicing the greens and offer them whole.
- Remove uneaten greens as new greens are added. Greens and grasses wilt quickly becoming undesirable to the rabbits and can mold in just a day or two.
- Provide drinking water in a shallow lid or a water bottle when young rabbits start to nibble on solid foods.
- Other solid food items include rabbit chow, rolled oats, wheat germ, corn, apple and carrot slivers, dry hay, or alfalfa fed free choice until released.
- Introduce new food items slowly and one at a time to allow their gut to adjust to the changes.
- Wean rabbits by 3–4 weeks.

Cottontail Rabbit Housing

- From 0–2 weeks use a small cardboard box or aquarium with secure lid.
- Use a heating pad on low under one-half of cage or heat light on one-half of cage.
- Supply soft, ravel-free cloth for bedding. Rabbits like layers to burrow into and prefer to be covered up.
- Once weaned remove heating pad and cloth bedding. Instead, bed with natural substrates such as hay, grasses, leaves, or pine straw.
- At 3 weeks move to a large plastic pet carrier or enclosed rabbit hutch. Rabbits need solid-sided cages and a quiet area to reduce stress.
- Do not overcrowd the cages.
- Littermates can be housed together but be careful mixing unrelated animals and do not mix different ages as they tend to fight and become stressed.
- Fatal enteritis can develop from environmental stress.
- Albon at 25–50 mg/kg PO SID × 5–14 days given to all rabbits initially may help prevent enteritis caused by stress-induced coccidiosis flare-ups.
- Be sure, there are no holes in the cage or cage door larger than $1/2$-inch square because infant rabbits can squeeze out of a 1 by 1 in. hole. Cover securely any questionable holes with burlap, netting, or screen.
- Acclimate to outside temperatures once rabbits are weaned.
- Provide hiding spots such as hay to burrow into, a cardboard or wooden nest box.

Cottontail Rabbit Release

- Ready for release by the end of 4 weeks.
- Many rabbits do not do well in captivity past 5–6 weeks old and should not be kept this long unless there is a medical reason.
- Rabbits ready for release should run and hide from all humans, pets, and noise.
- Release weight is between 100–200 g, ideally about 150 g.
- Find a site with open fields or pasture with nearby cover for a release site. Open cage door and allow rabbits to hop out by themselves or place them under cover and quietly leave the area.
- Cottontails do not need backup food if released in a proper habitat and they rarely return to release site.
- Release at dusk or dawn in mild weather.

Table A7.1 Raccoon care sheet.

Age (weeks)	Weights (g)	Age determinates	Diet	Amount	Frequency
0–1	50–100	Faint tail rings and mask, very lightly furred, ears pressed against head	KMR	Volume by B.W.	q 3 h, 1 PM feeding
1–2	100–150	Face mask furred, eye slit visible, crawling on belly	KMR		q 3.5 h, 1 PM feeding
2–3	100–200	Ear canals open, 18–24 d eyes open	KMR		q 3.5 h, no PM feeding
3–4	200–300	Fully furred tail rings, responds to sight and sound	KMR, add cereal		q 4 h
4–5	175–300	Able to walk, eyes open but cloudy blue, deciduous teeth	KMR, add soaked kibble		q 4 h
5–6	300–400	Able to run and climb, eyes darken			QID
6–7	400–600	Adult pelage begins (ends 12–14 weeks)			TID
7–8	600–650	2nd and 3rd premolars erupt, full sight and hearing	Start weaning		TID
8–9	650–675	1st permanent incisors erupt	Start dish feeding		BID
9–10	675–700	1st premolars erupt	No bottle feedings		SID
10–11	700–775	Wean 10–12 weeks	Weaned		
11–12	775–825				
12–13	825–875	3rd permanent incisors erupt			
13–14	875–900				
14–15	900–1,100				

Table A7.2 Flying squirrel care sheet.

Age (weeks)	Weights (g)	Age determinates	Diet	Amounts (mL)	Frequency
0–1	3–6	Pink, no fur, eyes closed, few whiskers	Esbilac	0.2–0.3	q 2 h, 2 PM feedings
1–2	6–10	Short hairs appear, toes separate	Esbilac	0.3–0.6	q 2 h, 1 PM feeding
2–3	10–15	Downy hair darkens, able to right themselves, ear canals open, lower incisors erupt	Esbilac	0.6–1.0	q 3 h, no PM feeding
3–4	17–23	Lateral tail hairs develop, responds to loud noises	Esbilac, add cereal	1.0–1.5	q 3 h
4–5	25–30	Fur covers body, upper incisors erupt, days 28–32	Esbilac, cereal, add solid food	1.5–2.0	q 4 h
5–6	30–38	Miniature version of adult	Weaning begins	2.0–2.5	TID
6–7	38–43		Add rodent pellets	2.5–3.0	BID
7–8	40–47		Add natural foods	3.0–5.0	SID-BID
8–10	47–53		Wk 8–9 weaned		
12–14	60	Ready for release			

Table A7.3 Opossum care sheet.

Age (Weeks)	Weights (g)	Age determinates	Diet	Amounts (mL)	Frequency
2		Whiskers start, blond nose hairs, pink skin	Tube—Esbilac	.50	q 2 h, 24 h
4	20	Blond belly hairs, pink skin	Same	1	q 2–3 h, 1 PM feeding
5–6	25–35	Slight bluish coloration, ears open	Same	1–2	q 2–3 h, 1 PM feeding
6–8	35–50	Furred, eye slits developed, mouth fully open	Same	2–3	q 3–4 h, 1 PM feeding
9	45–52	Eyes open, running around, lapping formula, teeth present, white-tipped guard hairs, ears erect	Bowl—Esbilac, add cereal	2.5–3	QID
10–11	50–75	Self-defecating/urinating; 3–6″ excluding tail	Bowl—Esbilac, cereal, add cat or puppy chow	2.5–4	QID
12	75–100	Thermoregulating; 4.5–6.5″	Start weaning	4	TID
13–15	100–500	Actively climbing; 6–10″	Weaned, dry chow	5	BID-TID
15–20	500–1,000	20 weeks—ready for release	Natural foods		BID

Table A7.4 Grey squirrel care sheet.

Age (weeks)	Weights (g)	Age determinates	Diet	Amounts (mL)	Frequency
0–1	15–25	Pink, no fur, eyes closed tight—bulgy	Esbilac	0.5–1.0	q 2 h, 1 pm feeding
1–2	25–35	Scant gray color to head, shoulder and back	Esbilac	1–2	q 2 h, 1 pm
		Day 10—lose umbilical cord			
2–3	35–60	Scant grayish fur, ears unglued, eyes less bulgy; Day 21—lower incisors emerge	Esbilac	2–4	q 2–3 h, no PM
3–4	60–90	Slick, shiny fur except under tail; ears open, eye slits relaxed and ready to open	Esbilac, add cereal	3–6	q 3–4 h
4–5	90–115	Downy white hair on belly, slight bush to tail, eyes open, may begin to walk	Esbilac, cereal, add rodent block	5–9	QID
5–6	115–175	Thicker hair, tail curling over back, upper incisors emerge, sitting up	Same; keep thickening	5–12	TID-QID
6–7	175–250	Furry all over, sleeping less, can sit up	Add small pieces fruit	9–15	TID-QID
7–8		Bushy tail, back molars come in	Rodent blocks	15–20	BID-TID
8–9		Looks like miniature squirrel	Begin to wean	20–25	SID-BID
9–10		Furred on underside except for 1″ at base tail, tail bushy	Wean	20–30	SID
10–11	300–425		Wean		
11–12		Tail completely furred	Weaned		
12–14		Ready for release			

Table A7.5 Cottontail care sheet.

Age (weeks)	Weights (g)	Age determinates	Diet	Amounts (mL)	Frequency
0–1	30–40	Pink, thin fur all over, eyes closed, ears flat and closed	KMR	0.5–1.5	3–4x/day
1–2	35–55	Fully furred, 7–10 days eyes open, ears erect	KMR, offer greens	2–6	2–3x/day
2–3	50–90	Ear length growth, 3 weeks self-defecating	Same	3–9	1–2x/day
3–4	60–120	Hopping, running, ears fully erect	Natural food; weaned		0–1x/day
4–5	150–190	Release			

Appendix 8

Biological Data of Selected North American Wild Mammals

Table A8.1 Biological data.

Animal	°F body temp	Pulse rate/min	Respiration rate/min	Weight at birth (g)	Adult weight (kg)	Weaning age (weeks)	Feeding formula	Eyes open (days)	Release age (weeks)
Armadillo	84–92			51–150.3	5–6	8	Esbilac	birth	
Badger	99–102			95	6–11	8–10	Esbilac	28–36	9–12
Bat (big brown)	95–102.2			3.3–4.0	11–16 g	6–8	Mother's Helper k-9	hrs after birth	6–8
Bat (red)	97–98.6			1.5–2.0	10–12 g	3–6		10	6–8
Bear (black)	100–102	60–90	15–30	170–227	90–214	22–26	Esbilac	35–42	1 yr.
Beaver	98–101	100	16	400–500	13–27	6–8	Esbilac	birth	10–12
Bobcat	99–102	110–140	26	283–340	6–15	8–9	KMR	3–11	16–20
Cottontail	100–103	130–325	32–60	35–45	0.9–2	2–3	KMR	6–8	3–4
Coyote	100–103	100–170		200–275	8.1–18	5–7	Esbilac	10–11	6 mo.
Deer (white tail)	101–102	70–80	16–20	2.5–4.0kg	M 34–180 F 22–112	8–12	lamb, doe, goat milk	birth	6–8 mo.
Fox (gray)	100–103			86	3–6	7–8	Esbilac	10–12	20
Fox (red)	100–103			71–119	5–7	8–10	Esbilac	8–9	24
E. Chipmunk	99–102	660–702		2.5–5.0	65–127 g	5–6	Esbilac	30–33	8
Hare (black-tailed jack rabbit)	99–102			60–180	1.8–3.6	3–4	KMR	birth	
Mink	99–103	250–300	18–20	6–10	0.5–1.4	5–8	Esbilac	21–30	8–10
Muskrat	98–101	148–306*	45	21	1–2	3–4	Esbilac	14–16	8–10
Opossum (Virginia)	90–99	120–140		.2	4–6	13–15	Esbilac	58–72	15
Otter (river)	99–102	130–178	20–60	132	5–11	12–16	Esbilac	21–35	9 mo.
Porcupine	99–100	280–320	100	400–500	5–12	3–5	Esbilac	birth	10–12
Raccoon	100–103	128–180	15–30	60–75	5–16	10–16	KMR	18–24	20
Skunk (spotted)	101–102			28	.340–1.2	6–8	Esbilac	28–32	
Skunk (striped)	101–102			33	3–6	6–8	Esbilac	14–28	9–12
Squirrel (S. flying)	98–102			3–6	50–79 g	8–9	Esbilac	29–40	12
Squirrels (fox)	98–102			14–18	0.5–1.4	8–9	Esbilac	28–35	12
Squirrel (grey)	98–102	390*		14–18	0.038–0.069	8–9	Esbilac	28–35	12
Weasel (least)	100–103	172–192		1.0–1.5	38–69 g	2–3		26–29	6–8
Wolf	100–102			454	23.5	6–8	Esbilac	11–15	
Woodchuck	99–100	180–264[a]		28.4–42.5	1.8–6.3	8–12	Esbilac	30	12

a)   Pulse rate under anesthesia.

Source: Information in part from Evans (1987), Fowler (1979), Stokes (1986), and Schwartz (1974).

Appendix 9

Glossary of Medical Conditions and Treatments

Bloat: Causes of bloat include a change in diet, internal parasites, improper diet, feeding a cold infant, overfeeding, or constipation. If an infant bloats, hold its belly down on a heating pad and gently but firmly massage its side from top to bottom of abdomen. Also use gas relief medications such as Di-gel, simethicone, activated charcoal, or powdered calcium carbonate dissolved in water orally in addition to warmth and massage. Long-term treatment is to eliminate the cause of the bloat.

Broken blood feathers: Feathers that are actively growing (pin feathers) contain a blood supply and when damaged may bleed. These feathers need to be removed by grasping the quill at the skin surface with hemostats, supporting the bone with the other hand, and pulling straight out. The entire feather must be cleanly removed from the follicle for the bleeding to stop.

Bumblefoot: A generalized inflammation of the foot that is most commonly seen in raptors but could occur in any bird. The condition usually starts out as a cut, puncture, swelling, bruising, crack, or abrasion on the bottom of the foot. Bacteria then enter the break in the skin and cause a generalized infection. The problem is often caused by improper or unclean perches and cages. Therapy must include topical cleaning and flushing of the wounds, proper bandaging, and often systemic antibiotics.

Constipation: In infant mammals, constipation may be due to overfeeding, change in diet, internal parasites, dehydration, intestinal obstruction, or too long since stimulation. If increasing the fluid intake and stimulating for a longer than normal time does not work, remove impacted feces in the colon by a warm water or mineral oil enema. A couple of drops of mineral oil or Laxatone orally may help alleviate constipation.

Crop stasis: "Sour crop" or crop stasis occurs when the contents of the crop fails to empty out. This sometimes occurs when the food was fed too cold, the crop was overfilled, foreign bodies are present or food was sour when fed. Crop infections such as trichomoniasis and systemic illness are other causes. Since the contents must be removed, administer a small amount of sterile water and gently massaging the crop. If the crop does not empty on its own within a few hours, the contents must be removed by drawing the material out with the tube and syringe used to feed the bird. Flush the crop with warm sterile water. Possible treatments consist of antimicrobial therapy and correction of dehydration and nutrition.

Dehydration: The excessive loss of fluid from the body. Dehydration is life-threatening and prevents every system in the body from functioning properly. The body cannot digest food, maintain body temperature, deliver proper oxygen or blood flow, or excrete toxins in a dehydrated state. The condition must be quickly assessed by determining the level of dehydration and the fluid treatment should be started immediately. Neonates need 2–3 times the fluid requirement of adults.

Maintenance: 50 mL/kg/day (OR) BW in g × .05 = daily mLs fluids

Replacement: Decimal value of % dehydration × BW in g = daily mls needed 0.10 = 10% (replaces fluid loss volume for volume e.g., diarrhea, hemorrhage)

Dehydration: 100 ml/kg/day (OR) BW in g × .10 = daily mls fluids (give ½ volume over 2–6 hrs; then ½ volume + maintenance over next 24 hours OR 50 mL/kg BID until rehydrated)

The daily volume must be divided by the number of times you wish to administer fluids. Use the least evasive method to resolve the dehydration. Oral is preferred for birds provided the animal is conscious and its bowels are functional. IV therapy is mandatory in cases of dehydration and shock, comatose animals, and starvation (Table A9.1).

Emaciation: Body weights and degree of muscle wasting are diagnostic. These animals should slowly be weaned onto solid food depending on category stage. First, offer a rehydrating solution such as LRS or LRS with 2.5% Dextrose orally. Then start with a diet such as Ultracal, Ensure, or Isocal. These liquid diets are high-calorie, low-volume, isotonic (requiring minimum energy for

Exotic Animal Medicine for the Veterinary Technician, Fourth Edition. Edited by Bonnie Ballard and Ryan Cheek.
© 2024 John Wiley & Sons, Inc. Published 2024 by John Wiley & Sons, Inc.
Companion Website: www.wiley.com/go/ballard/4e

Table A9.1 Method to determine degree of dehydration.

% Dehydration	Skin turgor in seconds	Clinical signs
6%	1–2	Tented skin; slight loss of skin elasticity
8%	2–3	Eyes slightly depressed; slow CRT; dry tacky mucous membranes
10%	3–5	Sunken eyes and cere; dry, tented, scaly skin; very slow CRT; wrinkling of foot, cere, and eyelid skin; pale oral membranes; feces dry
12%	>5	Early signs of hypovolemic shock; easily collapsible peripheral veins

Table A9.2 Method to determine degree of emaciation.

Category I	Category II	Category III
90–100% BW	75–90% BW	50–70% BW
Not eaten in 1 day	Not eaten in several days	Not eaten in 1 week
Hypoglycemic	Seizures	Near comatose
Mild muscle atrophy	Moderate muscle atrophy	Severe atrophy
Generally salvageable	Difficult to save	Few recoveries

digestion) food sources that can be fed to birds or mammals. Probiotics should be offered to help reestablish normal healthy gut flora. When the animal is hydrated and passing normal-looking stools, begin to offer diets for dehabilitated animals such as Clinicare, Hill's A/D, or Emeraid II.

The progression time period from fluids to solid foods will vary from category to category as well as from patient to patient. Always slowly mix new foods in with old diet to make the changes gradual (over several days) and easier on the animal. Meals should be small and as often as possible (weighed against frequent handling stress). These animals should be on vitamin supplementation to promote appetite. Supportive care should include heat and a stress-free environment (Table A9.2).

Fleas, ticks: Use VIP flea powder, 5% pyrethrin dust, or powder safe for kittens and puppies. Manually remove ticks.

Glue traps: Use a light sprinkle of cornstarch to neutralize the glue and prevent the animal from becoming more entangled. Cut away as much of the trap as possible. Warm Canola oil to 102–104°F and apply oil to stuck feathers or fur by gently working it in with your fingers. The warmed oil will soften the adhesive bond and after several minutes allow you to remove the animal from the trap. Work the soft gummy substance that forms up and off of the animal without pulling on the feathers or fur directly. After several more minutes, most of the glue should be soft enough to be removed or washed out. If the Canola oil leaves a residue you may need to do a Dawn bath and rinse as described under "soiled feathers."

Hyperthermia: Abnormally high body temperature. Factors that predispose animals to hyperthermia are fever, infection, excessive muscular exertion, exposure to high ambient temperatures, or high humidity. These patients need to be cooled down quickly. Submerge animals in a cold water bath and perform cold water enemas. Utilizing a circulating air fan will help provide evaporation cooling. The danger here is taking the body temperature down below normal levels so be sure to discontinue cooling methods once temperature nears normal.

Hypothermia: Abnormally low body temperature. Hypothermic animals must be warmed slowly. With temperatures 10–15° below normal, the animal is likely to become comatose and unable to respond or even shiver. At this point, it is critical that you understand why a heating pad will NOT be effective. Circulation is decreased in the peripheral parts of the body due to the body's attempt to conserve blood for the vital organs so contact heat from a heating pad is wasted. The body is not capable of carrying heat from the skin touching the warm pad into the rest of the body. The best sources of heat are heat lamps, incubators, or a warm water bath that supplies radiant heat evenly over the entire body at one time. Warm water enemas are helpful as well. Gradually increase the temperature and make sure the animal does not burn or get heated up too fast which is equally damaging.

Maggots: In small numbers, best removed manually. Heavy infestations may require flushing with peroxide to kill them. Applying cornstarch to the maggots dries them out and they often fall off. A dose of Ivermectin will kill any remaining maggots and any eggs that may hatch. If the infestation is advanced and they have entered the body cavities, euthanasia is recommended.

Malocclusion: Improper tooth alignment is most critical with rodents and lagomorphs. These animals have two upper and two lower incisors that continue to grow throughout the animal's life. They normally wear down from chewing on hard objects and grinding teeth. Maligned incisors may continue to grow and overgrow resulting in starvation (from not being able to chew food) or self-induced puncture wounds (from the lower teeth puncturing the roof of the mouth). The prognosis is poor with this condition but manually trimming the teeth biweekly or so may allow the teeth time to grow back normally after the animal has healed from the fractured jaw or other facial injury that caused the trauma.

Mites: Dust baby and adult birds with an avian mite powder. Ivermectin applied to the back of the neck will treat birds for mites but be sure to accurately measure dose by body weight not just by applying "a drop." Ivermectin is effective against mites in mammals by injecting one dose SQ.

Ruptured air sac: Appears like an air bubble under the bird's skin often caused by impact trauma such as falling from nest. Small SQ pockets that do not interfere with the bird's mobility or breathing can be left to heal on their own. Otherwise, clean the skin over the bubble and make a small incision about 1/8"–1/4" long with a sterile scissors to let the air out. Be sure to avoid the cutaneous blood vessels that can usually be seen through the skin.

Shock: The definition of shock is an acute failure of the heart to provide adequate blood flow to the tissues. Signs of shock include glassy eyes, a fixed stare, unresponsive pupils, rigidity of the limbs, paleness of gums, listlessness, decrease in blood pressure, increase in pulse, lower body temperature, or unresponsiveness to stimuli. Treatment is a combination of heat, fluids, medications, oxygen, and stress removal. Seek veterinary care for animals that come into the clinic in this condition.

Soiled feathers (oil, tar, dirt): Feathers need to remain clean and waterproof to provide insulation and flight. If a bird comes in with soiled feathers or becomes soiled during rehabilitation, a warm water bath (103–104°F) using Dawn dishwashing detergent followed by a clean warm water rinse will remove caked-on food, feces, oil, and glue. It is very important to keep the bird warm at all times until completely dry. Wash and dry under a heat lamp if possible. Fill a container with warm soapy water and dip the bird into the solution carefully wiping it with the grain of the feathers. Agitate the bird's body around in the solution being careful to keep the animal's head dry. Then dip bird into warm clean rinse water until all soap and residue are gone. Repeat if necessary until water beads on feathers. This procedure is very stressful and should only be done on stable animals.

Appendix 10

Wildlife Product Sources

Product Sources

Products	Manufacturer/Supplier	Products	Manufacturer/Supplier
Aviary netting	Memphis Net & Twine Co., Inc. Knotless seine netting—1/8 or 1/4 inch Phone: 888-674-7638 E-mail: www.memphisnet.net PetScreen® Dog and cat resistant screening Phifer.com/product/petscreen Home Depot	Live insects: mealworms, crickets	Grubo, Inc. Phone: 800-222-3563 www.grubco.com Rainbow Mealworms Inc. Phone: 310-635-1494 www.rainbowmealworms.net Nature's Way Phone: 800-318-2611 www.thenaturesway.com discount to rehabilitators
Nipples "Catac" (Latex rubber nursing nipples, 3 sizes,) fits on slip tip or catheter tip: syringes	Chris's Squirrels and More, LLC Phone: 860-749-1129 www.squirrelsandmore.com Upco Phone: 800-254-8726 www.upco.com	Bird vitamins	Lafeber's Avi-Era® bird vitamins Lafebers Company Phone: 800-842-6445 www.lafeber.com
Nipples "Mothering Kit" (Silicone small tapered nipples fits on slip-tip syringes)	Chris's Squirrels and More, LLC Phone: 860-749-1129 www.squirrelsandmore.com	Snuggle safe warming discs, digital scales, homeopathy remedies, reference books	Chris's Squirrels and More, LLC Phone: 860-749-1129 www.squirrelsandmore.com
powdered fly larva	All Bird Products Phone: 888-588-3892 www.allbirdproducts.com Fly Farm Products www.Skipio.biz.com ova musca 1# bag Lady Gouldian Finch www.ladygouldianfinch.com	O-ring syringes, canula tips, feeding tubes	Chris's Squirrels and More, LLC Phone: 860-749-1129 www.squirrelsandmore.com Medcare Phone: 800-433-4550 www.medcareproducts.com
		Animals for food: frozen rats and mice, Coturnix quail, eggs, chicks	Perfect Pets, Inc. Phone: 734-972-5324 www.frozenrodents.com Rodent Pro Phone: 812-867-7598 www.Rodentpro.com

Products	Manufacturer/Supplier	Products	Manufacturer/Supplier
Zoologic milk matrix products, Esbilac, KMR, Multi-Milk	Pet- Ag, Inc. Phone: 800-323-0877 www.petag.com	Rodent blocks	Kaytee Forti-Diet Prohealth Rodent Food® Kaytee Products, Inc., Phone: 1-800-KAYTEE-1 www.Kaytee.com
	Chris's Squirrels and More, LLC Phone: 860-749-1129 www.squirrelsandmore.com		Pet stores that sell Kaytee products
Mesh bird cages Reptilarium® & Butterfly cages	Educational Science Phone: 800-832-3596 Educationalscience.com		Mazuri Rodent Block Diet® Chris's Squirrels and More, LLC Phone: 860-749-1129 www.squirrelsandmore.com
Wildlife related Book sources— veterinary topics, specializing in: Natural history books, field guides, rehabilitation manuals	National Wildlife Rehabilitators Association (NWRA) www.nwrawildlife.com International Wildlife Rehabilitation Council (IWRC) www.theiwrc.com	Animal handling and restraint nets, traps, punch poles, handling gloves, blowpipes, darting equipment, ketch-all poles	Animal Care Equipment & Services, Inc (ACES) Phone: 800-338-ACES www.animal-care.com
	Chris's Squirrels and More, LLC Phone: 860-749-1129 www.squirrelsandmore.com	Snake hooks, etc.	Tomahawk Live Trap Inc. Phone: 800-272-8727 www.livetrap.com
Zupreem primate dry Chow® Monkey biscuits/chow	Jeffers, Inc. Phone: 1-800-533-3377 www.JeffersPet.com		Ketch All Company Phone: 877-538-2425 www.ketch-all.com
	Chris's Squirrels and More, LLC Phone: 860-749-1129 www.squirrelsandmore.com	Incubators, brooders	Thermocare Phone: 805-238-2259 www.thermocare.com
Hummingbird nectars	Nekton Nectar Plus® Chris's Squirrels and More, LLC Phone: 860-749-1129 www.squirrelsandmore.com		Brinsea TLC® Brooders Phone: 1-888-667-7009 www.Brinsea.com
	Roudybush Nectar® Hummingbird nectars Phone: 1-800-326-1726 www.roudybush.com	Plastic leg bands, tagging and supplies	Red Bird Products, Inc www.Redbird.coffeecup.com www.Birdbands.com
			Chicken Hill Store www.Chickencharm.com
Emeraid® diets:(Psittacine) (Carnivore) (Insectivore) (Carnivore Care®) (raptors, carnivores), Critical Care® diets (herbivores)	Lafeber Company Phone: 800-842-6445 www.lafeber.com Oxbow Pet Products Phone: 800-249-0366 www.oxbowanimalhealth.com	Pet store products: bowls, vitamins, foods, formulas, cages, water bottles, vaccines, Nutri-cal®, books, nest boxes, etc.	Upco Pet Supplies Phone: 816-233-8800 www.upco.com
			That Pet Place Phone: 888-842-8738 www.thatpetplace.com

Products	Manufacturer/Supplier	Products	Manufacturer/Supplier
Animal caging products: Cages, wire, netting, latches, watering systems, cage building supplies, incubators, brooders, heat lights, etc.	Stromberg's Phone: 800-720-1134 www.strombergschickens.com Global Pigeon Supply Phone: 1-800-449-0422 www.Globalpigeonsupply.com	Falconry equipment, raptor books, raptor handling gloves	Northwoods Limited Phone: 800-446-5080 www.northwoodsfalconry.com
Chicken/Duck starter crumbled balanced diet for growing ducks, chickens and geese	Feed stores and some larger pet stores	Reptile equipment: Tongs, hooks bags, heat lamps, U/V light	Mid-West Tongs Inc. Phone: 1-877-87TONGS www.tongs.com

Appendix 11

Additional Resources

Natural History: General

Chapman, JA. 1982. Wild Mammals of North America. Baltimore and London: Johns Hopkins University Press.

Elbroch, M, Rinehart, K. 2011. Behavior of North American Mammals. Boston: Houghton Mifflin Harcourt.

Peterson, RT. 1980. Peterson Field Guides. Boston: Houghton Mifflin Company.

Rue, LL, III. 1981. Furbearing Animals of North America. New York: Crown Publishers, Inc.

Stokes, D, Stokes, L. 1986. Stokes Nature Guides, A Guide to Animal Tracking and Behavior. Boston: Little Brown & Co.

Birds

Baicich, P, Harrison, C. 2005. Nests, Eggs, and Nestlings, 2nd edn. Princeton, NJ: Princeton University Press.

Eastman, J. 1997. Birds of Forest, Yard and Thicket. Mechanicsburg, PA: Stackpole Books.

Eastman, J. 1999. Birds of Lake, Pond and Marsh. Mechanicsburg, PA: Stackpole Books.

Eastman, J. 2000. Birds of Field and Shore. Mechanicsburg, PA: Stackpole Books.

Ehrlich PR, Dobkin DS, Wheye, D. 1988. The Birder's Handbook, A Field Guide to the Natural History of North American Birds. Fireside, Simon & Schuster.

Fox, N. 1995. Understanding the Birds of Prey. Blaine, WA: Hancock House Publishers.

Johnsgard, P. 1988. North American Owls, Biology and Natural History. Smithsonian Institution.

Rule, M. 2013. Songbird Diet Index. Pompano Beach, FL: Coconut Creek Publishing.

Sibley, David Allen. 2001. The Sibley Guide to Bird Life & Behavior. National Audubon Society. New York: Chanticleer Press, Inc.

Stokes, D, Stokes, L. 1979. Stokes Nature Guides, A Guide to Bird Behavior. Volumes 1–3. Boston: Little Brown & Co.

Terres JK. 1980. The Audubon Encyclopedia of North America Birds. New York: Alfred A. Knopf, Inc.

Tyrrell, EQ. 1985. Hummingbirds, Their Life and Behavior. New York: Crown Publishers, Inc.

Rodents

Allen, EG. 1938. The Habits and Life History of the Eastern Chipmunk (Tamias striatus lysteri). NY State Museum Bulletin.

Barkalow, F, Shorten, M. 1973. The World of the Gray Squirrel. New York: J.B. Lippincott Co.

Booth, ES. 1946. Notes on the Life History of the Flying Squirrel. J Mammal 27 (1): 28–30.

Costello, DF. 1966. The World of the Porcupine. New York: Lippincott Co.

Nichols, JT. 1958. Food Habits and Behavior of the Grey Squirrel. J Mammal 39 (3): 376–80.

Rue, LL, III. 1964. The World of the Beaver. Philadelphia: J.B. Lippincott.

Long, K. 1995. Squirrels: A Wildlife Handbook. Boulder, Colorado: Johnson Nature Series, Johnson Publishing Co.

Long, K. 2000. Beavers: A Wildlife Handbook. Boulder, Colorado: Johnson Nature Series, Johnson Publishing Co.

Steele, M, Koprowski, J. 2001. North American Tree Squirrels Smithsonian Institution.

Wells-Gosling, N. 1985. Flying Squirrels: Gliders in the Dark. Smithsonian Institution.

Lagomorphs

Laber-Laird, K, Swindle, M, and Flecknell, P. 1996. Handbook of Rodent and Rabbit Medicine. Tarrytown, NY: Elsevier Science.

Exotic Animal Medicine for the Veterinary Technician, Fourth Edition. Edited by Bonnie Ballard and Ryan Cheek.
© 2024 John Wiley & Sons, Inc. Published 2024 by John Wiley & Sons, Inc.
Companion Website: www.wiley.com/go/ballard/4e

Lockley, RM. 1964. The Private Life of the Rabbit. New York: Macmillan Publishing Co., Inc.

Opossum

Keefe, JF, Wooldridge, D. 1967. The World of the Opossum. Philadelphia: J.B. Lippincott.

McManus, J. 1974. Didelphis virginian. Mammalian Species, No. 40: 1–6.

Nave, P, Lacy, J. 1983. Rehabilitation notes: Opossum (Didelphis marsupialis). WRC J, Winter, pp. 7–10.

Canids

Fox, MW. 1971. Behavior of Wolves, Dogs and Related Canids. New York: Harper & Row.

Henry, David. 1986. Red Fox, The Cat Like Canine. Smithsonian Institution Press.

Rue, LL, III. 1969. The World of the Red Fox. Philadelphia: J.B. Lippincott.

Van Wormer, J. 1964. The World of the Coyote. Philadelphia: J.B. Lippincott.

Mustelids

Caine-Stage, M. 1990. American River Otter, Lutra canadensis. Wildlife J 13(1): 7–10.

Hall, RR. 1951. American Weasels. Lawrence: University of Kansas Press.

Kruuk, Hans. 2006. Otters Ecology, Behaviour and Conservation. New York: Oxford University Press Inc.

Park, E. 1971. The World of the Otter. New York: J.B. Lippincott.

Verts, BJ. 1967. Biology of the Striped Skunk. Urbana, IL: University of Illinois Press.

Procyons

Goldman, EA. 1950. Raccoons of North and Middle America. U.S. Department of Interior, U.S. Fish and Wildlife Services, North American Fauna 60. Washington, DC.

Rue, LL, III. 1994. The World of the Raccoon. Springville, CA: Wild Ones Animal Books.

Stuewer, FW. 1943. Raccoons: their habits and management in Michigan. Michigan Ecol Monograph, 13: 203–57.

Wildlife Rehabilitation Organizations

Basically Bats Wildlife Conservation Society, Inc. (www.basicallybats.org): Nonprofit organization devoted to bat rehabilitation, research, education and conservation; includes resources, contacts and promotes public awareness.

BCI—Bat Conservation International (www.batcon.org): Bat information, their conservation and how to get involved. **IWRC—International Wildlife Rehabilitation Council** (www.theiwrc.org): This site offers membership, training, education, and support for wildlife rehabilitators, literature catalogues, non-releasable animal placement, job line, symposium information, on line training, standards, rehabilitation links.

NOS—National Opossum Society, Inc. (www.opossum.org): Yearly Subscription Natural history, rehabilitation, medical management, husbandry, etc. for the Virginia Opossum.

NWRA—National Wildlife Rehabilitators Association (www.nwrawildlife.org): This site offers membership, training, education, and support for wildlife rehabilitators, NWRA/IWRC Minimum Standards, state and federal permit agency listings, career page, baby animal care, publications, literature order reprints, upcoming events, and symposiums.

Rehabilitation Books and Manuals

Many of these books can be purchased from the IWRC or NWRA web sites, downloaded from sources listed.

General Rehabilitation Topics

IWRC—Wildlife Rehabilitation: A Comprehensive Approach 2nd edn. An interpretation of existing biological and veterinary literature for the wildlife rehabilitator. Includes anatomy, physiology, calculating drug dosages, nutrition, housing, release, euthanasia, and more.

Wild Animal Care and Rehabilitation Manual, 4th edn. 1991 by Vicki Johnson. Editor Monica Evans, Beech Leaf Press. Kalamazoo Nature Center, 7000 North Westedge Ave. Kalamazoo, MI 49007.

Wild Mammal Babies, The First 48 hours and Beyond, 4th edn, pp 448 2007 by Irene Ruth & Deborah Gody.

Wildlife Care Basics for Veterinary Hospitals- Before the Rehabilitator Arrives, 2012 by Irene Ruth. Humane Society Veterinary Medical Association (HSVMA); free download.

Wild Neighbors: The Humane Approach to Living with Wildlife. 2007. Edited by John Hadidian, Guy R. Hodge, and John W. Grandy. The Humane Society of the United States. Free download.

NWRA Quick Reference 3rd edn. 2006 by E.A. Miller DVM. Includes a glossary, abbreviations, tables, calculations, drug dosing, fluid charts, infant developing, and anatomy pertaining to wildlife.

NWRA—Principles of Wildlife Rehabilitation, The Essential Guide for Novice and Experienced Rehabilitators 2nd edn. 2008. By Adele T. Moore and Sally Joosten. Printed by Burgess International Group Inc., Edina, MN.

NWRA/IWRC Standards for Wildlife Rehabilitation 5th edn. 2021. Miller, E. A, and J. Schllepes, editors. Includes basic housing requirements for mammals and birds, euthanasia standards, and disease transmission, much more. Available on IWRC and NWRA website.

Practical Wildlife Care, 2nd edn 2005 by Stocker, L. Ames, IA: Blackwell.

Wildllife Search and Rescue: A Guide for First Responders 2012 by Dmytryk, R. Hoboken, NJ: Wiley-Blackwell.

Answering the Call of the Wild 2010 by Luther, E. Toronto Wildlife Center. Reference manual to managing wildlife issue calls from the public. Available on the NWRA website.

Mammal Rehabilitation

Bats in Captivity. 1995. By Susan M. Barnard. Now available free of charge online at www.basicallybats.org/onlinebook.htm.

Complete Rehabilitation Guide for North American Bats. By Amanda Lollar, Barbara French, and Patricia Winters.

North American River Otter, Lontra canadensis, Husbandry Notebook, 3rd edn. 2008. By Janice Reed-Smith. John Ball Zoological Gardens, Grand Rapids, MI. Free online download; otterspecialistgroup.org.

Opossum Orphan Care Traininga Manual by Paula Taylor of the Opossum *Society of the U.*S., 14pp 1995; guides new opossum rehabilitators through the rearing process: Wildlife Publications.

Stinky Business: How to Rehabilitate Skunks by Share Bond, 5th edn. 2007, 151 pp. Scratch n sniff publishing.

Squirrel Rehabilitation Handbook by Shirley J and Allan M. Casey, 265pp 2003; sold only to permitted wildlife rehabilitators and subpermittees; order form available at www.ewildagain.org.

Rehabilitation and Release of the Eastern Cottontail by Orr, D. www.animaladvocates.us/bunnyrehabilitation-manual.pdf.

Avian Rehabilitation

Care and Rehabilitation of Injured Owls, 4th edn. 1987. By Katherine Mckeever. The Owl Rehabilitation Research Foundation, Vineland, Ontario, Canada.

Raptors in Captivity: Guidelines for Care and Management. 2007. By Lori R. Arent. The Raptor Center at the University of MN; NWRA website.

Raptor Rehabilitation: A Manual of Guidelines. By Mathias Engelmann, Pat Marcum. The Carolina Raptor Center (1993).

Hand-Rearing Birds, 2nd edn. 2020. by Laurie Gage DVM and Rebecca Duerr DVM, 456pp Wiley-Blackwell Publishing.

Rehabilitation and Conservation of Chimney Swifts 4th edn. 2004 by Paul and Georgean Kyle; www.chimneyswifts.org, Chimney Swift Conservation Association.

Passerine Fundamentals 4th edn. 2020 by Bowers, V. Sebastopol, CA: Native Songbird care & Conservation.

An Introduction to Aquatic Bird Rehabilitation by Bill, January et al 2012. Arcata, CA; Bird Ally X. www.birdallyx.net.

Wildlife Veterinary Topics

NWRA Wildlife Formulary 4th edn. 2017 by Erica Miller DVM. Available on the NWRA website.

Topics in Wildlife Medicine Vol 1 Clinical Pathology 2005 and Vol 2 Emergency and Critical Care 2007 by Florina S. Tseng DVM and Mark A Mitchell DVM, MS, PhD; NWRA website.

Topics in Wildlife Medicine Vol 3 Infectious Diseases 2009 by Karen Shenoy DVM; NWRA website.

Topics in Wildlife Medicine Vol 4 Orthopedics 2017 by Rebecca Duerr, DVM. Available on the NWRA website.

Medical Management of Birds of Prey: A Collection of Notes on Selected Topics. 1993. By Patrick Redig, D.V.M., PhD University of Minnesota.

Field Manual of Wildlife Diseases: National Wildlife Health Center www.nwhc.usgs.gov; available for free download (43MB).

Web Sites Useful to Rehabilitators

- **Wildlife Hotline Online**: Baby Bird ID. www.baby-birdid.com.
- **CDC**: Diseases and zoonotics: www.cdc.gov/ncezid.
- **National Wildlife Health Center**: Invaluable site for wildlife disease information, emerging diseases, wildlife health news updates: www.nwhc.usgs.gov.

- **Southeastern Cooperative Wildlife Disease Study (SCWDS)**: Current news on wildlife diseases, diagnostic services, education, zoonotics: www.vet.uga.edu/scwds.
- **Merck Veterinary Manual:** Free electronic manual online version: www.merckmanuals.com.
- **Internet Center for Wildlife Damage Management (ICWDM)**: Tips on dealing with urban wildlife and people conflicts, wildlife control and management: www.icwdm.org.
- **Urban Wildlife Rescue Inc**: Humane solutions to wildlife problems, conflicts, and humane removal. www.urbanwildliferescue.org.
- **Tri-State Bird Rescue and Research Center**: Wild bird care, tips on living with wildlife, oil spill response: www.tristatebird.org.
- **USF&W**: home page: www.fws.gov.
- **Songbird Diet Website**: Excellent site with detailed information on songbird Natural and captive diets: www.snowcrest.net/kellyj/wildbirdcare.
- **Animal Diversity Web**: University of Michigan Museum of Zoology: http://animaldiversity.ummz.umich.edu/site/index.html.
- **Squirrel Tales**: Squirrel rehabilitation, care and information sight: www.squirreltales.org.
- **The International Otter Survival Fund (IOSF)**: River Otter rehabilitation, care, conservation, and information: www.otter.org.
- **WildAgain Wildlife Rehab, Inc.**: Resources and tools for wildlife rehabilitators, teleclass training, seminars on wildlife homeopathy and squirrel rehabilitation, publications, squirrel care, articles for free download on wildlife rehabilitation and homeopathy: www.ewildagain.org.
- **The National Opossum Society**: Opossum care and information: www.opossum.org.
- **Urban Coyote Ecology and Management**: 2006, Cook County Illinois, Coyote Project. http://ohioline.osu.edu/b929/pdf/b929.pdf.
- **Beavers: Wetlands and Wildlife**: Co-existing with beavers and conflict resolution ideas. www.beaversww.org.

Appendix 12

Supplies Necessary for an Exotic Practice

3.5–5 red French rubber catheters
Dremel tool
Dental stand for rabbits
Drinking water bottles
Electrocautery unit
Avian feeding formulas
2–3.5mm endotracheal tubes
Endotracheal tubes, uncuffed
Feeding tubes
Gavage needles of various sizes
Gram scale
Gram stain kit
Heat lamps
Heated cages
Heating pads
Incubators
Induction chamber/Oxygen cage
Instrument pack with small hemostats, scissors, forceps, and needle holders
Isoflurane or sevoflurane precision vaporizer
Microdrip IV sets and pumps
Microtainer blood collection tubes
Mouth speculum (stainless steel and rubber)
Nasolacrimal cannulas
Chlorhexidine solution and scrub
Perches of different sizes
Quick stop
Raptor gloves
Rigid endoscope
Small anesthesia masks (cones)
Small hand towels
Small nonrebreathing circuit

Small rebreathing bag for an anesthesia machine
Sterile cotton tip applicators
Wing trimming scissors

Equipment and supplies needed for fish medicine

Air pumps
Air tubing
Assorted plastic totes/sweater boxes
Assorted glass aquaria
Assorted sizes of plastic fish bags
Assorted nets
Commercial dechlorinator
Rubber bands
Sea salt
Sponge filters
Water test kit
Water sample bottles (plastic, 250 mL)
5-gallon bucket(s)
Centrifuge
Complete dissecting kit
Compound microscope
Eugenol (clove oil) 1:9 with 95% ethanol (stock approx. 100 mg/mL)
Fish anesthesia machine
Gram scale (to 1 kg)
KG scale (to 10 kg)
MS-222 (10 mg/mL buffered stock solution)
Oxygen tank with regulator
Plastic surgical drapes
Refractometer
Sterile surgical pack(s)
(Fish medicine list courtesy of Dr. Greg Lewbart)

Exotic Animal Medicine for the Veterinary Technician, Fourth Edition. Edited by Bonnie Ballard and Ryan Cheek.
© 2024 John Wiley & Sons, Inc. Published 2024 by John Wiley & Sons, Inc.
Companion Website: www.wiley.com/go/ballard/4e

Appendix 13

Animal Training Documentation

ANIMAL TRAINING DOCUMENTATION

Individual Animal   Date:_____

Accession #: _____ **Trainer #1:** _____

House Name: _____ **Trainer #2:** _____

Length of Session: _____ **Weight:** _____

Change in:

☐ Reinforcement   ☐ Social Group
☐ Goal   ☐ Time of Session
☐ Trainer   ☐ Training Step from Plan
☐ Observer (vet, new person)
☐ Internal Factors (illness, estrus, and injury)
☐ External Factors (weather conditions, construction noise/visual, and enclosure modifications)

Describe Change:

_____

_____

Behaviors to track for this session: **Percentage to Goal**

_____   _____ %

_____   _____ %

_____   _____ %

_____   _____ %

_____   _____ %

Aggression:

_ 1. none
_ 2. mildly (attentive, but abrupt behavioral movements)
_ 3. moderately (intense, but not directed)
_ 4. very (intense, focused and directed)
_ 5. serious (intense, long-lasting, may result in physical consequence/injury)

    comment: _____

Animal's Attention Span:

_ 1. ignored trainer
_ 2. somewhat attentive; participating , 30% of session time
_ 3. moderately attentive; participating 30–60% of session time
_ 4. participating for 60–85% of session time
_ 5. very attentive; participating for 85–100 % of session time

Trainer Attitude Toward Session:

_ 1. did not go well   _ 2. went moderately well   _ 3. went extremely well

Today's goal/comment on session: _____

_____

_____

_____

Appendix 14

Animal Data Transfer Form

AMERICAN
ASSOCIATION
of ZOO KEEPERS

ANIMAL DATA TRANSFER FORM

1. Curator's copy of information on new arrival
2. Keeper's copy of information on new arrival   Date:
3. Copy for zoo files and/or veterinarian
Please send a copy of this form to shipping institution and state condition of animal(s)

Previous Institution (s) _____
Current Institution _____
Contact Person _____
Title _____
Email _____   Phone/Fax _____
Receiving Institution _____

Common name: Scientific name:

Zoo ID#	House Name	Sex	Hatch/Birth Date*	Tattoo Band/Tag#	Weight*	Transponder	Studbook # (Regional/International)

*Note if it is actual or estimated

DIET: Present diet and supplements, favored items, problem foods, feeding procedures.

BEHAVIORAL HISTORY and SPECIFICATIONS: Please list any unique behavioral traits, problems with aggression, safety concerns, or other behavioral problems that may affect management.
General Disposition (skittish, prefers males over females, imprinted, aggressive, etc.):

Stereotypic behavior (frequency, severity, duration, triggers)

Methods used for managing stereotypic behavior:

Does the animal have a history of aggression toward keepers and/or other animals? ☐ no   ☐ yes
          If yes, please explain:

What are the conditions and behavioral precursors to the aggression?

What successful strategies are used for dealing with the aggression?

General comments or describe other behaviors that require further explanation:

MEDICAL HISTORY OR PHYSICAL CONDITION: Medication techniques, immobilization techniques, chronic medical problems, Vet Contact.

ENCLOSURE DATA: Exhibit dimensions and description, disinfection/cleaning needs, temperature, and climate control needs.

Exhibit Features: *(When offered or provided, please list or check where applicable. Add comments where necessary)*

Substrates: sand ☐   gunite ☐   mulch ☐   leaf litter ☐   soil ☐   other ☐

Exhibit Furniture: deadfall ☐   live trees ☐   rockwork ☐   perching ☐   termite mounds ☐   other ☐

Water features:

Holding Area: indoor ☐   outdoor ☐   none (see above) ☐

Substrates: sand ☐   mulch ☐   leaf litter ☐   soil ☐   other

Holding Furniture:

How frequently rotated:

SOCIAL HISTORY *(check all that apply)*

Rearing type: ☐ dam, parent or family reared   ☐ hand reared (☐ with conspecifics ☐ without conspecifics) ☐ puppet
☐ supplemental ☐ foster reared (☐ by same species ☐ by different species) ☐ none ☐ autonomous
☐ colony/peer

Comments:

Animal housed:

☐ individually   ☐ with conspecifics (list #_____)   ☐ with mixed species [List species and # of each_____]
☐ other, please describe:

Housed on exhibit ☐   off-exhibit ☐   access to both ☐

Comments:

REPRODUCTIVE HISTORY: Relevant information, introduction techniques, behavior toward young, specific concerns.

ENRICHMENT HISTORY (Please attach any relevant schedules, approved item lists, sample calendars, etc.)

Goals for the enrichment:

Enrichment activities offered in exhibit:

Enrichment offered: daily ☐   weekly ☐   monthly ☐   scheduled ☐   other ☐

How frequently rotated:
Enrichment activities offered in holding (if different from those offered on
exhibit)

Food Enrichment
Diet Presentation:
  # of feedings per day: Varied times: ☐   When: Food scattered ☐   Hidden ☐
Novel Foods (please list or attach approved list of food items, frequency and amounts offered and presentation):

Enrichment Devices/Items

PVC feeders ☐   Tires ☐   Burlap/towels ☐   Plastic containers ☐   Puzzle feeders

☐ Cardboard boxes/tubes/bags ☐   Ropes/vines/fire hose ☐   Balls/kegs/barrels ☐   Toys (Kong®, dog chews, etc.)

Attachments methods used *(chain, rope, bungee)*:

Preferred enrichment for this animal (list):

Safety Concerns *(ingests cloth, has become impacted, displays at cage mates with large items, etc.)*:

General Comments (including expanding on any of the data entered, above):

TRAINING OR BEHAVIORAL CONDITIONING:
Training goals for this animal (list general behavioral goals and indicate which goals have been achieved and/or which goals were partially shaped but not complete at time of shipment):

How long has animal participated in a behavioral conditioning program?

Frequency and Duration of Training Sessions:
☐ once daily   ☐ twice daily   ☐ once weekly   ☐ twice weekly
☐ other, please specify:

Average length of training session (minutes):

Animal attitude/demeanor toward/during training:

Level of contact between the keeper and animal: ☐ free contact   ☐ protected contact

Social arrangement during training sessions:
☐ housed individually and trained individually ☐ separated from conspecifics for training
☐ trained with conspecifics present ☐ trained with mixed species present
☐ other, please describe:

Animal conditioned to enter crate/chute/cage for transport? (circle appropriate device*) ☐ No   ☐ Yes

        Length: Width: Height:

*Attach pictures if necessary to describe training area or device (crates, chutes, etc.).

Reinforcers: ☐ verbal   ☐ food   List type and amount used:
                  ☐ tactile   ☐ combination of all of the above

Bridging stimulus: ☐ clicker   ☐ verbal, describe:
                        ☐ whistle   ☐ other, describe:

How are undesirable behaviors addressed? ☐ Time-out   ☐ ignore ☐ re-direct ☐ incompatible behavior ☐ other (describe):

Which methods have been most successful?:

BEHAVIORS TRAINED (Please provide a brief summary – more detail can be added in subsequent section)

Behavior	Verbal cue/command	Visual cue	Criteria for reinforcement	Devices used

Please attach list of behaviors if more room is needed.

General Training Comments:

Appendix 15

Operating Protocols: Animal Training Request Form

Shaping Plan

Concept Phase:

Date:	Submitted by:
Area:	Species:
Behavior/Project Name:	Accession #:
Goal of training this behavior:	
Alternative applications for behavior:	
Predicted level of difficulty training this behavior:	
Primary trainer:	
Frequency of sessions:	Time of sessions:
Number of keepers for session:	Location of session:
Estimated start date:	Estimated end date:
Primary reinforcement:	Is it on approved list?
Projected veterinary assistance?	Material needed:

Shaping Plan:

1:
2:
3:
4:
5:
6:
7:
8:

Approved by Supervisor:	Date:

Actual training steps:

1:
2:
3:
4:
5:
6:
7:
8:
End date (behavior is placed in maintenance mode):

Appendix 16

Operating Protocols: Enrichment and Evaluation Form

Date:_____   Species:_____

Accession #'s: _____   Sex:_____

Enrichment Item:_____   Goal: _____

1.

Did you meet the set goal?	Was the schedule of delivery sufficient?	Health or safety concerns?
Comments:		

Continue use of item: yes/no
Makechanges to item: yes/no

2.

Did you meet the set goal?	Was the schedule of delivery sufficient?	Health or safety concerns?
Comments:		

Continue use of item: yes/no
Make changes to item: yes/no

3.

Did you meet the set goal?	Was the schedule of delivery sufficient?	Health or safety concerns?
Comments:		

Continue use of item: yes/no
Make changes to item: yes/no

Nashville Zoo at Grassmere
Operating Protocols
Enrichment Documenting Scale

Updated 12/24/2013

Enrichment Documenting Scale

<u>**Direct Evidence**</u>: keeper observes animal and assesses its level of interaction with enrichment initially

1	Animal runs/flees form enrichment
2	Animal appears to ignore enrichment
3	Animal orients to/looks at, but does not physically contact enrichment
4	Animal makes brief contact (e.g., sniffs/licks/pecks at enrichment)
5	Animal makes substantial or repeated contact with enrichment

<u>**Indirect Evidence**</u>: keeper is unable to observe animal's response to enrichment by directly observing interaction, but instead used indirect evidence of the animal's use of enrichment

A	No evidence of interaction (e.g., pristine, untouched cardboard box)
B	Minimal evidence of interaction (e.g., evidence of touching or brief contact with box)
C	Moderate evidence of interaction (e.g., box moved and urine marked)
D	Substantial evidence of interaction (e.g., box upside down, urinated on, and moved 8 ft.)
E	Significant evidence of interaction (e.g., box ripped to shreds and scattered everywhere)

Index

Note: Page numbers in *italics* refer to figures; those in **bold** to tables.

Exotic Animal Medicine for the Veterinary Technician, Fourth Edition. Edited by Bonnie Ballard and Ryan Cheek.
© 2024 John Wiley & Sons, Inc. Published 2024 by John Wiley & Sons, Inc.
Companion Website: www.wiley.com/go/ballard/4e